FUNDAMENTALS OF SURGERY

RICHARD D. LIECHTY, M.D.

Professor of Surgery and Associate Dean, Graduate Medical Education,
University of Colorado School of Medicine, Denver, Colorado

ROBERT T. SOPER, M.D.

Professor of Surgery, Director, Pediatric Surgical Services,
University of Iowa College of Medicine, Iowa City, Iowa

SIXTH EDITION

with 751 illustrations

The C. V. Mosby Company

ST. LOUIS   BALTIMORE   TORONTO   PHILADELPHIA   1989

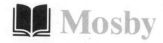

Editor: Terry Van Schaik
Assistant Editor: Pat Jusich
Project Manager: Karen Edwards
Design: John Rokusek
Editing and Production: Editing, Design & Production, Inc.

SIXTH EDITION

Copyright © 1989 by The C.V. Mosby Company

Previous editions copyrighted 1968, 1972, 1976, 1980, 1985

Printed in the United States of America

The C.V. Mosby Company
11830 Westline Industrial Drive, St. Louis, Missouri 63146

Library of Congress Cataloging in Publication Data

Liechty, Richard D., 1925-
    Fundamentals of surgery/Richard D. Liechty, Robert T. Soper.—
6th ed.
      p. cm.
    Rev. ed. of: Synopsis of surgery. 5th ed. 1985.
    Bibliography: p.
    Includes index.
    ISBN 0-8016-2962-4
    1. Surgery—Handbooks, manuals, etc. I. Soper, Robert T., 1925–
II. Liechty, Richard D., 1925– Synopsis of surgery.
III. Title.
    [DNLM: 1. Surgery, Operative. WO 500 L718s]
RD37.L53 1989
617—dc19
DNLM/DLC
for Library of Congress
                         88-38876
                            CIP

C/MV/MV   9 8 7 6 5 4 3 2 1

Contributors

William H. Baker, M.D.

Professor and Chief,
Section of Peripheral Vascular Surgery,
Department of Surgery,
Loyola University Medical Center;
Attending, Department of Surgery,
Foster G. McGaw Hospital of Loyola University,
Maywood, Illinois

Edward J. Bartle, M.D.

Assistant Professor,
Department of Surgery,
University of Colorado Health Sciences Center,
Denver, Colorado

Douglas M. Behrendt, M.D.

Professor and Chairman,
Division of Cardiothoracic Surgery,
University of Iowa College of Medicine,
University of Iowa Hospitals and Clinics,
Iowa City, Iowa

George Block, M.D.

Professor, Department of Surgery,
University of Chicago,
University of Chicago Hospitals,
Chicago, Illinois

Daniel Clarke-Pearson, M.D.

Professor, Department of Obstetrics and Gynecology,
Duke University Medical Center;
Director, Division of Gynecologic Oncology,
Duke University Medical Center,
Durham, North Carolina

Reginald R. Cooper, M.D.

Professor and Head,
Department of Orthopaedics,
University of Iowa College of Medicine
University of Iowa Hospitals and Clinics,
Veterans Administration Hospital,
Iowa City, Iowa

Albert E. Cram, M.D.

Associate Professor,
Department of Surgery,
University of Iowa College of Medicine;
Director,
Division of Plastic and Reconstructive Surgery,
University of Iowa Hospitals,
Iowa City, Iowa

Merril T. Dayton, M.D.

Assistant Professor,
Department of Surgery,
University of Utah College of Medicine;
Gastrointestinal Surgeon,
Department of Surgery,
University of Utah Medical Center,
Salt Lake City, Utah

Judith B. Dillman, M.D.

Assistant Professor,
Chief, Pediatric Anesthesia Group,
Department of Anesthesia,
University of Iowa College of Medicine,
Iowa City, Iowa

Ben Eiseman, M.D.

Professor, Department of Surgery,
University of Colorado Health Sciences Center,
School of Medicine,
Denver, Colorado

Adrian Flatt, M.D.

Chief, Department of Orthopaedics,
Baylor University Medical Center,
Dallas, Texas

David W. Furnas, M.D.

Clinical Professor,
Division of Plastic Surgery,
University of California, Irvine;
Chief, Division of Plastic Surgery,
UCI Medical Center,
Orange, California

Howard P. Greisler, M.D.

Assistant Professor,
Department of Surgery,
Loyola University Medical Center;
Attending Surgeon,
Department of Surgery, Section of Peripheral
Vascular Surgery,
Loyola University Medical Center,
Edward Hines, Jr., Veterans Administration Hospital,
Maywood, Illinois

Nelson Gurll, M.D.

Professor,
Director of Surgical Education,
Department of Surgery,
University of Iowa College of Medicine;
Surgical Residency Program Director,
University of Iowa Hospitals and Clinics,
Iowa City, Iowa

John F. Hansbrough, M.D.

Associate Professor,
Department of Surgery,
University of California, San Diego Medical Center,
San Diego, California

Claude L. Hughes, Ph.D., M.D.

Assistant Professor and Director of the Reproductive
Hormone Lab,
Division of Reproductive Endocrinology
and Infertility,
Department of Obstetrics and Gynecology,
Duke University Medical Center,
Durham, North Carolina

Mardi R. Karin, M.D.

General Surgery Resident,
Department of General Surgery,
University of Iowa Hospitals and Clinics,
Iowa City, Iowa

Gerald P. Kealey, M.D.

Assistant Professor,
Department of Surgery,
University of Iowa College of Medicine;
Director, Burn Treatment Center,
Department of Surgery—Burn Center,
University of Iowa Hospitals and Clinics,
Iowa City, Iowa

Ken Kimura, M.D.

Associate Professor,
Department of Surgery,
University of Iowa College of Medicine,
University of Iowa Hospitals and Clinics,
Iowa City, Iowa

Charles J. Krause,

Professor and Chairman,
Department of Otolaryngology,
University of Michigan Medical Center,
Ann Arbor, Michigan

John Lemmer, M.D.

Assistant Professor,
Division of Cardiothoracic Surgery
University of Iowa College of Medicine,
University of Iowa Hospitals and Clinics
Iowa City, Iowa

R.D. Liechty, M.D.

Professor of Surgery,
Department of Surgery,
University of Colorado Health Sciences Center
School of Medicine,
Denver, Colorado

Flavian M. Lupinetti, M.D.

Assistant Professor,
Division of Cardiothoracic Surgery,
University of Iowa College of Medicine,
University of Iowa Hospitals and Clinics,
Iowa City, Iowa

Donald E. Macfarlane, M.D., Ph.D.

Associate Professor,
Department of Internal Medicine,
University of Iowa College of Medicine,
University of Iowa Hospitals and Clinics,
Iowa City, Iowa

Harold R. Mancusi-Ungaro, Jr., M.D.

Associate Professor and Chief,
Division of Plastic Surgery,
University of New Mexico Medical School;
Director, Burn Center,
University of New Mexico Medical Center,
Albuquerque, New Mexico

Edward E. Mason, M.D., Ph.D.

Professor and Chairman,
Division of General Surgery,
University of Iowa College of Medicine,
University of Iowa Hospitals and Clinics
Iowa City, Iowa

Brian F. McCabe, M.D.

Professor and Head,
Department of Otolaryngology–Head and
Neck Surgery,
University of Iowa College of Medicine,
University of Iowa Hospitals and Clinics,
Iowa City, Iowa

J. Scott Millikan, M.D.

Staff Surgeon,
Department of Thoracic and Cardiovascular Surgery,
The Billings Clinic,
Billings, Montana

Jeffrey R. Mitchell, M.D.

Resident in Surgery,
Department of Surgery,
Medical College of Ohio Hospitals,
Toledo, Ohio

Hiro Nishioka, M.D.

Assistant Clinical Professor,
Department of Neurological Surgery,
Medical College of Wisconsin,
Milwaukee, Wisconsin;
Department of Surgery,
Bellin Memorial, St. Vincent Hospitals,
Green Bay, Wisconsin

Lawrence W. Norton, M.D.

Professor and Vice Chairman,
Department of Surgery,
University of Colorado Medical School;
Chief, Department of Surgery,
Veterans Administration Hospital,
Denver, Colorado

Nathan W. Pearlman, M.D.

Associate Professor,
Department of Surgery,
University of Colorado School of Medicine,
University of Colorado Health Sciences Center;
Chief of GI/Tumor Surgery Section,
Department of Surgery,
Denver Veterans Administration Hospital,
Denver, Colorado

Israel Penn, M.D.

Professor,
Department of Surgery,
University of Cincinnati Medical Center;
Chief, Department of Surgery,
Veterans Administration Medical Center,
Cincinnati, Ohio

Jack Pickleman, M.D.

Professor of Surgery,
Chief, Division of General Surgery,
Department of Surgery,
Loyola University Medical Center,
Maywood, Illinois

Joseph J. Piotrowski, M.D.

Chief Resident,
Department of General Surgery,
University of Colorado Health Sciences Center,
Denver, Colorado

Nicholas P. Rossi, M.D.

Professor, Department of Surgery,
University of Iowa College of Medicine,
University of Iowa Hospitals and Clinics
Iowa City, Iowa

Joseph D. Schmidt, M.D.

Professor of Surgery/Urology,
Department of Surgery,
University of California, San Diego,
School of Medicine;
Head, Department of Surgery,
Division of Urology,
University of California, San Diego,
San Diego, California

Siroos S. Shirazi, M.D.

Professor, Department of Surgery,
University of Iowa College of Medicine,
University of Iowa Hospitals and Clinics
Iowa City, Iowa

John T. Soper, M.D.

Assistant Professor,
Division of Gynecologic Oncology,
Department of Obstetrics and Gynecology,
Duke University Medical Center,
Durham, North Carolina

Nathaniel Soper, M.D.

Associate Professor, Department of Surgery,
Washington University School of Medicine,
St. Louis, Missouri

Robert T. Soper, M.D.

Professor, Department of Surgery,
University of Iowa School of Medicine,
University of Iowa Hospitals and Clinics
Iowa City, Iowa

Neil R. Thomford, M.D.

Professor and Chairman,
Department of Surgery,
Medical College of Ohio;
Chief of Surgery,
Department of Surgery,
Medical College Hospitals,
Toledo, Ohio

John H. Tinker, M.D.

Professor and Head,
Department of Anesthesia,
University of Iowa College of Medicine,
University of Iowa Hospitals and Clinics,
Iowa City, Iowa

Ivan M. Turpin, M.D.

Assistant Clinical Professor,
Division of Plastic Surgery,
University of California, Irvine,
UCI Medical Center,
Orange, California

Greg Van Stiegmann, M.D.

Associate Professor,
Department of Surgery,
University of Colorado School of Medicine,
University of Colorado Health Sciences Center;
Chief, Surgical Endoscopy,
Department of Surgery,
University of Colorado Hospital,
Denver, Colorado

Richard Weil III, M.D.

Professor of Surgery,
Department of Surgery,
New York University School of Medicine,
Chief of Transplantation,
Department of Surgery,
New York University Medical Center,
New York, New York

To
Valerie and Hélène

Preface

The first edition of this book was published in 1968, a tumultuous year. It marked the assassinations of Dr. Martin Luther King, Jr. and Robert Kennedy, the capture of the Pueblo by North Korea, the rioting at the Democratic Convention in Chicago, the announcement that President Johnson would not seek reelection, and the election of Richard Nixon as President. During the subsequent 20 years the world changed dramatically.

To the clinician, medical science has also changed dramatically. New scanning devices—computed tomography and magnetic resonance imaging—have revolutionized diagnosis. In some institutions, cardiac and liver transplantation have become routine procedures, and intensive care units have provided vital new dimensions to patient care.

Through all this evolution we have maintained our philosophy of writing for those students who are just beginning their clinical studies. Our coauthors have readily accepted the concept of ". . .a textbook carefully designed for a particular audience, the student, whether still in school or 15 years out of school. . ." (JAMA 197:133, 1966).

Although we have resisted the constant pressures to include more data, to make this a book for all readers, *Fundamentals of Surgery* has inevitably grown. We hope, nevertheless, that this sixth edition will continue to give students a broad grasp of surgical principles yet allow them some spare moments to think about other things—to gain perspective. "For perspective," said Will Durant, "is the secret of philosophy." And it well may be the secret to understanding this world of rapid change.

Richard D. Liechty, M.D.
Robert T. Soper, M.D.

Contents

I

Surgical Principles

1

Origin of Surgical Disease

Richard D. Liechty
Robert T. Soper

Obstruction
Perforation
Erosion
Tumors

Each day of the year our medical school libraries add the equivalent of three new *volumes* of medical literature to their already extensive collections. As in other scientific fields, the medical profession, and especially the medical student, faces an "information crisis." The volume and scope of medical literature dramatically emphasize the diversity of specialization. However, common bonds do exist across the specialty fields. Obstruction is still obstruction whether in the lacrimal duct, ureter, or spinal canal. We would like to begin by emphasizing some of the common concepts that link one specialty to another.

All somatic diseases, regardless of what specialties treat them, have their origins in the following six basic pathologic processes: congenital defects, inflammations, neoplasms, trauma, metabolic defects and degeneration, and collagen defects.

Four phenomena that result from these fundamental pathological processes are responsible for almost all surgical diseases and for many nonsurgical diseases as well. These phenomena are (1) obstruction, (2) perforation, (3) erosion, and (4) tumors or masses.

OBSTRUCTION

Cerebrovascular disease (strokes) and coronary heart disease (coronaries) are two of the leading causes of death in the United States. Both result from obstruction of vital arteries carrying blood to the brain or to the heart muscle, respectively. Glaucoma, one of the two leading causes of blindness in the United States also results from obstruction, in this case obstruction to the outflow of fluid from the anterior chamber of the eye.

Free flow of blood, urine, cerebrospinal fluid

Table 1-1. Diseases Resulting from Obstruction

System	Disease	Nature of Obstruction
CNS	Hydrocephalus	Congenital obstruction of cerebrospinal fluid
ENT	Middle ear infection	Eustachian tube obstruction
Eye	Glaucoma	Obstruction of aqueous humor
Lung	Atelectasis	Mucus plug in bronchus
Biliary tract	Cholecystitis	Cystic duct stone
GI	Appendicitis	Fecalith, appendix
GU	Prostatism	Prostatic hypertrophy
Extremity	Intermittent claudication	Arteriosclerosis

Table 1-2. Examples of Perforation

System	Disease	Nature of Perforation
CNS	Cerebral hemorrhage	Rupture of CNS artery
ENT	Perforation of tympanic membrane	Infection with pressure
Lung	Spontaneous pneumothorax	Rupture of bleb
Biliary tract	Rupture of gallbladder	Obstruction, distension, necrosis
GI	Duodenal ulcer	Perforation of ulcer
GU	Ruptured bladder	Obstruction and distension
Vascular	Aortic aneurysm	Rupture of aneurysm

Table 1-3. Examples of Erosion

System	Disease	Nature of Erosion
CNS	Meningitis	Erosion of abscess wall; mastoiditis
ENT	Pharyngeal carcinoma	Bleeding; erosion into blood vessels
Lung	Tuberculosis	Bleeding; granulomatous erosion into blood vessels
GI	Duodenal ulcer	Bleeding; ulcer erosion into blood vessels
GU	Bladder stone	Bleeding; erosion of bladder wall
Extremity	Raynaud's phenomenon	Digital ulceration; ischemic erosion of skin

(CSF), lymph, and other fluids, as well as air, is essential for health. Table 1-1 shows the wide variety of diseases that result from obstruction.

PERFORATION

Perforation, similarly, is the direct cause of many surgical diseases. Perforation is often such an intensely dramatic event that few medical students will forget the boardlike abdomen of the patient with a ruptured peptic ulcer or the shock that overwhelms the patient with a ruptured aortic aneurysm. Examples are given in Table 1-2.

EROSION

Erosion is a "partial perforation," a slower process of ulceration (i.e., a break in the continuity of a tissue surface). Examples of erosion are given in Table 1-3.

TUMORS

The most subtle of these four phenomena is a tumor, or mass. This explains in large measure why cancer is so often detected only after it induces one of the three processes (e.g., we occasionally see tumors of the breast that have grown to astonishingly large size). Because no vital flow is obstructed and perforation or erosion of the skin occurs very late, symptoms, and consequently diagnosis, are delayed, often tragically.

These four phenomena, *obstruction, perforation, erosion,* and *tumors,* are the underlying direct causes of most surgical diseases. Like the theme of a symphonic work, they recur in many different forms. Sometimes they appear unmistakably loud and clear; at other times they are soft, muted, and elusive. The able physician will learn to recognize and understand them. Such recognition and understanding are the chief concern of this book.

2

Wounds and Wound Healing

David W. Furnas
Richard D. Liechty

Although the healing of wounds is a vital part of surgery, it also plays an important role in other medical fields. For example, the fibrous healing of myocardial infarcts often leads to life-threatening arrhythmias or ventricular aneurysms, and fibrous vegetations threaten embolization from rheumatic valvular disease. In posthepatitis patients scar tissue infiltrates the liver and in some cases fatally encases the regenerating liver cells or produces portal venous hypertension. In these examples fibrous tissue healing in its exuberant, sometimes misdirected, growth may eventually prove fatal. Wound healing, the surgeon's constant concern, is of more than casual interest to other physicians as well.

Healing by regeneration in man is limited to simple tissues, such as epithelium, and one compound organ, the liver. All other organs (skin, bowel, heart, brain) heal by merely sealing or patching the wound. Paraplegia, for example, results from transection of the upper spinal cord. Scar tissue joins the severed cord ends but blocks all nerve impulses; the distal neurons, separated from their cell nuclei, degenerate and die. Unfortunately humans have, in their evolutionary past, virtually lost the ability to regenerate compound tissues. There remains, however, this remarkable process of sealing, or patching, on which humans depend to survive the hostile environment.

Tissues heal by three main processes: *epithelialization, fibrous tissue synthesis,* and the powerful force of *contraction*. Many surgical decisions depend on a clear understanding of these extraordinary phenomena. When to remove sutures, where to make incisions, when to release a postoperative patient for normal activities, when to splint a wound, when to close a wound primarily, and when to leave it open are practical applications that the student should keep in mind as

5

he or she studies the fundamental aspects of wound healing.

We first discuss the healing of *incised wounds, avulsed wounds,* and *contaminated wounds.* Pathological wound healing, wound complications, placement of incisions, suture materials, wound drainage, and drainage tubes complete this chapter.

INCISED WOUNDS AND SUPERFICIAL WOUNDS

A simple *clean incised wound* heals by *primary intention* after accurate surgical closure *(primary closure).* Within the first few hours of injury the cut edges of the wound are coapted by a fibrinous coagulum that serves as a scaffold for formation of granulation tissue. During the first day, leukocytes, mast cells, and macrophages enter the area to dispose of local debris and bacteria. The *epithelial cells* of the neighboring epidermis dedifferentiate, flatten out, multiply, migrate into and across the wound, and redifferentiate. In an incised and sutured wound, the epidermal surface is intact within 24 hours. This same sequence of fibrin deposition, granulation tissue, and epithelialization serves to replace and heal the surface of broader wounds, such as second-degree burns or light abrasions, within a few days or weeks.

During the first few days that an incision is healing, the *inflammatory phase,* almost no tensile strength is gained. Meanwhile, *capillary buds* begin to sprout from the wound edges and differentiate into functioning networks, and *fibroblasts* migrate into the wound area, probably from nearby loose connective tissue. These fibroblasts form *collagen,* the material that knits the wounded dermis and deeper structures and gives strength to the wound. First the fibroblasts secrete *tropocollagen,* which aggregates into large *procollagen* fibers. These herald the *collagen phase,* the earliest evidence of tensile strength. Procollagen, through polymerization and cross linkages, becomes collagen, and from the fifth through the fifteenth day there is a rapid gain in tensile strength.

The young collagen fibers mature, link with one another, and orient along lines of stress. The wound reaches almost its full strength within 6 weeks. Although a slight gain continues over a number of months, the scar seldom, if ever, becomes stronger than the surrounding skin and fascia.

The *rate of healing* is accelerated by a rich blood supply, and perhaps by warmth of the wounded part. Thus the face heals rapidly and sutures may be removed in a few days. In contrast, sutures must be left for 10 to 14 days in wounds of the lower leg because of its poorer blood supply.

As *wound maturity* progresses, the fibroblasts and capillaries greatly diminish in number and the resultant scar is composed chiefly of collagen connective tissue capped with epithelium. This progress is observed clinically as an initial red, raised, hard *immature scar* that molds into a flat, soft, pale *mature scar* over a period of 3 to 12 months or more, as collagen molecules and cross links rearrange.

An excised wound or defect closes more slowly but in identical fashion, except that contraction of the wound edges plays the principal role. The edges of the defect advance into the defect, probably owing to the action of contractile myofibroblasts. These recently described cells resemble *smooth muscle cells* and can be inhibited in experimental animals by smooth muscle antagonists. Wound contraction is a consistent, powerful force that all experienced surgeons respect (Figs. 2-3 and 2-4).

"EXCISED" OR AVULSIVE WOUNDS

If a wound cannot be closed primarily, it must heal by *secondary intention,* by means of the mechanisms of contraction and epithelialization. Examples are wounds that are excessively contaminated, wounds whose treatment has been delayed, and burns and other wounds that involve necrosis of large areas of skin. In a few days the raw, exposed area becomes filled with *granulation tissue* ("proud flesh"; Fig. 2-1) composed of sprouting capillaries and fibroblasts. The wound edges creep toward each other by *contraction* and *epithelial migration.* A mantle of necrotic skin that clings to the surface of the defect is called an *eschar.* Formed of coagulated collagen and debris, it is much thicker and

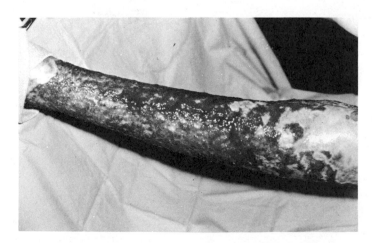

Fig. 2-1. Granulation tissue. Red, moist bed of fibroblasts and capillaries covering surface of leg that sustained full thickness burns 6 weeks before.

tougher than the scab of a superficial wound (Fig. 2-2). Tightly attached at first, it eventually separates from the underlying granulation tissue and falls away.

Healing is speeded by removal of dead tissue, debris, and secretions by surgical excision (débridement) and by intermittent application of dressings moistened with antibacterial solutions. The capillarity of the dressings drains away bacterial exudate. Dead tissue that adheres to the dressings is removed when the dressings are changed. There soon emerges a clean granulating surface that resists reinfection. If the wound edges can be apposed, wound closure can be hastened by *secondary closure* undertaken a few days after injury. Sutures are used to appose the wound edges, usually after the granulation tissue is first excised. Larger wounds are closed with split skin grafts. If the defect is too large, an unstable scar may result.

In many instances healing by *secondary intention* is convenient and desirable (Fig. 2-3); however, when the wound is located on the face or over a joint (where mobility of the part favors excessive displacement), contracture is likely which can result in diminished motion and sometimes grotesque deformity (Fig. 2-4). This is prevented by early closure of the wound with skin grafts or pedicles before contraction occurs. In addition, splints and physical therapy may help prevent skin grafts from contracting.

CONTAMINATED WOUNDS

Wounds received outside of the operating room are contaminated wounds. They may be *grossly clean* or *dirty, neat,* or *ragged,* and contused (*tidy* or *untidy* in British parlance).

A "golden period" of approximately 6 hours was cited several decades ago as the optimal time during which to close a contaminated wound; if closure was not accomplished by 6 hours, the wound should be left open to prevent infection. This concept should not be entirely ignored, but more important is the answer to the question: Can this *contaminated wound* be converted into a surgically *clean wound,* or is this a *con-*

taminated wound in which bacterial activity is already so advanced that it *cannot* be converted?

We now have antibiotics and more refined surgical techniques, so given *an excellent blood supply, we can take liberties with the golden period*. A 2-day-old wound of the foot that shows no sign of infection can be closed with appropriate preparation (not simply "putting in stitches") with little risk of infection. A grossly clean, neat wrist laceration, 12 hours old, can be repaired safely. However, a 3-hour-old wound of the lower leg received from a dirty barnyard source should probably be left open.

A contaminated wound is always converted to a *surgically clean wound* before early closure, by the following steps:

1. Take culture; start antibiotics if wound is large; administer tetanus prophylaxis.
2. *Clean* all foreign material and loose debris by use of syringes, scrub brushes, and curets; avoid traumatic tattoos.
3. Accomplish *hemostasis*.
4. *Irrigate* with several liters of sterile solutions (saline, hydrogen peroxide, benzalkonium chloride) to dilute the number of bacteria remaining in the wound and to carry away microscopic debris.
5. *Match* the landmarks of the wound so that a tentative plan for débridement, shifting of tissue, and closure can be made.
6. *Débride*—excise with scalpel ragged wound edges, all dead or questionably viable tissue, and tissues that contain embedded foreign material.
7. *Close* with sutures, grafts, or pedicle, *or* if there is heavy contamination or missing tissue.
8. *Dress* frequently with moist antibiotic dressings and carry out delayed closure several days later *or* dress and await secondary healing.

PATHOLOGICAL WOUND HEALING

At times an excessively hard, raised, red, itching, unsightly *hypertrophied scar* (Fig. 2-5) may result from excessive tension on the wound, unfavorable site, inaccurate wound closure, or unknown factors. Exuberant

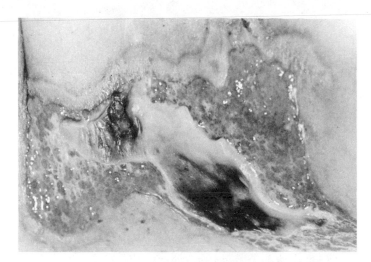

Fig. 2-2. Eschar. Deep burn coagulated full thickness of skin several weeks before. Eschar is in process of separating from underlying bed of granulation tissue. Copious exudate from local bacterial activity speeds process.

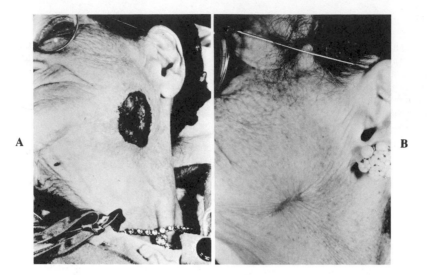

Fig. 2-3. Useful wound contraction. **A,** Wide removal of carcinoma of skin with electrocoagulation leaving open 3 × 4 cm. defect. **B,** Defect several months later after spontaneous closure by contraction and epithelialization.
(Courtesy Department of Dermatology, University of Iowa Hospitals.

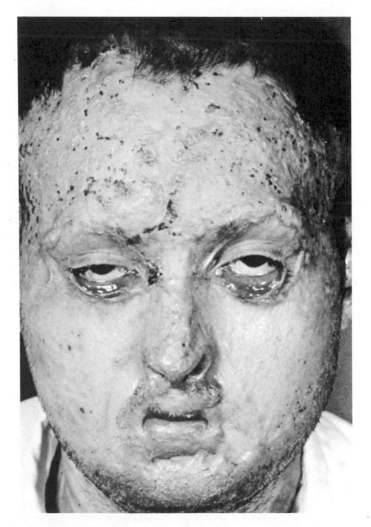

Fig. 2-4. Inimical wound contraction. Ectropion of eyelids and stenosis of mouth resulted from spontaneous closure of burn wounds of face by contraction and epithelialization.

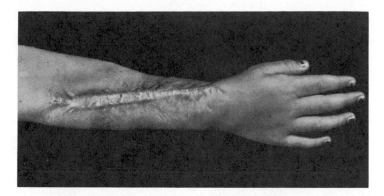

Fig. 2-5. Hypertrophied scar resulting from closure of forearm defect under tension.

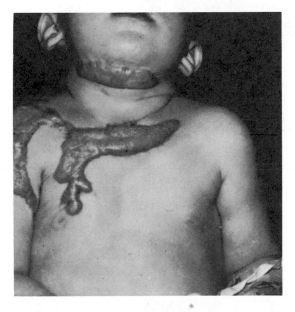

Fig. 2-6. Exuberant hypertrophied scar resulting from scalds (deep partial thickness burn).

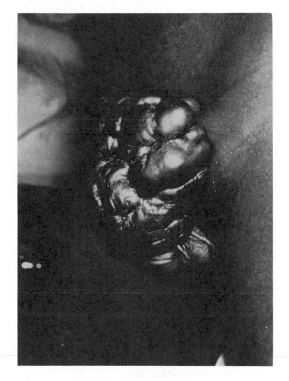

Fig. 2-7. Keloid in right inguinal hernioplasty wound.

hypertrophied scars sometimes result from partial-thickness burns in children (Fig. 2-6). Improvement usually occurs with time; surgical excision and revision of the scar may be necessary. The patient must understand that *scar "removal" can never eradicate scarring but can only minimize it.*

Occasionally a massive overgrowth of scar tissue invades the normal surrounding skin and creates unsightly, gnarled protuberances called *keloids* (Fig. 2-7). Keloids occur only in susceptible individuals, most often of the pigmented races. They have great propensity for recurrence when excised.

If a granulating wound defect is too large, closure by the process of contraction will be unsuccessful and will leave an open expanse of granulation tissue. In time the capillaries and fibroblasts diminish and the granulation tissue is gradually transformed into avascular scar tissue. Epithelial migration yields only a thin, fragile mantle over the scar. The result is an *unstable scar* that is prone to reinjury and chronic ulceration. If recurring ulceration proceeds for several decades, metaplasia and, finally, squamous carcinoma (Marjolin's ulcer) may occur at the site of the injury. To prevent an unstable wound, the surgeon converts exposed granulation tissue into a closed wound by application of a split-thickness skin graft or pedicle.

WOUND COMPLICATIONS

Healing of wounds is retarded by the *protein deficiency* seen in severely depleted patients (particularly deficiency of the amino acid methionine), but healing is not greatly affected in patients who have moderate deficiencies. *Ascorbic acid deficiency* interferes with formation of collagen from collagen precursors, and the wounds develop little tensile strength. Because all collagen, and especially wound collagen, is continually

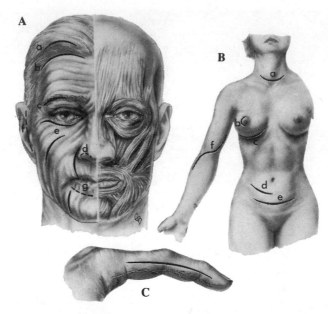

Fig. 2-8. A, Incisions camouflaged, *a,* in scalp, *b,* at scalp line, *c,* in eyebrow, *d,* in nostril, *e,* in wrinkle lines, *f,* in retroauricular area, and *g,* inside mouth. **B,** Incisions camouflaged in, *a,* neck creases, *b,* areolar border, *c,* submammary fold, *d,* skin creases of abdomen, *e,* wrinkle line and pubic hair of abdomen, and *f,* design of incision across the flexor surface of a joint to avoid contracture. **C,** Incision along neutral border of finger (where flexor skin creases meet extensor creases) to avoid contracture.

being built up and destroyed, lack of vitamin C can cause disruption of wounds that are years old. This explains the mystifying wound disruptions in scorbutic sailors, so well described in seafaring tales. Excessive levels of *adrenocortical hormones* suppress fibroblastic activity. *Diabetes mellitus* sometimes engenders poor healing. *Infection, excessive motion, hematomas, seromas, edema, venous stasis, foreign material,* and *heavily traumatized tissue* in the wound area all impede satisfactory healing. *Reduced vascular supply* from any cause retards or prevents wound healing (e.g., *excessive tension* on the wound edges, *radiation changes, heavy scarring,* or *arteriosclerosis*).

Meticulous attention to nutrition, antisepsis, operative technique, hemostasis, and postoperative care will favor satisfactory wound healing.

PLACEMENT OF INCISIONS

Minimal scar formation and maximal camouflage are most likely to result when incisions are placed in the *wrinkle lines* of Kraissl and Conway (Fig. 2-8). These lines fall at right angles to the direction of pull of the underlying muscles. On the face they are most easily identified by having the patient grimace and perform exaggerated expressions. Elsewhere they are found by close inspection of the skin. Sometimes incisions may be hidden at or above the hairline, in the eyebrows, behind the ears, in the mouth, or along the areolar border of the nipple (Fig. 2-8, *A* and *B*). If an incision must cross the flexor surface of a joint, it is important that it curve or zigzag, nearly parallelling the transverse joint crease for part of its distance. Access to the flexor surface of the finger is made through the midlateral line, or *neutral border,* of the finger (Fig. 2-8, *C*). Straight, longitudinal incisions across flexor surfaces of joints

are notorious for the contractures they cause. On the abdomen, transverse (wrinkle line) incisions generally offer superior healing, though the need for extensive exposure sometimes dictates vertical incisions. Because the main muscular pull is transverse, transverse incisions parallelling these tensions have less tendency to disrupt. Transverse incisions are preferable on the chest also. Vertical incisions on the sternal region are noted for their tendency to hypertrophy.

SUTURE MATERIALS

Catgut and *chronic catgut* are made from intestinal submucosa of sheep. They are *absorbed* by the tissues, an advantage in contaminated wounds. They cause more inflammatory reaction (i.e., they are more *reactive* than other suture materials), and they are not so easy to manipulate as sutures of natural fiber. *Polyglycolic acid sutures* are also absorbed.

Natural fiber sutures—silk, cotton, and linen—are *not absorbed,* are *much less reactive,* and have more tensile strength. They are the easiest of all sutures to handle, but if buried in a contaminated wound, they act as a nidus for bacteria and tend to cause small draining sinuses that persist for many months until the sutures are finally expelled or removed.

Synthetic fiber sutures—nylon, Dacron, polyester, polypropylene, etc.—are *not absorbed.* They are *stronger* and *less reactive* than silk, with much less tendency to cause draining sinuses after closure of contaminated wounds, particularly if they are *mono*strand rather than *poly*strand. The monostrand sutures are more difficult to handle than natural fiber sutures, but they have an advantage of minimal capillary action.

Wire sutures—stainless steel, silver, or tantalum— are *not absorbed,* have minimum capillarity and mini-

Table 2-1. Surgical Procedures Commonly Followed by Drainage

Procedure	Material to be Drained
Cholecystectomy	Bile from accessory bile ducts—from liver to gallbladder
Pancreatic resection	Pancreatic juice from many tiny pancreatic ducts
Parotidectomy	Secretions from transected parotid gland
Thoracotomy	Air or serous fluid drained from intrapleural space; important to keep lung expanded
Splenectomy	Pancreatic juice; tail of pancreas is often very close to splenic hilum
Nephrectomy	Perinephric fat, which is susceptible to infection
Incision and drainage of furuncles	Pus; allows wound to heal from bottom
Large flaps	Serum and blood are prevented from collecting with suction catheters

mum reactivity, and are the *strongest* sutures. They are more difficult to handle than the other materials and tend to cut through tissues.

WOUND DRAINAGE

Drains are placed in wounds only when *abnormal fluid collections* are present or expected. The purpose of drainage is to provide an exit for these fluids. Collections of body fluids can be harmful in the following ways:

1. Provide culture media for bacterial growth.
2. Cause tissue irritation or necrosis (as from bile, pancreatic juice, pus, urine).
3. Cause elevation of skin flaps with loss of vascularity and sloughing.
4. Cause pressure on adjacent organs.

In clean wounds, when no abnormal collection of fluids is expected, for example, after a thyroidectomy or hernia repair, drainage is unnecessary. Bleeding should seldom, if ever, be used as a rationale for draining. Hemostasis should be attained at the time of operation. Blood clots may obstruct drains and give the surgeon a false sense of security while bleeding proceeds in the wound. Surgeons vary somewhat in their indications for drainage. Table 2-1 lists surgical procedures in which drains are commonly used.

Typically, soft rubber or plastic drains are used for wound drainage; when large amounts of drainage material are expected or when a "dry wound" is important, suction applied to hollow tube drains is effective.

Drains act as foreign bodies. Granulation tissue forms about them and rapidly walls them off, thus the area in which drains are effective is soon limited by this isolating effect of healing tissue. Drains are usually removed slowly as the amount of drainage decreases over a period of days or, rarely, weeks.

T TUBES AND OTHER "FISTULA"-FORMING TUBES

Hollow drainage tubes are often used to form *fistulas* (hollow connections) from internal organs, either to drain a body fluid (bile) to the outside or to instill materials into body organs (feeding jejunostomy).

The short member of the T tube is placed in the common bile duct, and the longer member leads outside the body, thus providing a channel for the bile to the outside. It is also used to inject radiopaque dye for x-ray studies of the bile ducts. Granulation tissue soon forms a fibrous wall about the T tube, walling it off from the remainder of the peritoneal cavity: the rubber tube is a foreign body. After 9 to 10 days a T tube can be removed with no fear of internal bile leak; however, if a T tube is pulled out within 48 hours of its insertion, a bile leak invariably occurs into the peritoneal cavity with consequent bile peritonitis. This same walling off process occurs around *gastrostomy, jejunostomy, cecostomy, cystostomy,* and other tubes. If these tubes become displaced before the fibrous tract forms, extravasation almost always results, often with serious or fatal consequences. Because of their important function, these tubes are stitched securely to the skin and should seldom be removed earlier than 10 days after insertion.

Urinary catheters, nasogastric tubes, and rectal tubes pass through natural orifices that are lined by epithelium and, therefore, can be removed at any time because fibrous sealing off of the tube does not ensue. *Thoracotomy tubes* are discussed in Chapter 29.

3

Fluids and Electrolytes

Edward E. Mason

The subject of fluids and electrolytes is sometimes neglected because of both its simplicity and its potential complexity. Probably 95% of surgical patients require only short-term, routine replacement of fluids. When patients resume oral feeding, they regulate themselves. Furthermore, with short-term intravenous therapy, patients can withstand gross insults. Normal kidneys, by excreting excess fluids, readily compensate for most fluid overloads, and when fluid replacement is inadequate, the kidneys conserve fluids.

This chapter presents a simple scheme for rational analysis of the daily fluid requirements for all patients, whether the problem is simple or complex, and especially to the recognition, understanding, and logical analysis of requirements for the occasional difficult patient whose kidneys are not functioning well and whose life may depend on this portion of the treatment.

Three major questions must be answered in order to provide optimal parenteral fluids: (1) What metabolic fluids (urine and insensible loss) are needed? (2) What abnormal body fluids currently being lost (by vomiting, diarrhea) must be replaced? (3) What fluids are needed to correct accumulated fluid and electrolyte imbalances? The first two questions are commonplace. Serious, neglected illnesses and injudicious fluid therapy underlie the last question.

A clear comprehension of this chapter is best achieved by an initial rapid reading followed by methodical study with concentration on those areas the student finds most difficult.

COLLECTION OF INFORMATION

What information is required to answer these questions about a particular patient, and how is it obtained? Four major sources are used: history (including accurately maintained records of intake and output), physical examination, laboratory analyses, and diagnosis *ex juvantibus* (based on the response to treatment).

History

If a physician is seeing a patient for the first time, only an estimate may be available of the amounts of fluid loss in vomitus, liquid stools, and urine. Similar rough estimates should be made for fluid intake, in terms of containers familiar to the patient and relatives.

For the hospitalized patient whose intake and output are recorded, a table should be made of all the solutions that have been given, starting from the time fluids and electrolytes were last believed to be in balance. The total amounts of the following should be determined: intravenous electrolytes and water, excreted urine and electrolyte-containing fluids lost from the body by gastric suction or other routes. An estimate must also be made of the insensible loss by evaporation from skin and lungs. In the average adult, at normal temperatures and humidity, this loss totals about 800 ml/day.

Physical Examination

During the physical examination, an estimate should be made of the amount of subcutaneous extracellular fluid (ECF) present. This requires an awareness of the effect of varying amounts of subcutaneous fat and elastic tissue on skin turgor. One can evaluate skin turgor by pinching the skin into a fold and observing the rate of return to normal. In the very obese patient, severe depletion of ECF may be masked by fatty turgor of the skin. In the elderly, and often poorly nourished, patient with little fat and elastic tissue, poor skin turgor often *suggests* depletion of ECF even though the ECF volume is normal. In a young, lean, acutely ill adult, severe deficiency of ECF is characterized by skin that can be pinched up into a fold and remains in that position for several seconds.

Overexpansion of ECF is sometimes difficult to determine until the patient develops dependent edema along the back or buttocks or, if the patient has been in a standing or sitting position, pitting edema of the ankles. Sometimes, even though definite edema cannot be found, the jellylike movement of the tissues on percussion will be suggestive of waterlogged subcutaneous tissues. *Changes* in the findings are often much more helpful than the static findings at any single examination. These changes in ECF (skin turgor, edema, and ascites) are easier to detect than changes in total body water. *Rapid* changes in total body water—either overhydration or dehydration—do lead to mental confusion, coma, and convulsions (which may mimic the signs and symptoms of a poorly localized cerebrovascular accident); however, total body water abnormalities, in contrast to changes in ECF, produce no detectable changes in skin turgor.

Physical examination not only reveals signs of gross abnormalities of total body water and ECF volumes but also may provide clues to abnormal *chemical composition* of body fluids. A patient with suspected potassium deficiency will often have weakness of the muscles and distension of the bowel with poor bowel sounds. A high serum potassium may cause disturbances of the heart rhythm as the potassium approaches a lethal level of 8 to 10 mEq/L. High serum calcium levels cause mental confusion, nausea and vomiting, and profound weakness. Low calcium levels are accompanied by muscle spasm and neuromuscular irritability, so that tapping over the facial nerve causes contraction of the facial muscles (Chvostek's sign).

Central nervous system diseases, such as encephalitis and cirrhosis, often result in coma states. The consequent rapid ventilation causes "blowing off" of carbon dioxide, which results in *respiratory alkalosis*. This causes a decrease in ionized calcium and may be accompanied by the signs of calcium deficiency. Patients with metabolic acidosis breathe rapidly and deeply in an effort to blow off sufficient carbon dioxide to lower carbonic acid levels and, by virtue of this respiratory alkalosis, to compensate for the *metabolic acidosis*. The physician who is familiar with the patient's basic underlying disease is in an excellent position to recognize various physical signs of abnormal fluid and electrolyte balance. Reexamination of the patient is important. Changes in physical findings not initially evident are often recognized during repeated examinations. Changes in body weight, skin turgor, alertness, and breathing rate *during treatment* also contribute to the evaluation.

ANALYSIS OF DATA
Estimation of Body Fluid Volumes in Health

In the average healthy adult male who is well nourished but has a minimum of fat (fat contains almost no free water), about 60% of the body weight is made up of fluid components. Women have more fat than men. By finding out what an obese patient weighed before becoming obese (or, if necessary, by simply estimating what the patient should weigh after a satisfactory regimen of weight reduction) one can arrive at a rough idea of the patient's expected normal lean (nonfat) body mass. From lean body mass, estimates of the volume of fluids in the body compartments can be calculated easily.

The lean body weight is converted from pounds to kilograms by dividing by 2.2 (2.2 pounds/kg). The extracellular water is estimated by multiplying the lean body mass by 20%: 15% of the lean body mass as fluid between the cells, or interstitial fluid; and 5% as fluid in the circulating blood volume, exclusive of the blood cells. This leaves, therefore, 40% of the lean body mass as intracellular fluid; a 70 kg lean man should possess about 3.5 L of plasma; 7% to 8% of the lean body mass is the usual estimate of normal blood volume (plasma + cells).

VOLUME, TONICITY, AND BODY SOLUTES

Every solution has a characteristic solute curve, illustrated by Fig. 3-1, where the horizontal axis is the volume, the vertical axis is concentration, and the curving line represents a given amount of solute. Since the amount of solute is fixed, any volume increase causes a reciprocal decrease in concentration. Similarly, with decreasing volume the concentration rises.

The equation *Volume × Concentration = Total body solute* depicts this relationship mathematically. The body solutions share this relationship, but obvi-

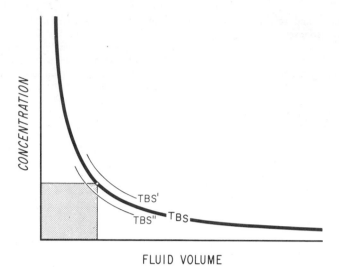

Fig. 3-1. Concentration-volume relationship. Concentration of electrolytes on vertical axis against fluid volume on horizontal axis. Because total body solutes *(TBS)* is a fixed amount of solutes, any point on the curving line equals any other point. Since concentration × volume = TBS, then if volume increases, concentration must decrease; if volume decreases, concentration must increase. *TBS´*, Increase in solutes (electrolyte overinfusion). *TBS´´*, Decrease in solutes (from vomiting and diarrhea).

ously life depends on these three variables remaining within a limited physiological range.

Body solutions differ from simple solutions in vitro because the body has two distinct fluid compartments (cellular and extracellular). Cells separate the body solutes by pumping sodium out and allowing potassium to replace the displaced sodium, but the concentration of solute in the cellular compartment *always equals* the concentration of solute in the extracellular compartment. This is the *law of osmotic equilibrium*. The concentration of intracellular cations (chiefly potassium) always equals the concentration of extracellular cations (chiefly sodium). Water diffusing freely between the two body compartments maintains this osmotic equality. Fig. 3-2 shows the concentration–volume–total solute relationship as it applies to man.

Although we depend on ECF (serum) samples for concentration measurements, we know they reflect intracellular concentrations as well. Despite the dual fluid compartments and the physiological segregation of cations in the body, the *Concentration*, × *Volume* = *Total body solute* relationship is equally valid in living organisms and in the test tube.

Concentrations of sodium, the dominant extracellular cation, holds the key to body tonicity and volume. Since sodium represents 92% of all extracellular cations, we can use it as if it were the only cation. The body zealously guards sodium concentration maintaining a level between 136 and 145 mEq/L. Despite wide individual variations in the intake of salt and water, control of thirst and antidiuretic hormone stabilizes sodium concentration within this narrow range.

Sodium concentration is a measure of *tonicity* of body fluids: sodium concentrations below 136 mEq/L denote *hypertonicity;* concentrations above 145 mEq/L indicate *hypotonicity.*

We can estimate acute body volume changes by determining weight changes, skin turgor, pulse rate, dryness of tongue, hematocrit, hemoglobin,* and other indicators. We can also accurately determine body tonicity (sodium concentration) in the laboratory. With the aid of these two measurements and clear understanding of the concentration–volume–total solute relationship, we can diagnose and treat most body fluid abnormalities. The six chief abnormalities are total body water loss, total body water gain, extracellular fluid loss, extracellular fluid gain, pure salt deficit, and malnutrition. I will discuss and illustrate these abnormalities in terms of the concentration–volume–total body solute diagrams.

BODY FLUID ABNORMALITIES
Total Body Water Loss

An estimate is made of the total body water deficit, incurred by lack of oral intake and the duration of desiccation from loss of urine and continued evaporation from skin and lungs. This number of liters of water is subtracted in the diagram when the line *E* is moved appropriately closer to *I*. For example, if a 70 kg man has

---

*Red blood cells and concentration defects: Another concentration measurement helpful in the diagnosis of ECF deficit is the concentration of red blood cells. Plasma is part of the ECF. Plasma volume contracts along with the interstitial fluid volume. The result is an increase in the hemoglobin concentration and hematocrit. Often a hemoglobin or hematocrit has not been determined before the patient loses ECF. An estimate can still be helpful, however, if the patient has not had signs or symptoms of anemia or polycythemia. Under such circumstances a hematocrit of 60 or above or a hemoglobin of 19 g/dl allows a strong presumption that contraction of the ECF volume has occurred. The single measurement is interpreted as *a change in concentration caused by a change in compartment volume.*

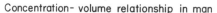

Concentration- volume relationship in man

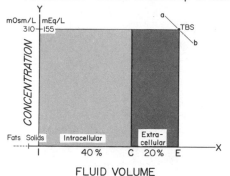

FLUID VOLUME

Fig. 3-2. Concentration of electrolytes on vertical axis against fluid volume on horizontal axis. Distribution of body fluids into, *I*, intracellular (40%) and, *E*, extracellular compartments (20%). Remaining 40% of body weight is composed of solids and normally distributed fat, Total body solutes, *TBS*, are depicted by a curving line, *a-b*, which is a *mathematical constant*. (Concentration × volume = total solutes in *any* solution.) This line naturally falls at the intersection of volume and concentration. Diagram depicts mathematical relationship of concentration × volume = total solutes. When one changes, another *must* also change. A clear understanding of these diagrams in health and in the disease states that follow is as fundamental to understanding fluid and electrolyte problems as are the multiplication tables to understanding mathematics.

been unable to drink for 2½ days and during this time has continued to evaporate water, he has an estimated loss of 2 L. Also, if during this time he has excreted 1 L of urine, his total body water deficit would amount to 3 L (approximately 7% of his lean body weight). This is depicted by a 7% decrease in the distance between *I* and *E* (Fig. 3-3).

The cells also participate in this loss, depicted by a 7% decrease in the distance between *I* and *C*. Any change in total body water is a change in both the *cellular volume* and the *extracellular fluid volume*. Water moves freely across the cell membranes, equalizing the osmotic pressure *outside* and *inside* the cell. Since no solutes are lost, the concentration rises.

Total Body Water Gain

If the patient has retention of water without any change in total body salt, concentration of salt decreases. Retention of 4 L in a 70 kg man (total body water is about 42 L) represents a 10% increase in total body water, and the concentration of solutes (as depicted by sodium) can be expected to decrease by 10% (Fig. 3-4). This means that the sodium should now be 129 mEq/L instead of 143.

Extracellular Fluid Loss

The ECF volume is altered when the patient loses electrolyte-containing fluids, as in vomiting and diarrhea or after a severe burn. In major trauma (as after prolonged and extensive operations or major hemorrhage), a decrease in ECF occurs. An effort should be made to estimate the actual number of liters of electrolyte-containing fluid lost: one depicts this by moving the line *E* to the left but with no change in the intracel-

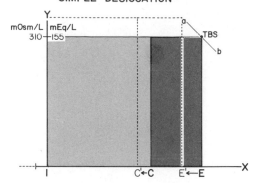

SIMPLE DESICCATION

Fig. 3-3. In simple desiccation, volume decreases, concentration increases, and total body solutes (the product of volume × concentration) remain the same. Remember, the curving line, *a-b*, is a constant. (Any point on this line equals any other point.) Both extracellular and intracellular compartments share in water loss.

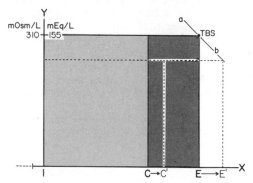

PURE WATER EXCESS

Fig. 3-4. In pure water excess (usually renal failure), fluid volume increases and concentration decreases. Total body solutes remain the same. Notice that this excess water is distributed throughout total body water.

lular fluid volume *IC* (Fig. 3-5). Sometimes, when the diagnosis of ECF deficit can be made, the data necessary for quantitation are deficient. The degree of ECF contraction must then be estimated from physical findings plus response to treatment. A loss of one fourth to one third of the extracellular fluid volume is sufficient to cause signs of circulatory disturbance such as a lowered blood pressure, especially when the patient is in a sitting position. Urinary output is low. A patient who has vomiting and diarrhea and who has very poor skin turgor may therefore need as much as 3 to 4 L of expansion of ECF before he begins to look well, to resume normal renal function, and to have a normal blood pressure and normal peripheral circulation.

Extracellular Fluid Gain

Patients with heart failure or with cirrhosis and increased aldosterone, or patients with decreased renal function who are given too much sodium-containing fluid, may develop edema, ascites, or pleural fluid.

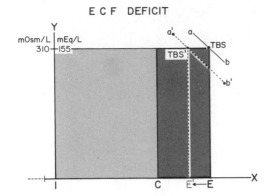

Fig. 3-5. Extracellular fluid deficit. Because body solutes are *lost* from body (vomiting, diarrhea, burns), *TBS* changes to *TBS´* (the new constant is parallel curving line *a´-b´*). Concentration stays the same, but volume of extracellular fluid decreases.

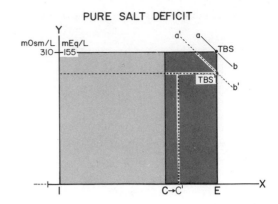

Fig. 3-6. Vomiting or diarrhea followed by drinking water is common cause of pure salt deficit. Volume stays the same; concetration decreases. Again, since body solutes have been lost, position of *TBS* changes to *TBS´*. The excess water distributes evenly between intracellular and extracellular compartments. Overall effect is shrinking of extracellular compartment. Hematocrit reflects this shrinkage by rising. Intracellular fluid volume is increased.

One can estimate this retention by knowing the increase in *total body weight,* and it should be depicted in Fig. 3-2 as an increase in ECF volume *(EC)* and a new *TBS* line, which is to the right of line *a-b*. Congestive heart failure and overtransfusion of blood and salt solutions are two common examples.

Pure Salt Deficit

The patient who loses ECF containing electrolytes and receives nonelectrolyte fluid may have a normal body weight and a normal total body water volume but reduced total body solute. This is depicted in Fig. 3-6 by *TBS´*. With simple loss of ECF (Fig. 3-5), the position of the cell membrane, *C,* does not change; however, in pure salt deficiency (with vomiting of electrolyte solution and replacement with water), an internal shift to *C´* (water goes into cells) occurs. Even though the patient's body weight is normal, the concentration of sodium is low and the hematocrit and hemoglobin are elevated. This paradoxical decrease in sodium concentration and rise in hematocrit and hemoglobin concentration strongly suggest a pure salt deficit. The white blood count is usually greatly elevated. This may be suggestive of infection, but the body temperature is usually below normal and when the salt is replaced the white count falls toward normal along with the hematocrit.

Total Body Water Excess Versus Pure Salt Deficiency

Sometimes the information from history and physical findings is insufficient to make a complete diagnosis in a patient with a *low* concentration of serum sodium, and the physician must determine whether the problem is total body water excess or pure salt deficiency. Examination of Figs. 3-4 and 3-6 reveals how this question can be settled. The lowered concentration of serum sodium indicates that if total body solute is normal (a simple total body water excess), ECF volume is increased *(E´* would now be opposite *b)*. With the increase in ECF volume, intracellular fluid volume (including red blood cells) would be equally increased.

The hematocrit would be normal. In contrast, if the problem is loss of electrolyte solution and replacement with nonelectrolyte solution (a pure salt deficiency), total body water and body weight are unchanged. There is, however, an internal shift of fluids into the cells depicted by an increase in *IC* and a decrease in *EC,* with *C´* the position of the cell membranes. Since the ECF volume is contracted, the hematocrit will be high. The rise in hematocrit with pure salt deficit distinguishes it from total body water excess in which the hematocrit is unchanged.

There is still another possible explanation for a low concentration of serum sodium—protein malnutrition. Under such circumstances serum albumin is decreased and plasma volume tends, therefore, to be inadequate. Retention of sodium occurs and water retention also occurs to the extent that an effective plasma volume is established by increase in ECF and total body water. A simplified summary of these changes is shown in Fig. 3-7. Because of the decrease in cellular tissue and potassium, total body solute is decreased.

Assessing Laboratory Data

Two concepts must be mastered regarding the interpretation of serum sodium concentration. These are the rules of *osmotic equilibrium,* which we have already discussed, and *electrical neutrality.* The second rule states that *total anions must equal total cations* in an electrolyte solution. It implies that any change in concentration of sodium must be accompanied by an equal change in concentration of anions.

Once the use of sodium concentration as an index of tonicity of body fluids and the rule of electrical neutrality are accepted, the clinician may evaluate the accuracy of a set of laboratory data (Fig. 3-8). The internal consistency of a set of laboratory data should be scrutinized carefully. If the concentration of chloride plus CO_2 (as bicarbonate) approaches or exceeds the value given for sodium, obviously a laboratory error in-

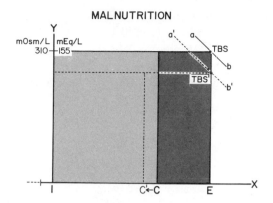

MALNUTRITION

Fig. 3-7. Chronically malnourished patient has low concentration of serum sodium but total body sodium is increased. Deficit in body solute is in exchangeable potassium. There is movement of sodium into cells as well as expansion of extracellular fluid and total body water. Plasma volume is actually above normal and hematocrit is reduced. History and physical findings should distinguish this condition from pure water excess. Low hematocrit distinguishes malnutrition from pure salt deficiency.

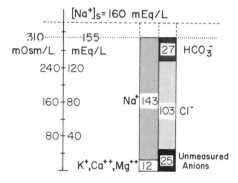

Fig. 3-8. Total anions must always equal total cations. Dilution or concentration of body electrolytes will affect both sides of Gamble diagram so that change in anion concentration is proportional to change in cation (sodium) concentration.

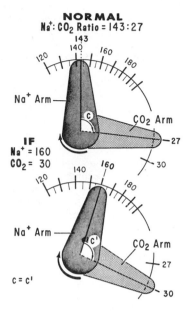

NORMAL
$Na^+: CO_2$ Ratio = 143:27

Fig. 3-9. Arms to circular slide rule are set as normal ratio of CO_2 to sodium. Arms with this fixed ratio are then moved to observed sodium, and expected CO_2 is read. Expected chloride for any observed sodium is determined in same fashion.

volves at least one of these ions. All three of the determinations must be repeated.

If the concentration of sodium is excessively high in comparison to the concentration of CO_2 plus chloride, there may be a laboratory error, but it may also indicate an abnormal accumulation of unmeasured anions as occurs in uremia, ketosis, severe infection, and circulatory insufficiency. If the patient has no disease or condition that would cause an elevation of unmeasured anions, laboratory error should be suspected.

Bedside Proportions

A small circular slide rule (Fig. 3-9) was once helpful for these proportions and for other calculations at the bedside. Today a wrist or pocket calculator is used, but the calculations remain the same. The ratio of normal concentration of chloride to sodium can be established (143 to 103), and then maintaining this ratio at a fixed angle, the sodium arm can be moved to the observed abnormal value, say 160. For such a patient,

with a relative deficiency in total body water (Figs. 3-3 and 3-9), the expected chloride would be 115. Changes in concentration of major anions should be proportional to changes in concentration of sodium unless an associated disturbance of electrolyte *composition* of the extracellular fluid exists.

The normal ratio of CO_2 content to sodium concentration is 27 to 143. This ratio (or fixed angle) is established on the arms of the slide rule (Fig. 3-9). As the sodium arm is moved over to 160, it is observed that the normal CO_2 content for the patient becomes 30. In this way the rule of electrical neutrality allows determination of the internal consistency of a set of data as well as determination of whether an observed chloride or CO_2 concentration is altered simply by virtue of the change in *total body water* or by a true change in the composition of the electrolytes in ECF.

A reciprocal relationship is also seen between CO_2 content (HCO_3 in Fig. 3-8) and chloride. A compositional change in which the concentration of one of the anions increases greatly cannot exist without a decrease in another of the anions. For example, when a patient with a peptic ulcer vomits acid gastric juice containing high concentrations of chloride, the remaining fluid in the body has a deficit of chloride (hypochloremia). This is a deficit of chloride in the entire ECF. The bicarbonate anion will be above normal. When the CO_2 content (bicarbonate) is normal or decreased and the chloride is greatly decreased, some cause for elevation of the unmeasured anions, such as phosphate, ketone bodies, or organic acids, must be sought. One of the more common causes of this is renal insufficiency; the blood urea nitrogen and creatinine will be elevated.

The other ions exist in such low concentrations that they do not participate in the reciprocity with total body water and are not influenced in a significant way by considerations of electrical neutrality. One trace cation is normally present in a concentration of 40 nm/L. This is the hydrogen ion, and in so-called *metabolic* disturbances of acid-base balance (diabetic acidosis, uremia) the serum CO_2 content in mEq/L may permit a very good estimate of the severity of hydrogen ion increase (acidosis) or decrease (alkalosis). If the patient has been vomiting, the resultant hypochloremia and an increase in the bicarbonate (or CO_2) content indicate a *hypochloremic alkalosis*. In situations in which chloride or other anions are increased in concentration and bicarbonate is decreased, a diagnosis of metabolic acidosis is made. Whether this is primary metabolic acidosis or is compensatory to respiratory alkalosis is a question that is discussed in the section on acid-base balance (p. 20).

WRITING THE PRESCRIPTION

The physician at the bedside who understands the concentration-volume relationships and the clinical status of his patient is well prepared to order replacement fluids. So that nothing is left out of this order, he should consider three items: *metabolic fluid losses, current abnormal fluid losses,* and *accumulated imbalances.*

Replacing Urine and Insensible Fluid Loss

First the patient needs *metabolic fluids* for urine and insensible loss. This fluid is relatively low in electrolyte concentration and can be supplied by the use of 5% glucose. The average patient will produce about 1000 ml of urine in 24 hours and will require some 800 ml of the same fluid for replacement of insensible loss from skin and lungs. This does not include sweat, which should be considered an abnormal fluid and would require some replacement with salt. This may approach 2000 or 3000 ml in hot weather or with fever. Accurate body weights are essential when losses occur that cannot be measured. They are indicated in all patients receiving intravenous fluids.

Replacing Abnormal Fluid Losses

The second type of fluid required depends on *ongoing abnormal losses*. Usually the orders are written on morning rounds. At this time about 8 hours of the day have passed, and it is a simple calculation to determine the amount of fluid in the gastric suction or drainage from other parts of the gastrointestinal tract and simply to multiply the amount of fluid by 3 to estimate total 24-hour requirements. If the patient has no abnormal fluid losses, this item can be ignored. If the fluid being lost is acid gastric juice, as determined by a quick bedside determination with pH-sensitive paper, replacement should be with 0.9% saline. If the intestinal juices are quite alkaline, as is the case with a fresh ileostomy or leakage from a duodenal fistula, replacement should be with saline and one-sixth molar sodium lactate in the ratio of two parts and one part. If the patient is losing extracellular-like fluid with a normal body fluid pH, e.g., the removal of a large volume of pleural or peritoneal fluid, it should be replaced with a fluid that has the composition of normal ECF. This can be approximated by use of isotonic saline and one-sixth molar so-

dium lactate in the proportions of 4 to 1, which is the ratio of the major anions in ECF—chloride and bicarbonate, 103 and 27.

Restoring Normal Balance

The third and most complex item to be considered is *correction fluids*. The concentration volume diagram is of great help in situations of imbalance. A few examples of the various abnormalities just discussed are given in the following paragraphs:

1. If the patient is deficient in *total body water* as evidenced by a 10% increase in sodium concentration (and weight loss of 8 pounds), he will require a 10% increase in total body water, which can be supplied as 5% glucose. This means that to change a sodium concentration from 158 to 143 in a lean 70 kg man, it would be necessary to provide 4 L of 5% glucose. Remember, this is *in addition to* the fluids required for metabolic purposes (urine and insensible loss) and replacement of current abnormal losses.

2. If the patient has a *deficit* of *extracellular fluid* estimated to be approximately one fourth of his normal expected extracellular volume, this can be replaced with lactated Ringer's solution or with a mixture of saline and M/6 sodium lactate in the proportions of 4 to 1. For the hypothetical 70 kg lean man, this would require 20% of 70, which is 14 L, times a one-fourth deficit, or 3.5 L of ECF replacement.

3. For the patient who has a *pure salt deficiency* and a normal total body water (Fig. 3-6), corrective salt replacement is calculated as follows: Given a serum sodium concentration of 121 mEq/L the deficency is 143 mEq/L − 121 mEq/L = 22 mEq/L. Since in this situation the "excess" water has shifted into cells (remember, water moves freely across cell membranes), the deficit in sodium (22 mEq/L) must be multiplied by the *total body water* (42 L) to give 924 mEq. This is the total deficit, which is the amount of salt contained in 6 L of ECF.

This much salt should never be given as a single order. Initially a hypertonic salt solution can be used, but not more than 9 to 10 g of salt should be given without reevaluating the patient. This is the amount of salt present in 200 ml of 5% sodium chloride or 300 ml of 3% sodium chloride. In such a severe ECF salt deficiency, this order may be repeated twice, but then the remainder of the deficit should be made up of isotonic electrolyte solution. Additional salt can thus be administered in the fluids needed for metabolic requirements for urine and insensible loss. Usually these are nonelectrolyte solutions, but in the patient with a salt deficit the entire intravenous fluid therapy can consist of giving electrolyte solution over a period of several days until the deficiency is corrected.

4. If the patient has a *hypochloremia*, the replacement solutions should be composed of 0.9% saline. *Saline is an acidifying solution* and will correct a metabolic alkalosis because saline has 155 mEq/L of chloride, in comparison with normal ECF, which has only 103 mEq/L. This means that in every liter of 0.9% saline approximately 50 mEq of extra chloride is provided to increase the chloride concentration. The *ECF total chloride deficit* and the number of liters of 0.9% saline required to supply this amount of excess chloride can be calculated.

If the metabolic alkalosis is severe, hydrochloric acid may be infused by use of a 0.1 to 1 N solution administered through a central venous catheter by gravity drip at 1 mEq per minute until two thirds of the calculated dose has been given. Such treatment is indicated only when two of the following three criteria are met: pH 7.45 or above, base excess 7 mEq/L or more, partial pressure of arterial CO_2 50 torr or higher.

5. If the patient has a *metabolic acidosis* with a bicarbonate of 17 mEq/L and one desires to increase this to 27, the deficit of 10 mEq/L is multiplied by the estimated liters of *ECF*, which in the 70 kg person should be 14 L for a total of 140 mEq. A molar solution of sodium lactate contains 1000 mEq/L of lactate. The lactate is metabolized, and the result is bicarbonate. One-sixth molar sodium lactate solution contains one-sixth as much bicarbonate as molar lactate, or 166 mEq/L. This means that some 850 ml of one-sixth molar sodium lactate would supply the required 140 mEq of bicarbonate.

Selecting and Administering Fluids

As the various requirements of fluid and electrolytes are added up, some of the electrolytes may be placed in metabolic fluids if necessary to avoid use of hypertonic electrolyte solutions. In a patient who has large current losses and an extensive past deficit (in addition to his metabolic needs), the administration of 8 to 9 L of fluid in 24 hours may be required. If this is the case, the order should be written so that the nurse will run the fluids at a rate to approximate 9 L in 24 hours. The size of drops varies, but the average is about 16 drops/ml; 9 L of fluid contain 144,000 drops. There are 60 minutes in the hour, and in 24 hours there are 1,440 minutes. A simple division reveals that the intravenous fluid should run at the rate of 100 drops per minute. Always specify the rate at which intravenous fluids should be infused.

Recording Intake and Output

The various bags of fluid ordered should be numbered. The nurse should write the numbers on the bags when they are prepared for the patient, so that they correspond with the physician's orders. When each bag is empty, it should be kept near the patient's bed—at any time the numbered bags can be reviewed to determine what fluids have been given and what fluids are yet to be given. At least once every 24 hours, usually at midnight, all the bags are gathered together and the total 24-hour urine volume is measured as well as the volume of gastrointestinal juices. This information must then be recorded accurately in the chart.

Bedside Tests

Much of the information is now available for writing a new set of fluid orders for the next 24 hours. Either the nurse or the physician can obtain additional useful information at the bedside by measuring the specific gravity of the urine. With color-coded test tape, pH should be measured in the urine and in all other fluids removed from the patient. A patient who is losing acid gastric juice will develop alkalosis, and his urine will tend to become more alkaline. A patient who is losing alkaline juices in excess of what is replaced will gradually develop metabolic acidosis, and his urine will become more acid. A patient who is not receiving enough water will produce urine with a high specific gravity. A patient who is receiving gavage feedings with a high-protein, high-calorie feeding and an inadequate amount of water may have 1 L of urine, but the specific gravity may be 1.035, indicating that the water intake is inadequate for this solute load.

Bedside tests are available for estimation of urine chloride (the Fantus test) or urine sodium (the zinc uranyl acetate precipitation test). These tests show whether the urinary salt excretion is normal, high, or low; for example, if a patient with a low or normal serum concentration has 8 to 9 g of salt in the urine continuously despite the fact that a seemingly adequate amount of salt is being given intravenously each day, either adrenal insufficiency or a salt-losing disease of the kidney should be suspected. Such a patient can be given 8 to 10 mg of desoxycorticosterone acetate (Doca). If this causes an immediate reduction in the salt excretion, the patient has adrenal insufficiency and will need treatment with corticosteroids. If steroids are ineffective, a renal abnormality exists, and the salt loss will have to be replaced as an abnormal loss in the same way that loss of electrolyte in gastrointestinal secretions is replaced.

Clinical Reevaluation

When the fluids have been ordered, the physician should examine the patient again periodically to make sure that the diagnosis is correct and that the patient is responding to the fluid therapy as anticipated. A patient with severe metabolic acidosis who is receiving one-sixth molar sodium lactate should have a progressive decrease in the rate and depth of respiration. A patient with a severe ECF volume deficit who is receiving 3 to 4 L of extracellular fluid should show improvement in skin turgor, pulse, blood pressure, and rate of urinary output. A patient with a total body water deficit should show improvement in sensorium and increase in output and decrease in specific gravity of the urine. If such a patient has an excessive amount of urine and seems to be losing urine as fast as 5% glucose is given, one should suspect diabetes insipidus and test for it by giving vasopressin (Pitressin). These are examples of *diagnosis ex juvantibus*. If the response to treatment is not as expected, the collection and analysis of information must be reviewed since the basis for the fluid orders may have been erroneous.

SPECIAL PROBLEMS

The healthy, young, thin patient with a surgical problem such as inguinal hernia or appendicitis receives parenteral fluids for a very short time and will tolerate gross errors of fluid therapy ranging from receiving no fluids to receiving only glucose solution or saline. Since the majority of patients do not require careful analysis, there is a real danger that a physician will become careless and fail to think through the logical analysis, which may be lifesaving in the critically ill patient. The general analysis has been presented, and after some experience in its use it actually requires only a few minutes to complete in the majority of patients. In addition to the preceding outline, the experienced physician will apply additional reasoning when he recognizes certain specific problems such as complicated acid-base imbalance, disturbances in potassium metabolism, acute trauma, and other problems, some of which will be discussed briefly.

Acid-Base Balance

The hydrogen ion concentration in body fluids plays a critical role in enzyme systems and other physiological processes (conservation of base by the kidneys and binding of oxygen by hemoglobin, for example). Remarkable *buffer systems* dampen or moderate any rapid changes in hydrogen ion concentration. The main buffer system, the bicarbonate ion–carbonic acid buffer, is aided first by pulmonary regulation of excretion of volatile acid as CO_2 and second by renal excretion of nonvolatile acids such as those of phosphate and ammonium. The ratio of bicarbonate ion to carbonic acid in body fluids is normally 20 to 1. The Henderson-Hasselbalch equation expresses this important relationship of body pH, bicarbonate ion (nonvolatile), and carbonic acid (volatile) in mathematical terms:

$$pH = pK + \log \frac{BHCO_3}{H_2CO_3}$$

In clinical concepts, this may be expressed as:

$$\text{Acid-base balance} = \text{Constant} + \frac{\text{Kidney function}}{\text{Ventilation}}$$

Primary diseases in the kidneys, which cause ineffective excretion of nonvolatile acids, are compensated for by increased excretion of volatile (carbonic) acid by the lung. The converse is also true. In assessment of acid-base disturbances, CO_2 content, which measures volatile and nonvolatile acids, is of limited value in patients with complicated metabolic, renal, and pulmonary problems.

Two pieces of data and a diagram (Fig. 3-10) are necessary to analyze acid-base disturbances more completely. These are pH and Pco_2. They are obtained rapidly and accurately from arterial blood samples.

Concept of pH

pH is the negative log of the hydrogen ion concentration and is a convenient way of stating a very small number. The normal arterial pH is 7.4. With increasing hydrogen ion concentrations, the pH decreases, and this is referred to as a state of *acidosis*. Hydrogen ion concentration decrease is associated with an increased pH and is called alkalosis.

Two types of pH disturbance are classified according to whether they are caused by a change in the body carbonic acid (respiratory disturbances) or whether they are caused by a change in concentration of nonvolatile, nonrespiratory substances, (metabolic disturbances). Whenever fluids that are excreted, secreted, or lost from the body differ in their hydrogen ion concentration from normal body fluids, an opposite change occurs in the hydrogen ion concentration of the fluids remaining in the body: if a patient loses acid gastric juice, the body changes toward alkalosis. If the patient excretes very alkaline urine, the body fluids change toward a state of acidosis. Acidosis and alkalosis (or basosis) are, for the clinician, terms signifying a deviation from a normal body pH of 7.4.

Concept of Pco_2

The second important datum is the partial pressure of CO_2 (Pco_2) in the body fluids and in the alveolar air, which is in equilibrium with these fluids. Usually the alveolar CO_2 concentration is about 5.6%. (Partial pressures, measured in torr, or mm Hg, vary with barometric pressure and vapor pressure.) A normal Pco_2 is usually about 40 torr. The rate of excretion of CO_2 by ventilation regulates the carbonic acid in the body. A Pco_2 above normal (hypercapnia, hypercarbia) indicates *respiratory acidosis*. If the ventilation is above normal so that the patient is blowing off excessive amounts of CO_2 (hypocapnia, hypocarbia), the Pco_2 will be below normal (respiratory alkalosis).

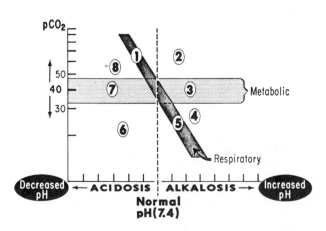

Fig. 3-10. All possible acid-base abnormalities in terms of Pco_2 and pH.
(Modified from Siggaard-Andersen, O.: The acid base status of the blood, Baltimore, 1964, The Williams & Wilkins Co.)

1. Respiratory acidosis
2. Mixed respiratory acidosis and metabolic alkalosis.
3. Metabolic alkalosis
4. Mixed metabolic and respiratory alkalosis

5. Respiratory alkalosis
6. Mixed metabolic acidosis and respiratory alkalosis
7. Metabolic acidosis
8. Mixed metabolic and respiratory acidosis

Types of Acid-Base Imbalances

Acid-base deviations can be classified as primary, compensatory, or mixed. A patient with a primary metabolic acidosis from retention of lactic acid (attributed to poor circulation or shock) will usually respond to the increased concentration of hydrogen ions by breathing more rapidly and increasing the rate of excretion of carbonic acid. This is *compensatory respiratory alkalosis*. *Primary respiratory alkalosis* may occur in a patient with portal hypertension and cirrhosis. Portacaval shunt may cause an increase in ammonia in the blood and, as a result of this, stimulation of the respiratory center. Increased ventilation results in "blowing off" carbonic acid, which eventuates in primary respiratory alkalosis. Sometimes a patient develops two primary conditions, one of which is respiratory and the other metabolic, and yet neither of these is compensating. Both are the result of some disease process or its complication; these are referred to as *mixed forms of acid-base imbalance*. For instance a patient with emphysema may be unable to excrete carbon dioxide normally and may develop an elevated P_{CO_2}, or a *primary respiratory acidosis*, from the retained carbonic acid. At the same time such a patient may have one of several different conditions that might also cause a *primary metabolic alkalosis*, such as an obstructing duodenal ulcer causing vomiting of acid gastric juice.

Graphic Summary of Acid-Base Abnormalities

The pH-P_{CO_2} diagram (Fig. 3-10) makes it possible to summarize all primary, compensatory, and mixed acid-base abnormalities. Pure abnormalities of nonrespiratory, or metabolic, origin are depicted in areas 7 and 3, and pure deviations from normal (caused by decreased or increased excretion of carbonic acid or respiratory abnormalities) are shown in areas 1 and 5. Areas 2, 4, 6, and 8 are all mixed areas. Area 6 is a common location for patients who have a primary metabolic acidosis and a compensatory respiratory alkalosis. Area 2 includes patients with mixed primary problems but also *respiratory compensation for a metabolic alkalosis*. If a patient with a primary metabolic alkalosis moves into area 2, it may signify that he also has a primary abnormality in his pulmonary function, and one should look for airway obstruction, pneumonia, pulmonary embolism, or another cause of impaired gas exchange.

Importance of Clinical Correlation

The preceding examples illustrate that *understanding a particular patient's acid-base problem requires more than just laboratory data*. The clinician must know what primary acid-base abnormalities might be present according to the disease process (i.e., increased ventilation may result because the lungs and the central nervous system function in a normal manner to compensate for a metabolic acidosis). If a patient has a high blood urea nitrogen and diseased kidneys fail to excrete excess organic acids, the retention of these acids will cause a metabolic acidosis. If the patient has severe ketosis, secondary to uncontrolled diabetes, and the lungs are clinically normal, then the excessive ventilation is compensatory, and the clinician knows, before he enlists the help of the laboratory, that the patient's P_{CO_2} and pH will converge somewhere in area 6.

With accurate clinical knowledge of the patient, measurement of P_{CO_2} and pH is often unnecessary. The CO_2 content of blood will provide a sufficiently accurate estimate of the abnormality in base excess. Normally the CO_2 content is 27 mEq/L in such samples, and in the patient described the CO_2 content might be 17, or even 7. The difference from normal in CO_2 content is -10 or -20 and is the deficit in base; thus, if the CO_2 content is only 7, this means a 20 mEq deficit. A 70 kg lean patient with 14 L of extracellular fluid would need 20 times 14, or 280, mEq of bicarbonate or lactate to bring the CO_2 content back to 27. This would require 1687 ml of one-sixth molar sodium lactate since 166 mEq is present in 1 L.

When pH and P_{CO_2} Measurements Are Necessary

Situations arise in which seriously ill patients (often found in postoperative and intensive care areas) probably have both metabolic and respiratory abnormalities. In these complex situations measurements of P_{CO_2} and pH are invaluable guides for determining whether the primary abnormality is metabolic, respiratory, or both.

From the examples given, simple calculations will determine the amount of one-sixth molar sodium lactate required for treatment of a metabolic acidosis or the amount of 0.9% saline, with its 50 mEq/L chloride excess, required to treat a metabolic alkalosis (provided that it is not secondary to potassium deficiency). Primary respiratory abnormalities of course, are best treated by measures to restore normal ventilation rather than by administration of any particular type of intravenous fluid. Alkaline solutions (one-sixth molar sodium lactate) may be necessary to correct a compensatory metabolic acidosis before sedation is given to correct the primary respiratory alkalosis (inappropriate overactivity of respiratory center).

Blood Gas Measurements

Arterial blood gas measurements may be needed frequently in patients who are seriously ill with abnormal cardiopulmonary function. Single samples can be obtained, or an indwelling arterial cannula may help to provide samples as needed. Allen's test consists of compressing the radial and ulnar arteries while the patient pumps blood out of the hand by fist clenching. Releasing only one artery at a time demonstrates whether there is adequate collateral blood flow should the radial artery become occluded. If the blood supply of the hand is dependent on the radial artery, other vessels should be used to obtain arterial blood samples, especially if an indwelling cannula is to be considered.

Arterial blood samples are frequently analyzed not only for P_{CO_2} and pH but also for partial pressure of O_2 (P_{O_2}), and not just to determine acid-base balance but to evaluate the adequacy of ventilation and oxygenation. Respiratory failure may occur suddenly without prior signs and symptoms but will usually be preceded by a progressive fall in Pa_{O_2}. Pa_{O_2} is normally 97 torr when a patient is breathing air. A value below 80 is abnormal and requires explanation and appropriate treatment. Oxygenation and ventilation are assessed separately by determination, respectively, of Pa_{O_2} and Pa_{CO_2}. Perfusion of areas of the lung that are not properly aerated causes a decrease in Pa_{O_2} because of the venous admixture or so-called shunt. Frequently ventilation is appropriate to maintain a normal $Paco_2$ even though there is a decrease in Pao_2. A rising $Paco_2$ indicates ventilatory failure. The focus of management then should be on the restoration of a more normal ventilation and not just on the administration of oxygen or correction of acid-base imbalance.

Oxygen therapy usually helps a patient with hypoxia, provided that ventilatory failure is not present. If $Paco_2$ is high and the respiratory drive is dependent on hypoxia, administration of oxygen alone will not help and may even exacerbate ventilatory failure. An endonasal endotracheal tube and ventilatory support may be urgently needed in addition to increased oxygen inhalation. The cause of CO_2 retention must be found and corrected. Blood gas analysis is the first step in recognition, evaluation, and determination of appropriate treatment of respiratory failure.

Potassium

Special thought must be given to potassium balance because potassium is the chief cation within cells (94% of total body potassium is in the cells). Young adult women have 2000 to 3000 mEq total potassium, and men have up to 5000 mEq. The correlation in humans between total exchangeable potassium and energy consumption (in calories per day with moderate activity) is around 0.90. The total exchangeable body potassium can be measured by dilution with radioactive potassium, but this is not a practical clinical test. The clinician must rely on analyses of serum potassium. There are only about 70 mEq of potassium in the ECF. The normal serum potassium ranges between 3.5 and 5 mEq/L. If as much as 70 mEq of potassium moves out of its location in cells into ECF or if this much potassium is retained in extracellular fluid during intravenous potassium administration, the patient will probably die of cardiac arrest.

Recognition of Potassium Abnormalities

Like the recognition of sodium deficiency, recognition of body potassium deficiency is dependent to a great extent on the suspicion of the clinician. Suspicion is raised by knowledge of circumstances that cause potassium loss. Potassium is continually excreted in urine. In contrast to sodium, despite cessation of potassium intake, the kidneys continue to excrete potassium (minimum rate, 10 to 20 mEq/day). It is also lost in gastrointestinal juices. If a patient has been losing large amounts of such fluids and the replacement solutions have contained no potassium, total body potassium deficiency will eventually occur, usually accompanied by a lowering of serum potassium concentration. The degree of lowering of serum potassium concentration, however, tells little about the magnitude of total body potassium deficiency.

Patients unable to take food by mouth and those who have suffered trauma, burns, or major operative procedures or were treated previously with steroids or diuretics are likely to have a potassium deficiency. The physical signs are nonspecific. Such patients have weakness (occasionally almost to paralysis), decreased deep tendon reflexes, and commonly ileus, abdominal distension, and a picture easily confused with chronic bowel obstruction. The electrocardiogram shows a flattening or even inversion of the T wave. These patients are quite sensitive to digitalis and may, if treated with digitalis, show signs of intoxication, with nausea and abnormal rhythm.

Patients with high serum potassium also may have muscle paralysis and complain of paresthesias. The electrocardiogram shows elevated and peaked T waves, and, at nearly lethal potassium levels, the electrocardiogram loses all of its normal components.

Potassium problems are divided into (1) those patients in whom the ECF potassium concentration is abnormal but without any intracellular deficit, and (2) those patients who have a total body potassium deficiency. The extracellular fluid potassium is affected by the rate of potassium absorption or absence of intake, the rate of loss from the body in various fluids, and the maintenance of a normal cellular metabolism. Sodium is continuously pumped out of cells, allowing a high concentration (or gradient) of potassium within the cells compared with the concentration of potassium in extracellular fluid. If the patient becomes severely ill so that metabolism is impaired and the sodium pump begins to fail, sodium tends to remain in cells and potassium tends to leak out; ECF potassium rapidly reaches a level incompatible with life.

Potassium excess. If a heavy object crushes large masses of muscle, potassium leaks out into the ECF along with myoglobin. The kidneys may become damaged from the pigment and from impaired circulation, and such a patient will die of potassium poisoning within 18 to 24 hours after the crushing injury. Severe burns and major operative procedures are also followed by elevation of serum potassium because of tissue damage and impaired renal function.

In most instances all that is required relative to potassium balance is to restrict potassium during the first 24 hours after a major operation or during the first few days after a burn. The patient with crush syndrome has to have vigorous treatment with peritoneal dialysis or use of the artificial kidney, and the dialyses may have to be carried on almost continuously during the first few days while large amounts of potassium are being lost from the crushed muscle. The patient in negative nitrogen balance who is burning his own cellular protein also loses potassium, and the amounts of potassium entering extracellular fluid can be reduced when 400 to 800 calories a day are supplied by the administration of glucose in the intravenous fluids so as to minimize protein catabolism.

Potassium ion and hydrogen ion concentration. The concentration of potassium in extracellular fluid is influenced by the hydrogen ion concentration. Increasing concentrations of hydrogen ion in the extracellular fluid (acidosis) cause hydrogen to move into cells and potassium to move out of cells, so that the serum potassium rises. If the acidosis is treated with sodium bicarbonate or sodium lactate, the serum potassium concentration will fall as the patient becomes less acidotic. If a patient has an alkalosis, this will cause the serum potassium to fall. The patient with severe diabetic acidosis may on initial examination have a serum potassium that is high and then in the course of treatment (and in a matter of hours if the acidosis is rapidly corrected) the potassium may fall to a very subnormal level, partly as a result of the change in acid-base balance and also because the patient may have a severe total body deficit of potassium.

Potassium deficit. Total body potassium deficit may arise in a variety of situations, but one of the classic examples is the patient who develops pyloric obstruction from a duodenal ulcer; vomiting produces a *hypochloremic alkalosis*. The physician prescribes an amount of saline that he believes should correct the hypochloremic alkalosis and, after treatment with this, finds that the patient still has a low chloride concentration and a high CO_2 content in blood. He may also observe that the patient has an acid urine, which seems inconsistent with alkalosis. In the days before the flame photometer, this was sufficent to justify a diagnosis of potassium deficiency,but with potassium analysis it is possible to document this by finding a low serum potassium.

For every 3 mEq of potassium lost from the cells, 2 mEq of sodium and 1 mEq of hydrogen ion enter the cells. The hydrogen, of course, is bound to protein and other buffers, but, as a result of this exchange, the cells become more acid. The cells lining the renal tubules participate in potassium deficiency and cellular acidosis so that the urine formed is acid (Fig. 3-11). Excretion of acid urine produces hypochloremic alkalosis in ECF. In the patient who has been vomiting acid gastric juice and also losing potassium, there are therefore two reasons for developing hypochloremic alkalosis. Both potassium and chloride are required to correct the potassium deficiency and the extracellular alkalosis.

Notice that two different problems related to potassium and hydrogen ion have been discussed. In the first situation a primary *extracellular acidosis* occurs and hydrogen ion moves into the cell forcing potassium out, causing an increase in concentration of serum po-

tassium. In the other situation the primary abnormality is an *intracellular potassium deficiency* and an increase in cellular hydrogen-ion concentration along with movement of sodium into the cell, followed by the production of an extracellular alkalosis. In the first situation the acidosis begins in ECF and also involves intracellular fluid. In the second situation, an intracellular acidosis initiates and sustains extracellular alkalosis. As you might expect, some patients who develop an extracellular acidosis, as in diabetic ketosis or with diarrhea, also develop a depletion of cellular potassium.

Treating Potassium Imbalances

The best treatment is prevention; potassium imbalance, like other fluid and electrolyte problems, can be prevented by replacement of abnormal fluid losses as they occur and provision of adequate calories and metabolic fluids together with 40 mEq of urinary loss potassium per day. The potassium requirements may be slightly higher if the patient is receiving steroids or diuretics. The requirements are nil if the patient is oliguric or acidotic or has recently undergone a major operation.

Gastrointestinal juice losses should be replaced in the same quantity and at the same rate as they are being lost. For each liter of intravenous electrolyte solution required, 40 mEq of potassium chloride should be added. Potassium should almost always be diluted in intravenous fluids so that 40 mEq is distributed in at least a liter of fluid. If, however, the serum potassium is below 3 mEq/L as much as 80 mEq can be placed in each liter of intravenous fluid. In some instances it will be necessary to give several hundred milliequivalents in a day, perhaps for a number of days, until the total body potassium deficit is repaired. This must be monitored with serum potassium analyses, and the treatment

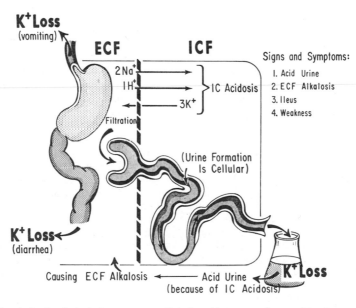

Fig. 3-11. Hypokalemic alkalosis is a common clinical problem seen after vomiting because of obstructing duodenal ulcer or pyloric stenosis with replacement of NaCl but *not* K^+. K^+ leaves cells. H^+ and Na^+ enter cells. Intracellular *acidosis* results from this exchange. Kidney cells are also acidotic and therefore secrete acid urine; ECF alkalosis is exaggerated. This situation is reversed only by correction of the K^+ deficit.

is tapered to maintenance levels as soon as the serum potassium reaches a normal range.

High potassium levels in patients who are severely acidotic and who have adequate renal function will return to normal as the patient's acidosis is corrected. In oliguria or acute renal failure a serum potassium of 7 mEq/L or above should be treated with emergency measures such as the administration of one-sixth molar sodium lactate to correct the acidosis, calcium to counteract the effect of potassium on myocardial irritability, and glucose and insulin to cause deposition of potassium along with phosphate and glycogen in the liver. If the patient can take sodium polystyrene sulfonate (an exchange resin) with sorbitol by mouth, it will remove potassium, but it should not be relied on in the emergency situation. The exchange resin can also be given as a retention enema. Peritoneal dialysis or hemodialysis is often required to restore the potassium to normal in the patient with renal failure; delay is deadly.

Calcium and Phosphate

Hypocalcemia

The administration of parenteral calcium or phosphate is infrequently required, but the circumstances in which it is required may be very dramatic. Tetany usually occurs within 2 days after parathyroidectomy or injury of the blood supply of the parathyroid glands during radical thyroidectomy. Recognition may be delayed for several weeks if the deficiency is mild. Hypocalcemia also occurs after removal of parathyroid adenomas or hyperplastic parathyroid glands and is to be expected if the patient has osteitis fibrosa cystica or other evidence of bone demineralization, such as an elevated alkaline phosphatase level.

Hypocalcemia is common in chronic acidosis and becomes manifest when the acidosis is treated. Acidosis tends to sustain a relatively high concentration of *ionized* calcium. When the acidosis is treated and the body fluids become more alkaline, rapid reduction in ionized calcium causes onset of symptoms. This is seen in patients with chronic renal insufficiency and occasionally in patients treated for acidosis from other causes such as diabetic ketosis or acidosis associated with chronic diarrhea. Patients with malabsorption and steatorrhea, such as that occurring after the removal of small bowel or sidetracking of small bowel for purposes of treating obesity, may lose calcium from bone but maintain normal serum calcium levels.

The symptoms of low serum calcium are tingling of the fingers and feet and paresthesias about the face, especially around the lips and tongue. Some patients have severe spasm of various muscles, more commonly the back muscles and the muscles of the hands and feet, so that the patient develops a characteristic flexion of the wrist and the metacarpophalangeal joint with extension of the distal phalangeal joints, referred to as carpopedal spasm. One can demonstrate the muscular irritability by tapping over the facial nerve and observing the contraction of the facial muscles, especially the orbicularis oris (Chvostek's sign). Production of carpopedal spasm by application of a tourniquet (Trousseau's sign) is less often demonstrable but is equally pathognomonic of hypocalcemia.

The muscle spasm and paresthesias cause anxiety, which commonly causes the patient to hyperventilate. The subsequent reduction in carbonic acid and respiratory alkalosis leads to a further decrease in the ionized calcium, which increases the symptoms and frightens the patient, causing further hyperventilation. This is similar to the hyperventilation syndrome with tetany occasionally seen in a patient who has a normal serum calcium, but it is much more likely to occur in a patient with hypoparathyroidism.

The suspected diagnosis is confirmed by a serum calcium below 8 mg/dl and, probably of even more importance, a serum phosphorus that is above 4.5 mg/dl. If both calcium and phosphorus are below normal, there may be a problem of inadequate nutrition rather than hypoparathyroidism. Patients with uremia have retention of phosphate and reduction of serum calcium so that the laboratory values may imitate primary hypoparathyroidism, and in the chronic forms of uremia, a compensatory hyperplasia of the parathyroid glands may result.

Treating hypocalcemia. Parathyroid tetany is safely and dramatically treated by intravenous administration of 10 ml of 10% calcium gluconate. This should be given slowly, and if the patient is not completely relieved of symptoms, a second 10 ml may be administered. This may have to be repeated several times in the first few days, and for the patient who has had hyperparathyroidism and depletion of bone minerals, it may be necessary to add up to 80 ml of 10% calcium gluconate to each liter of intravenous fluids and to run the intravenous infusion of 5% glucose continuously at a rate sufficient to keep the patient from having tetany.

Vitamin D_2 (calciferol) is given in oral doses of 50,000 units/day along with oral calcium gluconate. This calcium salt is rather insoluble and must be given in a saturated solution or a suspension. Vitamin D has a slow action, requiring at least a week for its full effect. If a patient still has hypocalcemia after several weeks, the dosage can be increased to 100,000 units. Occasional patients require as much as 200,000 units/day of vitamin D_2 to maintain a normal serum calcium. The patients are taught to test their own urine with Sulkowitch reagent, and they are advised to report immediately if the urinary calcium precipitation is too dense to see newsprint through. The hypoparathyroidism that occurs after thyroidectomy may be temporary, and it is important to avoid vitamin D poisoning. These are toxic doses of vitamin D for a patient whose parathyroid function returns to normal. The urinary calcium test is not very accurate, and serum calcium determinations are also required until the patient is well regulated. Even then the serum calcium should be measured several times a year. The use of calcium in the intravenous fluids should be discontinued as soon as the patient can get along without the medication for several days without any signs or symptoms of tetany. Mild tetany is not dangerous. Prolonged hypocalcemia should not be tolerated, however, because such patients develop cataracts.

Hypercalcemia

Hypercalcemia causes many nonspecific symptoms that are related to the gastrointestinal tract, the kidneys, and the neuromuscular and skeletal tissues. Patients complain of anorexia, nausea, vomiting, constipation, diarrhea, abdominal pain, nocturia, polyuria, thirst, headache, backache, bone pain, aching thigh muscles, weakness, lethargy, loss of interest, exhaustion with mild physical effort, dizziness, fainting, and confusion, as well as symptoms of acute peptic ulcer, pancreatitis, renal stones, and kidney infection. Hyperparathyroidism has been referred to as "a disease of stones, bones, abdominal groans, and psychic moans with fatigue overtones." Despite all these symptoms the diagnosis was often not made for months or years, and many patients developed parathyroid crisis with serum calcium levels of 14 mg/dl or above and serum phosphorus levels below 3 and often in the range of 1.5 mg/dl. We now almost routinely measure serum calcium and phosphorus levels in hospital patients. This practice detects hyperparathyroidism before severe complaints or serum chemical alterations have had time to develop. An elevation of parathyroid hormone confirms the diagnosis.

There are no typical physical signs. The patients are irritable, seclusive, distracted, and dull. They often have laxity of their joints, which makes them able to put their feet behind their head and also causes them to have a peculiar and unsteady gait. The diagnosis is made from the typical serum calcium elevation and extremely low serum phosphorus. Once these chemical abnormalities are found, a differential diagnosis arises that involves hyperparathyroidism, multiglandular adenomas, cancer of the breast and other cancers with bone metastases (or cancerous production of parathormone), sarcoidosis, and milk-alkali syndrome. The last condition is infrequent but results when a patient with peptic ulcer drinks several quarts of milk a day and ingests large amounts of alkaline powders in the treatment of the ulcer.

Treating hypercalcemia. Albright suggested in 1932 that sodium phosphate might be used in the treatment of hyperparathyroidism, since excessive excretion of phosphates by the kidney and a consistently low serum phosphorus were found in those patients who had not yet developed uremia. The retention of phosphorus is greatly in excess of the observed rise in serum phosphorus during the recovery of patients who have had hyperparathyroidism, and this has suggested that these patients probably have a great deficit of phosphate in extraskeletal tissues. Acute hypercalcemia has been treated successfully by isotonic disodium phosphate and monopotassium phosphate. This causes a prompt reduction in serum calcium levels from the dangerous areas above 14 mg/dl to normal levels and is effective whether the hypercalcemia is caused by hyperparathyroidism or cancer. Improvement in stupor, nausea, renal function, and other symptoms and signs of hypercalcemia is usually rapid.

This treatment should not take the place of appropriate diagnostic measures and surgical treatment of the underlying cause of the hypercalcemia, but it does solve the emergency problem and allows the surgeon to perform a necessary operation under more favorable conditions. High serum calcium also causes renal damage. In animals even 24 hours of hypercalcemia will cause calcification in the kidney, with resultant decrease in glomerular filtration rate and elevation of blood urea nitrogen. Myocardial and brain damage may also occur during prolonged and severe hyperparathyroidism.

Magnesium
Magnesium Deficiency

Magnesium deficiency is likely to be present in patients with delirium tremens, in patients with cirrhosis in whom fluid and salt retention require the use of diuretics, and in patients with ulcerative colitis and chronic diarrhea. The signs and symptoms of magnesium deficiency in such patients may be mimicked by other deficiencies likely to be present at the same time. Prolonged parenteral fluid therapy without magnesium supplement is a common precedent now to magnesium deficiency, just as in similar patients a few years ago prolonged parenteral fluid therapy without addition of potassium was a common antecedent to hypokalemia. Another similarity between potassium and magnesium deficiencies is their occurrence in patients with chronic renal disease who have a high urine output, but without uremia. Magnesium deficiency may appear in the patient who has been operated on for severe hyperparathyroidism. The serum magnesium concentration tends to fall parallel to the decrease in calcium concentration during the early hypocalcemic phase of recovery from hyperparathyroidism. This is undoubtedly related to the repletion of magnesium in the bones. Magnesium is also localized in cells, particularly in the mitochondria. The intracellular fluid magnesium is around 28 mEq/L, whereas the serum levels normally range between 1.5 and 2.5 mEq/L.

Deficiency of magnesium causes central nervous system and neuromuscular hyperirritability with hallucinations, jerking, plucking at the bedclothes, and movements of the hand that simulate the so-called hepatic flap of liver failure. Convulsions may occur. The reflexes are usually hyperreactive, and the patient may develop nystagmus or a positive Babinski sign and other signs suggestive of central nervous system disease. This picture is easily confused with water intoxication, which can also cause convulsions and coma. Treatment is usually given intramuscularly with 50% magnesium sulfate in doses of 2 ml at a time, repeated every 6 hours until the serum magnesium is again normal. One gram a day of magnesium sulfate is sufficient for maintenance, but in the majority of patients parenteral fluids are not required over a long enough period of time so that a significant magnesium depletion would develop.

Magnesium Excess

Magnesium intoxication is difficult to separate from hyperkalemia and other associated abnormalities that occur in uremia. A patient with acute renal failure who is treated frequently with peritoneal or extracorporeal dialysis should not develop magnesium intoxication.

Extracellular Fluid Loss

Internal sequestration of sodium-containing fluids is a common circumstance in the surgeon's practice and is difficult to recognize or to treat quantitatively because the fluid is hidden. ECF loss occurs in patients with burns, intestinal obstruction, peritonitis, serum sickness, and multiple soft-tissue injuries. It also occurs in connection with hemorrhage if the blood is not replaced immediately. Since bleeding is a part of major operations and extensive fractures, such patients require a mixed type of replacement with both blood and extracellular-like fluid. Physicochemical changes occur in the collagen in burned skin and cause it to swell by taking up ECF. Anyone who has seen an obstructed bowel with its severe edema or exudate of peritonitis involving large surface areas, including both visceral and parietal peritoneum, can readily understand the mechanism of sodium fluid sequestration.

Trauma and Hemorrhage

If blood is lost by simple hemorrhage and is replaced immediately and if no tissue damage occurs either from the injury or from a period of shock, no electrolyte solution is required. If a few hours transpire during or after the hemorrhage before treatment, sodium-containing fluids become sequestered in the body. The resultant reduction in effective ECF volume requires both replacement of the blood and restoration of the effective ECF volume. In the average adult one should give as much as 2 L of extracellular-like fluid while waiting for the blood to be cross matched. If more than 1000 ml of blood is required, some additional electrolyte solution may also be given.

During prolonged major operations, a reduction in effective volume of 15% to 20% often occurs. Administration of this fluid during the operation will reduce the amount of blood required to maintain normal vital signs. This does not obviate replacing lost blood. The electrolyte fluid should be given in addition to blood.

In all of these patients with burns, trauma, hemorrhage, and operative procedures lasting longer than 2½ hours, the extracellular-like fluid can be made up of 0.9% saline and one-sixth molar sodium lactate in the proportions of 4 to 1. In most hospitals lactated Ringer's solution is available and has the composition of ECF.

When ECF is sequestered as a result of a burn, trauma, or shock-induced tissue injury, and the patient receives appropriate electrolyte solutions to replace this fluid, mobilization and excretion of such fluid must follow. If the kidneys do not function well and the fluid is retained, pulmonary edema may occur. After resuscitation, electrolyte-containing solutions should be withheld, and, if necessary, diuretics should be given until the fluid overload is corrected.

Patients should be prepared for major operative procedures by having blood volume and hemoglobin levels restored to normal before the operation. Severe depletion of blood proteins should also be corrected by the administration of either plasma or human serum albumin. The normal patient has approximately 60% of total body volume in the veins, including the large veins leading into the right side of the heart; 1 to 1.5 L of blood may be lost before hypotension sets in simply because the constriction of these veins maintains venous return.

The normal patient also has about 60% of his albumin in extravascular areas and can lose this much of his total body albumin before he begins to show the signs and symptoms of reduced plasma volume. If a patient with reduced blood volume and reduced body albumin is subjected to a major operation and does not have more than his operative blood loss replaced, he may in the postoperative period demonstrate failing renal function, poor peripheral circulation (even with the appearance of arterial thromboses in major vessels), and an extremely high hematocrit. If the problem is not recognized and treated vigorously with electrolyte solution, plasma, and blood, such a patient will die. Deficiencies of albumin and whole blood should be repaired before the operation.

Replacement of Gastrointestinal Fluid Loss

Much of the imbalance in fluid and electrolytes could be avoided if gastrointestinal fluids were properly replaced at the time of their loss. This requires ECF, of course; accurate records of the type and volume of fluid lost. In the adult this is a loss of isotonic fluid and it is simply replaced with isotonic fluid, such as 0.9% saline or saline plus one-sixth molar sodium lactate. Since all the fluids lost and the two replacement solutions have the same concentration of electrolytes, the chief difference relates to the anion composition, and therefore the pH (Table 3-1). The pH of the fluid being lost can be determined at the bedside with pH paper. If acid juice is lost from the stomach (not all juice aspirated from the stomach is acid gastric juice), the fluids remaining in the body are more alkaline. Fluid lost from the upper small bowel (through a long intestinal tube or a duodenal fistula) is alkaline, resulting in acidosis. If the loss is a balanced loss of gastric and intestinal juices having a pH of approximately 7.4, the acid-base balance of the patient is unchanged.

If the juice being lost is acid with an excess of chloride, the replacement solution should be isotonic saline, which has an excess of 50 mEq/L of chloride as compared with the chloride concentration in normal ECF. If the fluid being lost is alkaline, the replacement solution should be made up of only 2 parts saline and 1 part one-sixth molar sodium lactate. If the solution lost is approximately that of ECF, the proportions of isotonic saline and one-sixth molar sodium lactate should be 4 to 1, which is the proportion of bicarbonate to chloride in ECF.

A few physicians stubbornly maintain that the kidney will take care of any imbalance and that any elec-

Table 3-1. Effects of Treatment of Acid-Base Disturbances

Type of Fluid Loss	Resultant Acid-base Disturbances	Intravenous Fluid Ratio (0.9% NaCl:M/6 Na lactate)		
		Neutral (4:1)	Acidifying (1:0)	Alkalinizing (2:1)
Balanced loss	None	Balance	Acidosis	Alkalosis
Acid juice loss	Alkalosis	Alkalosis	Balance	Severe alkalosis
Alkaline loss	Acidosis	Acidosis	Severe acidosis	Balance

trolyte loss may be treated by the administration of 0.9% saline. If a patient loses alkaline intestinal juices and therefore has a metabolic acidosis and is then treated with saline solution, which causes its own hyperchloremic acidosis, even a normal kidney cannot correct this condition. In a patient with severe acidosis the kidneys do not function normally.

The patient with ulcerative colitis who has a total colectomy and ileostomy illustrates the need for continuous monitoring of the type of intestinal fluids lost. During the early postoperative period, the loss is primarily one of acid gastric juice from the stomach that tends to produce alkalosis and requires treatment with saline. As the intestine begins to function several days after the operation and acid gastric suction fluid loss ceases and alkaline ileostomy fluid loss begins, a large loss of alkaline intestinal juices results in acidosis. At this time the treatment must suddenly be changed from the administration of the acidifying saline solution to an alkalinizing replacement solution containing 2 parts saline and 1 part one-sixth molar sodium lactate. In the replacement of all intestinal fluid loss, 20 to 40 mEq of potassium should be added for each liter of fluid lost. Gastric juice potassium concentration is usually around 8 to 10 mEq/L. Intestinal juices may contain as much as 50 or 60 mEq/L potassium.

Acute Renal Failure

Kidney shutdown is usually the result of a combination of several factors such as hypotension, intravenous hemolysis (infusion of mismatched blood or distilled water), dehydration, extensive trauma, crushing of muscle, and release of myoglobin. *Ischemia* is the common denominator of most causes of acute renal failure.

All degrees of injury from mild tubular injury to complete renal cortical infarction are seen. In most patients there is a lysis of tubular cells with varying numbers of breaks in basement membranes. The latter results in permanent tubulovenous fistulas or obstructed nephrons. Tubulolysis is a reversible lesion, analogous to a burn, with remaining islands of viable cells from which regeneration occurs. Recovery of function requires a few days to as long as 3 weeks. During the period of regeneration, the patient remains oliguric. As the nephrons begin to retain the glomerular filtrate, polyuria develops. As the living cells mature and begin to show subcellular organelles such as mitochondria, normal concentrating function is restored and the diuretic phase of recovery is replaced by normal renal function.

Prevention of acute renal failure requires adequate and early replacement of blood and extracellular fluid. A traumatized patient requiring four units of blood replacement may, in addition, need 3 or 4 L of lactated Ringer's solution before the urine output is adequate.

Mannitol or furosemide may restore urine flow even though there is a persistent inadequacy of blood and ECF volume, but it will not correct, and may obscure, the circulatory insufficiency at fault.

Progressive decrease in urine volume to less than 500 ml/day or a rising blood urea nitrogen and creatinine with greater urine output indicates probable acute renal failure. Persistent circulatory insufficiency must be ruled out, and a trial of blood or lactated Ringer's solution may be given to see if normal urine volume can be restored. Simple retention must be ruled out by catheterization or irrigation of an indwelling catheter. The urine is examined for blood cells and casts; tests for urea, creatinine, and electrolytes in the urine are not usually necessary. With renal failure, the chemical composition of urine approaches that of blood.

Acute renal failure causes a retention of any fluids that are administered to the patient; the dilution of total body solute depends on the magnitude of accumulated water, as illustrated in Fig. 3-4. The percent decrease in serum sodium concentration will be equal to the percent increase in lean body mass calculated from change in body weight. If acute renal failure is recognized early and if fluid is restricted adequately, serum sodium concentration remains normal.

Potassium and organic acids accumulate with a resultant progressive fall in CO_2 content. If the patient vomits or loses acid gastric juice by nasal gastric suction, the CO_2 may remain normal while the serum chloride decreases. This is ideal, since retained *organic acids* do not cause acidosis. A low serum chloride never requires treatment if the CO_2 content is normal. As phosphate is retained, the serum calcium falls. Death occurs after about 10 to 12 days from high potassium, from retained fluids and pulmonary edema, or from pneumonia. Death may occur in 24 hours with crushing injuries, as mentioned on p. 22. No patient should die from renal failure.

Emergency treatment of high serum potassium requires *glucose and insulin* to force potassium into glycogen stores, *correction of the acidosis* to force potassium into cells, *elevation of serum calcium* to counteract the effect of potassium on myocardial irritability, and dialysis as soon as possible.

Patients who have not had recent abdominal operations can be subjected to peritoneal dialysis within a very short time. Peritoneal dialysis or hemodialysis is required at intervals of every few days to maintain reasonably normal body chemistries while the kidneys are recovering. Peritoneal dialysis is less efficient than hemodialysis with an artificial kidney, and it must be used more frequently and for longer periods of time, but peritoneal dialysis can be used when an artificial kidney is not available.

In addition to the treatment of hyperkalemia, management of acute renal failure should include replacement of only insensible and renal water losses, weighing the patient daily—about 1 pound is the anticipated daily loss—giving calories in the form of sugar-sweetened butterballs for protein-sparing effect, and oral administration of ion exchange resins that bind potassium and increase its excretion in the stool.

SUMMARY

The surgeon is a physician who operates. He is responsible for the complete day-to-day care of his patients and should make a habit on rounds of asking himself what each patient needs for metabolic fluids, replacement of abnormal loss, and restoration of any imbalance. The latter should be defined on the basis of the data available from history, physical findings, intake and output records, and any laboratory analyses of abnormalities of volume, tonicity and chemical composition, and acid-base balance. The diagrams—(1) volume versus concentration, (2) bar graph of ECF cations and anions, and (3) P_{CO_2}-pH—should be drawn in the patient's chart (progress notes) together with appropriate modifications from normal. One should adjudicate inconsistencies in the analyses by collecting additional data, repeating examinations of patient and laboratory tests, and reviewing the logic of the diagnostic analysis. Finally the needs for fluids, electrolytes, and nutrients should be totaled for the day and incorporated into a simple prescription that the nurse can supply, with prepared intravenous solutions.

4

Disorders of Hemostasis: Diagnosis and Treatment

Donald E. MacFarlane

PHYSIOLOGY OF HEMOSTASIS

Mechanisms to bring about the arrest of bleeding from ruptured blood vessels have evolved in parallel with the increasing complexity of cardiovascular systems. These mechanisms usually function rapidly and efficiently at the site of an injury, and they are carefully regulated to ensure that they do not operate at the wrong time or in the wrong place, which might cause ischemic injuries such as myocardial infarction or thromboembolic stroke. Hemostasis involves three interconnected mechanisms—vascular contraction, formation of a hemostatic plug, and blood coagulation. *Vascular contraction* is a process that has received little attention but is to be responsible for the fact that a gratifyingly large proportion of small blood vessels cut by the surgeon's knife do not bleed and do not need to be tied or cauterized.

Hemostatic Plug and Platelet Aggregation

The second process is the formation of a *hemostatic plug,* which is initially composed of aggregates of blood platelets adhering to the fibrillar proteins exposed at the edges of the ruptured vessels. Platelets have receptors on their surfaces that detect the presence of a variety of aggregating agents such as collagen, thrombin, adenosine diphosphate (ADP), epinephrine, thromboxanes, and prostaglandin endoperoxides. These receptors activate the hydrolysis of certain membrane lipids, yielding two intracellular messengers (diacylglycerol and inositol trisphosphate) that activate protein phosphorylation and mobilize calcium. A contractile event follows that changes the shape of the platelet from a disk to a sphere bearing pseudopods, and receptors on these transformed platelets appear which bind fibrinogen and von Willebrand's factor, thereby sticking platelets to each other and to the cut blood vessels. A few seconds later these platelets begin to synthesize prostaglandins and release ADP and other factors from specific storage organelles. These products recruit more platelets to the hemostatic plug. The surface of activated platelets accelerates the action of several of the *blood clotting enzymes,* so that the hemostatic plug is soon stabilized by a retracted network of polymerized fibrin. The platelets also secrete factors that attract inflammatory cells and promote the growth of smooth muscle cells and fibroblasts. This starts the process of normal healing or (if the hemostatic plug forms inappropriately in an intact artery) accelerates atherosclerosis.

Blood Coagulation

Blood clotting occurs when two peptides are cleaved by thrombin from fibrinogen, inducing it to polymerize into fibers, which are further stabilized by the cross-linking enzyme, factor XIII. These events are the culmination of the *clotting cascade,* so named because this biochemical system is rather similar to a multistage photomultiplier tube, in which the impact of a single photon on the surface of the first stage discharges a few electrons each of which dislodges a few more electrons in the next stage. After several such stages of logarithmic amplification, the original impact of the photon causes the flow of an easily detectable number of electrons in the last stage. In the clotting cascade (Fig. 4-1) the activation of few molecules of factor XII by surface contact causes the activation (with high-molecular-weight kininogen) of many molecules of factor XI by proteolytic cleavage, each of which activates several molecules of factor IX. Activated factor

IX, assisted by factor VIII, cleaves factor X on the surface of the platelet (or on a phospholipid surface) to an active enzyme, which, in a similar reaction with factor V, activates prothrombin to thrombin. Tissue factor generated in injured tissues enables factor VII to activate factor X. The enzymes in this system have reactive serines in their active sites, and factors II (thrombin) VII, IX, and X have calcium binding sites generated by a vitamin K–dependent carboxylation of glutamic acid. Factors V and VIII are large molecules whose cofactor activity is greatly enhanced by thrombin, thereby generating a positive feedback loop.

Anticoagulant Systems

Negative feedback (in the form of destruction of activated factors V and VIII) is provided by an endothelial protein (thrombomodulin) that enables thrombin to activate protein C (a vitamin K–dependent enzyme which requires protein S for full activity). The coagulation system is damped by several inhibitors of proteases (serpins) including antithrombin III, which forms an irreversible enzyme complex with thrombin and activated factor X. This complexation is accelerated by heparin. The system is reversed by lysis of the clot, which occurs when a plasminogen activator converts plasminogen incorporated into the clot at its formation to plasmin. Deficiencies in one or more of these factors are found in a substantial proportion of patients who have unusual or frequent venous thromboses, especially if they have a family history of similar events.

Prothrombin Time and Partial Thromboplastin Time

The performance of the clotting cascade (see Fig. 4-1) can be evaluated in the laboratory by performing a prothrombin time (PT) test in which a reagent is added that activates factor VII and, hence, the extrinsic pathway, or by the performance of an activated partial thromboplastin time (PTT) test, in which the initiating event is the activation of factor XII by surface contact (the intrinsic pathway). The schematic diagram in Fig. 4–1 gives a reasonable representation of what happens during these tests *in virtro* laboratory, but it fails to account for two conflicting clinical observations. Patients who are congenitally deficient in factor XII have markedly prolonged PTTs, but they do not bleed abnormally, whereas patients deficient in factor VIII or IX have severe spontaneous hemorrhages (hemophilia). Quite clearly, factors VIII and IX must be involved in hemostasis to a much greater extent than is factor XII.

PREOPERATIVE EVALUATION
History

Before surgery is performed, the surgeon must make an evaluation of the likelihood that the patient will either bleed excessively or have a thromboembolic event. By far the most important part of this evaluation is the taking of an *accurate personal and family history.* This is done by inquiring into the bleeding that followed each challenge to the hemostatic system (circumcision, tonsillectomy, tooth extractions, menstruation, childbirth, trauma, and other operations) or which apparently occurred spontaneously (epistaxis, joint hemorrhage, soft tissue bleeds, hematuria, bruising, purpura, etc.). An attempt should be made to determine

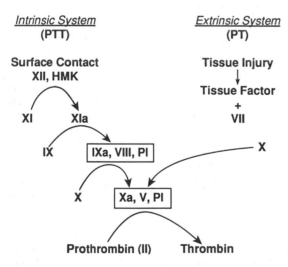

Fig. 4-1. The coagulation cascade. *PL* refers to specific binding sites on the surface of activated platelets, for which phospholipid is substituted in most laboratory clotting assays. Thrombin coagulates fibrinogen and potentiates the activity of factors VIII and V in the blood. In the presence of normal endothelium, thrombin activates protein C, which destroys activated factor V and VIII. Calcium ions are required for the activation of factor X and prothrombin.

the amount and duration of blood loss at each episode and whether blood transfusions were given or special tests performed. Similar inquiries should be made about possible venous thrombosis, determining whether there was an inciting event, what investigations (e.g., venograms) were performed, and whether anticoagulants were prescribed.

If other bleeders or clotters are identified in the family, their relationship to the patient must be carefully noted. X-linked disorders such as hemophilia are inherited by a boy from his mother, and the disease is likely to be expressed in either the mother's father or her brothers, and in her sisters' boys. All of the girls fathered by an affected man are carriers, and all of his boys are normal. Autosomal-dominant disorders occur with equal probability in both sexes and in each generation. Autosomal-recessive disorders are rare and can occur sporadically or in the children of consanguineous marriages with no family history.

The taking of this history is not easy, and it can be time consuming. Young patients often are not knowledgeable of their family histories, and second- or third-hand accounts of bleeding or thrombotic episodes are often inaccurate. Good judgment is needed to decide whether an episode of bleeding is sufficiently abnormal to justify further investigation. A telephone call can often be very helpful, especially if placed to the office of a physician who already has made a definitive diagnosis in the patient or a family member.

The history may also reveal evidence of an acquired hemostatic deficit, manifested by the recent onset of bruising, purpura, gum bleeding, or gastrointestinal hemorrhage. Acquired defects are particularly dangerous because their severity cannot be judged by the history. It is important to determine whether the patient has taken aspirin in the previous week and whether or not the patient is anticoagulated or is likely to be deficient in vitamin K because of a combination of poor dietary intake and the administration of antibiotics. The effects of drugs other than aspirin which influence platelet function (including nonsteroidal antiinflammatory drugs [NSAIDS] and high-dose semisynthetic penicillins) reverse in a day or two. Excessive use of alcohol, as in binge drinking, causes defective platelet function at the time and thrombocytopenia a few days later. Hemostasis is adversely affected by malnutrition by several mechanisms.

Physical Examination

The *physical examination* of patients with bleeding disorders may be normal if the defect is fairly mild, or it may be strikingly abnormal. Patients with hemophilia (factor VIII or factor IX deficiency) frequently have obvious skeletal deformities caused by repeated hemarthroses and deep muscle bleeds. Patients with disorders of platelet function or with von Willebrand's disease may have bruises following trivial trauma, and patients with thrombocytopenia may have a petechial rash (purpura) on the lower legs, the mucous membranes of the oropharynx, or in the retina. Oozing of blood or extensive ecchymoses around venipuncture sites suggests the presence of bleeding disorder. Patients with amyloidosis may have a bleeding tendency, and deposits in the skin, tongue, or elsewhere may be revealed by physical

exam. Joint laxity and increased skin elasticity in some types of Ehlers-Danlos syndrome is associated with bleeding.

Laboratory Screening

Laboratory testing is of value to confirm or reject specific diagnoses, but if the history and physical examinations do not reveal evidence of a bleeding diathesis, the use of a battery of screening tests will be more likely to mislead than to illuminate. The normal range quoted by the laboratory is usually set so that it includes about 95% of the values observed with normal specimens. Thus, a small percentage of normal people have "abnormally" high PTTs. On the other hand, the probability that an adult male patient has undiagnosed, mild hemophilia or von Willebrand's disease with a negative history is rather low (probably less than 1 in 20,000). If 20,000 people are tested, a few hundred will have an abnormal PTT and will require further testing, but only one will have a congenital bleeding disorder, and even he may be missed because the PTT is frequently normal in such a patient. Long PTTs detected by screening normal patients are more likely to be due to improper specimen collection, contamination of the sample with heparin, insignificant abnormalities of factors XII or XI, or the presence of a nonspecific (lupus-type) anticoagulant (which predisposes to thrombosis, not bleeding) than to the presence of a congenital bleeding disorder (deficiencies of factor VIII, IX, or von Willebrand's factor). The investigation of a long PTT can be expensive because it is likely to delay operation. Similar problems of specificity and selectivity apply to the other available screening tests (such as the prothrombin time, thrombin time, fibrinogen, and euglobulin lysis time). It is therefore a reasonable policy not to use screening tests on otherwise healthy patients with no bleeding history who are to have elective surgery. It is sensible to freeze a plasma sample from such patients preoperatively so that if they do bleed the sample can be thawed and used to make the correct diagnosis.

On the other hand, a high proportion of patients who undergo emergency surgery or who have been sick or hospitalized for a few days do indeed have bleeding problems, most of which are correctable. The use of screening tests before surgery in these patients is essential. The PT test is sensitive to vitamin K deficiency. PT and PTT are both prolonged in patients with poor synthesis or rapid consumption of clotting factors, and a long thrombin time or low fibrinogen with elevated fibrin degradation products suggest a consumption coagulopathy. A short euglobulin lysis time may be seen in patients with circulating plasmin causing fibrinolysis. Thrombocytopenia may occur for a variety of reasons, including sepsis, liver disease with hypersplenism, bone marrow suppression, disseminated intravascular coagulation, idiopathic thrombocytopenic purpura, or the use of heparin.

CONGENITAL BLEEDING DISORDERS
Hemophilia and Christmas Disease

Two types of molecular defects result in identical clinical syndromes—hemophilia, which is caused by the absence or reduced activity of factor VIII, and

Christmas disease (or hemophilia B), which is caused by the absence or reduced activity of factor IX. These proteins function together to activate factor X in the clotting cascade. The genes of these molecules have been cloned and sequenced, and the diseases arise because of a variety of mutations (deletions, insertions, point mutations) in the coding or noncoding regions of these genes.

Both genes are carried on the X chromosome, so the disease is expressed far more commonly in males than in females. About one male in 7000 has factor VIII deficiency. Christmas disease is less common. The severity of the disease correlates with the factor activity measured by clotting assay using factor-deficient substrate plasmas. Some patients are found to synthesize a functionally defective protein, but other mutations result in genes incapable of generating stable mRNA, so that no protein is secreted; these patients may generate antibodies to infused factor, a feared and not uncommon complication of the management of hemophilia.

Natural History

Patients with *severe* hemophilia (1% or less of normal activity) have a lifelong bleeding disorder manifested by frequent spontaneous hemorrhages into joints resulting (when untreated) in a crippling arthropathy, and bleeds into muscle masses. These soft tissue bleeds can result in expansile hemorrhagic pseudotumors, especially if periosteum is involved. Severe hemophiliacs bleed at operation or tooth extraction in an uncontrolled fashion, and they may bleed for days after minor injuries, producing only an unstable friable clot at the site. Before effective treatment was available, these patients had life expectancies of less than 20 years, most deaths being caused by intracranial or other hemorrhages. Laboratory investigation reveals a prolonged PTT (2 to 3 times normal), normal PT, and (usually) normal bleeding time. The prolonged PTT is corrected when the patient's plasma is mixed with normal plasma (unless an inhibitor is present). Specific factor assays reveal the diagnosis of factor VIII or factor IX deficiency.

Hemophilia in patients with factor levels of 1% to 5% of normal is classified as *moderate*. Their spontaneous hemorrhages are less frequent, but they are likely to bleed at operation. Patients with *mild* disease (5% to 50%) may avoid spontaneous bleeds completely, and they may not be diagnosed until late adulthood. Close questioning of these patients usually reveals some historical evidence of a bleeding diathesis and they do bleed extensively at surgery.

Surgery and Hemophilia

The management of hemophiliacs at the time of surgery requires the services of a number of specialists working together as a team, such as exists at designated regional hemophilia centers. This team consists of the surgeon, anesthesiologist, hematologist, laboratory coagulationist, social worker, physical therapist, psychologist, and pharmacist or blood banker. The team is best organized by a nurse coordinator.

The members of this team must be involved early in the planning process. The preparation required includes establishing the correct diagnosis of the bleeding disorder; checking for the presence of inhibitors that would greatly complicate the management of the patient; deciding whether the patient is presently infected with human immunodeficiency virus (HIV) and non-A, non-B, or another hepatitis virus; choosing the type of factor replacement that will be used; establishing whether the patient has adequate financial resources with or without public assistance; and planning pain management, psychological support, and physical therapy. Concerns that the hospital personnel may have about having HIV-positive patients in their care should be discussed openly in advance of the patient's admission.

As a result of this preparation, a decision as to whether the operation is warranted can be discussed with the patient and his family. Unnecessary surgery should not be performed on hemophiliac patients, but operations of any type can be performed safely on patients with factor VIII deficiency who have no inhibitors. The management of patients who do have inhibitors is difficult, and some patients with Christmas disease may develop thrombosis or consumption coagulopathy when given factor concentrates, so surgery on these patients is more dangerous.

Do's and Don'ts with Hemophilia Patients

Do *not* give intramuscular injections. The trauma of injections is sufficient to cause hematomas, which can develop into hemorrhagic cysts. Pain management is best effected by continuous intravenous infusions of morphine. Bolus intravenous injections of opiates increase the probability of opiate abuse after discharge.

Do *not* prescribe aspirin or other nonsteroidal analgesics. Moderate doses of nonsteroidals are sometimes useful in the management of arthritic pains, but they should be avoided perioperatively.

Do use blood precautions. Assume that every hemophiliac who used commercial concentrates in the period from 1980 to 1985 is infected with HIV and with non-A and non-B hepatitis viruses. Many patients have elected not to have HIV serologies recorded in their medical record.

Do allow hemophiliacs to administer their own factor. Hemophiliacs on home therapy are taught to give themselves factor when they need it.

When in doubt, give factor replacement immediately. Do *not* delay therapy in the emergency room pending the outcome of imaging studies or consultations.

DDAVP

The therapeutic options for factor replacement in hemophiliacs are becoming rather numerous. The infusion of 1-desamino-8-D-arginine vasopressin (DDAVP, desmopressin, 0.3 µg/kg body weight infused over 20 minutes) causes the release of factor VIII into the circulation, thereby increasing the level twofold to threefold. If the preinfusion level is above about 10%, this increase may be enough to enable minor surgery and tooth extractions to be performed without exposing the patient to blood products. The increased factor level lasts for about 8 hours. A second infusion of DDAVP can be given the following day, but the response to this and subsequent infusions may be attenuated.

Cryoprecipitate

When blood plasma is frozen and thawed, certain proteins do not immediately redissolve. These cryoprecipitated proteins include factor VIII (carried on von Willebrand factor) and fibrinogen. The cryoprecipitate from one donation of blood contains about 100 units of factor VIII coagulant activity (normal plasma contains an average of 1 unit/ml by convention). The distribution volume for infused factor VIII is 40 to 50 ml/kg (the same as the volume of plasma) and its half-life is 8 to 12 hours. Complete correction (to 100% of normal) requires 40 to 50 units/kg, or the cryoprecipitate from 35 bags of blood for a 70 kg patient. This level can be maintained by infusing about half this amount each 8 to 12 hours. Cryoprecipitate is prepared locally, and it is just as likely to contain infectious viruses as the blood from which it was derived. It can be prepared with greater yield and safety by plasmapheresis of specially selected DDAVP-treated donors (a typical example would be the father of a hemophiliac child). Cryoprecipitate can be price competitive with commercially prepared factor concentrates, but it is less easy to store and reconstitute. The volume administered (about 20 ml/bag) is acceptable for most purposes.

Further purification of factor VIII from cryoprecipitate is not practical on a small scale. Instead, pools of plasma from thousands of donors are processed commercially, yielding a stable, lyophilized powder. Factor concentrates usually contain little or no functional von Willebrand's factor. A variety of techniques have been used to reduce the infectivity of contaminating HIV and hepatitis viruses, with increasing degrees of success. Factor VIII concentrates purified by monoclonal antibody absorption are now available, and genetically engineered factors VIII are in the early stages of testing. Both products are likely to be much more expensive than earlier concentrates, but they will become price competitive as the technology involved in their production improves.

Dosing Schedules

Factor VIII should be replaced to 80% to 100% of normal before major operations (40 to 50 units/kg), and maintained at 40% to 50% (about 20 units/kg every 8 to 12 hours by bolus or continuous infusion) until wound healing is well advanced (7 to 21 days). Despite adequate factor levels, bleeding may occur at about 10 days after surgery, particularly after joint replacement. Minor operations, spontaneous muscle bleeds, and severe hemarthroses need replacement to about half the extent necessary for major surgery.

Tooth extractions can be managed with a single bolus of factor VIII to give 50% replacement before the extraction, followed by oral ε-aminocaproic acid (EACA, Amicar, 6 grams every 6 hours) or tranexamic acid (1 gram t.i.d.) for 7 to 10 days. These inhibitors of fibrinolysis are of little value for other bleeds, and their use is contraindicated in patients with hematuria from a kidney. Minor hemarthroses are treated with one or two boluses of 15 to 25 units/kg factor VIII.

Inhibitor with Patients

Inhibitors (antibodies) to factor VIII both neutralize the activity of the factor and accelerate its clearance. If the titer of the antibody is low (less than 10 Bethesda units), it may be possible to overwhelm the inhibitor by giving high doses of factor VIII. This will result in an anamnestic response in high-responder patients, which may make further factor VIII administration futile. These antibodies often cross react only weakly with porcine factor VIII, which can then be used as factor replacement for a period of weeks (or sometimes longer) before antibodies to the animal factor appear. Some patients can be rendered tolerant to Factor VIII by combinations of immunosuppression, high-dose γ-globulin, and prolonged infusion of factor VIII.

Preparations of prothrombin complex (typically containing factors II, VII, IX, and X) prepared for the treatment of patients with Christmas disease contain an activity that bypasses the need for factor VIII. The spontaneous hemarthroses and other minor bleeds in patients with factor VIII deficiency with inhibitor often can be managed by giving these preparations (75 units factor IX activity per kg, every 8 hours). There is no general agreement as to which commercial product is the most cost effective for this use.

Christmas Disease

Patients with Christmas disease require replacement to slightly lower plasma levels than do hemophiliacs. The distribution volume of infused factor IX is about 100 ml/kg (twice the plasma volume), and the half-life for elimination is about 24 hr. Major operations can be performed after the infusion of 50 units/kg, giving about 50% replacement, followed by 12 to 20 units/kg twice daily by bolus injection to maintain a level of about 25%. Minor surgery requires half these doses, and minor hemarthroses often respond to a single infusion of 30 units/kg. Factor IX concentrates contain a thrombogenic material that causes life-threatening thromboses or consumption coagulopathy if infused into patients with liver disease or if given by continuous infusion. Patients with liver disease (cirrhosis) should receive (by plasma exchange if necessary) fresh frozen plasma (which contains 1 unit of factor IX/ml) to achieve adequate levels. The thrombogenic effect of factor IX concentrate may be reduced—but is certainly not completely prevented—by mixing it with heparin (5 units for each milliliter of reconstituted factor).

von Willebrand Disease

The common form of von Willebrand disease (type I) gives rise to a rather mild and variable bleeding diathesis characterized by bleeding at surgery and after trauma, menorrhagia, and excessive bruising, especially if the patient takes aspirin. It is inherited as an autosomal-dominant trait, and it is about as prevalent as hemophilia. Spontaneous joint or deep muscle bleeds do not occur. Laboratory testing reveals a prolonged bleeding time, a slightly prolonged (or upper range of normal) PTT, normal PT, factor VIII coagulant level of about 50% of normal, von Willebrand antigen of about 50% of normal, and ristocetin cofactor activity (the ability of the patient's plasma to support

ristocetin-induced agglutination of fixed washed platelets) of 50%. The disease is caused by the partial lack
of the multimeric protein (von Willebrand factor) that
mediates the adherence of blood platelets to the edges
of damaged blood vessels and also carries the factor
VIII coagulant molecule. A number of variants of the
disease occur (type II), which are due to abnormalities
in the multimeric structure of the protein, either in the
plasma or in platelets, and which may be associated
with a more obvious bleeding diathesis.

An extreme form of von Willebrand disease arises
when the individual inherits two defective von Willebrand genes (the autosomal-recessive form, sometimes
referred to as type III). These patients have a hemophiliac pattern of bleeding with spontaneous joint hemorrhages, and their circulating factor VIII coagulant activity is a few percent of normal because of absence of
the von Willebrand factor to carry the factor VIII molecule.

Patients with mild type I von Willebrand disease
can undergo minor surgery after administration of
DDAVP (see above), which increases the factor levels
by 2 to 3-fold and shortens the bleeding time. Patients
with type II variants may or may not get a useful response to DDAVP and can even get a transient thrombocytopenia (type IIB) with this hormone. Patients
should be challenged with DDAVP well before operation to determine whether a useful response is obtained.

Patients with severe disease or who are to undergo
major operation should receive replacement with cryoprecipitate using the same initial dose as is used for hemophilia (½ bag/kg; each bag contains about 100 units
of factor VIII activity). Patients with von Willebrand
disease display a prolonged rise in factor VIII level after infusion of cryoprecipitate, so that the interval of
treatment required to maintain an adequate therapeutic
level is longer than with hemophilia.

Other Coagulation Disorders

Congenital defects have been described for each of
the known clotting factors. In comparison with deficiencies of factor VIII and IX, these deficiencies are
rare and may cause the patient little or no problem. Patients with defects of factor XII have markedly prolonged PTTs but no bleeding diathesis. The bleeding in
patients with low factors XI, X, VII, V, and prothrombin does not correlate well with the factor level and is
generally mild. Patients with afibrinogenemia may
bleed. Patients with functional defects of fibrinogen
that impair its clotting often do not have a bleeding tendency, and paradoxically, these patients may have a severe thrombotic tendency.

Platelet Disorders

Severe platelet disorders such as Glanzmann's
thrombasthenia (caused by defective glycoproteins in
the fibrinogen receptor) or Bernard-Soulier disease
(caused by a defective von Willebrand factor receptor)
are exceedingly rare. Patients have a lifelong bleeding
tendency with a prolonged bleeding time and normal
PT and PTT. Platelets of patients with these disorders
fail to aggregate with physiological aggregating agents
and ristocetin, respectively. A variety of congenital defects in the granules in which ADP and serotonin, are

stored have been described, and these defects may be
associated with other syndromes, such as albinism or
absent radii. These "storage pool defects" are uncommon. Defective release of these granules are, however,
not rare. Both defects cause a mild bleeding tendency
with easy bruising. Laboratory testing reveals an absence of the "second wave" of platelet aggregation.
Platelet defects can be managed with platelet transfusion.

ACQUIRED BLEEDING DISORDERS
Coagulation Defects

The majority of patients who have bleeding disorders have acquired them, and in hospitalized patients
they may be multifactorial in origin. The most severe
type of acquired bleeding disorder in adults is the appearance of an antibody to factor VIII in a previously
normal person. This autoimmune disease may occur after pregnancy or after the administration of penicillin;
more often it is spontaneous. These unfortunate patients have catastrophic deep muscle bleeds and spec-
tacular ecchymoses. Their PTT is prolonged, and it
does not correct on mixing with normal plasma. The
diagnosis is made by demonstrating reduced factor VIII
activity and an inhibitor with activity specifically directed against added factor VIII. The inhibitor may
fade in months or a few years, and its disappearance
may be hastened by immunosuppression.

Patients with paraproteins (such as occurs in Wal-
denstrom's macroglobulinemia or multiple myeloma)
have a variety of bleeding disorders, as do patients with
liver disease. Severe bleeding can also be seen in patients (who are frequently health professionals) who
surreptitiously poison themselves with coumadin or
heparin. Such patients (who are health professionals)
have bizarre histories and wildly fluctuating laboratory
data.

Thrombocytopenia

Petechial hemorrhage (a nonblanching pinpoint rash
on the lower leg) is the hallmark of severe thrombocytopenia from many causes. Patients with *idiopathic
thrombocytopenic purpura* have normal bone marrow
examination and are otherwise healthy. The disease is
caused by a disordered immune system which causes
platelets to be removed rapidly by the spleen. It frequently responds to a burst and taper of corticosteroids
followed (if necessary) by splenectomy. Their bleeding
disorder is much less marked than would be expected
from the platelet count. Patients with *bone marrow diseases,* particularly acute promyelocytic or monocytic
leukemia (in which disease disseminated intravascular
coagulation [DIC] is common), present with bleeding
due to thrombocytopenia. The hematologic diagnosis is
made by examination of the blood smear and the bone
marrow.

Thrombotic thrombocytopenia purpura carries a
high mortality. Patients present with bleeding, thrombocytopenia, a brisk hemolytic anemia with fragmented
red cells (schistocytes), mild fever, and multisystem
(including central nervous system) disease. This syndrome merges with the *hemolytic uremic syndrome,* in
which renal failure is more prominent. The diagnosis is
made by examination of the blood smear and exclusion

of other causes of red cell fragmentation. Immediate plasma exchange is effective therapy, for unclear reasons.

Thrombocytopenia with or without bleeding can be seen in autoimmune disease, infectious diseases (particularly infectious mononucleosis, rickettsial disease, overwhelming bacteremia, and a variety of tropical diseases such as malaria and Dengue fever), liver disease and other causes of hypersplenism, acute alcoholism and pernicious anemia.

Acquired Platelet Disorders

Platelet function is decreased in patients with uremia, liver failure, acute alcohol ingestion, myeloproliferative disorders, and in some patients with paraproteinemia. Aspirin irreversibly inhibits the synthesis of prostaglandins by platelets, which reduces their ability to release their granule contents, resulting in a slight prolongation in the bleeding time. Other non-steroid anti-inflammatory drugs (such as ibuprofen) reversibly inhibit prostaglandin synthesis. Semisynthetic penicillins inhibit platelet function when present in high concentrations. Ticlopidine specifically inhibits platelet aggregation and prolongs the bleeding time. Large lists have been prepared of other medications that are alleged to inhibit platelet function, but documentation that such effects are significant in clinical practice is usually inadequate.

PERIOPERATIVE BLEEDING

Hospitalized or sick patients frequently have bleeding tendencies that may be life threatening, are multifactorial in origin, and may be difficult to diagnosis and treat. The combination of antibiotics and poor dietary intake regularly causes *vitamin K deficiency,* which causes a prolonged PT and which can be corrected by parenteral administration of the vitamin. Generalized malnutrition contributes to poor synthesis of clotting factors, giving rise to a prolonged PT and PTT.

Against this background of mild disorders, a number of more severe syndromes occur intraoperatively which may require specific intervention (Table 4-1).

Massive Transfusion

Massive blood transfusion in the face of brisk hemorrhage will result in a "washout" of clotting factors if plasma expanders and red cells are used in place of whole blood or red cells plus fresh frozen plasma. Laboratory testing reveals a reduction of most of the clotting factors and platelets. This can lead to the impression that a particular patient is bleeding because of a coagulopathy, when in fact the coagulopathy is due to inappropriate blood product replacement. If the patient continues to bleed after correction of the coagulopathy with fresh frozen plasma (6 to 8 units), cryoglobulin (10 to 15 bags to correct a low fibrinogen), and platelets, the bleeding site should be identified and managed surgically.

DIC (Disseminated Intravascular Coagulation)

Consumption of clotting factors occurs during surgery for a variety of reasons, especially during cardiopulmonary bypass or when there has been extensive tissue damage. Such consumption is usually self-limited and does not cause much of a coagulopathy. The concept of disseminated intravascular coagulation (DIC) is a difficult one, because in the vast majority of cases in which the diagnosis is entertained the process that gives rise to a consumption of clotting factors is not disseminated, does not occur in the intravascular compartment, or does not involve the coagulation of fibrinogen. A consumption coagulopathy caused by DIC that requires intervention to prevent bleeding or continued thrombosis is not a particularly frequent event.

In the full-blown picture of DIC, activation of the clotting cascade triggers the fibrinolytic system, which results in the production of fibrin degradation products (FDPs, which can act as an anticoagulant) from fibrin-

Table 4-1. Common Postoperative Findings

Finding	Exam	PT	PTT	Fibrinogen	FDPs	Platelets	Comment
Insignificant DIC	Normal	↑	↑	→	↑	→	Common
Liver disease	Evidence of cirrhosis, etc.	↑	↑	↑	↑	↓	High factor VIII, fibrinogen low in severe disease
Sepsis	Low systemic vascular resistance, ARDS	↑	↑	→↓	↑	↓	
Vitamin K deficiency	Bleeding at surgical site	↑	→	→	→	→	Common in patients with inadequate diet
Heparin contamination of sample	Normal	→	↑↑	→	→	→	Common in intensive care setting
Washout	Bleeding at surgical site	↑	↑	↓	→	↓	Massive transfusion without plasma replacement
Consumption coagulopathy	Generalized oozing	↑	↑	↓↓	↑	↓	Rare

Note: If the patient is bleeding only at the site of the operation, a local cause should be sought by reoperation.

ogen, and the consumption of clotting factors and antithrombin III. Clinically, the patient shows clear signs of a bleeding diathesis with oozing from intravenous sites (IV), ecchymoses, and bleeding at the surgical site. In its fulminant form, microthrombi may be detected in a variety of vascular beds. Laboratory testing reveals a long PT and PTT, low fibrinogen, elevated FDPs, low platelet count, and a short euglobulin lysis time suggesting circulating plasmin. Factors VIII and V and plasminogen are typically low.

This syndrome is much feared in obstetrics, in which it can be seen after amniotic fluid embolism or abruption of the placenta. An acute DIC may occur with mismatched blood transfusion, hyperpyrexia, snake bite, and some overwhelming infections. There seems to be synergy between DIC and shock. DIC also occurs in a more chronic form in most patients with acute promyelocytic leukemia, and occasionally in patients with widely metastatic adenocarcinoma, prostatic tumors, aortic aneurysms with false channels, and in patients with hemangiomas or retained dead fetus. Fibrinolytic agents such as streptokinase cause consumption of fibrinogen.

Unless the event that triggered the DIC is self-limited, or can be reversed, aggressive measures must be taken to correct the coagulopathy. The mainstay of treatment of chronic consumption coagulopathy is the infusion of heparin at rates that slightly prolong the PTT (400 units/hour is a reasonable starting dose, but much more may be required), followed by the administration of fresh frozen plasma (4 to 6 units) and sufficient cryoprecipitate (10 bags initially) to restore the fibrinogen level to about 100 mg/100 ml. In the most acute forms of DIC, the blood may be incoagulable, in which case a bolus of heparin (15,000 units has been recommended) should be given. If fibrinolysis continues after adequate heparinization, Epsilonaminocapric acid EACA (1 g every hour) can be added to the regimen.

The majority of hospitalized patients who have only laboratory evidence of DIC (elevated fibrin degradation products, slight prolongation of PT and PTT, mild thrombocytopenia) do not have a consumption coagulopathy that requires intervention. These patients do not have ooze from IV sites, and their fibrinogen and factor VIII levels are in or above the normal range. These patients frequently have liver disease (which delays the clearance of fibrin degradation products and compromises the patients' ability to synthesize clotting factors) or bacterial infection. Septicemia should be strongly suggested by thrombocytopenia and elevated degradation products in postoperative patients with low systemic vascular resistance who are having difficulty with oxygenation. Such patients should be treated aggressively with antibiotics after appropriate cultures have been taken, rather than with heparin and clotting factor replacement.

Thrombocytopenia

Mild thrombocytopenia is common in severely ill patients and is probably caused by a number of coexisting factors, including infections, the use of indwelling lines, autoimmune phenomena, and poor bone marrow response. Heparin frequently causes an approximately 30% reduction in the platelet count, which often escapes attention. Less frequently it causes a drop in the platelet count to the 50,000 to 100,000 range, and it should be discontinued if this occurs. Dextran can be used in its place if necessary. Very rarely, previously sensitized patients treated with heparin develop an acute onset of massive thrombosis with profound thrombocytopenia (the white clot syndrome) resulting in gangrene of the limbs and renal failure.

Other drugs such as quinidine and sulphonamides occasionally cause profound thrombocytopenia with purpura, and the same can occur 10 days after blood transfusion in a small proportion of patients who lack the PL^{A1} antigen. Amrinone frequently causes a dose-related thrombocytopenia. A wide range of drugs are reported to cause mild thrombocytopenia, but clear evidence of cause and effect is usually not available.

HYPERCOAGULABLE STATE

All patients undergoing surgery are liable to develop deep venous thrombosis (DVT) and pulmonary embolism. A few patients have repeated episodes of venous thromboembolism without such an identifiable precipitating event. About one third of these hypercoagulable patients have familial partial deficiencies of antithrombin III, protein C, protein S, plasminogen, or plasminogen activators or a dysfibrinogenemia, and some others have acquired disorders such as the lupus or nonspecific anticoagulant (autoantibodies directed against phosphodiester groups which prolong the PTT by binding to the phospholipid reagent in the test) or myeloproliferative disorders. Malignancies may present with thromboembolic events (such as thrombophlebitis migrans), but indulging in an extensive hunt for an "occult" malignancy in patients with DVT is unlikely to be worthwhile.

The management of patients with a continuing hypercoagulable state is determined by the history. Patients who have had two or more documented venous thromboses in different sites with no inciting cause (with or without pulmonary emboli) should be anticoagulated for life with coumadin, unless their lifestyle or other medical condition makes coumadin therapy more dangerous than average. Anticoagulated patients can be switched to heparin during surgery.

Patients who have had one episode of thromboembolism or who are at high risk for thromboembolism at the time of surgery because of advanced age, debility, the type of surgery performed, or other predisposing factors should receive prophylactic therapy with subcutaneous minidose or adjusted dose heparin.

Thromboembolism occurring in hospital is frequently not diagnosed unless it is specifically sought. Data from dozens of prospective studies show that the mortality from pulmonary emboli in general surgical patients over the age of 40 approaches 1%. Even higher figures are published for surgical specialties. Each surgeon should have a consistent and well-thought out policy in effect to prevent thromboembolism, and this policy should be consistent with the recommendations of the various deliberative bodies which have addressed this problem.

CONCLUSION

The management of bleeding patients is difficult, and the interpretation of laboratory data is a confusing business, to say the least. Surgeons should be ready to consult a hematologist as soon as any markedly abnormal bleeding is detected, because arriving at the correct diagnosis and instituting effective therapy becomes progressively more difficult with time. Patients with a lifelong bleeding diathesis usually have a positive history, and patients who acquire a bleeding diathesis perioperatively usually bleed from more than one site. As a corollary to these two statements, patients with a negative history who bleed only at the operative site deserve the close attention of the surgeon (including reoperation if necessary) to be sure that the bleeding cannot be arrested by the time-honored method of tying off a pumper.

5

Shock

G.P. Kealey
M.R. Karin

The intact organism must have a circulatory system that provides for nutrient flow to peripheral cells and organs and removal of toxic metabolic biproducts. Vertebrates, in order to allow individual mobility and tolerance of diverse environments, have developed a closed cardiovascular system and neuroendocrine control mechanisms to modulate nutrient distribution to their highly diverse and specialized organ systems. Shock is the result of either inadequate flow of nutrients to meet the metabolic needs of various organs or the failure of these organ systems to utilize effectively the nutrients available to them. The effects of shock may be manifested as failure of certain cellular functions within an organ, organ failure, or death of the organism.

There are many inciting causes of the shock state; however, the final common result is reduced tissue blood flow resulting in cellular hypoxia anaerobic metabolism, and metabolic acidosis, which may progress to cell death. No single diagnostic test determines unequivocally the adequacy of tissue perfusion or cellular metabolic status. Therefore, the diagnosis of shock must be deduced by evaluating the clinical findings exhibited by the patient and the results of laboratory studies and invasive monitoring. Accurate diagnosis of the shock state and reversal of the underlying cause is vital to patient survival.

NORMAL PHYSIOLOGY

Oxygen and other nutrients are pumped by the heart in a pulsatile flow to peripheral tissues. The blood pressure is maintained by pumping a relatively fixed volume of blood through a vascular bed capable of variable peripheral resistance. A variable peripheral vascular resistance allows for local and systemic control of organ and local cellular perfusion. Neuroendocrine control mechanisms and local metabolic requirements serve to modulate vascular resistance and to direct local arterial blood flow. The precapillary sphincters maintain peripheral vascular resistance and control blood flow through the capillary beds (Fig. 5-1). Normally only 20% of the capillaries in the body are perfused at any one time (the other 80% are closed). All capillary beds are periodically perfused with oxygen and nutrients at a flow rate compatible with local metabolic needs. Metabolic by-products (hydrogen ions, lactic acid, etc.) are absorbed across the capillary bed and returned to systemic circulation by the venous system. Normally, there is only a small decrease in pH of the blood across the capillary bed due to the presence of effective acid-base buffers and the rapid blood flow across the capillary beds. Excess arterial blood may be shunted away from the capillary beds into arteriovenous shunts, which returns the blood to the central venous circulation.

Maintenance of a functional circulatory system involves many complex macrophysiologic and microphysiologic interactions. Disequilibrium can occur at any level and in various combinations. Knowledge of the pathophysiology of shock is necessary for the proper recognition and management of the shock state.

PATHOPHYSIOLOGY

Acute blood loss, acute cardiac failure, and decreased peripheral vascular resistance all can lead to hypotension. A decrease in mean arterial pressure triggers the carotid baroreceptor reflex and release of catecholamines (epinephrine and norepinephrine). By constricting peripheral arteries, catecholamines selectively divert available cardiac output to those organs critical for immediate survival—heart, central nervous system, and respiratory muscles. The sympathetic autonomic discharge also results in a reduction of venous capacity, which may compensate for a reduction in blood volume of up to 25%. α-Adrenergic and β-adrenergic humoral stimulation increase myocardial contractility and heart rate to maintain adequate cardiac output.

Renal blood flow is reduced, and urine output falls proportionately to the glomerular filtration rate. Hyperventilation occurs and represents respiratory compensation for metabolic acidosis caused by peripheral tissue anoxia. Reduced pulmonary capillary blood flow causes increased physiological dead space in the lung (due to alterations of the ventilation-perfusion ratio) and results in tachypnea. Decreased capillary blood flow results in an increased plasma oncotic pressure. Subsequently, up to 1 L of interstitial extracellular fluid (ECF) shifts into the intravascular space. This hemodilution is manifested by a decrease in hematocrit and electrolyte changes.

Inadequate tissue perfusion deprives the affected cells of oxygen and nutrients essential to normal cell function. A series of complex chemical transformations is necessary for the synthesis of adenosine triphosphate (ATP), the ultimate source of energy of life processes. In the absence of oxygen, ATP is inefficiently produced. Anaerobic metabolic conditions produce 2 moles of ATP per mole of glucose, while aerobic metabolic conditions produce 38 moles of ATP per mole of glucose. Lactic and pyruvic acids accumulate in the tissues during anaerobic metabolism, producing metabolic acidosis. As stored high-energy phosphate bonds decrease, cellular enzyme systems become inefficient leading to cellular dysfunction.

Organ dysfunction results from cell dysfunction. Gastric and intestinal ischemia result in the destruction of the mucosal intestinal barrier, with secondary bleeding, sepsis, diarrhea, and hematochezia. Renal failure due to acute tubular necrosis occurs. Capillaries become more permeable, resulting in peripheral and pulmonary edema, and possibly adult respiratory distress syndrome (*ARDS*). Cerebral dysfunction is manifested as confusion and stupor.

In later stages of shock, as cellular anoxia increases, microsomal breakdown occurs with release of proteolytic enzymes, the most powerful being bradykinin. These potent vasodilators expand the vascular bed, increasing the intravascular space to well above what could be filled even by a normal circulating blood volume. This phenomenon generally worsens the relative hypovolemia.

In the final stages of shock intracellular edema develops due to sodium-potassium membrane pump failure. This results in further disruption of cell and organ function and the accumulation of metabolites and vasoactive substances. There is stagnation of capillary flow and a tendency to develop a disseminated intravascular

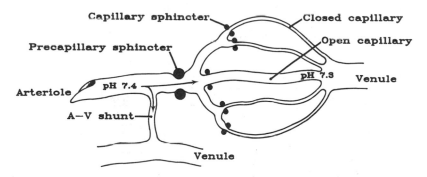

Fig. 5-1. Diagram of normal microcirculation. Precapillary sphincter is partially constricted, diverting some arterial blood directly to veins through the arteriovenous shunt. Blood entering capillary system is perfusing only about 20% (one out of five capillaries in diagram) of cells nourished by this system at any given time. Intermittent opening and closing of capillary sphincters assure periodic perfusion of all tissue.

coagulopathy (DIC). The factors of stagnation of flow, acidosis, and capillary thrombosis are a vicious cycle that leads to cell death, organ failure, and the demise of the patient.

CLASSIFICATION

Circulatory shock occurs when cardiac output and blood pressure are not adequate to perfuse peripheral tissues. Division of shock into subcategories is useful in understanding the etiology and characteristics of the shock state and the therapeutic approach.

1. *Hypovolemic shock:* hemorrhage, fractures, burns, intestinal obstruction, diarrhea, dehydration
2. *Distributive shock:* septicemia, anaphylaxis, neurogenic, vasodilator drugs
3. *Cardiogenic shock:* myocardial infarction, dysrhythmias
4. *Obstructive shock:* pericardial tamponade, pulmonary embolism, large peripheral embolism, valvular disease, dissecting aortic aneurysm, intracardiac tumors, tension pneumothorax, acute diaphragmatic rupture

Hypovolemic Shock

Hypovolemic shock occurs when there is a significant loss of circulating blood volume, extravascular fluid, or both. This is the most common type of shock seen in surgical practice and is characterized clinically by cold skin, tachycardia, lowered blood pressure, decreased central venous pressure, decreased cardiac output, decreased urine flow, and increased arterial blood lactate level. Whole blood loss may occur either externally, due to surface injury, or internally into tissue planes, as with crush injuries, burns, pancreatitis, major fractures, and peritonitis. Bleeding into the lumen of the gastrointestinal tract is another major cause of hypovolemic shock in the surgical patient. External blood loss is easy to recognize, quantitate, and treat, whereas internal bleeding or third space sequestration of fluid is frequently more difficult to recognize, quantitate, and manage.

When the arterial blood pressure falls from any cause, the compensatory response is mediated primarily through the sympathetic nervous system by increasing peripheral resistance (arteriolar constriction through α-adrenergic receptors) and increasing cardiac output (through β-adrenergic receptors). In addition, venous capacitance is decreased to deliver more blood from venous reservoirs to the heart. The vessels of the heart, brain, and respiratory muscles are not involved in arteriolar constriction and thus receive available cardiac output. Renin is released from the juxtaglomerular body in the kidney in response to decreased mean arterial pressure. This proteolytic enzyme forms angiotensin I from plasma precursors. Angiotensin I is converted to angiotensin II in the lung. Angiotensin II increases the production and release of aldosterone from the adrenal gland. Antidiuretic hormone is released from the pituitary gland in response either to changes in serum osmolality or decreased blood volume. The renal response to increased levels of aldosterone and antidiuretic hormone is retention of salt and water. This in turn increases the circulating plasma volume.

When plasmalike fluid is the primary constituent of the blood that is sequestered in tissues, as occurs in burns, cellulitis, or trauma, there is hemoconcentration and increased blood viscosity. Under these circumstances, blood sludging and thrombosis occur in the microcirculation, with the added risk of intravascular coagulation. In contrast, when whole blood is lost, fluid shifts from the extravascular to the intravascular space, resulting in hemodilution. Therefore, the additional deleterious effects of sludging in the microcirculation do not occur.

Hypovolemic shock may be classified on the basis of both the volume of blood loss and the symptoms produced. The initial signs and symptoms of decreased perfusion are caused by baroreceptor reflex initiation of increased sympathetic nerve tone. Hypotension is a late sign and is seen consistently only in class III and IV shock (see Table 5-1).

Distributive

Distributive shock is a clinical state in which the patient is normovolemic, usually has increased cardiac output, but has inadequate tissue perfusion secondary to decreased peripheral vascular resistance. This is commonly caused by bacterial sepsis. The vasodilatory effect of bacterial exotoxins and endotoxins on peripheral arterioles and precapillary sphincters results in the maldistribution of arterial blood flow. Arterial blood is shunted past the capillary beds, resulting in low capillary flow and cell anoxia.

The clinical signs of septicemia are rigors, fever, leukocytosis, decreased platelets, hypotension, coagulopathy, and end organ dysfunction (lungs, kidneys, heart, liver, and skin). Initially, tachycardia, increased cardiac output, a widened pulse pressure, and normal or low blood pressure may be observed. In advanced

Table 5-1. Physiologic Changes in Hypovolemic Shock

	Class I	Class II	Class III	Class IV
Blood loss (ml)*	≤750	1000-1250	1500-1800	2000-2500
Blood loss	≤15%	20%-25%	30%-35%	40%-50%
Pulse rate	72-84	>100	>120	≥140
Blood pressure	118/82	110/80	70-90/50-60	<50-60 systolic
Respiratory rate	14-20	20-30	30-40	>35
Urine output (ml/hr)	30-35	25-30	5-15	Negligible
CNS-mental status	Slightly anxious	Mildly anxious	Anxious and confused	Confused, lethargic
Lactic acid	Normal	Transition	Increased	Increased

*Adult 70 kg body weight

septic shock, hypotension, decreased cardiac output, narrow pulse pressure, increased pulmonary vascular-resistance, and variable systemic vascular resistanceoc-cur. The infecting organisms release a variety of exo-toxins and endotoxins into the bloodstream that directly affect cellular membrane function, causing changes in peripheral and pulmonary vascular resistance, cardiac function, the release of endogenous vasodilators, com-plement activation, and release of myocardial and vas-cular depressive factors.

Septic shock may be caused by gram-positive or, more commonly, gram-negative bacteria. Immunosup-pressed patients are more prone to develop invasive in-fection and, therefore, septic shock. Two factors con-tribute to the decreased peripheral vascular resistance present in septic shock. The precapillary arteriolar-venous shunts are opened and arteriolar vasodilation occurs secondary to the bacterial toxins. Therefore, the septic patient may have pink skin and warm extremities in the early stages. Since the size of the vascular bed is increased by vasodilation, *relative hypovolemia* occurs, which triggers the carotid baroreceptor reflex to pro-duce tachycardia and increased cardiac output.

When the body's ability to compensate by increas-ing cardiac output is insufficient, hypotension and de-creased capillary perfusion occur leading to cellular hy-poxia, anaerobic metabolism, and lactic acidosis. De-creased oxygen extraction and utilization at the cellular level results in damage to the cell membranes. The shift to anaerobic metabolism reduces the metabolic ca-pabilities of the cell. Eventually lysosomes break down and release hydrolytic enzymes, causing further dam-age inside the cell. The cell is eventually destroyed, re-leasing other toxic factors, initiating a vicious cycle of activated enzyme release and diminished cellular func-tion in the immediate area and in distant organs. Re-sponse to the stress hormones (glucagon, growth hor-mone, and catecholamines) is diminished in the preter-minal stage of septic shock.

A similar type of precapillary shunting, diminished peripheral vascular resistance, and inadequate cellular perfusion may be seen in patients who have received an overdose of vasodilatory drugs or high spinal anesthe-sia or who have traumatic spinal cord transection. Re-duction of sympathetic nervous activity results in va-sodilation, hypotension, and maldistribution of avail-able cardiac output during spinal shock.

Cardiogenic Shock

Cardiogenic shock occurs when there is inadequate tissue perfusion secondary to a decreased cardiac out-put despite a normal blood volume. The most common cause is myocardial infarction with resultant ventricular dysfunction. Other causes are myocardial contusion and cardiomyopathy. Cardiogenic shock occurs when more than 40% of the myocardium is damaged or there is a significant conduction defect with dysrhythmias re-sulting in low cardiac output.

Decreased cardiac output and systemic arterial hy-potension result in a compensatory increase in periph-eral vascular resistance. When cardiac failure ensues, pulmonary edema and peripheral edema usually de-velop. Elevated cardiac filling pressure and elevated peripheral vascular resistance initiate a degenerative cy-

cle of increasing cardiac work in the face of diminish-ing myocardial blood flow. This leads to increasing myocardial ischemia and infarct extension. Treatment includes reduction of cardiac preload and afterload by means of diuretic drugs and vasodilators, as well as cardiac inotropic agents to support myocardial contrac-tility and optimize cardiac output. Intraaortic balloon counter pulsation is occasionally used to improve coro-nary circulation and reduce cardiac afterload in cardio-genic shock.

Obstructive Shock

Cardiovascular collapse in obstructive shock is due to mechanical factors that decrease cardiac output inde-pendent of the intrinsic myocardial functional capabil-ity. This may result from vena cava obstruction, intra-cardiac tumors, pericardial tamponade, cardiac valvular disease, pulmonary embolism, dissecting aortic aneu-rysms, peripheral arterial embolism, positive pressure ventilation, tension pneumothorax, or diaphragmatic rupture with visceral herniation into the thoracic cavity. The decreased cardiac output leads to reflex tachycardia and an increase in peripheral vascular resistance. Ther-apy must be based on a careful differential diagnosis.

Expansion of blood volume to augment cardiac fill-ing provides temporary support. Inotropic and chrono-tropic agents should be applied cautiously prior to ac-curate diagnosis as they may be detrimental in the case of pulmonary embolism or aortic dissection. Acute val-vular dysfunction results in overload of the ventricles with subsequent decreased myocardial contractility and congestive heart failure. Therapy must be directed at the relief of the inciting cause. Until the underlying cause can be corrected, circulatory support must be maintained by appropriate adjustment of vascular vol-ume and peripheral vascular resistance to optimize car-diac output.

DIAGNOSIS

The early diagnosis of shock and the simple state-ment "This patient is in shock" do more to speed treat-ment and enhance care than any other factor. The most difficult aspect of shock management is its diagnosis. Although several specific types of shock have been listed, the clinical setting for each of these is very non-specific. Recognition of the presence of shock or its manifestations becomes critical. The classic signs of shock are metabolic acidosis, systolic pressure below the range of 80 to 90 torr, oliguria, and poor tissue per-fusion; however, if the diagnosis is delayed until these signs are present, treatment will be too late in many cases.

The early diagnosis of shock depends on a high level of clinical suspicion and careful observation of the patient's vital signs. Early in shock the pulse pres-sure (the difference between the systolic and diastolic pressures) will be reduced, indicating a decrease in stroke volume; the patient will also have tachycardia. Before major changes in urine volume are observed, urine concentration increases, and urine sodium de-creases. When there is a major drop in blood pressure or renal blood flow, urine output may decrease or stop. Another early sign of shock is tachypnea with associ-ated respiratory alkalosis. Metabolic acidosis is a very late sign and reflects the severity of cellular damage and decreased metabolism. Changes in mental state and signs of poor peripheral perfusion (cold, clammy skin) are also helpful diagnostic signs.

The following priorities are assigned to organ systems relative to the order in which they are deprived of adequate blood flow in hypovolemic shock: (1) skin and subcutaneous fat, (2) intestinal and skeletal muscle, (3) major viscera such as kidney and liver, and (4) heart, brain, and respiratory muscles. Clinical criteria and bedside tests roughly parallel the selective perfusion of tissues noted above. *Pale, cold* and *clammy skin* and mucous membranes reflect the skin and subcutaneous vasoconstriction, *muscle weakness* and *paralytic ileus* reflect reduction in blood flow to muscle and intestine, *oliguria* results from renal vasoconstriction and changes in distribution of renal blood flow, and alterations in the state of *consciousness* roughly reflect cerebral blood flow.

USE OF SWAN-GANZ CATHETER IN DIAGNOSIS AND CLASSIFICATION

The Swan-Ganz catheter is a valuable aid in diagnosing shock, determining the type of shock present, and guiding therapeutic measures. When more than one mechanism of shock is present in a given patient, the Swan-Ganz catheter is essential for accurate diagnosis and proper therapy in complex clinical situations. Its principal usefulness is in determining left and right heart filling pressures, peripheral and pulmonary vascular resistance, and cardiac output. Patients in shock also require intraarterial lines for continuous monitoring of blood pressure. A central venous pressure (CVP) monitor alone provides insufficient information for proper management of such complex clinical problems.

In all types of shock there is inadequate tissue perfusion, generally reflected by systolic hypotension. Decreased cardiac output and increased peripheral vascular resistance (PVR) occur in all types of shock except distributive shock. The unique feature of distributive shock is inadequate tissue perfusion in the presence of decreased PVR and increased cardiac output. Table 5-2 demonstrates how these cardiovascular measurements

obtained with the Swan-Ganz catheter usually vary in different types of shock, thereby aiding diagnosis. It is important to note, however, that often the trends that develop as these parameters change can be more reflective of the underlying shock state than any single value. Once appropriate therapy is instituted, the trends in these parameters are also very useful in monitoring the physiological response to treatment.

MANAGEMENT

The shock state must be recognized and the etiology established in an expeditious manner (see Table 5-2). A primary survey, including evaluation of airway patency, adequacy of breathing, and circulatory status is rapidly performed. Baseline vital signs, including temperature, pulse rate, blood pressure, and level of consciousness are rapidly determined. Life support measures including cardiopulmonary resuscitation, cardiac dysrythmia control, placement of large-bore intravenous lines, supplemental oxygen with the patient in supine position, and application of MAST trousers are initiated as necessary. Bleeding is controlled by direct pressure, splinting of fractures, or appropriate surgical therapy.

A secondary survey of the patient is then performed in an orderly, careful, head-to-toe fashion that ensures the diagnosis of concomitant injuries or preexisting illness. A nasogastric tube is passed to evacuate stomach contents and to determine whether there is blood in the upper gastrointestinal tract, and a urethral catheter is passed and urine output is monitored. Life-threatening derangements are thus rapidly identified, and supportive measurements are undertaken. An adequate minute ventilation is assured, the blood volume is expanded, and cardiac function is restored. Laboratory and x-ray studies are obtained at this time. These usually include a complete blood count (CBC) with platelet count, arterial blood gases, electrolytes, blood urea nitrogen (BUN), and creatinine. Electrocardiograms should be obtained if there is any evidence of myocardial ischemia or a history of thoracic trauma. X-ray studies include an upright chest film, cervical spine films, and views of all fractures.

Table 5-2. Important Characteristics of Different Types of Shock

Type of Shock	BP	CVP	PCW	CO	PVR	Therapy
Hypovolemic	↓	↓	↓	↓	↑ ↑	Intravenous fluid
Distributive	↓	↓ or ↔	↓ or ↔	↑ ↑	↓ ↓	Direct at underlying cause; administer fluid as tolerated without producing pulmonary edema, then pressors
Cardiogenic	↓ ↑ or ↔	↑	↑	↓ ↓	↑	Inotropic agents, adjust preload and afterload to optimize CO: intraaortic balloon pump
Obstructive	↓	↑	↑ ↓ or ↔	↓	↑ ↑	Direct at underlying cause; intravenous fluid to increase filling pressures of heart and increase CO

BP = Blood pressure
CVP = Central venous pressure
PCW = Pulmonary capillary wedge pressure
CO = Cardiac output
PVR = Peripheral vascular resistance

Evaluation and Therapy of Shock

Recognition of shock, differential diagnosis
Primary survey—check ABC's (airway, breathing, circulation, and C-spine)
Secondary survey—complete head-to-toe evaluation
Basic life support—O_2 delivery, ventilation, control bleeding, MAST suit

The immediate and long-term goal is a patient who is alert, has stable vital signs, adequate systemic perfusion as evidenced by warm, dry skin, and a satisfactory urine output.

Specific Measures

Hypovolemic shock is treated by fluid administration. This is begun when a patent airway and adequate ventilation are established. Two large-bore peripheral intravenous lines are placed, and a balanced salt solution (lactated Ringer's) is given initially. A blood loss of up to 20% may be treated with lactated Ringer's solution alone. A blood loss of 20% to 40% responds best to a balanced administration of lactated Ringer's and blood to restore the circulating blood volume and red cell mass to ensure adequate oxygen-carrying capacity. A blood loss of greater than 40% is a life-threatening situation and requires aggressive immediate transfusion therapy and volume resuscitation (see Table 5-1).

Control of hemorrhage is mandatory in all patients. MAST trousers raise the peripheral vascular resistance and are an adjunct to fluid resuscitation. The patient should be placed in Trendelenburg's position to maximize return of venous blood to the heart. Fluid therapy of nonhemorrhagic hypovolemic shock is determined by the type and volume of fluid deficit. Generally, a balanced salt solution is administered at a rate necessary to restore peripheral organ perfusion.

Distributive shock due to septicemia results from vasodilation and maldistribution of available cardiac output. These patients require aggressive therapy and invasive physiologic monitoring to optimize survival. Fluid resuscitation using a balanced salt solution (lactated Ringer's) can establish an effective circulating blood volume in the presence of peripheral vasodilation. Bacterial culture specimens must be obtained from all appropriate sources prior to the institution of broad-spectrum antibiotics. Surgical debridement of all necrotic tissue and drainage of all septic foci is mandatory. An intraarterial catheter and a Swan-Ganz pulmonary artery catheter are necessary to determine cardiac output, cardiac filling pressure, and pulmonary and peripheral vascular resistance patterns. The utilization of vasoactive adrenergic drugs is based upon invasive physiologic monitoring. Like most patients in shock, these patients are best treated in an intensive care setting.

Patients who develop distributive shock due to spinal cord dysfunction or drug overdose should initially be placed supine or in Trendelenburg's position and volume resuscitated with a balanced salt solution. Respiratory insufficiency, acute gastric dilatation, and urinary retention frequently occur in these patients. These sequelae must be anticipated and the appropriate sup-

Hypovolemic Shock

Rapid volume resuscitation—two large IVs, lactated Ringer's, blood products if needed
Control blood loss—pressure, splinting, MAST, surgery
Maintain O_2 transport—Hb >10 g/dl
Support cardiac output—invasive monitoring, pharmacologic agents

Distributive Shock

Sepsis
  Volume resuscitation—raise PCWP to 15-18 cm H_2O
  Obtain cultures
  Broad-spectrum antibiotics
  Control of septic focus (debridement, abscess drainage)
  Optimize distribution of CO-vasoconstrictors, vasodilators
Spinal cord dysfunction
  Volume resuscitation
  Supine or Trendelenberg position

Obstructive Shock

Volume resuscitation
Careful differential diagnosis and appropriate diagnostic studies
Specific corrective therapy (e.g. tap, chest tube, surgery)

Cardiogenic Shock

Careful differential diagnosis
Dysrhythmia control
Possible fibrinolytic therapy
Invasive monitoring-preload and afterload adjustment to optimize CO
Inotropic and chronotropic agents
Intraaortic balloon pump

Modified from Chernow B and Roth BL: Pharmacologic manipulation of the peripheral vasculature in shock: clinical and experimental approaches, Circ Shock 18:141, 1986.

port measures must be taken—ventilatory support, nasogastric tube insertion, or Foley catheter insertion.

The cause of obstructive shock is a mechanical blockade of blood flow. Intravenous fluid therapy provides volume expansion and augments cardiac output, giving temporary support to the patient. A careful diagnostic evaluation is essential to direct corrective therapy. After the patient has been examined and the history taken, diagnostic steps may include pericardiocentesis, thoracocentesis, upright chest film, echocardiography, angiography, or cardiac catheterization. Care should be taken before instituting inotropic pharmacologic support therapy, as these agents may be detrimental in the presence of pulmonary embolism, peripheral embolism, or dissection of the aorta.

Cardiogenic shock usually occurs after a myocardial infarction. The decrease in cardiac output may be due to a loss of more than 40% of the myocardium or to cardiac arrhythmias. Diagnosis is based on examination of the patient and the electrocardiographic findings. Life-threatening dysrhythmias must be suppressed by appropriate intravenous drugs or by electrocardioversion. Swan-Ganz and intraarterial catheters should be placed in order to determine and to optimize cardiac preload and afterload. Intravenous fluids, diuretic drugs, vasodilators, and inotropic agents such as Dopamine or dobutamine may be necessary to optimize cardiac output and control pulmonary edema. Occasionally the intraaortic balloon may be used for temporary support. Cardiac surgery has been shown to be efficacious in patients who develop acute mitral valve insufficiency or ventricular septal defects after a myocardial infarction. In spite of all these aggressive and exotic therapies cardiogenic shock continues to have a high mortality (see box).

Monitors and Guideposts to Adequate Treatment

The appearance of the patient is important in judging therapeutic adequacy. The patient should be alert and communicative. Skin should be dry, pink, and of normal temperature. Nail bed capillary refill should be prompt. Vital signs (pulse, arterial blood pressure, respiratory rate) are monitored frequently. The stable patient should have normal vital signs: pulse rate of less than 120/minute in an adult, respirations of less than 28/minute, and systolic blood pressure greater than 90 torr.

Urinary output is one of the most sensitive monitors of cardiac output and peripheral perfusion. Hourly measurements of urinary output are especially valuable for determining the rate of fluid replacement in patients who do not require invasive physiologic monitoring. A urinary catheter is placed in any patient who is judged to have significant shock. Hourly urine output should be as follows: 2 ml/kg/hour in an infant or child, 30 ml/hour in a normal adult, 20 ml/hour in the elderly patient. The urine specific gravity and pH are measured in each of the hourly specimens.

Left and right atrial pressures may be measured with a Swan-Ganz pulmonary artery catheter. These catheters also allow determination of cardiac output by the thermodilution technique. An intraarterial line allows the beat-to-beat measurement of arterial pressures and ready access to the arterial blood for arterial blood gas determination and frequent serum sampling. This combination of invasive physiologic monitoring enables the physician to manipulate the preload and afterload of both the right and left ventricles to determine oxygen delivery and consumption by the patient and can be a valuable aid in the resuscitation and management of the shock patient. Laboratory studies such as arterial blood gases, serum electrolytes, BUN, creatinine, and clinical blood counts are invaluable in determining the course and response to therapy of the shock patient.

The preceding parameters are used to determine the severity of shock and the response to therapy. None of them may be used alone, and frequent careful evaluation of the patient is essential in determining the response to therapy. The goal of appropriate management of shock is restoration of adequate tissue perfusion.

6

Surgical Infection

Merril T. Dayton

Definition
Host Defense Mechanisms
Pathogenesis of Infection
Infection Prevention
Diagnosis of Surgical Infections
General Principles in Treating Surgical Infections
Specific Surgical Infections
AIDS Infections in Surgery

Serious infections remain an important cause of complications threatening surgical patients in spite of advances made in the understanding of preoperative nutrition, the development of more potent and broader-spectrum antibiotics, and improvements in surgical technique. In addition to being life-threatening on occasion, surgical infections cause significant morbidity, result in enormous increases in hospital costs, which total billions of dollars per year, and cause a significant increase in the work load on surgical services. The pattern of complicating infections has changed in the last two decades from one dominated by gram-positive cocci to one of nosocomial infections that over half the time are due to gram-negative bacilli; nevertheless the attendant morbidity, mortality, and financial impact of serious infection have not changed and remain a formidable problem for the surgeon.

DEFINITION

Any definition of the term *surgical infection* must stress the unique relationship between a given infection and the primary etiologic or therapeutic role of an operative procedure with regard to its outcome. "Medical infections" generally are associated with a single type of bacteria, have minimal local tissue reaction, manifest with constitutional symptoms, and, by definition, can usually be successfully treated with antibiotics alone. On the other hand, "surgical infections" are those that are either the direct result of an operative procedure (complication) or those that can be successfully treated only by surgical intervention. They are usually polymicrobial, are associated with significant local tissue reaction such as erythema, fluctuation, and point tenderness, will not respond to antibiotics alone, and eventually require either incision and drainage or excision for resolution. Common examples are abscesses, necrotizing fasciitis, cholangitis, wound infections, empyema, gas gangrene, and appendicitis.

HOST DEFENSE MECHANISMS

Man is surrounded by a multitude of potentially pathogenic bacteria, fungi, and viruses, which remain harmless because of a delicate immunologic balance between the host and these potential pathogens. Any perturbation of this balance such as a breakdown of host defenses or an increase in pathogen inoculum results in a potentially serious infection.

Because of their invasive nature, operative procedures often interrupt these defense barriers (skin, bowel wall, peritoneum) and render the host more liable to infection. Reports from the Communicable Disease Center underscore this liability to infection by demonstrating that the highest infection rates among hospitalized patients are found on surgical services. Paradoxically, while operations sometimes predispose the patient to infection, in other circumstances the patient may recover from a serious infection (abscess, gas gangrene, necrotizing fasciitis) only after aggressive surgical treatment.

One irony of modern medical progress is the further compromise of host defenses related to implementation of new apparatuses, surgical techniques, and mechanical equipment such as endotracheal tubes, Foley catheters, and vascular cannulas used in monitoring and treating such patients.

Successful defense of the host against microbial invasion thus depends on properly functioning immune mechanisms. Intact skin and mucous membranes play an invaluable role in protecting the host; the high infection rates in burn patients confirm the importance of this tough, reliable protective layer. Normal cell and humoral function are imperative in preventing serious infections; the neutropenic or agammaglobulinemic patient is easy prey for microbes that ordinarily are not pathogenic.

Upon penetrating the host's first line of defense, the pathogen triggers a complex array of humoral and cellular defense mechanisms (Fig. 6-1). Commonly the invasion is associated with tissue injury, which stimulates an inflammatory vascular response mediated by the kinin system and other vasoactive substances. The result is increased capillary permeability and capillary sphincter tone and vascular dilation. Consequently, plasma proteins ooze into the interstitium along with neutrophils and monocytes by diapedesis.

Two general mechanisms now play complimentary roles in the defense process. Humoral factors, including antibody-antigen aggregates, activate the complement system promoting chemotaxis, increased adherence, and anaphylactoid substances. This results in amplified phagocyte function and eventual bacterial cell wall lysis. Similarly, cellular factors make critical contributions after opsoninization leads to phagocyte attachment to the bacterium, followed by engulfment and

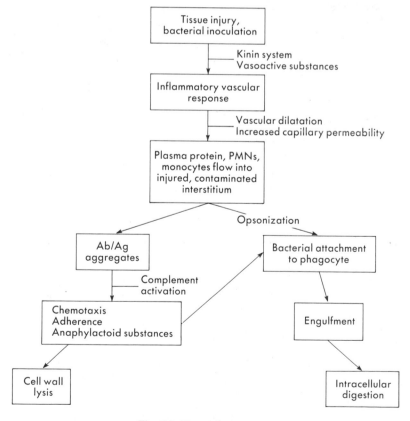

Fig. 6-1. Host defense system.

subsequent intracellular digestion of the bacterium. Although both neutrophils and lymphocytes are capable of phagocytosis, the neutrophil plays the most important role in early defense against invading pathogens.

PATHOGENESIS OF INFECTION

Any imbalance of the host defense system whether from *overloading, intrinsic abnormalities,* or *host defense interference* results in infection. In addition, the type of bacteria invading the host plays a role in whether an infection develops; some types inhibit phagocytosis because of cell surface structures, others produce potent exotoxins, and still others are toxic because of surface components.

Overloading occurs when the inoculum is large or continued; unresolved contamination simply overwhelms the host's defense capabilities. Intrinsic abnormalities relate to systemic conditions that suppress the humoral and cellular limbs of host defense. Examples include malnutrition, alcoholism, steroid administration, diabetes, poor tissue perfusion, anemia, obesity, chronic renal failure, malignancy, immune suppression, and hypoproteinemia. Host defense interference is usually caused by local factors in surgical patients. Devitalized or necrotic tissue, foreign bodies, excessively tight sutures interfering with blood supply, dead space with hematoma or seroma, and rough tissue handling resulting in injury are all known deterrents of wound healing. Large clinical studies have clearly shown the correlation between the factors aforementioned and an increased risk of wound or surgical infection (Table 6-1).

INFECTION PREVENTION

Without question the most effective, least expensive, and most desirable method of dealing with infection is to prevent it from ever occurring. Systemic conditions that suppress normal host defenses should be dealt with preoperatively. Malnourished patients should be appropriately alimented before surgery, steroid use should be minimized if possible, diabetes should be carefully controlled, anemia should be corrected, and weight loss for obese patients is highly desirable.

Bacterial contamination intraoperatively can be minimized by careful antiseptic preparation of both the patient and surgical team members. Breaks in technique (e.g., glove tears) should be rectified immediately, devitalized tissue should be debrided, all foreign bodies should be removed or kept to a minimum (e.g., suture), and any time a contaminated organ is entered or transected, the remainder of the field should be carefully excluded. Careful hemostasis and wound closure without tension are of paramount importance in successful wound healing without infection. Other important factors include minimizing the length of the operative procedure and limiting the length of the preoperative and postoperative hospital stays.

Prophylactic antibiotics are another important weapon in the armamentarium of infection prevention. Whereas multiple studies have clearly demonstrated the efficacy of prophylactic antibiotics in high-risk surgical patients, other studies have shown that prophylaxis regimens need not be prolonged or expensive to be effective. Similarly, little benefit is derived when prophylactic antibiotics are used in low-risk patients; on the contrary, improper use results in increased patient cost, the development of drug-resistant bacteria, and serious complications such as pseudomembranous colitis. Determinants of surgical patients with high risk of wound infection have been previously described, and surgical procedures have been classified according to degree of bacterial contamination, as follows:

Table 6-1. Factors Increasing Incidence of Surgical Infections

Factors	X-fold Increase in Infection
Host Intrinsic Factors	
Malnutrition	3
Alcoholism	
Steroids	2
Diabetes	2
Poor tissue perfusion	
Anemia	
Obesity	2
Chronic renal failure	
Malignancy	
Immune suppression	
Hypoproteinemia	
Infection at nonrelated site	3
Age over 60 years	3
Local Wound Factors	
Contaminated wound	6
Foreign body	
Devitalized or necrotic tissue	
Preoperative hospitalization	4
Excessively tight sutures	
Emergency operation	3
Excessively long operation (over 3 hours)	2
Hematoma, seroma	
Electrocautery	2
Penrose drain use	2

1. Clean
    No hollow viscus entered
    Primary wound closure
    Elective procedure
    No breaks in septic technique
    No inflammation
    Infection incidence 2%
2. Clean-contaminated
    Hollow viscus entered but controlled
    Primary wound closure
    Mechanical drain used
    Minor break in aseptic technique
    No obvious inflammation
    Infection incidence 10%
3. Contaminated
    Uncontrolled spillage from hollow viscus
    Open, traumatic wound
    Major break in aseptic technique
    Inflammation apparent
    Infection incidence 20%
4. Dirty
    Uncontrolled, untreated spillage from hollow viscus

Open, suppurative wound
Pus present in operative field
Severe inflammation, patient toxic
Infection incidence 50%.

The procedures requiring prophylactic antibiotics are as follows:

High infection rate or high risk
  Colon and rectum surgery
  Vaginal hysterectomy
  Vascular procedures involving prostheses
  Biliary procedures at risk (acute cholecystitis, cholangitis, common duct obstruction)
  Procedures for gastric obstruction, bleeding, cancer, or ulcer with achlorhydria
  Appendectomy (nonincidental)
  Major head and neck resections
  Urethra and bladder surgery in females
  Noncardiac thoracic surgery (lung and esophageal resections)
  Open heart procedures
Presence of indwelling prosthesis
  Cardiac valve
  Arterial graft
  Artifical joint
  Ophthalmic implant
  Ventricular shunt
  Synthetic mesh

In summary, proper prophylactic therapy is short term, inexpensive, properly timed (i.e., started before the incision is made), and used only in high-risk patients.

DIAGNOSIS OF SURGICAL INFECTIONS

Physical examination remains the most effective modality in diagnosing surgical infection. The majority are associated with local erythema, fluctuation, crepitus, calor, induration, or point tenderness. Radiography may be helpful in the diagnosis of the intraabdominal infections; flat plate and upright films of the abdomen may show an elevated hemidiaphragm (subphrenic abscess), a soap bubble pattern (lesser sac abscess), obliterated psoas margin (appendiceal abscess), pneumoperitoneum (perforated ulcer), and air-fluid levels outside the bowel lumen (abscess secondary to gas-forming organism). Soft tissue radiographs often show subcutaneous air associated with clostridial infection. Ultrasound is particularly helpful in identifying large fluid collections or cystic spaces; it is limited when there is excessive bowel gas. Computed tomography (CT) also helps identify pancreatic and other abdominal fluid collections, even in the face of significant bowel gas. Labeled leukocyte scans are becoming increasingly helpful in identifying occult infection and are replacing gallium scans for that specific indication.

GENERAL PRINCIPLES IN TREATING SURGICAL INFECTIONS

Incision and drainage are indicated in virtually all abscesses wherever encountered in the body (exceptions include amebic liver abscesses and lung abscesses). Because of altered local blood supply, inadequate antibiotic levels, closed spaces under pressure, and overwhelming inoculum, conservative therapy is normally doomed to failure. Adequate surgical therapy involves widely opening the abscess cavity, draining its contents, breaking up loculations, and leaving a drainage tube.

Excision of the diseased organ or source of infection is often definitive therapy, and no further treatment, including drainage or antibiotics, may be necessary. Not infrequently antibiotics and excision are used concomitantly to provide optimal therapy.

Débridement is an important principle in treatment of surgical infections that is applied when necrotic tissues are present or a virulent, progressive tissue infection threatens the patient's life. Débridement is surgical resection of devitalized, necrotic, heavily contaminated, or severely injured tissue using a scalpel or scissors. Occasionally, coarse gauze may be used to débride a contaminated wound; after gently packing a wound with gauze, débridement occurs as the dressing is changed, when nonviable tissue adheres to the gauze.

Diversion of the fecal stream is often helpful in treatment of bowel perforation, fistulas, and severe perianal infections.

For small localized abscesses without attendant septicemia, incision and drainage may be all that is required for adequate treatment of the condition; however, when there is a large abscess with adjacent organs involved, bacteremia and obvious systemic manifestations such as hypotension, tachycardia, high fever, decreased urine output, and respiratory deterioration, antibiotics become a crucial ally of surgical therapy for optimal patient management. Selection of the appropriate antibiotic should initially be made after Gram stain of the pyogenous drainage or after detection of the diseased organ responsible for the contamination; further modification of the antibiotic regimen can be made after carefully collected aerobic and anaerobic specimens are cultured and organism sensitivity to the various antibiotics is determined (Table 6-2).

SPECIFIC SURGICAL INFECTIONS
Cellulitis

Cellulitis, a nonsuppurative infection of soft tissue, is often the earliest host response to bacterial invasion. Pathophysiologically it is characterized by bacterial invasion and multiplication with concomitant capillary dilation, leukocyte infiltration, and increased capillary permeability and edema of the dermal and subcutaneous layers. It manifests clinically as a diffuse erythema that is palpably warm and often tender. There is usually a trauma or wound site, which is the portal of entry, and the patient often has a fever. Frank abscess rarely occurs, and the disease is mentioned here primarily because it may be confused with the true surgical infections that have attendant inflammation. It is most commonly caused by streptococci and should be treated with large doses of penicillin given intravenously, warm soaks, elevation, and immobilization of the involved area, if possible.

Lymphangitis

A previously established infection serves as a nidus for the disease process called lymphangitis, which results when bacteria invade the lymphatic system draining a local infection. Clinically, one sees a tender, edematous extremity with linear erythematous streaks

Table 6-2. Preferred Antibiotics for Serious Surgical Infections

Organism	First Choice	Second Choice
Streptococcus viridans	Penicillin G	Cephalosporin
Streptococcus pyogenes	Penicillin G	Cephalosporin
Streptococcus sp., group B	Penicillin G	Cephalosporin
Streptococcus as enterococcus form	Ampicillin	Penicillin G or vancomycin
Staphylococcus aureus		
penicillinase (−)	Penicillin G	Cephalosporin
penicillinase (+)	Oxacillin, nafcillin	Cephalosporin
Peptostreptococcus	Penicillin G	Clindamycin
Streptococcus pneumoniae	Penicillin G	Erythromycin
Clostridium perfringens	Penicillin G	Chloramphenicol
Clostridium tetani	Penicillin G	Tetracycline
Clostridium difficile	Vancomycin	Metronidazole
Bacteroides, oral strains	Penicillin G	Clindamycin
Bacteroides, GI strains	Metronidazole	Clindamycin
Enterobacter	Gentamicin or tobramycin	Amikacin
Escherichia coli	Gentamicin or tobramycin	Amikacin, ampicillin
Klebsiella	Gentamicin or tobramycin	Amikacin
Proteus mirabilis	Ampicillin	Gentamicin
Proteus indole (+)	Gentamicin or tobramycin	Amikacin
Serratia	Gentamicin or amikacin	Cefotaxime
Pseudomonas aeruginosa	Gentamicin or tobramycin and carbenicillin or ticarcillin	Amikacin and carbenicillin
Providencia	Amikacin	Cefotaxime
Candida	Amphotericin B	—

in the distribution of the lymphatic channels leading to the regional lymph nodes. In the prepenicillin era this condition was known as "blood poisoning" and was a harbinger of serious complications related to the infection. Treatment is identical to that for cellulitis, because streptococci are usually the offending organism.

Furuncle/Carbuncle

In contrast to the spreading, diffuse nature of streptococcal infections, staphylococcal infections are usually localized and indurated and have a central cellulitic area that necroses and forms a cutaneous abscess. Furuncle is an example of a staphylococcal infection that starts most commonly when a sebaceous gland at the base of a hair follicle becomes obstructed and the normally colonized follicle develops a localized abscess. This may then enlarge, extend into subcutaneous tissues, and even rupture spontaneously. Clinically the patient will complain of a local, raised lesion that is tender, fluctuant, and inflamed. A carbuncle is a necrotizing infection of dermis and subcutaneous tissues originating as a cluster of furuncles. As the lesion progresses, multiple pus-draining sinuses develop, central suppuration occurs, and occasionally existing skin bridges slough. Treatment of an uncomplicated furuncle is incision and drainage; for more advanced furuncles with surrounding inflammation or multiple lesions, antibiotics with incision and drainage are required. The procedure involves opening the lesion widely, evacuating pus, breaking up loculations, and either packing the wound open or "saucerizing" it (removing a superficial ellipse of skin) to prevent superficial wound closure before deep tissues have healed. Treatment of carbuncles involves appropriate antibiotics given intravenously and aggressive surgical therapy consisting of incision,

drainage, and even excision of sinus tracts on occasion. A penicillinase-resistant agent such as oxacillin or nafcillin should be used to treat this family of infections.

Postoperative Wound Infections

Postoperative wound infections occur in 3% to 10% of patients undergoing operative procedures. Their development is the result of a complex interaction between (1) surgical technique and wound care, (2) bacterial contamination during surgery, and (3) the relative efficacy of the host's immune system. Risk factors and patients at high risk for developing postoperative wound infections were previously discussed in this chapter. Importantly, the two most common sources of bacterial contamination are the patient's skin and any colonized hollow organ of the patient entered during the operation (e.g., colon, trachea, gallbladder). Exogenous sources such as operating team members and operating room environment play a minor etiological role in postoperative infections. The most common pathogens isolated from postoperative wound infections remain *Staphylococcus aureus* and gram-negative rods. With the exception of *Clostridium* and β-hemolytic streptococci wound infections, which may manifest within 24 hours postoperatively, the majority become evident some 5 to 7 days postoperatively. The clinical picture is one of low-grade fever, wound pain, erythema, local edema, and drainage. Treatment consists in widely opening the wound by removal of skin stitches or clips, evacuating purulent material, appropriately débriding, and loosely packing the wound open to heal by secondary intention. Antibiotics usually are not required but may be added if systemic symptoms are present.

Tetanus

Tetanus is a disease that manifests primarily with neurological symptoms directly related to a potent bacterial exotoxin called tetanospasmin. The etiologic agent *(Clostridium tetani)* is a gram-positive, anaerobic, spore-forming rod, which is usually introduced into the injured area as a spore. Under conditions of warmth and low tissue oxygen tension, the spores convert to the vegetative form, which produces the toxin. Wounds that are predisposed to develop tetanus include deep stab injuries, injuries with massive tissue necrosis, and farm injuries. The incubation period is 3 to 21 days, and when symptoms occur, they do so in one of three ways: (1) generalized tetanus with trismus, local spasm, lethargy, irritability, dysphagia, abdominal cramps, and laryngeal spasm; (2) local tetanus with persistent muscle rigidity near the injury site; and (3) cephalic tetanus, a rare condition characterized by involvement of cranial nerves. The most common form is generalized tetanus, which has a mortality of 50%.

The most important principle in treating tetanus is prevention by appropriate wound care and primary immunization. The latter consists of three sequential doses of tetanus toxoid followed by a booster dose 1 year after the third dose. Further booster doses should be repeated every 10 years. Wound care involves copious irrigation and aggressive débridement of skin injuries, usually with the skin being left open to heal by secondary intention. Determining adequate immunization in the recently injured patient may be difficult; treatment guidelines are indicated in Table 6-3. When the diagnosis of tetanus is made, treatment should include aggressive débridement of the surgical wound, high doses of intravenously administered penicillin, intramuscular doses of human tetanus immune globulin, and supportive care including sedation and use of paralytic agents. With the latter, endotracheal intubation and ventilatory support are necessary.

Clostridial Infections

Clostridial organisms cause a wide spectrum of disease ranging from simple contamination to an aggressive, invasive myonecrosis. *Clostridium perfringens* is causal in 80% of cases. The organism is a gram-positive rod that requires a low redox potential and anaerobiosis for optimal growth. Trauma, ischemia, foreign body, or pyogenic infection causes conversion of spores to the vegetative forms, which produce the toxin responsible for the clinical manifestations. The toxins include fibrinolysin, lecithinase, collagenase, and hyaluronidase. Although not common, different diseases in the spectrum must be differentiated because their treatments are vastly different. Examples are clostridial cellulitis and clostridial myonecrosis.

Clostridial cellulitis is usually initiated by a puncture wound of an extremity. The first symptom occurs after 3 or 4 days. Thereafter, multiple blebs occur extruding foul-smelling, reddish brown fluid; frank necrosis of the skin and subcutaneous tissue then completes the cycle. The dissection develops immediately above the deep fascial planes and is often associated with skin discoloration. Crepitus is always a prominent feature, with gas being both extensive and easily demonstrable; muscle is not involved, however. The patient usually has few constitutional symptoms, a finding that helps distinguish this form from myonecrosis. Gram stain of aspirated, watery pus usually confirms the diagnosis. Therapy involves radical incision, drainage, débridement, high-dose intravenously administered penicillin, and wound packing. Later skin grafting may be necessary.

Clostridial myonecrosis, or "gas gangrene," is the most severe form of clostridial infection and usually occurs after extensive lacerations or muscle devitalization, ischemia, gross soil contamination, or delayed wound treatment. Incubation is usually 3 days, and the disease onset is acute, the initial symptoms being a sense of increasing weight and deep pain. Progression of the disease is rapid, and the patient becomes pale, diaphoretic, and often delirious. Tachycardia and hypotension follow, and shock may develop at any point in the course. The wound has a profuse serosanguineous discharge that has a sweet, musky odor initially; overlying skin is white, shiny, and tense. Gas bubbles may be seen at the wound entrance, and exposed muscle is edematous and noncontractile; crepitus is often noticed when the disease is advanced. A Gram stain of the drainage confirms the diagnosis though the clinical picture is strongly suggestive. Radiographs also demonstrate subcutaneous air. Treatment includes radical débridement of nonviable muscle and opening of fascial compartments; if the disease is extensive and far advanced, amputation of the extremity may become necessary. Ancillary treatment includes high-dose intravenously administered penicillin and hyperbaric oxygenation; although the method is somewhat controversial, some also advocate the administration of clostridial antitoxins. Inadequately treated, clostridial myonecrosis invariably has a lethal outcome. Overall mortality is 20%.

Necrotizing Fasciitis

Necrotizing fasciitis is one of the most common serious surgical infections. It may complicate either traumatic or surgical wounds, especially when an abdominal hollow viscus has been opened. The condition is a mixed infection caused by a synergistic combination of aerobic gram-negative rods and anaerobes plus microaerophilic streptococci or hemolytic staphylococci. The disease is a rapidly invasive infection of superficial fascia with associated thrombosis of penetrating vessels from the deep system to the skin. The latter results in skin necrosis along with impressive fascial dissection (Fig. 6-2).

Clinically one sees lymphedema extending in all directions associated with mottled, reddish purple skin. As the disease progresses, blebs filled with serosanguineous fluid form followed by skin necrosis in 30% of cases. The fascia is a grayish, nonviable color ("dishwater appearance") and easily separates from the subcutaneous layer without pain. The patient is most frequently profoundly toxic with fever, hypotension, tachycardia, tachypnea, and mental confusion. Aggressive fluid resuscitation is necessary before the patient is taken to the operating room; hypocalcemia and anemia may also occur and mandate correction before anesthesia induction.

Treatment involves radical excision of all nonviable

Table 6-3. Guidelines for Tetanus Prophylaxis in Injured Patients

	Previously Immunized				Not Previously Immunized	
	Immunized More than 10 Years Ago		Immunized Less than 10 Years Ago			
	Minor Wound	Tetanus-prone Wound	Minor Wound	Tetanus-prone Wound	Minor Wound	Tetanus-prone Wound
Wound	Wash, removal of foreign body	Débridement, irrigation, removal of foreign body	Wash, removal of foreign body	Débridement, irrigation, removal of foreign body	Wash, removal of foreign body	Removal of foreign body, aggressive débridement, removal of devitalized tissue, copious irrigation
Tetanus toxoid	0.5 ml tetanus toxoid intramuscularly	0.5 ml tetanus toxoid intramuscularly	If no booster within 5 years, tetanus toxoid	If no booster within 1 year, tetanus toxoid	Basic immunization starting with 0.5 ml tetanus toxoid intramuscularly	0.5 ml tetanus toxoid intramuscularly; then continue immunization
Human tetanus immune globulin	No	250 units of tetanus immune globulin intramuscularly, contralateral side	No	No	No	250 units tetanus immune globulin intramuscularly, contralateral side
Antibiotics	No	Penicillin intravenously	No	No	No	High dose of penicillin intravenously

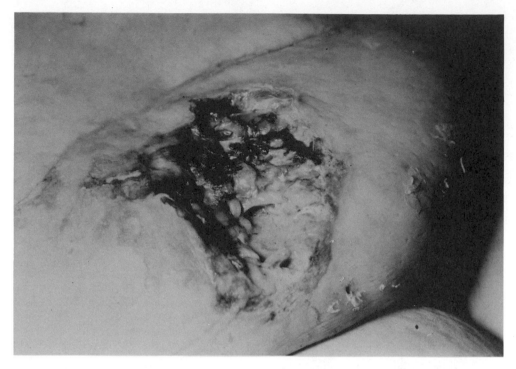

Fig. 6-2. Postoperative necrotizing fasciitis with obvious skin necrosis, mottling, and fascial dissection.

fascia and skin back to healthy tissue. Where necrotic fascia undermines viable skin, long parallel incisions may be made for removal of all nonliving fascia and preservation of overlying skin. Antibiotics are supplementary and should include an aminoglycoside and penicillin initially with appropriate adjustments made after culture and sensitivity tests are completed.

Serious Streptococcal Infections

Streptococcal hemolytic gangrene (necrotizing cellulitis) is produced by hemolytic streptococci, usually after a minor skin wound. Clinically the patient develops a low-grade temperature along with edema, warmth, erythema, and pain in the skin region involved. Over a 2- to 3-day period, even with antibiotics, the skin becomes dusky and forms large, dark, serous blebs; in contrast to clostridial infections, the fluid in the blebs has no odor. The last stage in the disease is cutaneous necrosis and gangrene (Fig. 6-3). Treatment includes emergency incision and drainage beyond involved tissue longitudinally and deep to underlying fascia; undermining skin flaps usually is not necessary. The incision releases skin tension, prevents ischemia, and allows wound packing, elevation, and débridement of necrotic skin.

Streptococcal myositis is caused by anaerobic streptococci and is characterized as a massive infection of muscles with skin discoloration, edema, local pain, crepitation of muscle, and generalized toxemia. In contrast with clostridial myositis, cutaneous erythema is more pronounced, involved muscle, while edematous, is still alive and contractile, the odor is distinctly different, and Gram stain shows no gram-positive ba-

cilli. Management consists in incisions, drainage, and occasionally excision of necrotic muscle.

Progressive Bacterial Synergistic Gangrene

Also known as Meleney's synergistic gangrene, this infection develops 2 weeks after an operative or skin wound and is caused by a nonhemolytic streptococcus and a hemolytic staphylococcus. The wound has a characteristic appearance typified by three zones: peripherally, a wide area of edema and erythema adjacent to a zone of purplish, painful skin, and a central zone of necrosis and ulceration (Fig. 6-4). Low-grade fever, anemia, and weakness are occasionally present; systemic manifestations may occur early and should be treated with fluids and intravenously administered antibiotics. Definitive treatment, however, is radical excision of all nonviable layers extending well into viable tissue. Skin grafting may become necessary later.

Nonclostridial Gangrene

Gangrenous lesions with associated subcutaneous gas are usually classified as clostridial in origin. However, a host of gram-negative organisms can produce gas with extensive soft-tissue dissection; these are probably more common and less severe than gas gangrene from clostridial organisms. *Escherichia coli,* anaerobic streptococci, *Bacteroides* species, and *Enterobacter* species have all been associated with this infection. Commonly the infection occurs after wet gangrene of an extremity develops; crepitus is then detected on physical examination or radiograph. A lack of systemic toxicity with extensive air dissection is suggestive of the diagnosis. Therapy involves débridement

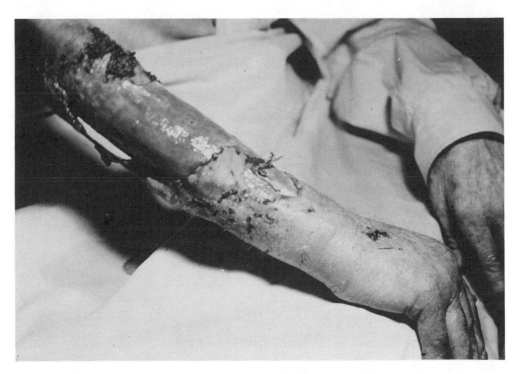

Fig. 6-3. End-stage streptococcal hemolytic gangrene with cutaneous necrosis evident.

and local wound care; the extensive gas dissection can generally be ignored.

Fungal Infection

Actinomycosis is caused by a gram-positive fungus that branches into filamentous structures; it is anaerobic and is often part of the normal oral flora. Three major clinical types of the disease are described: cervicofacial (which is the most common), thoracic, and abdominal. It is characterized by firm, nodular granulomas that break down, suppurate, and discharge pus through multiple sinuses (Fig. 6-5). Gram stain reveals "sulfur granules" that are aggregates of mycelia. Long-term treatment with penicillin is necessary as well as occasional excision of the sinus tracts.

Nocardiosis is caused by *Nocardia,* a gram-positive aerobic fungus that has become an important complication of immune suppression or immunodeficiency. It presents as a chronic, suppurating, draining sinus tract resembling actinomycosis. It may also extensively involve the central nervous system or respiratory system and present with systemic manifestation of low-grade fever, lethargy, weakness, weight loss, and irritating cough. Primary treatment involves administering sulfonamides, but surgical therapy, in the form of sinus tract excision and abscess drainage, may be necessary.

AIDS INFECTIONS IN SURGERY

In the late 1970s clinical description of a previously unrecognized syndrome was reported that was characterized by overwhelming opportunistic infections, malnutrition, and the development of Kaposi's sarcoma. Intensive research in the subsequent years established a retrovirus infection of human T cell lymphocytes by the human T cell lymphoma virus (HTLV-III) as the cause of the disease. Further characterization of the disease caused widespread concern because it was usually fatal and because no cure was known. The disease, now known as acquired immunodeficiency syndrome (AIDS), occurs primarily in two high-risk groups, male homosexuals and abusers of intravenous (IV) drugs. Over 37,000 cases of AIDS have now been reported, 21,000 of them fatal. Without question, AIDS is one of the most virulent and devastating infections in the history of humanity.

HTLV-III has been isolated from a host of body fluids including blood, tears, saliva, semen, urine, and cervical, amniotic, and cerebrospinal fluids. The disease causes special concern to surgeons primarily because (1) they frequently come into contact with the above-mentioned body fluids during therapeutic and diagnostic maneuvers and (2) they frequently transfuse blood or blood products into their patients. A surgeon's greatest concerns center around the possibility that he or she may be innoculated with the virus during an inadvertent needle stick, scalpel cut, splash of contaminated fluids into the eyes, or contact of contaminated fluids with a break in the skin. There is also concern that a patient may acquire the virus during the course of a blood transfusion. Fortunately, the likelihood that HTLV-III will be acquired through a single exposure by accidental needle stick or cut is remote. In a recent study of 640 health care workers reporting exposure to the virus by needle stick, cut, or mucous membrane, only 2 tested positive for anti–HTLV-III antibodies *and* denied having any AIDS risk factors. Similarly,

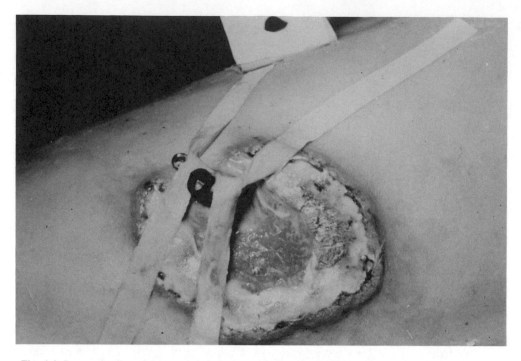

Fig. 6-4. Progressive bacterial synergistic gangrene with three characteristic zones: peripheral erythema, purplish skin in the middle, and central necrosis.

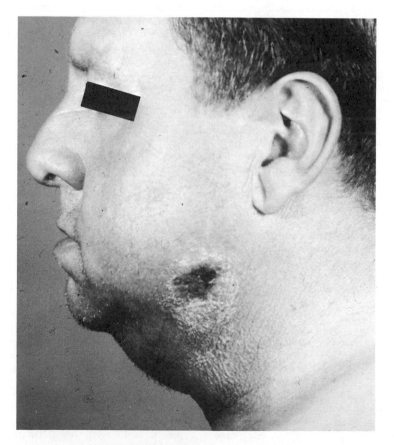

Fig. 6-5. Draining sinus of actinomycosis of jaw.

the risk of contracting the disease during blood transfusion has been greatly diminished because donated blood units are now screened for IITLV-III antibodies.

While the risk of accidental transmission of the AIDS virus is low, the Center for Disease Control has recommended the following precautions for health workers involved in invasive procedures: (1) routine barrier precautions (gloves, masks, gowns, protective eye wear) should be used to prevent skin or mucous membrane exposure when contact with blood or body fluids of an AIDS patient is anticipated; (2) hands should be washed immediately after contamination with blood or body fluids or after glove removal; (3) all health care workers should take extra precautions to prevent injuries from sharp instruments during invasive procedures; (4) in resuscitation areas, mouthpieces, resuscitation bags, or other ventilation devices should be available to avoid emergency mouth-to-mouth resuscitation; (5) health care workers with weeping, exudative lesions should refrain from direct patient care until the condition resolves, and (6) pregnant health care workers should be especially familiar with and strictly adhere to precautions to minimize AIDS transmission.

7

Surgical Nutrition

Nathaniel J. Soper
Robert T. Soper

Basic Metabolic Considerations
Delivery of Nutritional Support
Conclusion

A well-balanced diet has long been recognized as necessary for good health; however, the fact that disease states, trauma, and operations increase nutritional requirements has been appreciated and documented only during the past half century. Further, the materials and delivery systems that have allowed these increased demands to be met in patients who, for one reason or another, are unable to eat ordinary diets have evolved only during the past 2 or 3 decades. The purpose of this chapter is to review current concepts of basic nutritional requirements, the manner in which they are affected by disease and operations, and different techniques by which these increased nutritional demands may be met.

BASIC METABOLIC CONSIDERATIONS
Energy Requirements

Carbohydrate and protein (4 kcal/g each) and fat (9 kcal/g) supply dietary energy. The daily energy requirements can be calculated when the energy requirements for activity are added to those demands required for basal metabolic purposes. Basal energy demand varies with size and age. Thus an infant requires approximately 100 kcal/kg/24 hours to meet the enormous metabolic demands for growth and development, whereas a young adult male needs only 20 to 30 kcal/kg/24 hours to meet his basal energy requirements. Generally, 1 ml of fluid is required for each calorie of energy that is expended. Fig. 7-1 graphically portrays a simple method of estimating maintenance body fluid and calorie requirements, based on body weight. Many other formulas for calculating basal energy requirements are available, including the Harris-Benedict equation, which is presented later in this chapter.

Energy requirements are increased by a number of

factors, including fever (7% per 1° F), major long bone fractures, severe burns, body growth and development, healing of wounds, pregnancy, hyperthyroidism, and physical activity.

Protein Requirements

Protein needs must be considered separately from calorie requirements. Protein cannot be stored except in functional tissue, as somatic and visceral protein. Normal daily protein requirements vary from 2 g/kg/day in infants to 40 to 60 g/day in adults. If inadequate calories are supplied, structural proteins will be "cannabalized" to produce energy, a process termed *gluconeogenesis*. This accelerated protein breakdown is reflected by increased urinary nitrogen excretion. Stressed or injured patients should receive twice the normal daily protein requirements. Such severe injuries as major thermal burns may increase the protein requirements to 300 g/24 hours in adults.

An important characteristic of the supplied diet is the calorie-to-nitrogen ratio. Energy is required to incorporate protein into tissue protoplasm. Dietary protein will be converted to glucose and used for energy rather than to form structural proteins if less than 150 nonprotein calories are supplied per gram of nitrogen. Depletion of body protein in surgical patients results in impaired wound and anastomotic healing, increased infection rate, anemia, edema, and weakness.

Carbohydrate and Fat

These substances are the body's primary energy substrates. Certain tissues (brain, myocardium, erythrocytes, and phagocytes) require glucose as their principal energy source. Many of these tissues can, however, adapt during the course of starvation to use ketone bodies from the oxidation of fat. Thus, during the initial period of fasting, much protein will be catabolized to form glucose, whereas later the demand for gluconeogenesis decreases. The initial period of catabolism can be minimized by adding as little as 100 g of carbohydrate per day to the patient's intake.

There are ample stores of energy in the body under normal circumstances in the form of body fat—10 to 15 kilograms, representing 90,000 to 135,000 kilocalories in an average adult. In sharp contrast, carbohydrate storage in the form of glycogen is minimal. Approxi-

mately 500 g (2,000 calories) of glycogen is available in liver and muscle, but it is quickly exhausted during stress.

There is a specific requirement for essential fatty acids, so-called because they cannot be manufactured or stored in the body. For example, approximately 2% of the caloric intake must be linoleic acid to prevent deficiency states. Essential fatty acid deficiency may quickly become apparent in infants, but it is uncommon in adults; it can be prevented when intravenous fat emulsion (Intralipid or Liposyn) is supplied once or twice per week.

Requirements for Vitamins, Minerals, and Trace Elements

In order for the body to utilize optimally these nutrients, certain additives such as fat- and water-soluble vitamins, minerals, and trace elements (zinc, copper, manganese, iodine, magnesium) are required. Commercial solutions of water-soluble vitamins and trace elements are available and should be routinely supplemented during prolonged nutritional therapy. Vitamin K (as indicated by clotting studies) and iron (given as intramuscular iron dextran or blood transfusion) may also be necessary during prolonged nutrition therapy.

Effects of Stress and Trauma

Stress and trauma activate the sympathoadrenal axis to release catecholamines, glucocorticoids, and glucagon. These hormones stimulate gluconeogenesis, glycogenolysis, and the release of free fatty acids, with the resulting hyperglycemia leading to the so-called diabetes of stress. This hypermetabolic pattern may greatly increase caloric requirements (Table 7-1).

Catecholamines trigger protein catabolism for gluconeogenesis, and explain why protein demands are so much greater during stress than with unstressed starvation. Great amounts of protein may be lost, particularly with coexistent trauma and infection. In excess of 30 g of urinary nitrogen may be excreted daily, which equals the loss of 190 g of protein or 1 kg of wet muscle. Even when large quantities of protein and calories are provided, it may be difficult to reverse nitrogen wasting. Therefore nutritional support should be instituted early after trauma and in adequate amounts to patients such as those with extensive burns, which are known to trigger a prolonged catabolic state.

Consequences of Malnutrition

Recent studies have documented quite clearly why we need to be concerned about the nutritional status of patients. These studies have shown that as many as 50% of hospitalized surgical patients suffer from protein-

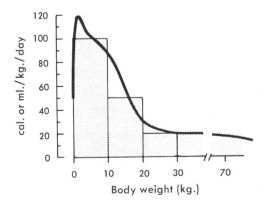

Fig. 7-1. Maintenance needs, caloric or fluid.

Table 7-1. Metabolic Response to Stress in Adults

Clinical Status	Calorie Requirements (kcal/kg/day)
Unstressed starvation	20
Basal metabolism	25-30
Elective surgery	35
Trauma	40
Severe infection	50
Major burns	50-70

calorie malnutrition. In turn, malnutrition is associated with increased mortality and morbidity (primarily infectious), retarded healing rates, and depressed in vivo and in vitro parameters of immunity. Furthermore, optimal nutritional support has been shown to reduce mortality and lower the sepsis rate in surgical patients.

Measuring Nutritional Status

A thorough history and physical examination are the primary screening tests to determine which patient needs nutritional support. There are many clinically utilized tests by which nutritional status can be estimated: (1) anthropometrics (triceps skin fold, etc.), (2) biochemical tests (creatinine-height index, serum albumin, and prealbumin, plasma transferrin, nitrogen balance determinations), and (3) tests of immune competence (total lymphocyte count, delayed hypersensitivity skin testing). Multivariant analysis of various nutritional parameters was used by Mullen and colleagues to provide a Prognostic Nutritional Index which identifies surgical patients at greatest risk for morbidity and mortality due to malnutrition. Factors that they found to be related to perioperative complications were serum albumin, plasma transferrin, triceps skin fold thickness, and delayed cutaneous hypersensitivity. The tests that we have found most useful to evaluate the adequacy of nutritional therapy are serial measurements of caloric intake and body weight, and frequent determinations of albumin level and nitrogen balance. Useful nutritional constants and equations follow:
Harris-Benedict equation to calculate basal energy expenditure (BEE):

$$\text{BEE (men)} = 66.47 + 13.75 \times \text{Weight (kg)} + 5.0 \times \text{Height (cm)} - 6.76 \times \text{Age}$$

$$\text{BEE (women)} = 655.10 + 9.56 \times \text{Weight} + 1.85 \times \text{Height} - 4.68 \times \text{Age}$$

$$\text{BEE (infants)} = 22.10 + 31.05 \times \text{Weight} + 1.16 \times \text{Height}$$

$$\text{Nitrogen balance} = [\text{Administered protein (g)} \div 6.25]$$
$$- [\text{Urinary urea nitrogen (UUN; 24-hour sample)}$$
$$+ 3\text{g (stool losses, nonurea urinary nitrogen)}]$$

$$\text{Protein catabolized} = \text{UUN} \times 6.25$$

$$\text{Muscle broken down} = \text{UUN} \times 30$$

$$(\text{Muscle} = 73\% \text{ water, } 23\% \text{ protein})$$

DELIVERY OF NUTRITIONAL SUPPORT
Total Parenteral Nutrition

Total parenteral nutrition (TPN) is a technique whereby all the required proteins, calories, and essential minerals are delivered intravenously. TPN can be administered either into a small peripheral vein or into a large central vein. When given peripherally, the fluid can be only mildly hypertonic, thus requiring large volumes to satisfy nutritional needs; new venipunctures are required daily or more often. On the contrary, when infused centrally, the solution can be quite hypertonic, since it is delivered into a large vascular channel where blood flow is rapid. This dilutes the solution quickly to isotonic concentrations, before it is disseminated throughout the body.

TPN is generally indicated for anyone who is unable

to take enough nutrition by way of the gastrointestinal tract and who has no prospect for improvement for a predictable, but variable, time interval; 1 week of starvation is sufficient to render newborns malnourished, and 2 weeks of starvation will initiate the process in previously healthy adults. TPN is especially indicated when there are excessive calorie demands due to illness or injury, as after major thermal injuries, in sepsis, or after multiple trauma.

TPN can provide the prolonged gastrointestinal rest that is required by certain medical problems, such as prolonged diarrhea, disaccharidase deficiencies, protein-losing enteropathies, severe gastrointestinal allergies, or inflammatory bowel disease. However, the majority of diseases for which parenteral hyperalimentation is indicated fall within the surgical realm and include massive bowel resection, prolonged or multiple intestinal obstructions, gastroenteric fistulas, prolonged paralytic ileus, or wound dehiscence; the prospect of lengthy and debilitating chemotherapy or x-ray therapy is also an indication.

The TPN Formula

Most hospitals stock a standard TPN solution that consists of 25% dextrose, 3.5% to 4.5% amino acids, and appropriate electrolytes. This mixture results in a calorie-to-nitrogen ratio of 150 to 1 to 225 to 1. Water-soluble vitamins and trace elements are provided daily, and heparin may be added to each bottle to inhibit venous thrombosis. Emulsified fat solution should be administered at least twice weekly.

Meticulous attention to sterility must be maintained by the pharmacy when the TPN solutions are being made, because the high glucose content makes it an excellent culture medium. The solutions should be prepared in a laminar airflow hood with appropriate quality control precautions.

Special clinical situations may require that the standard TPN formula be altered. Patients who are in renal failure require a higher calorie-to-nitrogen ratio which can be supplied either by 35% dextrose or exclusive delivery of essential amino acids (Nephramine solution). Carbon dioxide retention in patients with chronic lung disease may be lessened when an increased percentage of calories is supplied as fat, to lower the respiratory quotient. Recently there have been marketed branched-chain-enriched amino acid solutions, which are claimed to improve the clinical outcome in patients with hepatic failure or major trauma.

The TPN Delivery System

Because TPN formulas are hypertonic compared to serum, they must be delivered into a high-flow part of the venous system for rapid dilution and to minimize endothelial damage and thrombosis. The superior vena cava is well suited for this purpose. The inferior vena cava can be used, but the problems with sterility and immobilization of the catheter in the lower venous compartment make it less desirable.

In the short-term hospitalized adult patient the catheter can be introduced percutaneously into the subclavian vein from just inferior to the midpoint of the clavicle, the catheter being threaded into the superior vena cava. However, in the infant and younger child it is safer to insert the catheter by a surgical cutdown into either the external jugular vein or a branch of the internal jugular vein through which the tip is threaded into the superior vena cava (Fig. 7-2). The fact that the tip of the catheter has been accurately placed into the superior vena cava must be confirmed by fluoroscopy or x-ray examination, since malposition is common and dangerous.

For sterility purposes, it is best to separate the point where the catheter penetrates the skin as far as possible from the place where the catheter enters the vein. In the infant and young child the catheter can be tunneled subcutaneously to exit from the skin over the flat portion of the mastoid bone behind the ear (Fig. 7-2), or alternatively it can be tunneled down the chest wall to exit at midsternum. The entire procedure is carried out in the operating room under strict aseptic technique.

In infants and for long-term venous access in any patient, we prefer an intravenous catheter that is constructed of Silastic (silicone rubber) that has been impregnated with silver to render the catheter radiopaque. Silastic is much softer than conventional plastic catheters. It is nonirritating and nonreactive and can lie in the venous system for years without provoking phlebitis. The catheter is anchored by a suture at the point where it penetrates the vein so as to discourage inadvertent removal. The Broviac and Hickman catheters have a Teflon felt cuff affixed to the subcutaneous part of the catheter, which has obviated the need for suture fixation at the point where the catheter exits from the skin. These catheters are commonly tunneled around the rib cage to exit over the midsternum. Granulation tissue "grows into" the Teflon felt cuff to anchor the catheters in place. These catheters are now available with a double lumen so that, in selected patients, one lumen can be used for infusion of TPN and the other for venous sampling.

The entire system, including the tubing from the formula bottle to the Silastic catheter, is changed daily under aseptic conditions and must be maintained as a completely closed system. Under no circumstances should this venous line be violated for drawing blood,

administering other intravenous fluids, or determining central venous pressure. A small sterile dressing (Opsite or Tagaderm) covers the Silastic catheter where it exits from the skin. This dressing is changed three times weekly by specially trained nurses. The skin is defatted with acetone and cleaned with an appropriate antiseptic, and povidone-iodine (Betadine) ointment is placed over the exit site.

The formula is usually administered at a constant hourly rate over each 24-hour period. A gravity drip will suffice if monitored closely by skilled personnel, but an infusion pump is generally preferable. Nurses specially trained in TPN techniques can teach catheter care and infusion techniques to either the patient or his family to allow the patient to be discharged home when lengthy periods of nutritional support are anticipated. Under these circumstances, it is often possible to limit the nutritional infusions to the nocturnal hours so as to allow the patient greater freedom and activity during the waking hours of the day. Some patients have been managed at home with TPN successfully for years provided that proper catheter care is maintained.

Special Considerations of TPN

During the first few days of hyperosmolar intravenous feeding, amino acids and sugar are commonly lost in the urine, posing the threat of osmotic diuresis and dehydration. This problem is minimized by use of a half-strength TPN solution the first day, a three-fourths solution the second day, and then the full-strength TPN formula the third day. During this period of TPN initiation, frequent examinations of the urine for sugar may justify administration of exogenous insulin to prevent serious hyperglycemia and glycosuria. After several days of parenteral hyperalimentation, endogenous insulin production increases so that blood and urine glucose levels may be maintained within normal limits. By the same token, the hyperalimentation infusion should not be discontinued abruptly as hypoglycemia will ensue.

When TPN is first started, the body weight, fluid balance, serum electrolytes, and blood and urine glucose and serum osmolality are monitored daily. When

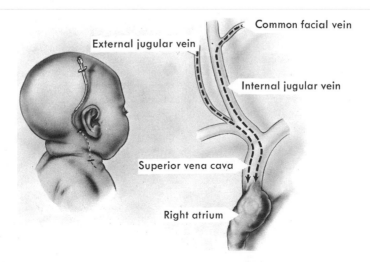

Fig. 7-2. Insertion of delivery-system catheter into external or internal jugular vein in infant.

the patient has stabilized on TPN, weekly checks of these parameters suffice for proper monitoring, except that urine glucose levels should be measured four times daily while therapy is initiated, and it is wise to make spot checks of urine glucose levels daily until therapy is discontinued. During TPN infusion the body is in an anabolic state, and potassium and phosphate requirements are often increased above maintenance needs. Potassium, like nitrogen, is incorporated intracellularly and usually is given in direct ratio to the amount of administered nitrogen (10 to 15 mEq/g of nitrogen).

As the patient recovers, oral feedings are begun and gradually increased as tolerated. TPN administration is reduced proportionately in a stepwise manner. As the patient approaches normal oral feedings, the TPN solution is diluted in concentration and gradually diminished in volume before being terminated.

Complications of TPN

Thrombosis around the catheter is a common complication of lengthy TPN administration and may be minimized by use of Silastic catheters and the addition of dilute heparin to the formula. Catheter misplacement and occult pneumothorax are avoided by x-ray or fluoroscopic evaluations carried out along with catheter placement.

Septicemia is unquestionably the most serious complication of TPN. It ultimately will occur when any foreign body, such as the TPN catheter, dwells in the vascular system for lengthy periods of time, especially in debilitated patients who frequently have other sites of infection associated with their surgical problem. However, the rate of infection is directly proportional to the care that is exercised during the initial catheter placement, the length of the subcutaneous tunneling of the catheter, and the subsequent day-to-day care of the catheter. With careful attention to these points, infection can be minimized. We have frequently had a single catheter in place for a period of several months without infection.

Ultimately, however, infection will occur with lengthy superior vena cava or inferior vena cava catheterization. Under these circumstances, sepsis often is caused by bizarre organisms such as fungi or yeast or by skin bacteria that are usually not considered to be pathogenic.

At the first sign of infection (unexplained temperature elevation, leukocytosis, hyperglycemia, or simply an unexpected deterioration in the patient's general condition) serial blood cultures are drawn; if these return positive, the TPN catheter is withdrawn and cultured. Whether changing the catheter over a guidewire is adequate therapy for TPN line sepsis is controversial. The patient's general condition is assessed carefully for possible infection elsewhere, and antibiotic therapy is directed by results of Gram stain and culture. After appropriate treatment of septicemia is under way, a catheter can be placed in another vein within 24 to 48 hours.

Metabolic complications, frequently seen during administration of TPN, necessitate changes in the formula or its rate of administration. These complications include azotemia, hypophosphatemia, trace metal deficiency, and carbon dioxide retention. Hepatobiliary problems may also arise during TPN therapy. Fatty liver and cholestasis, manifested by elevated liver enzymes and serum bilirubin, may be corrected when one lowers the glucose content of the solution. Acalculous cholecystitis, presumably attributable to biliary stasis, has recently been recognized as a potential complication of long-term TPN administration in fasting patients. Recent studies suggest that biliary stasis may be minimized by administering patients either small amounts of oral fat or intravenous cholecystokinin daily, to stimulate gallbladder emptying.

Peripheral Vein Hyperalimentation

Recently, solutions have been formulated that are low enough in tonicity (less than 600 mOsm/L) to allow their safe infusion into small peripheral veins without provoking phlebitis. Because of lower glucose concentration, large volumes must be given to satisfy nutritional needs. Alternatively, amino acids or amino acids and 5% dextrose may be given as "protein-sparing" therapy during periods of fasting that are predictably relatively short. The main advantage of peripheral hyperalimentation is to eliminate the major complications of thrombosis and sepsis of centrally placed catheters.

The basic solution used in peripheral hyperalimentation is 3% to 4.25% amino acids in a 10% dextrose solution. Fat emulsion is added to supply 50% to 60% of the nonprotein calories as fat. Electrolytes and vitamins are added to satisfy daily requirements. Dilute heparin may be added to discourage phlebitis. Obviously, larger volumes of this fluid must be infused to satisfy nutritional needs than the more hypertonic fluid that is used in central infusion. Renal failure, cardiac failure, and overhydration are indications to shift to a central infusion. Because of the need for frequent venipunctures, peripheral vein hyperalimentation is limited to the hospitalized patient.

Enteral Nutrition

If the patient's condition allows, enteral tube feeding is preferable to either peripheral or central nutrition for the following reasons: lower cost, fewer catheter-associated complications, hepatic and gastrointestinal "integrity" can be maintained better, and possibly the provision of greater resistance to intraabdominal infection. Enteral alimentation is indicated in patients who have an intact gastrointestinal tract but who are unable or unwilling to consume adequate nutrients; it is useful in patients with swallowing problems and those who have psychiatric inanition, in patients suffering oropharyngeal or esophageal disturbances or diseases, and in patients with burns or multiple trauma. Tube feedings may be administered through nasoduodenal tubes, gastrostomy tubes, or tubes placed transmurally into the jejunum during celiotomy.

Tube Feeding Formulas

Commercial diets vary widely in calorie density, osmolality, protein source, and cost. Patients with normal gastrointestinal tracts can utilize meal replacement formulas that consist of casein or soy protein isolates, oligosaccharides, and long-chain fatty acids. Examples of these diets include Ensure, Osmolite, and Isocal.

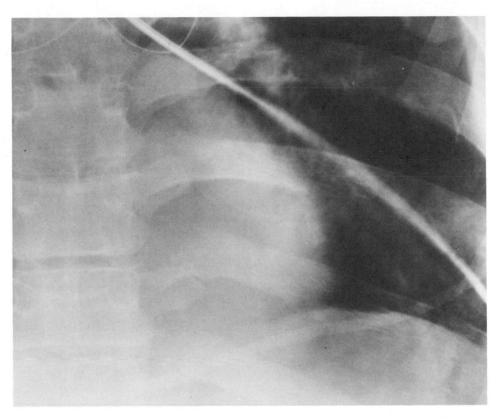

Fig. 7-3. Spot film taken to check placement of radiopaque feeding tube. Patient was asymptomatic, even though feeding tube traverses left lower lobe bronchus. Had feedings been given, a pulmonary disaster would have ensued.

Patients with short bowel syndromes, selective malabsorption, or fistulas often require elemental diets. These contain crystalline amino acids or protein hydrolysates, glucose, oligosaccharides, and medium-chain triglycerides, and therefore need minimal digestion. Because of their rich carbohydrate content, these diets are generally higher in osmolality. Examples of elemental formulas include Vivonex and Vital.

Techniques of Enteral Feeding

Feedings administered through nasogastric tubes are often complicated by gastroesophageal reflux and aspiration. Silastic tubes of 7 to 9 Fr have recently been introduced which bear a mercury-weighted tip; these tubes can be passed transnasally into the distal duodenum for drip feeding into the small bowel. Passage of these flexible tubes into the stomach may be facilitated by a guidewire. With the patient positioned on his right side, gravity and peristalsis will commonly propel the tube through the pylorus and around the duodenum. If the tube does not pass spontaneously, metoclopramide may be given to stimulate gastric emptying, or the tube can be manipulated through the pylorus and into the duodenum under fluoroscopic control.

If the need for enteral nutritional support is recognized at laparotomy, a standard or needle catheter jejunostomy tube may be inserted at that time. Feedings can generally be started within 48 to 72 hours postop-

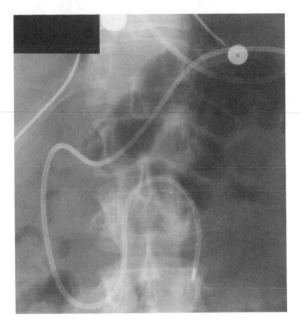

Fig. 7-4. Plain abdominal roentgenogram showing correct position of radiopaque feeding tube. Tube has a single loop in stomach and then traverses duodenal C-loop; mercury-weighted tip of tube lies in jejunum just beyond ligament of Treitz.

eratively, after the injection of water-soluble contrast material has verified correct catheter placement.

It is mandatory to verify tube position every time a feeding tube is passed. Small tubes may be inadvertently passed into the bronchus without triggering respiratory symptoms (Fig. 7-3), and the simple auscultation of injected air may be misleading. Tube position can be verified by plain films or fluoroscopy (Fig. 7-4) or by aspiration of gastric contents and bile.

Bolus feedings can be given directly into the stomach; however, when the feedings are administered into the duodenum or jejunum, continuous infusions controlled by pumps are desirable. Half-strength feedings are initiated at 50 ml/hour in adults, with 25 ml/hour increases every 8 hours until the volume goal is achieved. The solution strength is then gradually increased to meet calorie requirements.

Complications of Enteral Feedings

Metabolic complications of tube feedings are similar to those seen with TPN and mandate intensive glucose, electrolyte, and metabolic screening, particularly early in therapy. Mechanical problems include nasopharyngeal irritation, tube displacement, and aspiration. Gastrointestinal disturbances that are related to tube feedings include cramping, distension, and diarrhea and are the most common complications of enteral nutrition. The strength or infusion rate of the solution should be decreased, and the possibility of lactose intolerance must be considered.

CONCLUSION

Parenteral hyperalimentation, whether infused into a peripheral or central vein, is a very useful and sometimes life-saving technique to prevent or treat serious malnutrition in patients whose medical or surgical illness precludes enteral feedings. Tube feeding can often be used in patients with intact gastrointestinal tracts who are unable or unwilling to consume adequate nutrients. When adequate nutrients are provided by any of these modalities, the following objective evidence of nutritional improvement will occur: weight gain, prompt wound healing, closure of intestinal fistulas, reversal of severe inflammatory gastrointestinal disorders and improvement in serum albumin concentration. Many patients enjoy a general feeling of well-being. It is no longer necessary for a patient to starve simply because he temporarily is unable to eat.

8

Preoperative Care

Edward Bartle

The Patient
The Disease
The Treatment

Judging precisely which patient will survive, or succumb to, any specific operation for a disease, or diseases, is impossible. The many obvious variables such as age, seriousness of the primary disease, and coexisting diseases, account for the intangible nature of risk in any operation. Healthy, good-risk patients have died after simple operations, and aged, poor-risk patients have eased through procedures of astonishing magnitude. Therefore estimation of surgical risk is at best an educated guess based on experience. When asked to guarantee an operation (and this happens not infrequently), the experienced surgeon refuses to guarantee anything but his professional concern and competence. Sound surgical judgment, nevertheless, requires an estimation of surgical risk, especially in difficult cases when surgical risk must be cautiously weighed against any expected benefit from the operation. Surgical risk involves three main elements—the patient, the disease, and the treatment:

The patient + The disease + The treatment =
Surgical risk

THE PATIENT
Age

Infant prematurity and extreme old age are associated with increased operative risk. Little difference is seen, however, in operative mortality in the third decade as compared to the eighth decade for *brief procedures* that disturb physiological functions minimally, such as thyroidectomy or hernia repair; with operations of greater magnitude, involving increased physiological stress, the mortality is substantially greater in older patients. The mortality of combined abdominoperineal resection, for example, rises strikingly with age.

Heart

"A man is as old as his arteries," according to an old adage. We could add, "especially his coronary and cerebral arteries." For example, more than half of the patients who survive major arterial reconstructions (femoroiliac, internal carotid) and who have diabetes or coronary disease die within 5 years after these procedures, most from myocardial infarction.

In addition to recent myocardial infarction (less than 6 months) Goldman lists eight other factors that increase life-threatening cardiac complications in the postoperative period:

1. An S_3 gallop or distended jugular veins prior to operation
2. Myocardial infarction in the preceding 6 months
3. Rhythm other than sinus or premature atrial contractions on the preoperative electrocardiogram
4. More than five premature ventricular contractions per minute at any time before operation
5. An intraperitoneal, intrathoracic, or aortic operation
6. Age greater than 70 years
7. Important valvular aortic stenosis
8. An emergency operation
9. Poor general condition

The New York Heart Association ranks patients with cardiac symptoms from Class I (no symptoms) to Class IV (symptoms at rest). More than half of the deaths come from within Class IV.

When life-threatening disease arises in a patient with serious cardiac disease, even a few hours of intensive cardiac care—to control hypertension, arrhythmias, or heart failure—can increase survival.

The risk of venous thrombosis and pulmonary embolism, which are more common in patients with chronic heart disease, may be decreased by low-dose heparin (5,000 units subcutaneously every 12 hours). Many believe that this prophylactic therapy lowers mortality, especially in older persons.

Lungs

Pulmonary dysfunctions—inability to move air in and out of the lungs, to clear the bronchial tree by coughing, and to perfuse the lungs—often underlie postoperative pulmonary complications. Heavy cigarette smoking is often a precedent cause. We can anticipate pulmonary problems by asking simple clinical questions. How many flights of stairs can the patient climb? How many blocks can he walk without dyspnea? Can he comfortably carry out routine tasks? If normal exertion prompts shortness of breath, pulmonary ventilation tests (vital capacity, forced expiratory volume in 1 second) and arterial blood gases, before and during exercise, will help quantitate the deficit and indicate the urgency for postoperative respiratory support.

Kidneys

Chronic renal failure increases operative risk. A useful screening test for renal function is serum and urine creatinine levels. Urine creatinine concentrations should exceed by 10-fold the normal serum levels (<1.6 mg/dl). Meticulous attention to fluid and electrolyte replacement can prevent problems in patients with compromised renal function. Dialysis (peritoneal or he-

modialysis) should precede all elective operations in patients with chronic renal disease and elevated blood urea nitrogen (BUN) and creatinine levels.

Liver

Jaundice and ascites usually indicate severe liver disease. Unremitting, progressive jaundice signals a need for urgent remedial operation for the jaundice, if the jaundice is "surgical." A negative history for jaundice and normal serum bilirubin, proteins, alkaline phosphatase, transaminases, and prothrombin time usually indicate an adequate liver. Abnormalities in any of these tests should indicate the need for further investigation of liver functions. The type of liver disease will often influence the choice of anesthetic.

Blood

A diffuse organ, the blood and blood-forming tissues can be the limiting element in any surgical procedure. Anemia, with fewer red cells to carry oxygen, lowers oxygen delivery to tissues. Clinical and experimental studies show that a hematocrit of 30% will provide adequate oxygen transportation during surgical procedures. (However, it must fall to 7%, a level that barely sustains life, before wound healing is substantially impaired.) Platelet activity, essential for blood clotting, depends on platelet counts above 50,000/ml (normal values are 150,000 to 300,000/ml). Counts below this level require preoperative or intraoperative platelet transfusions, or both.

White blood cells and macrophages defend against infections. Leukemia, Hodgkin's disease, diabetes, acquired immune deficiency syndrome (AIDS), and immunosuppressive drugs will impair these first-line defenses. In addition, remember that general anesthesia agents and major operations interfere with the body's immune responses. Broad-spectrum antibiotics can help such patients withstand the additional stresses from surgical procedures.

Endocrine System

Endocrine factors are discussed in Chapters 14, 15 and 16. *Diabetes* coexists with many surgical problems. Uncontrolled diabetes, a distinct hazard, must be treated vigorously before induction of anesthesia.

Preoperative Treatment of Diabetes

Carbohydrate (minimum of 200 g) and insulin must be given together in order for the body to utilize the carbohydrate. In general, hypoglycemia (coma, convulsions) is more hazardous than hyperglycemia. Blood glucose levels of 200 to 250 mg/dl are innocuous in the absence of ketoacidosis. For moderate diabetes, the usual regimen includes the following:

1. Giving half the patient's usual insulin (NPH or lente) dose subcutaneously at the beginning of the operative procedure along with 1000 ml of 10% glucose in water
2. Repeating the same dose at the end of the procedure while infusing 10% glucose solution (total 2000 to 3000 ml in 24 hours)

For poorly controlled diabetes, start with 10 units of subcutaneous crystalline insulin every 6 hours and give

5 to 10 additional units for each 50 mg/dl increase in blood glucose above 200 mg/dl (or for each 3+ or 4+ urine glucose reaction).

Dehydration States

Varying states of simple desiccation, extracellular fluid loss, hemorrhage, or loss of specific electrolytes can appreciably affect operative risk. They are discussed at length in Chapter 3.

Nutritional Status

Chronic disease and subsequent malnutrition impede wound healing. Surgeons now have the tools, given adequate time, to improve a patient's nutritional status before operation. Parenteral hyperalimentation can provide proteins, amino acids, calories (glucose), vitamins, minerals, and fats—in short, total nutritional needs. Infusing these hypertonic solutions into high-flow veins (superior vena cava) has made this life-saving procedure possible.

Lacking time to reverse preoperative malnutrition in emergency situations, such as a perforated colon cancer, the surgeon begins hyperalimentation during the operation and continues it postoperatively (see Chapter 7).

Obesity is associated with renal disease, pulmonary problems, diabetes, hypertension, cerebrovascular diseases, and orthopedic problems. As a consequence, morbidly obese patients (100 pounds more than ideal weight) lose about 10 to 15 years of life expectancy. Because obesity increases operative time, this adds to the risk of septic, pulmonary, and vascular complications. Obese patients require brief operative procedures, intensive respiratory support, rapid mobilization, and sometimes antibiotics and heparin.

THE DISEASE

The variability of the physical status of patients parallels the wide range of diseases that may afflict them. The nature of the disease (malignant or benign, infected or sterile), the physiological disturbances it causes, the site, and the length of time the disease has been present are all important factors that affect surgical risk.

With critical disorders (cancers or diseases causing exsanguinating hemorrhage), consideration of surgical risk becomes a clear, hard question of life or death. When the alternative to operative treatment is so obvious, most surgeons (and patients) would choose an operation with even the slight probability of saving life as the hoped for reward.

Malignant Versus Benign Disease

Operations on specific organs are, by and large, more hazardous for malignant diseases than for benign diseases. A gastric operation for cancer, for example, carries a higher mortality than one for benign gastric ulcer. Operations for thyroid nodules are less hazardous than those for thyroid cancer.

Septic Versus Sterile Disease

Septic diseases are more complicated, with a higher mortality, than sterile or relatively sterile diseases are.

Perforated appendicitis has a higher mortality than early acute appendicitis. Septic cholecystitis is more often fatal than aseptic, uncomplicated cholecystitis.

Site of the Disease

The site of the disease is an important determinant of surgical risk. In descending order of operative risk, the sites are heart, thoracic esophagus, brain, rectum, colon, stomach, and lung. The nature and extent of the disease is, of course, an important factor in each site.

Time Element

The longer the patient has had the disease, the poorer the operative risk. For example, the complication rate from a septic source (e.g., a perforated appendix) varies directly with the time interval between perforation and treatment. Debilitating effects from cancer that has lurked undetected for long periods also increase surgical risk.

THE TREATMENT

Treatment strongly influences both the *patient* and the *disease*. This is the only one of the three factors of surgical risk over which the surgeon has much control. Knowledge of the patient's overall status and the disease that afflicts him is the key to successful management. After assessing the patient and the disease as completely as possible, the surgeon plans the operative treatment.

Magnitude of the Operation

After restoring the ill patient to as near normal condition as possible, the extent of the operation must be considered. One thought should be clearly in mind: *surgical risk increases with the magnitude of the procedure.* Blood loss, trauma to the patient, and operating time are all cofactors. Replacement of an intracardiac valve is obviously more hazardous than the comparatively simple mitral valvulotomy. Cholecystostomy is a shorter, simpler, and safer procedure than cholecystectomy for acute cholecystitis. A wide variety of other examples illustrate the importance of surgical judgment. In choosing among the possible therapeutic options, the surgeon must weigh this critical factor of surgical magnitude carefully. In most instances decisions are relatively easy; in a few they are immensely difficult.

An additional important but largely unassessable factor is the skill of the surgeon and the team. What can be performed expeditiously with a well-trained team in a modern hospital may, unfortunately, become catastrophic under less favorable conditions

Postoperative Care

The quality of postoperative care is another important, yet variable, factor in operative risk. Experienced nurses in intensive care units have reduced postoperative mortality more than any other factor. Their efficiency, skill, and dedication are more important than electronic monitors, suction and inhalation equipment, or any of the other mechanical devices that aid in the postoperative care of the patient. Their continued training is the responsibility of the surgeons who work with them.

Operative risk is an intangible yet invaluable and practical concept. The spectrum of variables inherent in the *patient,* the *disease,* and the *treatment* defies precise analysis. Eventually computers may help assess operative risk; at the present time valid statistical analyses of the many variables (to program a computer) exist only as research projects. Estimation of surgical risk must, as always, be based on experience, intuition, and a generous measure of common sense.

9

Anesthesia

Judith B. Dillman
John H. Tinker

Before the 1840s, "surgery" was limited to procedures that could be accomplished in seconds or minutes in concert with screams of agony from the patient. The development of anesthesia changed all this and is variously credited to Crawford Long's use of ether in 1842, or Horace Wells' 1845 report of nitrous oxide rendering the patient pain free but still moving on the table, or William Morton's use of ether in 1846 (under public scrutiny) to prevent both pain and movement. Diethyl ether gained early supremacy in the United States, whereas chloroform became popular in Europe. Anesthesia was "discovered" many years before hypodermic needles, electrocardiography, blood pressure measurement (in man), and intravenous fluid therapy. Regional anesthesia developed with use of cocaine during the 1880s and procaine before 1910. Cyclopropane (1929) and thiopental (1935) were both in widespread use before penicillin was. In the mid-1950s, halothane gained worldwide acceptance because of potency, ease of administration, and nonflammability. It was followed by several other nonflammable fluorocarbon potent volatile agents, plus new potent narcotics and other injectables. Now anesthetics are administered to over 20 million Americans yearly.

The objectives of surgical anesthesia are fourfold: (1) to prevent perception of pain, (2) to obliterate awareness of surroundings (unless regional anesthesia is employed), (3) to provide muscle relaxation if needed, and (4) to obtund untoward autonomic reflexes. Clearly anesthesia satisfying these requirements is not sleep! The state we call anesthesia must be a subtle set of alterations of physiologic function. It must be readily reversible: it must not constitute significant physiologic or pharmacologic trespass. Xenon, a noble gas, that does not enter into conventional chemical reactions, is an anesthetic. Anesthesia, thus, does not necessarily have to be attributable to a drug binding to a specific receptor. Removal of pain, awareness, muscle tone, and many protective reflexes places squarely on the anesthesiologist the responsibility of maintaining safe circulation, respiration, metabolism, and other functions. Producing anesthesia in a patient is not difficult. Keeping that now helpless patient safe while providing adequate conditions to permit effective and expeditious surgery is another matter.

There is a strange conundrum that because anesthesia is seldom if ever directly therapeutic, it must necessarily be inherently *safe,* and that any and all untoward outcomes must, of necessity, be caused by poor practice. Not so. Anesthetics and accompanying adjuvants are potent and dangerous drugs; many of their actions and interactions are neither explored nor explained. Why such safety should be demanded of these agents and techniques is a mystery, since all other drugs and procedures are accepted to have risk-benefit ratios. Patients who would not have been considered viable candidates just a few years ago today are presented for major operations. They are often taking a variety of other potent drugs and have complex fluid or electrolyte disturbances, metabolic derangements, and multiple organ failure. Some form of "anesthetic" can almost always be given to even the most moribund patient, but always there is a price.

PHYSIOLOGIC AND TOXIC DERANGEMENTS DURING ANESTHESIA
Ventilatory and Respiratory Effects

Ventilation is gas exchange, whereas respiration is adequacy of oxygen delivery to tissues. The anesthetist must often take over, control, and monitor both. The *airway,* glibly mentioned as important in cardiopulmonary resuscitation courses, becomes crucial to the anesthesiologist. Beginners are amazed and dismayed at (1) how rapidly the patient loses ability to maintain his or her airway and (2) how difficult it can be to obtain and maintain an unobstructed safe airway. General anesthesia results in loss of muscle tone to produce nearly complete inspiratory obstruction (snoring is but a hint). Various maneuvers, such as tilting the head backward, lifting the mandible anteriorly, placing artificial oral and nasopharyngeal airways, adding positive pressure to inspired gases, and inserting an endotracheal tube are all airway maintenance and protection procedures. Securing the airway and providing adequate ventilation in a patient who has a bronchopleurocutaneous fistula, wherein positive pressure ventilation causes most of the gas to take the path of least resistance through the fistula is an extreme example, but it does serve to point out the range of difficulties with the airway that can be encountered during anesthesia.

Just ventilating the lungs may indeed adequately remove carbon dioxide from the blood, but it does not necessarily assure adequate oxygenation of the blood or tissue delivery thereof. During anesthesia, especially when muscle paralysis is added (with neuromuscular blocking agents), gradual increases often occur in regional pulmonary ventilation-perfusion mismatch, especially in patients with diseased lungs. This can result in decline, sometimes to alarmingly low levels, in arterial oxygen partial pressure, unless careful monitoring is performed. Precise mechanisms causing this problem are not known, but there often (not necessarily) is a gradual decrease in lung functional residual capacity (FRC), sometimes to the point where airway closure ("closing capacity") may occur during tidal breathing. Maintaining a clear airway is not all that is necessary to assure adequate tissue oxygen delivery during anesthesia.

Cardiovascular Effects

With the exception of some narcotics, anesthetics are *all direct myocardial depressants.* This includes agents like ketamine and cyclopropane, which also excite the sympathetic nervous system (and may raise the blood pressure). An agent like ketamine, which usually results in sympathetic activation, may still produce myocardial depression in a patient whose cardiac muscle has been depleted of endogenous catecholamines (as in severe myocardial failure). Certain narcotics, notably fentanyl, are not direct myocardial depressants, though they are not complete anesthetics either. Other narcotics, such as meperidine *are* myocardial depressants. Is this direct myocardial depression necessarily harmful? Not always. Judicious myocardial depression may decrease cardiac oxygen demand and be protective if there is severe coronary artery disease. If myocardial depression and the peripheral vasodilation that usually accompanies it are carried too far, the resultant hypotension may compromise pressure-dependent areas in myocardium or brain and produce infarction. Furthermore, peripheral vasodilation may trigger undesirable reflex tachycardia—again compromising a diastolic time-dependent coronary artery-diseased heart.

Not only do anesthetics cause varying degrees of myocardial depression and arteriolar vasodilation, but also there is often venodilation and decreased venous return. All these effects may combine to produce hypotension. Dysrhythmias may occur from direct anesthetic-catecholamine interaction (usually seen with halothane), or from insufficient sympathoadrenal suppression.

Circulatory *hyperdynamism* may also occur, from anesthetic levels that are insufficient to counteract the effects of sudden or gradual surgical stimulation. The resultant hypertension or tachycardia may result in sufficient myocardial regional oxygen supply and demand imbalances to produce ischemia or infarction. Clearly, monitoring and controlling of hemodynamics play a major role in anesthesia management.

Central Nervous System Effects

Anesthesia itself implies suppression of at least some activity in the central nervous system (CNS), whether it is by blocking major nerve trunks or spinal cord (via spinal or epidural anesthesia) or the entire CNS. The student should clearly understand that "anesthesia" is *not sleep* but just as clearly that it is *not coma.* Such selective depression of the CNS must preserve vital integrity, namely, basal (often medullary) functions. All modern potent anesthetics can be fatal in high enough concentrations simply by causing massive CNS depression. Anesthetics in reasonable concentrations do spare vital CNS functions while suppressing awareness (cortical function). The reverse corollary to this is that sympathetic stimulation during surgical maneuvers often *will* get through; that is, the CNS is not sufficiently depressed to prevent some activation of the sympathetic system. This results often in "roller coaster" blood pressure, heart rate, and systemic vascular resistance during actual anesthesia and operation, and this effect is a continual problem for anesthesiologists. The student should realize that many of these major stimuli do "get through." Hypnosis studies have even shown that voices and other happenings in the operating room are getting through also, at least at a subconscious level. Actual conscious subsequent recall of events during anesthesia has concerned anesthesiologists who care for critically ill patients for whom high concentrations of anesthetics might prove too depressant to compromised cardiovascular systems. Another group of patients in whom "too-light" anesthesia may result in awareness are pregnant patients, in whom the clinical objective is to administer sufficient anesthesia to obliterate maternal awareness without dangerously depressing the delivered infant. Awareness under anesthesia can be a problem, for example, during emergency cesarean section.

Renal Effects

If anesthesia decreases arterial blood pressure, renal blood flow will decrease, usually proportionally. The formerly used anesthetic methoxyflurane underwent approximately 50% metabolic degradation. The most frequent by-product of that agent, inorganic fluoride, occasionally caused nephrotoxicity, which resulted in a form of high-output renal failure. The only modern anesthetic metabolized into appreciable inorganic fluoride is enflurane. Careful studies in animals and in patients with mild to moderate renal failure have shown that fluoride levels do not increase sufficiently to produce nephrotoxicity with enflurane.

Another side of the renal effect question comes when the anesthesiologist tries to protect the kidney against postoperative acute renal failure. These situations often occur during major vascular surgery, whether aortic cross clamping occurs above or below the renal arteries. Which anesthetic technique is best to optimize renal protection is not known. Whether to administer loop or osmotic diuretics before the expected renal insult is also controversial. Anesthesiologists often give a "prophylactic" dose of mannitol before aortic cross clamp, but valid, controlled outcome studies are not available. Whether any particular rate of urine formation is any more protective against postoperative renal failure than any other is not known. Postoperative renal failure is a devastating, often fatal complication to which a satisfactory solution has not yet been found.

Hepatic Effects

Chloroform, first used as an anesthetic in 1847, is clearly a hepatic toxin. When halothane was introduced in 1956, anesthesiologists were concerned that it might also be hepatotoxic because its chemical structure is similar, as shown below:

$$F-\overset{\overset{\displaystyle F}{|}}{\underset{\underset{\displaystyle F}{|}}{C}}-\overset{\overset{\displaystyle Cl}{|}}{\underset{\underset{\displaystyle Br}{|}}{CH}}$$

Halothane

Halothane is a potent, nonflammable, extremely clinically useful anesthetic. It became immensely popular and has been given to millions upon millions of patients throughout the world. Reports of rare but devastating fatal postoperative hepatic necrosis began to appear shortly after the introduction of halothane. This prompted the massive National Halothane Study in 1961. In that study, halothane was clearly the safest anesthetic then in use, but there *were* several unexplained cases of massive hepatic necrosis after halothane anesthesia. Most experts today do believe there is a clinical entity called "halothane hepatitis." Unfortunately, today some internists (and laywers) blame halothane for many (most?) postoperative hepatic difficulties despite the fact that there is absolutely no way in which "halothane hepatitis" can be distinguished pathologically from other causes of centrilobular hepatic necrosis. Indeed, numerous cases of "halothane hepatitis" have been "diagnosed" despite the record-proved fact that the patient in question did not receive halothane at all!

Can we make sense out of all this? There are animal models (rats) wherein postanesthesia hepatic centrilobular necrosis can be reproducibly obtained. With halothane as the anesthetic, this model requires all of the following together: (1) hepatic microsomal mixed function oxidase (cytochrome P_{450}) *induction,* with either barbiturates or polychlorinated biphenyl (PCB), (2) a *hypoxic* gas mixture of less than 14% oxygen, and (3) halothane in low doses, approximately 0.5%. The situation gets complicated, however, by the fact that both enflurane and isoflurane (the two other volatile anesthetics in use today) can be substituted for halothane in the above model and hepatic centrilobular necrosis still results. With the other two anesthetics, lower oxygen levels (about 10%), higher anesthetic dosages (1.5% to 2%), and *fasted* (24-hour) animals are required. Probably, postanesthesia hepatic necrosis is real and is related to a complex series of events, including diminution of oxygen delivery to the liver. It is likely that the halothane is somewhat more likely to be associated with this toxicity than either enflurane or isofluorane is, but the syndrome is rare. There *are* situations wherein halothane is a nearly ideal choice, for reasons that are beyond the scope of this chapter. Halothane should not disappear from the anesthesiologists' armamentarium. Clearly, hepatic effects of general anesthetics are important, controversial, and interesting. Surgical stress itself affects liver function in many ways discussed in other chapters.

HOW ANESTHESIA IS PRODUCED

General anesthesia is often (but not necessarily) *induced* with a rapidly acting intravenously administered drug, such as sodium thiopental, ketamine, midazolam, or sodium methohexital. The uptake and distribution characteristics of these drugs make them difficult to use, continuously or intermittently, to *maintain* lengthy anesthesia. A "sleep dose" of sodium thiopental, for example, may wear off in approximately 17 minutes. It is not metabolized or eliminated in that short period; instead, a *redistribution* of the agent away from the brain occurs. A significant percentage of the administered dose originally lodges in brain tissue simply because about 15% of the resting cardiac output goes to that organ. The fatty tissues elsewhere, though poorly perfused, constitute a vast reservoir into which these highly lipophilic drugs will eventually be redistributed. Thus the patient awakens after a "sleep dose" of thiopental because of redistribution. *Maintenance* of general anesthesia may be achieved with gaseous or volatile agents whose concentrations in blood and brain can normally be rapidly changed via the *lungs*.

Therefore general anesthesia often is *induced* with a rapidly acting intravenous agent but then *maintained* with volatile or gaseous anesthetics. Today, the term "volatile" applies to a liquid that is vaporized. Halothane, enflurane, and isoflurane are the three such agents currently in use. "Gaseous" applies to nitrous oxide, in use since 1845. Nitrous oxide is relatively impotent, requiring high concentrations; consequently, it almost always is considered an adjunct to an anesthetic technique employing other agents. For example, if nitrous oxide is used as a supplement to volatile agent anesthesia, the procedure is generally considered to be volatile agent–based anesthesia. If, by contrast, nitrous oxide is used to supplement intravenous agents, including narcotics such as morphine or fentanyl, or hypnotics such as diazepam or barbiturates, the anesthesia is said to be a *balanced* type.

During general anesthesia, *muscle relaxation* may be desirable for surgical exposure and manipulation during some procedures, such as intraabdominal operations. Relaxation formerly was provided by administration of high concentrations of agents such as diethyl ether. These "deep" anesthetics carried risks of severe circulatory and respiratory depression. Since the advent of specific neuromuscular blocking drugs, beginning with curare in 1942, "lighter" planes of anesthesia could be maintained with the inhaled anesthetic while muscle relaxation was provided by the specific intravenous agent, undoubtedly rendering them safer. Certainly not all general anesthetics require addition of muscle relaxants.

Regional anesthesia offers a wide range of choices. Many believe that regional anesthesia is "less" anesthesia and, therefore, inherently safer. There is little evidence that this is true. A major regional anesthetic might very well result in severe hypotension, for example. On the other hand, an axillary block of the upper extremity may be an ideal choice for a patient with a full stomach who requires emergency hand surgery. Spinal (intrathecal drug injection) or epidural (local anesthetic injected into the epidural space) are commonly chosen to try to lessen the amount of anesthetic drug absorbed by the fetus during labor or delivery. Herniorrhaphy is well performed under the nearly cadaveric abdominal muscle relaxation that results from spinal anesthesia.

Many times, a combination of regional and general anesthesia seems reasonable. For instance, for a cholecystectomy, it is possible to first perform bilateral intercostal nerve blocks at T6 through T12, administer a light general anesthetic by intravenous induction, and then maintain it with nitrous oxide plus narcotic supplementation, with ventilation controlled through an endotracheal tube. There are as many potential nerve blocks as there are points at which nerves can be reasonably approached with local anesthetics.

Patient acceptance of regional anesthesia is not always enthusiastic. Patients who object to being "awake" often can be given a light general anesthetic in addition to the regional block. Patients who believe friends or relatives have been injured by regional anesthesia are not likely to be impressed with the mathematics of event psychology (the fact that random occurrences associated with—before or after—a significant event are anecdotally likely to be causally associated with it). Patients should never be coerced into accepting either an anesthesiologist's or a surgeon's preconceived ideas about the ideal anesthetic for a particular procedure.

The idea that the sickest patients should get regional anesthesia is also not necessarily logical. General anesthesia may result in less hypotension and better oxygenation, carbon dioxide elimination, and airway control. On the other hand, a small dose of local anesthetic, deposited in the subarachnoid space, does provide a large area of superb surgical anesthesia, with little drug to be metabolized or excreted. Regional anesthesia has perhaps received best acceptance during labor and delivery because of the objective of avoiding fetal depression.

CLINICAL ANESTHESIA MANAGEMENT
Preoperative Evaluation

Anesthesia management is complex *medical* care. A thorough evaluation of the patient before anesthesia is mandatory. This must include detailed knowledge of the patient's medical history, including details of prior cardiac and cerebrovascular events, specific systemic disease, drug reactions, current drug therapies, difficulties with prior anesthetics, and all other relevant vital organ problems. Specific areas of further interest include potential for difficult airway management, problems with dentition, neck and jaw ranges of motion, and potential difficulties in obtaining vascular access.

In addition to a medical work-up, plus determining that the patient's ongoing medical diseases or problems are in optimal control, plus the specific anesthesia-related problems mentioned above, the preoperative visit serves the additional extremely useful purpose of allaying patient fear and uncertainty to a considerably greater degree than any pharmacologic premedicant. Patient and family questions can be answered, and unknowns are replaced by expectancies. Media publicity about risks associated with anesthesia have increased public awareness to the point where careful explanations and achievement of trust are often demanded by the patient before informed consent is given to induce anesthesia and perform surgery. The reasonably foreseeable risks associated with the anesthetic, as well as the risks of any invasive monitoring which the anesthesiologist chooses to employ, need to be explained to the patient (or in the case of a minor child, to the parent or legal guardian) and his understanding and agreement must be documented in the medical record.

Preoperative preparation includes a suitable nothing-by-mouth (NPO) period (not necessarily "NPO past-midnight") to try to attain gastric emptying. Premedication may include a drying agent (atropine or scopolamine), an analgesic (morphine, meperidine), and a sedative (diazepam, lorazepam, barbiturate). The sedatives should be given by mouth with a sip of water whenever possible. Premedication is difficult at best. Heavy sedation, with airway and respiratory compromise resulting in hypercarbia may severely increase intracranial pressure in patients with space-occupying intracranial lesions. Too-light premedication plus anxiety may trigger an angina episode indistinguishable (without work-up) from a beginning myocardial infarction. No combination or recipe works well all the time. Personal contact and trust are often most important.

Selection of Monitoring

The anesthesiologist must plan carefully the degree to which the patient's physiologic responses to anesthesia and surgery are to be monitored. Few patients today are, or should be, anesthetized without continuous monitoring of at least one lead of the electrocardiogram. Ventilation and circulation are continuously monitored by the anesthesiologist through a variety of means ranging from simple precordial or esophageal stethoscope auscultation of heart tones and breath sounds to more sophisticated technologies of continuously monitoring end-tidal carbon dioxide levels and hemoglobin oxygen saturation via pulse oximetry. Blood pressure is monitored by cuff, automated oscillometry, or invasive arterial catheter through a strain gauge transducer, depending on the degree to which major blood pressure fluctuations are expected *plus* a careful estimate as to whether such fluctuations will likely be dangerous to that particular patient.

Estimates of *right* ventricular preload by central venous pressures give some idea of dynamic blood volume status in patients with healthy hearts undergoing procedures wherein major ($\pm$ 15%) blood loss is expected or has occurred. Thermistor-equipped flow-directed pulmonary artery catheters permit measurement of cardiac output, calculation of systemic and pulmonary vascular resistances, and estimates (by use of pulmonary artery wedge pressures) of *left* ventricular preload. Such invasive, and potentially hazardous, monitoring equipment is reserved for *patients undergoing major surgery in whom myocardial dysfunction is known to exist or is suspected*. The pulmonary artery catheter has been controversial because it is expensive, complex, and potentially hazardous. It is not proper to use it always for certain procedures and never for others, without taking into account the degree of the patient's myocardial dysfunction. It is extremely useful during anesthesia and well into the critical postoperative period.

The *brain* can be monitored by an electroencephalograph, computerized EEG analysis, somatosensory cortical evoked potentials, and verbal contact during regional anesthesia. EEG monitoring is often performed during carotid endarterectomy. Evoked potential monitoring may find use as a monitor of spinal cord integrity during scoliosis repair and thoracic aortic aneurysmectomy.

Pulmonary function monitoring consists in constant observation for color changes, arterial and mixed venous blood gases, and various devices to guard against delivery of hypoxic gas mixtures or ventilator failure. Special pulmonary artery catheters with fiberoptic infrared sensors are available for detection of changes in mixed venous oxygen saturation.

Renal function monitoring usually consists in measuring urine output, but more sophistication can be lent by measurement of urinary electrolytes or osmolarity, or both. *Liver function* monitoring generally is not done during anesthesia. *Endocrine function* monitoring may be especially important in diabetic patients (serial blood glucoses). *Coagulation* monitoring during operation can range from simple activated coagulation times to all-out efforts by sophisticated coagulation laboratories. Electrolyte disturbances of all types can occur during anesthesia, and Na^+, K^+, ionized Ca^{++} plus serum osmolarity can all be easily measured.

Conduct of the Anesthesia

The patient generally is not anesthetized outside the operating room, though induction rooms are used for regional anesthesia and induction of general anesthesia in pediatric patients in some institutions. Once the patient is in the operating room, induction by inhalation, intravenous agents, or regional anesthesia is accomplished after planned monitors have been attached and validated. It is not always necessary to have an intravenous catheter established for a short minor procedure in a healthy patient (e.g., myringotomy in a healthy NPO 5-year-old child).

The decision to maintain the airway using a mask, an oral or nasal airway, endotracheal tube, or tracheostomy is complex and outside the scope of this chapter. Every "long" case does not necessarily mandate an endotracheal tube. Anesthesia, whether regional or general, *should never be performed without the presence of someone experienced in airway management,* someone who can obtain and maintain airway patency throughout the procedure. A deadly trap, for example, is to induce local or regional anesthesia in a situation where airway maintenance is dubious or no one present is sufficiently skilled. Such a patient might undergo collapse for various reasons and need immediate airway maintenance by someone highly skilled. The student's respect for the difficulty of airway maintenance will grow, no matter what field he or she chooses.

Special Techniques

In addition to special monitoring, several special techniques are available to facilitate anesthesia or surgery. *Deep hypothermia* with subsequent deliberate circulatory arrest during certain cardiac and cerebral operations requires forethought and skill. *Deliberate arterial hypotension,* achieved by direct vasodilation or other ways may reduce blood loss, provide better exposure of tumor margins, or reduce risk of transfusion hepatitis. *Deliberate hypertension* is often employed during carotid endarterectomy. *Deliberate hyperthermia* for cancer treatment requires numerous anesthesia skills. *Autotransfusion* of shed blood, often after centrifugal "washing," is now commonplace. Endotracheal *jet ventilation* can facilitate laser excision of laryngeal lesions. *High-frequency ventilation* may be useful in surgery for bronchopleural fistulas. Intraaortic *balloon counterpulsation, left ventricular assist devices,* and *optimal pacing* are all employed in cardiac surgery.

Subspecialty Anesthesia

Cardiovascular, neurosurgical, pediatric, obstetric, orthopedic, and other surgical specialties have developed highly technical procedures. Anesthesiologists have also specialized in trying to provide optimal management of these special cases. Just a few examples should suffice. The coronary artery bypass operation is often relatively straightforward, but a difficult emergence from bypass in a patient with severe ventricular dysfunction requires skills best (perhaps only) developed through frequent and extensive experience. Neurosurgical sitting-position craniotomies pose severe air embolism hazards, requiring Doppler monitoring and special treatment techniques. Operations on tiny infants may pose severe size-related metabolic or respiratory problems. The student should not be taken in by the "glamour" of these highly specialized situations. Anesthesia management of major abdominal surgery in a heavy smoker with cardiac disease may be a considerably greater challenge than a coronary artery bypass procedure.

Problems During Anesthesia

Arterial hypotension can occur suddenly and at life-threatening levels during anesthesia. Possible causes include anesthetic overdose, hypoxemia, major blood loss, surgical positioning, retractor obstruction of venous return, myocardial ischemia or cardiac arrhythmias or both, various drug-to-drug interactions, anaphylaxis, and other drug or transfusion reactions. The anesthesiologist often does not have the luxury of an extensive work-up but must make rapid therapy decisions, objectively evaluate the ongoing results of those decisions, and be willing to alter therapy if subsequent events indicate.

Problems with *airway management* are common. Examples include inadvertent disconnection of the breathing circuit, secretions plugging the endotracheal tube, and endobronchial intubation and tube cuff over-inflation. Again, diagnosis and therapy must be prompt, for these are potentially humbling and disastrous experiences.

In addition to problems with circulation and respiration, the anesthesiologist must try to prevent pressure injuries, electrocautery ground return plate burns, dental damage, peripheral nerve injuries from malpositioning of extremities, and injuries to the eyes, ears, and vocal cords.

"Vigilance" is an easy word to write in a chapter such as this, and is, with good reason, the official motto of the American Society of Anesthesiologists. It implies discipline and dedication. The minute-to-minute care during anesthesia and surgery is one of the few times any physician personally renders such continuous care. Improper drug administration, technical maneuvers, and incorrect therapies are often as immediately apparent as the results of poor surgical technique.

Postoperative and Intensive Care

The period during which patients recover from anesthesia is one of rapid fluctuations in vital signs and mental status and may therefore be quite hazardous. Recovery room nursing is a recognized subspecialty of that profession, with good reason. Rapid assessment of deteriorating neurological function in a postoperative neurosurgical patient may, for example, signal the need for immediate reoperation. Assessments of circulation, respiration, renal status, and neurologic status are crucial. Outpatients who have undergone general or major regional anesthesia need informed critical evaluation to determine their ability to leave the hospital. In large hospitals, the recovery room is a fast-changing, sometimes chaotic-looking place. Professionalism must reign if safe anesthesia and surgery are to be carried out.

Critically ill postoperative patients who will require extended care are often transferred directly to the surgical intensive care unit from the operating room. Here, all manner of difficult acute and chronic medical and surgical problems must be managed. Nursing personnel again bear the brunt of the front-line action. Morale and organization have much to do with the success, or lack of it, of such a unit. Jurisdictional disputes among various physician specialists must be solved with professionalism in the patient's best interest. It is important for all to remember that these are critically ill patients, outcomes are not always going to be rosy, and occasionally treatments will fail. Physicians facing such failures must *deal effectively with their own anxieties and insecurities* regarding these difficult patients. Those insecurities must not be defended by arrogance, dogmatism, or arbitrary and capricious behavior. Successful care of these patients really does require a dedicated, professional *team* approach.

Involvement of anesthesiologists in intensive care activities is natural because of their expertise in ventilatory and circulatory support, airway management, and respiratory care. Critical care specialists now come from anesthesiology, pulmonary medicine and other areas of internal medicine, pediatrics, and surgery backgrounds. If these persons are to become true critical care experts, none must assume that their original backgrounds confer the requisite totality of expertise.

PAIN MANAGEMENT

Acute pain can prolong recovery from surgery by delaying ambulation and inhibiting good respiratory efforts in the postoperative patient. Many anesthesiologists utilize intrathecal or epidural narcotics after selected surgical procedures to eliminate or reduce pain for up to 24 hours following a single injection. The side effects of this form of narcotic therapy, namely nausea, pruritus, urinary retention, and late respiratory depression, have limited its general application.

Many patients have *chronic* pain syndromes of various sorts. Therapies such as repeated peripheral nerve blocks with local anesthetics, intrathecal or epidural steroid or narcotics, and even ablative therapy with nerve blockade using ethanol or phenol are sometimes successful. Many anesthesia departments have established or have participated in pain clinics. Sometimes these are multidisciplinary, with psychological, psychiatric, neurologic, and surgical support. These are difficult patients to help. They may be taking large dosages of numerous drugs, may be addicted, may have numerous secondary gains, and may be litigation prone. Nonetheless, many can be helped to return to gainful employment. Furthermore, in-hospital pain management services may provide better acute pain care. Pain therapy research is currently very active. Knowledge about these hitherto poorly understood disorders is burgeoning. Anesthesiologists have therapy to offer and are participating.

CONCLUSION

Anesthesiology has been said to be "hours of boredom and moments of sheer terror." Not true. Competent anesthetists are in tune with their patient's physiology. When perturbations occur, decisive, logical, previously thought out steps are taken to obtain a diagnosis, administer treatment, objectively evaluate results, and alter therapy accordingly. Anesthesiology is, in other words, the detailed, technical, and critical *practice of medicine*.

10

Postoperative Care

Richard D. Liechty

Complications may occur after almost any operation, regardless of its magnitude. Even simple, routine diagnostic procedures (with catheters or needles, drugs, or various contrast media) may cause complications and even death.

In the study of surgical complications, *anticipation* and *early recognition* keynote successful treatment. The majority of all postoperative complications are signaled by one of two signs: *fever* or *shock* (cardiovascular collapse). Pain and tenderness, so important preoperatively, are often masked by operative pain or suppressed by sedation, especially in the first few hours after operation. Because sedation dulls the patient's responses, the surgeon must develop exceptional sensitivity to the *signs* of postoperative complications. In this chapter we outline a general overview of postoperative complications and refer the reader to other chapters that discuss specific problems in detail.

PATTERN OF SURGICAL COMPLICATIONS
Chain Reaction

Fortunately, surgical complications usually appear singly, but all too often, especially in the older, debilitated patient, they occur as *chain reactions*—one complication begets another: Prolonged ileus requires gastrointestinal suction and intravenous feeding. The patient is shackled to his bed for prolonged periods by a tube in the nose and a needle in the arm. Thus the stage is set for thrombophlebitis from inactivity or for pneumonitis from irritation of the upper respiratory areas with sepsis. These secondary and tertiary complications are serious, and occasionally fatal. Any number and variety of chain reactions may arise, but they almost invariably begin with one complication. Anticipation and prevention of the initial complications can thwart the sinister chain reaction. Predisposing factors in surgical complications are discussed in Chapter 8.

RECOGNIZING SURGICAL COMPLICATIONS

Fever is the most common evidence of postoperative complications. *Cardiovascular collapse,* though less common, is more dramatic and emergent. Together these two signs forecast at least 90% of postoperative complications. Since early recognition is so important, we will discuss complications in association with these two signs that tell us something is wrong.

Fever

Mild transient fevers appear after most operations from tissue necrosis, hematoma, or cauterization. Higher sustained fevers arise with the following four most common postoperative complications: (1) atelectasis (collapse of portions of the lung), (2) wound infection, (3) urinary infection, and (4) thrombophlebitis. These frequent causes of fever should be committed to memory as the *Four W*'s: "wind, wound, water, and walk." When fever occurs, the student should think first of these four common sources.

Lung Problems (Wind) Within the First 48 Hours

Lung complications commonly occur after operations for the following reasons:

Endotracheal tubes; oxygen and ether irritate the respiratory tree and increased secretion results.
Atropine causes inspissation of bronchial secretions.
The position of the patient cannot be changed on the operating table, and secretions tend to fill the lung and thereby encourage the growth of organisms.
An anesthetized patient cannot cough to clear secretions.
In the immediate postoperative period the patient, because of sedation or pain, cannot move or cough to clear secretions adequately; obstruction (from secretions) and atelectasis result.
Abdominal distension impairs diaphragmatic excursion.

Fever, tachypnea, and (when large portions of the lung are affected) cyanosis characterize atelectasis. Pneumonitis may result from sustained obstruction. Coughing, deep breathing, moving percussion of the chest wall, and humidified air help clear the respiratory tree of these secretions. If large areas of lung are involved by pneumonia, the patient becomes confused, with few other signs and symptoms. Confusion means poor oxygenation of the brain and should prompt the physician to order a chest film. In the older male with chronic disease of the lung or heart, gram-negative rod pneumonia is common. In certain outbreaks in hospitals *Staphylococcus aureus* is the prime cause of pneumonia in elderly postoperative patients. Bronchoscopy or tracheal catheterization with aspiration of mucus plugs can stimulate patients who have difficulty in coughing. These procedures themselves may introduce new bacteria into the lung, bypassing the usual host resistance barriers.

Respiratory Distress Syndrome

Adult respiratory distress syndrome (ARDS, posttraumatic lung, shock lung) follows massive trauma, burns, sepsis, shock, or multiple blood transfusions. In a complex reaction to these many possible insults the injured pulmonary capillary endothelial cells leak fluid and proteins into the lung interstitium, perivascular lymphatic spaces, and alveoli. The flooded alveoli collapse creating pulmonary shunts, which lower arterial (Po_2)—the hallmark of ARDS. Postmortem studies show grossly heavy lungs (3 to 6 times normal), chiefly from edema fluid and some fibrosis.

The syndrome usually appears 1 or 2 days after correction of the circulatory problems. Restlessness and respiratory distress accompany the radiographic picture of increasing patchy opacification of the lung fields. The Pao_2 progressively decreases, and hyperventilation keeps the $PaCo_2$ low. Pulmonary studies show falling lung compliance, decrease in functional residual capacity, and increase in respiratory work. The patchy lung lesions may become confluent. Without ventilatory support the patient succumbs.

Mechanical ventilation and positive end-expiratory pressure (PEEP) keynote the treatment. The added pressure increases functional capacity, opens collapsed alveoli, and prevents further collapse. The Swan-Ganz catheter, monitoring left atrial filling pressures and cardiac output, helps to guide therapy. Any source of sepsis should be treated concurrently (see Chap. 11).

Wound Infections (Wound)

Wound infections may occur after any operation. Except for *Clostridium* or β-hemolytic streptococcis, which may become evident within 24 hours, most surgical infections become obvious within 5 to 7 days. They are most common, however, after gastrointestinal operations. Drying of tissues by long exposure, operation on contaminated structures, gross obesity, diabetes, malnutrition, immunosuppression, or operations on very young or very old patients are directly related to an increase in sepsis rate. Experiments on medical students by Elek show that the infection rate from inoculated staphylococci increases 1000-fold with a foreign body (suture).

Patients who harbor infections remote from the operative site are likely to have greater wound infection rates than those without such remote infections. Wound infection rates rise proportionally with the duration of operative procedures. Any lapse in aseptic technique can contribute to wound infections during operations or with later dressing changes.

Heat, redness, and tenderness in a wound demand investigation and surgical drainage. Most surgical wound infections feature *Staphylococcus aureus,* gram-negative rods, or a mixed flora. Mixed infections have become more frequent in the past decade. A prudent plan of treatment should proceed as follows: wound culture and sensitivities, antistaphylococcal penicillin (penicillinase-resistant) or cephalosporins (both are lipophilic agents), change in antibiotics according to the patient's response, and laboratory evidence of sensitivity (see Chap. 6).

Abdominal wound dehiscence. Heralded by a serosanguineous discharge about 5 to 6 days postoperatively, the abdominal incision opens and viscera usually protrude through it. Hematomas, seromas, infection, excessive coughing, retching, distension, or poor nutrition (diabetes, uremia, starvation, immunosuppression) often underlie this catastrophe. Inadequate sutures or excessively tight closures that compromise blood supply are the chief technical offenders.

In most cases immediate operative closure with through-and-through wire or other strong materials solves the urgent problem. In the presence of infection or immunosuppression our transplant surgeons have re-emphasized an invaluable technique: they pack these wounds open and let them heal secondarily, with surprising success.

For a discussion of other wound problems, see Chapter 2.

Urinary Infection (Water) 5 to 8 Days

Postoperative patients often have difficulty voiding and sometimes require catheterization. Although urinary infections occur without catheterization, the usual initiating factor is the introduction of a catheter that mechanically carries organisms into the bladder. Single catheterizations are associated even under the best of circumstances with a 4% infection rate. Irrigation of the anterior urethra with bacitracin or neomycin, frequent catheter changes, and constant irrigation with 0.25% acetic acid or neomycin-bacitracin-polymyxin mixtures help prevent sepsis. A round pad of plastic foam about 2 inches in diameter and about 1 inch thick, threaded on a Foley catheter and pushed up to rest against the external urinary meatus, helps anchor the catheter. Subsequently the pad can be moistened with an antiseptic or with antibiotic solution or cream.

Experimental work with *Serratia marcescens* has shown that these organisms migrate into the bladder in the fluid (urine and exudate) that forms alongside the catheter. Thus these local procedures help prevent the upward migration of organisms. Patients with infection develop dysuria, frequency, urgency, hesitancy, and fever. Systemic antibiotics can control generalized sepsis but cannot control localized urinary infections as long as the catheter is in place. Recent experience shows that intermittent catheterization, under rigorous aseptic precautions, carries less risk than continuous (Foley) catheterization.

Thrombophlebitis (Walk) 7 to 14 Days

We do not understand all the factors that lead to spontaneous thrombosis in the deep leg and pelvic veins of certain postoperative patients; however, *stasis* and *increased coagulability* of blood are two important factors. Obesity, birth control medications, immobility, advanced age, cardiac problems, and abdominal malignancies are associated factors. Thrombophlebitis is characterized by fever, pain, tenderness, and redness along superficial veins. Pain and edema occur with thromboses in deep veins. The great hazard of blood clots in deep veins rests in the possibility of the clots moving to the lungs (pulmonary emboli). About 25% of patients who develop pulmonary emboli die from one or more of the following: arrhythmias, bronchoconstriction, pulmonary edema, or inadequate return of blood to the left side of the heart (which causes right ventricular failure). Early movement, pneumatic stockings, ambulation, and wrapping of the legs help prevent stasis. Most thromboses respond to rest, elevation of the legs, and chemotherapy with heparin and fibrinolytic agents. Ligating or narrowing the lumen of the inferior vena cava can prevent subsequent emboli if patients develop emboli while on full heparin anticoagulation (Fig. 10-1; see Chaps. 29 and 32.)

Third-Day Fever

The "third-day surgical fever" comes from inflammation surrounding intravenous catheters. Removal and antibiotic therapy bring rapid relief.

Cardiovascular Collapse

The signs of cardiovascular collapse—a cold, clammy, pale patient, decreased blood pressure, and a rapid, thready pulse—usually occur with alarming suddenness in the postoperative patient. Table 10-1 is a helpful guide into rapid detection and treatment of postoperative shock. The cited chapters discuss these causes of shock in detail. The student should think of

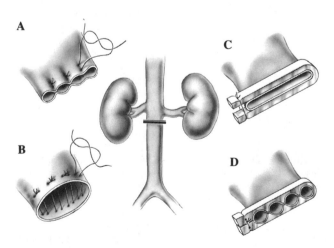

Fig. 10-1. Vena cava narrowing to prevent emboli. **A,** Multiple channel method. **B,** Suture sieve method. **C,** Slit Teflon clip. **D,** Serrated Teflon clip.

Table 10-1. Postoperative Shock

Cause	Diagnosis	Treatment
Bleeding Usually in peritoneal or pleural cavities or retroperitoneal areas	Check wounds, drain sites, open wounds, or use diagnosis aspiration if necessary; CVP is low.	Blood and immediate ligation of bleeding vessel (see Chaps. 3 and 5).
Cardiac shock Myocardial infarction or arrhythmias, arrest	Check for pulse irregularities, electrocardiogram, absence of pulse and cyanosis suggest cardiac arrest; SGOT aids diagnosis of infarction; CVP is high	Dependent on diagnosis general measures, oxygen, sedation, cardiopulmonary resuscitation (see Chaps. 5, 11, and 30).
Pulmonary embolus	No specific signs; chest pain, hemoptysis suggest diagnosis; angiography, ventilation, and perfusion scans can make diagnosis; obesity, previous cardiac difficulties, cancer and pelvic operations, immobility, and increased age are associated factors.	Embolectomy; heparin, fibronolytic agents to dissolve clots are promising (see Chaps. 11, 29, and 32).
Transfusion reaction (contaminated blood)	Smears of blood show gram-negative organisms; shock rapidly follows blood administration; usually fatal.	Discontinue blood; corticosteroids; massive doses of antibiotics intravenously (see Chap. 4).
Sepsis	Culture of blood or suspicion of gram-negative bacterial source of septicemia; symptoms often subtle: tachycardia, hypotension, oliguria, fluid retention, respiratory failure—"silent signs of sepsis."	Massive intravenous antibiotics, fluids, corticosteroids, drainage of pus (see Chaps. 5 and 6).
Toxic shock syndrome	Fever, erythroderma, shock, multiorgan failure; associated staphylococcal infections usually are vaginal or localized.	Fluids, antibiotics; treat organ failures; drain abscesses.
Adrenal failure	Must be diagnosed by suspicion or history of steroid therapy, lack of other causes.	Intravenous corticosteroids (100 to 300 mg hydrocortisone; see Chap. 16).
Anaphylactic shock	Obscure clinical picture; history of drug sensitivities is vitally important; urticaria and edema may aid diagnosis	Epinephrine, antihistamines, corticosteroids.
Fat embolism	Tachycardia, dyspnea, hypotension, increased CVP; nodular pulmonary infiltrates.	Ventilatory support, heparin, dextran, steroids, immobilization of fractures (see Chaps. 29 and 33).

bleeding and cardiac disease (myocardial infarction) as the two most common causes.

LESS COMMON COMPLICATIONS
Acute Parotiditis

Acute parotiditis is a rare complication that occurs in older, debilitated patients. An acute, painful, tender swelling of the parotid gland is an unmistakable sign. Dehydration may cause inspissation and obstruction in the duct, with a secondary staphylococcal invasion. This is one of the few instances in which x-ray therapy is used for benign disease. It is effective in the early stages. Surgical incision and drainage may be necessary if x-ray therapy fails to halt suppuration.

Postoperative Cholecystitis and Pancreatitis

Postoperative cholecystitis and pancreatitis are rarely seen; consequently they are often overlooked.

Dehydration may engender these conditions, as in parotiditis. Treatment is conservative (fluids, gastrointestinal suction, atropine, and rest). Occasionally, cholecystostomy or cholecystectomy is required.

Fat Emboli

See Chapter 33.

GASTROINTESTINAL COMPLICATIONS

A high percentage of anesthetized patients are nauseated and vomit in the postoperative period. Such a common phenomenon cannot be considered a complication.

Aspiration of Vomitus

Aspiration of vomitus is a serious complication that must be prevented by emptying the stomach before inducing anesthesia (with a nasogastric tube when necessary). Turning the patient on his side with the head lowered when vomiting occurs may prevent this complication.

Paralytic Ileus

Temporary cessation of peristalsis of the gastrointestinal tract occurs after anesthesia, trauma, and abdominal operations. If it becomes sustained, electrolyte imbalance, wound infections, or some metabolic disturbance (myxedema or adrenal failure) may be the cause. Nasogastric suction and fluid replacement will correct most cases.

Acute Gastric Dilation

Acute gastric dilation is an uncommon complication that may follow abdominal, chest, spine, or central nervous system procedures. The precise cause is obscure. An astonishing amount (several liters) of gas and dark, foul material may collect in the stomach. Vomiting and distension are the main diagnostic points. The vomiting, which is seldom accompanied by retching, features an overflow type of regurgitation that, curiously, may not be attended with nausea.

The distension may rapidly progress to fatal cardiovascular collapse within hours. Immediate intubation of the stomach and aspiration of its contents and fluid and electrolyte replacement may be life saving. Aspiration of 2 liters or more of gas and liquid material virtually assures the diagnosis of acute gastric dilation. Continuous decompression will usually relieve the gastric dilation immediately and reverse the gastric atony within 48 hours. The surgeon can safely discontinue aspiration at that time if no mechanical obstruction coexists.

Hiccup

Hiccuping in the postoperative patient may indicate some potentially serious underlying problem; this is its chief significance. Most commonly hiccups are a short-lived nuisance and nothing more. Abscesses near the diaphragm, uremia, gastric dilation, paralytic ileus, peritonitis, anxiety, and acidosis are the more common conditions that cause these spasms of the diaphragm. Rarely hiccups may persist for days or weeks and utterly exhaust the sufferer. Correcting the associated disease is the obvious and logical treatment. Vagal pressure, rebreathing air or carbon dioxide, sedation, or tranquilization may bring symptomatic relief.

OTHER URINARY COMPLICATIONS
Retention of Urine

Anesthesia, narcotics, anticholinergic drugs (atropine), operative trauma, advanced age, and diseases of the urinary system (an enlarged prostate) contribute to urine retention. Having the patient sit or stand to void is helpful. Sterile catheterization of the bladder must be done to prevent overdistension of the bladder if the patient cannot void.

Acute Renal Insufficiency

Acute renal insufficiency is a rare condition that may occur after operative procedures. The urine output decreases despite adequate intake. Precise replacement of fluids will often be sufficient therapy, and the patients will begin excreting urine within 7 to 10 days in most cases (see Chap. 3).

Peritoneal lavage with fluids designed to collect and remove nitrogenous wastes and potassium provides a "substitute kidney" in severe cases. Because peritoneal dialysis is relatively simple, it has largely replaced more complicated renal dialysis with the artificial kidney for short-term therapy.

ANAPHYLACTIC REACTIONS AND SERUM SICKNESS

In addition to shock, anaphylactic reactions are characterized by urticaria, angioedema, rhinitis, conjunctival congestion, wheezing, dyspnea, or any combination of these manifestations. An injection of foreign material induces an antigen-antibody response; subsequent exposure triggers the reaction. In humans the cardiorespiratory system (nose, glottis, pulmonary artery, bronchioles, and right ventricle), the hepatic venules, and renal glomeruli are specific targets for these reactions. A generalized urticaria often covers the patient.

Almost any organic substance, such as blood proteins, enzymes, horse serum, glues, and many foods (fish, chocolate, egg whites) may cause anaphylaxis. Penicillin, dextran, local anesthetics, contrast media, and dyes are proved offenders.

Serum sickness is a close relative of anaphylaxis but with onset 4 to 10 days after administration of the causative serum or drug. Adenopathy, arthralgia, fever, leukopenia, neuropathy, and rash characterize serum sickness.

When systemic anaphylactic symptoms appear, 0.25 ml of 1:1,000 epinephrine is given immediately and repeated every 5 minutes until nervousness or tachycardia appears. Asthmatic symptoms may be relieved by intravenous aminophylline. Antihistamines and corticosteroids are slower acting but may curtail advancement of symptoms. Tracheostomy may be required to bypass obstructing glottic edema. Since serum sickness is much less violent than anaphylaxis, symptomatic treatment with aspirin or corticosteroids will prove adequate in most instances.

BEDSORES

Bedsores (decubitus ulcers) are caused by *pressure* over bony areas (sacrum, elbows, heels). Ischemia is induced by compression of the blood vessels that supply these areas. Since decubiti can form within hours in living tissues, but not in cadavers, some surgeons hypothesize a lytic factor arising from ischemic, compressed, viable tissue. Ischemia (arteriosclerosis) and anesthesia (paraplegia) are precedent factors in most cases. The disease affects the older, debilitated patient or the younger patient who has a neurologic disease; paraplegics are extremely susceptible to bedsores.

Protection and *frequent movement* are the key words in prevention of bedsores. The nurse plays the principal role in prevention.

POSTOPERATIVE NEUROSES AND PSYCHOSES

When a surgical procedure has been successful and nonmutilating, most patients react with mild euphoria. They feel an inner satisfaction in having overcome a hazardous experience. *Depression* normally occurs after loss of any important part of the body, whether it be functionally or cosmetically deforming. Anxiety for an uncertain future in the patient's new state adds to the depression. Most patients, fortunately, adapt to these changes and resume a reasonably normal life. Severe depression characterized by withdrawal, restlessness, insomnia, expressions of hopelessness, and the desire for death should arouse suspicion of suicidal intent. The surgeon's responsibility includes listening to his patient, reassuring him, and closely following a patient with symptoms of depression. Much aid can be given to the patient with a colostomy, for example. Being introduced to a colostomy club can mean an abrupt change of attitude. A patient who sees others who have accepted their colostomies and lead successful, normal lives, adjusts rapidly and gratifyingly to a colostomy. With amputees early positive emphasis on physical therapy and rehabilitation is one of the most important factors in a successful recovery.

Major personality disturbances are, fortunately, un-common in the postoperative period. The stress of the illness, the intensity of therapy, and previous emotional makeup are the important underlying factors. A sudden, acute onset of symptoms, especially when the patient seems to overreact to the stresses, often bodes a good prognosis. The immediate problem lies in physically restraining and sedating the patient. Psychiatric consultation should be obtained for these reactions as well as for severe depressions, suicidal tendencies, or any other aberrant behavior that may threaten a normal recovery.

Dehydration and other disturbances in fluid and electrolyte balance may cause severe personality changes (the problems are discussed in Chap. 3). Sepsis, uremia, alcoholism, barbiturates, and other drugs are also known offenders in producing aberrant behavior patterns. History, physical examination, or specific chemical tests can uncover most of these causes.

SPECIFIC COMPLICATIONS

The purpose of this chapter has been to discuss complications that may arise after any operative procedure. Specific complications that arise only in certain circumstances, such as thyroid storm or hypoparathyroidism, are discussed in later chapters.

Each of the many highly technical operative procedures has its own technical complications. In shunting procedures for hydrocephalus, for example, a variety of technical failures result from attempts to shunt excess cerebrospinal fluid from the brain through man-made conduits to other parts of the body. As new operative techniques evolve in any field, a new set of technical complications will follow. Of necessity, these complications must be managed by those trained to recognize and treat them.

11

Intensive Care

J. Scott Millikan

Joseph J. Piotrowski

A system of treating patients who have serious and often life-threatening trauma or illness, intensive care uses special resources, manpower, and technology. The intensive care unit (ICU) is an *area* where patients requiring this specialized care are concentrated and where these resources, technology, and expertise are developed and maintained. Here the physician's knowledge, judgment, and skills are often tested, and critical decisions are frequently made. In this context, the ICU also provides an excellent forum for the medical student to study physiologic principles in the treatment of surgical disease (Fig. 11-1).

HISTORY

Centralization of health care is an old concept. The so-called Nightingale wards of the early 1900s allowed a single nurse to simultaneously care for many patients. This style of hospital care set the stage for specialized treatment centers. During World War II, "shock units" were developed to handle the increasing numbers of injured soldiers who were saved by improved methods of medical evacuation. These units grouped specialized equipment and staff with those patients who were most seriously injured.

Stimulated by reports of increasing numbers of postanesthesia deaths, many hospitals in the 1940s designated postoperative observation areas where patients were closely monitored until the effects of anesthesia had dissipated. Before 1950, these "recovery rooms" were usually the only specialized care areas in hospitals. Subsequent technologic advances led to increasingly complex operations requiring prolonged recovery and extensive monitoring that could not safely be carried out on regular wards. The solution to this problem was a natural extension of the recovery room concept—the intensive care unit.

Once principles of intensive care proved successful, ICUs became subspecialized. Surgical intensive care in some medical centers diversified into burn, trauma, cardiovascular, neurosurgical, pediatric, and general surgical units. Medical ICUs have become similarly specialized as pulmonary, general medical, and coronary care units.

PROS AND CONS

Advantages of intensive care are numerous. The ICU allows for placement of a patient into an environment containing the most expertise in dealing with his particular problems. In addition, when patients with similar problems are concentrated in one area, the experience of a few highly trained staff members, both medical and nursing, is enhanced. The ICU also provides for efficient utilization of the technology and equipment available to a hospital. Several studies have demonstrated improved survival among patients treated in an intensive care setting.

Disadvantages of ICUs include increased risk of cross contamination and subsequent infection. ICU patients, often immunosuppressed, are more susceptible to infection, sources of which include mechanical ventilators, open and contaminated wounds, and indwelling catheters. Cross contamination is all too frequent, and miniepidemics have on occasion nearly wiped out entire ICU populations. Sleep deprivation and lack of privacy are also notable problems.

MAINTENANCE OF CELLULAR AND ORGAN SYSTEM FUNCTION

Perhaps the most important purpose of the intensive care unit is to monitor, correct, and maintain normal cellular and organ system function throughout a patient's illness. This demands a thorough knowledge of basic physiologic principles. Cellular homeostasis requires adequate delivery of oxygen and nutrients, normal removal of waste products, and correction of metabolic abnormalities.

Oxygen Substrate Delivery

Optimal delivery of oxygen to tissues requires adequate pulmonary, cardiac, and vascular function. Enough oxygen must be presented to the patient and delivered to the alveoli for diffusion across the pulmonary capillary membrane. Sufficient hemoglobin should then be available for oxygen binding. In addition, effective cardiac function is required to transport blood to the tissues. Finally, resistance to arterial flow must allow delivery of blood to the capillaries. There, after oxyhemoglobin dissociation, oxygen and metabolic substrates diffuse into tissues.

Waste Product Removal

Removal of carbon dioxide and acid metabolites also requires proper pulmonary, cardiac, and vascular function. Delivery of these metabolites to the lungs, liver, and kidneys, critically important in maintaining normal cell physiology, requires normal venous and arterial vascular function.

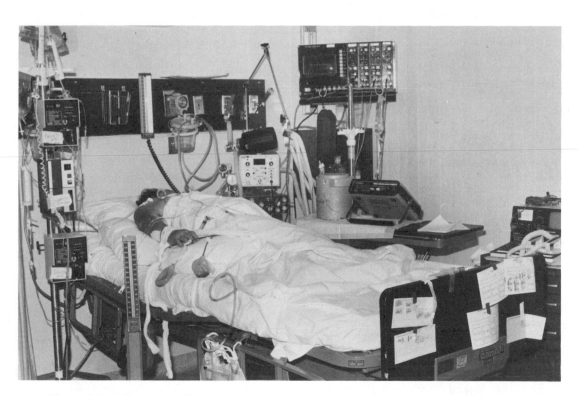

Fig. 11-1. Intensive care unit illustrating the complex monitoring and life-support systems necessary for moment-to-moment care.

Although these pathways seem simple, any defect along the way may result in end organ dysfunction, which often triggers a vicious cycle eventually leading to death. Numerous variables in this framework of oxygen substrate delivery and byproduct removal must be monitored and controlled by the ICU physician in order to optimize end organ function.

The Pulmonary System

The initial step in ensuring normal cell physiology is evaluation and correction of abnormalities in pulmonary function. Pulmonary failure results from defects in gas exchange and is manifest initially as irregularities in arterial blood gases and later as organ and tissue failure. Pulmonary failure is heralded by an arterial partial pressure of oxygen (Po_2) below 50 torr or an arterial partial pressure of CO_2 ($PaCO_2$) above 50 torr in patients who are not chronic CO_2 retainers. Ventilation and oxygenation are the two principal components of pulmonary function. They may fail separately or together and must be individually evaluated when pulmonary abnormalities are suspected.

Ventilatory failure results when an inadequate amount of gas is actively exchanged with pulmonary venous blood. The degree of ventilation at the alveolar level is inversely proportional to the Pco_2 in arterial blood. Ventilatory failure is present when the Pco_2 is greater than 50 torr. Alveolar ventilation can be increased and the Pco_2 decreased by improvement in minute ventilation, which is directly proportional to respiratory rate and tidal volume of each breath.

Hypoventilation may be attributable to alterations in central nervous system (CNS) function (narcotics, anesthetics, stroke, head or spinal cord injury), defects in neuromuscular activity (tetanus, aminoglycoside antibiotics, Guillain-Barré syndrome), or ineffective diaphragm and chest wall motion (pain after abdominal or thoracic surgery, hemopneumothorax, flail chest, scoliosis). Impairment in ventilation may also result from defects in the pulmonary airways (asthma, foreign body, mucus plug, laryngospasm) or lung parenchyma (atelectasis, aspiration, fluid overload). On the other hand, hyperventilation most often results from improper management of the mechanical ventilator but may also be secondary to CNS dysfunction.

Oxygenation failure is manifest by a decrease in arterial Po_2 (<50 torr) and an abnormally low percentage of oxygen saturation of hemoglobin. Causes of hypoxemia include (1) decreased inspired oxygen fraction (Fio_2), (2) alveolar hypoventilation, (3) abnormalities of oxygen diffusion across the alveolar capillary membrane, and (4) regional mismatching of pulmonary ventilation and blood flow, the most frequent cause of hypoxemia among ICU patients. Mismatching occurs when pulmonary blood flows across nonventilated alveoli. Unoxygenated blood then mixes with normally oxygenated blood, and the overall oxygen content of systemic arterial blood diminishes. The percentage of blood that shunts through the pulmonary vascular circuit without being oxygenated (shunt fraction) can be calculated and is normally less than 5%. Hypoxemia from pulmonary shunting is often poorly responsive to increases in Fio_2. Treatment usually involves correction of underlying causes, which may include atelectasis,

pneumonia, aspiration, and adult respiratory distress syndrome (ARDS). Another, though infrequent, cause of hypoxemia is a right-to-left central vascular shunt in which desaturated systemic venous blood flows directly into the systemic arterial circuit, usually subsequent to congenital anomalies of the heart or great vessels. This type of hypoxemia is unresponsive to oxygen therapy and generally requires operative correction.

Depending on the clinical situation, oxygenation may be improved by augmentation of Fio_2, or by an increase in the ventilation (respiratory rate × tidal volume). Oxygenation can also be improved by maximizing the number of open and functioning alveoli, thus limiting pulmonary vascular shunting. In most patients, vigorous pulmonary toilet and deep breathing exercises will achieve this; however, the patient on a mechanical ventilator may have alveolar collapse, particularly after expiration. When one increases the amount of air remaining in the lungs at the end of a breath (i.e., the functional residual capacity, FRC), alveolar collapse may be limited resulting in less ventilation-perfusion mismatching and improved oxygenation.

This result is attained clinically by use of positive end-expiratory pressure (PEEP), which maintains positive airway pressure throughout the respiratory cycle, thereby increasing FRC. Usual amounts of PEEP range from 5 to 20 cm H_2O. Although PEEP improves oxygenation, this maneuver can reduce cardiac output because increased intrathoracic pressure can lead to decreased venous return to the heart and myocardial dysfunction. The net result may be an actual *decrease* in total oxygen delivery to the tissues.

Pulmonary Support

Most ICU patients adequately ventilate, oxygenate, and clear tracheobronchial secretions spontaneously. Effective respiratory therapy, including incentive spirometry exercises, chest physiotherapy, and sufficient hydration, often prevent major pulmonary problems. Many patients also benefit from supplemental oxygen (given by nasal cannula or face mask).

Critically ill patients often require endotracheal intubation. Indications for artificial airway placement include (1) relief of airway obstruction, (2) protection from aspiration, (3) control of tracheal secretions, and (4) pulmonary failure with the need for mechanical ventilation. The first three goals are achieved with a T-piece system whereby humidified and heated gas of preset oxygen concentration flows across the end of an endotracheal tube. The fourth indication, pulmonary failure, requires endotracheal intubation and mechanical ventilation.

The indications for intubation and mechanical ventilation are as follows:

Decompensation of chronic lung disease
CNS disorders
Chest wall or diaphragm dysfunction
ARDS
Pulmonary aspiration
Severe pneumonia

Ventilators open airways, improve oxygenation, increase alveolar ventilation, and reduce the work of breathing. There are two basic types of ventilators: pressure cycle and volume cycle.

Pressure cycle. A pressure cycle ventilator delivers gas to the patient until a preset airway pressure is obtained. The amount of gas given is difficult to control, varying with the compliance of the lungs and the airway resistance to gas flow. Inaccuracy of ventilation management has led many centers to abandon its use.

Volume cycle. A volume cycle machine delivers a fixed volume of gas to the lungs with each breath. Pressure subsequently generated within the tracheobronchial tree and alveoli varies depending on the compliance (distensibility) of the lungs and chest wall. Low peak inspiratory pressures imply easily distensible (highly compliant) lungs, whereas high peak inspiratory pressures imply poor compliance and "stiff lungs." Poor chest wall compliance, mucous plugging of the ventilatory circuit, and PEEP may also increase peak inspiratory pressures.

Abnormally elevated airway pressure during mechanical ventilation is potentially dangerous. Increased pressure may overinflate alveoli causing rupture. Gas may then dissect the visceral pleura from the contiguous tissues and move into the mediastinum, abdominal cavity, and subcutaneous tissues of the chest and neck causing crepitus on palpation. Gas can also migrate into the pericardial space. Tension pneumopericardium, seen most often in infants, may precipitate cardiovascular collapse. In addition, gas escaping from ruptured alveoli may penetrate the visceral pleura and enter the pleural space causing pneumothorax with complete or partial collapse of the lung. If a "flap valve" effect occurs in the lung, whereby gas is forced into the pleural space but cannot escape, pressure increases in that hemithorax causing complete collapse of the lung and eventual shift of the mediastinum away from the affected side (tension pneumothorax). Severe mediastinal shift may cause a sudden decrease in venous return to the heart and cardiovascular collapse. Pneumothorax or tension pneumothorax, a surgical emergency, must be treated immediately by evacuation of the air from the pleural space, thus allowing the lung to reexpand and the mediastinum to resume normal position. This is achieved by placement of a chest tube through the thoracic wall and into the pleural space. The tube is then attached to a suction drainage system (Fig. 11-2).

Because of the potential dangers, volume cycle ventilators are equipped with a pop-off valve, which limits peak inspiratory pressure by diverting additional tidal volume away from the patient. Activation of this valve should sound an alarm and receive prompt attention. If excessive volume is shunted away from the patient, hypoventilation and hypoxemia may occur.

Ventilator Mode

The type of mechanical support required by patients in pulmonary failure varies, depending on the clinical setting. Most ventilators are equipped to deliver several types, or modes, of ventilatory assistance.

Continuous mandatory ventilation delivers gas at a set tidal volume and rate regardless of the patient's respiratory activity. Patients who lack functional respiratory drive and require total support need this mode of ventilation.

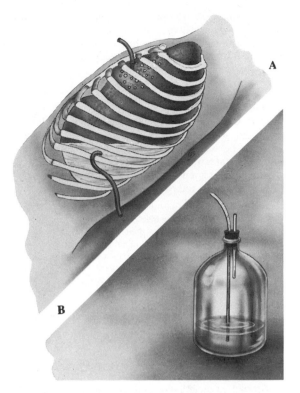

Fig. 11-2. Intercostal chest tubes with underwater-seal drainage. **A,** Tube to remove air from pleural space is introduced through second intercostal space at midclavicular line; tube to remove liquid (blood, pus, and postoperative fluid collection) is introduced through eighth intercostal space at anterior axillary line. **B,** Tubing is connected to glass rod on bottle that is covered with sterile water; pleural air bubbles into bottle and escapes to outside, while fluid collects in bottle.

Intermittent mandatory ventilation (IMV) allows the patient to breathe at his own rate and volume but also delivers additional breaths of fixed volume and rate. This mode can be adjusted to deliver the mandatory breaths synchronously with the patient's own inspirations (synchronous IMV, or SIMV). This type of ventilation permits the patient to exercise his own respiratory muscles. The amount of support may be varied according to the patient's needs, and as the number of machine-delivered breaths is decreased, the patient can increase his own respiratory activity and be slowly weaned from the ventilator.

Assist control delivers a fixed volume of gas each time the patient initiates an inspiratory effort. This mode is used in patients with an intact respiratory drive and virtually eliminates any work of breathing. Patients, however, can hyperventilate and develop respiratory alkalosis if not carefully monitored.

Ventilator Adjustments

All the parameters previously discussed including tidal volume, respiratory rate, FIO_2, PEEP, and peak inspiratory pressure are adjustable on mechanical ventilators. The ratio of inspiratory to expiratory phases, as well as inspiratory and expiratory patterns, may also be adjusted on newer models. By properly modulating these variables the ICU physician in most cases ensures effective oxygen delivery and carbon dioxide removal at the alveolar level. Careful monitoring including chest films and arterial blood gas analysis should detect most abnormalities in pulmonary function and guide any necessary corrections.

Ventilator Weaning

Once the underlying cause of pulmonary failure is diagnosed and successfully treated, the ventilator patient can be weaned from mechanical support. If the patient tolerates this and fulfills the following criteria ("spontaneous parameters") for extubation, the endotracheal tube can be removed:

1. Vital capacity greater than 10 ml/kg.
2. Tidal volume greater than 3 to 5 ml/kg.
3. Inspiratory force greater than 25 cm H_2O
4. Respiratory rate less than 25 breaths/minute
5. Intrapulmonary shunt measurements less than 20%
6. Stable T-piece trial for 30 minutes
   a. Normal or usual arterial blood gases
   b. FIO_2 at 40%
   c. No PEEP
   d. Hemodynamic stability: normal pulse and blood pressure
   e. In patients with good "spontaneous parameters," the T-piece can be omitted.
7. Patient can protect his own airway.

Arterial gases and close monitoring are essential after extubation. If the patient fails weaning, mechanical support is reinstituted until the patient's condition improves.

Cardiovascular System

The cardiovascular system also requires frequent evaluation and correction of abnormalities to assure adequate oxygen-substrate delivery along with carbon dioxide-metabolite removal at the tissue level.

Hemoglobin

Efficient oxygen transport requires adequate amounts of hemoglobin, which should be maintained at greater than 10 g/dl. Hematocrit should be kept greater than 30%. These values may fluctuate depending on the patient's state of hydration. An abnormally elevated hematocrit may increase blood viscosity and cause capillary sludging and decreased oxygen delivery.

Cardiac Function

Cardiac output, the amount of blood pumped by the heart and, theoretically, delivered to the tissues each minute, depends on two parameters: heart rate and stroke volume. Heart rate is easily monitored and can be manipulated to improve cardiac output; usually with pharmacologic agents that have a chronotropic effect or with pacemakers that stimulate the myocardium. Stroke volume, the other determinant of cardiac output, is less easily measured and depends on numerous variables including (1) the amount of left ventricular filling and subsequent myocardial fiber stretching (preload) as described by the Frank-Starling hypothesis, (2) the degree of impedence to left ventricular ejection (afterload), which is related to arterial vascular resistance, and (3)

the performance of the heart independent of preload and afterload (i.e., contractility). Preload, afterload, and cardiac contractility along with heart rate are the parameters that the intensive care physician must monitor and vary to achieve optimal cardiovascular function.

Preload. Cardiac preload is best approximated by measuring left ventricular volume at the end of diastole, just before systolic ejection. Direct measurement of this volume is not currently feasible in clinical practice; however, given certain assumptions, left ventricular *volume* is directly related to left ventricular diastolic *pressure,* which, at the end of diastole with the mitral valve open, is directly related to left atrial pressure. Therefore, measurement of left atrial pressure approximates measurement of preload, or end-diastolic left ventricular filling.

Indirect measurement of left atrial pressure was also difficult until 1970, when Drs. Swan, Ganz, and Forrester developed a flow-directed pulmonary artery catheter. This catheter (Fig. 11-3) is introduced into the central venous system. An inflated balloon near its tip carries the catheter by venous flow into the right atrium and then through the right ventricle and into the pulmonary artery. As it advances, pressures are recorded from the aforementioned vascular spaces. As the catheter moves along the pulmonary artery, the inflated balloon eventually "wedges" into and occludes the arterial segment. The "pulmonary wedge pressure" is that recorded just beyond the occluded pulmonary artery and reflects pulmonary capillary pressure, which in turn approximates left atrial pressure. The Swan-Ganz catheter thus allows for bedside estimates of cardiac preload. In addition, these devices contain various blood-drawing ports for evaluation of venous blood gases. They are also equipped with thermistors that allow direct calculation of cardiac output by temperature-dilution curves. A measured amount of cold 5% dextrose of known temperature is injected into the proximal port, and the distal thermistor records temperature variations in the pulmonary artery. A computer calculates the cardiac output from the Steward-Hamilton equation.

Normal pulmonary capillary wedge pressure, or ventricular filling pressure, is 5 to 10 torr. However, a damaged or sick heart may require greater filling pressures (10 to 15 torr) to generate optimal cardiac output. Ventricular filling pressure is augmented by intravenous fluid (or blood) infusion. Abnormally elevated wedge pressure (over 20 torr) indicates fluid overload and impending pulmonary edema. In addition, excessive ventricular filling may overstretch myocardial sarcomeres and decrease stroke volume and cardiac output. For fluid overload, diuretics remain the key treatment. However, nitroglycerin dilates venous capacitance vessels and decreases ventricular filling as well.

Afterload. Decreased stroke volume may be related to abnormally elevated peripheral vascular resistance (afterload). Although only infrequently required in clinical situations, afterload reduction by arterial vasodilation may dramatically improve stroke volume and cardiac output. Pharmacologic agents most frequently used include chlorpromazine, trimethaphan camsylate,

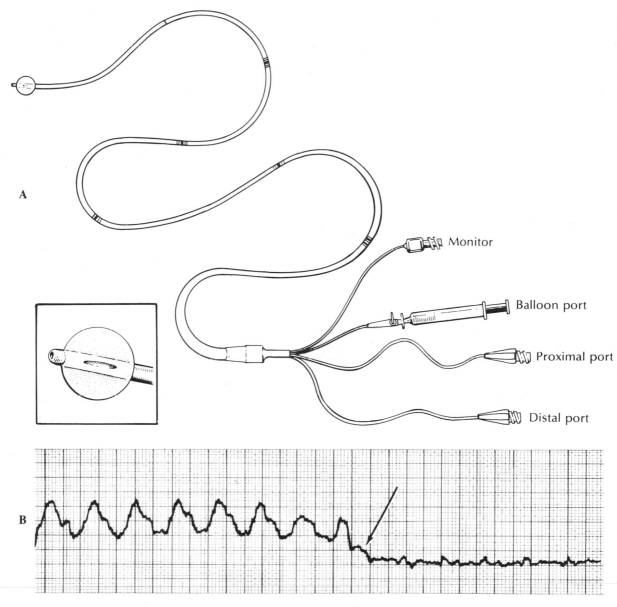

Fig. 11-3. A, Swan-Ganz catheter has a major lumen and a smaller lumen within wall of major lumen. Latex balloon at top of catheter contains a side hole that enters minor lumen. Proximal lumen terminates about 30 cm from catheter tip so that its lumen is in right atrium when distal lumen is in pulmonary artery. Proximal lumen can be used to obtain central venous pressure measurements and right atrial pressures. Major lumen is attached to pressure transducer. **B,** Pulmonary artery pressure becomes wedge pressure with inflation of balloon *(arrow)*. With deflation one should see return of pulmonary artery pressure tracing.

(From Moore, E.E., Eiseman, B., and Van Way, C.W.: Critical decisions in trauma, St. Louis, 1983, The C.V. Mosby Co.)

and sodium nitroprusside. Blood pressure must be closely monitored during vasodilator therapy because hypotension is a frequent and often serious sequela.

Contractility. Stroke volume is also directly related to the contractility state of the heart at any given end-diastolic volume and afterload. Contractility is affected by numerous commonly used drugs. Myocardial depressants include lidocaine, barbiturates, and local and general anesthetics. Myocardial ischemia, acidosis, and myocardial depressant factors that probably occur in certain disease states, such as sepsis, also decrease contractility. Myocardial infarction also hinders the effectiveness of cardiac contraction and must be considered when poor cardiac output is evident. Cardiac contractility is augmented by many pharmacologic agents. Cardiac glycosides (digoxin), ionized calcium, catecholamines, and xanthines (theophylline) have a positive inotropic effect on heart muscle.

Treatment Plan

Inadequate cardiovascular function may become clinically manifest in numerous ways, including hypotension, acidosis, poor peripheral perfusion, and abnormal end organ function, such as low urine output and confusion. All clinical signs, unfortunately, are nonspecific; thus accurate evaluation of cardiac output requires direct measurement with a Swan-Ganz catheter. As mentioned previously, skilled physicians can insert this device at the bedside with little morbidity.

If measured cardiac index is normal (over 2.4 L/min/m^2), other causes of end organ dysfunction should be actively sought out. Potential sources include pulmonary dysfunction, low hemoglobin, sepsis, and other metabolic abnormalities.

If cardiac output is low, optimize preload by fluid administration. If cardiac dysfunction continues, measure peripheral vascular resistance. If vascular resistance is abnormal, pharmacologic correction may be warranted. After preload and afterload are optimized, continuing poor cardiac output requires inotropic agents to improve cardiac contractility.

Oxyhemoglobin Dissociation

The final checkpoint in the oxygen substrate delivery scheme is transfer of oxygen from the hemoglobin molecule to tissues. Metabolic abnormalities that impair oxygen delivery at the cellular level, including hypothermia and alkalosis, should be monitored frequently and corrected.

Once pulmonary and hemodynamic functions are optimized, end organ dysfunction can safely be evaluated and treated on a system-by-system basis.

DAILY CARE OF THE ICU PATIENT

The critically ill patient is often in a state of flux. Changes occur rapidly and delay in the diagnosis of developing problems often can lead to a tragic outcome. The ICU physician must continually know the patient's status. This requires frequent bedside *examination* and *evaluation* of the patient by the physician, intensive care nurses, respiratory therapists, and consultants.

ICU Monitoring

The critically ill patient requires close attention to vital signs and organ system function, often on a second-to-second basis. Advances in technology have engendered numerous monitoring systems that, when combined with frequent physical examination, help one to recognize physiologic instability.

Vital Signs

Temperature is recorded at regular intervals, depending on the patient's condition. The most accurate measure of core temperature is obtained by use of a central venous thermistor on a Swan-Ganz catheter, though rectal probes are also satisfactory. Oral temperatures, often inaccurate, should not be used. Both hypothermia and fever are important findings requiring careful appraisal.

Respiratory rate is calculated by observing chest wall motion. Not only rate but also quality of respiratory effort should be noted. As discussed previously, hyperventilation and hypoventilation must be evaluated promptly. Physical exam and chest radiography, as well as blood gas analysis, are helpful in sorting out pulmonary problems.

Pulse and rhythm pattern are usually recorded continuously on an electrocardiogram monitor. Normal pulse and rhythm pattern displayed on a monitor must, however, be interpreted properly. They do *not* necessarily imply normal cardiovascular function. The patient with electromechanical dissociation may have a normal-looking monitor but no stroke volume or cardiac output. An effective pulse is best verified by both precordial auscultation and confirmation of peripheral blood pressure transmission (established by palpation, or a monitored indwelling arterial pressure catheter).

Cardiac rhythm disturbances are frequent in ill patients. Dysrhythmias are often secondary to easily treated underlying conditions such as electrolyte abnormalities (hypokalemia), acid-base disorders, volume problems (fluid overload), or hypoxia. Some dysrhythmias require specific drug therapy. All rhythm disturbances demand immediate diagnosis and appropriate treatment because many benign dysrhythmias may, if uncorrected, degenerate into life-threatening rhythm patterns. Once diagnosed, malignant dysrhythmias require aggressive therapy, often pharmacologic, and correction of the underlying cause. Dysrhythmias can be categorized into atrial or ventricular, depending on the source of the abnormal impulse. Ventricular dysrhythmias are generally more serious. The categorization and treatment of the numerous dysrhythmias, however, is beyond the scope of this chapter.

On occasion, a patient with a severe cardiac conduction defect may require a *temporary pacemaker* to support a rhythm and pulse. These devices consist of an electrical current generator and a conduction cable (lead) to the myocardium. The pacemaker leads can be placed percutaneously into a large central vein and maneuvered into the right ventricle, which can then be stimulated to produce regular cardiac contractions. These leads also can be placed under emergency conditions directly through the anterior chest wall into the epicardium. Transcutaneous pacemakers are new additions for emergent pacing. Temporary pacemaker cables are often placed during cardiac surgery, since rhythm disturbances may arise both intraoperatively and postoperatively. Patients who remain pacemaker dependent require conversion to a permanent pacemaker (Chap. 30).

Blood pressure is also measured frequently, depending on the patient's condition. The sphygmomanometer is most accurate but cumbersome and time consuming. The seriously ill patient who requires potent cardiovascular agents or demonstrates unstable blood pressure needs continuous monitoring by a pressure line placed into a peripheral artery. The pressure wave form is transmitted through fluid-filled tubing to a transducer that converts pressure changes to electrical signals. These signals are displayed as an arterial wave form on a monitor with continuous systolic and diastolic pressure readings (Fig. 11-4). The radial artery is most frequently utilized, followed by brachial or femoral arteries. Catheter sepsis and ischemia distal to the arterial

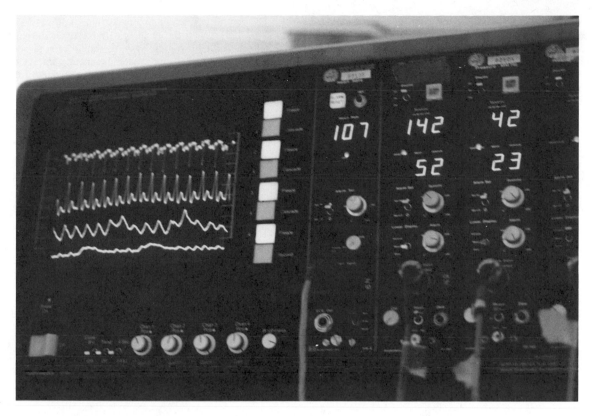

Fig. 11-4. Monitor showing, *top to bottom,* electrocardiographic pattern, systemic arterial pressure, pulmonary arterial pressure, and central venous pressure wave forms. Digital readout of pulse, systemic arterial pressure, and pulmonary arterial pressure is illustrated on right side of monitor.

catheter are potential serious complications. Arterial catheters also provide access for blood samples, including arterial blood gas analysis.

Volume Status

The injured or postoperative patient often experiences major changes in intravascular, intracellular, and interstitial fluid volumes (Chap. 3). *Total body fluid status* must be calculated at least on a shift-to-shift (8-hour) basis. Physical exam including evaluation of skin turgor, mucous membranes, and the presence or absence of edema, pulmonary rales, or perspiration gives a rough estimate of hydration status. Careful recording of all fluid given to the patient (the "ins") and all fluid removed (the "outs"), including urine output and drainage from all tubes, is mandatory. In addition, one must estimate unmeasured or insensible losses, taking into account increased losses with fever or other hypermetabolic states and decreased losses among patients on mechanical ventilators. Body weight measured daily on the same scale gives an accurate estimation of total body fluid changes.

Intravascular fluid status, as previously discussed, is an important element in maintaining hemodynamic stability and adequate organ function. Inadequate intravascular volume may lead to tachycardia, hypotension, and poor tissue perfusion (hypovolemic shock). Intravascular fluid overload may cause pulmonary edema

and myocardial dysfunction. The most readily available ways to monitor intravascular volume include physical exam (e.g., jugular-venous distension) and end-organ evaluation (e.g., mental status, urine output). Other methods include measurement of pulmonary wedge pressure or central venous pressures (CVP).

CVP, obtained by placement of a catheter in the superior vena cava near its junction with the right atrium, measures filling pressure of the right ventricle (just as the pulmonary wedge pressure reflects the filling pressure and volume of the left ventricle). If pulmonary vascular resistance and cardiac ventricular function remain stable, changes in CVP generally reflect variations in intravascular volume. CVP measurements are reliable, safe, and easy to obtain.

Intracellular and interstitial fluid status is clinically less significant and rarely measured. An exception occurs when so-called third-space interstitial fluid accumulation is large and must be considered in the patient's overall fluid status evaluation. Examples of third-space losses include abdominal ascites, pleural effusion, fluid sequestration in the gastrointestinal tract, and massive tissue swelling.

Diagnostics

Information generated from the hospital laboratory, nuclear medicine, and radiology departments is important in evaluation of the ICU patient. Unfortunately, these services are often overutilized, representing a common source of mismanagement of health care funds. Each patient should be evaluated daily. Laboratory and radiologic tests are then carefully ordered, as needed. "Shotgun monitoring" of a patient with unnecessary lab data and imaging is wasteful.

The ICU Flow Sheet

Data collected by the nurses and technicians are recorded on a flow sheet. Data include vital signs, fluids "in" and "out," hemodynamic measurements, and mechanical ventilator parameters. These data can help the physician evaluate the patient's status and adjust therapy, but only in concert with physical examination of the patient and close communication with the nursing staff.

Systems Management

Once information is gathered from careful questioning of the patient; communication with the ICU nurses and technicians; physical examination of the patient; evaluation of flow sheet data including vital signs, ins and outs, fluid status, hemodynamic and pulmonary data; and consideration of laboratory and other special test results, each organ system and phase of the patient's support should be evaluated.

The central nervous, pulmonary, and cardiovascular systems and as well the renal, gastrointestinal, musculoskeletal, and hematologic systems should be assessed individually, and the appropriate therapeutic interventions should be taken to ensure ongoing recovery. In addition, daily attention must be given to the patient's nutritional and infection status (see Chaps. 6 and 7). Metabolic problems, including endocrine derangements, fluid and electrolyte disorders, and acid-base abnormalities must similarly be evaluated and treated. The physician who deals with the patient on a system-to-system basis is less likely to overlook details regarding the patient's care. In the ICU attention to detail best ensures a successful outcome.

SUMMARY

The ICU is unique in the hospital environment. Its main concern often leads to dissociation of the patient into groups of cells and systems that ultimately integrate into a functioning organism. Care in this somewhat dehumanized environment should, however, go beyond treating kidneys, hearts, and lungs. Amidst all the technology, the ICU physician must never forget the ultimate aim—restoring the patient to full functioning.

II

General Surgical Problems

12

Malignant Neoplasms

Nathan W. Pearlman

In 1988, there will be about 1 million new cases of cancer in the United States (Table 12-1). More than three quarters of these will be solid, nonhematologic, malignancies, and most will be treated surgically at some time in their course. Since the incidence of many of these cancers continues to increase (Figs. 12-1 to 12-3), surgery is likely to remain an important part of treatment. This chapter reviews the general concepts of surgery, radiotherapy, chemotherapy, and immunotherapy in the management of solid tumors.

EPIDEMIOLOGY—THE GLOBAL PERSPECTIVE

Cancer is a worldwide problem with poorly understood but intriguing racial, ethnic, sex, age, and geographic differences; for instance, carcinoma of the stomach has been rapidly decreasing in the United States but increasing in Japan. On the other hand, female breast cancer, so common in the United States (1 in 11), is rare in Japan.

Burkitt's lymphoma, a curious malignancy frequently affecting children in tropical Africa, may be caused in part by a DNA virus (Epstein-Barr virus, EBV) and perhaps by impairment of the victim's resistance by malaria, acquired immunodeficiency syndrome (AIDS), or other environmental factors. Another strange tumor, nasopharyngeal cancer, is frequent in China and localities in the Mideast and has a causative relationship with EBV.

There are many myths about special places that are cancer free. Usually there are no health facilities in such places and, thus, few authentic diagnoses; also the inhabitants usually die at an early age. In brief, no multicellular animal species are free of cancer. Environmental and genetic factors alter the development of various kinds of cancer, but unknown factors predominate.

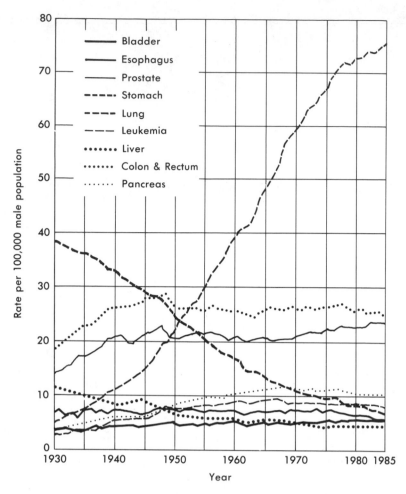

Fig 12-1. Cancer death rates for selected sites, males, United States, 1930 to 1985, adjusted to the age distribution of the 1970 U.S. Census population. (Data from National Center for Health Statistics and U.S. Bureau of the Census.)

Table 12-1. Estimated New Cases of Cancer in 1988

Head and neck	42,000
Lung	152,000
Digestive tract	227,000
Breast	136,000
Female genital	71,000
Male genital	106,000
Urinary tract	69,000
Leukemia/lymphoma	77,000
Melanoma	27,000
Other	77,000

Cancer of the lung, the leading cancer in men, is about five times more common in male than in female Americans. However, women (who started smoking heavily about two decades after men) are beginning to catch up. Breast and uterine cancer are the most common female cancers, but lung cancer will soon be more common. Most of these excessive cancer deaths from tobacco use (affecting cells of the lung, mouth, throat, esophagus, bladder, and pancreas) could be prevented.

Despite the association of cancer and aging, malig-

nancies can occur at any age. Malignancies are now a major cause of death in children (see Chap. 39). The development of cancers may take from 5 to 40 years, and the host's ability to destroy or restrain cancer cells may lessen with age.

ETIOLOGY

The causes of some of the 150 kinds of human cancer are known; causes of others are complex or unknown. Genetic factors and susceptibilities are associated with both precancerous and cancerous growths; some examples follow:
Hereditary neoplasia
Retinoblastoma
Nevoid basal cell carcinoma
Trichoepithelioma
Multiple endocrine adenomatosis
Chemodectoma
Gardner's syndrome
Genetic factors
Polyposis coli
Albinism or light skin and blue eyes

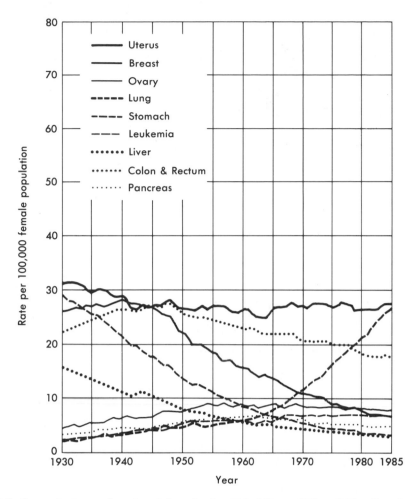

Fig. 12-2. Cancer death rates for selected sites, females, United States, 1930 to 1985, adjusted to the age distribution of the 1970 U.S. Census population. (Data from National Center for Health Statistics and U.S. Bureau of the Census.)

Immune deficiencies
Chromosome abnormalities

Cancers develop more frequently in patients with suppressed immunity, such as organ transplant recipients and patients who have acquired immune deficiency syndrome (AIDS). Breast cancer is more frequent in daughters whose mothers or maternal grandmothers had breast cancer, especially if it developed before menopause. Persons with red hair, blue eyes, and light skin are far more likely to develop skin cancers and malignant melanoma. In certain areas (Australia, southern United States) increased exposure to sunlight has probably brought about the marked increase in malignant melanomas.

Some known and suspected causes of cancers are listed in Table 12-2. There are also "promoting agents" that by themselves do not cause cancer but increase the carcinogenicity of causal factors by stimulating the growth of the cancer cells.

Cancer cells exhibit permanent genetic changes and, often, both increased numbers of chromosomes and ab-

normal chromosomes. Cancer cells escape many but not all the normal restraints of the body.

CLARIFICATION OF TERMS

Cancer is an emotionally charged word. Perhaps because of this, use of inaccurate terms easily creates misunderstandings between patient and physician. *Inoperable* is a term often used to describe cancer; yet, its meaning is vague. Operations vary from simple to complex—biopsy, laparotomy, thoracotomy, removal, or bypass of a tumor. It is almost always possible to carry out some operation to benefit a cancer patient. Few are really inoperable. *Resection*, in contrast, entails removal of tissue. Patients may be operable or inoperable, but tumors are *resectable* or *unresectable*. The cancer may be unresectable for *anatomic* reasons (the extent of the tumor is beyond that of the operation), or *physiologic* reasons (the patient cannot withstand the stress of surgery required for removal). Experience has shown that when the terms *inoperable* or *unresectable* are critically reviewed, many patients can, in fact, undergo removal of their cancer. This may

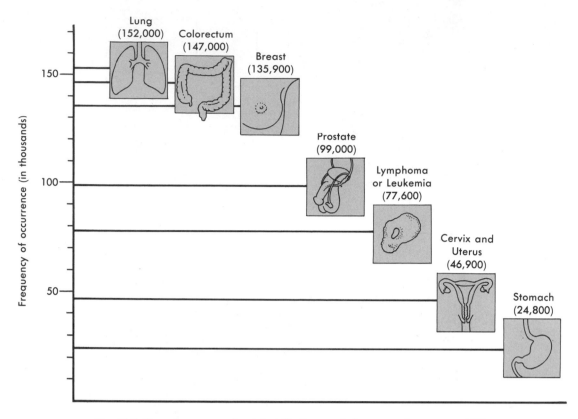

Fig. 12-3. Sites of new cancer in adults of both sexes, in frequency of occurrence, 1988.

be the result of better preoperative preparation, better counseling, or better procedures.

Curative resections entail removal of the tumor, a margin of histologically normal surrounding tissue, and, with some exceptions, regional lymph nodes. *Palliative* resections remove that segment of the cancer that is causing symptoms but leaves other asymptomatic segments intact. An example is palliative gastrectomy in a patient with gastric cancer and liver metastases. The stomach is removed to relieve gastric obstruction or stop bleeding, whereas the liver metastases are left alone and treated later, perhaps by chemotherapy. Palliative resections require grossly normal resection margins to be effective, although it is acceptable on occasion for such resections to have microscopic involvement of the margins. In contrast *debulking procedures,* also intended to palliate, cut through gross tumor and rarely palliate. With few exceptions, debulking has no place in the treatment of solid tumors.

Lymph node dissections are formal procedures designed to remove most of the nodes in a regional drainage basin. *Therapeutic* dissections remove enlarged, hard, *clinically positive* nodes felt to be involved with cancer. *Prophylactic* dissections remove nodes that are *clinically negative* (not suspicious for metastases) but may be *histologically positive* (harboring microscopic metastases). Lymph node *sampling,* in contrast, is not a formal procedure and removes only some nodes from a regional node basin for staging, leaving others behind.

Cure results from eradication of the tumor and of any metastases it may have generated. Cure may be an ephemeral goal, because after apparently successful treatment residual occult foci of disease may remain. While recurrence of most solid tumors occurs within 2 to 3 years after treatment, some recur 4, 6, and even 10 years after treatment. Patients who survive one malignancy are at increased risk of developing another, and suspected metastases in such individuals may not be recurrence but a new primary cancer. Given this unpredictability in the behavior of cancer, we prefer to use the term *cure* sparingly. Instead, patients are informed of their chance of tumor recurrence, advised of the need for close follow-up (so as to diagnose and treat recurrence or new cancer early), and the issue of cure is left indeterminate. In every case, optimism and concern for the patient are keynotes of the surgeon's approach.

STAGING

Not infrequently, solid tumors are described in such vague terms as fist-sized, egg-sized, or inoperable. A staging system is designed to standardize tumor descriptions. Such a system has several advantages. (1) Different types of treatment are better evaluated when all patients have the same extent of disease. (2) It is easier to determine the most appropriate form of treatment when the stage is known. (3) Survival figures are more relevant for particular stages of disease than for the disease as a whole.

The most commonly used staging system at present is the TNM (tumor, nodes, metastases) system. Pri-

Table 12-2. Selected Human Carcinogens

Carcinogens	Organ System
Chemical (occupational and social)	
Chimney soot	Scrotal skin
Asbestos (usually with smoking)	Lung (mesothelioma)
Tobacco smoke	Lung, bladder, larynx
Aniline dyes	Bladder
Hydrocarbon compounds	
Benzene	Bone marrow
Coal tar and pitch, creosote	Skin, scrotum, lip
Mineral oils, other petroleum	Skin, scrotum
Halogenated hydrocarbons	Various tumors
Ethylene dibromide (EDB)	
DDT, DBDP, heptachlor, etc.	
Vinyl chloride	Liver (hemangiosarcoma)
Arsenic	Skin, lung, liver
Chromium, nickel, cadmium	Lung, nasal cavity
Physical	
Ionizing radiation	Many organs, bone marrow, thyroid, connective tissue
Particulate:	
Thorotrast etc.	
Ultraviolet radiation	Skin (basal and squamous cell carcinoma, and melanoma)
Dietary	
Aflatoxins	Liver
Nitrosamines	Gastrointestinal tract
Toxic plants: cycad, bracken, safrole	Small and large bowel, liver
Alcohol	Oral cavity, esophagus, liver
Immunosuppressive agents and antineoplastic drugs	Reticulum cell sarcoma, epithelial malignancies of skin and viscera
Antilymphocyte serum	
Corticosteroids	
Anticancer agents (many)	
Hormones	
Estrogens (prenatal)	Vagina, cervix
Androgenic steroids	Liver
Hypohormone, e.g., thyroid	Thyroid
Biological viruses	Over 300 malignancies, many species
Epstein-Barr virus	Burkitt's lymphoma (?), nasopharynx (?)
Human immunodeficiency virus (HIV)	Kaposi's sarcoma
Oncogenes	Many tissues

mary tumors are given a T status (T1 to T4), regional nodes an N status (N0 to N3), and distant metastases an M status (M0, M1). The various T, N, and M categories are then combined to give a stage of disease (I to IV). For example, a T2N1M0 head and neck cancer would be stage III. Clinical staging involves evaluating the tumor externally (breast, head and neck, uterine cervix, and prostate cancer). Histologic staging follows removal of the tumor and nodes, (gastric, colorectal, bladder, and lung cancer). Criteria for each T and N category vary somewhat from cancer to cancer because of their different natural histories. Thus, a 6 cm tumor may be considered T3 in some cancers, T2 in others. Although TNM criteria now exist for virtually all cancers, this has not always been the case. Certain cancers, such as colorectal, prostate, and bladder, historically have been staged with an alphabetical system (A, B, C, D). Many practitioners who are more familiar with these alphabetical systems than with the newer TNM system prefer to use the former, feeling it provides equally valid information. As long as accurate staging is carried out, the system used is immaterial. Further details of the staging system(s) can be found in the *American Joint Committee Manual on Staging of Cancer*.

PRINCIPLES OF SURGICAL MANAGEMENT

The present surgical approach to cancer is based on the concept that most solid tumors begin in one site and spread in a centrifugal fashion to regional nodes before disseminating to distant sites. This concept is not universally accepted, however, and has been a source of contention since Roman times. Although surgeons of that era removed some breast and lip tumors, Galen, about 200 AD, declared cancer to be a systemic disease, incurable by operation, and this view went relatively unchallenged for the next 1600 years. In the seventeenth century, Valsalva, LeDran, and Morgagni argued that clinical and autopsy studies showed solid tumors were more of a local-regional problem than a systemic disease, but their opinions were ignored. In the mid-nineteenth century, introduction of inhalational anesthesia allowed cancer operations of increasing magnitude. Initially, operations consisted of little more than local excision of primary tumors and isolated removal ("berry-picking") of any enlarged lymph nodes. Local and regional recurrence of disease was extremely common, and cures were virtually unknown. In 1867, Moore, of Great Britain, advocated wide resection of the breast and lower axillary lymph nodes to prevent recurrences of mammary cancer. In 1880, Gross, of the United States, reported a 9% cure rate of breast cancer with this approach. These authors went relatively unnoticed in their home countries, but they did attract attention on the continent. Surgeons in the great German clinics of the day began to carry out wide "radical," en bloc, resections for cancer in various sites. Halsted and Meyer, impressed with this approach while touring these clinics, adopted radical mastectomy for treatment of breast cancer after their return to the United States. In 1894, both authors independently reported fewer local-regional recurrences and better survival with this operation. Support for radical surgery grew after publication of Crile's 1904 article describing the technique and results of radical neck dissection for metastatic cervical lymph nodes. Further support was provided by Miles' description of abdominoperineal resection for rectal cancer in 1908 and Wertheim's account of radical hysterectomy for cancer of the uterine cervix in 1911. From that point until the mid-twentieth century, cancer came to be regarded as a local-regional disease, which, if diagnosed early enough, could be cured in a high percentage of patients by radical surgery encompassing the primary site and regional lymph nodes. Improving cure rates seemed to justify this position, as did the relative rarity of distant metastases in the absence of regional node metastases. Prognosis appeared to reflect not only lymph node involvement but size and number of involved nodes as well. It seemed logical to remove nodes when only microscopic involvement was present, and prophylactic dissection came into widespread use.

In the latter half of the twentieth century, the basis for this approach to malignancy came under increasing question. Long-term follow-up studies, particularly in breast cancer, began to show an increasing number of distant metastases in patients who had been cured of local-regional disease by radical surgery. While such distant spread occurred most often in those with metastases to regional nodes, it also occurred when nodal metastases were absent. Another disturbing finding, again in breast cancer, was that local and regional recurrence of disease often proved to be a harbinger of distant metastases, and not, as previously held, the result of an insufficiently radical operation. Prospective studies of prophylactic lymph node dissection during this time failed to demonstrate any benefit. Outcome was the same whether nodal metastases were removed when only microscopic (prophylactic dissection) or later, when the nodes were obviously involved (therapeutic dissection). In addition, studies of conservative resection of early cancer showed results that were essentially the same as those of more traditional radical resection. Finally, adjuvant chemotherapy (systemic treatment) achieved better survival in breast and testicular carcinoma metastatic to lymph nodes than did any form of radical local-regional surgery. A second school of thought began to emerge, one which viewed solid tumors as a local disease only at inception, and as a systemic disease once cancer had spread to lymph nodes. Advocates of this position considered radical surgery overtreatment for localized disease and futile for nodal metastases. Surgical therapy, therefore, should consist of "conservative" removal of the primary tumor and sampling of regional nodes. If nodal metastases are found the patient is considered a candidate for chemotherapy, immunotherapy, or other systemic measures, but not further resection.

These two schools of thought explain some of the behavior of solid tumors, but not all. Most neoplasms stimulate growth of new blood vessels to support their growth, and the walls of these vessels are highly permeable. Given cancer's ability to infiltrate local tissues, a tumor can easily enter the circulation by direct invasion of these vessels and need not spread through lymph nodes to gain such access. In fact, direct invasion of veins adjacent to cancer has been noted by pathologists since 1829. Nevertheless, the fate of malignant cells once in the circulation is uncertain. Some may become established metastases in distant sites such as liver or lung; others may leave the vascular space, enter a lymphatic compartment, and eventually migrate to lymph nodes. Most die. In experimental animals, fewer than 1% of tumor cells injected directly into a vein survive to become metastases. Several animal models exist wherein a progressively growing primary tumor is accompanied by demonstrable circulating tumor cells but no metastases. Circulating cancer cells in humans correlate poorly with prognosis. Why this is so remains unknown—it may be due to metabolic, inflammatory or immunologic factors—but the mere existence of these circulating cells does not mean that distant metastases inevitably result.

Tumors can also invade lymphatic channels directly and spread to regional nodes by that route. Once again, their fate is uncertain. Some experimental studies show that tumor cells pass rapidly through lymph nodes into the circulation via lymphaticovenous connections. Others, which used a different tumor strain, show trapping of cells in these nodes. The outcome is also unpredictable if a tumor does become trapped in a node: it may die (for reasons listed above), it may lie dormant, or it may become established and grow. If it grows, the cancer may spread to other nodes or invade the circulation.

Because the behavior of cancer can vary, so should the surgical approach. Given what we presently know about the disease, a policy of small operations for small tumors, and extensive procedures for large lesions seems reasonable. The type of tumor being treated should also be taken into account. Sarcomas and parotid carcinomas, for example, tend to recur locally after conservative treatment, and metastases usually occur in distant sites before regional nodes. Because of this, radical local treatment of such tumors is logical; routine lymph node dissection is not. In contrast, squamous head and neck cancers, and most colorectal cancers tend to spread in an orderly manner through the lymph node chain before disseminating to distant sites. Both tumors also have a tendency to recur locally when excised conservatively. Thus, the traditional radical local-regional resection is probably the best approach to these lesions. A third group of malignancies, such as breast cancer, melanoma, and teratoma, generally do not recur locally (unless very large initially) but frequently spread to distant sites, whether or not there is regional nodal metastasis. In this group conservative local resection, lymph node sampling, and frequent use of adjuvant chemotherapy or immunotherapy make the most sense. Formal regional node dissection cures many of these patients with fewer than three nodal metastases; however, because of this, radical treatment of these cancers should not be totally abandoned. A final group of tumors, best characterized by oat cell lung cancer, are virtually always systemic diseases at the time of diagnosis. Treatment, therefore, is primarily systemic: chemotherapy, with local therapy—surgery or radiation—added as needed for control or palliation of the primary lesion.

As newer treatment modalities emerge, these options undoubtedly will change. Surgery may come to play a more important role in treatment of some cancers, and a less important role in others. Current operations may be replaced by new ones. In spite of these changes surgery will continue to keynote solid tumor therapy for some time to come.

RADIATION THERAPY

Surgery treats cancer by removing it; radiation therapy tries to kill it with ionizing radiation. X-rays were first described by Roentgen in 1895, and by 1899 they had already been used to treat some skin cancers, often with dramatic results. The equipment of the time was unreliable, however, and of limited energy. It could treat only superficial lesions. In addition, early therapists had little understanding of radiation biology and used massive exposures aimed at eradicating the tumor in one treatment. As a result, the morbidity and mortality of treatment was substantial, and partial or complete regression of tumors was often followed by recurrence. In the 1920s and 1930s, studies by Regaud and Coutard in France demonstrated that fractionation of treatment into successive daily doses would cure more tumors and produce fewer side effects than would a single massive exposure. Introduction of more powerful (200 kilovolt) machines during this time also improved cure rates. Nevertheless, it was difficult, if not impossible, to treat deep-seated tumors with this equipment because of energy loss and scattering as the beam passed through skin. Skin tolerance usually limited the total dose to less than the cancericidal dose. Following World War II, the modern era of megavoltage irradiation began with cobalt teletherapy and linear accelerators. The beams from these machines produced maximal damage at significant depths below the skin and had sharply defined edges that could be focused. Skin tolerance, therefore, no longer limited the total dose, and the ability to focus the beam allowed more radiation to be delivered in close proximity to vital structures. Cure rates for tumors treated primarily by irradiation improved markedly, and more cancers could be treated by this modality than ever before.

Ionizing radiation damages tumors and normal tissue by causing breaks in strands of chromosomal DNA. Some of these breaks are quickly repaired by cellular enzymes (sublethal damage), whereas others are irreversible (the cell dies). Work by Puck, Elkind, and Phillips in the 1950s and 1960s showed an exponential relationship between radiation dose and cell survival. A "shoulder," or flat region, in the initial part of the curve presumably reflects repair of sublethal damage in the low-dose range. On the basis of this information alone, one would expect a single large radiation dose to kill more tumor cells than multiple small doses, but other factors also influence injury from radiation. In the 1950s and 1960s, Gray found that oxygenated cells are about three times more sensitive to radiation injury than are hypoxic cells. Oxygen helps convert initially reversible chemical alterations induced by ionization to irreversible changes, thus fixing the radiation damage. Most tumors have a relatively hypoxic core that is resistant to even large doses of radiation. With only one, or a few treatments, this core lives on after destruction of the periphery of the tumor, and eventually begins to grow again. Theoretically, fractionated treatment allows the hypoxic core to reoxygenate and regain radiosensitivity as the periphery gradually dies. Whether this actually occurs is still unclear; however, fractionated treatment is clearly more effective than a single exposure or a few massive ones. Fractionation has become an integral part of most radiotherapy regimens, generally consisting of five to six treatments each week for a period of 4 to 6 weeks.

Radiation therapy has a variety of purposes. At medium and high doses, it cures a high proportion of patients with Hodgkin's disease and those with early head and neck or cervical cancer. At lower doses, it effectively palliates bone and brain metastases from a number of malignancies. It also can be combined with surgery, where surgery or radiotherapy alone is followed by an unacceptably high incidence of local recurrence (advanced head and neck or rectal cancer). The rationale behind combined therapy is to remove the gross, radioresistant, disease surgically and treat residual microscopic, radiosensitive disease with radiotherapy. This approach improves local control rates, with less morbidity than if surgical resection were extended to include all possible areas of microscopic metastases. Finally, radiation therapy can be combined with chemotherapy, as is frequently done in lymphomas, leukemias, and oat cell cancer of the lung. In these cases, chemotherapy is the main line of treatment and radiotherapy is added to treat bulk disease that has failed to respond or sites, such as the brain, where chemotherapy penetrates poorly.

CHEMOTHERAPY

The use of drugs to treat cancer is as old as the use of surgery. Colchicine, a drug that arrests mitosis in metaphase, was noted to have antitumor effects in the first century AD. Arsenic, which uncouples oxidative phosphorylation, was found to be effective against leukemia by Lissauer in 1865 and was used for this condition until the early twentieth century. In the 1940s, studies of chemical warfare agents led to the discovery that nitrogen mustard, an alkylating agent, caused shrinkage of lymphosarcoma in animals and humans. Other research programs in nutrition, arthritis, nucleic acid metabolism, and tuberculosis in the 1940s and early 1950s found antitumor activity in certain antimetabolites (aminopterin, methotrexate, 6-mercaptopurine), corticosteroids, and antibiotics (actinomycin-D). From this background, an organized and intense effort to find more and better anticancer drugs was initiated in 1955; the effort continues today. Anticancer drugs can be grouped in categories as follows:

Alkylating agents
  Nitrogen mustard
  Cyclophosphamide
  Phenylalanine mustard
  Thiotepa
  Nitrosoureas (BCNU, CCNU, Me-CCNU)
  Dacarbazine (DTIC)
Antimetabolites
  Methotrexate
  6-Mercaptopurine
  6-Thioguanine
  5-Fluorouracil (5-FU)
  Floxuridine (FUDR)
  Cytarabine (Ara-C)
Antibiotics
  Dactinomycin
  Doxorubicin (Adriamycin)
  Daunorubicin
  Bleomycin
  Mithramycin
  Mitomycin-C
  Streptozotocin
Alkaloids
  Vincristine
  Vinblastine
Hormones
  Estrogens
  Androgens
  Corticosteroids
  Thyroxine
Antihormones
  Antiestrogens (tamoxifen)
  Antisteroids (aminoglutethimide)
Miscellaneous
  Procarbazine
  Hydroxyurea
  Cisplatin
  Epipodophyllotoxins (VP-16)

These agents act in different ways. Alkylating agents and epipodophyllotoxins produce breaks and abnormal cross linking of DNA similar to that seen with ionizing radiation. Antimetabolites and hydroxyurea replace normal metabolites in key molecules, or compete with normal metabolites for places in key enzymes, rendering the molecule or enzyme inoperative. The antibiotics and cisplatin bind to DNA by interposition between base pairs; antibiotics may also create damage by forming free radicals, chelating important metal ions, or directly poisoning the cell membrane. Vinca alkaloids bind to microtubular proteins that make up the mitotic spindle and arrest mitosis. Metabolites of procarbazine depolymerize DNA. Hormones and antihormones compete with each other for binding sites on cell receptor proteins. If the hormone or antihormone competes with the usual stimulating agent (estrogens in breast cancer, androgens in prostate cancer), the tumor fails to grow or actually regresses. Aminoglutethimide blocks formation of all adrenal steroids (a "medical adrenalectomy").

In all cells, whether normal or malignant, the cell cycle begins with mitosis (Fig. 12-4). This is followed by a rather quiescent period, or G_1 phase. G_1 is fol-

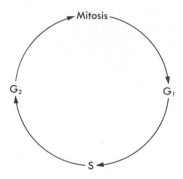

Fig. 12-4. Cell cycle.

lowed by the S phase, during which there is active synthesis of DNA, and the DNA content of the cell is doubled. Once this has occurred, the cell enters the G_2 phase and undergoes RNA and protein synthesis required for cell division. Some chemotherapeutic agents affect only a part of the cell cycle and are termed *phase specific;* others work throughout the cycle and are called *phase nonspecific.* The alkylating agents, antibiotics, hormones and antihormones, procarbazine, cisplatin, and epipodophyllotoxins are all *phase nonspecific.* Methotrexate, 6-mercaptopurine, 6-thioguanine, cytarabine, and hydroxyurea are *phase specific,* damaging only cells in S phase. The vinca alkaloids are also *phase specific* and affect cells undergoing mitosis. Floxuridine and 5-FU, designed to be phase-specific antimetabolites, act more like *nonspecific* agents, for reason unknown.

The effects of chemotherapy are far from specific. While these agents damage malignant cells, they also harm normal tissue, especially rapidly dividing cells (gastrointestinal mucosa hair follicles, bone marrow). Side effects of treatment limit the dose or frequency with which the drugs can be used. Some of the more common side effects are nausea and vomiting, anorexia, oral and intestinal mucositis, hair loss, bone marrow suppression, nerve damage, and kidney damage. In addition, while chemotherapy has been very effective in curing hematologic malignancies and lymphomas, it has cured few solid tumors. The principal uses for chemotherapy in solid tumors at present are palliative (to shrink symptomatic lesions when surgery or radiotherapy cannot be used) or adjuvant (to prevent or delay onset of distant metastases). Another increasingly common use is "neoadjuvant" therapy. Response rates in many cancers are much higher when chemotherapy is given before, rather than after, surgery or irradiation. Because of this, treatment of certain advanced cases begins with chemotherapy, in hope of shrinking the tumor prior to definitive surgery or irradiation, making definitive therapy more effective. Chemotherapy may in the future, become the major treatment for some solid tumors; however, at present, it has not reached this goal.

IMMUNOTHERAPY

Surgery, radiation therapy, and chemotherapy all damage normal tissue. Furthermore, surgery and radiation therapy are regional treatments, useless against disease outside the area being treated. Immunotherapy, in contrast, holds out the promise of specifically killing malignant cells wherever they reside while leaving adjacent normal cells intact. Several observations indicate that the immune system influences the natural history of at least some tumors. Spontaneous regression of cancer is a rare but well-documented event. Circulating tumor cells, while commonly found in many patients, appear to have little relationship to prognosis or development of distant metastases. The incidence of cancer is much higher than expected in patients with congenital or acquired immunodeficiency states. Tumor-associated antigens have been found in many human neoplasms, and many patients mount at least some degree of immune response to these antigens. Furthermore, in numerous animal models, manipulation of the immune system leads to rejection of tumor cell inoculums.

Most human tumor-associated antigens described to date are weak immunogens with limited ability to induce host resistance. The major aim of treatment at present is stimulation of the immune system to augment the immune response. One means of doing this is nonspecific stimulation with agents such as bacillus Calmette-Guerin (BCG), *Corynebacterium parvum*, or levamisole. BCG, an attenuated strain of *Mycobacterium bovis* used as a vaccine against tuberculosis, and *C. parvum*, a heat-killed microorganism, are both potent stimulators of host defense mechanisms. Each agent can prevent growth of inoculated tumor cells in animals, and each will cause regression of cutaneous malignancies in humans when injected directly into lesions. Levamisole, an oral synthetic antihelminthic agent, also has nonspecific immunostimulatory properties. Subcellular fractions of lymphocytes (immune RNA or transfer factor) or combinations of lymphokines such as interleukin 2 with infusions of cultured lymphokine-activated natural killer lymphocytes (LAK) can stimulate any existing host resistance. Although pilot studies with each of these approaches have shown promise, larger trials have shown only slight increases in survival. Thus, the potential of immunotherapy is, at present, an unrealized ideal.

GENERAL TREATMENT OF CANCER PATIENTS

A majority of cancer patients will suffer from advanced disease. The physician must combine his technical skill with a vitally important sensitivity and sympathy. He must sustain some degree of hope for the patient yet not mislead him. The cancer patient often goes through phases of rage (Why me?), denial (I don't believe it), and antagonism toward those caring for him before progressing to an acceptance of his serious and possibly fatal disease. The physician must guide the patient through these emotionally grueling periods. The patient will sense that he is in the hands of an aggressive yet sympathetic therapist who is knowledgeable about new therapies. Optimal care and support of the patient require the skills of internist, radiologist, surgeon, physiotherapist, nurse, social worker, and, of great importance, the informed close relatives. In addition to this desirable team effort, a patient should have a single physician to whom he can relate his hopes and fears.

Patients with cancer, even when far advanced, do not necessarily have severe pain. The discomfort is often a minimal physical stimulus (fatigue, loss of interest) with maximum overlay of anxiety and the loss of normal activity and work patterns. The loss of independence and increasing dependence on others is frustrating. There are many methods of controlling pain without narcotics. Local or regional pain, can be controlled by peripheral nerve blocks with alcohol, epidural instillation of phenol, and other modifications of local and regional anesthesia (see Chap. 35). Early addiction of a cancer patient induces tolerance, which reduces the effectiveness of narcotics when they are most needed. Combination of tranquilizers, sleep-inducing drugs, and programs of activities all aid in minimizing the use of narcotics. Oral forms of many drugs permit the competent patient to adjust his medications to meet his individual needs.

In addition to the psychological and painful aspects of malignant disease, other manifestations of distant and local involvement demand treatment. Effusions of the pleural and peritoneal cavities can be controlled by drainage, systemic chemotherapy, local instillation of drugs, sodium restriction, and diuretics. Pleural effusions are particularly distressing because they slowly suffocate patients. Patients who cannot tolerate cytolytic agents because of bone marrow depression may require quinacrine injections (50 mg initially, and daily increments of up to 200 or 250 mg). Peritoneal effusions may be shunted back into the venous system through catheters with one-way valves (the Denver shunt).

Metastases to the central nervous system are common from lung and breast cancer and melanomas. Craniotomy may be worthwhile to remove a single mass that causes symptoms. Steroids and radiotherapy also may relieve increased intracranial pressure.

Metastasis can collapse vertebral bodies, with subsequent pressure on the spinal cord or spinal nerves. Epidural metastases may impinge on nerves without bony involvement. When symptoms of compression rapidly progress, emergency laminectomy and radiotherapy may prevent paralysis.

Bony metastases occasionally result in pathological fractures. The pain of bone metastasis can often be controlled with radiation therapy, and pathological fractures often heal. Fractures of weight-bearing bones often require immobilization by the use of intramedullary devices followed by radiation therapy. If possible, these techniques should be applied before the fracture occurs.

The superior vena cava may be selectively obstructed in patients with lymphomas and lung cancer. Simultaneous chemotherapy and radiation therapy may be palliative for these patients.

The patient with bowel obstruction may benefit from a resection, intestinal bypass, gastrostomy, ileostomy, or colostomy. Cervical esophagostomy (which prevents accumulation of secretions in the pharynx and bronchial aspiration) can be palliative for patients with high esophageal obstruction. By supplying calories and other nutritional elements, hyperalimentation aids healing, extends palliation, and supports the patient during chemotherapy (see Chap. 7).

The prompt treatment of the cancer-endocrine syndromes such as hypercalcemia in association with breast cancer can prolong and improve vitality.

Adrenocortical steroids, mithramycin, restriction of calcium, and increased fluid intake with diuretics may lower hypercalcemia. Adrenalectomy or o,p'-DDD may palliate ectopic Cushing's syndrome. Bromocriptine mesylate, aminoglutethimide, 5-FU, and other newer drugs may inhibit hormone synthesis.

13

Skin

David W. Furnas
Ivan M. Turpin

The Epidermis and Its Adnexal Structures
The Dermis
Pigment-Producing Cells
Nerve Tissues
Vascular Tissues
Subcutaneous Fat

The skin is the largest organ of the body and is the device that allowed our distant forebears to emerge from the sea without fear of desiccation or bacterial ambush. The skin is composed of several different structures, each giving rise to characteristic disease processes. Only the few that have surgical significance are considered here.

THE EPIDERMIS AND ITS ADNEXAL STRUCTURES

Hair follicles, sebaceous glands, and sweat glands (eccrine and apocrine) are formed by labile epithelial cells that can quickly regenerate to repair any superficial injury. (See discussion on skin grafts in Chap. 34.) Infections and tumors are common in these structures.

Infections

Furuncles, or boils, are caused by *Staphylococcus aureus* infections of hair follicles; they respond to surgical incision, drainage, and antibiotics. *Carbuncles* are staphylococcal infections of the back or of the posterior part of the neck that burrow and branch into the deep dermis and subcutaneous fat. Adequate drainage requires wide and deep incisions. *Hidradenitis suppurativa* is a chronic infection of apocrine sweat glands in the axilla or the perineum. If far advanced, this disease is treated by excision of the involved skin and repair of the resultant defect with skin grafts or pedicles. The surgical importance of *acne vulgaris,* a recurring pustular infection of the skin follicles of the face, arises from the need to improve resulting scars with excision, dermabrasion, or collagen injections.

Benign Conditions

Rhinophyma, a grotesque hyperplasia of the nasal skin, is treated simply by sculpting a more desirable

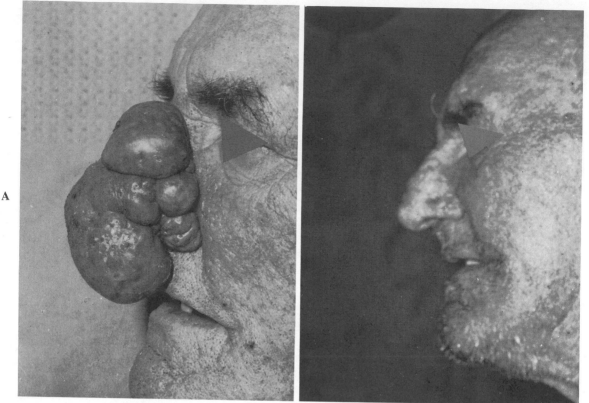

Fig. 13-1. Rhinophyma. **A,** Preoperative condition. **B,** Nasal bulk reduced by simple surgical paring.

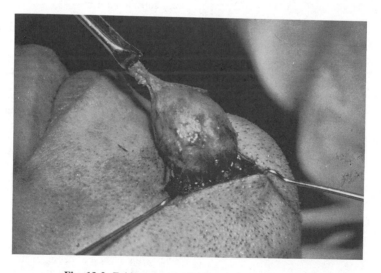

Fig. 13-2. Epidermal cyst of chin exposed at operation.

shape with a scalpel; it arises after years of the chronic inflammatory process *acne rosacea* (Fig. 13-1).

Epidermal cysts (sebaceous cysts, or wens) occur anywhere on the body but particularly on the face, neck, or scalp (Fig. 13-2). They may result from bits of epidermis implanted in the depths of the skin by sharp objects (see discussion on implantation cyst, Chap. 40), or possibly from a blocked hair follicle or sebaceous gland. They are lined by epidermis and are filled with epidermal debris. Rarely, a *true sebaceous cyst* is

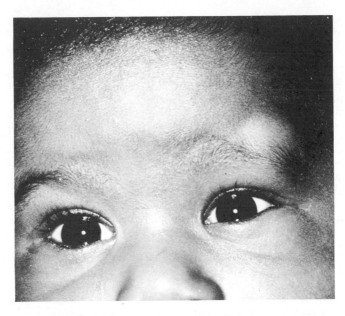

Fig. 13-3. Dermoid cyst of upper lateral part of left orbital rim. Cyst caused indentation in frontal bone.

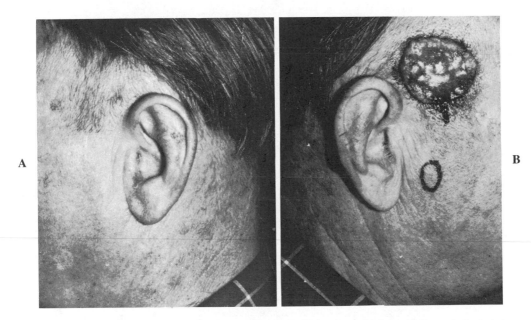

Fig. 13-4. Progress of precancerous change to cancer. **A,** Senile keratoses of left temple (just anterior to hairline) and scaphoid fossa of external ear. **B,** Frank squamous epidermoid carcinoma of right temple of same patient with metastasis to preauricular lymph nodes *(inked circle)*.

encountered that is lined by sebaceous cells and filled with sebum. The lining of *dermoid cysts* contains not only keratinizing epidermis but also adnexal structures. They presumably arise from primordial islands of skin that were displaced during embryonic development. They are common around the eyes (Fig. 13-3) and nose, and sometimes they extend into the cranial vault; therefore the surgeon undertaking their excision should

be properly armed. *Seborrheic keratoses* are brownish, raised, velvety-feeling blotches, common in elderly patients. They have no malignant potential. Because of their superficial purchase on the skin, they can be shaved off with a knife, and the wound will epithelialize. Sometimes they are so numerous that excision is impractical. There are numerous types of *benign adenomas, papillomas,* and *polyps* of epidermal and adnexal origin for which excision (or dermatological removal) is performed to obtain a diagnosis and to improve appearance.

Premalignant Lesions

There are numerous premalignant lesions of the skin that develop into squamous cell or basal cell carcinomas decades after the initial inciting insult (Fig. 13-4). *Senile* or *actinic keratoses* result from years of exposure to sunlight (e.g., in farmers and sailors). The solar radiation responsible for the malignant degeneration in skin is ultraviolet radiation with wavelengths between 290 and 320 nm (UV). *Keratotic radiation changes* result from repeated small doses of ionizing radiation (e.g., hands of dentists) or from therapeutic doses of radiation received many years before (Fig. 13-5). Long-term treatment for syphilis or psoriasis with Fowler's solution or other arsenical drugs results in premalignant *arsenical keratoses,* which are found on palmar or plantar surfaces. Chronic contact with certain hydrocarbon compounds, accompanied by irritation or sunlight, may result in keratoses such as those that lead to the scrotal carcinoma in chimney sweeps. *Chronic unstable burn scars* or *chronic draining osteomyelitis*

causes premalignant changes that lead to *Marjolin's ulcer,* a squamous carcinoma. The unfortunate children who inherit *xeroderma pigmentosum* through an incomplete sex-linked recessive gene have an exquisite sensitivity to ultraviolet radiation, causing keratoses and ultimately multiple squamous cell carcinomas, basal cell carcinomas, and even sarcomas and melanomas. They are doomed to die before adulthood. Patients with *lupus vulgaris* (tuberculosis of the skin) develop keratoses and frequent basal or squamous carcinomas (lupus carcinoma) in their later years. *Nevus sebaceus* is an ovoid, hairless, yellow-brown plaque with a verrucous surface that is present at birth or develops in childhood. Such nevi are associated with epilepsy, mental retardation, and secondary neoplasms such as basal cell carcinoma and syringocystadenoma.

Most of the skin cancers that arise from these predisposing lesions are prevented if one avoids exposure to the various inciting causes. Diagnosis is confirmed by histological examination of suspicious lesions. Either *excisional biopsy* (complete removal of suspicious lesions including margins of normal tissue on all sides) or *incisional biopsy* (removal of only a sample of the lesion) with a knife or punch is done. Premalignant le-

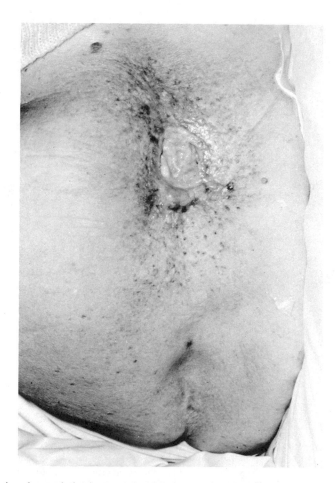

Fig. 13-5. Radiation changes in lumbar area caused by radiation received for "lumbago" 35 years previously. Central area of necrosis is surrounded by atrophic keratotic skin. Many basal cell and squamous cell carcinomas were found on microscopic examination.

sions may be treated by excision, shaving, dermabrasion, electrodesiccation, topical chemotherapeutic agents, or careful observation.

Malignant Lesions

Basal cell carcinomas and *squamous cell carcinomas* that arise in the epidermis (sometimes called *epitheliomas*) are the *most common of all malignant tumors*. They arise from the epidermis because of the

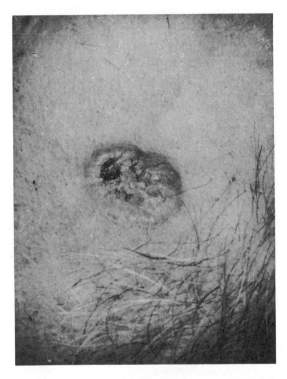

Fig. 13-6. Basal cell carcinoma. Translucency, mild lobulation, delicate vasculature, and slight ulcerations are seen.

previously mentioned factors or from no obvious cause. Of the predisposing factors, sunlight is by far the most important. Light-complexioned male outdoor workers in hot climates receive the most solar radiation and are therefore the most frequent victims. Hands, faces, and necks are the most common sites. The most superficial epitheliomas are *multicentric basal cell carcinoma, intraepidermal squamous cell carcinoma,* and *Bowen's disease.*

Basal cell carcinoma (basal cell epithelioma) (Fig. 13-6) of the skin is most common on the face, particularly the cheeks, eyelids, nose, and lips (nonvermilion surface). Northern European ancestry strongly predisposes to basal cell carcinoma. It has a raised, pearly, translucent appearance and a delicate capillary network, frequently without ulceration. Ulceration develops as the lesion increases in size. It almost never metastasizes, but if inadequately treated, it relentlessly erodes through soft tissues, cartilage, and bone until death ensues from invasion of arteries, brain, or airway (hence the name *rodent ulcer*). If the patient is seen early and excision and histological study are carried out properly, the cure rate should approach 100%.

Squamous cell carcinoma (squamous cell epithelioma; see Fig. 13-4, *B*) of the skin has the power to metastasize to regional lymph nodes; however, it is a well-differentiated carcinoma, and metastases occur late. Antecedent trauma such as radiation injury (see Fig. 13-5), chronic chemical exposure (hydrocarbons, arsenic), burns from plastic or hot metal, or unstable scars (as well as sunlight) predispose to squamous cell carcinomas. They are horny, crusted lesions and frequently show rolled margins surrounding an area of ulceration. The ears, temples, upper parts of the face, and dorsum of the hands are the most common sites. Squamous cell carcinoma is almost as common as basal cell carcinoma, but it affects an older group of patients. Wide excision or radiation of early lesions yields a 5-year survival rate of over 90%. The outlook is gloomier for patients with very large lesions and lymph node me-

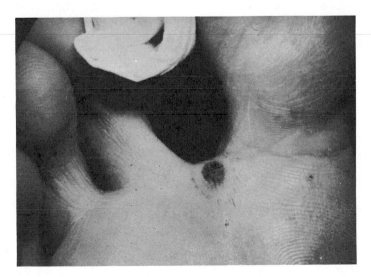

Fig. 13-7. Junctional nevus. Flat, hairless, brownish gross appearance (proposed incision line marked with ink).

tastases. Regional lymphatic dissection is carried out when lymphatic metastases are suspected.

Keratoacanthoma (self-healing epithelioma, molluscum sebaceum) grows rapidly from a small papule to a sizable raised tumor with an umbilicated, necrotic center in 6 to 8 weeks and then subsides, leaving a scarcely visible mark. It has the microscopic picture of a well-differentiated squamous cell carcinoma. Rarely, it fails to regress, behaving like an invasive squamous carcinoma. The numerous types of neoplasms of the adnexal structures of the skin will not be discussed because of their rarity.

For certain spindle cell and poorly differentiated carcinomas of the skin, electron microscopy or immunoperoxidase procedures may be of help in making the diagnosis.

THE DERMIS

Excessive proliferation of dermal fibroblasts occurs in hypertrophied scars and keloids (see Chap. 2), and in some rare lesions such as desmoids.

PIGMENT-PRODUCING CELLS

The surgically important pigmented lesions, nevi and melanomas, arise from pigment-producing cells of neuroectodermal origin (melanocytes, Schwann cells, or both). Freckles and lentigines are pigmented but are not composed of pigment-producing cells.

Pigmented Nevi

Junctional nevi (Figs. 13-7 and 13-9), in which the nevus cells are clustered at the junction of the dermis and the epidermis, are flat and hairless and can give rise to malignant melanomas. *Intradermal nevi* (Figs. 13-8 and 13-9) are formed of nests of nevus cells buried in the dermis, deep to the dermoepidermal junction. They are usually raised, may be hairy, and do not become malignant. The *compound nevus* (Fig. 13-9) has both junctional and intradermal elements and has the same malignant potential as the junctional nevus (Table 13-1).

Junctional nevi are much more common in children than in adults (70% of nevi in children under 15, but only 20% in adults), yet, paradoxically, malignant melanoma is almost unknown in children. (*Juvenile melanomas,* which microscopically resemble malignant melanomas, occur in children but are not malignant.) Curiously, almost all nevi below the knee in adults are junctional nevi.

There are so many nevi and such a minute percentage of them turn into malignant melanomas that it is impractical to excise every flat, hairless mole. However, nevi at points of constant irritation (foot, belt line, neck, bearded area) and nevi that show any sort of change, such as increase in size, deeper pigmentation, itching, or bleeding, should be excised and examined microscopically.

The uncommon *blue nevus* (benign dermal melanocytoma) derives its color (sometimes a striking deep blue) from intense pigmentation plus its location deep within the dermis. Occasionally the regional lymph nodes become pigmented, but metastases are almost unknown.

The *giant hairy nevus* and *"bathing trunk"* nevus appear at birth and may cover half of the body surface. These sometimes give rise to true malignant melanomas in childhood. Removal by dermabrasion before 10 months of age has been promising (Fig. 13-10).

Malignant Melanomas

Malignant melanomas (Fig. 13-11) are highly malignant pigmented skin lesions (rarely nonpigmented) found anywhere on the skin, especially in areas exposed to the sun. The most common sites are the head, neck, and lower limbs. They can metastasize through both the lymphatic system and the bloodstream and may spread to any organ of the body. Small islands of microlymphatic spread near the primary lesion are called *satellites.* Other foci of spread may outline the course of regional lymphatic vessels. About half the malignant melanomas arise from junctional or compound nevi, and half arise de novo. They occur particularly in young adults and throughout the adult years. The blotchy *Hutchinson's spot* or *malignant lentigo,* seen on the facial skin of elderly patients, is a relatively indolent melanoma and metastasizes only at a late date. It has a proclivity to local recurrence.

Malignant melanomas are radioresistant and must be treated by wide local excision, frequently combined with removal of the regional lymphatics. Chemotherapy or immunotherapy is sometimes a useful adjunct (see Chap. 12). Prognosis depends on clinical type, level of invasion, and metastasis. *Lentigo malignant melanoma* commonly afflicts the aged and has the best prognosis. *Superficial spreading malignant melanoma* and *nodular malignant melanoma* arise in youth and middle age and carry an intermediate and a poor prognosis, respectively. Clark classifies malignant melano-

Table 13-1. Description of Nevi

Junctional Nevus	Compound Nevus	Intradermal Nevus
Flat	⟶	Raised
Hairless	⟷	Often hairy
Often present below knee		Rarely present below knee
Present in most young children		80% of nevi in adults
70% of nevi in children under 15 years		Rarely present in young children
Nevus cells in clumps at dermoepidermal junction	Nevus cells at both sites	Nevus cells in nests within the dermis
Precursor to malignant melanoma	Same significance as junctional nevus	Not premalignant

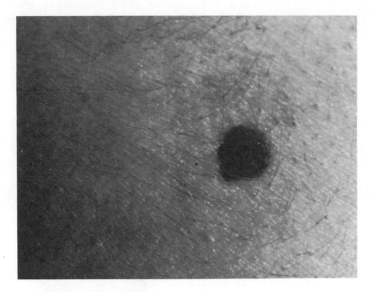

Fig. 13-8. Intradermal nevus. Notice elevated contour.

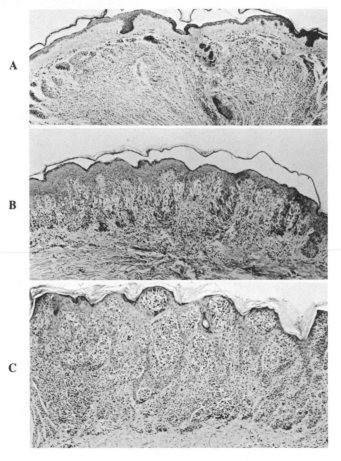

Fig. 13-9. Nevi. **A,** Intradermal nevus. Nevus cells are all well below dermo-epidermal junction and occupy the entire lower four fifths of pictured specimen. **B,** Junctional nevus. Nevus cells are found only in clusters at junction area between dermis and epidermis. **C,** Compound nevus. Nevus cells are seen in nests at dermo-epidermal junction and also throughout much of dermis. (Courtesy Dr. James H. Graham, Department of Dermatology, University of California, Irvine, Calif.)

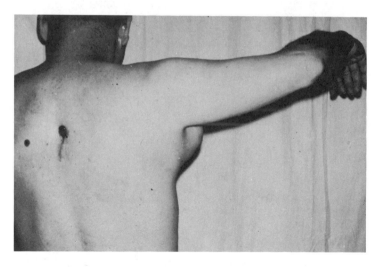

Fig. 13-10. A, Congenital hairy nevus. **B,** Five years after treatment by dermabrasion.

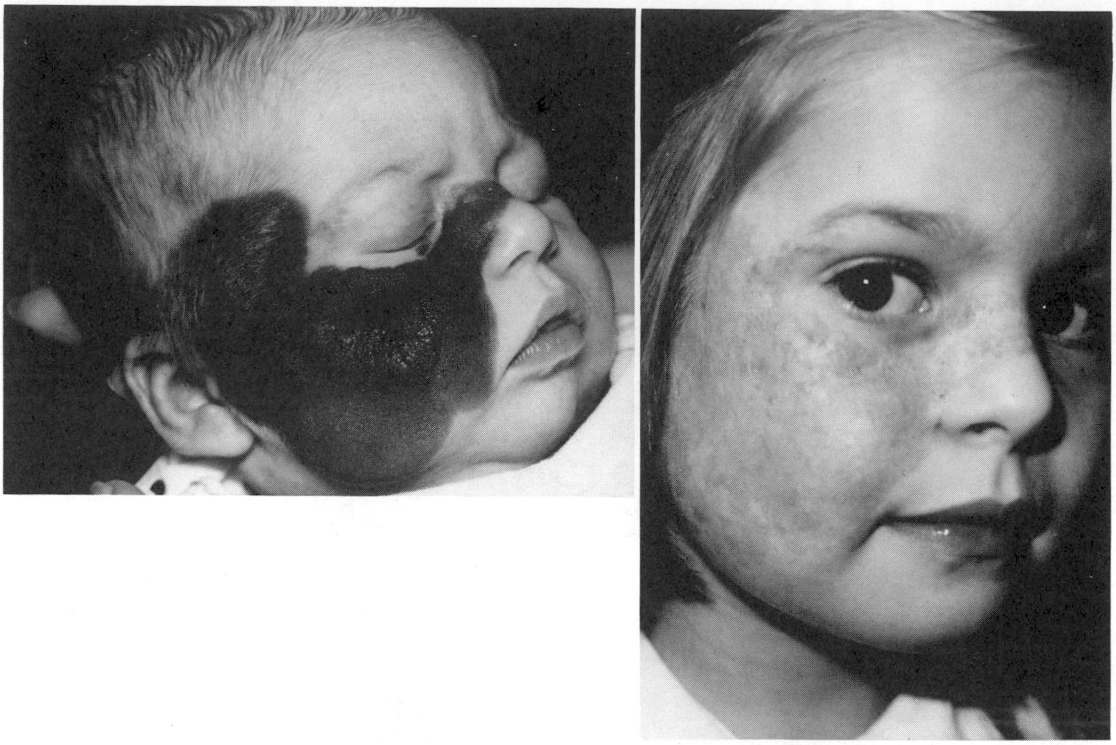

Fig. 13-11. Malignant melanoma. Malignant melanoma of back has metastasized to right axillary lymph nodes, causing large axillary mass.

Clark's levels of invasion by melanoma

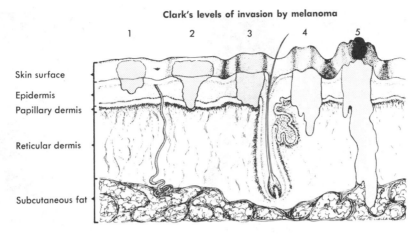

Fig. 13-12. Clark's five levels of invasion by melanoma.

mas in five levels (Fig. 13-12): (1) in situ, above basal lamina of epidermis; (2) extension through basal lamina into papillary layer; (3) tumor fills papillary level to the junction of the reticular dermal layer; (4) invasion into the reticular layer; and (5) invasion of subcutaneous fat. Breslow measures the thickness directly. Lesions less than 0.86 mm thick rarely metastasize. Depending on type and level, the prognosis for localized malignant melanomas ranges from 20% to 100% 5-year survival. Lymphatic spread reduces the expected survival to 15% or less, and bloodstream seeding cuts it to practically zero.

NERVE TISSUES

A *neuroma* (traumatic neurilemmoma) is an outgrowth of Schwann cells and axons mixed with scar tissue located at the proximal cut end of a severed nerve. (See discussion on benign tumors of the hand, Chap. 34.) A *neurilemmoma* is a discrete, encapsulated, benign tumor arising from the Schwann cells of peripheral nerves. It is usually solitary, but it may occur in neurofibromatosis. A *neurofibroma* (Fig. 13-13) is a benign, nonencapsulated, diffusely infiltrating benign tumor, usually found in multiple sites. At times neurofibromas cause strikingly grotesque deformities. They are usually associated with café-au-lait spots and are part of the hereditary disorder *von Recklinghausen's syndrome*. The multiplicity and permeation of the lesions can make a mockery of ablative surgery, though often the patient's appearance can be improved. Sarcomatous degeneration is a late complication.

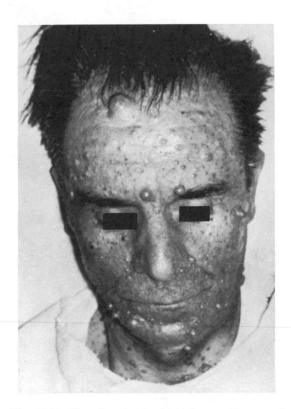

Fig. 13-13. Neurofibromatosis. Multiple neurofibromas of face in patient with von Recklinghausen's syndrome.

VASCULAR TISSUES

Capillary Hemangioma

The port-wine stain, or nevus flammeus, commonly appears as a large, flat, purplish blotch on the face or neck with no disruption of normal contour. It is present at birth, does not regress, and is important only because of its appearance. It can be camouflaged with skillful makeup. The argon laser is now the treatment of choice (Fig. 13-14). "Stork bites" are purplish areas of delicate capillary dilation on the nape of the neck, eyelids, or glabella of newborn babies, and they sub-

side before the child reaches 1 or 2 years of age. Strawberry mark (or nevus vasculosus; Fig. 13-15) is a highly cellular capillary hemangioma that appears as a raised, bright red lesion anywhere on the body. It regresses spontaneously.

Cavernous Hemangiomas

Involuting cavernous hemangiomas appear shortly after birth as small, blue-red lesions, commonly on the face or neck, which rapidly grow into large space-occu-

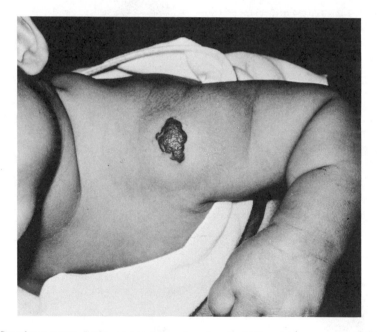

A   B

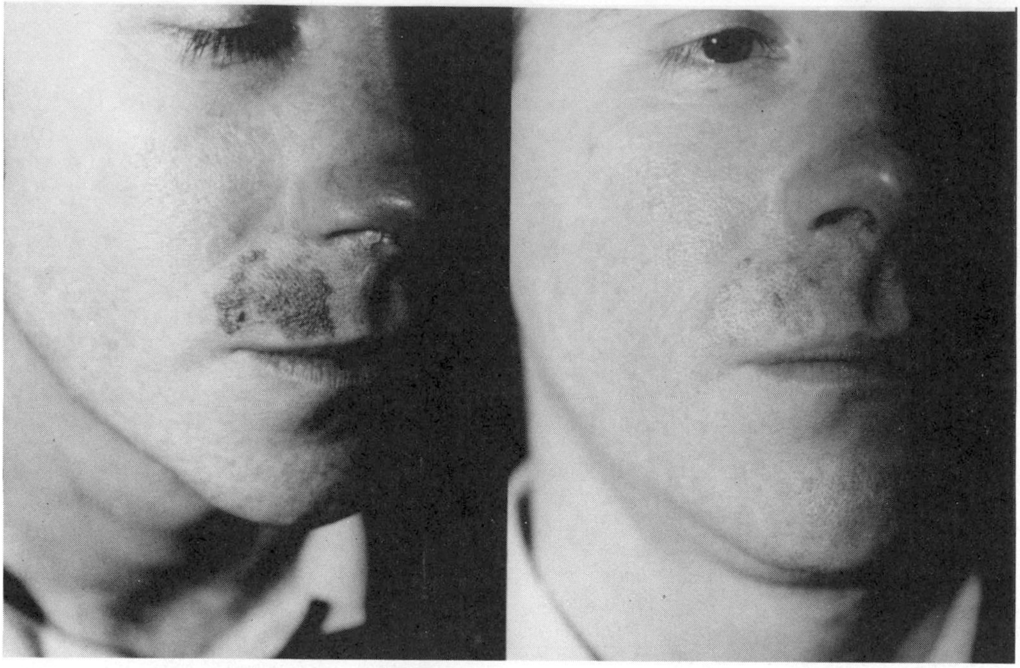

Fig. 13-14. A, Capillary hemangioma involving the right upper lip. **B,** Appearance after treatment with the argon laser. (Courtesy Dr. Bruce M. Achauer, University of California, Irvine Medical Center, Orange, Calif.)

Fig. 13-15. Strawberry nevus. Lesion appeared several weeks after birth and spontaneously subsided before 2 years of age.

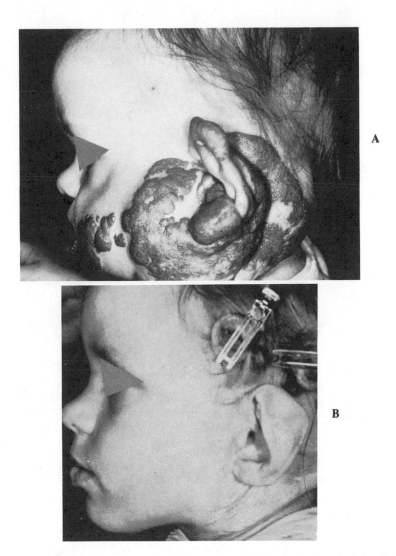

Fig. 13-16. Involuting cavernous hemangioma. **A,** Appearance at height of growth cycle during first year of life. **B,** Appearance several years after spontaneous involution. (Courtesy of Dr. Richard Caplan, University of Iowa Hospitals, Iowa City, Iowa)

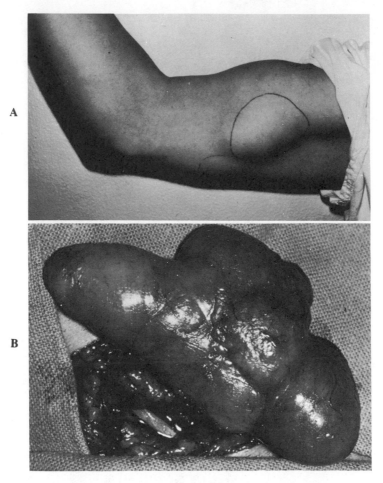

Fig. 13-17. Lipoma. **A,** Preoperative lumps on right arm, suspected to be lipomatous. **B,** Operative specimen showing fat lobulations of lipoma in contrast to pattern of adjacent subcutaneous fat.

pying masses that may cause grotesque disfigurement (Fig. 13-16). They usually involute before the age of 2 or 3 years, but they may leave in their wake distortion and displacement of facial features, which necessitates reconstructive surgery. Early excision may be needed to prevent amblyopia or airway obstruction. Pressure devices and steroid therapy may accelerate involution.

Ordinary cavernous hemangiomas may be of any size, shape, or location, may be multiple, and may be associated with arteriovenous fistulas, hemorrhage, or infection. Treatment is usually excision. At times location or size may make surgical attack impractical. Injection of sclerosing agents or steroids may be of help.

Malignant tumors of vessels are very rare and are highly malignant.

SUBCUTANEOUS FAT

Lipomas are soft, multilobulated, benign lumps of fat that have a color and texture different from that of immediately surrounding subcutaneous fat (Fig. 13-17). They are treated by excisional biopsy in order to differentiate them from malignant soft tissue tumors such as *liposarcoma, fibrosarcoma,* or *rhabdomyosarcoma.* If the mass is large, hard, and truly suspicious for malignancy, an incisional biopsy with study of permanent microscopic sections is the best prelude to definitive surgery.

14

Thyroid Gland

Richard D. Liechty

Physiology
Thyroid Medications
Diseases of the Thyroid

The normal human thyroid gland weighs only 20 to 30 g. As is true of other endocrine glands, its hormonal activity is far greater than one would expect from its size.

Thyroid hormones have three vitally important functions in man: (1) they control metabolism within the cells, (2) they have a profound effect on growth and development, and (3) they strongly influence tissue differentiation.

The cellular actions of these hormones remain poorly understood, but the clinical consequences of excesses or deficits of thyroid hormones are well known and most important. The diseases of function and structure of the thyroid gland are the main concern of this chapter.

PHYSIOLOGY

The thyroid gland is the only tissue in the body with the ability to store significant amounts of iodine. It combines the trapped iodine with tyrosine to form two active hormones, thyroxine tetraiodothyronine, (T_4), and triiodothyronine (T_3). These hormones, stored in the thyroid as thyroglobulins, are released into the circulation and are immediately bound to thyroid-binding globulin. The concentration of serum T_4 is about 40 times that of T_3. But the more potent T_3 accounts for at least half the total metabolic effect. Some researchers believe that T_4 is converted to T_3 and that T_3 is the only active hormone intracellularly.

Hypothalamic-Pituitary-Thyroid Triangle

The pituitary gland controls the thyroid gland through its thyroid-stimulating hormone (TSH), which is released by thyrotropin-releasing hormone (TRH) from the hypothalamus and which incites thyroid cells to produce and release thyroid hormones. Without the

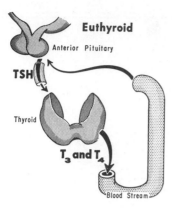

Fig. 14-1. Normal pituitary-thyroid relationship.

TSH stimulus, the thyroid gland (the target gland) is absolutely powerless to function, and it consequently atrophies.

The thyroid hormones, as they increase in the blood in response to TSH, inhibit or stop production of TSH. This negative feedback control system monitors the amount of thyroid hormones at a steady level. This level is "set" in brain centers (probably the hypothalamus), and TRH conveys this message to the responsive thyrotropic cells in the anterior pituitary (Fig. 14-1).

Understanding this hypothalamic-pituitary-thyroid feedback relationship is vital to understanding thyroid disease: whenever functioning thyroid tissue is ablated, thyroid hormones decrease and TSH increases (the blocking action of thyroid is removed). The increased TSH, in turn, stimulates any remaining thyroid tissue to grow.

On the other hand, when thyroid hormones are added, they block TSH and place the thyroid gland at rest. This latter effect explains the action of thyroid hormones in suppressing growth of goiters, nodules, and even some cancer, all of which theoretically arise in response to increased TSH. Exogenous thyroid hormones, acting much like a cast on an extremity, "splint" and rest the thyroid gland.

THYROID MEDICATIONS

Probably no other common drug is more misunderstood or misused than desiccated thyroid. The active substances in *desiccated thyroid* are T_4 and lesser amounts of T_3 purified from animal thyroids. It has a long action (up to 2 months) that peaks in 10 to 14 days. The normal daily requirement in adults is 120 to 180 mg. Giving subnormal amounts for losing weight or "pepping up" patients is worthless; 30 mg a day will suppress the production of TSH "30 mg worth." The feedback system goes into action, TSH drops, thyroid production decreases, and the consequent level of thyroid hormones remains the same.

Synthetic thyroid substances offer more predictable physiologic effects than desiccated thyroid does. T_3 (cytomel in its sodium form) acts rapidly (within hours) and probably is cleared from the body within a week (25 μg of T_3 is equal to 65 mg of desiccated thyroid). L-Thyroxine (Synthroid, T_4) acts less rapidly than T_3. The usual daily dose is 100 to 200 μg.

Normal adults require full replacement doses of any thyroid drug. The only valid indication for smaller doses is in beginning treatment of myxedema. These patients are sensitive to thyroid hormones, and the dosages must be increased gradually, especially in those with cardiac disease and in the elderly.

DISEASES OF THE THYROID

Thyroid disease may be divided into two main types: functional diseases and anatomical, or structural, diseases.

Functional Diseases
Hyperthyroidism (Graves' or Basedow's Disease, Thyrotoxicosis)

Hyperthyroidism is probably caused by an immunologic process; an abnormal protein mimicking TSH releases excess T_3 and T_4 (Fig. 14-2). At the present time thyrotoxicosis is best thought of as a runaway thyroid gland. TSH is low. The onset may be preceded by sudden emotional shock, such as the death of a loved one. Thyrotoxicosis is four times more common in women than in men. Secondary hyperthyroidism attributed to increased pituitary TSH secretion is rare.

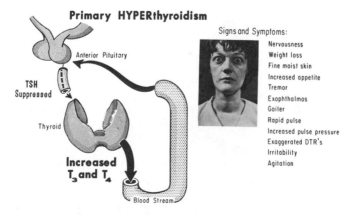

Signs and Symptoms:

Nervousness
Weight loss
Fine moist skin
Increased appetite
Tremor
Exophthalmos
Goiter
Rapid pulse
Increased pulse pressure
Exaggerated DTR's
Irritability
Agitation

Fig. 14-2. Primary hyperthyroidism. Excess thyroid hormones released by overactive thyroid gland. TSH is suppressed.

Clinical picture. The clinical picture of hyperthyroidism includes the following: nervousness, weight loss, fine moist skin, increased appetite, tremor, exophthalmos, goiter, rapid pulse, increased pulse pressure, exaggerated deep tendon reflexes, irritability, agitation, heat intolerance, and pretibial myxedema. Older patients show fewer signs and symptoms of hyperthyroidism; occasionally only refractory congestive heart failure or arrhythmias indicate thyrotoxicosis in older patients (masked hyperthyroidism). Severe hyperthyroidism in time may also appear paradoxically as a decrease in activity and appetite ("apathetic hyperthyroidism"). Such a state must be aggressively treated, even to forced feeding.

T_3 thyrotoxicosis appears rarely (1%) as a variant of thyrotoxicosis. The usual laboratory values remain low or normal, but elevated serum T_3 levels and failure to suppress (positive Werner's test) are diagnostic.

Laboratory tests. The most dependable thyroid screening tests are the serum T_4 level and the T_3 uptake test (Table 14-1).

The *serum thyroxine test* (T_4 test) measures the total serum T_4 (by displacement with radioactive T_4 or radioimmunoassay). Increased serum proteins, (chiefly thyroid-binding globulin (TBG)), cause falsely elevated T_4 values. Pregnancy and contraceptive agents are common causes of abnormally elevated serum proteins and, consequently, of falsely increased levels of serum T_4.

The *T_3 uptake test* measures thyroid function based on the binding capacity of the patient's serum proteins for a known amount of radioactive T_3. The patient's serum is incubated with a measured amount of radioactive T_3. The patient's unbound proteins bind the T_3. The excess or unbound radioactive T_3 is taken up on a resin sponge where it is measured by a radiation counter. A hyperthyroid patient, for example, will have fewer binding sites available on his TBG, thus the radioactive T_3 will be taken up in larger amounts by the resin sponge.

Conditions that cause increased serum proteins (pregnancy, contraceptive agents) will cause falsely depressed T_3 values, but these same conditions falsely elevate the T_4 test. Thus, by obtaining both T_4 and T_3 uptake tests and free T_4 index, the physician can evaluate a patient's thyroid function despite abnormal serum proteins.

The *^{131}I uptake test* measures the amount of radioactive iodine taken up by the thyroid in 4 hours and 24 hours. A scintillation counter records the uptake in percentages of radioactivity given. In addition to measuring thyroid activity, the radioactive iodine in the thyroid gland can be mapped by a scintillation scanner to show the size and shape of the gland *(a thyroid scan)*.

The *TSH test* measures plasma TSH. It is elevated with hypothyroidism, after total thyroidectomy, or with any disease that lowers T_4 or T_3. Conversely, hyperthyroidism or exogenous thyroid depresses TSH. *TSH response to TRH* is an extremely sensitive test that is often blunted in early hyperthyroidism even before T_3 and T_4 levels rise. An excellent test for incipient hyperthyroidism, it has largely replaced the T_3 suppression test.

Treatment of thyrotoxicosis. Three methods for treatment of thyrotoxicosis are commonly employed:

antithyroid drugs, surgery, and radioactive iodine (^{131}I). Surgery and ^{131}I permanently *ablate* thyroid tissue; antithyroid drugs only *block* thyroid function by blocking hormone synthesis by thyroid tissue (Table 14-2). Unfortunately, thyrotoxicosis often recurs when drug therapy is discontinued. Therefore in most instances ablation of thyroid tissue is the preferred treatment. Many physicians do not favor using ^{131}I in young (or pregnant) women or children because of fear of irradiation. Before surgical removal of the thyroid gland, thyrotoxicosis *must* be controlled by antithyroid drugs to prevent *thyroid storm*. Thyroid storm is probably caused by massive release of thyroid hormones at operation or during other stress. A frighteningly rapid pulse, high fever, and rapid fluid loss can result in death. Fluids, steroids, antithyroid drugs, hypothermia, and adrenergic blocking agents, especially propranolol, headline the current therapy. Prevention by proper patient preparation is the best treatment. Advantages and disadvantages of the three treatment methods are summarized in Table 14-3.

Prognosis. The treatment of hyperthyroidism is most gratifying. All the signs and symptoms of thyrotoxicosis predictably diminish with treatment, except for exophthalmos.

Exophthalmos. A most distressing symptom, exophthalmos is usually accompanied by chemosis. Leukocytic infiltration and retroorbital mucopolysaccharide deposition characterize the underlying pathology. Treatment includes rapid control of the hyperthyroidism, wearing dark glasses, and prednisone. In most cases, the exophthalmos gradually recedes over months or years. For severe or malignant exophthalmos, tarsorrhaphy and, rarely, orbital decompression may be necessary to prevent optic nerve injury and blindness.

Hypothyroidism (Myxedema)

Cause. The most common cause of myxedema is *spontaneous atrophy* of the thyroid gland (Fig. 14-3). An autoimmune mechanism (sensitization to thyroxine) may play a role in this process. The second leading cause of myxedema is treatment of hyperthyroidism with ^{131}I. In some series the incidence approaches 50% of patients treated in follow-up studies of 10 years or more. TSH serum levels are usually increased. Failure of TSH production (secondary myxedema) because of pituitary failure is rare. Hypothyroidism may vary from mild signs and symptoms to the full-blown picture of myxedema.

Clinical picture. The clinical picture of myxedema includes coarse thick hair, dry skin, puffy face, deep voice, yellow skin (carotenemia), sluggish reflexes, and constipation. In more severe cases ascites, pleural and pericardial effusions, paralytic ileus, hypothermia, and coma appear. The diagnosis is strongly suggested by a serum T_4 below 4 μg/dl, a T_3 uptake below 25%, a decreased ^{131}I uptake below 5% and 10% (4 hours and 24 hours), and elevated serum TSH levels.

Treatment. Perhaps no other disease responds to treatment more successfully than myxedema. Small doses of thyroid substances initially, increasing to full replacement doses (100-150 mg synthroid) restore normal function in almost all patients.

Table 14-1. Important Diagnostic Thyroid Tests

Test	Normal Values	Theory	Comments
Serum thyroxine	4-11 μg/dl	Measures total thyroxine in serum	Neither inorganic nor organic iodides interfere; increased serum proteins elevate values; decreased serum proteins depress values
T_3-resin uptake test (T_3RU)	25%-35%	Measures excess radioactive T_3 that becomes absorbed on resin; in toxic patients the protein molecules are "saturated"; thus radioactive T_3 will be absorbed on resins	Radioactive T_3 is incubated with patient's blood in vitro; can be used in pregnancy; not affected by I_2 or antithyroid drugs; thus can be used to check patients treated with these drugs; low serum proteins cause falsely increased values; increased serum proteins cause falsely depressed values
Free thyroxine index	4.6-16	Multiplying $T_4 \times T_3$ resin uptake (and dividing by mean value of T_3RU) gives artificial number that corrects for increases or decreases in thyroid binding proteins.	Excellent screening test for thyroid function; especially useful in pregnancy or patients taking birth control medications
Radioactive iodine (^{131}I) uptake	15%-40% at 4 and 24 hours	Measures amount and rate that thyroid takes up ^{131}I in 4 and 24 hours	A reliable test; not used during pregnancy; I_2 and antithyroid drugs block this test
Serum T_3	96-172 ng/dl	T_3 may be ultimate, active product of T_4	Valuable in diagnosing T_3 thyrotoxicosis; other tests usually normal
Scintiscan	Normal glands show an even distribution of ^{131}I throughout gland	^{131}I map of thyroid	Cysts, nodules, and cancer may be "cold"; little help in picking out malignant nodules; one definite asset is recording thyroid metastases to other areas (neck, bones, etc.)
Suppression test	4- and 24 hour ^{131}I uptake is depressed by 50% (after suppression with 5 day course of T_3)	The pituitary-thyroid axis is tested by oral exogenous T_3 to suppress TSH; normal patients suppress by 50%; toxic patients do not suppress	Very useful in determining the borderline hyperthyroid patients, when other laboratory values are equivocal
TSH	Values vary with laboratory	Elevated with any disease that depresses thyroid function; decreased with hyperthyroidism or exogenous thyroxine	Excellent method to check adequacy of thyroid suppression
TSH response to TRH	Values vary with laboratory	Tests hypothalmic-pituitary-thyroid triangle Exaggerated response in hypothyroidism Flat response in thyrotoxicosis Flat response, with normal or low TSH, points to pituitary failure	Completed in 2-3 hours Gradually replacing suppression test Extremely sensitive; will detect hyperthyroidism before T_4 rises

Anatomic or Structural Diseases
Goiters and Nodules

A *goiter* is, by definition, an enlargement of the thyroid gland. A goiter may be diffusely enlarged (simple goiter) or nodular (nodular goiter). A nodule may occur in an otherwise normal gland; these are called solitary thyroid nodules.

The most common cause of goiter is a deficiency in iodine ingestion or metabolism (endemic goiter). The thyroid responds by increasing in size in an effort

Table 14-2. Antithyroid Drugs—Dosage and Action

Drug	Dosage	Action
Thiocarbamides		
Propylthiouracil	100-300 mg q.6-8 hours	Blocks organic binding of iodine and prevents conversion of T_4 to T_3
Methimazole (Tapazole)	5-30 mg q.6-8 hours	Blocks organic binding of iodine
Iodine (Lugol's solution)	5-10 drops daily	Decreases blood flow to thyroid
Propranolol	40-720 mg/day, divided doses	β-Receptor blocking agent relieves toxic symptoms

Table 14-3. Comparison of Three Common Methods of Treatment of Hyperthyroidism

Method	Action	Advantages	Disadvantages
I. Antithyroid drugs	Block thyroid hormone synthesis	1. Avoids surgery and irradiation	1. High incidence of drug reaction, blood dyscrasias, skin reaction 2. Frequent visits to physician necessary 3. Recurrence rate high when therapy discontinued
II. Surgery	Removal of functioning tissue	1. Most rapid method of permanent control 2. Avoids irradiation	Complications of surgery 1. Damage to recurrent laryngeal nerves 2. Damage to parathyroid glands (1%) 3. Wound complications 4. Permanent hypothyroidism (<10%; leaving 10 g remnants of thyroid)
III. ^{131}I	Radioactive destruction of thyroid cells	1. Avoids surgery 2. Permanent control 3. Avoids drug reaction	1. Danger of irradiation 2. Hypothyroidism rate is high, 50% or more in 10 years; probably 100% in 20 years 3. Often treatment period is lengthy (up to 2 years) 4. Contraindicated in pregnancy and in very young patients

to produce the necessary thyroid hormones. Nodules and cysts may form as a consequence of thyroid enlargement.

Another cause of goiter is the ebb and rise of metabolic stress such as menstrual cycles and pregnancy. This explains why women have five times more goiters and nodules than men do.

Thyroiditis and malignancy also cause thyroid enlargement and will be discussed separately.

Solitary thyroid nodules (Fig. 14-4 and Table 14-4) are suggestive of malignancy because they arise in a gland otherwise normal to palpation. About 50% of these "solitary" growths are really dominant nodules in a multinodular goiter; the other nodules are too small to be palpated clinically. Some of them are "new growths"; thus all solitary nodules should be evaluated for malignancy by fine needle aspiration biopsy or large cutting needle biopsy. These tests yield cells for cytologic study and tissue specimens for histologic study. They are most accurate in the diagnosis of papillary

Table 14-4. Pathology of Solitary Nodules of Thyroid (From Composite Studies)

Multinodular goiters	50%
Adenomas	20
Cancer	20
Thyroiditis	5
Cysts	5
TOTAL	100

cancer (psammoma bodies and ground-glass nuclei) and lymphocytic thyroiditis (lymphocytes and fibrous trabeculas). They are least accurate in the diagnosis of follicular cancer. The most helpful of all preoperative tests, needle biopsies give more definitive information than scintiscans or ultrasound imaging. Scintiscans may show "cold" nodules, but these are usually cysts or benign adenomas rather than cancer. Similarly, ultrasound may differentiate cystic from solid lesions, but so will needle aspiration, and at far less cost.

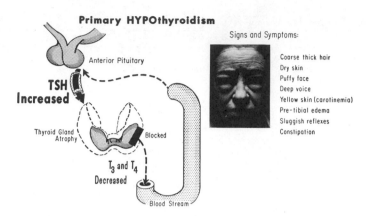

Fig. 14-3. Primary hypothyroidism. Most common cause is spontaneous atrophy. Thyroid hormones are diminished. TSH and TRH are increased.

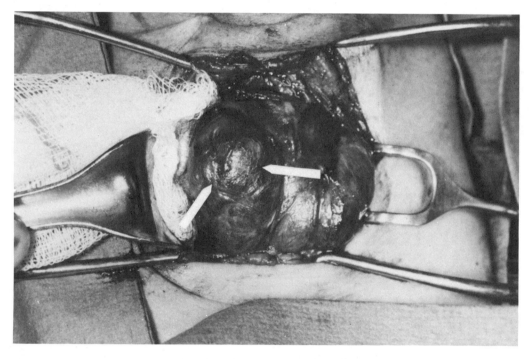

Fig. 14-4. Solitary nodule in right lobe of thyroid.

Treatment of goiters and nodules. As a useful rule, all *solitary nodules are considered malignant* until proved benign; all *multinodular goiters are considered benign* until some evidence is suggestive of malignancy. The incidence of malignancy in *clinically solitary* thyroid nodules is about 20% nationwide. No infallible test short of microscopic diagnosis can detect the dangerous nodules. If needle biopsy specimens are abnormal or equivocal, the nodules should be excised with margins of surrounding normal tissue (lobectomy). Many soft nodules that occur in pregnancy will regress in response to suppressive doses of desiccated thyroid or after the pregnancy is terminated; thus these nodules can be treated conservatively.

Diffuse and multinodular goiters are not removed routinely. Small, palpable nodular goiters are very common (5% to 10% of adults); thyroid cancer is uncommon. Thus operative mortality for routine thyroidectomy would likely exceed any saving of life from thyroid cancer. We operate only on suspicious goiters, rapidly growing nodules, hard or fixed lobes or nodules within the goiter, or evidence of cervical metastasis. Goiters are removed also for cosmetic reasons or for obstruction of the trachea or esophagus. Since nodules occurring in children carry a high risk of malignancy, all such nodules should be excised and examined.

Thyroiditis

Thyroiditis is a general term that describes the five types of inflammatory diseases of the thyroid gland. The lymphocytic type is by far the most common.

The five types of thyroiditis and the approximate relative incidence are as follows:

	Number of cases
Lymphocytic type (Hashimoto's struma, struma lymphomatosa)	100
Viral type (subacute, granulomatous, de Quervain's)	10
"Silent" type	1
Riedel's (woody)	0.1
Suppurative (acute, bacterial)	<0.1

Clinical characteristics

Lymphocytic type. Lymphocytic thyroiditis is probably caused by an autoimmune mechanism. Thyroid tissue becomes sensitized to its own hormones, resulting in an invasion of lymphocytes and fibrous tissue. A diffuse, rubbery, nontender goiter results. The thyroid and mesenchymal antibody titers are usually elevated. Although chiefly afflicting woman 20 to 50 years of age, it is the most common cause of goiter in children. Many believe it eventually leads to myxedema. Biopsy and replacement of thyroid (T_3 or T_4) keynote the treatment.

Viral type. Viral thyroiditis causes a tender, diffuse enlargement or occasionally a tender nodule, mild fever, increased sedimentation rate, and general malaise. Bed rest, sedation, aspirin, and, in extreme cases, steroids to reduce inflammation are the usual methods of treatment. Biopsy diagnosis is rarely necessary for the skilled clinician.

"Silent" thyroiditis. This new form of thyroiditis mimics Graves' disease at first. It features both lymphocytes and granulomas. Self-limiting, it may result in persistent goiter, hypothyroidism, or both.

Riedel's type. Riedel's type is very rare. Associated with fibrosclerosis elsewhere (mediastinum, retroperitoneum), the gland becomes woody hard. Because it mimics the firmness of cancer, it demands biopsy and treatment with replacement doses of T_3 or T_4.

Acute suppurative thyroiditis. Acute suppurative thyroiditis is a medical oddity. Having seen only one case, I mention this entity last to emphasize its rarity. The source of bacterial thyroiditis is most often abscessed teeth. Treatment, as with any abscess, includes drainage and antibiotics.

Cancer

Cancer of the thyroid has an extremely wide range of behavior. It is rivaled in this respect only by breast cancer among the common malignancies. Most differentiated types grow slowly over years. The undifferentiated types grow rapidly and may be lethal within weeks or months. Since most undifferentiated types afflict older adults, advanced age often signals an ominous prognosis. Cancer of the thyroid may be classified as follows:

Differentiated 80%	Intermediate 5%	Undifferentiated 15%
Papillary	Medullary	Small cell
Follicular		Large cell
Mixed papillofollicular		Sarcomas

Papillary cancer occurs in children and young adults of the third and fourth decade, often with a history of prior irradiation to the neck area. It is the most common thyroid malignancy. For small lesions (1.5 cm) with no metastases, lobectomy alone is often adequate treatment. With progression of the tumor, metastases usually appear in the neck and grow slowly. Total thyroidectomy and excision of regional metastases form the basic treatment. Total thyroidectomy accomplishes two objectives: it removes thyroid tissue that competes with tumor for ^{131}I and it removes possible multicentric foci of tumor. When cervical spread has occurred, most surgeons prefer conservative removal of only the involved tissues. The patient is allowed to become hypothyroid. If residual tumor is shown to take up iodine, ^{131}I is given in large therapeutic doses. TSH, or a thiouracil drug to increase the body's TSH, often increases the ^{131}I uptake in the metastases. Suppressive doses of thyroid are administered for the remainder of the patient's life.

Follicular cancer tends to metastasize distantly and occurs in a slightly older age group (fifth decade). Before ^{131}I treatment, total thyroidectomy prepares the patient by removing tumor and allowing any remaining metastases to pick up ^{131}I more effectively.

Mixed type is a commonly occurring composite of the preceding two types. A variant of papillary cancer, it is treated accordingly.

Medullary cancers contain varying amounts of amyloid and carry an intermediate prognosis. The 10-year survival rate exceeds 60% in resectable cases. Medullary cancers tend to be familial and are associated with pheochromocytomas, hyperparathyroidism, and neurofibromatosis. Some medullary cancers produce calcitonin. Elevated levels of serum calcitonin have predicted medullary cancers, preoperatively, in family members who carry this trait.

Undifferentiated thyroid cancer is aggressively malignant. It occurs in older people and rarely takes up [131]I. Radical surgical excision, chemotherapy, and external irradiation are the only, and usually ineffective, treatment.

Sarcomas of various types are rare. Occasionally, wide excision will offer a favorable prognosis.

15

Parathyroid Glands

Richard D. Liechty

A multihormonal system regulates calcium, magnesium, and phosphate homeostasis in all vertebrates. The organs involved in this regulation are bone, kidney, and gut, and the major hormones are parathyroid hormone (parathormone, PTH), calcitonin (CT), and vitamin D. In general PTH and vitamin D act in concert with (but opposing) CT to maintain serum calcium between 9.0 and 10.5 mg/dl. Calcium regulates neuromuscular excitability, blood coagulation, membrane function, secretory processes, and many enzyme reactions; to maintain these vital functions, nature zealously keeps calcium within these narrow limits.

ANATOMY AND EMBRYOLOGY

Man normally has four parathyroid glands situated close to the posterior surface of the thyroid, one gland near each pole. Each gland should weigh no more than 70 mg. Their weight and their location make the parathyroid glands liable to accidental removal or damage during thyroid surgery. The parathyroid glands, derived from the third and fourth branchial pouches, differentially migrate caudally so that the lower pair come from the third pouch and the upper pair from the fourth. About 10% of parathyroid glands are ectopically located within the thyroid, thymus, superior mediastinum, and even pericardium. Histologically, parathyroid glands contain cords of chief and oxyphilic cells. Chief cells, subdivided into water-clear and dark cells according to their content of secretory granules, secrete PTH. Most adenomas feature dark cells; hyperplastic parathyroid glands arise from either cell.

Calcitonin comes from C-cells (for calcitonin) derived from the ultimobranchial body. These cells disperse into thyroid, thymus, and parathyroid tissues in man. They resemble adrenal medullary cells and pan-

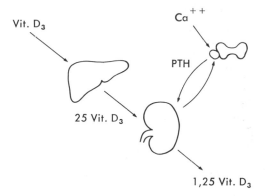

Fig. 15-1. Vitamin D_3, a hormone. Renal parenchymal cells convert vitamin D_3 to 1,25-$(OH)_2$ vitamin D_3 under influence of two stimuli: (1) elevated PTH or (2) lowered serum PO_4. PTH and 1,25-$(OH)_2$ vitamin D_3 form feedback control system. Kidney is endocrine organ and 1,25-$(OH)_2$ vitamin D_3 is hormone.

creatic alpha cells, with which they probably share a common origin.

PHYSIOLOGY (Figs. 15-1 and 15-2)

PTH, a polypeptide hormone, elevates plasma calcium levels in three ways. First, it shifts calcium from bone to plasma, probably by stimulating osteoclasts. Second, it inhibits tubular resorption of phosphate, thus promoting phosphaturia, while enhancing calcium reabsorption. Third, it stimulates the conversion of 25-OH vitamin D_3 to 1,25-$(OH)_2$ vitamin D_3 (1,25-dihydroxycholecalciferol) in the kidney. In turn, 1,25-$(OH)_2$ vitamin D_3 incites the intestinal absorption of calcium and phosphorus. This potent metabolite of vitamin D_3 also helps shift calcium from bone to plasma, but only in the presence of PTH. Low phosphorus and high PTH levels turn on the kidney's 1-hydroxylation mechanism; high phosphorus and low PTH levels turn it off. This dual control provides the body with a constant supersaturated solution of calcium and phosphorus, ions vital to cell metabolism (cardiac conduction, ATP) and bone metabolism.

Calcitonin, by suppressing osteoclastic activity, will antagonize any sudden rise in calcium levels. Thus these three hormones, coupled with their classical feedback systems (PTH and calcium; PTH and vitamin D_3; calcitonin and calcium), maintain plasma calcium and phosphorus concentrations at remarkably constant levels. They control these levels precisely despite widely varying intakes and body demands.

Calcium circulating in blood and extracellular fluid represents less than 1% of the total body content. About half is in an active, or ionized, form; the rest is protein bound or un-ionized and therefore biochemically inactive. Calcium binds chiefly to albumin; lesser amounts bind to globulins. To correct for variations in serum proteins, they should be measured along with serum calcium levels. About 0.9 mg calcium is bound per gram of protein, allowing for a rough estimation of the ionized calcium level. The binding of calcium to albumin is enhanced by alkalosis (e.g., the tetany of hyperventilation) and decreased by acidosis.

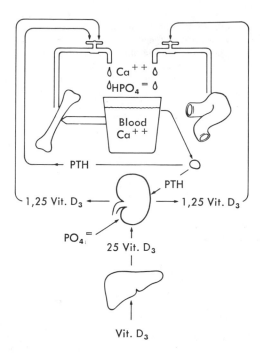

Fig. 15-2. PTH-vitamin D interaction. Vitamin D_3 is hydroxylated in liver to 25-OH vitamin D_3. Kidney adds another hydroxyl group to make 1,25-$(OH)_2$ vitamin D_3. This sterol stimulates intestinal absorption of Ca^{++}. It also releases calcium from bone but only when PTH is present. High PTH + low $PO_4^=$ levels turn on 1-hydroxylase mechanism.

HYPERPARATHYROIDISM
Primary Hyperparathyroidism

Clinical features. About one case of primary hyperparathyroidism emerges from every 900 carefully screened hospital admissions. Ionizing radiation, postmenopausal state, sunless climates, and thiazide therapy have all been linked to hyperparathyroidism. It rarely afflicts children and is most common in women, especially older women. This disease results from the autonomous and increased secretion of PTH, usually from neoplastic transformation (Fig. 15-3). About 80% of patients with hyperparathyroidism have as the cause a single parathyroid adenoma; hyperplasia, multiple adenomas, or a mixture of the two (and rarely cancer) account for the rest. Most pathologists agree that distinguishing hyperplastic from adenomatous tissue, especially on frozen section, is unreliable, if not impossible.

Cancers of other organs commonly elevate serum calcium, chiefly from osteolytic metastases, but some tumors (notably in the lung and kidney) secrete a PTH-like substance and thus mimic primary hyperparathyroidism.

The nonspecific symptoms of muscle weakness, fatigue, nausea, anorexia, constipation, mental changes, polyuria, polydipsia, and renal colic and infections characterize hypercalcemia. Between 60% and 75% of patients have detectable renal involvement including stones or gravel, repeated infections, hematuria, nephrocalcinosis, and azotemia. About 5% to 10% of all patients with renal stones prove to have hyperparathyroidism. Clinical bone involvement caused by excessive resorption is found in about 20% of patients. Most often this is diffuse, resembling osteoporosis. Less frequently seen now are the classical lesions of osteitis fibrosa cystica. Fig. 15-4 shows subperiosteal resorption, which is diagnostic. This resorption usually involves the fingers and lateral third of the clavicles. Hypertension accompanies hyperparathyroidism with greater than expected frequency (about 40%).

Hyperparathyroidism, usually featuring chief cell hyperplasia or adenomas, runs in some families. Pheochromocytomas and medullary thyroid carcinomas, multiple endocrine neoplasia (MEN II), and pituitary and pancreatic islet tumors (MEN I), characterize these syndromes of multiple endocrine neoplasia. Peptic ulcer, pancreatitis, and hypertension increase in incidence with hyperparathyroidism and often defy therapy until the adenoma is removed. All patients with these diseases should have a serum calcium determination. Occasionally the serum calcium will become acutely and severely elevated, leading to a life-threatening coma—a *parathyroid crisis*.

Diagnosis. The causes of hypercalcemia in hospitalized patients are as follows:

Bone metastases	55%
Hyperparathyroidism	20%
Ectopic PTH	15%
Other causes	10%
Thiazide ingestion	
Sarcoidosis	
Vitamin D poisoning	
Milk-alkali syndrome	
Thyrotoxicosis	
Adrenal failure	

Differential diagnosis. Asymptomatic patients with mild hypercalcemia for a year or more who deny excessive intake of milk products and vitamins and have no family history of endocrine disorders virtually all have hyperparathyroidism. Elevated serum PTH levels (Fig. 15-5), depressed phosphorus levels, and a chloride-to-phosphorus ratio of more than 33 further confirm the diagnosis. In addition, elevated serum alkaline phosphatase indicates the degree of bone destruction. Hyperchloremia, mild metabolic acidosis, and hyperuricemia often coexist. Hypercalciuria is common, but the total calcium excretion is usually less than 400 mg/day because PTH promotes calcium resorption.

A long duration of hypercalcemia without weight loss eliminates malignant disease, both osteolytic and ectopic. The lack of familial hypercalcemia, of hypocalciuria, and of early onset (before age 10 years) rules out familial hypocalciuric hypercalcemia (FHH). The absence of symptoms and signs of the other causes of hypercalcemia effectively eliminates them from consideration. The tests used in the differential diagnosis of hyperparathyroidism (listed in order of importance) are as follows:

Serum
    Calcium
    PTH
    Phosphate
    Chloride
    Alkaline phosphatase
    Uric acid
    Total protein/albumin
    Hematocrit (HCT)
    Sedimentation rate
    pH
    Blood urea nitrogen (BUN)
    Creatinine
Other tests
    Urinary calcium, urinalysis, chest film, kidney-ure-

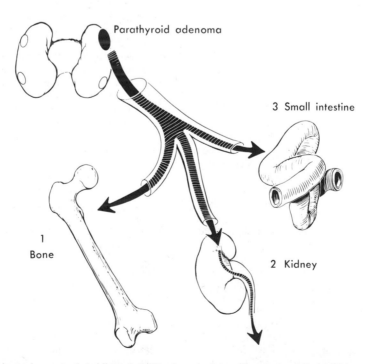

Fig. 15-3. Primary hyperparathyroidism. *1*, PTH releases calcium from bone while inhibiting new bone formation. *2*, PTH promotes renal reabsorption of calcium and inhibits tubular reabsorption of phosphate, *3*, PTH stimulates 1,25-$(OH)_2$ vitamin D_3 secretion, and this hormone increases intestinal absorption of calcium.

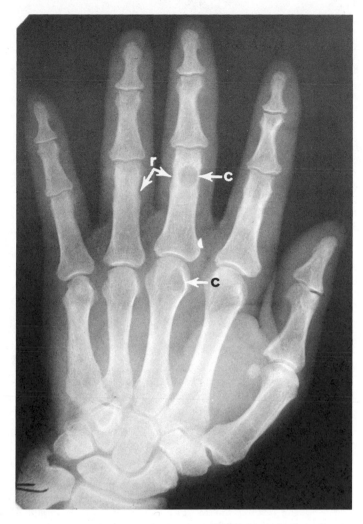

Fig. 15-4. Radiologically diagnostic lesions of subperiosteal resorption, *r,* and associated cysts, *c.* Such lesions are more likely demonstrable in patients with large adenomas.

ter-bladder (KUB) abdomen, or intravenous pyelogram, hydrocortisone suppression test, urinary or nephrogenous cAMP

LOCALIZING PROCEDURES

The thallium–technetium 99m (^{99}Tc) pertechnectate scan is based on the finding that both thyroid and parathyroid glands take up thallium but only the thyroid takes up ^{99}Tc. Image subtraction usually identifies enlarged parathyroid glands with an accuracy of about 50% to 75%. Ultrasound best detects tumors in or near the thyroid gland. The overall accuracy is about 75%. Computed tomography (CT) is not as accurate as ultrasound in picking up tumors near the thyroid gland, but it often outlines larger glands in distant locations. Arteriography (Fig. 15-6) and venous sampling for PTH can sometimes be helpful, but they are invasive procedures.

Before the initial operation, most experienced surgeons forego these costly procedures since the operation will be curative in 95% of cases. With repeat operations, however, these tests become extremely helpful.

Therapy

Three problems complicate surgical treatment: there may be more than the normal four glands; 10% of adenomas arise ectopically (Fig. 15-6); and frozen section diagnosis often fails to distinguish between hyperplasia and adenoma. Knowing that the initial operation allows him the golden chance to evaluate the pathologic parathyroid condition, the surgeon must plan the operation methodically.

Because 3% of patients will have multiple adenomas and 15% hyperplasia, the surgeon must attempt to identify all four glands, no matter how tedious and time-consuming this may prove. The one enlarged gland must be removed if three other normal or atrophic ones are found, and if only three glands are found, the thyroid and thymus on the side of the missing gland is resected. Parathyroid glands may lie totally within thyroid or thymus tissue. Subtotal parathyroidectomy (three and one-half glands removed) is the procedure of choice (1) for gross enlargement of more than one gland, (2) if all glands appear normal or minimally en-

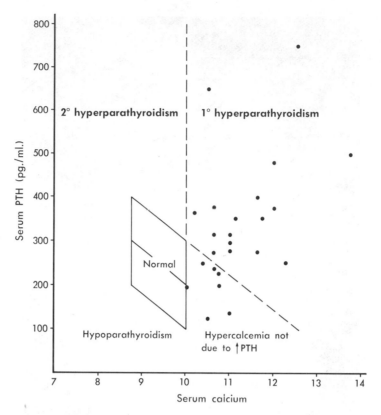

Fig. 15-5. PTH levels help differentiate causes of hypercalcemia. High levels of both calcium and PTH indicate primary hyperparathyroidism. Low levels of PTH with high levels of calcium point to some other cause. (See causes listed under "Differential diagnosis.")

larged with no evidence of a fifth gland, (3) for familial parathyroid disease, or (4) for chronic, mild renal insufficiency. An alternative procedure involves removing all glands and transplanting a remnant (about 50 to 70 mg) into neck or arm muscle. The remnant must be divided into 1 mm to 2 mm fragments that are dispersed into muscle pockets. Some surgeons use subcutaneous pockets. These plans offer the greatest chance for permanent cure with minimal risk of permanent hypoparathyroidism or recurrence.

Parathyroid crisis (Ca^{++} 15 mg/dl or higher) calls for immediate action, including intravenous phosphates, saline diuresis, and mithramycin or calcitonin infusions. These measures aim at lowering the serum calcium before *urgent* exploration.

When operative removal is not feasible, chronic medical treatment with oral phosphate-phosphorus (2 to 5 g/day) can normalize serum calcium levels in most patients. Many physicians prefer mithramycin because they fear renal precipitation of calcium phosphates.

Secondary Hyperparathyroidism

In chronic renal failure the kidney's 1-hydroxylation mechanism fails, causing 1,25-$(OH)_2$ vitamin D_3 levels to drop. To compensate, PTH increases, and in time the stressed parathyroid glands become hyperplastic. The elevated levels of PTH, if sustained, produce renal osteodystrophy, a painful, often crippling, bone disease. Because the diseased kidneys lose their ability to

excrete phosphorus, plasma phosphorus levels increase. This elevation further suppresses 1-hydroxylation and favors ectopic calcifications. Although calcium levels tend to remain normal or even low, increased phosphate levels (exceeding the solubility coefficient) favor deposition of calcium phosphate salts, which can obstruct vital arteries (coronary, renal). Thus *renal osteodystrophy* and *ectopic calcifications* characterize advanced renal failure with secondary hyperparathyroidism. PTH remains under feedback control but only by higher levels of calcium. The treatment of secondary hyperparathyroidism includes (1) treatment of the renal disease, (2) 1,25-$(OH)_2$ vitamin D_3 to bypass the defective 1-hydroxylation mechanism, and (3) low-phosphate diet. In almost all instances this regimen, which on occasion includes renal transplantation, will control the secondary hyperparathyroidism.

Tertiary Hyperparathyroidism

Occasionally, the normal feedback controls fail. Hyperplastic parathyroid glands become autonomous, causing calcium levels to rise to dangerous levels. These conditions of tertiary hyperparathyroidism call for subtotal parathyroidectomy. In advanced stages the glands can enlarge to 50 times their normal weight or more. In our hospital we resect all but 50 to 70 mg of tissue. By transplanting this remnant in forearm muscles, we can check its viability, monitor the amount of PTH produced, and, if necessary, easily

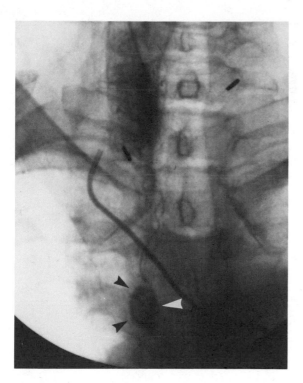

Fig. 15-6. Arteriogram showing ectopic parathyroid adenoma in mediastinum.

gain access to resect more tissue should it continue its hyperplastic growth.

HYPOPARATHYROIDISM
Classification and Clinical Features

Hypoparathyroidism, characterized by hypocalcemia and hyperphosphatemia, can result from loss of glandular function or from end organ resistance to PTH action. Hypoparathyroidism most commonly occurs after removal of the glands or damage to their blood supply during thyroid surgery. Within a few hours neuromuscular irritability emerges as muscle spasms or cramps and paresthesias, particularly of the hands, face, and feet. Tapping the facial nerve results in facial muscle contractions (Chvostek's sign), whereas application of an inflated blood pressure cuff leads to carpal spasm (Trousseau's sign). Pronounced hypocalcemia can induce laryngeal spasm and convulsions. This syndrome can be transient or permanent. Hypocalcemia often occurs in the 24 to 48 hours immediately after removal of a parathyroid adenoma. Although usually transient, this relative hypoparathyroidism can require treatment for months, especially when the bones have suffered chronic calcium "starvation" from extensive dissolution.

Treatment

For acute hypocalcemia, intravenous calcium gluconate will bring immediate relief. This is later changed to oral calcium carbonate (5 to 15 g/day) or other calcium salts.

Vitamin D remains the keystone of long-term treatment. The most effective form, $1,25\text{-}(OH)_2$ vitamin D_3, has distinct advantages: small doses (daily dose about 0.5 to $1\mu g$), rapid action (within hours), and similarly rapid withdrawal. This final active metabolite of vitamin D_3 remains independent of renal conversion and, therefore, effective regardless of renal function. Permanent hypocalcemia requires careful treatment to prevent cataracts and basal ganglia calcification, which causes Parkinson-like symptoms.

Idiopathic Hypoparathyroidism

The rare disease idiopathic hypoparathyroidism attacks in childhood or middle age. Cataracts, basal ganglia calcification, mental retardation, and cutaneous involvement such as candidiasis, brittle nails, and patchy hair characterize the childhood disease. Usually the glands are absent or atrophic. Symptoms often are chronic and insidious in onset, particularly in the adult.

Pseudohypoparathyroidism

Pseudohypoparathyroidism is an interesting example of end organ (kidney) resistance to the effects of a hormone. These patients have all the chemical and clinical features of hypoparathyroidism yet have elevated PTH levels. The kidneys of these patients fail to give the normal phosphaturic response to PTH. This genetic disease also includes peculiar skeletal abnormalities (stunting, short metacarpals) that distinguish it from the idiopathic form.

16

Adrenal Glands

Richard D. Liechty

Physiology
Diseases of the Adrenal Cortex
Diseases of Adrenal Medulla

Nature has fashioned the mammalian adrenal gland in a curious way. Taking two separate embryonic tissues, it has fused them, as adrenal cortex (mesoderm) and medulla (ectoderm), into one gland. Despite this anatomic merger that allows the cortex to bathe the medulla with the body's richest concentration of steroids, man and other mammals do perfectly well without the medulla. Perhaps nature, in our evolutionary past, has devalued the biologic ties indicated by the anatomic fusion of adrenal cortex and medulla. Whatever the reason, most scientists today believe that the adrenal medulla (which secretes epinephrine and norepinephrine in a ratio of 4 to 1) has no more physiologic significance than other sympathetic ganglia that secrete catecholamines. In contrast, the cortex maintains critically important functions. Together, man's two adrenal glands weigh only about 14 g, but without the functioning cortex and its hormones, man dies.

PHYSIOLOGY
Adrenal Hormones

The adrenal medulla is the body's chief source of epinephrine. Epinephrine and norepinephrine together increase cardiac rate and stroke volume (B receptors). They increase depth and rate of respiration and constrict cutaneous and renal vessels (A receptors). In addition to these cardiovascular and respiratory effects, catecholamines regulate body fuels. They suppress insulin and stimulate glucagon, thus elevating blood glucose. They also release fatty acids from fat deposits. Consequently, they provide immediate calories (glucose) and begin the body's anticipated conversion to long-term calories (fats). In the fight-or-flight reaction catecholamines have an initial and crucial role.

Three main types of hormones are secreted by the adrenal cortex: glucocorticoids, mineralocorticoids, and sex steroids. All three originate from the cholesterol molecule. Enzymes within the cells of the adrenal cortex change the chemical structure of cholesterol to produce corticosteroids.

Hypothalamic-Pituitary-Adrenal Triangle

Both the glucocorticoids and the sex steroids are under hypothalamic-pituitary control. Adrenocorticotropic hormone (ACTH) released by the pituitary gland, in response to corticotropin-releasing factor (CRF) from the hypothalamus, stimulates the adrenal cortex to produce both glucocorticoids and sex steroids. (Mineralocorticoids are largely independent of pituitary control.) Glucocorticoids (chiefly cortisol), in turn, block ACTH secretion at the pituitary and CRF at the hypothalamic level. This is the reciprocal, negative feedback mechanism (similar to the pituitary-thyroid relationship) that is vital to understanding adrenal physiology.

Corticosteroid Hormones
Glucocorticoids

The chief glucocorticoid in the body is cortisol (hydrocortisone). Glucocorticoids increase glycogenolysis (breakdown of glycogen to glucose), convert proteins to glucose, and have an antiinflammatory action. In large amounts they increase fat deposition and cause weakness (from destruction of muscle protein) and water retention. Their most important action is protecting the body against stress. The exact mechanism of glucocorticoids in response to stress is not known. They probably act on the vascular tree by dilating small vessels, thus increasing blood volume. They make energy available in the form of glucose and free fatty acids. Some believe that protection of lysosomal membranes is a vital cell function. Another theory relates glucocorticoid action to their inotropic effect on myocardium, which increases cardiac output.

Mineralocorticoids

Aldosterone is secreted chiefly in response to decreased blood volume mediated by renal receptors. It acts to retain sodium and water and to excrete potassium. In concert with ADH (antidiuretic hormone) and renin-angiotensin, it maintains body fluid volume at a constant level.

Aldosterone and water balance. In the normal person the adrenal gland secretes aldosterone, the body's main mineralocorticoid, chiefly in response to decreased blood volume. The kidney's juxtaglomerular apparatus senses the volume deficit and secretes renin, which in turn releases angiotensin I. Enzymes, chiefly in the lungs, rapidly convert angiotensin I to angiotensin II. Angiotensin II, a powerful vasoconstrictor by itself, stimulates the adrenal gland to synthesize and release aldosterone. Acting on the distal convoluted tubule, aldosterone retains Na^+ (and H_2O) and excretes K^+. Thus in normal man the kidney and adrenal gland combine two mechanisms to ensure normal blood volumes through varying states of hydration, electrolyte concentration, and position. Although low Na^+, high K^+, and ACTH also stimulate aldosterone, the most powerful influence is angiotensin II. Acting as a feedback, the aldosterone build-up and increased water volume suppress or turn off renin secretion.

Antidiuretic hormone (ADH). The aldosterone-angiotensin mechanism has a powerful ally in the hypothalamic–posterior pituitary area. Responding chiefly to dehydration (increased osmolality), osmoreceptors in the hypothalamus stimulate release of pituitary-stored ADH. ADH, acting on the renal collecting ducts, causes reabsorption of water. Severe volume deficits (sensed in the heart and large arteries) also elevate ADH, since nature attempts to protect volume at all costs even in the face of hypo-osmolality. Coupled to the osmoreceptor cells, a third center signals severe thirst synchronous with water conservation. Thus two main neurohormonal centers, in the brain and paravertebral gutters, protect the body's water balance.

Sex steroids

Androgens, estrogens, and progesterone are produced by the adrenal cortex in small amounts. When they are secreted in excess, they cause virilization (the adrenogenital syndrome) or, rarely, feminization. They do not suppress ACTH, and they are not essential to life.

Adrenocortical Hormone Similarities and Differences

In the confusing welter of steroid hormones occurring in the body (more than 30 have been isolated) and the dozens of commercial steroid preparations, many students feel lost. Certain principles will help clear their understandable confusion:

1. All steroids have one of three basic actions: (a) "metabolic," or glucocorticoid, (b) mineralocorticoid, or (c) sex steroid.
2. Some overlapping of actions occurs with most corticosteroids. For example cortisol, primarily a glucocorticoid and the "mother steroid" in the body, will produce mineralocorticoid effects (water retention) and sex steroid effects (acne, hirsutism) if given in large enough amounts.
3. Suppression of ACTH is primarily a function of glucocorticoids. New synthetic anti-inflammatory steroids with advertised "decreased side effects" produce less water retention and masculinizing effects, but their glucocorticoid properties are very much evident and they strongly suppress ACTH.

A "triangle of steroid activity" is a helpful device for understanding basic steroid physiology (Fig. 16-1). All steroid preparations may be placed somewhere in this triangle corresponding to their action.

DISEASES OF THE ADRENAL CORTEX
Addison's Disease (Adrenocortical Failure)

Any process that destroys or suppresses the adrenal cortex (or the hypothalamic-pituitary ACTH centers) will cause Addison's disease. Adrenocortical infections (meningococcosis, tuberculosis), cortical atrophy (probably of autoimmune origin), and surgical adrenalectomy can cause Addison's disease. One of the most common causes is suppression of ACTH from long-term steroid therapy. Other causes are hereditary and congenital, hemorrhage (from sepsis, from anticoagulants, or during pregnancy), or pituitary insufficiency.

Clinically, Addison's disease appears in the adult as *chronic insufficiency, acute adrenal failure,* or an intermediate state between these two.

Chronic addisonian patients have dark pigmentation, weakness, hypotension, apathy, nausea, vomiting, weight loss, abdominal pain, hyponatremia, hypoglycemia, and hyperkalemia. They show decreased plasma cortisol levels and urinary 17-hydroxycorticosteroids (OHCS) excretion. *Inflexibility* best describes these patients. Any stress, such as an operation or potent drugs, can throw them into shock. Infections will cause critically high fevers with subsequent shock and death unless patients receive vigorous steroid replacement.

Acute adrenal failure comes on suddenly with fever, abdominal symptoms, coma, and shock. Sudden discontinuance of steroids after long-term administra-

tion is a common cause of acute adrenal failure. This critical condition demands immediate treatment with intravenous cortisol, 300 mg, (or more) in the first 24 hours, with gradual tapering doses. Maintenance cortisol doses average 25 to 50 mg/day orally.

Patients receiving steroids for long periods of time often pose problems for the surgeon. Some can receive large doses of steroids for several months and still maintain an effective adrenal stress response, whereas others receiving smaller doses over shorter intervals may not. In any emergency situation (lacking time to evaluate pituitary-adrenal integrity) the surgeon should support these patients with full "stress doses" of ste-

Table 16-1. Laboratory Methods Used to Differentiate the Causes of Cushing's Syndrome*

	Normal	Hyperplasia	Tumor	Ectopic *ACTH*
Plasma cortisol	10-25 µg/dl Rhythmic	↑ No rhythm	↑ No rhythm	↑ No rhythm
Plasma ACTH	0.1-0.04 mU/dl	↑	↓	↑
17-OHCS In 24-hour urine collection	5-10 mg/24 hours	↑	↑	↑ ↑
Urinary free cortisol	80-400 µg/24 hours	↑	↑	↑
Stimulation 25 Units ACTH IV over 8 hours	↑	↑ ↑	↔	↔
Suppression Dexamethasone by mouth 0.5 mg q.6 hours for 48 hours	↓ >50%	↔ or ↓	↔	↔
Dexamethasone by mouth 2 mg q.6 hours for 48 hours		↓ >50%	↔	↔, occasionally ↓
Metyrapone (SU-4885) 30 mg/kg IV over 4 hours	↑	↑ ↑	↔	↔
24 hour urine collections are completed: ACTH: 24 hours after ACTH begun Dexamethasone: in the second 24-hour period of dexamethasone administration Metyrapone: 24 hours after metyrapone begun				

*Key: ↑ increased; ↓ decreased; ↑ ↑ greatly increased; ↔ unchanged.

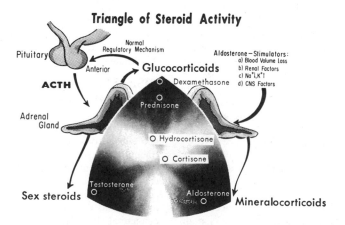

Fig. 16-1. Adrenocortical hormone activity is demonstrated by triangle with three main types of cortical hormones at apices. Overlapping of functions (glucocorticoid, mineralocorticoid, and sex steroid) occurs with most steroid compounds. Approximate overlapping of functions is illustrated by several steroids placed within this triangle.

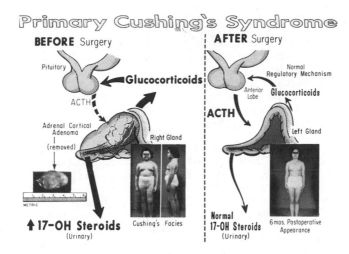

Fig. 16-2. Cushing's syndrome caused by adrenal adenoma. ACTH is suppressed by excess glucocorticoids. After tumor was removed, normal pituitary-adrenal balance resumed. Insets show cushingoid effects in 9-year-old girl and postoperative appearance 6 months after removal of benign adrenal adenoma.

roids (300 mg cortisol/day). Little harm comes from short-interval "burst" therapy, but catastrophe may follow if the surgeon overlooks the vital importance of steroid replacement in patients with marginal adrenal reserves.

Cushing's Syndrome

Cushing's syndrome is caused by excess quantities of glucocorticoids, mainly cortisol. It may occur from any of the following causes:

1. Adrenal hyperplasia secondary to excess ACTH stimulation from a pituitary tumor (either a basophilic or chromophobic adenoma) or functional pituitary overactivity probably caused by excessive hypothalamic activity. This is called *Cushing's disease.*
2. Ectopic Cushing's syndrome—some extra-adrenal cancers (of the lung, pancreas, thyroid gland, parotid gland, liver, and thymus) secrete large amounts of ACTH that cause Cushing's syndrome. These cancers are usually inoperable.
3. A functioning tumor (Fig. 16-2), either an adenoma or a carcinoma, of the adrenal cortex.
4. Administration of large quantities of glucocorticoid drugs (such as cortisone).

About 70% of all spontaneous cases of Cushing's syndrome result from hyperplasia, 20% from tumors, and 10% from ectopic ACTH.

The clinical picture is the same: amenorrhea, moon face, truncal obesity, muscle loss and weakness, hirsutism, acne, diabetes mellitus, skin atrophy, hypertension, abdominal striae, ecchymoses, osteoporosis, and mental disturbances (depression to frank psychoses).

Laboratory Tests

Diagnosing Cushing's syndrome. The *overnight dexamethasone suppression test* is the most valuable single screening test for Cushing's syndrome. Dexamethasone, 1 mg taken at midnight, will lower morning plasma cortisol levels below 5 µg/dl in normal people (normal values, 5 to 20 µg/dl). Patients with Cush-

ing's syndrome usually have values above 10 µg/dl after suppression.

Urinary 17 OHCS average 5 to 10 mg/24 hours in normal people. High levels, especially when they fail to suppress with dexamethasone, indicate Cushing's syndrome (Table 16-1).

Urinary free cortisol (normal: 80 to 400 µg/day) correlates more closely than 17-OHCS with cortisol secretion rates. It is becoming the most dependable test.

Loss of diurnal plasma cortisol variation is a sign of Cushing's syndrome. Normal people show elevated plasma cortisol levels in morning blood samples and depressed levels in the afternoon. Patients with Cushing's syndrome show little or no diurnal variation.

Differentiating the cause of Cushing's syndrome. The physician who makes the diagnosis of Cushing's syndrome with one or more of the previously mentioned tests should attempt to define the cause. Table 16-1 summarizes the tests. ACTH will invariably stimulate the normal and hyperplastic glands but will stimulate tumors variably since their output is largely autonomous. The lower dose (2 mg/24 hours) dexamethasone suppression test differentiates normal patients from those who have *any form* of Cushing's syndrome. The higher dose (8 mg/24 hours) test differentiates adrenal hyperplasia from adrenal tumors.

The metyrapone test checks the integrity of the hypothalamic-pituitary-adrenal triangle, thus providing another good differentiation between adrenal hyperplasia and adrenal tumors. Metyrapone blocks the final step in cortisol production in the normal or hyperplastic cortex while allowing the precursors of cortisol to be produced. (These precursors are measured as 17-OHCS in the urine.) But these precursors cannot block ACTH; only cortisol has this ability. Thus metyrapone removes cortisol suppression of ACTH. Normal patients and those with hyperplasia respond by excreting increased amounts of urinary 17-OHCS. Patients with adrenal tumors, given metyrapone, continue to secrete excess cortisol unabated, therefore they show no variation in 17-OHCS excretion. Patients with ectopic ACTH-producing tumors continue to secrete the same excessive amounts of ACTH, despite metyrapone. Large amounts of exogenous ACTH will suppress pituitary ACTH; ectopic ACTH production acts similarly. They have lost the normal hypothalamic-pituitary-adrenal triangle. Therefore patients with ectopic Cushing's syndrome, given metyrapone, will not produce increased amounts of urinary 17-OHCS.

Plasma ACTH measurements (by radioimmunassay) also reliably separate the causes of Cushing's syndrome. Patients with adrenal tumors have low ACTH plasma levels; those with hyperplasia or ectopic ACTH production have high levels. Petrosal venous ACTH samplings when elevated indicate a pituitary source for the ACTH.

X-ray examination. Although skull films with tomograms will show large pituitary lesions computed tomography (CT) is more precise in detecting smaller (<10 mm) tumors. In detecting adrenal lesions scintigraphy with iodocholesterol (NP-59) and CT are the most useful diagnostic procedures. Echography, venography, and arteriography are less popular now. The latter two share the disadvantages of invasive procedures. Magnetic resonance imaging (MRI) provides images similar to those of CT but with better resolution.

Treatment. The treatment of Cushing's *syndrome* caused by adrenal tumors is clear cut—excision of the tumors, if possible—but treatment of Cushing's *disease* is controversial.

Irradiation of the pituitary. Conventional irradiation often takes several months to control the disease, and recurrences are common. High-energy proton beam irradiation, available in only a few centers, is more effective. Irradiation may, of course, destroy other pituitary cells.

Pituitary microsurgery. Some reports indicate a high incidence (80%) of microadenomas and excellent responses from transsphenoidal excision of these minute tumors. Other pituitary functions can often be simultaneously preserved. Pituitary microsurgery has become the first-line therapy.

Surgical adrenalectomy. Adrenalectomy controls excess cortisol but not excess ACTH. After adrenalectomy, about 10% to 20% of the patients will develop symptomatic pituitary enlargement (Nelson's syndrome). Thus all postadrenalectomy patients require periodic reassessment of pituitary status. Bilateral adrenalectomy has three main advantages: it can rapidly control florid Cushing's disease, it does not directly threaten other pituitary functions, e.g., fertility, and it is more widely available.

Drug therapy. Several agents are effective in treating Cushing's disease. *Cyproheptadine* blocks release of CRF at the hypothalamus. Relapses, however, are common after discontinuance of the drug. *Bromocryptine* inhibits CRF secretion, but responses vary. Because of its unpredictability and side effects, it is seldom used as initial treatment. *Aminoglutethimide* inhibits the conversion of cholesterol to pregnenolone, thus blocking the synthesis of all adrenal steroids. Although it has no effect on ACTH levels, it can palliate hypercorticolism. *Metyrapone* also blocks cortisol synthesis,

by blocking the 11-β-hydroxylation step. It has been used with aminoglutethimide to lower excess cortisol levels. Like the previous three drugs, metyrapone is not definitive therapy. *Mitotane* lyses adrenal cortical cells, usually sparing the glomerulosa (mineralocorticoid) layer. Although it has frequent side effects (nausea, vomiting, diarrhea, leukopenia) it is the only agent of proven value in treating adrenocortical cancer.

Aldosteronism

Hyperplasia, or tumors, can arise from any of the three cortical cell types. Although the glomerulosa layer may become hyperplastic, it usually forms single adenomas that secrete excess aldosterone. Hypertension results and, although uncommon, is surgically curable.

Hyperaldosteronism and hypertension coexist in two clinical situations: *primary aldosteronism,* which usually responds to adrenalectomy, and *secondary aldosteronism,* from extra-adrenal causes.

Primary aldosteronism. Accounting for about 1% of all cases of hypertension, primary aldosteronism gives the following clinical picture: hypertension, headaches, polydipsia, polyuria, muscle weakness, electrocardiographic partial paralysis, and the ECG changes of hypokalemia. Sodium retention and excessive potassium excretion are the two underlying mechanisms responsible for these symptoms and signs.

Laboratory tests show elevated serum Na^+, alkalosis, depressed K^+, increased serum and urine aldosterone, and low serum renin. Increased blood volume and aldosterone levels suppress serum renin.

The pathologic changes of primary aldosteronism occur in the outer, glomerulosa layer of the adrenal cortex as (1) solitary aldosterone-producing adenomas (APA), (2) idiopathic adrenal hyperplasia (IAH), or (3), rarely a dexamethesone-suppressible form. APA accounts for about 75% of primary aldosteronism and IAH for most of the remainder (Fig. 16-3).

Ruling out secondary aldosteronism. Any disease that stimulates renin also elevates aldosterone: renal artery stenosis, intrinsic renal ischemia, juxtaglomerular hyperplasia, etc. Secondary aldosteronism always involves increased renin levels; pure primary aldosteronism, never. Thus renin and aldosterone determinations help select those patients (from the millions of hypertensives) who have potentially curable, aldosterone-induced hypertension (Table 16-2).

Differentiating adenomas from hyperplasia. Because patients with adenomas respond well to excision and those with hyperplasia respond poorly, attempts to separate them become vitally important. The characteristics in Table 16-3 help differentiate these two pathologic causes.

Table 16-2. Serum Renin and Urinary Aldosterone Relationships in Three Main Types of Hypertension*

Cause of Hypertension	Serum Renin	Urinary Aldosterone
Renovascular	↑	↑
"Essential"	↔	↔
Aldosteronism	↓	↑

*Key: ↑ increased; ↓ decreased; ↔ unchanged.

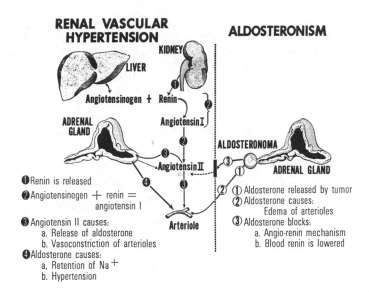

Fig. 16-3. Comparison of mechanisms causing renal vascular hypertension and primary aldosteronism.

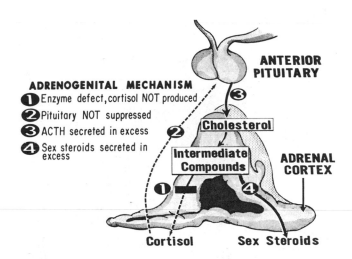

Fig. 16-4. Mechanism of adrenogenital syndrome.

Table 16-3. Aldosteronism: Adenomas *vs.* Hyperplasia

Clinical & Laboratory Data	Aldosterone-Producing Adenomas (APA)	Idiopathic Adrenal Hyperplasia (IAH)
Blood pressure ↑	Often severe	Moderately high
Aldosterone levels after standing	Decreased	Unchanged or increased
CT	Single tumor	Bilateral enlargement
Iodocholesterol scan	Uptake in single tumor	Bilateral uptake
Venous sampling (aldosterone)	Unilateral increase	Bilateral increase

Treatment. With more than 95% accuracy, the above clinical and laboratory data differentiate APA from IAH. After excision of an aldosteroma, 50% of patients become normotensive and an additional 25% require less hypertensive medication. In almost all, the potassium returns to normal. Patients with hyperplasia respond best to spironolactone. Since bilateral adrenalectomy fails to relieve hypertension in many patients, it should be reserved for patients who are refractory to medical treatment.

Adrenogenital Syndrome

In the steps of cortisol synthesis a branching chain is responsible for the formation of the sex steroids (Fig. 16-4). In some children a defective enzyme system allows the sex steroids to be produced while cortisol pro-

duction is blocked. One can anticipate the chain of events that ensues. In the absence of cortisol, the main inhibitor of ACTH from the anterior pituitary, the anterior pituitary produces excess amounts of ACTH and thus stimulates the secretion of more sex steroids (that cannot suppress ACTH). The overall result is a masculinizing effect. In children the treatment is simply giving cortisol or other glucocorticoids that supply bodily needs while blocking the secretion of excess ACTH. This cuts off all stimulation to the abnormal pathway for sex steroid production. Virilizing symptoms that appear in adult life are strongly suggestive of an adrenal or ovarian tumor.

DISEASES OF ADRENAL MEDULLA
Pheochromocytoma

Pheochromocytoma is a rare tumor arising from the nervelike tissue of the adrenal medulla. Bilaterality, malignancy, and extra-adrenal location each occur in roughly 10% of the cases, and it has been called the "10% tumor." Extra-adrenal pheochromocytomas usually arise from the abdominal sympathetic ganglia, but they may originate within the chest, cranium, or even the bladder wall. Increased production of epinephrine and norepinephrine is responsible for the clinical picture that features the two main types of symptoms—*hypermetabolic* and *neurologic*. These symptoms (and signs) are nervousness, sweating, palpitations, headache, weakness, weight loss, syncope, psychic distur-

Pheochromocytoma

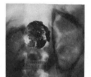

SYMPTOMS:
BP 280/160
Headache
Nervousness
Sweating
Personality Changes

Retroperitoneal Air Outlines
Tumor on X-ray Film

Fig. 16-5. Left adrenal pheochromocytoma outlined by retroperitoneal CO_2 insufflation.

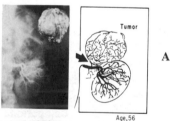

ADRENAL TUMOR (Pheochromocytoma)
Outlined by Selective Renal Arteriography

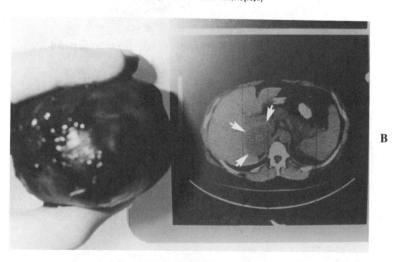

Fig. 16-6. A, Left adrenal pheochromocytoma outlined by dye injected into left renal artery. **B,** Right adrenal tumor *(outlined by arrows)* on CT scan.

bances, and hypertension (Fig. 16-5). The tumors have been reported in all age groups from the newborn to the aged. The patients are usually thin, and about 50% show abnormal glucose tolerance curves or glycosuria. Neurofibromas coexist in some patients with pheochromocytomas. The symptoms occur as "attacks" in about half the cases. Pheochromocytomas tend to be familial. Coappearing with medullary thyroid cancers, parathyroid adenomas, and a Marfan-like body build, they form a multiple endocrine neoplasia (MEN II) with autosomal-dominant transmission.

Diagnosis. The most difficult problem is diagnosis. Among the many patients with hypertension, the patient with a pheochromocytoma is sometimes hopelessly obscured. Diagnostic work-ups are costly and time consuming. Thus suspicion and selection are vital diagnostic requisites. Hypertension associated with childhood, glycosuria, pregnancy, orthostatic hypotension, neurofibromas, paroxysmal sweating and headaches, and wide variations in blood pressure recordings should evoke suspicion.

Laboratory tests. Elevated urinary metanephrines, vanillylmandelic acid (VMA), and free catecholamines provide a diagnostic accuracy of over 90%. Quantification of these metabolic products of the epinephrines has largely replaced the more hazardous histamine provocative test and the adrenergic blockade test. Intravenous pyelograms, computerized tomography (CT), and selective arteriography help localize these tumors (Fig. 16-6).

A new specific radionucleotide, ^{131}I-*meta*-iodobenzylguanidine (MIBG), concentrates in chromaffin cells and has localized pheochromocytomas within the adrenal glands and in ectopic sites. Because it tests adrenal medulla *function*, it can distinguish functioning from nonfunctioning tissue. This provides the surgeon with vital preoperative data. For example, in adrenal medullary hyperplasia, the medulla enlarges at the expense of the adrenal cortex. Even a 10-fold medullary enlargement can be missed by ultrasound or CT scans, whereas MIBG will show it clearly.

Treatment. Surgical excision is usually curative. Because 10% of these tumors are bilateral and 10% are extra-adrenal, most surgeons prefer the abdominal approach. Preoperative preparation (for 10 to 14 days) with α-blocking agents (phenoxybenzamine [Dibenzyline]), which decrease blood pressure, increase blood volume, and reverse myocardial damage, provide a smoother operative and postoperative course. β-Blockade with propranolol is added (but only after alpha blockade) for tachycardias, arrhythmias, or both.

Some metastatic tumors have responded to MIBG, an exciting new development that simulates the response of thyroid cancer to radioactive iodine.

Bilateral Medullary Hyperplasia

Bilateral medullary hyperplasia, a rare occurrence, can mimic the clinical characteristics of pheochromocytoma.

17

Breast

Lawrence W. Norton

Breast disease, common among women, is usually benign and self-limited. The discovery of a lump in the breast can be frightening, however, because of the threat of cancer. Most women want to be examined, diagnosed, and treated as soon as possible. The surgeon must deal with the patient's anxiety as well as her disease. This chapter describes the detection, nature, and management of benign and malignant breast disease.

ANATOMY

The glands of the breast arise from the skin and are similar to sweat or sebaceous glands. Between 15 and 25 branching epithelial channels, or ducts, form in early life (Fig. 17-1, *A)*. At puberty, a resurgence of growth results in the formation of lobes, with each main duct emptying into the nipple. Lymphatics within the breast drain into axillary nodes, internal mammary nodes, supraclavicular nodes, and, via the rectus sheath, abdominal nodes (Fig. 17-1, *B)*.

Supernumerary breasts or nipples may occur along the milk line (Fig. 17-2). Cancer may originate in extra breast tissue in the axilla. Such tissue is often removed for diagnostic or cosmetic reasons. Neonatal hypertrophy occurs commonly in both male and female infants because of estrogenic stimulation. It usually subsides within 6 months.

DETECTION OF BREAST DISEASE
Breast Examination

A quarter of breast masses are detected by physicians during routine physical examinations. The technique of breast examination begins with observation of the breasts while the patient is sitting. Asymmetry, nipple or skin retraction, edema, abnormal venous pattern, skin redness or an obvious mass may be apparent. Raising the arm tightens skin in the lower half of the breast to reveal abnormalities in that area. As the pa-

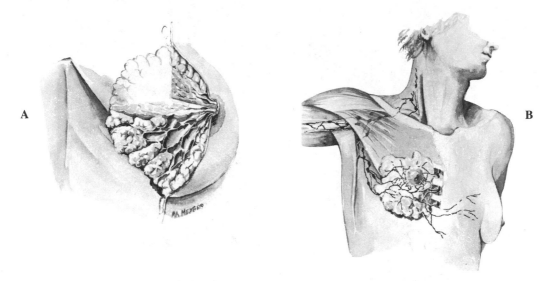

Fig. 17-1. A, Cross-section of breast illustrating lobes and ducts. **B,** Main lymphatic channels of breast.

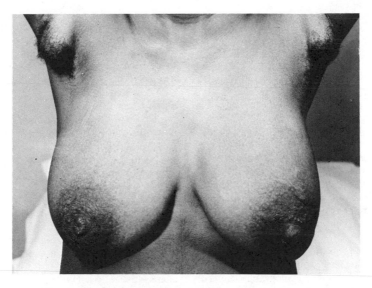

Fig. 17-2. Bilateral breast tissue in axillae of 22-year-old woman.

tient pushes her hands against her hips, the pectoralis major muscles contract. This accentuates any skin retraction. Palpation is performed with the patient sitting and supine. In the latter position, the ipsilateral area is elevated by having the patient place her hand behind her head. This spreads the breast over the chest wall and improves accuracy in assessing breast tissue. Gentle pressure by the fingers is applied in a pattern designed to cover the entire breast. Findings may range from tenderness alone to vague densities, irregular masses, or dominant lumps. The examination ends by palpating carefully for axillary and supraclavicular lymph nodes.

Breast self-examination is recommended for all adult women. The value of this exercise in terms of improving survival from breast cancer is controver-

sial, but the presumed benefit of early detection supports the practice. Despite efforts to instruct women in the technique, breast self-examination is not practiced widely.

Mammography

Screening mammography is the best available means to detect occult breast disease. It is recommended for all women within certain age categories (Table 17-1). The current dose of irradiation used for mammography is unlikely to cause cancer in more than one of a million women so studied. While mammography can detect early, impalpable breast disease, it does not demonstrate all breast cancers and is, therefore, a complementary study to physical examination. Mammography cannot diagnose cancer of the breast, but it

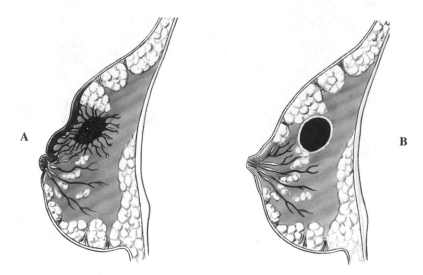

Fig. 17-3. Mammography. **A,** Malignant mass—ragged borders, skin thickening, stippled calcifications, and nipple retraction. **B,** Benign mass—smooth borders, no calcifications, and normal skin.

Table 17-1. Recommendations for Screening Mammography

Age	Frequency
35-39	Baseline
40-49	Every 1-2 years
Over 50	Every year

can demonstrate lesions within breast tissue that may represent cancer.

Two common lesions found by mammography are occult masses and microcalcifications. Certain characteristics, such as spiculated margins of a mass and clusters of microcalcifications, raise the level of suspicion for cancer (Fig. 17-3). Confirmation of cancer requires histologic examination.

The value of screening mammography in improving the outcome of breast cancer treatment is debated. Early experience with screening mammography showed improved 5-year survival rates after mastectomy. Subsequent studies confirm this improvement but suggest that the advantage may be merely lead-time bias. Ultrasonography can differentiate cystic breast masses from solid ones. Thermography, transillumination, and computed tomography (CT) are not as useful as mammography.

DIAGNOSIS OF BREAST MASS

Palpable mass

A solitary or dominant breast mass must be evaluated. The first step in the management of a palpable mass is needle aspiration. If fluid is aspirated and the mass disappears entirely, biopsy is unnecessary. When the mass is not cystic, tissue is sampled by one of three techniques. Lesions 5 cm or less in diameter are amenable to excisional biopsy (Fig. 17-4). This techinque has the advantages of supplying the maximal amount of tissue for pathologic examination and of removing the

mass. It is usually performed on an outpatient basis using local anesthesia. The excised specimen is placed in ice to perserve hormone receptors. Some tissue is used to determine ploidy of cells by the technique of flow cytometry.

When a mass is greater than 5 cm in diameter, incisional rather than excisional biopsy is recommended. A portion of tissue is obtained for histologic diagnosis by either direct incision or by the technique of core needle biopsy. The latter has the advantage of being a relatively simple office procedure. Its disadvantages lie in the small volume of tissue obtained and in the possibility that tumor is not sampled.

When a palpable breast mass is suspected of being cancerous, diagnosis can be obtained with reasonable confidence by fine needle aspiration and cytology. Accuracy in identifying malignant cells is approximately 90%. The procedure is not recommended to diagnose nonproliferative benign disease because such tissue is characteristically acellular.

Nonpalpable Mass

Occult lesions detected by mammography may require removal by the technique of needle localization biopsy. Because the target lesion cannot be palpated, it is localized by means of a needle inserted into the breast under mammographic control. The tip of the needle is positioned as close as possible to the target lesion. The needle is then used as a guide by the surgeon to remove the occult disease. Success is evaluated by a specimen radiograph and is achieved in about 90% of attempts. The average yield of cancer in such specimens is 15% to 20%.

BENIGN BREAST DISEASES

The incidence of benign breast disorders can only be estimated. Symptoms referable to the breast occur in about 50% of American women. Of breast masses removed for histologic examination, at least 80% are benign. Risk factors for benign disease include a history

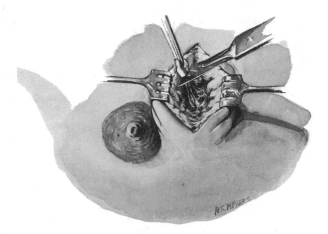

Fig. 17-4. Open excision biopsy of breast mass. Frozen section microscopy done immediately for specific diagnosis.

of premenstural breast discomfort, irregular menses, spontaneous abortions, small breasts, and late menopause. Use of oral contraceptives is inversely related to risk.

A common explanation of the cause of benign breast disease is neuroendocrine imbalance. Estrogen is responsible for development of ductal epithelium while progesterone causes lobular proliferation. One thesis suggests that dysovulation or an inadequate corpus luteum reduces the ratio of progesterone to estrogen. Such change occurs during menarche and menopause, two periods of life in which the incidence of benign breast problems is high.

The clinical features of benign breast disease range from premenstrual swelling and tenderness to dominant breast masses. Nodularity or lumpiness of breast tissue and mastalgia (breast pain) occur frequently. Nipple discharge and infection are less common. The variety of presenting symptoms and signs makes precise diagnosis by physical examination difficult.

Fibrocystic Disease

A number of different histologic conditions are included in the traditional term "fibrocystic disease." A better expression for this spectrum of normal variants and pathologic conditions is "fibrocystic changes." Some pathologists use the terms "fibrocystic disease" and "mammary dysplasia" interchangeably; others prefer to label each lesion as a specific pathologic entity. In an effort to standardize classification and to eliminate the vague term fibrocystic disease, a division of benign breast disease into clinically relevant types is useful.

Nonproliferative Lesions

This category includes cysts, papillary apocrine changes, mild hyperplasia, microcalcifications associated with epithelium, and fibroadenomas. A cyst may be large or microscopic, single or multiple (Fig. 17-5). Frequently, a cyst is surrounded by fibrous stroma and lined by flattened epithelial cells. It may appear blue in color in tissue (blue dome cyst). A cyst is rarely associated with cancer (relative risk 1.5). If a mass persists

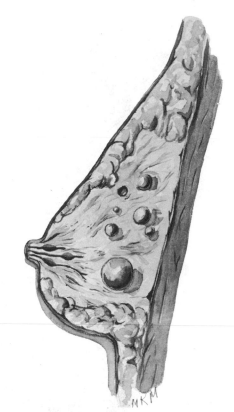

Fig. 17-5. Cross-section of breast with mammary dysplasia, showing multiple cysts and excessive fibrous tissue.

after aspiration of a cyst, excisional biopsy should be performed. Because the yield is low, cyst fluid usually is not analyzed cytologically. An exception is made if the fluid is tinged with blood.

Proliferative Disorders without Atypia

This category includes sclerosing adenosis, ductal involvement with cells characteristic of atypical lobular hyperplasia, ordinary hyperplasia, and intraductal papilloma. These lesions may or may not present as a palpable mass. Areas of adenosis frequently contain microcalcifications that mimic carcinoma. Moderate and florid hyperplasia of the usual type are the commonest forms of proliferative breast lesions. So long as atypia is not present, hyperplasia does not increase the risk of developing carcinoma.

Atypical Proliferative Lesions

These include atypical hyperplasia that has some, but not all, of the features of ductal or lobular carcinoma in situ. Its significance is an increased risk of developing invasive carcinoma. This risk is 4.4 compared to a reference population. If cancer occurs in patients with atypical hyperplasia, it may occur in any part of the breast or be bilateral.

Treatment of Benign Breast Symptoms

Breast pain and parenchymal masses attributed to benign disease often defy therapy. A number of agents are used for these conditions, and they may or may not be effective in an individual patient. The use of progesterone is based on the assumption that progesterone levels are low in comparison to estrogen. Bromocriptine is prescribed because it antagonizes the effects of prolactin. Danazol, a synthetic androgen, appears to decrease mastodynia but has side effects such as menstrual irregularities, facial hirsutism, and voice changes. Dietary restriction of methylxanthine, reported to improve symptomatic benign breast disease, does not offer advantages over a placebo in controlled, prospective studies. Vitamin E, although widely used, is not effective therapy for breast pain.

Fibroadenoma

This is a nonproliferative benign breast lesion that occurs principally in young women. Fibroadenomas typically are firm, spherical, well-defined masses that seem, on physical examination, to be encapsulated (Fig. 17-6). In fact, they are only pseudoencapsulated, and they sometimes fuse with adjacent tissue to suggest carcinoma. Rarely, carcinoma occurs in association with fibroadenoma, but the benign tumor does not become carcinoma. For this reason, excision is not required if the diagnosis is certain. Most lesions are removed, however, to confirm the diagnosis or simply to eliminate the mass and the anxiety it causes.

Intraductal Papilloma

A solitary intraductal papilloma is a tumor of a major lactiferous duct that occurs in women age 30 to 50 and is associated in 50% of cases with nipple discharge of serous or bloody fluid. The lesion is often small (< 1 cm) and may not be palpable. Its presence is detected by applying fingertip pressure concentrically from the nipple outward. Pressure over the site of the papilloma

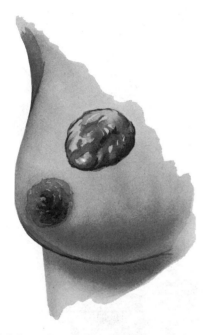

Fig. 17-6. Large fibroadenoma of breast.

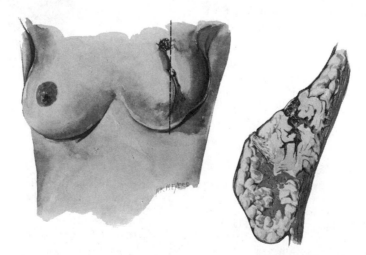

Fig. 17-7. Advanced breast cancer showing skin ulceration, nipple retraction, deformity of breast contour, and fixation to chest wall.

can release a jet of fluid from the nipple. Treatment is excision of a wedge of tissue at the site.

Mammary Duct Ectasia

The combination of dilated subareolar ducts and inflammation may lead to discharge of purulent or bloody fluid from the nipple. Whether duct dilation or infection is primary is unknown. Mammary duct ectasia occurs most often in perimenopausal or postmenopausal women. A mass may be palpable deep to the areola and skin. Nipple retraction is not unusual. Changes in the skin of the nipple can be confused with Paget's disesae of the breast. Treatment of mammary duct ectasia is local excision of involved breast tissue.

Fat Necrosis

This benign lesion can simulate breast cancer on physical examination and in mammograms. It occurs most often in large, pendulous breasts. Fixation to skin can cause retraction. Half of patients with fat necrosis have a history of breast trauma.

Gynecomastia

The most common benign lesion in the male breast is a firm, flat subareolar mass that is composed primarily of fibrous tissue and breast parenchyma. It is properly described as mammoplasia but is commonly called gynecomastia. It occurs typically during the neonatal period, puberty, and senescence, suggesting a hormonal etiology. Gynecomastia can result from testicular failure, testicular tumors, drugs, and systemic diseases. Chronic liver disease is sometimes associated with bilateral gynecomastia.

BREAST CANCER
Epidemiology

The breast is the most common site of cancer among American women. One in 10 women is affected. The incidence of breast cancer is increasing at a rate approaching 2% per year. About 135,000 new cases were diagnosed in the United States in 1988. Despite its prevalence, breast cancer is second to lung cancer as a cause of death among women.

Risk factors for the development of breast cancer are listed in the box below. The peak occurrence of disease is ages 55 to 75. Risk is increased sharply if a patient's mother or sister had bilateral or premenopausal breast cancer or if more than one first-degree relative has breast cancer. The importance of endocrine influences in the etiology of breast cancer is suggested by the association with early menarche, late menopause, and late first childbirth. A role for both obesity and increased dietary fat in the etiology of breast cancer is likely but still unproven.

Clinical Presentation

Breast cancer presents as a lump in 80% of cases. Pain is uncommon (10%). Nipple discharge is rare. Advanced disease, seen infrequently today, can cause nipple or skin retraction, prominent venous pattern, or breast enlargement (Fig. 17-7). Neglected cancer may become ulcerated with a foul discharge from necrosis (Fig. 17-8). Breast cancer originates most often in the upper outer quadrant (40%) or in the subareolar area (25%). The absence of palpable axillary nodes does not exclude regional metastases. About 40% of patients without adenopathy have microscopic nodal involvement.

Breast cancer is staged on the basis of the initial physical examination for tumor size (T), axillary dissection for nodal involvement (N), and imaging procedures for metastases (M). The TNM system of staging

---

Breast Cancer Risk Factors

Major
    Age
    Family history
    Previous breast cancer in patient
Minor
    Early menarche
    Late menopause
    First child after age 30
    Obesity
    Radiation
    Atypical hyperplasia

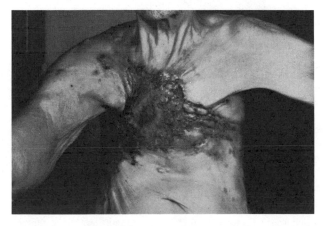

Fig. 17-8. Far-advanced, untreated, ulcerating breast cancer in elderly female.

Table 17-2. TNM Breast Cancer Staging System

T—Primary tumor diameter

TIS	Preinvasive carcinoma
T1	Tumor < 2 cm
T2	Tumor 2-5 cm
T3	Tumor > 5 cm
T4	Chest wall extension

N—Axillary lymph node status

N0	No nodes involved
N1	Movable axillary nodes
N2	Fixed axillary nodes
N3	Supraclavicular nodes

M—Distant metastases

M0	Absent
M1	Present

Table 17-3. Histologic Types of Breast Cancer

Type	Frequency %
Infiltrating ductal	74.0
Lobular invasive	6.0
Intraductal	3.5
Lobular in situ	3.0
Medullary	2.7
Cystosarcoma	2.5
Paget's disease	2.3
Mucinous	2.0
Papillary	1.5
Inflammatory	1.5
Tubular	1.5

is summarized in Table 17-2. In general, stage 1 disease is any tumor mass less than 2 cm in diameter with negative axillary nodes and no metastases. Stage II disease is usually a mass under 5 cm with positive nodes. Stage III represents advanced local disease, and stage IV implies distant metastases.

Pathology

Most breast cancers are infiltrating ductal carcinoma (Table 17-3). Carcinoma arising in lobules is less frequent but more likely to be bilateral (20%). Medullary, mucinous, tubular, and other forms of breast cancer are perhaps slightly less virulent than ductal carcinoma but are managed in the same way.

Inflammatory carcinoma is invasive ductal carcinoma that obstructs subcuticular lymphatics and presents clinically as skin redness and edema (*peau d'orange*). It usually involves a large area of the breast skin when discovered. Because of a high rate of local recurrence and low rate of survival when treated primarily by mastectomy, inflammatory carcinoma is best managed by administering chemotherapy or irradiation before mastectomy is attempted.

Paget's disease of the nipple is an eczematoid change of the skin associated with crusting, erosion, and discharge. It often (40%) represents a variant of ductal carcinoma. Whether cancer begins in the nipple epidermis or in deeper ducts is unknown. A mass in the breast may or may not be palpable. Because of the possibility of cancer, any lesion of the skin of the nipple must be biopsied.

Male breast cancer occurs less than 1% as often as female breast cancer. Hyperestrogenism (e.g., Klinefelter's syndrome) is a risk factor. The median age of onset is 60 years. A firm painless mass is usually present. It may be confused with gynecomastia. Treatment by modified radical mastectomy is usually adequate despite proximity of the tumor to the pectoralis major muscle. Chemotherapy is advised if regional lymph nodes are involved. Metastatic disease can respond to orchiectomy or the antiestrogen drug tamoxifen.

Cystosarcoma phylloides is a rare fibroepithelial tumor of the female breast that can be either benign (75%) or malignant (25%). It may arise from a pre-existing fibroadenoma. Excision of the benign tumor is followed by local recurrence in 20% of patients. Reexcision is then required. Total mastectomy is adequate treatment for malignant disease because regional lymph node metastasis is extremely rare.

An important consideration in the pathophysiology of breast carcinoma is doubling time of the tumor mass. Doubling times vary, but an average interval is 100 days. At this rate, the time required for a single malignant cell to grow to a clinically detectable 1 cm mass would be more than 8 years.

Breast cancer diagnosed during pregnancy traditionally is associated with a poor prognosis; in fact, 5-year survival of patients with negative axillary nodes approaches that of nonpregnant women. Unfortunately, lymph node metastases are 50% more common in pregnant than in nonpregnant patients. This may reflect delay in diagnosis of the primary tumor. Such delay may be due to gestational breast changes or physician procrastination. Treatment of breast cancer in pregnant or lactating patients is usually mastectomy. The risk of radiation is uncertain. Chemotherapy may also be unsafe, particularly during the organogenesis period. Therapeutic abortion may be recommended if chemotherapy or irradiation must be used. Subsequent pregnancy does not appear to shorten survival after treatment for gestational breast cancer.

Primary Treatment

The choice of primary treatment for early breast cancer is determined by pathology (in situ versus invasive), tumor size, and patient preference. Invasive carcinoma that is less than 4 cm in diameter can be treated with equal effectiveness by modified radical mastectomy or by a combination of partial mastectomy (lumpectomy), axillary dissection, and irradiation ("breast conservation treatment"). The evidence that rates of survival, local recurrence, and distant metastases are similar after each treatment comes from prospective randomized studies in Milan (10-year follow-up) and the National Surgical Adjuvant Breast Project in the United States (5-year follow-up).

The advantage of lumpectomy and irradiation is preservation of the breast. A disadvantage of this option is the time required to complete irradiation (5 to 6 weeks). Modified radical mastectomy offers shorter treatment time but at the cost of losing the breast. Reconstruction by means of a breast prosthesis can follow

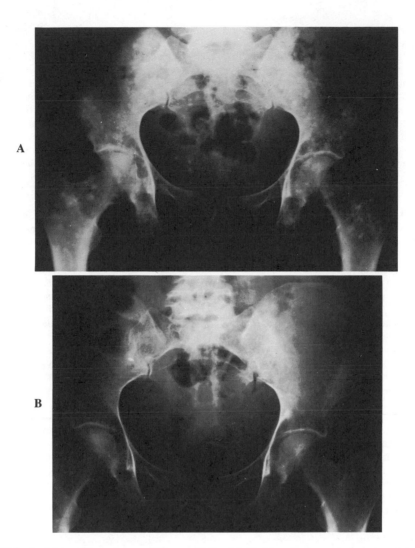

Fig. 17-9. A, Advanced breast cancer (52-year-old female). Notice extensive metastases to pelvis. **B,** Same patient 2½ years later after steroid therapy. Metastases have almost vanished. Patient died 1 year later.

mastectomy immediately or be delayed for several years. Modified radical mastectomy, unlike the classical radical mastectomy, preserves the pectoralis muscle. This results in less chest wall deformity and facilitates breast reconstruction. Results of treatment by the classical and the modified radical mastectomy are the same in terms of overall and disease-free survival (DFS).

When tumor diameter exceeds 4 cm, modified radical mastectomy is indicated because prospective studies have not been done to determine whether irradiation is as effective as mastectomy in these circumstances. When cancer is adherent to pectoralis major muscle, a portion of muscle is excised in preference to performing classical radical mastectomy.

Axillary dissection, whether performed as part of a modified radical mastectomy or as a separate procedure prior to irradiation, is important in two respects. First, it determines prognosis. The number of positive axillary nodes correlates with survival. Second, the presence of even one positive node is indicative of systemic

disease and justifies the use of adjuvant chemotherapy or hormones.

Primary treatment of carcinoma in situ is controversial. Intraductal carcinoma (ductal in situ) can be cured by total masectomy alone. This procedure removes the breast but not axillary nodes. Primary irradiation of the breast may be equally effective, although local recurrence of disease in the form of invasive cancer has been reported. Lobular carcinoma in situ requires neither mastectomy nor irradiation. After excisional biopsy, the patient is followed by mammography and physical examination.

Outcome of Primary Treatment

Ten year disease free survival (DFS) of patients treated by either mastectomy or irradiation for stage I invasive breast cancer is 80%. When lymph nodes are involved, DFS at 10 years is only 25%. Results of treatment for advanced breast cancer are dismal. Stage III and IV patients rarely survive 10 years.

Adjuvant chemotherapy in patients with positive

nodes benefits some patients. Several studies show a prolongation of DFS and overall survival in premenopausal women. A few studies show benefit in both premenopausal and postmenopausal patients. Currently, the National Cancer Institute recommends adjuvant therapy for *all* patients with invasive breast cancer. The chemotherapy is usually a combination of drugs and may include cytoxan, methotrexate, 5-fluorouracil (5-FU), vincristine, or prednisone. Tamoxifen significantly prolongs DFS when used as single adjuvant therapy regardless of menopausal, nodal, or hormone receptor status.

Recurrent Cancer

Except for stage 1 disease, breast cancer recurs after primary treatment in the majority of patients. Relapse can occur after any interval, occasionally as much as 30 years. Most local recurrences are noted within 2 years. Predictors of recurrence are axillary node and hormone receptor status and DNA activity in cancer cells. Positive nodes, negative receptors, and aneuploidy of cells correlate with risk of recurrent disease.

Recurrent breast cancer may be local or metastatic. After mastectomy for cure, local or regional recurrence is seen first in 10% to 30% of patients who relapse. The first sign of such disease is often a mass in the surgical scar. Half of patients with incisional recurrence have concurrent demonstrable metastatic disease. Local recurrence, therefore, may result from widespread metastatic disease rather than inadequate surgical excision. Treatment of chest wall recurrence consists of a combination of techniques that may include excision, chemotherapy, hormonal therapy, irradiation, and immunotherapy. Permanent cure after treatment of recurrent breast cancer is unusual. Recurrence of cancer in a breast treated primarily by irradiation carries a less ominous prognosis than incisional recurrence after mastec-

tomy. Treatment by salvage mastectomy is only slightly less effective than initial mastectomy would have been.

Bone is most often the first site of distant metastases (50%; Fig. 17-9). The incidence of bone involvement in stage I and II disease is low, making bone scan a low-yield screening technique in these patients. The second most common site of distant metastases is lung or pleura (15% to 30%). Other sites of relatively frequent involvement are liver, central nervous system, and skin. Once metastases occur, the outlook for survival is grim. Median survival with treatment is 1 to 2 years. An exceptional patient survives 10 years or longer.

Chemotherapy and/or hormone therapy is used to treat metastatic breast cancer. A number of variables influence the response to therapy, and, in all cases, treatment is palliative. Systemic therapy is useful to relieve symptoms and to decrease tumor bulk. It can temporarily reverse fatal progression of disease in some patients. Treatment of asymptomatic metastases does not appear to influence survival and is usually withheld.

Radiotherapy is helpful in managing both advanced and recurrent breast cancer. If local disease is bulky and cannot be excised adequately, irradiation provides a means of control, and, rarely, cure. It is especially effective in healing ulcerations. Symptomatic metastatic disease in bone may be particularly benefited by irradiation.

A final form of surgical treatment for advanced or recurrent breast cancer is ablation of ovarian, adrenal, or pituitary function. Oophorectomy, adrenalectomy, and hypophysectomy are seldom performed today. The effect of oophorectomy can be simulated by administration of tamoxifen and that of adrenalectomy by aminoglutethimide.

18

Liver and Biliary Tract

Robert T. Soper

Nelson J. Gurll

Anatomy
Physiology
Surgical Diseases of the Liver
Surgical Diseases of the Biliary Ducts and
  Gallbladder

The liver and biliary ducts form a functional unit that directs numerous metabolic and excretory processes that are essential to life. The liver has many unique features: It is the largest internal organ in the body, weighing 1.5 kg in the adult. It is the chemical center regulating at least 40 to 50 metabolic processes ranging from detoxification to synthesis and excretion (and probably many others that are presently unknown). Its unusual blood supply provides inflow of both arterial (hepatic) and venous (portal) blood from two different vascular systems (systemic and portal, respectively). The liver, therefore, is the only organ that has large inflow arteriovenous shunts, an admixture that occurs in the hepatic sinusoids. It is composed of two lobes, right and left, with a different boundary line separating the anatomical lobes (at the falciform ligament) from the functional lobes (entirely within the right anatomic lobe, at about the position of the gallbladder fossa). Finally, the liver possesses an enormous functional reserve and prodigious regenerative capability. In the experimental animal 80% of the liver can be removed without detectable impairment of function, and regeneration virtually to normal size occurs in 3 to 4 weeks. These unusual features make the liver and biliary tract one of the organ systems most vital to life and largely dictate the role played by the surgeon in caring for patients with hepatic disease.

ANATOMY
Liver

The liver, one of the best protected organs in the abdominal cavity, is guarded anteriorly and laterally by the lower rib cage and superiorly by the muscular diaphragm. Furthermore, it is anchored superiorly and inferiorly by the ramifying vascular and ductal structures that pass vertically through it. Quite dense peritoneal ligaments attach the superior and posterior surfaces of the liver to the inferior surface of the diaphragm, encompassing a large triangular area of liver devoid of peritoneum known as the "bare area"; the bare area is attached directly to the diaphragm by areolar tissue and also contains the hepatic veins, which return blood to the inferior vena cava. The falciform ligament, which contains the ligamentum teres and divides the liver into its anatomic right and left lobes, anchors the liver to the anterior abdominal wall down to the umbilical level. The lesser omentum connects the inferior surface of the liver with the duodenum and stomach, and the hepatorenal ligament attaches the inferior and posterior surfaces of the liver to the right kidney, adrenal gland, and inferior vena cava. All these ligaments and tubular structures tend to anchor the liver securely to the surrounding structures and prevent rapid dislocation during trauma.

The blood supply to the liver comes from two sources (Fig. 18-1). Venous blood returns from the entire gastrointestinal tract through the portal vein, which accounts for 75% of the blood flow to the liver, delivered with a relatively low pressure (5 to 15 cm water) and oxygen content but rich in products of digestion.

The arterial inflow comes through the hepatic artery under high arterial pressures and rich in oxygen but delivers only 25% of the afferent blood to the liver. Both of these vessels enter the inferior surface of the liver in juxtaposition to the major bile duct (Fig. 18-1, *A*), comprising a triad of structures of extreme importance to the surgeon during operations on the duodenum, stomach, and biliary system. Each of these structures divides into a right and left branch to supply the two functional lobes, the dividing line of which lies entirely within the right anatomical lobe in the area of the gallbladder fossa.

The microscopic anatomy of the liver is epitomized by the smallest functional hepatic unit, the lobule (Fig. 18-2). It is composed of a central vein that contains venous blood efferent from the liver to the inferior vena cava and thence to the right side of the heart. Surrounding the central vein are radially arranged polygonal hepatic cells that perform most of the chemical and excretory work of the liver. Between the radiating cords of liver cells are the hepatic sinusoids, which are lined by endothelial and specialized Kupffer cells of the reticuloendothelial system; these sinusoids are supplied by tiny lobular end branches from both the portal and hepatic vessels. The bile canaliculi likewise are juxta-

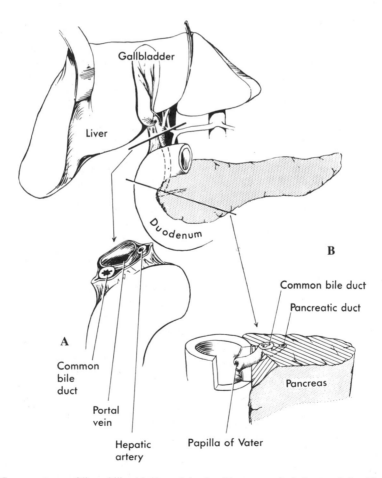

Fig. 18-1. Gross anatomy of liver, biliary ducts, and duodenal loop area. **A,** Intimate relationship of common bile duct, portal vein, and hepatic artery. **B,** Relationships of common bile duct, pancreatic duct, pancreas, and duodenum.

posed between the cords of liver cells and coalesce in the perilobular spaces into cholangioles and tiny biliary ductules. These in turn converge to form the right and left hepatic ducts, which emerge from the inferior surface of the liver with hepatic and portal vessels.

Biliary Ducts

The two main biliary ducts emerging from the inferior surface of the liver join to form the common hepatic duct, which becomes the common bile duct when joined by the cystic duct from the gallbladder (see Fig. 18-1). The common bile duct then enters the head of the pancreas and empties into the medial or concave surface of the second portion of the duodenum through a thickening in the muscle of the duodenal wall known as the sphincter of Oddi (see Fig. 18-1, *B)*. The ampulla of Vater is a dilation of the terminal portion of the common bile duct just proximal to the sphincter of Oddi, and it is the site of entry of the main pancreatic duct when a so-called common channel (of bile and pancreatic juice) exists. The main pancreatic duct may empty independently into the duodenum.

The common bile duct is 6 to 8 mm in diameter and occupies the free edge of the lesser omentum, lying anterior to the aperture into the lesser sac known as the foramen of Winslow. The hepatic artery lies medial to the common duct, its right hepatic branches crossing posterior to it in transit to the right lobe of the liver. The cystic artery is a branch of the right hepatic artery. The portal vein lies posterior and between the common duct and hepatic artery. Abnormalities of positions and relationships of these ducts and vessels are common.

The gallbladder is a pear-shaped, hollow organ with a normal capacity of approximately 50 ml. It lies within the depression on the inferior surface of the right lobe of the liver known as the gallbladder fossa, roughly marking the division between the *functional* right and left hepatic lobes. The rounded fundus of the gallbladder protrudes below the sharp edge of the right

liver lobe and is continuous with the slightly larger body, which then narrows into the neck of the gallbladder. Often the neck of the gallbladder is sacculated into a structure known as *Hartmann's pouch,* where stones are commonly sequestered.

The cystic duct connects the gallbladder to the common bile duct and is characterized by a tortuous and narrow channel filled with spiraling mucosal folds known as the valves of Heister. It is understandable why gallstones so frequently become impacted in the cystic duct when one considers its tortuous and relatively small lumen.

The gallbladder wall has serous, fibromuscular, lamina propria, and mucosal layers from without inward. The biliary duct walls are thinner and contain few, if any, muscular elements. The bile duct serves as a simple conduit. Bile flow is the result of pressure produced by elaboration of bile from the hepatocytes and contractions of the gallbladder. The colicky pain of obstruction results from distention of the bile duct. Veins and lymphatics of the gallbladder may enter the liver directly.

PHYSIOLOGY
Liver

The polygonal liver cell is responsible for the majority of the important metabolic, detoxifying, and secretory functions of the liver. The Kupffer cells are mainly concerned with phagocytosis but also produce γ-globulin, which is important in immune defense mechanisms.

Bile Formation

Bile is excreted by the liver at an irregular rate, averaging approximately 40 ml/hr. Liver bile is a dilute, slightly alkaline, and only mildly pigmented material composed largely of water (97%), bile salts (2%), bilirubin, cholesterol, phospholipids, and minute amounts of calcium and other electrolytes.

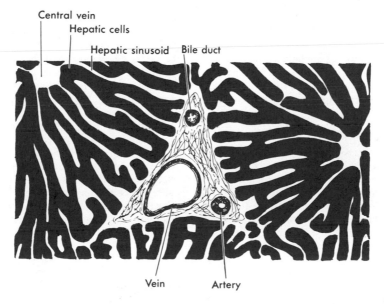

Central vein
Hepatic cells
Hepatic sinusoid   Bile duct

Vein   Artery

Fig. 18-2. Microscopic anatomy of the liver.

Bilirubin is formed from the catabolism of hemoglobin in mature erythrocytes by the reticuloendothelial system, especially spleen and bone marrow. The bilirubin, bound to albumin, is transported in the circulation to the liver, where it is conjugated. After conjugation, the water-soluble bilirubin diglucuronide is excreted into the bile canaliculi and passes into the biliary ducts.

Bile salts are water-soluble substances formed by liver cells from cholesterol and are conjugated to glycine or taurine. Cholesterol is excreted into bile by the liver cells. Cholesterol is totally insoluble in aqueous systems and would immediately precipitate were it not acted on by the bile salts and phospholipids. Lecithin, the chief phospholipid in bile, combines with cholesterol to form liquid crystals. In turn, bile salts exert a detergent-like effect to break these insoluble liquid crystals into small soluble aggregates called mixed micelles. The hepatic secretion of cholesterol, lecithin, and bile salts in ideal ratios prevents cholesterol from precipitating in bile as stones. Bile salts are conserved by their reabsorption from the intestine (mainly distal ileum) into the portal system where they are reexcreted into the bile (enterohepatic circulation).

If the ductal system is obstructed, bile is regurgitated into the general circulation. Conjugated bilirubin is excreted by the renal glomerulus to lend to the urine the golden yellow color so characteristic of obstructive jaundice. Unconjugated bilirubin cannot pass the glomerular endothelium; therefore the jaundice associated with excessive breakdown of red blood cells (hemolytic jaundice) is acholuric (colorless urine). Excessive levels of bile salts in the serum are precipitated in the skin, causing pruritus associated with obstructive jaundice and biliary cirrhosis.

Carbohydrate Metabolism

The liver converts monosaccharides absorbed from the intestine into glycogen, the chief form of carbohydrate storage in the body. Glycogen can be broken down into glucose and pentoses, which can be utilized for energy and synthesis of nucleic acids, fats, and proteins.

Fat Metabolism

Fatty acids and neutral fats are both synthesized and catabolized by the liver. The liver is the principal site of cholesterol synthesis and esterification. Production and degradation of phospholipids and lipoproteins also occur in the liver.

Protein Metabolism

Amino acids are transported from the intestine to the liver, where new protein molecules are formed and different amino acids are created; some of the amino acids are deaminized and converted into carbohydrate or fat. Most clotting factors are made in the liver. Serum albumin, prothrombin, and fibrinogen are three important proteins manufactured by the liver cell. The ammonia resulting from deaminization is synthesized to urea for excretion by the kidney.

Steroid Synthesis and Metabolism

Steroids containing the phenanthrene ring (cholesterol, estrogen, cortisone, bile acids) are synthesized (cholesterol, bile acids) and metabolized (estrogen, cortisone) to inert metabolites by the liver.

Detoxification

Ammonia from protein metabolism is converted to urea. Morphine and barbiturates are metabolized to inactive forms and excreted by the liver.

The bile is the major excretory pathway for iodinated phenolphthalein compounds (iopanoic acid [Telepaque] or iodipamide [Cholografin]), certain dyes (sulfobromophthalein [Bromsulphalein], rose bengal), and some enzymes (alkaline phosphatase) to form the basis for diagnostic tests of hepatic and biliary tract function.

Biliary Ducts

Approximately 1 L of bile is produced each day by the liver at a pressure of 25 to 30 cm water (Fig. 18-3). The sphincter of Oddi maintains this head of pressure by tonic contraction. During periods of fasting, much of the bile is diverted into the cystic duct for storage within the gallbladder. Here the bile is concentrated 10 to 15 times by absorption of water and electrolytes such that the solid content of the gallbladder bile approaches 10% to 15% in contrast to 2% to 3% in the bile as it is excreted by the liver. With the entrance of hydrochloric acid and food into the duodenum during a meal, the hormone cholecystokinin is excreted, which causes the sphincter of Oddi to relax and the gallbladder to contract, emptying its bile into the common duct for delivery to the duodenum.

Bile is important to normal digestion principally because it emulsifies and saponifies ingested fats to improve their digestion and absorption from the intestine; fat-soluble vitamins A, E, D, and K require emulsification for normal absorption. Lipolytic and proteolytic enzymes within the succus entericus are activated by bile. Bile increases the absorption of iron and calcium, increases intestinal motility, and is bacteriostatic for many gastrointestinal tract organisms.

Colon bacteria reduce bilirubin to urobilinogen and then to stercobilin, to give the brownish pigmentation characteristic of normal stools. Some of the urobilinogen and more than 95% of bile salts are reabsorbed into the portal circulation from the intestine (so-called enterohepatic circulation) where much of it is conserved to produce more bile, and a fraction enters the general circulation; small amounts of urobilinogen are normally excreted in the urine.

Obstruction of the biliary tract (obstructive jaundice) prevents bile from reaching the intestine, producing gray-colored stools that are bulky and fatty because of the poor digestion and absorption of dietary fat; reduced absorption of the fat-soluble vitamin K will cause a hemorrhagic tendency if it persists long enough. Anorexia, weight loss, osteoporosis, and an iron-deficiency anemia are commonly seen with long-standing absence of bile from the intestine.

Tests of Liver and Biliary Tract Function

Literally dozens of different tests on blood, urine, duodenal drainage, and stool measure, directly or indirectly, different aspects of hepatic and biliary tract function (Table 18-1). Because of the enormous func-

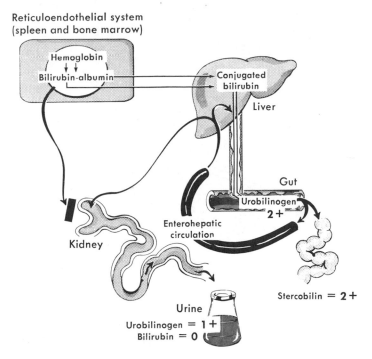

Fig. 18-3. Normal bilirubin metabolism.

Table 18-1. Liver Function Tests

Liver Function Tests	Normal	Hemolytic Jaundice	Parenchymal Jaundice	Obstructive Jaundice
Bilirubin				
Serum				
Direct	0.2-0.5 mg/dl	Normal	Increase	Pronounced increase
Indirect	0.2-0.5 mg/dl	Increase	Increase	Normal early
Urine				
Urobilinogen	1+	4+	1+	0
Bilirubin	0	0	2+	4+
Stool stercobilin	2+	4+	1+	0
Serum alkaline phosphatase	30-120 mU/ml	Normal	Increase	Pronounced increase
Serum albumin	4-5 gm/dl	Normal	Decrease	Normal early
Prothrombin time	12-14 sec or 85%-100% of normal control	Normal	Prolonged	Normal early Prolonged late
Bromsulphalein	3%-5% remains in 45 min	Normal	Increase	Increase
Serum aspartate aminotransferase (AST)	7-40 mU/ml	Normal	Increase	Normal to slight increase

tional reserve of the liver, widespread and far-advanced liver disease may occur before distinctive changes are seen in many of these tests. Furthermore, the results of the tests vary from time to time as the disease waxes and wanes, and some functions of the liver may be severely curtailed while others proceed normally, at least according to our limited ability to measure them.

Liver function tests are most commonly performed to differentiate among the three major types of jaundice: parenchymal hepatic disease, extrahepatic biliary ductal obstruction, and hemolytic jaundice. They help measure advanced degrees of hepatic insufficiency and indicate the trend of hepatic disease or the residual liver damage after recovery. Tests of liver function help in evaluating the risk that liver or biliary surgery imposes on the patient. A few of the more commonly employed tests are described in some detail in the paragraphs that follow.

Tests of Liver Excretory Function

Serum bilirubin. Total serum bilirubin normally varies from 0.4 to 1 mg/dl. The direct-acting fraction

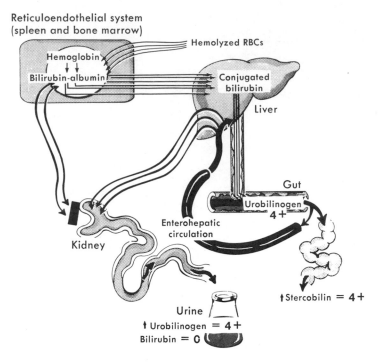

Fig. 18-4. Bilirubin metabolism in hemolytic jaundice.

represents bilirubin that has been conjugated with glucuronic acid in the liver, and the indirect fraction represents bilirubin tied to albumin before conjugation. A normal total value is dependent on normal rates of red blood cell break-down, conjugation, and excretion by the liver, and passage through the biliary ducts to the intestine. Abnormalities of any one of these three steps involved in bilirubin metabolism might alter these levels. *Extrahepatic* obstruction classically produces elevation of the total and direct bilirubin, whereas *hemolytic* jaundice elevates the total and indirect fraction. *Parenchymal* liver disease is asssociated with elevation of total bilirubin and generally both its direct and indirect fractions.

Serum alkaline phosphatase. The normal value of this enzyme is less than 120 mU/ml. The enzyme is released by rapidly metabolizing cells in many organ systems of the body, especially in bone, pancreas, and liver. It is excreted by the liver into the bile and is ultimately lost from the body in the stool. Elevation of serum alkaline phosphatase occurs with extrahepatic biliary tract obstruction and, to lesser degrees, with hepatic cellular disesae, liver metastases, hyperparathyroidism, bone tumors, and Paget's disease of bone. Differentiation from bone disease may be helped by determination of 5'-nucleotidase or leucine amino peptidase.

Urine and stool bile and urobilinogen. Urobilinogen is partially reabsorbed in the enterohepatic circulation and partially excreted in the stool; small amounts are normally present in both the stool and the urine. Urobilinogen may be measured by simple, gross or fairly sophisticated quantitative tests. Extrahepatic obstruction of the biliary ducts is associated with no urobilinogen or bilirubin in the stool (acholic stool) and no

urobilinogen but increased amounts of conjugated bilirubin in the urine. With increased hemolysis, the amounts of both urobilinogen and bilirubin are increased in the stool, whereas in the urine the urobilinogen is increased; there is no bilirubin in the urine, since unconjugated bilirubin is not excreted by the kidney.

Metabolic Function Tests

Serum albumin. Serum albumin is one of the proteins manufactured by liver cells. The normal serum albumin level is 4.5 to 5 gm/dl of serum, and the albumin-globulin ratio in the serum is generally above 1. Chronic liver cell damage is associated with a lowering of the serum albumin and a decrease or reversal of the albumin-globulin ratio.

Prothrombin time (PT). Prothrombin is manufactured by the liver cells when adequate amounts of vitamin K are present. A deficiency of vitamin K occurs with prolonged obstructive jaundice (no bile to emulsify and aid in the absorption of the fat-soluble vitamin K) or chronic hepatocellular disease, resulting in inadequate production of prothrombin and prolongation of the PT. Normal PT is about 12 to 14 seconds. An elevated prothrombin time signals the need for parenteral vitamin K administration in the preoperative patient, a return to normal indicating adequate liver cell reserve and perhaps a less bloody operation.

Bromsulphalein test. Bromsulphalein, a dye, is metabolized by the liver cell and excreted in the bile very rapidly; only 3% to 5% remains in the serum 45 minutes after intravenous administration. Elevation of the amount of Bromsulphalein present 45 minutes after administration is a rather sensitive indicator of hepatocellular damage.

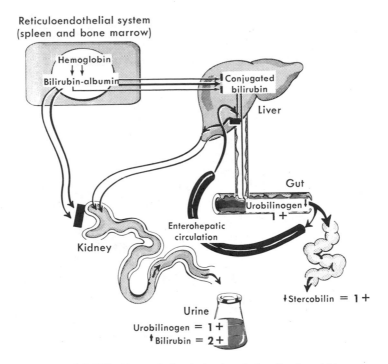

Reticuloendothelial system
(spleen and bone marrow)

Hemoglobin

Bilirubin-albumin

Conjugated bilirubin

Liver

Gut

Urobilinogen 1 +

Enterohepatic circulation

Kidney

↓Stercobilin = 1 +

Urine

Urobilinogen = 1 +
↑Bilirubin = 2 +

Fig. 18-5. Bilirubin metabolism in intrahepatic jaundice (hepatitis).

Serum AST. AST is present in liver, heart muscle, skeletal muscle, kidney and pancreas and may be elevated after injury to any of these organs. In reference to the liver, greatest elevations of this enzyme occur with hepatocellular injury (parenchymatous jaundice), and very slight elevations accompany hemolytic or obstructive jaundice.

Jaundice

Jaundice is a yellowish discoloration of the skin, sclera, body surfaces, and secretions. It can be detected on clinical examination when the serum bilirubin rises above 2.5 mg/dl. Three major classifications of jaundice are based on the nature and site of the disturbance of bilirubin metabolism: (1) *excessive hemolysis* of red blood cells (hemolytic, acholuric, prehepatic jaundice); (2) *hepatocellular (parenchymatous) disease,* which inhibits bilirubin conjugation (hepatocellular, retention, intrahepatic, or medical jaundice), and (3) *obstruction* of bile flow occurring anywhere from the canaliculi on down the biliary tract into the intestine (obstructive, regurgitation, posthepatic, extrahepatic, or surgical jaundice).

In *hemolytic jaundice* (Fig. 18-4) an excessive lysis of red blood cells causes increased production of bilirubin by the reticuloendothelial cells in the spleen and bone marrow; more bilirubin is produced than can be excreted by the normally functioning hepatic excretory mechanisms. The excess of nonconjugated bilirubin in the serum cannot be excreted in the urine but elevates the *indirect* fraction of bilirubin in the serum, with normal *direct*-acting fraction. The tests for hepatocellular function are normal, but excessive amounts of *urobilinogen* in the urine and stool and bilirubin (stercobilin) in the stool are diagnostic. Hemolytic jaundice is seen in congenital spherocytosis, thalassemia, septicemia,

transfusion with mismatched blood, and after certain venomous snake bites. Treatment is directed at the cause of the hemolysis rather than the jaundice per se, and it is nonsurgical except for the definitive treatment of congenital spherocytosis (splenectomy).

Intrahepatic or *parenchymatous jaundice* (Fig. 18-5) is seen with liver infections (hepatitis), exposure to hepatotoxic agents (chloroform, arsenicals, occasionally chlorpromazine), and in the terminal stages of liver failure. Acute viral hepatitis is characterized by elevated AST and alanine aminotransferase (ALT) in the serum, but with chronic hepatic disorders the liver function tests are seldom diagnostic. There is a moderate elevation of both the direct and indirect serum bilirubin with decreased serum albumin levels, a mild increase in the alkaline phosphatase, and prolongation of the prothrombin time (with a poor response to vitamin K). Treatment is nonsurgical and largely supportive until the disease has run its course.

Obstructive jaundice (Fig. 18-6) results from interference of bile flow somewhere within the biliary ductal system. Most of these obstructions occur within the extrahepatic ducts and are amenable to surgical bypass or removal of the obstruction; therefore differentiation from the other two major types of jaundice becomes very important. In obstructive jaundice the stool is clay colored or very lightly pigmented, the stool and urine urobilinogen are diminished or absent, and the bilirubin (chiefly the direct fraction) is elevated. The hepatocellular tests are normal early, but with increasing duration of jaundice liver cell damage occurs.

Stones within the common bile duct (choledocholithiasis) are the most common cause of extra-hepatic obstructive jaundice, generally associated with pain and fluctuation in the intensity of the jaundice. Strictures of

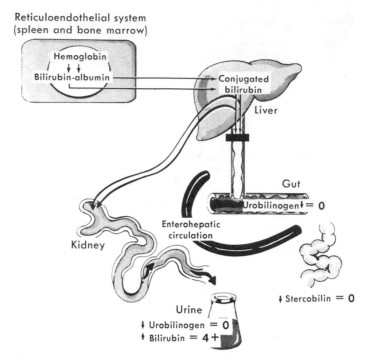

Fig. 18-6. Bilirubin metabolism in obstructive (surgical) jaundice.

the bile ducts most commonly result from duct injury during cholecystectomy. The resulting jaundice tends to be fluctuating, essentially painless, and often associated with fever and cholangitis. Cancers of the bile ducts, ampulla of Vater, and head of the pancreas characteristically produce a progressively deepening and painless jaundice. Jaundice can also result from acute or chronic pancreatitis. Congenital atresia of the bile ducts is one of the two chief causes of *jaundice in the newborn*. It must be distinguished from neonatal hepatitis by early laparotomy.

Occasionally with the administration of certain drugs (chlorpromazine, arsenicals), with sepsis, and during the acute course of hepatitis, the intra-hepatic cholangioles becomes obstructed by edema and inflammation to produce a variety of obstructive jaundice indistinguishable biochemically from extrahepatic obstructive jaundice, the so-called *cholestatic* jaundice. Furthermore, the longer obstructive jaundice from any cause persists, the more damage to liver cells will ensue from back pressure, regurgitation of bile, and infection; tests of hepatocellular function become progressively altered, and the laboratory tests therefore become less helpful in distinguishing obstructive from parenchymatous jaundice.

The type of jaundice can be diagnosed correctly in 75% to 80% of patients by a carefully taken history, complete physical examination, and a few simple tests performed on the patient's urine, stool, and blood. In the remaining 20% the more sophisticated liver function tests, cholangiography, liver biopsy, or even exploratory laparotomy may be necessary to make a correct diagnosis.

Although not an emergency, the work-up of a jaundiced patient should proceed expediently, and a decision regarding the need for surgical exploration should be made as early as possible. The complications of untreated and long-standing jaundice are biliary cirrhosis, cholangitis, bile nephrosis, and, ultimately, both hepatic and renal failure. All have high morbidity and mortality.

SURGICAL DISEASES OF THE LIVER

Although the liver is often *damaged* by surgical disease (extrahepatic obstructive jaundice) or becomes secondarily involved by surgical disease (liver metastases from a primary intestinal neoplasm), and although liver disease can produce secondary changes that require surgical treatment (splenectomy, esophageal varices ligation, and portalsystemic shunts for portal hypertension), few diseases *of* the liver are treated by operations *on* the liver.

Trauma

The liver is commonly injured by penetrating wounds of the abdomen and chest (stabbings, high-velocity missiles), and it ranks third among the intraabdominal organs injured by nonpenetrating abdominal trauma. Even minor trauma may severely damage a liver enlarged by disease. The right anatomic lobe of the liver is larger and more exposed than the left and is therefore more frequently traumatized. Associated injuries to the right rib cage and other intraabdominal organs often overshadow the hepatic injury.

Traumatic rupture of the liver results in intraabdominal spillage of blood and bile with signs of shock and peritoneal irritation proportionate to the volume and speed of extravasation. Pain is initially localized to the right upper abdominal quadrant, then it becomes more generalized, and often is referred to the right shoulder tip. Abdominal tenderness and guarding follow the pain, with percussion dullness, and occasionally a palpable mass (hematoma). Paralytic ileus with abdominal distension occurs late.

Flat and decubitus plain films of the chest and abdomen may reveal fractured ribs, a mass, or elevation of the right hemidiaphragm—all suggestive of liver injury. Peritoneal lavage should be performed and computed tomography (CT) of the abdomen may be invaluable in determining which injuries can be followed nonoperatively.

Treatment of minor degrees of hepatic trauma is nonsurgical—bed rest, analgesics, and supportive care. Occasionally delayed subcapsular liver hematomas may rupture; thus observation of the patient for 1 to 2 weeks is advisable. The surgical goals in the treatment of more serious liver injuries are to debride devitalized tissue and to control bleeding. Actively bleeding lacerations are best stopped by direct suture of identifiable vessels. Control may require exploration of the laceration and even hepatic artery ligation. Parenchymal damage resulting from stellate lacerations and blunt injuries is treated by wide debridement. Lobectomy is rarely required, and mortality is higher than with debridement. Extensive drainage of the damaged area is of paramount importance. T-tube decompressions of the biliary tree is associated with complications and is generally not indicated.

Surgical Infections of the Liver
Pyogenic Liver Abscess

Better diagnosis and treatment of infections have greatly reduced the incidence, morbidity, and mortality of pyogenic liver abscesses. Most begin as small microabscesses in the portal triads, which then progress to destroy liver cells and coalesce into gross abscesses. Selective antibiotic therapy administered during the microabscess stage probably reverses the infection and is the best explanation for the lowered incidence of frank abscesses.

The origin of 10% to 20% of pyogenic liver abscesses is unknown; the majority of the remainder originate in some portion of the gastrointestinal tract with spread to secondarily involve the liver. The most common cause is infection in the biliary tree associated with obstruction or manipulation. Acute suppurative appendicitis, diverticulitis, ulcerative colitis, and enteritis are less common contributors. Coliform organisms are responsible for most pyogenic liver abscesses. Staphylococcal liver abscesses arise from systemic infections (osteomyelitis, carbuncles) and reach the liver through the hepatic artery.

The early clinical features are dominated by signs and symptoms of the causative extrahepatic infection. Right upper quadrant distress heralds hepatic abscess progressing to pain, spiking fever, sweating, shaking chills, and a palpably enlarged and tender liver. Mild jaundice may complicate the picture late in the clinical course and in general is an unfavorable prognostic sign.

The laboratory tests show anemia and leukocytosis with a shift to the left in the differential white blood cell count. Radiographs reveal an elevated and relatively immobile right hemidiaphragm with an enlarged hepatic shadow. Blood cultures are positive unless antibiotics have been given. Liver scintiscans may disclose a filling defect if the abscess is more than 2 or 3 cm in size and is located fairly near the surface. Selective hepatic arteriography may reveal defects smaller than the resolution of a scintiscan. The defects are avascular in contrast to most hepatic tumors.

Diffuse bacterial insults to the liver are critical diseases. Antibiotics and supportive care are always indicated. Pyogenic liver abscesses are treated by needle aspiration guided by CT or ultrasound combined with specific antibiotics. Surgical (open) drainage may be required if the abscesses are multiple or loculated.

Amebic Abscess

Acute amebic colitis is common in tropical and less developed countries; about 10% of cases are complicated by amebic liver abscesses if not properly treated. There is no history of dysentery in one half of patients with amebic liver abscess. Trophozoites of the parasite *Entamoeba histolytica* gain access to the portal venous tributary through the involved colon wall and migrate to the liver, where liquefactive necrosis of liver tissue occurs with coalescence into larger cavities. These abscesses are composed of necrotic liver tissue of a chocolate-red color often likened to anchovy paste. The offending parasite can usually be found in the wall of the abscess cavity, and with proper treatment it becomes encapsulated and calcified in time. If untreated, the abscesses may enlarge and perforate into the abdominal cavity or burrow through the diaphragm and empty into the thoracic cavity.

The clinical and laboratory findings resemble those of pyogenic liver abscesses except that the white blood cell count is lower, with less of a shift to the left in the differential count. Eosinophilia may be present. The liver complication may occur weeks after the colonic phase, which is often minor and unrecognized. Sigmoidoscopic examination and scrapings from the superficial mucosal ulcerations and warm stool examinations will usually reveal the amebas.

When the diagnosis of amebic hepatitis is made or suspected, the patient should be treated with metronidazole (Flagyl), 750 mg orally three times a day for 10 days. A dramatic improvement in the patient's condition confirms the diagnosis and is therapeutic as well. Large amebic abscesses can be aspirated percutaneously. If the signs of liver infection worsen, laparotomy is necessary for confirmation of diagnosis; aspiration of the amebic abscess is preferable to open drainage for fear of a more general contamination of the peritoneal cavity by external drainage.

Cysts and Tumors of the Liver
Simple Cysts

Liver cysts may be associated with cysts of the kidneys and may be multiple and small or single and large. They are thin-walled and filled with watery, colorless fluid. The larger cysts are treated by total or partial excision or drainage into the peritoneal cavity or intestine. Their main importance lies in distinguishing them from neoplasms, primary or metastatic, to the liver.

Echinococcus Cysts

Echinococcal cysts of the liver are common in sheep-raising countries of the world where man serves as the intermediary host in the life cycle of the dog tapeworm *(Echinococcus granulosus)*. The tapeworm within the dog intestine sheds eggs that are excreted and ingested by sheep or man (especially children), with secondary involvement of the liver and lung from intestinal migration. Echinococcus liver cysts, usually slow-growing, may reach a large size with rupture into the free peritoneal cavity, lung, or bile ducts.

Eosinophilia occurs frequently, and complement fixation tests are specifically diagnostic. Plain films often reveal calcification in the cyst wall. Surgical treatment consists of excision after careful evacuation of the cyst contents by aspiration and injection of 20% to 30% sodium chloride or 0.5% sodium hypochlorite to kill the scoleces.

Benign Tumors of the Liver

Hemangiomas, fibromas, and hamartomas occasionally arise in the liver and must be distinguished from metastatic or primary malignant neoplasms. Large hemangiomas of the liver are removed if they are traumatized (hemorrhage) or sequester large amounts of blood.

Hepatic adenomas are benign tumors whose incidence seems to be increasing because of the use of oral contraceptives. These lesions should be resected (usually by hepatic lobectomy) because they are frequently attended by life-threatening complications such as rupture and bleeding.

Malignant Tumors of the Liver

The most common malignant tumor of the liver is *metastatic* from a primary neoplasm in the stomach, colon, breast, or pancreas. The gastrointestinal tract metastases reach the liver through the portal vein, and others reach the liver through the hepatic artery. Direct spread from primary malignancies of the gallbladder, stomach, and other organs adjacent to the liver also occurs.

The majority of liver metastases are multiple and involve both lobes; only rarely are metastases localized so that resection can be considered. The exceptions to this treatment rule are liver metastases from malignant carcinoids or the Zollinger-Ellison type of pancreatic neoplasm, in which partial resection of the liver metastases is indicated to palliate the functional hormonal effects of the metastases. Radiotherapy of hepatic metastases is rarely indicated because of the severe symptoms (anorexia, nausea, vomiting) that occur when liver tissue is irradiated and because of the relentless (and hopeless) course of liver metastases. Chemotherapeutic agents occasionally produce palliation, especially when delivered directly into the portal vein or hepatic artery by indwelling catheters.

Primary malignant lesions of the liver are rare in the United States but are common among certain ethnic groups such as the Chinese and the African Bantu. Hepatomas arise from the liver cells and are almost invariably preceded by years of cirrhosis, hemochromatosis, or some other such chronic primary inflammatory liver disease. Cholangiocarcinomas arise from the intrahepatic bile duct cells and are not necessarily a sequela of chronic liver disease.

Symptoms of primary malignant liver tumors are insidious and nonspecific at first, including weight loss, anorexia, and low-grade fever. Liver enlargement (nodular or localized) follows with ultimate development of ascites and jaundice. The serum alkaline phosphatase is characteristically high. Treatment is usually futile. Although cholangiocarcinomas localized to one lobe are amenable to hemihepatectomy, the prognosis is poor. Chemotherapeutic agents may offer some palliation.

Portal Hypertension

The pressure within the portal vein varies between 5 and 15 cm of water, depending on position, exertion, and other variables. Portal venous pressure consistently above 20 cm of water pressure indicates portal hypertension. Portal hypertension occurs whenever the flow of blood within the portal vein is impeded or obstructed; such obstruction can occur at three principal sites:

Intrahepatic obstruction. Intrahepatic obstruction is the most common cause of portal hypertension and is almost always caused by cirrhosis (of varying types) of the liver. Alcoholism generally precedes cirrhosis among adults in this country, though among nondrinkers and children previous severe hepatitis with *postnecrotic cirrhosis* is the most likely precursor. The fibrosis and scarring that occur with any type of cirrhosis inhibit the transport of blood into the central veins of the hepatic lobules, leading to stasis and increased pressure within the portal venous system.

Subhepatic obstruction. Obstruction of the portal vein is the most common cause of portal hypertension among children and very young adults. Portal vein obstruction may result from an extension of the normal postnatal obliterative mechanisms in the umbilical vein and ductus venosus, neonatal septic pylephlebitis (from omphalitis), sepsis of other origin, or occasionally a congenital malformation (cavernous transformation) of the portal vein. Whatever the cause, the portal vein obstruction inhibits passage of its blood *to* the liver.

Suprahepatic obstruction. Obstruction within the hepatic veins or the vena cava itself results in stasis of blood within the liver that is transmitted to the portal venous system leading into the liver. The obstruction may result from thrombosis *(Budd-Chiari syndrome)* or from tumors. It is the least common of all causes for portal hypertension, accounting for about 1% of cases.

Regardless of the site of the block in the venous drainage, the increasing volume and pressure of blood within the portal venous system produce a nonspecific group of secondary clinical disorders that are grouped together under the rubric of *portal hypertension*.

The most serious symptoms are caused by enlargement and collateralization of the vessels that connect the portal and the systemic venous systems. Normally these collateral veins are small and carry minute amounts of blood under low pressure. The naturally occurring portasystemic venous shunts are as follows: *esophageal veins* (which carry portal blood into the azygos system), *hemorrhoidal veins* (which carry portal blood into the pudendal and iliac veins), and *umbilical veins* (which carry portal blood to the anterior abdominal wall veins). There are innumerable other unnamed collaterals in the retroperitoneal spaces adjacent to the kidneys and spleen. The dilation and increase in venous pressure within all of these systems may then result in several conditions.

Esophageal varices. Esophageal varices protrude into the lumen of the esophagus, where ulceration results from irritation of food, tubes, or acid-peptic factors. Massive and potentially lethal upper gastrointestinal bleeding is a dreaded result. Diagnosis is confirmed by esophagogram (Fig 24-2) and esophagoscopy.

Hemorrhoids. Hemorrhoids may prolapse and bleed.

Caput medusae. In this condition the abdominal wall collaterals may increase in size, radiating outward from the umbilicus.

A second major effect of portal hypertension is on the spleen (see Chap. 20). It is characterized by splenomegaly and hypersplenism with anemia, leukopenia, and thrombocytopenia.

The final effect of portal hypertension is increased production of ascites fluid, associated with the suprahepatic or intrahepatic blockage. Poor drainage of the lymphatics of the liver capsule with "bleeding" of this lymph fluid into the free peritoneal cavity is the probable cause. There is also increased formation of hepatic and splanchnic lymph. Additional causes for ascites often accompany portal hypertension associated with primary liver disease and include hypoalbuminemia and sodium and water retention because of endocrine and renal factors.

Portal hypertension attributed to primary liver disease may be complicated by hepatic coma from liver decompensation. This is especially likely to occur when large amine loads are thrust on a poorly functioning liver (by massive gastrointestinal tract hemorrhage from gastritis, ulcer, or esophageal varices). The liver cells are incapable of handling the amine load resulting from the bacterial digestion of blood proteins in the gastrointestinal tract, or these amines are shunted through portasystemic collaterals into the systemic circulation without passage through the liver. Resulting hyperammonemia may be responsible for many central nervous system manifestations of hepatic failure (coma, liver flap). Other possible mechanisms for hepatic coma involve the production of certain amines and amino acids that can act as false neurotransmitters.

Clinical features. Massive upper gastrointestinal tract bleeding is the most frightening manifestation of portal hypertension, especially as the vomiting of blood (hematemesis). Consequent hypovolemia and hyperammonemia superimposed on severe liver disease may be lethal. Bleeding from esophageal varices in patients with subhepatic obstruction (normal liver function) is tolerated much better. Caput medusae is an interesting diagnostic adjunct to the diagnosis of portal hypertension but is not clinically significant. The enlarged and bleeding hemorrhoids, often a nuisance, are not a serious threat to the patient's life and are seldom treated surgically.

Signs of impending liver failure can often occur after gastrointestinal tract bleeding in patients with liver disease; concurrent jaundice is a grave prognostic sign. Ascites may be the outstanding clinical feature of patients with suprahepatic obstruction.

Diagnosis and differential diagnosis. Massive upper gastrointestinal tract bleeding from esophageal va-

rices must be distinguished from blood originating within the stomach and duodenum (Chap. 24). Peptic ulcer of the stomach or duodenum and gastritis are the most common lesions to be differentiated, though carcinoma of the stomach in the older patient must also be ruled out. Distinguishing a bleeding peptic ulcer from esophageal varices is difficult, especially if the patient has cirrhosis, since cirrhotic patients have a 7 to 10 times greater incidence of peptic ulcer than the general population does. To complicate the picture further, peptic ulcer or gastritis and esophageal varices may coexist.

If most of the blood is effortlessly vomited and little appears rectally, esophageal varices are likely to be the site of bleeding; on the other hand, bleeding that occurs mainly as tarry stools (melena) with little blood in the stomach is most likely to be duodenal (and peptic) in origin. Hemorrhage originating in the stomach may present with significant hematemesis and tarry stools concomitantly. Differentiation among these three sites of bleeding is important because of the different approaches in management.

Careful attention to the history of previous acid-peptic diathesis plus a history of current or prevous alcoholism or hepatitis is important. Children and non-drinkers who have never had hepatitis most likely have subhepatic blockage. Physical examination should be directed toward finding stigmas of liver disease such as jaundice, reddened palms, spider hemangiomas, caput medusae, ascites, hepatosplenomegaly, and hemorrhoidal varices.

PT, Bromsulphalein retention, and serum ammonia tests may be helpful. If they are abnormal, the diagnosis of cirrhosis can be presumed, and treatment with vitamin K is begun. Gastric intubation and lavage are helpful in assessing the volume of blood loss. Emergency esophagogastroscopy is indicated, since patients with varices are often found to be bleeding from other sites. Emergency upper gastrointestinal barium studies are performed if the patient's condition stabilizes. Central venous pressure and urinary output should be monitored.

Emergency treatment. The initial treatment of bleeding esophageal varices is aimed at stabilization of the circulating blood volume with fluid and blood. Fresh blood is preferable to bank blood because of its higher platelet content and other support of the blood coagulation mechanism. Control of bleeding can be attempted by balloon tamponade, vasopressin infusion, injection sclerotherapy or operation.

A triple-lumen rubber tube *(Sengstaken-Blakemore tube; Fig. 24-3)* is helpful in both differential diagnosis and treatment of bleeding esophageal varices. The tube is passed into the stomach, and the gastric balloon, inflated with 250 ml of air, is pulled up snugly against the esophagogastric junction. Compression of the gastroesophageal collaterals by this maneuver commonly arrests bleeding from esophageal varices. The inner lumen of the tube allows continued gastric aspiration and lavage. If bleeding ceases, its origin from esophageal varices is confirmed. Also, if blood continues to well up into the hypopharynx with the gastric balloon in place, esophageal varices are probably responsible. These can be tamponed temporarily by inflating the esophageal balloon with air to a pressure of 30 to 40 torr. The Sengstaken-Blakemore tube is left inflated for 24 to 36 hours. This respite allows time for diagnostic work-up and stabilization of the patient. The esophageal and gastric balloons must be deflated gradually. The tube is removed if bleeding does not recur in the next 24 hours. Pressure necrosis of gastric or esophageal surfaces may result if the Sengstaken-Blakemore tube remains in place for longer than 48 to 72 hours.

Treatment of the patient during the period of tube inflation should include blood transfusions, vitamin K, neomycin to reduce the bacterial flora (responsible for liberating the amines from the blood proteins), lactulose, and vigorous laxation and enemas to remove the residual blood from the gastrointestinal tract. Intravenous glucose and vitamin B support the diseased liver. Peritoneal dialysis or exchange blood transfusions may be helpful if liver failure seems imminent.

If bleeding from the esophageal varices resumes after deflation of the tube, the gastric and esophageal balloons are quickly reinflated and preparations are made for emergency sclerotherapy or portasystemic shunting. The constant intravenous infusion of vasopressin is extremely effective in controlling variceal bleeding during preparation for definitive operation and sometimes is followed by long-term cessation of bleeding. It should not be used concurrently with balloon tamponade because of the cumulative morbidity and mortality.

Emergency portasystemic venous shunting procedures carry a high mortality, and every effort is made to control acute bleeding, followed by intensive medical treatment, preparation for elective portasystemic shunting. Injecting the esophageal varices through an endoscope with an agent that rapidly induces clotting (sclerotherapy) has been resurrected, is effective in controlling bleeding, and has achieved widespread use as an alternative to emergency operation.

Definitive treatment. Surgical procedures are available for prophylactic and more definitive treatment of good-risk patients with hypersplenism and portal hypertension. Patients with serious liver disease who have already had one episode of major hemorrhage from esophageal varices run a 50% risk of being dead within a year from a second massive hemorrhage. On the other hand, patients with subhepatic portal obstruction almost never die from major esophageal hemorrhage provided that adequate blood replacement and supportive care are available.

The mortality for the major portasystemic venous shunt operations (Fig. 18-7) is about 10%; the highest mortality is seen in patients with intrahepatic block with a serious degree of liver impairment. Good-risk patients have a serum bilirubin less than 3 mg/dl, serum albumin greater than 3 gm/dl, Bromsulphalein retention less than 30%, and PT more than 50% of normal after the administration of vitamin K; they will not have ascites and should be less than 60 years of age. These are useful guidelines in the selection of candidates for portasystemic shunt procedures.

Work-up of a patient who is a candidate for operation includes careful esophagogastroscopy to verify the presence of varices and the absence of concomitant peptic ulcer, selective arteriography with careful attention to the venous phase to visualize vascular anomalies and the patency of the portal system, and percutaneous splenoportography in selected patients in whom the question of portal pressure or the state of the portal venous system is unclear. This information is vital in both the timing and the selection of the proper shunting operation.

Definitive operations. The only portasystemic shunts possible for patients with subhepatic obstruction are splenorenal and mesocaval shunts (see Fig. 18-7). Splenectomy is often done at the time of side-to-side splenorenal shunt (see Fig. 18-7, *C*) but is seldom indicated as the sole treatment of portal hypertension because the thrombosis of the splenic vein that inevitably occurs obviates later splenorenal shunt should that become necessary. After successful portasystemic shunting, the spleen decreases in size and returns to normal function.

Five types of portasystemic venous shunts are commonly used in patients with intrahepatic portal block (see Fig. 18-7). The end-to-side or side-to-side anastomosis of the portal vein just below the liver to the inferior vena cava is a commonly used shunt. When the portal vein is thrombosed, the splenorenal shunt may be performed. The mesocaval shunt has the advantage of relative technical simplicity (as compared to side-to-side splenorenal and portacaval shunts). The distal splenorenal shunt has a lower incidence of death from encephalopathy than other portasystemic shunts but is less effective in preventing further bleeding.

Prognosis. The benefit of any of the shunting procedures depends on maintained patency of the anastomosis, since thrombosis is followed by a recrudescence in the portal hypertension and its serious sequelae. After a successful portasystemic shunt, the prognosis in patients with subhepatic block is excellent, whereas that in patients with intrahepatic obstruction and cirrhosis is dependent on the liver disease itself. Survival is better in alcoholic cirrhosis patients who manage to abstain from alcohol.

SURGICAL DISEASES OF THE BILIARY DUCTS AND GALLBLADDER

Operations on the gallbladder and biliary tree rank next to hernia repair and appendectomy in frequency of abdominal operations performed in the United States. Most of the biliary tract disorders arise from the complications of gallstones. Many Americans harbor gallstones at autopsy; the frequency reaches 30% in females and 10% in males about 65 years of age.

Meticulous dissection in a bloodless operative field and absolute identification of anatomic structures are laudable principles in any surgical procedure, but never are they so vital as in gallbladder and biliary tract operations (Fig. 18-1). The closeness to the portal vein, hepatic arteries, and other structures vital to life, the propensity for congenital anatomic variations, and the obliteration of landmarks imposed by inflammation combine to emphasize the need for strict adherence to these general principles. Biliary tract surgery in the infant and young child is further complicated by a spectrum of diseases different from that in the adult, plus the additional technical problems imposed by size.

Congenital Anomalies

The liver and biliary tree arise embryonically as a diverticulum from the ventral aspect of the foregut at

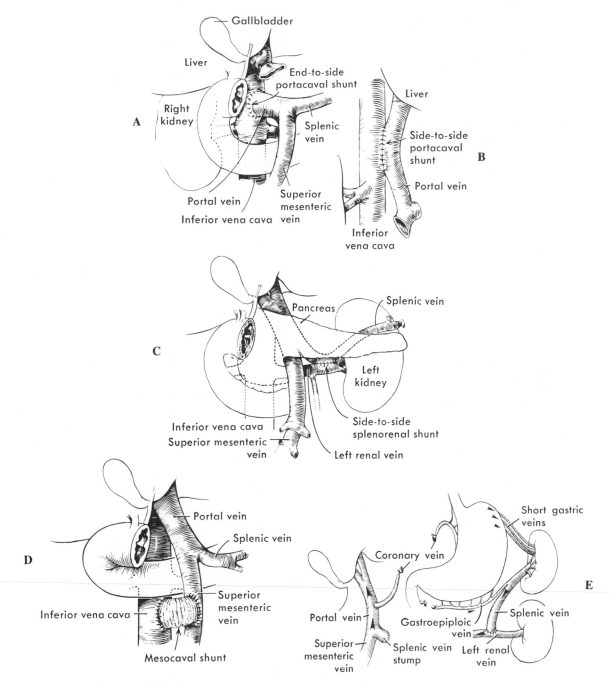

Fig. 18-7. Major types of shunting operations performed for portal hypertension and esophageal varices bleeding. **A,** End-to-side portacaval shunt (end of divided portal vein anastomosed to side of inferior vena cava). **B,** Side-to-side portacaval shunt (portal vein not divided, some blood flows retrogradely from liver into inferior vena cava). **C,** Side-to-side splenorenal shunt (splenic vein anastomosed to left renal vein). **D,** Mesocaval shunt (superior mesenteric vein connected to inferior vena cava by knitted Dacron graft 18 to 20 mm. in diameter, 5 to 8 cm. in length). **E,** Distal splenorenal or Warren shunt (with portoazygous disconnection to ensure drainage of esophagogastric variceal blood through spleen and splenic vein into left renal vein).

the 3 mm embryo stage; the lumen early becomes solidified by cellular accumulations but later recanalizes. Liver cells and supporting mesenchymal tissue proliferate beneath the developing diaphragm. Abnormalities in development are common; hence the anatomical variations of the biliary ducts and their relationship to the hepatic artery, portal vein, and pancreatic ducts that are encountered at operation.

Neonatal jaundice is apparent clinically in about 50% of term babies and 80% of premature babies. In almost all of them, fortunately, it is transient and insignificant. The age of onset of jaundice has some bearing on cause and prognosis:

Jaundice beginning on the *first day of life* generally results from intrauterine hemolysis, most often with Rh incompatibility (erythroblastosis fetalis) and less frequently with major ABO blood group incompatibility between the fetus and the mother.

Jaundice that is first apparent on *the second or third day* of life is almost always "physiological" and resolves rapidly and spontaneously.

Jaundice arising on *days 3 to 7* of life most commonly caused by infections (sepsis, syphilis, toxoplasmosis, cytomegalovirus) and drugs (vitamin K, sulfonamides), but occasionally it may result from hematoma absorption and thrombocytopenic purpura.

Jaundice becoming apparent *at or beyond 2 weeks* of life may be caused by neonatal hepatitis, infections (sepsis, syphilis, herpes, toxoplasmosis), metabolic storage disorders (Gaucher's disease, Niemann-Pick disease), or galactosemia. Extrahepatic obstructive jaundice occurs less often and results from bile inspissated within the ducts, atresia of the ductal system, or choledochal cyst.

Differential diagnosis of jaundice arising at 2 to 3 weeks of age rests between hepatitis and obstructive jaundice. The other medical causes for jaundice can generally be diagnosed or ruled out. Differentiation between hepatitis and extrahepatic obstructive jaundice is difficult (if not impossible) by physical examination or laboratory tests; therefore, if the jaundice persists for 4 to 6 weeks, exploratory laparotomy is required. Open liver biopsy with frozen section evaluation will quickly establish the diagnosis of hepatitis on the basis of giant cells and lack of bile duct proliferation, and no further exploration is necessary. If the liver biopsy is not diagnostic, the surgeon must determine ductal patency by cholangiograms and surgical dissection.

The *inspissated bile syndrome* results from a plug of tenacious, thick bile somewhere within the ductal system. Some cases are associated with previous hemolytic disorders, and others complicate neonatal hepatitis. Cholangiograms obtained after the ductal system is flushed with saline introduced through a needle or catheter in the fundus of the gallbladder are both diagnostic and therapeutic.

Congenital atresia of the bile ducts is characterized by partial or complete obliteration of some portion of the biliary tree. In only about 10% will the obstruction be correctable: a block in common bile duct or gallbladder with dilated proximal ducts draining bile. Surgical bypass is carried out by means of choledochojejunostomy. Until recently, the other 90% of babies with biliary atresia died of liver failure within 2 years. However, Japanese surgeons have developed the Kasai operation (hepatic portoenterostomy), which cures 20% to 40% of these patients. A button of tissue is removed from the liver hilum where the intrahepatic bile ducts converge, to which the jejunum is anastomosed. The operation succeeds if there are bile-containing ducts within the liver hilum but not if the intrahepatic ducts are sclerosed or nonexistent.

Choledochal cyst is a cystic dilation of the supraduodenal portion of the common bile duct contain-

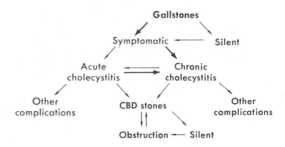

Fig. 18-8. Natural history of gallstones. *CBD,* Common bile duct.

ing stagnated bile (and often stones). A tiny and poorly functioning connection to the duodenum at the ampulla of Vater is usually seen. Whether the cyst is truly congenital (because of developmental difficulties) or arises secondary to abnormal ductal anatomy, which allows pancreatic juice to enter the common bile duct, is unknown. In any event, the complications of gallstone formation, cholangitis with biliary cirrhosis, and perforation have all been reported.

Choledochal cyst commonly presents as a right upper quadrant abdominal mass in a child or young adult associated with recurrent bouts of mild jaundice and attacks of right upper abdominal pain. Oral cholecystography reveals displacement of the gallbladder; upper gastrointestinal tract barium studies reveal a downward and medial displacement of the duodenum. Use of ultrasound is diagnostic. These cysts are best treated by excision and biliary-enteric drainage, since their malignant degeneration has been described.

Gallstones

Gallstones produce the majority of surgical diseases of the gallbladder and bile ducts (Fig. 18-8). The incidence of gallstones varies with different races, geographic locations, and dietary habits. All autopsy studies have shown a distinct relationship to age, with frequency increasing with advancing age. A striking sex relationship is also noted; women harbor stones three times more often than men and at a younger age. Gallstones almost invariably arise within the gallbladder and only secondarily involve the common bile duct. A higher than normal incidence of gallstones occurs with pregnancy, diabetes, pancreatitis, cirrhosis, obesity, and hypothyroidism. About 10% to 15% of gallstones are radiopaque.

Two main types of gallstones are recognized: *Cholesterol stones.* Stones containing 60% to 95% cholesterol by dry weight are the most common type of gallstones (75% of all). The noncholesterol component of such gallstones is predominately inert material with small amounts of bile pigment and calcium. They are generally multiple, faceted by indentations created by their neighbors, and firm, and they contain concentric laminae suggestive of periodic deposition. Occasionally cholesterol stones present as a single, large, smooth, soft, yellow-white stone containing almost pure cholesterol arranged in a radiating manner. *Cholesterosis of the gallbladder* is a specific pathologic entity in which many tiny plaques of cholesterol are present within heaped-up mucosal folds in the gallbladder dotting its interior lining; since they resemble the seeds of a ripe strawberry, the term *strawberry gallbladder* is often used.

Pigment stones (25%). Pigment stones are multiple, soft, and black and resemble fine particles of sand. They are composed of bilirubin or biliverdin and may develop from antecedent cirrhosis, chronic hemolysis, or bile stasis with or without infection. Whereas cholesterol stones are most common in Western civilizations, pigment stones are more frequent in countries where thalassemia, congenital spherocytosis, sickle cell anemia, and certain parasitemias are common.

Etiology

Although the precise cause of gallstones is poorly understood, four etiologic factors are present, to varying degrees, in most patients with cholelithiasis.

Metabolic. Cholesterol stones are commonly associated with diabetes mellitus, obesity, pregnancy, and hypothyroidism. Although these same conditions are associated with increased levels of cholesterol in blood, hypercholesterolemia itself has not been clearly established as the cause of cholesterol stones in these patients. Pigment stones are associated with hemolytic disorders such as thalassemia, congenital spherocytosis, and sickle cell anemia.

Chemical. Cholesterol is insoluble in water and is held in emulsion by combining with lecithin and bile salts to form tiny soluble micelles. Thus the concentration of bile cholesterol, lecithin, and bile salts control cholesterol solubility. Chronic elevation of bile cholesterol (as seen in native Americans or the morbidly obese) or reduction of bile salts (as seen in ileal resection and inflammatory bowel disease) frequently result in cholesterol gallstone formation. Once a nidus of cholesterol is present, additional cholesterol will be precipitated during those periods of each day when bile is supersaturated with cholesterol even in normal persons.

Stasis. Stagnation of bile flow favors precipitation of the emulsified solids. Stasis of bile occurs during pregnancy and proximal to tortuous or narrowed portions of the ductal system.

Inflammation. Inflammation is almost always associated with cholelithiasis. The inflammatory exudate of mucus, cellular debris, and fibrin is believed to be incorporated within the substance of developing stones; inflammatory edema also can narrow the ducts, thereby encouraging stasis and obstruction to perpetuate the cycle. β-Glucuronidase released by certain gram-negative organisms leads to deconjugation of the soluble bilirubin diglucuronide to insoluble bilirubin, which can precipitate and form the nidus for precipitation of cholesterol or more bilirubin with resultant stone formation.

Acute Cholecystitis

Acute cholecystitis is triggered by *obstruction* to the outflow of bile from the gallbladder (Fig. 18-9). The point of obstruction is commonly within the tortuous cystic duct, most often because of stone impaction. Less common causes of cystic duct obstruction are inflammatory edema, neoplasm, and, rarely, volvulus of an abnormally formed gallbladder suspended from a mesentery. Acute cholecystitis is basically a *chemical*

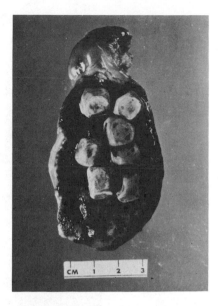

Fig. 18-9. Large gallstones causing acute cholecystitis.

inflammation. Bacterial inflammation may occur secondarily from coliform organisms in the bile or organisms that reach the gallbladder through lymphatics and vessels.

Early in the course of acute cholecystitis the gallbladder becomes distended with bile and later develops mucosal ischemia from pressure. Its wall becomes thickened, edematous, and injected, and an acute cellular inflammatory reaction develops rapidly. The cycle is self-perpetuating until and unless the obstruction to outflow is relieved. Migration of the omentum and adjacent organs to the inflamed gallbladder occurs, with fixation of the serosal surfaces to each other by vascular adhesions. These serve as tampons to prevent the inflammation from reaching the general peritoneal cavity. *Empyema of the gallbladder* is a descriptive term applied to the acutely inflamed, totally obstructed gallbladder to which bacterial contamination (with a purulent exudate) has been added. Complications occur rapidly unless the obstruction is relieved.

Complications of acute cholecystitis occur in 10% to 15% of cases if treatment is inadequate or delayed. Increasing intraluminal pressure of the inflamed gallbladder produces ischemia, ulceration, necrosis, and perforation of its wall. Pericholecystic collections of bile or pus will result if the walling-off processes are adequate, or contamination of the general peritoneal cavity will result if progression is unduly rapid or if the defense mechanisms are lacking.

In the other 85% to 90% of patients with acute cholecystitis, the cystic duct obstruction is relieved spontaneously (by a "ball valve" disimpaction of the stone) to abort the current attack. However, the stage is set for recurrent abdominal pain.

Clinical features. Acute cholecystitis is often preceded by a rather nondescript history of postprandial bloating, indigestion, food intolerance, and varying degrees of right upper quadrant abdominal pain.

The acute attack begins suddenly, often a few hours

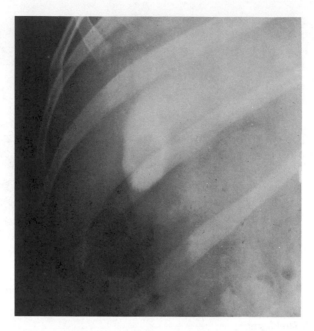

Fig. 18-10. Large, solitary gallstone producing filling defect in functioning gallbladder on oral cholecystography.

after ingestion of a large or fatty meal. The chief symptom is pain, initially colicky but later sustained. It is located in the epigastric or right subcostal region but is frequently referred to the tip of the right scapula. The pain is aggravated by pressure, but unlike in many other inflammatory intraabdominal conditions the patient is often more comfortable when up and about. Nausea, bilious vomiting, abdominal distension, and belching or flatulence are commonly associated. Later in the attack fever and mild jaundice are often noticed.

Physical examination reveals an acutely ill patient with upper abdominal tenderness and guarding, most pronounced in the right subcostal area. Gentle palpation of this area may suddenly stop the patient's inspiratory effort (positive *Murphy's sign*). The tender, globular gallbladder with adherent colon and omentum can be palpated in almost one third of the patients with adequate relaxation and analgesia.

Urinalysis is normal unless dehydration with ketosis is present. The white blood count is elevated to 15,000 mm^3 or above, with a pronounced shift to the left in the differential count. The serum bilirubin level may be elevated to 2 to 3 mg/dl, the borderline of scleral icterus, and occasionally as high as 6 mg/dl. Plain films of the abdomen often show localized paralytic ileus, and 10% to 15% of patients have calcified stones.

Differential diagnosis. The differential diagnosis of acute cholecystitis may be difficult. Acute appendicitis must be considered, but in this disease the evolution of the acute episode is slower, and the maximal signs of inflammation are anatomically lower than in acute cholecystitis. Right lower lobe pneumonia and pleurisy are extremely difficult to differentiate. Rales, a pleural friction rub, or radiographic evidence of pneumonia are suggestive of pulmonary disease. Acute pancreatitis

can be especially confusing and occasionally is associated with acute cholecystitis. Radiation of pain to the back, elevated serum amylase level, maximal tenderness in the epigastrium or left upper abdominal quadrant, pronounced tachycardia, and shock favor the diagnosis of pancreatitis. Confusion about the diagnosis can be resolved in favor of acute cholecystitis with an abdominal ultrasound (showing a gallbladder with a thick wall and gallstones) or a biliary scintiscan (technetium-labeled derivatives of iminodiacetic acid, IDA) showing technetium in the biliary ducts and not in the gallbladder, since acute cholecystitis is attributable to obstruction of the cystic duct, usually by stone, in 95% of cases; the obstruction prevents the flow of radioisotope medium into the gallbladder. Duodenal ulcer, pyelonephritis, and myocardial infarction are sometimes confused with acute cholecystitis.

Treatment. The treatment of acute cholecystitis is cholecystectomy, provided the inflammatory reaction is limited enough to allow meticulous and orderly anatomic dissection of the ducts. Intraoperative cholangiography should be performed to rule out common duct stones, which may be asymptomatic. Common bile duct exploration is undertaken if a common duct stone is found. Should the acuteness of the inflammatory reaction make dissection difficult, simple tube drainage of the gallbladder (cholecystectomy) is preferable to cholecystectomy

Chronic Cholecystitis

Over 90% of patients with chronic cholecystitis have stones in the gallbladder. The gallbladder is generally rather small and invariably has fibrosis and other evidence of chronic inflammation in its wall. Many previous episodes of indigestion, food intolerance, and

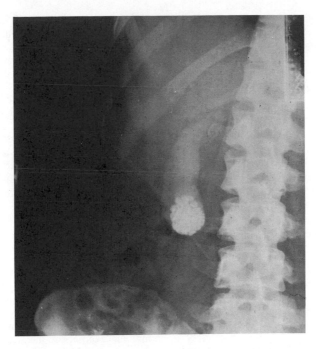

Fig. 18-11. Multiple, calcified gallstones.

acute or subacute attacks of right upper abdominal pain characterize chronic cholecystitis.

Occasionally the cystic duct becomes totally obliterated by fibrous scar tissue. In the absence of infection the bile pigment is absorbed during the ensuing weeks, and the gallbladder becomes slowly and progressively more distended with secreted mucus *(white bile)*. This phenomenon is called *hydrops of the gallbladder* and may be thought of as the "sterile" and slowly evolving counterpart of emphyema of the gallbladder. It is the only variety of chronic cholecystitis in which the gallbladder is palpable on physical examination. *White bile,* devoid of pigment, is characteristic of any long-standing and complete obstruction of the biliary tree.

Physical examination of the patient with chronic cholecystitis is seldom diagnostic. Blood and urine studies are of little help. Oral cholecystography commonly fails to visualize the gallbladder. If it is still functioning, the nonradiopaque stones will stand out as filling defects (Figs. 18-10 and 18-11). Sonography may reveal gallstones or evidence of chronic gallbladder disease (thick wall or shrunken gallbladder). In some patients laboratory support for the clinical diagnosis comes only from duodenal drainage (showing cholesterol crystals or bacteria) and cholecystokinin (CCK) cholangiography (the visualized gallbladder fails to contract normally or the patient's pain recurs after CCK). Because the majority of the patients are middle-aged or elderly, barium studies of the upper and lower gastrointestinal tracts are often performed to rule out peptic ulcers, gastric and colonic neoplasm, hiatus hernia, and other conditions that may mimic the nondescript clinical features of chronic cholecystitis. Electrocardiographic examination should

be performed in patients with a history of heart disease.

Treatment of symptomatic chronic cholecystitis is clearly surgical. Cholecystectomy is curative and gives the surgeon the opportunity to palpate the common bile duct carefully or evaluate it by means of dye injected through the cystic duct at the time of the operation *(operative cholangiography)* to rule out common bile duct stones.

Silent Gallstones

People who are incidentally found to harbor gallstones without symptoms are said to have silent gallstones. The incidence of silent gallstones is increasing as our population ages and as screening examinations become routine. They pose a treatment dilemma, inasmuch as they are potentially dangerous and yet not immediately or invariably so. Recent studies have suggested that they can be followed nonoperatively until they become symptomatic (2% per year) since they almost never produce complications without first producing symptoms.

Common Bile Duct Stones (Choledocholithiasis)

Overall, about 15% of patients with gallbladder calculi also have stones within the common bile duct, though this association will be found in nearly 50% of those over 80 years of age. They are believed to originate within the gallbladder and to subsequently pass into the common duct. Therefore common duct stones found months or even years after cholecystectomy were probably overlooked at the time of the initial operation.

The fear of overlooking common duct stones has been mitigated by the development of successful techniques to treat these stones by retrieval using endoscopic retrograde cholangiopancreatography (ERCP) and pulverization using extracorporeal shock wave lithotripsy (ESWL). Primary common duct stones originate in the common duct, are usually pigmented, and suggest the presence of obstruction and infection.

The classical indications for common bile duct exploration (choledochotomy) are (1) existing or recent jaundice, (2) a dilated (> 1 cm) common bile duct, (3) palpable stones within the common bile duct, (4) small stones in the gallbladder with a large cystic duct, (5) filling defects or other abnormalities in the preoperative or operative cholangiograms, and (6) pancreatitis in association with biliary tract disease.

Common bile duct stones cause symptoms from impaction within the distal duct at the ampulla of Vater. A "ball valve" effect produces intermittent obstruction with stagnation and increase in pressure of the bile, colicky pain (from hyperperistalsis), and obstructive jaundice. As the obstruction abates, so do the symptoms and signs. During total obstruction, the stool is acholic or only lightly pigmented and the urine is dark. Secondary infection may produce cholangitis with shaking chills and fever (Charcot's fever) and intrahepatic abscesses. Biliary cirrhosis results if the obstruction is chronic.

The clinical features of choledocholithiasis wax and wane with the obstruction. Up to 50% of patients harboring common duct stones have no obvious symptoms. If the gallbladder is present, cholecystitis may dominate the physical findings; *Courvoisier's sign* is negative: the gallbladder is usually not palpable with extrahepatic obstructive jaundice caused by gallstones since a chronically inflamed gallbladder is contracted.

The work-up of the jaundiced patient should include evaluation of the stool for bilirubin and the urine for urobilinogen and bilirubin. The serum bilirubin is elevated, mainly the direct fraction, as well as the serum alkaline phosphatase. Plain abdominal radiography may reveal a radiopaque stone. If the serum bilirubin is above 2 mg/dl oral cholecystography is futile because the biliary tract will not be visualized. Abdominal sonography or CT is used to show dilated ducts; then cholestatic jaundice can be ruled out.

Percutaneous transhepatic cholangiography (PTC) (Fig. 18-12), with injection of radiopaque dye through a long needle inserted into the liver after aspiration of bile, will clearly show the biliary duct anatomy and point of obstruction. The use of the "skinny" (Chiba) needle has obviated the previous problems of blood and bile leak into the peritoneal cavity with resultant peritonitis, and the procedure can be done without the obligation of immediate laparotomy.

ERCP. The advent of the fiberoptic duodeno-scope has made it possible to cannulate the ampulla of Vater in the awake patient. Contrast material injected through the cannula will identify the cause and site of obstruction.

Choledocholithiasis must be differentiated from the other causes of obstructive jaundice: ductal strictures and carcinomas of the extrahepatic biliary duct, am-

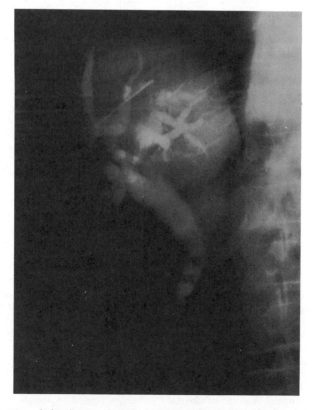

Fig. 18-12. Percutaneous cholangiogram showing multiple stones (filling defects) in dilated common bile duct.

pulla of Vater, and head of the pancreas. Progressive and unrelenting jaundice associated with fatty stools, hyperglycemia, and an enlarged palpable (Courvoisier) gallbladder is suggestive of carcinoma of the pancreas. Intermittent jaundice associated with occult blood in the stool and a filling defect in the duodenal concavity on upper gastrointestinal tract barium studies favor carcinoma of the ampulla of Vater. Unrelenting jaundice with an enlarged gallbladder but with no evidence of pancreatic exocrine or endocrine dysfunction is suggestive of carcinoma of the extrahepatic biliary tree. Intermittently painful and repeated episodes of jaundice with no palpable gallbladder indicate choledocholithiasis. Strictures of the common bile duct occur after accidental injury to the duct structures at the time of cholecystectomy; the jaundice is obstructive in type, generally painless, and associated with cholangitis. The history of preceding biliary surgery sets choledocholithiasis apart clearly from other causes of obstructive jaundice. Since laparotomy is necessary for diagnosis and treatment of all these conditions, it should not be delayed.

The treatment of choledocholithiasis can be by retrieval at ERCP, destruction using ESWL, or surgical removal of stones and temporary drainage of the common bile duct. If the patient is seriously ill, preoperative treatment with vitamins K and B complex, intravenous fluids, electrolytes, and glucose and other supportive measures for a short period of time may be needed. If the gallbladder is present, cholecystectomy should be performed in addition to choledochotomy and all the common bile duct stones should be removed. The common bile duct is explored both proximally and distally and is irrigated with saline until the bile is free of debris. A probe is passed through the ampulla and into the duodenum, and the duct is carefully palpated around this probe to be certain that no stones remain. The incidence of overlooked common duct stones is significantly reduced by the routine use of operative cholangiography during cholecystectomy and endoscopic visualization of the biliary tree (choledochoscopy) for choledocholithiasis. The duct should be closed snugly around a T tube, the short limbs of which are placed into the common bile duct and the long limb exteriorized through a separate stab wound. Operative cholangiograms should then be done through the T tube (Fig. 18-13) to be certain that the common bile duct contains no additional filling defects and that it empties freely into the duodenum. The T tube serves as an external vent for drainage of bile during the first few postoperative days. Cholangiograms are repeated through the T tube before its removal after the tenth postoperative day to assure once again that the biliary ducts are free of stones. A biliary-enteric anastomosis is done if the patient has had a previous common duct exploration.

Postcholecystectomy Syndrome

In about 5% to 10% of patients who have had cholecystectomy, some or all of the symptoms that the patient had before the operation (originally ascribed to cholelithiasis) persist or recur. This is referred to as the *postcholecystectomy syndrome*. It has a number of causes, including an erroneous original diagnosis, an unduly long and dilated cystic duct stump, residual common bile duct stones, biliary dyskinesia, and conditions outside the biliary tract with similar symptoms (hiatus hernia, duodenal ulcer, pancreatitis). Intravenous or percutaneous cholangiography is helpful in sorting out this problem, often accompanied by barium studies of the upper gastrointestinal tract. Repeat operation is necessary should a dilated cystic duct remnant or residual common duct stone be found.

Carcinoma of the Gallbladder and Biliary Ducts

Carcinomas of the gallbladder and extrahepatic bile ducts are generally associated with cholelithiasis and chronic inflammatory disease of the gallbladder and ducts, but it is not known whether the carcinomas are the cause or the result of the stones and inflammation. The cancers arise from the mucosal surfaces as adenocarcinomas.

Carcinomas of the gallbladder spread early to the liver by direct invasion and to the periportal lymph nodes. Because these carcinomas are silent and spread before discovery, surgical cure is possible only when the carcinoma is an incidental finding at the time of operation.

Neoplasms of the bile ducts are even more rare than those of the gallbladder, but because they cause symptoms earlier, the prognosis is better. The duct lumen is abruptly narrowed at the point of the neoplasm with proximal dilation, stagnation, and ultimately obstructive jaundice. Spread occurs locally to the contiguous viscera and to the liver through the periportal lymphatics and portal vein.

Neoplasms of the extrahepatic bile ducts are the

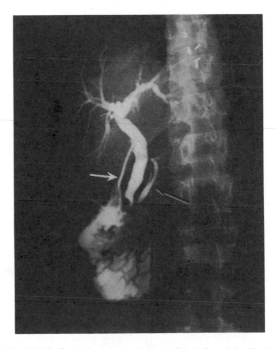

Fig. 18-13. Operative cholangiogram. Dye injected by T tube *(white arrow)* fills entire biliary system and pancreatic duct *(black arrow)* and enters duodenum inferiorly. Faint shadow in center of common bile duct is a retained stone.

cause in a small fraction of cases of total obstructive jaundice. When localized to the distal ductal system and if spread has not occurred, they are amenable to treatment by pancreaticoduodenectomy (Whipple procedure, Chap. 19). The 5-year cure rate with this operation in treatment of carcinomas of the distal biliary ducts (15%) is better than that for carcinoma of the head of the pancreas (5%) but not nearly so good as that for carcinoma of the ampulla of Vater (40%). If incurable surgically, bypass of the obstructed bile duct is carried out by anastomosis of the duct to the jejenum when possible. For tumors located more proximally, effective palliation can be obtained by dilation and transhepatic intubation of the tumor.

19

Pancreas

Jack Pickleman

Diseases of the pancreas are among the most serious and challenging that the surgeon is called on to treat. Because of its retroperitoneal location, the pancreas has remained relatively secure from radiographic investigation until recent years, when a wide variety of complex studies have completely revolutionized our management of patients with pancreatic disorders. These tests include ultrasound and abdominal computed tomography (CT), endoscopic retrograde cholangiopancreatography (ERCP), percutaneous transhepatic cholangiography (PTC), and arteriography. Recently, magnetic resonance imaging (MRI) has been added to this list, but it is presently too early to verify its advantages over CT. Today, the diagnosis of most pancreatic conditions can readily be made by a combination of these studies.

Treatment, however, has lagged behind diagnostic capabilities. The retroperitoneal location of the pancreas and its proximity to so many vital structures have thwarted many attempts to ameliorate both benign and malignant diseases, and morbidity and mortality of pancreatic procedures remain high, especially in the hands of the occasional pancreatic surgeon. This chapter focuses on the current state of our knowledge of the diagnosis and treatment of the more common pancreatic disorders.

ANATOMY

The pancreas lies obliquely across the upper abdomen running from the sweep of the duodenum, lying in front of the second lumbar vertebra and ending in the splenic hilum (Fig. 19-1). The distal common bile duct lies within the head of the pancreas, explaining the presence of obstructive jaundice when disease is present in the head of the gland. Diseases in the head of the pancreas can also obstruct the duodenum, giving rise to vomiting. The neck of the pancreas overlies the portal vein, which may be invaded by carcinoma, rendering such a lesion unresectable. The body overlies the vertebral column, and in blunt abdominal trauma, the pancreas can be crushed. The tail of the gland lies in proximity to the spleen and can be injured during splenectomy.

Upon opening the abdomen, the pancreas cannot be directly visualized, and several operative maneuvers are required to assess the gland. Incising the peritoneum lateral to the duodenal sweep (Kocker's maneuver) allows the surgeon's hand to pass posterior to the gland and anterior to the aorta and vena cava. This allows bimanual palpation of the gland. The body may be exposed by dividing the gastrocolic omentum and entering the lesser sac. The tail may be examined by mobilizing the spleen anteriorly and to the right. Following exposure of the pancreas, biopsy may be carried out by excising a small wedge of tissue, inserting a cutting needle directly, or inserting a cutting needle through the duodenal wall into the gland.

The blood supply of the pancreas is mainly from the superior and inferior pancreaticoduodenal vessels which provide numerous collaterals between the celiac vessels and superior mesenteric artery. Removal of the head of the pancreas also entails removal of the distal stomach, duodenum and common bile duct (Whipple's procedure) with reconstruction as noted in Fig. 19-9.

EMBRYOLOGY

The pancreas develops from the ventral and dorsal pancreatic buds, which protrude from the primitive gut in the third and fourth weeks of gestation. The ventral bud rotates posteriorly around the duodenum taking with it the distal common bile duct to join with the dorsal bud. The ventral bud becomes most of the head and duct of Wirsung. The dorsal bud contributes to the head and forms the remainder of the gland and duct system. If the ventral and dorsal buds fuse incompletely, the ducts will not cross-communicate (Fig. 19-2). Because of this variable embryonic development, several different patterns of ductal anatomy result (Fig. 19-3). Ectopic pancreatic tissue can occur anywhere in the gastrointestional tract but is usually found in the stomach or duodenum or in a Meckel's diverticulum. Complications of abnormally located pancreatic tissue include obstruction, bleeding, and intussusception.

ANNULAR PANCREAS

Pancreatic tissue surrounding the duodenum is a rare cause of duodenal obstruction in the infant. The probable embryonic explanation is anterior, rather than posterior, rotation of the ventral pancreatic anlage, which constricts the duodenum (see Fig. 19-2, see C_2). Air in the stomach and first portion of the duodenum on radiographs, the "double bubble" sign, is pathognomonic of duodenal obstruction. The ring of pancreatic

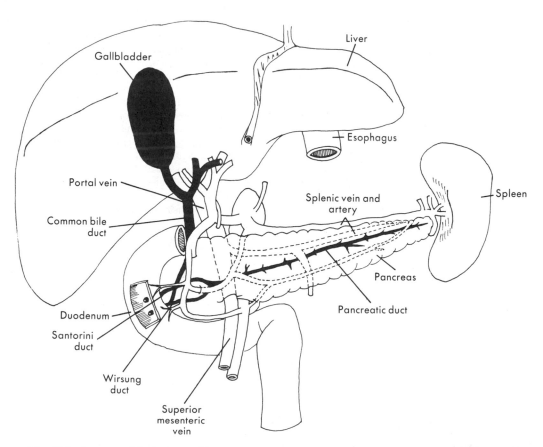

Fig. 19-1. Anatomy of the pancreas. The stomach and transverse colon are not shown because they would obscure gland. Notice intimate association of blood vessels with pancreas.

tissue is intimately associated with the duodenal musculature and contains ductal structures. Therefore, division of the constricting pancreas is contraindicated owing to the high incidence of postoperative pancreatitis, pancreatic fistula, and injury to the duodenal wall. Bypass operations, such as a duodenoduodenostomy or duodenojejunostomy are indicated. Gastrojejunostomy should be avoided because of the potential for formation of a stomal ulcer.

PANCREAS DIVISUM

Pancreas divisum results when the ductal systems of the ventral and dorsal pancreatic buds fail to fuse, causing independent drainage of the main and accessory pancreatic ducts into the duodenum. (Fig. 19-3). This condition may result in recurrent acute pancreatitis and is reliably cured by sphincteroplasty.

DISEASES OF THE PANCREAS
Acute Pancreatitis

In the United States, the majority of cases of acute pancreatitis are associated with gallstones or alcohol-ism. However, other causes exist and must be considered—trauma, peptic ulcer, hyperparathyroidism, hyperlipidemia (types I and V), ischemia, carcinoma, embryonic malformations (pancreas divisum), viruses, and drugs (corticosteroids, thiazides, azathioprine, furosemide). Although the exact pathophysiology of acute pancreatitis is not understood, the resultant local tissue injury is mediated by numerous enzymes. Trypsin not only destroys tissue but also activates other destructive enzymes such as elastase and lecithinase. Vasoactive substances including kinins, kallikrein, and histamine lead to cardiovascular dysfunction and collapse. In the full-blown picture, blood pressure falls and respiratory, renal, and myocardial failure supervene, accounting for the approximate 10% mortality noted in many series.

The presenting clinical features of acute pancreatitis are epigastric pain, often radiating to the back, associated with nausea, vomiting, and fever. Local tenderness is common, but frank peritoneal signs are less usual. Ileus is prominent. Unfortunately, several other acute abdominal conditions may give rise to similar signs and symptoms, including perforated duodenal ul-

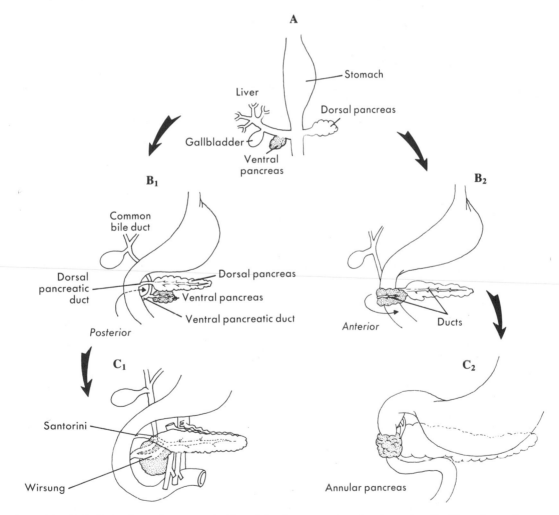

Fig. 19-2. Embryology of pancreas. **A,** Normal development at 4 weeks of gestation. **B₁,** Normal posterior rotation of ventral pancreas. **C₁,** Shaded area represents contribution of ventral pancreas. **B₂,** Abnormal anterior rotation of ventral bud. **C₂,** Final product of abnormal rotation and fusion is annular pancreas.

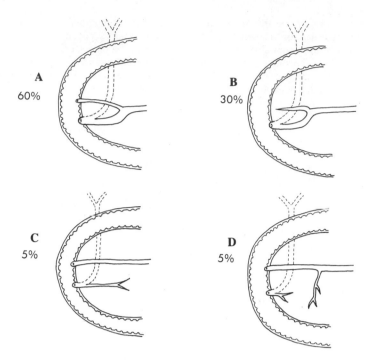

Fig. 19-3. Variations of pancreatic ducts. **A** and **B,** Most common patterns of duct anatomy. **C** and **D,** Two forms of pancreas divisum resulting from incomplete fusion of the ventral and dorsal pancreatic anlage.

cer, acute cholecystitis, and small bowel obstruction: therefore, the diagnosis may be difficult. The hallmark of acute pancreatitis is elevated serum amylase. This is not specific for acute pancreatitis, however, and many other acute abdominal conditions may be associated with amylase elevation. Further refinements in diagnosis have been sought such as the amylase-creatinine clearance ratio, but this has yielded mixed results. Urinary amylase levels may likewise be elevated, but this merely reflects increased serum levels. Serum lipase is also elevated, but, as this test takes considerably longer to perform than the serum amylase, it is less useful clinically. To further complicate the issue, the recent analysis of amylase isoenzymes has disclosed that many patients admitted with abdominal pain and hyperamylasemia with the presumptive diagnosis of acute pancreatitis have only elevation of the nonpancreatic fraction of amylase and, in reality, do not have pancreatitis.

In the usual situation, the presumptive diagnosis of acute pancreatitis is made in a patient with the above clinical signs whose serum amylase is elevated and who has no evidence of free air or small bowel obstruction on abdominal films. Hypocalcemia, hyperglycemia, and hypertriglyceridemia may accompany the amylasemia. Abdominal films usually show only localized ileus (sentinel loop) or less often left-sided pleural effusion.

The treatment of acute pancreatitis is medical; the cornerstone is adequate fluid replacement to replenish extracellular volume. Large quanitites of third-space fluids may be lost initially and must be aggressively replaced to prevent complications. A Foley catheter, central venous pressure catheter, and sometimes a pulmo-

nary artery catheter will be required. The resuscitative end points are normalization of vital signs and urinary output. Although the need for nasogastric suction has been questioned as a routine measure, it is probably indicated for all patients with severe acute pancreatitis to decrease hydrochloric acid stimulation of secretin secretion. On the other hand, empiric administration of calcium, anticholinergic drugs, and antibiotics has no apparent effect on morbidity. In severe cases, the early institution of total parenteral nutrition may prove beneficial.

Prognosis in patients with acute pancreatitis depends on whether the inflammation is of the edematous variety or the condition has progressed to the hemorrhagic stage, in which mortality rates of up to 90% may be noted. Death may come early from multiple organ system failure or later after the development of pancreatic abscess and resultant systemic sepsis. A number of prognostic signs tend to predict those patients whose course will be complicated or fatal. These signs have been described by Ranson and are commonly referred to as "Ranson criteria" for the severity of pancreatitis:

Excessive fluid requirements
Falling hematocrit
Elevated white blood cell count
Elevated blood glucose
Elevated lactate dehydrogenase and AST; SGOT
Elevated blood urea nitrogen (BUN)
Hypocalcemia
Hypoxemia
Acidosis

Indications for operation in patients with acute pancreatitis are obscure diagnosis, worsening clinical picture, trauma, pancreatic cyst, pancreatic abscess, and

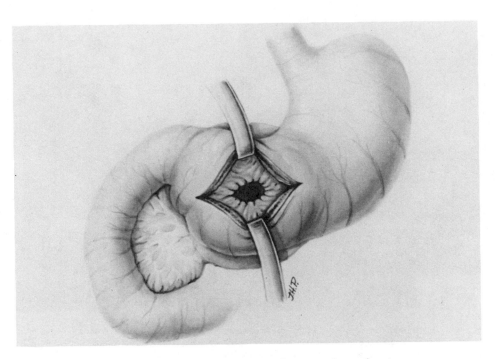

Fig. 19-4. Pancreatic cystogastrostomy for pancreatic pseudocyst.

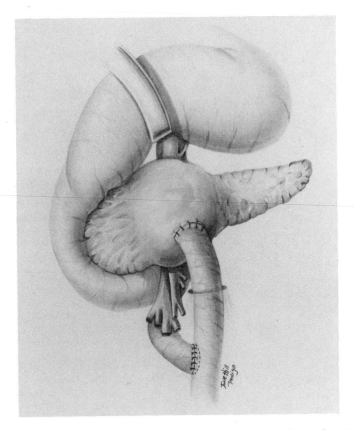

Fig. 19-5. Roux-en-Y pancreatic cystojejunostomy for pancreatic pseudocyst.

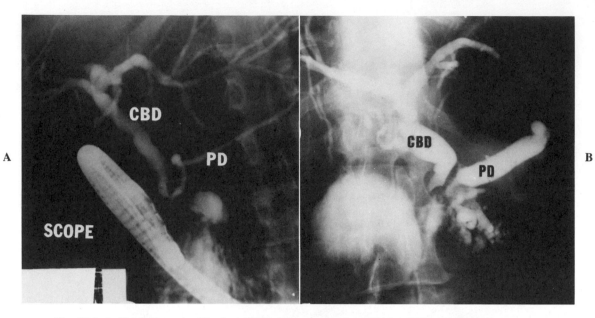

Fig. 19-6. A, Normal common bile duct (CBD) and pancreatic duct (PD) by ERCP (endoscopic retrograde cholangiopancreatography). **B,** Chronic pancreatitis with fibrosis and scarring. The common bile duct (CBD) is obstructed, the main pancreatic duct (PD) is greatly dilated, and there is pronounced ectasia of Wirsung's duct.

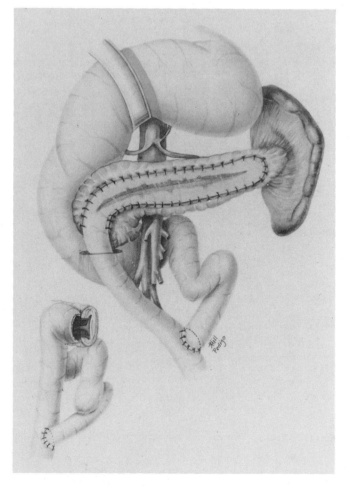

Fig. 19-7. Longitudinal pancreatic cystojejunostomy for chronic pancreatitis (Puestow procedure).

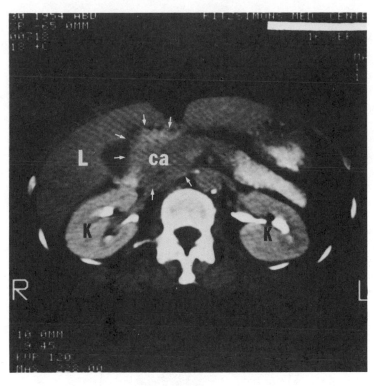

Fig. 19-8. CT scan of cancer in head of pancreas. *L,* Liver; *K,* kidney; *ca,* cancer.

pancreatic ascites. Although most authorities would agree that operation is needed in these circumstances, there is significant disagreement regarding the procedure of choice. Peritoneal lavage, either percutaneous or by catheters inserted at celiotomy, appears to dramatically improve some patients, resulting in decreased fluid requirements, improvement in vital signs, and elimination of the need for vasopressor support. Necrotic pancreatic tissue noted at celiotomy requires debridement and extensive sump drainage. Other surgeons, especially in France, have championed emergency pancreatectomy in these circumstances, but most authorities believe that this is unduly hazardous. Some form of intervention seems to benefit the acutely ill patient with multiple system failure, but late deaths from pancreatitis and its complications continue to occur.

The commonest complications of acute pancreatitis are pancreatic abscess, pseudocyst, and, less commonly, pancreatic ascites. Pancreatic abscess is heralded by sepsis in a patient recovering from an attack of acute pancreatitis and is easily diagnosed by either ultrasound or CT. Treatment includes celiotomy with extensive débridement and sump drainage of the pancreas. Despite optimal treatment, complications are common, redrainage is frequently required, and death occurs in at least 20% of patients. Recent attempts at percutaneous catheter drainage of these abscesses has been disappointing, probably because the cavities contain large pieces of necrotic material which require operative evacuation.

Pancreatic pseudocysts are lesser sac collections of pancreatic fluid arising during the course of an attack of acute pancreatitis. They are heralded by abdominal pain and a persistent or rising serum amylase level. Diagnosis is readily made by ultrasound. Unless complicated by sepsis, a rising bilirubin, or progressive increase in cyst size, acute pseudocysts may be observed, since 20% to 30% will resolve without treatment. Persistence beyond 4 to 6 weeks makes spontaneous resolution unlikely and calls for operative therapy. Internal drainage through a cyst gastrostomy or Roux-en-Y cyst jejunostomy (Figs. 19-4, 19-5) is the treatment of choice, depending on the location of the cyst. Should operation be required before 4 to 6 weeks for the above indications, external sump drainage alone will be required because the immature cyst wall may be too friable for internal anastomosis.

Pancreatic ascites afflicts patients who are recovering from an attack of acute pancreatitis. Because many of these patients are alcoholics, the development of ascites in the past has often been attributed to liver cirrhosis; however, analysis of the ascitic fluid demonstrating an elevated amylase or lipase and a total protein greater than 3 g/dl will point to the true cause. Many cases resolve spontaneously; other patients will require internal drainage of the associated leaking pseudocyst or pancreatic duct through a Roux-en-Y loop.

Gallstone Pancreatitis

One of the most serious complications of gallstones occurs when stones pass into the common duct with resultant impaction at the sphincter of Oddi, causing pancreatic duct obstruction and acute pancreatitis. Clini-

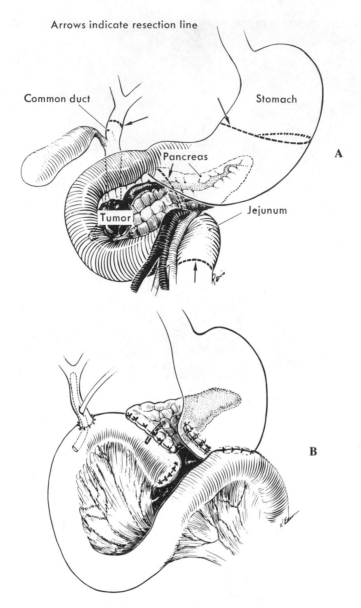

Arrows indicate resection line

Common duct

Stomach

Pancreas

A

Tumor

Jejunum

B

Fig. 19-9. Pancreaticoduodenectomy. **A,** Anatomical resection lines. **B,** Completed operation. Three anastomoses; pancreatojejunostomy, choledochojejunostomy, gastrojejunostomy.

cally, these patients have acute pancreatitis; serum amylase levels tend to be in the very high range (> 1500 IU), and this finding plus gallstones noted on ultrasound are diagnostic.

Conservative management brings about rapid improvement in over 90% of patients with a cessation of pain and normalization of serum amylase levels within 3 or 4 days. After this, cholecystectomy is performed along with operative cholangiography and common bile duct exploration as needed. About 85% of patients who undergo such treatment have no common bile duct stones at the time of cholecystectomy, indicating successful passage of the stones through the ampulla into the duodenum. Studies showing recovery of the stones in carefully strained stool specimens have documented this event. Advocates of early operation for gallstone

pancreatitis (during the attack of acute pancreatitis) base their approach on evidence that some patients have impacted common duct stones and will not recover without manual removal of the stones; however, the consensus of current studies indicates that early operation leads to significantly increased mortality rates and is therefore to be avoided.

If a patient does not promptly recover with conservative treatment, endoscopic papillotomy may be attempted; this will cause passage of the impacted stones, and cholecystectomy can be carried out electively a few days later. Patients who have spontaneously recovered from an attack of gallstone pancreatitis should clearly be advised to undergo cholecystectomy before discharge from the hospital, as 30% to 50% of such patients will develop recur-

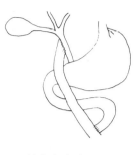

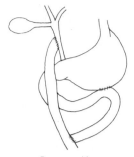

Roux-en-Y choledochojejunostomy

Roux-en-Y
choledochojejunostomy
with gastrojejunostomy

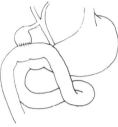

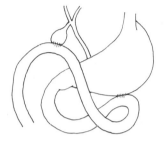

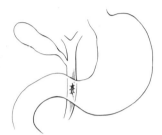

Loop cholecystojejunostomy

Gastrojejunostomy and
loop cholecystojejunostomy

Choledochoduodenostomy

Fig. 19-10. Methods used to bypass unresectable pancreatic cancer. A gastrojejunostomy is added if duodenal obstruction by the cancer is imminent.

rent gallstone pancreatitis during the next 6 months if cholecystectomy is deferred.

Chronic Pancreatitis

In this country, chronic pancreatitis generally accompanies alcohol abuse, the percentage being from 60% to 100% in reported series. Other less common causes include gallstones, trauma, and congenital problems. The overriding symptom is pain, often constant and requiring narcotic analgesics for control. Perhaps 20% of these patients manifest some degree of exocrine insufficiency and over one third have diabetes. Multiple calcifications throughout the pancreas are typical on abdominal films. Medical treatment is frequently unsuccessful in this alcoholic population, and operation may be necessary.

The operative procedure depends on the ductal anatomy noted on ERCP. For patients with a dilated duct system (Fig. 19-6), a longitudinal pancreaticojejunostomy (Puestow's procedure) is utilized (Fig. 19-7). The absence of duct dilation dictates subtotal pancreatic resection. Resection entails removal of 80% to 95% of the gland, with sparing of a small remnant in the duodenal sweep to preserve duodenal blood supply. Recently, vagotomy and antrectomy has also been successfully utilized in the treatment of patients with chronic pancreatitis. Approximately three fourths of patients benefit from any of these operations, with decreased or no pain. Permanent diabetes mellitus and exocrine insufficiency may accompany surgical treatment; therefore operation is reserved only for those patients with incapacitating pain.

Cancer of the Pancreas

The incidence of cancer of the pancreas is steadily increasing, and it truly deserves its notoriety as a major unsolved lethal disease (Fig. 19-8). With a 5-year survival rate of only 1% to 2%, pancreatic cancer is the fourth leading cause of cancer deaths (behind lung, colon, and breast). Symptoms of epigastric pain, weight loss, anorexia, and jaundice appear late, rendering early diagnosis difficult. Thus only 15% to 20% of patients have resectable disease at celiotomy. This tumor should be clearly differentiated from the less common periampullary tumors, such as carcinoma of the duodenum, ampulla, or common bile duct which similarly can present with obstructive jaundice, in which the prognosis is distinctly better and radical pancreaticoduodenectomy can be curative.

The advent of modern techniques for diagnosing pancreatic carcinoma has brought little improvement in outcome. Treatment of resectable lesions consists of a radical pancreaticoduodenectomy (Whipple's procedure, Fig. 19-9). Because of frequent local recurrences after this procedure, total pancreatectomy has been advocated to eradicate all foci of a possibly multicentric neoplasm and also to eliminate the tenuous pancreaticojejunal anastomosis. However, no evidence as yet indicates that patients who receive this operation have an improved outcome. In patients who present with jaun-

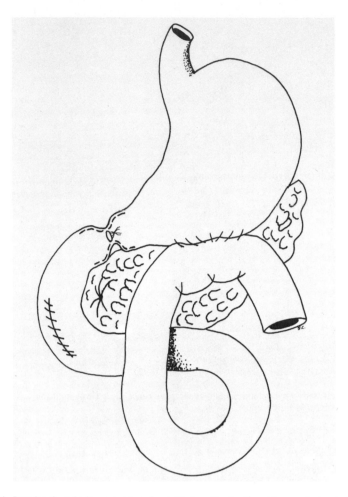

Fig. 19-11. Duodenal exclusion procedure for patients with significant trauma to head of pancreas.

dice and whose cancer is not resectable, biliary bypass (cholecystojejunostomy, choledochoduodenostomy or Roux-en-Y choledochojejunostomy) provides palliation of the jaundice and relief of pruritis (Fig. 19-10). Some of these patients also present with vomiting and signs of gastric outlet obstruction and require a concomitant gastrojejunostomy.

Endocrine Tumors of the Pancreas

Both hormonally functional and nonfunctional tumors can originate from the pancreatic islets. Although some of these tumors are malignant, the major clinical problems arise from the systemic effects of excessive hormone secretion.

Insulinoma

Arising from islet β-cells, insulinomas represent the commonest islet cell tumor. Over 90% of them are benign, and symptoms result from insulin excess and consist of weakness, trembling, sweating, hunger, palpitations, and sometimes incoherence and convulsions. In response to this, many patients learn to eat excessive amounts of sugar-containing foods to both prevent and treat the symptoms. Most patients demonstrate Whipple's triad: (1) hypoglycemia symptoms produced by

fasting; (2) symptoms associated with a blood glucose of less than 50 mg/dl; and (3) relief of symptoms by glucose administration.

The diagnosis can be confirmed by the presence of fasting hypoglycemia in the presence of inappropriately high levels of insulin. In general, fasting beyond 72 hours is unnecessary. If this test is equivocal, various provocative tests have been attempted utilizing tolbutamide or calcium infusions, but in general these tests are not necessary. Preoperative localization of these tumors is important, as they may be very small and can escape detection at celiotomy. Both CT and arteriography may be useful. More recently, intraoperative ultrasound has been utilized with good results in some centers. Some patients do not have a dominant tumor but rather islet cell hyperplasia or microadenomas, and in these patients no tumor will be palpable. In this circumstance, a subtotal resection of the gland may be necessary, especially in patients whose symptoms failed to respond preoperatively to diazoxide.

Glucagonoma

Mild diabetes, anemia, venous thrombosis, blackout spells, and necrotizing migratory erythema characterize this rare syndrome. Elevated plasma glucagon levels confirm the diagnosis. Most of these tumors are malignant, and resection should be carried out, if possible, followed by adjunctive chemotherapy.

Somatostatinoma

Somatostatinomas are rare and manifest a nonspecific clinical picture that includes diabetes, gallstones, steatorrhea, indigestion, and anemia. Elevated blood levels of somatostatin with decreased insulin and glucagon levels confirm the diagnosis. Most of these tumors are malignant.

Gastrinoma

(See Chap. 23.)

Vipoma

The ectopic islet cell tumor called vipoma (VIPoma, watery diarrhea syndrome) produces profuse watery diarrhea, dehydration, profound weakness, and sometimes tetany. The basic humoral cause is probably vasoactive intestinal polypeptide (VIP) hypersecretion, which mimics the actions of enterotoxic cholera. The massive secretions from small intestine and pancreas overwhelm the absorptive capacity of the colon. Elevated levels of VIP confirm the diagnosis. Excision of localized tumors or subtotal pancreatectomy for hyperplasia keynote the treatment.

PANCREATIC TRAUMA

Because of its retroperitoneal location, injuries to the pancreas are less frequent than injuries to other intraabdominal viscera. Both penetrating and blunt injuries, however, can prove fatal unless treatment is prompt and appropriate. Injuries to the pancreas are equally divided among head, body, and tail, and association with other visceral injuries is common. In patients with penetrating injuries, the pancreatic component is readily detected at celiotomy. The patient who sustains blunt trauma, however, poses a distinct diagnostic problem. Elevation of serum amylase is inconstant in pancreatic trauma. In one review of 74 patients with blunt pancreatic injury, only 71% had an elevated amylase. Likewise, an elevated amylase level in a trauma patient indicates pancreatic injury in only 15% of patients. With wider use of abdominal CT scanning in trauma cases, this should improve diagnostic accuracy and lead to earlier operation. Similarly, peritoneal lavage may be falsely negative in pancreatic injury, so information obtained from lavage must be carefully evaluated.

Treatment depends on the location and severity of the injury. Simple contusions and lacerations are readily managed by sump drainage. Distal resection is reserved for patients who have transection of the gland or severe distal injury. Patients with injuries to the head of the gland associated with major pancreatic duct injury may be managed by some form of duodenal exclusion, one example of which is shown in Fig. 19-11. In this procedure, the pylorus is ligated with absorbable suture material through a gastrotomy incision and a gastroenterostomy is fashioned. Extensive sump drainage completes the procedure, and within a few weeks the pylorus recanalizes. For extensive injuries of the head of the gland involving the duct and also somtimes the duodenum, a pancreaticoduodenectomy (Whipple's procedure) may be necessary. Complications of pancreatic injury are common and include fistula, abscess, and hemorrhage. Death from these complications occurs in 5% to 20% of patients.

20

Spleen

Robert T. Soper
Ken Kimura

Anatomy
Function
Surgical Disorders of the Spleen

The spleen is part of the reticuloendothelial system, filtering blood rather than lymph. At least in the adult it is not vital to life, though it does have important immune functions. Traditionally the only operation ordinarily performed on this organ has been its removal, splenectomy.

ANATOMY

The anatomic peculiarities of the spleen dictate much of its importance to the surgeon (Fig. 20-1). It is held loosely in the depths of the left hypochondrium by dense ligaments to surrounding organs (greater curvature of stomach, splenic flexure of colon, inferior surface of left diaphragm). When these ligaments are retracted during operations (on adjacent organs) or stretched suddenly when the spleen is rapidly displaced by external trauma, the fragile splenic capsule may tear. The splenic vein receives many short branches from the adjacent pancreas, anatomic features that generally require splenectomy when the distal part of the pancreas is removed. A portion of the lymphatic drainage of the stomach is through nodes in the splenic hilum, and splenectomy is necessary when curative gastrectomy is performed for carcinoma of the body of the stomach. The splenic vein contributes about one fourth of the portal blood; since this is a two-way street, any increase in portal pressure is transmitted to the splenic pulp. This results in splenomegaly and hypersplenism, which, at times, are the earliest manifestations of portal hypertension.

FUNCTION

The splenic capsule contains elastic fibers that allow considerable fluctuation in size of the organ. In lower animals the spleen acts as a blood reservoir; it stores up to one third of the blood volume for release back into circulation when additional blood is required, as in response to stress or epinephrine release. This is not an important function of the human spleen.

Red blood cells are destroyed in the spleen as they approach the end of their 120-day life span, with degradation of hemoglobin and salvage of iron. This destruction probably occurs because of increased osmotic and mechanical fragility of the cells with aging. Red blood cells that are excessively fragile for other reasons (spherocytosis) also are trapped and destroyed in the spleen. It is a curious paradox that red blood cells can also be manufactured (extramedullary hematopoiesis) in the spleen, normally during fetal life and abnormally in the adult with chronic bone marrow failure (fibrosis). Extramedullary hematopoiesis produces splenomegaly; bone marrow smears are done before elective removal of a large spleen so that marrow failure can be ruled out as the cause for splenomegaly. In addition to entrapping particles (particularly bacteria) and as part of its reticuloendothelial function, the spleen produces antibodies, lymphocytes, plasma cells, opsonins, tuftsin, and immunoglobulins (IgM, IgG). Splenic IgM is the first antibody produced in response to a new particulate antigen, such as a bacterium. Persons who are asplenic for whatever reason (congenital, sickle cell anemia, or after splenectomy) are subject to bouts of overwhelming sepsis, generally caused by mucopolysaccharide-encapsulated organisms (pneumococci, meningococci, and less commonly *Haemophilus influenzae*) that multiply rapidly and are normally filtered out of circulation by the spleen. This overwhelming sepsis has a 50% to 80% mortality within 24 to 36 hours of onset. Although its incidence is inversely related to age (the younger the asplenic patient the greater the risk) and is more likely to occur within 2 to 3 years after splenectomy, it has been reported in adults up to 15 years after removal of the spleen. Statisticians have calculated that persons without a spleen have a chance of developing overwhelming sepsis 50 times greater than that of the normal population.

Appreciation of these facts has prompted considerable change of attitude toward splenectomy in the past 2 decades. Splenectomy should be avoided when possible during childhood and is undertaken in adults with care. If splenectomy is necessary, prophylactic penicillin or pneumococcal vaccines should be considered postoperatively. All splenectomized patients need to be made aware of the overwhelming postsplenectomy infection (OPSI) syndrome.

SURGICAL DISORDERS OF THE SPLEEN
Splenic Rupture and its Causes

The most common indication for splenectomy is hemorrhage after rupture (Fig. 20-2). In descending order of importance splenic rupture is caused by (1) trauma, (2) surgical traction, and (3) softening and enlargement of the spleen because of disease, with subsequent spontaneous rupture.

Trauma

Despite the relatively small size of the spleen, its mobility, and protection afforded by the left lower rib cage, the spleen is the intraabdominal organ most susceptible to rupture by trauma. The spleen is more susceptible to injury in the child because of the greater flexibility of the overlying ribs and the relatively large size of the spleen.

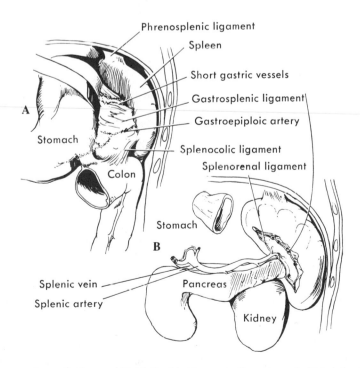

Fig. 20-1. Gross anatomy of spleen and its relationships to surrounding organs. **A,** Note intimate attachments of spleen to diaphragm, stomach, and colon. **B,** Cutaway section showing relationship of spleen to pancreas.

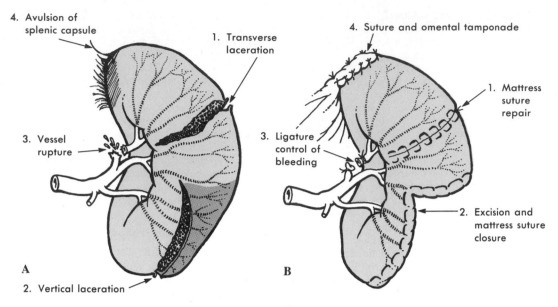

Fig. 20-2. A, Four types of splenic trauma are shown in left diagram: *(1)* Transverse laceration of splenic pulp parallels course of intrasplenic vessels; bleeding is minor and no splenic pulp is devascularized, *(2)* Vertical laceration cuts across vessels; bleeding is brisk and peripheral pulp (shaded) is devascularized, *(3)* Brisk bleeding from major hilar vessels, *(4)* Avulsion of splenic capsule by blunt force, usually by retraction during surgical procedure. **B,** Repair of four types of trauma is depicted in right diagram: *(1)* Mattress suture repair, *(2)* Excision and mattress suture closure, *(3)* Ligature control of bleeding, *(4)* Suture and omental tamponade. Splenectomy is not mandatory.

The trauma may be direct or indirect, by a penetrating or a nonpenetrating force. Associated injury to surrounding organs (stomach, colon, pancreas, left kidney) is common, and often splenic rupture is associated with multiple injuries to other parts of the body. The signs and symptoms of splenic injury may be masked by these other injuries. Splenic penetration by missiles is often seen in combat military practice. Nonpenetrating multiple system injury is more common in civilian automobile accidents or falls.

Surgical Traction

Iatrogenic tears in the splenic capsule by excessive traction on the tough capsular ligaments are occasionally produced during operations on adjacent organs. Downward traction on the stomach (during transabdominal vagotomy, Nissen fundoplication, or hiatus hernia repair) injures the spleen in about 5% of cases. Better exposure and more gentle traction reduce the frequency of this misadventure.

Spontaneous Rupture of a Diseased Spleen

An enlarged spleen from any cause will be more exposed and therefore subject to rupture by lesser degrees of trauma. A spleen softened by disease, such as malaria or lymphomatous involvement, on occasion ruptures spontaneously. Awareness of this possibility, especially in children subjected frequently to minor trauma, justifies early treatment of the primary disease.

Clinical manifestations. Multiple injuries to other body systems commonly complicate and mask splenic injury. The signs and symptoms of splenic rupture in

turn depend on the amount and rate of blood loss (Fig. 20-2). Thus a complete rupture of the major artery or vein in the splenic hilum produces massive blood loss signaled by profound shock. Lesser degrees of blood loss, as with a transverse laceration of the splenic pulp, are associated with gradually appearing signs of shock, often accompanied by abdominal pain, tenderness, percussion dullness, and an expanding hematoma mass in the left upper abdominal quadrant. The pain is more severe with breathing and may be referred via the phrenic nerve to the left shoulder tip (Kehr's sign, noted in 15% of cases). The left hemidiaphragm is elevated and restricted in its movement. Free blood in the peritoneal cavity may cause loin bulging and shifting dullness and is suggested on rectal examination by a fullness in the rectovesical space. Deepening pallor, rising pulse rate, narrowing pulse pressure, and serial diminution in the hemoglobin and hematocrit reflect the resultant hypovolemia.

In about 15% of patients with traumatic rupture of the spleen, the bleeding is controlled by intrinsic tamponade by the omentum or diaphragm to produce a perisplenic hematoma, or else the hemorrhage is confined beneath the splenic capsule. In this situation the signs of hypovolemia may be minimal or lacking and the abdominal signs may be more localized to the left upper abdominal quadrant. In time this hematoma may resolve entirely, may remain as a splenic cyst, or rarely may rupture secondarily into the free peritoneal cavity with a return of the progressive signs of hypovolemia and spreading hemoperitoneum. Delayed rupture has been reported up to 50 days after injury.

Exploratory laparotomy is the safest and most deci-

Table 20-1. Primary Hypersplenism

Disease	Blood	Marrow	Benefit by Splenectomy (%)
Idiopathic thrombocytopenic purpura	↓ Platelets	↑ Megakaryocytes	80
Congenital spherocytosis	↓ RBCs	↑ Erythroid elements	100
Primary neutropenia	↓ Neutrophils	↑ Myeloid elements	80
Primary pancytopenia	↓ Formed elements	↑ All precursor elements	80

Key: ↓, lowered; ↑, elevated.

sive way to confirm the diagnosis of splenic rupture. Abdominal paracentesis may help confirm the diagnosis of intraperitoneal hemorrhage before laparotomy. Supportive therapy should begin immediately, followed by laparotomy if the patient's condition is unstable.

When bleeding is slower, additional diagnostic study of the patient is possible. Computed tomography (CT) of the spleen is the most expedient noninvasive way to identify splenic injury. A radionuclide scan of the spleen is also useful. Leukocytosis of 15,000 to 20,000/mm^3 is an early but nonspecific sign of splenic rupture. Serial hemoglobin and hematocrits, which reflect dilution of circulating blood with extracellular tissue fluid to compensate for lost blood, are sometimes helpful. Plain films show elevation of the left hemidiaphragm, medial displacement of the gastric air bubble with serration of its greater curvature, and inferior displacement of the air within the splenic flexure of the colon associated with a "ground-glass" tissue density in the left upper abdominal quadrant.

Treatment. Splenic trauma requires splenectomy when the splenic pulp is smashed beyond repair, when the spleen is devitalized by avulsion of its hilar vessels, or if the patient's general condition is poor owing to concurrent injuries. However, because of recent studies that have documented the immunologic importance of the spleen at all ages (but especially in children), judicious attempts should be made to salvage traumatized spleens when possible. Avulsion injuries can be safely tamponaded by Gelfoam, Avitene, or omentum. Transverse lacerations are closed by simple mattress sutures. Devascularized segments are excised, and the raw splenic surface is sutured and covered by omentum (Fig. 20-2). Splenic bleeding can cease spontaneously or be arrested surgically; many traumatized spleens need not be removed.

Hypersplenism

The term *hypersplenism* is nonspecific and implies abnormal splenic sequestration of one or more of the formed elements of the blood (RBCs, WBCs, or platelets), (Table 20-1). It is almost always associated with spenomegaly, a depression of the sequestered blood elements, and increased bone marrow production of those elements that are diminished in the peripheral blood.

Hypersplenism may be primary or secondary. In *primary hypersplenism* no other known disease process induces the exaggerated splenic function. Examples include idiopathic (primary or essential) thrombocytopenic purpura, idiopathic (primary) splenic neutropenia or pancytopenia, and congenital spherocytosis.

Splenectomy is generally quite effective in the treatment of primary hypersplenism.

In *secondary hypersplenism* the overactivity is caused by another disease process involving the spleen and other portions of the reticuloendothelial system (leukemia, lymphomas, Hodgkin's disease, sarcoidosis, tuberculosis, β-thalassemia major, and the metabolic storage diseases). Splenectomy may temporarily improve the hematologic picture in secondary hypersplenism, but it does not affect the course of the primary disease per se. Hypersplenism associated with portal hypertension is the most common form of secondary hypersplenism.

Idiopathic Thrombocytopenic Purpura

Idiopathic thrombocytopenic purpura is an autoimmune disorder characterized by pronounced diminution in circulating platelets with a resultant bleeding diathesis. It must be distinguished diagnostically from thrombopenia and purpura associated with toxic bone marrow depression (and diminished platelets) caused by a wide variety of agents such as tuberculosis, excessive radiation, leukemia, widespread bony metastases, and bone marrow sensitivity to drugs such as sulfonamides, chloramphenicol, arsenicals, and benzol. Secondary thrombocytopenic purpura is not helped by splenectomy.

Idiopathic thrombocytopenic purpura is more common in females, children and young adults. As the name suggests, the basic cause is unknown. However, it is clearly an immunologically related disorder in which antiplatelet antibodies (formed within the spleen?) damage and shorten the life span of platelets.

Clinically the disease is characterized by periodic exacerbations of abnormal bleeding manifested by the appearance of petechiae, ecchymoses, and hematomas, which appear either spontaneously or after minor trauma. Surface bleeding can occur into the intestinal or urinary tract, and menorrhagia is seen in the menstruating female. Hematomas in the intestinal wall can produce obstruction or can serve as the lead point in intussusceptions. The most crippling and lethal bleeding occurs intracranially, and its prevention compels early treatment of this disorder. Large hematomas or hemarthroses are uncommon. This is the only form of hypersplenism that is not commonly (in only about 20% of cases) associated with splenomegaly; furthermore, if thrombocytopenia and splenomegaly are associated, it is likely that one is dealing with a secondary type of thrombocytopenic purpura.

The diagnosis of idiopathic thrombocytopenic purpura is suggested by a positive Rumpel-Leede test: petechiae are produced distal to sphygmomanometer cuff inflated above venous pressure. The bleeding time is prolonged and the clot retraction is poor, though the coagulation time is normal. Platelet count in the peripheral blood is below 40,000/mm^3, and the few platelets that are seen are usually large and bizarre in shape. Bone marrow smear contains increased numbers of platelet precursors (megakaryocytes).

Initial treatment often consists of steroids and transfusion of platelets or fresh blood collected in a siliconized container; this temporarily prevents additional bleeding. Remissions occur spontaneously and are often induced by steroid therapy, especially in children. The remissions may be permanent.

Splenectomy is indicated if a remission is not achieved or if the disease exacerbates while under steroid maintenance therapy. Splenectomy generally produces a thrombocytosis that reaches its peak between 2 and 12 days postoperatively, followed by a return of the platelet count to near normal ranges. Improvement in clot retraction and bleeding time will likewise occur promptly. Some patients are relieved of their bleeding tendencies even though the platelet count is unchanged.

Splenectomy is curative in about three fourths of patients with idiopathic thrombocytopenic purpura. It will prevent further serious bleeding episodes or will make steroid management easier in the majority of the other patients, even though the platelet counts remain low.

Idiopathic Splenic Neutropenia and Pancytopenia

In the rare *primary* disorders, idiopathic splenic neutropenia and pancytopenia, there is a deficiency in one or all of the formed blood elements within the peripheral blood, associated with an increase in marrow activity in the element or elements deficient peripherally. Further, no other diseases contribute to these changes. Splenectomy is curative.

Much more commonly, these varieties of hypersplenism occur *after* other primary disorders including infections (malaria, sarcoidosis), neoplasms (leukemia, lymphosarcoma, Hodgkin's disease), metabolic storage diseases (Gaucher's disease, Niemann-Pick disease, Hand-Schüller-Christian disease, Letterer-Siwe disease), β-thalassemia major, and portal hpertension. Progressive splenomegaly is characteristic of secondary splenic pancytopenia, and treatment should be directed at the primary disease rather than the spleen. Occasionally splenectomy is indicated when the massive size of the spleen itself produces symptoms or poses a threat to life because of ease of injury. Splenectomy is also done to improve the hematologic picture when the latter changes are extreme. Portal hypertension is the most common cause of secondary splenic pancytopenia; the hypersplenism improves with lowering the portal pressure by portasystemic venous shunts (Chap. 18).

Hemolytic Anemias

Hemolysis of red blood cells associated with anemia can be produced in many ways, including transfusion of mismatched blood, septicemia, and exposure to various hemolysins, such as certain snake venoms. Apart from these is a group of disorders in which the spleen is instrumental in destroying red blood cells to cause anemia and splenomegaly. Sickle cell anemia and β-

thalassemia major are not often benefited by operation and will not be considered further here.

Congenital Spherocytosis

Congenital spherocytosis is the best understood of these so-called hemolytic anemias. In this disorder the red blood cells are morphologically altered to a spheroid rather than a biconcave disk shape. This is genetically determined as a mendelian dominant trait transmitted by either parent. About 20% of cases seem to arise spontaneously, presumably by mutations, but the remainder show a strong family history of anemia and jaundice. However, the gene responsible for the hemolysis exhibits varying degrees of penetrance. Some members of the family have spherocytosis with little evidence of anemia or splenomegaly, whereas others have the full-blown clinical picture with the same degree of spherocytosis. In this disorder, the reticulocytes (red blood cell precursors) are *not* spherocytic. Their abnormal shape is acquired by the influx of fluid into the red cell, which in turn is due to a failure of its sodium pump and reduction in its adenosine triphosphate (ATP) energy levels. The spherocytic shape of the red cell increases its mechanical and osmotic fragility and renders it more susceptible to splenic entrapment and hemolysis.

Characteristically, mild anemia and jaundice with a slightly enlarged spleen are apparent in the first decade of life. Patients with mild forms of the disease may live a normal life span, though a significant proportion (25%) ultimately develop gallstones because of the chronic hyperbilirubinemia.

Aplastic crises. Patients with more severe forms of spherocytosis will develop intermittent crises, sometimes precipitated by infections. Such crises are characterized by abdominal pain, fever, nausea and vomiting, progressive anemia, acholuric jaundice, and splenomegaly. The peripheral blood reveals spherical erythrocytes on smear with an anemia that reflects the severity of the disorder. Reticulocytosis is expected during the recovery period after a crisis, but the reticulocyte count may fall to zero during a crisis. Recent theory ascribes the crisis to cessation of red blood cell formation in the bone marrow rather than to an increase in hemolysis within the spleen. A splenic hormone may be involved in this mechanism.

The red blood cell fragility test (preferably interpreted after 24 hours of incubation) is the most effective diagnostic study. Hemolysis of the spherocyte begins in 0.75% saline rather than in the 0.45% saline concentration necessary to lyse normal red blood cells. Hemolysis is completed at 0.4% rather than 0.3% saline in the normal person. The indirect serum bilirubin level is elevated and stools are more darkly pigmented than normal, though no bile is present in urine in keeping with the unconjugated nature of the bilirubin. The results of Coombs' test are negative, and a bone marrow smear reveals erythroid hyperplasia.

Initially treatment is directed at tiding the patient over the acute crisis by cautious blood transfusions. Splenectomy cures the serious hemolysis and prevents future crises but does not alter the red blood cell's shape or fragility. All patients who are symptomatic should have splenectomy as an elective procedure, since there is no known medical treatment, and spontaneous remissions do not occur when symptoms are pronounced. Cholecystectomy or cholecystotomy with stone removal should be carried out at the same time if the patient's condition allows and if cholelithiasis is present.

Acquired Anemias

The *other hemolytic anemias* are acquired (or secondary) and are not of particular sugical interest. Idiopathic acquired hemolytic anemia is a condition that belongs among the autoimmune family of disorders with spontaneously arising agglutinins and hemolysins that damage otherwise normal red blood cells. Splenomegaly, hemolysis, and anemia result. The results of Coomb's test are usually positive, the morphologic appearance of the red blood cell is generally normal (though cases are reported that do have some spherocytosis), and there is no family history of hemolytic anemia. Steroids are the preferred treatment. Splenectomy is indicated only for those who fail nonoperative treatment.

Miscellaneous

Primary neoplasms of the spleen are extremely rare and generally of mesenchymal tissue origin. Secondary splenic involvement is common in the leukemias and lymphomas, but metastases from carcinomas are almost unheard of.

Cysts of the spleen are rare and may be congenital, associated with liquefaction of old hematomas or parasitic infestations such as hydatid cyst, or caused by a solitary dermoid cyst.

Accessory spleens are miniature duplications of splenic tissue found on routine postmortem examination in about 10% of the population. They are usually located near the splenic hilum or the gastrocolic ligament and are darker than lymph nodes. Interestingly enough, accessory spleens are found in 20% of people with hypersplenism. Hypertrophy probably allows easier detection in hypersplenism. Accessory spleens must be removed at the time of splenectomy for hypersplenism—if left behind, they may undergo hyperplasia and assume the function of the parent spleen. Missed accessory spleens are occasionally a reason for failure of splenectomy in the treatment of hypersplenic conditions.

21

Peritoneal and Acute Abdominal Conditions

Neil R. Thomford
Jeffery R. Mitchell

Evaluation of the Patient
The Peritoneum and Peritonitis

The term *acute abdomen* endures as a valuable method for signaling an apparent intraabdominal crisis and indicating the diagnostic protocol to be followed. Neither the patient nor untrained observers may perceive the problem as being acute or of serious potential, but for the responsible physician the acute abdomen demands prompt if not immediate evaluation of the patient, a working diagnosis, and early, clear decisions regarding subsequent study and management.

A great number of illnesses have the capacity to produce acute abdomen. In most instances the syndrome is the result of a local disease process within the abdomen or pelvis. The following are possible causes:

Gastrointestinal
    Appendicitis
    Cholecystitis
    Perforated peptic ulcer
    Pancreatitis
    Diverticulitis of the colon
    Meckel's diverticulitis
    Mechanical obstruction of the intestine
    Granulomatous enterocolitis
    Ulcerative colitis
    Acute gastritis
    Acute hepatitis
    Gastrointestinal hemorrhage
    Gastroenteritis
Gynecologic
    Ectopic pregnancy
    Torsion or rupture of ovarian cyst
    Pelvic inflammatory disease
    Gonococcal perihepatitis
    Painful ovulation (mittelschmerz)

Regurgitation of menstrual blood into peritoneal cavity
Vascular
  Dissecting aneurysm of the abdominal aorta and its
    branches
  Embolic occlusion of visceral branches of the abdom-
    inal aorta
  Nonocclusive mesenteric infarction
  Ruptured aneurysm of the abdominal aorta or one of its
    intraabdominal branches
Genitourinary
  Urinary tract infection
  Urinary tract calculus
Systemic disease
  Diabetic acidosis
  Hyperlipidemia
  Porphyria
  Sickle cell anemia
  Henoch-Schönlein purpura
Neurogenic
  Tabetic crisis
  Spinal nerve root compression
  Herpes zoster
Other
  Primary peritonitis
  Mesenteric lymphadenitis
  Intraabdominal hemorrhage associated with trauma
  Intraabdominal hemorrhage associated with anticoag-
    ulants
  Acute lead poisoning
  Acute adrenal insufficiency
  Rectus sheath hematoma
  Black widow spider bite

In other cases the primary disease is systemic, with abdominal or pelvic manifestations of the illness causing the symptoms and signs. Finally, thoracic diseases may cause symptoms and signs suggesting an intraabdominal catastrophe:

Thoracic diseases
  Myocardial infarction
  Acute pericarditis
  Pneumonia
  Diaphragmatic pleurisy
  Pulmonary infarction
  Spontaneous pneumothorax
  Acute mediastinitis

To arrive at the correct diagnosis the examiner must know the anatomy and innervation of the abdominal tissues and organs, have a thorough understanding of the pathology and pathophysiology of the many causes of the acute abdomen, and be aware of both the potential and limitations of available diagnostic studies. The rapidity with which the evaluation and decision-making process is accomplished must match the urgency of the situation. The course of action when encountering a patient who is in profound shock from rupture of an abdominal aortic aneurysm will differ from that with a 20-year-old whose symptoms and signs are suggestive of early appendicitis. If the evaluation does not provide the diagnosis, clinical judgment must choose between observation, repeated or added diagnostic studies, and an exploratory operation.

EVALUATION OF THE PATIENT
The History

Acute disease or injury of organs and tissues in the abdomen and pelvis results in inflammation, obstruc-

tion of a hollow viscus, hemorrhage, or combination of any. These changes produce one or more symptoms that lead to the patient-physician encounter and the beginning of the evaluation and management of the patient with an acute abdomen.

Pain

Pain is the most common symptom of patients with a clinical picture of acute abdomen. Sensory nerve pathways from the abdomen include both spinal nerves and the autonomic nervous system. The intercostal branches of spinal nerves 5 through 11 innervate the parietal peritoneum. In addition the phrenic nerve provides sensory innervation to the peritoneal surface of the diaphragm. The innervation of the visceral peritoneum and the abdominal and pelvic organs is provided by the autonomic nervous system.

Because the gastrointestinal tract develops from the midline in the embryo, pain from lesions of the stomach and duodenum is epigastric in location, pain from the midgut is felt in the periumbilical area, and pain from the left colon and rectum is often localized to the hypogastric area. Since the gallbladder and appendix are also of midline derivation, the initial pain from disease of these structures is epigastric and periumbilical, respectively.

Pain may shift position, radiate, or occur as referred pain. When the periumbilical pain of appendicitis "localizes" in the right lower quadrant of the abdomen, this is an example of pain shifting. In this instance the shift results from extension of the inflammatory process through the wall of the appendix to involve the parietal peritoneum, with pain mediated through spinal nerves. Other mechanisms may cause pain to shift location. Severe epigastric pain from perforation of a peptic ulcer may shift to the right lower quadrant as gastric and duodenal contents spill into the peritoneal cavity and drain into the lower abdomen along the ascending colon. An example of radiating pain is the pain of a ureteral calculus, which often extends from the lumbar region and flank to the inguinal region and the scrotum. Finally, referred pain is the result of two separate anatomic areas being innervated by the same nerve trunk. The brain may then erroneously interpret the site of origin of the pain impulses. Because the phrenic nerve provides sensation for the peritoneal surface of the diaphragm and the skin of the top of the shoulder, subdiaphragmatic irritation may cause shoulder pain.

The character of the pain provides valuable diagnostic clues. Persistent uninterrupted pain characterizes strangulated intestine, whereas "waves" of pain often indicate acute pancreatitis. Intermittent cramps point to mechanical obstruction of the intestine. The severity of the pain may also assist in identifying the disease. Patients with dissecting aneurysms of the abdominal aorta are in agony and in many instances unable to control themselves and communicate with the physician. Renal colic also causes severe pain, whereas the pain of cholecystitis, pancreatitis, appendicitis, and diverticulitis is less incapacitating. Some significance may also be attached to the patients' response to their pain. Patients with cholecystitis usually "walk the floor," while persons with localized or generalized peritonitis from appendicitis, diverticulitis of the colon, or pelvic inflammatory disease prefer to lie still. When queried, patients with peritonitis often report that their pain increases with any sudden movement or jarring of the body.

Vomiting

The presence or absence of vomiting and the character of the vomitus may help determine the diagnosis. Vomiting is relatively common with biliary colic and mechanical obstruction of the gastrointestinal tract. When obstruction occurs in the proximal gastrointestinal tract, vomiting begins early; with obstruction of the distal small intestine or colon, vomiting begins late, if at all, and the vomitus often has fecal qualities. Vomiting is uncommon with perforated ulcer, appendicitis, and pelvic inflammatory disease. The presence or absence of red blood in the vomitus is of critical importance. The significance of occult blood in the emesis or gastric aspirate is often more difficult to assess.

Bowel Function

Diarrhea is suggestive of gastroenteritis or one of the inflammatory diseases of the colon. Yet some children with appendicitis and patients with hyperperistalsis caused by mechanical obstruction of the small or large intestine have frequent small liquid bowel movements. Cessation of flatus signifies intestinal obstruction. A history of the passage of bright or dark red blood or black, tarry stools must be considered together with the patient's other symptoms. In general, black, tarry stools are suggestive of hemorrhage proximal to or near the ileocecal valve. The passage of significant quantities of red blood through the rectum usually indicates hemorrhage from the colon but may occur with *massive* bleeding from the proximal gastrointestinal tract.

Syncope

Syncope occurs most often with acute abdominal disease when hemorrhage is the major complication of the illness. Syncope *without* pain often accompanies occult hemorrhage into the gastrointestinal tract. Syncope *with* abdominal pain should alert the examiner to probable intraperitoneal or retroperitoneal bleeding.

Menstrual History

No history of an abdominal or pelvic illness in the female is complete without a menstrual history. When did the last menstrual period occur? Was it normal? Is the patient pregnant? Acute pelvic inflammatory disease often occurs at the termination of the menstrual flow; mittelschmerz may be expected at the midpoint of the menstrual cycle, whereas the pain of endometriosis classically occurs during the last 2 to 3 days of the menstrual cycle. Small amounts of blood leaking from endometrial and functional cysts of the ovaries may be accompanied by pain in the pelvic region. When 500 to 1000 ml of blood is lost into the peritoneal cavity from rupture of an ectopic pregnancy, blood in the pelvis often results in the urge to urinate. Blood irritating the undersurface of the left hemidiaphragm may cause referred pain to the left shoulder.

Past Medical History and System Review

The more acutely ill the patient, the more rapidly the physician must act. Under emergency conditions the physician should inquire early about the past medical history. If the patient has had attacks of renal colic, has a history of peptic ulcer, or has known gallstones, this information is vital for quick arrival at a working diagnosis. If the patient presents symptoms suggestive of intestinal obstruction, the diagnosis becomes more likely if he has had a previous abdominal operation. Similarly, if the patient has had an abdominal aortic prosthesis inserted and now has hemorrhage from the gastrointestinal tract, he is presumed to have an aortaenteric fistula until proved otherwise.

A general review of systems should cover all areas not reviewed when the history of the illness is obtained. Special attention should be given to the cardiovascular and genitourinary system.

The Physical Examination

The physical examination must be complete. To exclude any area of the body or any particular part of the physical examination invites diagnostic error. Even in the emergency situation the accomplished clinician who is a keen observer may complete an adequate examination of the patient in a few minutes.

General Observations

The patient's posture, mental status, vital signs, and skin color and temperature, together with inspection of any emesis or rectal discharge, will allow a preliminary opinion as to whether or not the patient's acute abdomen is the result of inflammation, distension of a hollow viscus, or hemorrhage.

Examination of the Abdomen

Inspection of the abdomen will identify abdominal distension, asymmetry of the abdomen, an obvious mass, scars from previous operations, bruises or other abnormalities suggestive of trauma, or evidence of a hernia. In rare instances visible peristalsis will be strongly suggestive of a diagnosis of mechanical intestinal obstruction. A bluish discoloration of the navel (Cullen's sign) may indicate blood in the peritoneal cavity, whereas a dusty bluish hue in one or both flanks (Grey Turner's sign) may indicate retroperitoneal hemorrhage.

When time permits, the physician should auscultate the abdomen for a minimum of 1 minute, and preferably for 5 minutes, to assess accurately the degree and character of peristaltic activity. Hyperactive, high-pitched peristaltic sounds, rushes, and tinkles indicate mechanical obstruction of the intestine, whereas silence as a result of cessation of peristaltic activity points to intraabdominal inflammatory diseases. Auscultation should include a search for bruits. Percussion may identify tender areas and differentiate between air and fluid as a cause of abdominal distension. Percussion can identify the large liver of acute fatty infiltration or alcholic hepatitis, the enlarged spleen, and the distended urinary bladder.

Palpation of the abdomen ordinarily is the most informative method of evaluating the area. Gentleness is essential to distinguish between voluntary guarding and an area of involuntary muscle spasm caused by local irritation of the inner aspect of the abdominal wall. Rebound tenderness, a sign of inflammation of the parietal peritoneum, is elicited when the hand depressing the abdominal wall is quickly removed and pain occurs with the sudden return of the abdominal wall to its normal contour. Palpation should identify organ enlargement or a mass, rule out hernias of the abdominal wall and groins, and assess the aorta and the iliac and femoral arteries.

Examination of the rectum should include both digital examination of the rectum and bimanual palpation of the pelvis and lower abdomen. The pelvic examination of the female patient should include a speculum examination of the vagina and cervix to determine the patency of the cervical os, the nature of the cervical discharge, and the position of the uterus. The bimanual examination should determine the size, contour, and position of the uterus and ovaries. The finding of a purulent discharge from the cervix together with thickening, tenderness, or enlargement of the adnexa signifies pelvic inflammatory disease, whereas a tender mass of one adnexa may represent an endometrioma or an ectopic pregnancy. A number of special physical tests and signs are used by physicians evaluating patients with suspected abdominal or pelvic disease. These tests and signs are described in standard textbooks of physical diagnosis.

Examination of the head, neck, chest, back, and extremities will assist in ruling out causes of the acute abdomen outside the abdomen and pelvis.

Diagnostic Procedures

The nature and urgency of the situation as assessed by the examiner will determine which diagnostic studies are done and in what order. The following sequence is appropriate when the patient's condition is stable and adequate time is available.

Bedside Procedures

If gastrointestinal disease is suspected, a nasogastric tube may be inserted to determine the nature of the gastric aspirate and the presence or absence of gross or occult blood. Samples of the stool obtained at the time of rectal examination should be examined for gross or occult blood. If the examination indicates the need, a central venous catheter or Swan-Ganz catheter should be inserted to allow monitoring of central pressures and cardiac function.

Abdominal paracentesis in one or more sites may reveal hemoperitoneum or may identify bile, feces, or other contaminants of the peritoneal cavity associated with intraabdominal accidents. If simple paracentesis is not diagnostic, lavage of the peritoneal cavity with saline and microscopic examination of the aspirate may provide a more definite answer. Today, in the evaluation of the patient with blunt abdominal trauma, peritoneal lavage has become an especially valuable tool.

Laboratory Procedures

Minimum laboratory procedures should include hemoglobin concentration, hematocrit, white blood count, differential count, and urinalysis. Added selected laboratory tests may include serum sodium, potassium, and chloride concentrations, serum glucose, serum pregnancy test, serum amylase determination, arterial blood gas analysis, stools for ova and parasites, smears and cultures of the cervical discharge, an electrocardiogram, and studies of blood coagulation, hepatic function, and renal function.

Roentgenograms

Plain films of the chest and abdomen with the patient in both the supine and the erect position are essential. The chest x-ray examination assists in identifying thoracic causes of the acute abdomen and sometimes reveals specific x-ray findings of intraabdominal catastrophes (e.g., free air under the diaphragm associated with perforation of the gastrointestinal tract). In addition, the chest film often shows abnormalities that reflect subdiaphragmatic disease, such as a left pleural effusion from pancreatitis.

Radiographs of the abdomen are perhaps most essential in patients suspected of having mechanical obstruction of the intestine. The history and physical examination may be equivocal, and the results of laboratory studies are often within normal limits. In contrast, radiographs will show dilated segments of intestine with air-fluid levels. When the mechanical obstruction involves the small intestine, the absence of gas in the colon is often as important a diagnostic sign as the dilated loops of small bowel.

Radiographs of the abdomen made with the patient in the upright position show free air in the peritoneal cavity in 60% to 75% of patients who have a perforation of the gastrointestinal tract. Other potential findings with plain films of the abdomen include a fecalith of the appendix, a renal calculus (90% are radiopaque), calcifications in the pancreas suggestive of chronic recurrent pancreatitis, and curvilinear calcification of the left wall of the infrarenal aorta suggestive of an abdominal aortic aneurysm. Biliary tract disease may be identified in a small number of patients by identifying calcified gallstones (10% to 15% have sufficient calcium to be seen on plain films).

Other Diagnostic Studies

Several diagnostic methods are available for the evaluation of patients with abdominal pain suspected to be of gastrointestinal origin. Examination of the esophagus and gastrointestinal tract using barium sulphate as a contrast medium is safe unless one suspects perforation of the gastrointestinal tract with the potential for barium to enter the peritoneal cavity. The upper gastrointestinal, small bowel, and barium enema examinations may provide a definitive diagnosis of intestinal obstruction or identify fistulae, ulcers, varices, or other lesions responsible for the patient's symptoms and findings.

Endoscopy (including esophagogastroduodenoscopy, endoscopic retrograde cholangiopancreatography, proctosigmoidoscopy, and colonoscopy) is a rapid, direct, and often definitive method of identifying the cause of acute abdominal symptoms and signs. As with other diagnostic methods, patients must be properly selected for each of these endoscopic studies.

Angiography can disclose embolic occlusion of the superior mesenteric artery or other branches of the abdominal aorta or the origin and identity of hemorrhagic lesions of the gastrointestinal tract. The injection of radionuclide-tagged red blood cells into a peripheral vein or their injection into a selected artery via an intraarterial catheter represents another method of identifying the site of gastrointestinal hemorrhage. Radionuclide-tagged albumin may also be used as a peripheral venous injection.

The development of ultrasound instruments and computed tomography has provided physicians with noninvasive tests capable of identifying gallstones, cysts of the pancreas and ovary, aneurysms of the abdominal aorta, and other intraabdominal abnormalities. When clinical findings indicate a possible acute pelvic condition, one of the first diagnostic studies should be an ultrasound examination of the pelvis. Ultrasound is also of special value in identifying gallstones in patients suspected of having acute cholecystitis. Ultrasound and the more recently introduced biliary radionuclide scans can confirm the diagnosis of acute cholecystitis and thereby allow more specific medical therapy and earlier surgical intervention. The role of magnetic resonance imaging (MRI) in the evaluation of patients with acute abdominal symptoms and signs has yet to be defined.

Laparoscopy and minilaparotomy are formal surgical procedures. Although local anesthesia may be used, the surgeon must be prepared to proceed with general anesthesia. Finally, for patients who have an acute intraabdominal problem of unknown nature and whose symptoms, signs, and laboratory findings are suggestive of a threat to life, laparotomy remains the most prudent diagnostic procedure.

THE PERITONEUM AND PERITONITIS

The peritoneum is a single layer of mesothelial cells overlying a loose layer of connective tissue. The parietal peritoneum lines the abdominal cavity and is reflected onto the abdominal viscera as the visceral peritoneum or serosa. Organs and tissues of the abdomen and pelvis lie either within the peritoneal cavity or in the retroperitoneum.

Peritonitis is a response of the visceral or parietal peritoneum, or both, to irritation or injury. The local defense reaction includes hyperemia with increased capillary permeability and an influx of leukocytes and fibroblasts. In addition there is a more generalized response of the abdominal tissues to the injury, including "walling off" of the inflamed area by omentum, loops of intestine, and other tissues and organs. To help isolate inflammation, peristalsis decreases.

Primary peritonitis, an uncommon diffuse inflammation of the peritoneum, has no intraabdominal cause. Principally an illness of infants and children, it is almost always caused by a single pathogenic organism, usually *Pneumococcus, Streptococcus,* or *Escherichia coli*. Bacteria presumably enter the peritoneal cavity via the genital tract or the bloodstream, or by migration through the wall of the intestine.

The diagnosis of primary peritonitis depends on the analysis of fluid from the peritoneal cavity. A leukocyte count greater than $300/mm^3$ with more than 30% neutrophils is diagnostic of intraperitoneal infection. Isolation of a *single* organism is strongly suggestive of primary peritonitis.

Secondary peritonitis of varying degrees is common, accompanying most acute intraabdominal disease. Bacterial contamination leads all causes. Others include bile, pancreatic juice, blood, or acid released into the peritoneal cavity as a result of intraabdominal disease or injury.

There is great variation in both the symptoms and the physical findings of secondary peritonitis. With perforation of a duodenal ulcer, the pain is sudden in onset, and rigidity of the muscles of the abdominal wall is soon apparent. In contrast, the pain and tenderness of the common inflammatory conditions of the lower abdomen and pelvis are often insidious in onset. Fever and an increase in the pulse rate are present in most patients. Pain is the premier symptom. When there is generalized peritonitis, the pain is diffuse. With localized inflammation of the peritoneum, the pain will often allow identification of the site of the peritonitis. With the more localized variety, the point of maximum tenderness and the palpation of a mass are other findings that may allow identification of the origin of the peritonitis. These classical findings of peritonitis may be difficult to interpret in patients who have recently had an abdominal operation and may be absent in immunodepressed patients. Laboratory studies often include leukocytosis and evidence of dehydration. Radiographic examinations may show free air below the diaphragm from a ruptured viscus and adynamic ileus of both the small and large intestine secondary to the peritonitis. When the need for an exploratory operation is in question, needle aspiration or lavage of the peritoneal cavity may confirm the presence of peritonitis but cannot identify localized areas of inflammation.

22

Abdominal Hernias

Robert T. Soper

Ken Kimura

Inguinal
Femoral
Umbilical
Epigastric Hernia
Incisional Hernia
Lumbar Hernia
Respiratory Diaphragmatic Hernias
Internal Hernia
Rare External Hernias

A *hernia* is an abnormal protrusion of an organ or tissue through an aperture, or opening. Thus the brain may herniate through the foramen magnum or the lung through a thoracotomy incision. Usually, however, the word is restricted to describe an abdominal hernia, an abnormal opening in the abdominal wall through which protrusion of intraabdominal viscera occurs.

Hernial apertures, or openings, generally represent defects in the musculofascial tissues surrounding and supporting the abdominal cavity. These defects may be congenital or acquired. A pouch of peritoneum (the hernial sac) pushes through the fascial defect (the hernial ring) and then abdominal contents enter this sac because of continuity with the intraabdominal cavity. The neck of the hernia sac is that portion protruding through the musculofascial defect and defining its narrowest dimension. The omentum, small bowel, large bowel, stomach, and urinary bladder are the organs that most commonly herniate into hernia sacs, in roughly descending frequency.

The status of the contents of the hernia sac is of extreme clinical importance and is defined by the following descriptive adjectives: A *reducible* hernia is one in which the organs contained within the hernia sac can be returned to the abdominal cavity. An *irreducible* hernia is one in which the hernia sac contents cannot be returned to the abdominal cavity without operative reduction. An *incarcerated* hernia (Fig. 22-1, *B*) is synonymous with an irreducible hernia. Neither of these terms implies intestinal obstruction or vascular interference. A *strangulated* hernia is one in which the blood supply to the herniated viscus is compromised. Infarction of the viscus occurs if surgical reduction is not carried out promptly. If intestine is involved, obstruction is generally present. A strangulated hernia is generally irreduc-

185

ible or incarcerated, but an irreducible hernia is generally *not* strangulated.

Further definitions might clarify certain points about hernias for the student: A *ventral* hernia is one that occurs through the ventral abdominal wall and generally includes umbilical, epigastric, and incisional hernias.

An *incisional* hernia is one that occurs through an incision wound that fails to heal completely. Thus an incisional hernia may also be a ventral hernia, provided that the incision is made through the ventral abdominal wall.

Richter's hernia (Fig. 22-1, *A*) is herniation of only a part of the circumference of bowel through a fascial defect; it is especially dangerous because strangulation can occur *without* complete mechanical intestinal obstruction. It is most commonly found in femoral hernias because of the small size and sharp and relatively inflexible nature of the fascial ring in this area. *Littre's* hernia appears to be similar to Richter's hernia, but it should be restricted to herniation of Meckel's diverticulum through a fascial ring.

A *sliding* hernia (Fig. 22-2) is one in which a portion of the sac of a hernia is made up of the herniating viscus itself. Its importance lies in the fact that attempts at surgical removal of the entire sac will, of course, remove or injure the viscus that is "sliding." The most common sliding hernias involve the bladder in direct inguinal hernias, the sigmond colon in left indirect inguinal hernias and the cecum in right indirect inguinal hernias.

The anatomical location of a hernia is a convenient method of identification or classification. The following is a list of the more common hernias according to *location*:

Inguinal (indirect or direct)
Femoral
Umbilical (infantile, adult, or omphalocele)
Epigastric

Incisional (postoperative, ventral)
Pelvic
Lumbar
Diaphragmatic (congenital or hiatal)

INGUINAL

The surgical treatment of inguinal hernia is the most common major operation performed in the United States. Twenty four percent of people develop inguinal hernias during their life times. Inguinal hernias are several times more common in males than in females because of the defect in the abdominal wall occasioned by descent of the testis into the scrotum in the male and also perhaps because of the protection to the inside of the lower ventral abdominal wall afforded by the uterus in females.

Inguinal hernias are of two types: *indirect* and *direct*. The fascial defect in an indirect inguinal hernia (Fig. 22-3) lies *lateral* to the inferior deep epigastric artery, and the defect in the direct hernia (Fig. 22-4) lies

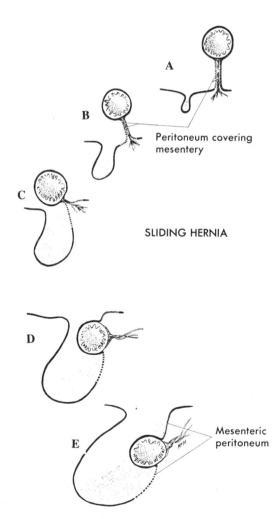

Fig. 22-2. Sliding hernia. Simple hernia evolves in **A** and **B**. It begins to "slide" with one mesenteric leaf in **C** and the bowel itself in **D**. In its final evolution in step **E**, bowel and both mesenteric leaves are part of hernial sac.

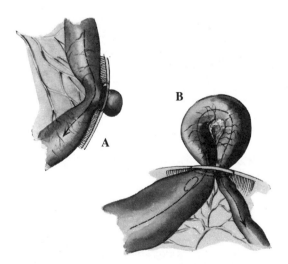

Fig. 22-1. A, Richter's hernia. Only a portion of bowel passes through hernial ring; arrow indicates that bowel need not be obstructed mechanically even with strangulation. **B,** Incarcerated hernia. Distended bowel in hernia cannot return to abdomen through narrow fascial defect.

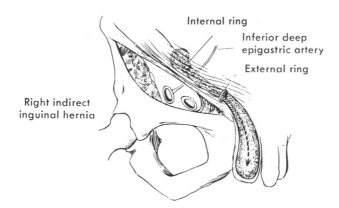

Fig. 22-3. Right indirect inguinal hernia. Hernial sac begins at internal (deep, or abdominal) inguinal ring lateral to inferior deep epigastric artery and exits from inguinal canal at external (subcutaneous) ring to descend into scrotum. Sac lies anteromedial to cord structures.

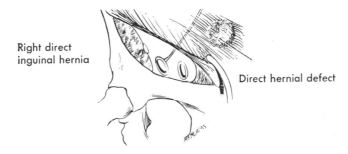

Fig. 22-4. Right direct inguinal hernia. Hernial sac arises in Hesselbach's triangle medial to inferior deep epigastric artery and just above pubic tubercle. It does not descend into scrotum.

medial to this structure. Usually the indirect type has a preformed, or congenital, sac, occurs in the infant to young adult, and is more symptomatic and more prone to develop complications; in contrast, the direct inguinal hernia is much less common, is seen in the elderly male as part of the "wear and tear" process of aging, almost never becomes complicated by strangulation, is generally less symptomatic, and is almost unheard of in females. The distinction between the two is perhaps academic in the good-risk patient, since both should be corrrected surgically at an elected time. However, in a poor-risk elderly patient the distinction between the two becomes important in the selection of the appropriate treatment; a low-risk direct hernia in a high-risk patient might better be treated by a well-fitted truss or other conservative methods.

Indirect

Etiology. Most indirect inguinal hernias arise because of retention or imperfect obliteration of the *processus vaginalis,* the embryonic outpocketing of peritoneum that precedes testicular descent into the scrotum. The testis originates along the urogenital ridge in the retroperitoneum and migrates caudal during the second trimester of pregnancy to arrive at the internal inguinal (abdominal) ring at about the sixth month of intrauterine life. During the last trimester, it proceeds through the abdominal wall via the inguinal canal and descends into the scrotum, the right slightly later and less far

than the left. The processus vaginalis then normally obliterates postnatally, except for the portion surrounding and serving as a covering for the testicle *(tunica vaginalis)*. Failurc of this obliterative proccss results in an indirect inguinal hernia at birth or during the first few months or years of life (coincident with the highest age peak of incidence of this hernia). The incidence then diminishes to rise again in young adult males. Herniation at this age probably results when the stress of muscular activity and the increase in intraabdominal pressure force open a previously imperfectly obliterated processus vaginalis. Indirect inguinal hcrnias seldom arise after 40 years of age, underscoring the importance of this congenital, or preformed, sac in its genesis.

A *hydrocele* is an unobliterated processus vaginalis in which the communication with the peritoneal cavity is large enough to allow peritoneal fluid to enter but not large enough to admit bowel. About 15% of inguinal hernias in infants and children are preceded by a hydrocele, but most hydroceles in the very young disappear spontaneously as the continuing obliterative process closes off the peritoneal connection. Hydroceles do not require treatment unless they persist into childhood; surgical treatment involves simply dividing and ligating the communicating tract.

Diagnosis. Early complaints of indirect inguinal hernia include a bulge or swelling in the groin that appears only when the patient strains, cries, or assumes an upright position and that disappears when reclining.

Commonly the bulge is associated with a nagging, dull discomfort locally. Occasionally forceful straining or lifting precipitates an acute hernia, heralded by sudden groin discomfort and a bulge in the area. With time, the groin bulge increases in size and pursues an oblique course from the internal inguinal ring downward and medially along the course of the inguinal canal, and when it descends to the bottom of the scrotum it becomes a *complete* or *scrotal* hernia.

Physical examination is the key to diagnosis. An oblong swelling in the groin that appears with standing and straining and extends downward and medially into the scrotum, disappearing in a reverse direction on assumption of the supine position, is the classical finding. Inversion of scrotal skin by the examining index finger confirms that the external (subcutaneous) inguinal ring has been dilated by the hernia. Asking the patient to cough or strain (cough impulse) will bring the bowel or the end of the sac down against the end of the examining finger. After an indirect inguinal hernia has been completely reduced, finger pressure over the internal (abdominal) inguinal ring (located 1 cm superior to the midpoint of a line drawn from the anterosuperior iliac spine to the pubic tubercle) prevents recurrence unless a direct hernia coexists (so-called *pantaloon* hernia).

Treatment. Indirect inguinal hernias should be repaired surgically unless specific contraindications exist because of the discomfort that they evoke, the certainty that once established they will persist and even become larger with time, and the constant threat of complications of the hernia. In the infant and young child adequate surgical treatment (Fig. 22-5) consists of simple division of the sac with high ligation of the sac neck. There is usually no need for fascial reconstruction, since the basic defect is the sac itself rather than a deficiency of the supporting musculoaponeurotic structures. The distal sac can be left in situ as normal cord and testicular coverings.

In the older child or young adult division and closure of the neck of the sac are carried out after reduction of the herniated viscera. In addition, the abdominal ring (aperture in the transversalis fascia) is snugged up closely around the carefully identified (and undamaged) cord structures over the top of the ligated sac. In those hernias that through neglect have grown to enormous proportions, destroying a good part of the supporting transversalis fascia and displacing the inferior deep epigastric vessels medially, a more extensive fascial repair is necessitated after the sac has been ligated. Reattachment of the fresh superior edge of transversalis fascia to Cooper's ligament and the prefemoral fascia (McVay's operation) is one of the more popular operations designed to restore the integrity of the musculoaponeurotic support. Recurrence of the hernia is seen in only 1% to 2% of the smaller hernias of infancy and childhood and in up to 5% of the very large hernias of adulthood.

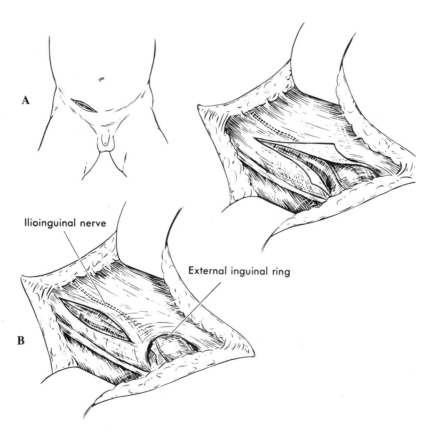

Fig. 22-5. Repair of right indirect inguinal hernia in infant. **A,** Groin-crease skin incision. **B,** Incision in external oblique aponeurosis exposes hernia and cord structures; ilioinguinal nerve should be protected.

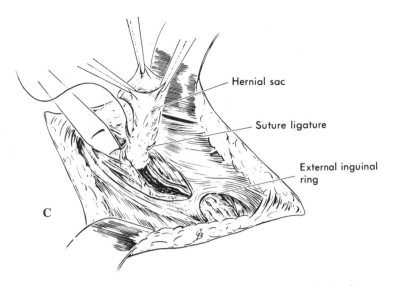

Hernial sac

Suture ligature

External inguinal
ring

C

Fig. 22-5, cont'd. C, Hernial sac has been separated from cord structures and divided, and contents have been reduced; suture-ligature is closing neck of sac.

Complications

Incarceration. Acute incarceration of a previously reducible hernia is associated with local pain, and, if not reduced promptly, it may produce edema and increased pressure at the narrowed sac neck with strangulation of the herniated viscera. Acute incarceration sometimes heralds the onset of inguinal hernia, especially in the infant and young child. Nonoperative reduction may be attempted, provided that the irreducibility is only a few hours in duration and there is no localized tenderness, redness, or signs of intestinal obstruction to suggest early strangulation. To accomplish mechanical reduction, the patient should be placed in the supine position with the hips flexed and the foot of the bed elevated; a sedative or analgesic agent will help produce relaxation, after which gentle pressure over the hernia is applied.

If gentle attempts at manual reduction are unsuccessful or there is any suggestion of early strangulation, surgical correction of the hernia must be carried out as an emergency procedure. The techniques of repair are the same, namely, opening the sac, careful inspection of the herniated viscera to assure their viability, after which they are reduced into the intraperitoneal cavity, high ligation and division of the sac neck, and fascial repair if indicated.

A long-standing hernia often becomes less completely reducible and ultimately may be completely irreducible or incarcerated. A chronically incarcerated hernia is not likely to be symptomatic, nor does it carry the threat of immediate strangulation. It often indicates that the hernia is really a sliding hernia (Fig. 22-2) rather than the more common nonsliding type. Surgical repair of a sliding hernia is more complicated in that complete sac dissection and division and closure of the sac neck are impossible because a portion of the sac wall itself is composed of the sliding viscus. Only that portion of the sac not made up of viscus can be excised, and the entire remaining sac and its sliding

viscus must then be reduced *en masse;* repair of the musculoaponeurotic supporting tissue can then be made superficial to the sac to prevent its recurrence. The morbidity, mortality, and recurrence after surgical repair of a sliding hernia are all higher than with a nonsliding hernia and justify early hernia repair before the sliding hernia has time to develop.

Strangulation. A hernia is more likely to strangulate if it has a capacious sac with a rather narrow sac neck surrounded by a rigid and unyielding fascial ring. Pressure at the ring first slows venous return, producing stasis and edema, thereby ensuring irreducibility. An inflammatory response adds to the vicious cycle and culminates with impedance of arterial inflow to the strangulated viscus with necrosis and gangrene. Small intestine is the most commonly strangulated viscus and is, of course, associated with mechanical intestinal obstruction at this point. Delaying surgical repair by attempts at forceful reduction will further traumatize the friable viscus, often resulting in perforation and spreading peritonitis. Surgical treatment should be undertaken promptly by resection of the strangulated organ, followed by anatomic repair of the hernia. The morbidity, mortality, and recurrence after strangulated hernias are understandably higher than for nonstrangulated types.

Direct

Direct inguinal hernia (Fig. 22-4) is only about one fifth as common as the indirect counterpart, originates after 40 years of age, and is almost never seen in females. The bulge is medial to the inguinal canal just above the pubic tubercle and is likely to be circular and diffuse, rather than distinct and elongated as the bulge in the indirect variety is. The fascial edges are indistinct in keeping with its origin as a gradual and diffuse weakening of the fascia transversalis in Hesselbach's triangle, associated with aging and increasing intraabdominal pressure from coughing (asthma), straining to micturate (prostatism), obesity, constipation, and nutritional defects. This very fact, however, is the reason direct inguinal hernias, though uncomfortable, rarely become complicated by incarceration. As they get larger, the bladder commonly "slides" into the medial edge of the direct hernia sac, a factor that must be remembered at the time of surgical repair.

On physical examination the distinction between indirect and direct hernias is not difficult. When the examining finger is placed through the external (subcutaneous) ring and then directed posteriorly, the weakness in the fascia transversalis forming the floor of the inguinal canal is the most distinctive finding. After reduction, finger pressure over the internal (abdominal) ring does not prevent a direct hernia from appearing immediately when the patient strains or stands. Direct hernia sacs have no direct relationship to the testicular cord structures, nor do they commonly descend into the scrotum. In view of the low complication rate, a direct inguinal hernia may be treated conservatively in a high-risk, debilitated patient. A well-fitted truss, though cumbersome, can relieve the symptoms.

The more expedient treatment consists of surgical repair. Direct inguinal hernia sacs are simply reduced, and the defect in the floor of the inguinal canal is repaired when one brings down the strong superior margin of fascia transversalis and reattaches it by suture to Cooper's ligament medially and to the prefemoral fascia laterally (McVay's repair). Recurrence rates are twice as high as with indirect hernias.

FEMORAL

A femoral hernia (Fig. 22-6) is one that occurs through an enlarged femoral ring, the medialmost compartment of the femoral canal. The femoral canal lies below the inguinal (Poupart's) ligament and above the pubic bone and is bounded medially by the rather unyielding lacunar ligament. The contents of the femoral canal from lateral to medial spell out the word *nave* (standing for femoral *n*erve, *a*rtery, *v*ein, *e*mpty space). It is through this empty space that a femoral hernia occurs.

Femoral hernias are more common in women than in men and are probably acquired rather than congenital. The narrowness of the sac neck and the rigidity of its boundaries predispose to its high incidence of irreducibility, strangulation (up to 20%), and Richter's type of strangulated hernia (see Fig. 22-1, *A*). It is understandable why symptoms occur earlier and why prompt surgical treatment should be carried out more urgently than with inguinal hernia.

Initially the bulge of a femoral hernia lies below the inguinal (Poupart's) ligament medial to the femoral arterial pulse. However, as the sac enlarges with time, it is likely to turn upward anterior to the inguinal (Poupart's) ligament and then present as an inguinal swelling difficult to distinguish from an indirect inguinal hernia. Careful inspection will often reveal that its neck is located low and that reduction occurs in a different direction from the indirect inguinal hernia.

Table 22-1. Inguinofemoral Hernias

	Femoral	*Indirect Inguinal*	*Direct Inguinal*
Age at onset	Young to middle-aged adult	Infant, child, young adult	Middle to old age
Sex	Female > male	Male 10:1	Almost always male
Cause	Acquired (?)	Congenital	Wear and tear
Incidence	Uncommon	Most common	Second most common
Origin	Femoral canal	Internal inguinal ring	Hesselbach's triangle
Neck size	Small, rigid	Small to medium	Large
Course of sac	Variable	Oblique to scrotum	Local protrusion
Incarceration	Common	15%-20%	Rare
Strangulation	Common	5%-10%	Hardly ever
Sliding	Rare	Common if longstanding; right-cecum, left sigmoid	Common (bladder)
Treatment	Always surgical	Always surgical	Surgical if symptomatic

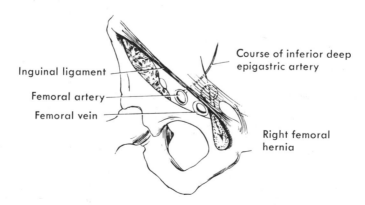

Fig. 22-6. Right femoral hernia. Hernial sac arises below inguinal ligament and medial to femoral vein.

Surgical repair is the only recommended treatment for femoral hernia, preferably undertaken before complications occur. The surgical approach is through the same skin incision (inguinal crease) as that used for the two more common types of inguinal hernias, and the essentials of repair are the same, namely, opening of the sac, reduction of the herniated contents, ligation and high closure of the sac neck, and reattachment of the fascia transversalis to Cooper's ligament to close off completely the empty space in the femoral canal without compromise to the femoral vein.

Table 22-1 compares and contrasts the three varieties of inguinofemoral hernias.

Differential Diagnosis of Inguinofemoral Masses

The three types of inguinofemoral hernias (direct inguinal, indirect inguinal, and femoral) can often be distinguished from one another on careful physical examination, and they *must* be distinguished carefully from other disorders that produce swelling in the same general area. A few of the more common considerations in differential diagnosis of inguinofemoral masses are discussed briefly:

Hydrocele of the cord or testis or both is distinguished from indirect inguinal hernia by the fact that it cannot be quickly reduced, is not attended by discomfort, transilluminates brilliantly, and often is associated with a thickening of the cord structures above the hydrocele.

Undescended testis. Careful palpation of the scrotal sac should make the diagnosis of cryptorchidism clear. When the testis is within the inguinal canal, it is palpated as a firm mass that cannot be brought down by traction to within the scrotum; this distinguishes it from a simple high-riding or retractile testis that, with gentleness, persistence, and often exposure to warm water, can be brought down into the scrotum and is not truly undescended. Cryptorchidism is almost invariably associated with an indirect inguinal hernia that in itself commonly justifies early surgical treatment of the hernia and concomitant replacement of the testis within the scrotum.

Inguinal lymphadenitis. Enlarged inguinofemoral lymph nodes generally are multiple rather than solitary and sometimes are tender. The site of infection within the extremity or perineum resulting in the inguinal node enlargement should be apparent on examination. The nodes do not become reduced or transmit a cough impulse.

Varix of upper greater saphenous vein. A localized varix, or thin-walled enlargement, of the proximal portion of the greater saphenous vein presents as a soft swelling below the inguinal ligament that is commonly confused with femoral hernia. It is generally associated with varicosities of the rest of the saphenous system. It transmits a cough impulse that is felt in the remainder of the dilated vein, and percussion of the veins transmits a percussion thrill to the varix to distinguish it clearly from femoral hernia. The varix swelling promptly disappears when the patient is recumbent.

Lipoma of the cord. A lipoma surrounding the cord structures is difficult to distinguish from indirect inguinal hernia. It occasionally is associated with a hernia and constitutes part of the inguinal canal swelling. Lipoma of the cord is not reducible, is not painful, and does not transmit a cough impulse.

UMBILICAL

There are three general types of umbilical hernia that differ greatly in causation, prognosis, and treatment: omphalocele, infantile hernia, and adult hernia (Table 22-2).

Omphalocele

An *omphalocele* is not a true hernia because its covering is made up of amniotic sac, it has no true inner peritoneal lining or skin covering its outer surface; it really represents a failure of the extracoelomic midgut to return to the peritoneal cavity after the tenth to twelfth week of intrauterine existence. The prognosis of an omphalocele is grave because of its propensity to rupture, a high incidence of associated congenital anomalies elsewhere, and extreme difficulty in reducing the herniated viscera even at operation. Surgical treatment is aimed at excision of the sac and closure of the abdominal wall in layers, when the contents can be reduced without tension and the defect in the abdominal wall is not large.

If the viscera cannot be safely reduced, even after the abdominal cavity has been enlarged by manual stretching of the abdominal wall, it is best to suture a Dacron-reinforced sheet around the defect and over the herniated viscera. This so-called silo affords a physio-

Table 22-2. Umbilical Hernias

	Omphalocele	*Infantile*	*Adult*
Age at onset	Newborn (premature)	Newborn (premature)	Middle to elderly
Sex	Equal	Equal	Female > male
Race	Equal	Black > white	Equal
Incidence	Rare	Very common	Common
Cause	Congenital	Congenital	Wear and tear
Skin cover	None	Intact	Intact
Other anomalies	Frequent	Average	Average
Neck size	Large	Small to large	Often small
Incarceration	Rare	Rare	Frequent
Strangulation	Rare	Rare	Frequent
Treatment	Surgical	Observation	Surgical

logic covering to the viscera, allowing their staged reduction into a gradually expanding abdominal cavity. Complete reduction is achieved by 7 to 10 days of age, allowing safe skin and fascial closure after removal of the silo.

Infantile

Infantile umbilical hernia is very common, occurring in upward of 5% of white infants and 20% of black infants. The incidence is higher among premature than among term infants. It represents protrusion of a hernia sac through an aperture created when the umbilical vessels thrombose and rapidly involute at the time of delivery. Because the infantile type of umbilical hernia almost never becomes complicated by incarceration or strangulation and almost always disappears spontaneously by the seventh year of life, the indications for surgical repair are few. Trusses do not speed resolution of an umbilical hernia and may even entrap and irritate herniated intestine; their use is therefore discouraged. In the occasional case that is symptomatic, becomes incarcerated or strangulated, or is so large as to predispose to external trauma, surgical repair is indicated.

Adult

The adult type of umbilical hernia occurs more commonly in the obese and multiparous female. It originates through a dilated and weakened umbilical ring or through a weak spot in the linea alba just above the umbilicus. Adult hernias in this region are dangerous because, like the femoral hernias, the neck remains small and unyielding despite often a very capacious hernia sac. This results in a high incidence of incarceration and strangulation, a feature that demands early surgical repair.

The surgical treatment of umbilical hernias is carried out through a curving infraumbilical incision; the sac is opened, the contents are reduced, and the neck of the sac is closed flush with its entrance into the abdominal cavity. The fascia surrounding the resultant defect is then brought together and often overlapped (imbricated) for a two-layer repair.

EPIGASTRIC HERNIA

Epigastric hernias occur in the linea alba between the xiphoid process and the umbilicus. These hernias are probably initiated by properitoneal fat protruding through apertures created by perforating vessels, which then gradually enlarge with continuing stress (a rise in intraabdominal pressure) to allow a peritoneal sac to protrude. They cause local pain and tenderness, even though small in size, and are generally seen in middle-aged men doing manual labor. The pain can mimic other types of intraabdominal surgical disease that must be ruled out before elective hernia repair is undertaken. The repair consists in excision and closure of the sac and repair of the defect in the fascia.

INCISIONAL HERNIA

An incisional hernia is one that occurs through an old operative incision in the abdominal wall that has become partially dehiscent. Incisional hernias develop more commonly in vertical than in transverse incisions and in patients with poor wound healing, *postoperative wound infections*, or conditions that cause increased intraabdominal pressure. Poor wound healing may occur because of faulty surgical technique (placement of sutures too close to the edges being apposed, use of too small or too large suture material, knots tied so tightly as to necrose abdominal wall layers, knots becoming untied, or interruption of a running suture that then unravels for the length of the incision). Hematomas and infections of the wound produce delayed and imperfect healing; foreign bodies brought through the wound (drains, catheters) prevent sound approximation of wound edges and are associated with a high incidence of herniation. Postoperative cough, distension, and hiccups all greatly elevate intraabdominal pressure and place undue strain on the sutures, which may then give way to initiate an incisional hernia.

The symptoms are those of a variable-sized swelling in an old incision line, generally attended by only mild symptoms of local discomfort. Incarceration is fairly common, but strangulation is rare because of the large size of the sac neck.

Treatment is generally surgical, though satisfactory control of moderate-sized hernias can be afforded by girdles or trusses for the poor-risk patient. Small and symptomatic hernias should be repaired surgically because of danger of strangulation, and the large and diffuse ones should be repaired surgically because of danger of strangulation, and the large and diffuse ones should be repaired because of failure of control by binders or girdles. In the large hernias with attenuated fascia, fascial grafts and prosthetic replacement to bridge gaps in the fascia are commonly necessary.

LUMBAR HERNIA

Most lumbar hernias are really incisional hernias occurring in old nephrectomy incisions. However, occasionally they occur spontaneously, either just above the iliac crest posteriorly or just below the twelfth rib. The hernias generally remain reducible, do not tend to strangulate, and can usually be controlled by a corset or belt.

RESPIRATORY DIAPHRAGMATIC HERNIAS

The respiratory diaphragm separates the thoracic from the abdominal cavity and is breached by the esophagus, the aorta, and the inferior vena cava. It is an extremely important muscular organ that assists in respiratory efforts and can remarkably affect pressures within the thoracic and abdominal cavities and vessels. It is formed embryonically by peripheral muscularization of the septum transversum. Hernias occur either through apertures resulting from imperfect development (congenital) or are acquired by increases in intraabdominal pressure, rupturing weakened points, or enlargement of the preexistent apertures.

Congenital

Congenital diaphragmatic hernia (Fig. 22-7) is one of the true surgical emergencies of the newborn period of life; 80% occur through the left posterolateral foramen of Bochdalek, and 20% occur through a similar defect on the right side—presumably the tamponade effect of the liver on the right side accounts for this difference in incidence. Most Bochdalek hernias have no sac. Since the aperture in the diaphragm occurs early during intrauterine life, before rotation of the midgut has occurred, it is commonly associated with malrotation; for the same reason, the involved lung is frequently immature and incapable of immediate normal expansion after surgical correction.

Rapid respiratory decompensation demands urgency in diagnosis and treatment of congenital diaphragmatic

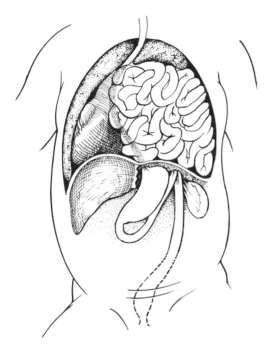

Fig. 22-7. Typical left-sided Bochdalek hernia with air-filled midgut in left pleural cavity. Midline structures (esophagus, heart) are displaced to right side and both lungs are compressed. Liver underlies right hemidiaphragm, accounting for lower incidence of right-sided Bochdalek hernia.

hernia. The sequential pathophysiology is as follows: the intestine rapidly fills with swallowed air postnatally, which expands the size of the herniated viscera in the chest, producing progressive mediastinal shift to the contralateral side with interference in respiratory exchange in the normal lung and impedance of venous return to the heart. The diagnosis is established by a plain upright radiograph that demonstrates gas-filled loops of bowel in the chest with a contralateral mediastinal shift. Emergency endotracheal intubation and assisted respiration temporarily stabilize the child. Nasogastric suction halts the lethal ingress of swallowed air before early laparotomy with reduction of the abdominal viscera from the chest and suture approximation of the edges of the defect in the diaphragm.

Even with early diagnosis and proper management, less than half the babies with Bochdalek hernia *who become symptomatic within the first 24 hours of life* survive. In sharp distinction are afflicted infants diagnosed after 24 hours of age, virtually all of whom survive surgical correction. Factors that adversely affect survival in the symptomatic neonate include severe preoperative hypoxemia, hypoplasia and immaturity of the lungs, persistent fetal circulatory shunts, postoperative contralateral pneumothorax, and elevated intraabdominal pressure.

Hiatal

Acquired diaphragmatic hernias (Fig. 22-8) generally involve the stomach, herniating either through an enlarged esophageal hiatus (the sliding type of esophageal hiatal hernia) or through a defect in the diaphragm just lateral to the diaphragmatic crura encircling the esophagus (paraesophageal or parahiatal type). The sliding hiatal hernia is many times more common than the paraesophageal; since it increases the acute esophagogastric angle, there is free reflux of stomach contents into the esophagus to produce the outstanding symptoms of esophagitis: regurgitation, heartburn, mild bleeding, and later scarring with stricture formation and dysphagia. Hiatal hernias are seen either in infants or in middle-aged to elderly patients with obesity and increased intraabdominal pressure for

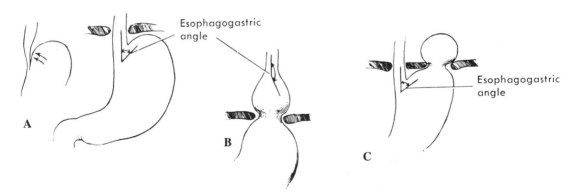

Fig. 22-8. A, Normal relationship of stomach and esophagus to diaphragm; acute esophagogastic angle helps prevent reflux from stomach into esophagus *(inset).* **B,** "Sliding" type of esophageal hiatal hernia; esophagogastic junction above diaphragm; obtuse esophagogastric angle favors reflux. **C,** Paraesophageal hiatal hernia; esophagogastric angle is normal, and no reflux into esophagus occurs.

one reason or another. The symptoms are aggravated by lying down and are improved by sitting up. Often an acid-peptic diathesis is associated.

Treatment is tailored to the severity of symptoms and the patient's general operative risk status. Hiatal hernias that are small and only mildly symptomatic or that occur in very poor-risk patients can be managed satisfactorily by restriction of the patient to an upright position postprandially, elevation of the head of the bed while sleeping, and introduction of histamine (H_2) blockers and/or antacid medical regimen. Reduction of body weight and other factors that reduce intraabdominal pressure also assist in the treatment program. Hiatal hernias that are large, progressively more symptomatic, or associated with complications of ulceration, bleeding, or stenosis should be treated surgically: the stomach is pulled down below the diaphragm, and usually the hiatal aperture is closed around the esophagus. Usually some sort of antireflux operation is then performed (Fig. 22-9) to further discourage gastroesophageal reflux. If an acid-peptic diathesis is present or the patient has an actual peptic ulcer, truncal vagotomy and an appropriate gastric drainage procedure are commonly added. The poor-risk patient who must be treated surgically because of complications can be improved by simple suture fixation of the reduced stomach to the anterior abdominal wall.

The less common parahiatal diaphragmatic hernias produce symptoms of vague epigastric and lower anterior chest pain aggravated by increases in intraabdominal pressure and recumbency. Since the esophagogastric junction is undisturbed, none of the symptoms of esophagitis is present. Complications include ulceration and bleeding within the herniated stomach, incarceration and strangulation, and progressive enlargement until most of the stomach is intrathoracic (giving an upside-down radiographic appearance to the stomach).

Treatment principles are similar to those of the sliding type of hiatal hernia: surgical reduction and repair of the aperture in the diaphragm.

Indirect or direct trauma to the diaphragm may produce tears or weak areas through which hernias develop. These are almost always on the left side, because of the protection afforded by the liver to the right side of the diaphragm. Respiratory and gastrointestinal symptoms coexist, and the diagnosis is confirmed by plain films of the chest and by barium studies of the upper and lower intestine demonstrating loops of intestine within the thorax. Surgical reduction and closure of the diaphragmatic rent prevent complications (intestinal obstruction, strangulation, atelectasis).

INTERNAL HERNIA

Internal hernia is the name given to the herniation of the intestine through an aperture (natural or acquired) within the abdominal cavity. Thus small bowel herniation through the foramen of Winslow into the lesser sac would be termed an internal hernia. There are recesses in the paraduodenal and paracecal areas in which internal hernias may occur. Postoperative adhesions may form an aperture through which an internal hernia occurs.

Internal hernias are dangerous because they may remain undiagnosed until complications of intestinal obstruction or strangulation occur that necessitate emergency surgical exploration. Treatment is directed at relieving the obstruction or strangulation by appropriate means and then closing the aperture through which herniation occurred.

RARE EXTERNAL HERNIAS
Obturator hernia

A hernia may accompany the obturator vessels and nerve into the thigh through the obturator foramen. *Obturator hernias* are uncommon at any age but more often occur in elderly women. They can be diagnosed by a swelling in the upper and medial aspect of the thigh associated with pain radiating to the medial aspect of the knee, aggravated by sudden increases in intraabdominal pressure but not by hip or knee movements. Hypesthesia in the area of pain radiation indicates irritation of the sensory component of the obturator nerve. The neck of the sac may be palpable on vaginal or rectal pelvic examination. Strangulation and incar-

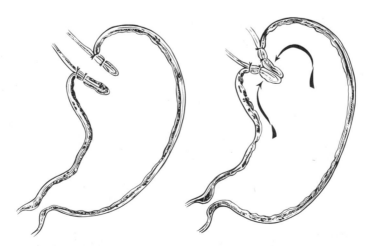

Fig. 22-9. Fundoplication. *Left,* Gastric fundus is wrapped around lower esophagus. *Right,* When stomach fills, pressure closes gastroesophageal function, preventing reflux.

ceration are common, and morbidity and mortality remain high because of delay in diagnosis. Treatment is reduction of the viscera at the time of exploratory laparotomy with closure of the peritoneum over the aperture.

Sciatic hernia

Sciatic hernias can occur through either the greater or lesser sciatic notches as bulges inferior to the gluteus maximus muscle. They become symptomatic by pro-ducing either intestinal obstruction or pain that has a sciatic nerve distribution.

Spigelian hernia

A *spigelian hernia sac,* by definition, originates at the junction of the semilunar and semicircular lines just lateral to the rectus muscle in its lower fourth. As the hernia sac enlarges, it may track from this location interstitially in almost any direction to present a most puzzling clinical picture. Strangulation may occur.

23

Stomach and Duodenum

Israel Penn

Peptic Ulcer
Gastric Cancer
Miscellaneous Conditions of Stomach and
Duodenum

Three disorders of the stomach and duodenum—peptic ulcer, gastric cancer, and hypertrophic pyloric stenosis—completely overshadow all other diseases that involve these important digestive organs. The main concerns of this chapter are peptic ulcer and gastric cancer. Hypertrophic pyloric stenosis is discussed in Chapter 39. The less common diseases of the stomach and duodenum are mentioned at the end of this chapter, as also is gastric surgery for the treatment of morbid obesity.

PEPTIC ULCER

A peptic ulcer is any gastrointestinal ulcer caused by contact with acid-pepsin secretions. Patients with pernicious anemia (total anacidity) very rarely get peptic ulcers. Although acid-pepsin secretions link the three main types of peptic ulcers, important differences separate them. The student should envision these three main classifications as follows: (1) duodenal ulcer diathesis (duodenal, pyloric channel, and synchronous gastric and duodenal ulcers); (2) chronic gastric ulcer; and (3) acute gastric mucosal ulcerations.

Peptic ulceration may also occur in the lower esophagus in patients with reflux esophagitis; in the jejunum in severe cases of the Zollinger-Ellison syndrome (see below) or after anastomosis of the stomach to the jejunum; or in the ileum in patients who have a Meckel's diverticulum containing ectopic gastric mucosa.

Gastric Physiology
Stimulation of Gastric Secretion

A combined vagal-antral phase increases gastric secretion as follows. Stimuli from the brain (hunger—thought, sight, smell, and taste of food) travel along the vagus nerves to incite the gastric parietal and chief cells to secrete acid and pepsin, and to stimulate the antral G cells to release gastrin, a secretory hormone that also stimulates the parietal and chief cells. Thus neural stimuli trigger a dual mechanism that heightens gastric secretion. Distension of the antrum by food also stimulates gastrin release, as do various secretagogues (peptones and amino acids from food). These overlapping mechanisms of gastric secretion potentiate one another.

Inhibition of Gastric Secretion

As digestion in the stomach ceases, several factors inhibit gastric secretion. Vagal activity decreases, and as the stomach empties, antral distension, an important stimulus to gastrin release, subsides. The low pH reached in the antrum also inhibits gastrin release. The acid contents of the stomach, as they flow into the duodenum, trigger release of a hormone (secretin) that inhibits both gastric secretion and motility. Acid, fat, and hypertonic solutions, as they enter the duodenum, all suppress gastric secretion (possibly by release of enterogastrone or gastric inhibitory peptide). Thus in normal people a remarkable mechanism stimulates gastric secretion during hunger and food intake and shuts it off as the food leaves the stomach.

The Mucosal Barrier

The answer to the question, Why doesn't the corrosive gastric content digest the stomach wall? rests on the concept of a gastric mucosal barrier, a secreting, dynamic "containing wall" capable of maintaining an H^+ hydrogen ion gradient (stomach to blood) of about 2,000,000 to 1.

This wall features a layer of mucus that acts chiefly as a lubricant and weak buffer and, most important, a layer of highly specialized, tightly joined, columnar cells that prevent back-diffusion of acid. A rich blood supply supports both of these layers and allows the mucosal cells to replace themselves within 48 hours, if injured. Several prostaglandins increase gastric mucosal blood flow and mucus production and decrease free acid production. They also increase the migration of basal cells toward the lumen to repair mucosal injury. Disruption of the integrity of the mucosal barrier, inhibition of prostaglandin synthesis, or inhibition of bicarbonate or mucus secretion may explain how gastric ulcers arise in tandem with low gastric acidity and why acute gastric mucosal ulcers accompany shock and stress.

Duodenal Ulcer

Incidence. The incidence in different parts of the world varies from 1% to 20% of the population. Duodenal ulcers occur in all age groups. Men are more frequently affected than women, especially in the younger age groups (Fig. 23-1).

Cause. Excess secretion of acid and pepsin keynotes the pathogenesis of duodenal ulcer. This is attributable in part to an increased number of functioning parietal cells, which may be hereditary, or to hyperplasia as a result of chronic stimulation. Hypersecretion may also result from a high secretory drive or from an increased sensitivity of the parietal cells to a normal drive. Reduction of duodenal buffers may contribute to ulceration.

Most experienced clinicians accept psychological factors as the most common link in the genesis of duodenal ulcers. Chronic psychic stress (e.g., the hard-driving, ambitious person) undoubtedly augments gastric secretion through brain centers and the vagus nerves. Duodenal ulcer traits run through families, especially those members sharing blood group O. The role of diet (e.g., coffee drinking) remains debatable. Excess alcohol intake may increase gastric secretion and the incidence of duodenal ulcer. For unknown reasons patients with pulmonary emphysema suffer a threefold increase in duodenal ulcers.

Clinical features. The classical symptom is a gnawing pain in the upper abdomen an hour or two after meals, sometimes radiating to the back and relieved by food. Some patients complain only of vague discomfort—a feeling of hunger or cramps. The pain frequently awakens patients from sleep and is relieved by milk or antacids. An important feature is periodicity of the pain. Attacks lasting for several weeks are interspersed with months of complete freedom from symp-

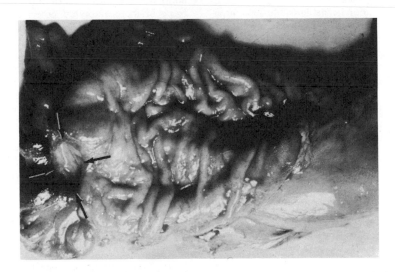

Fig. 23-1. Duodenal ulcer. Opened stomach on right; duodenal ulcer with sharply demarcated edges on left.

toms. An occasional patient will bleed severely yet deny any prior pain. The only common physical finding is mild tenderness in the right upper abdomen.

Laboratory examination. Overnight collections of gastric secretions show a two- to fivefold increase in volume and concentration of acids (Table 23-1). Barium x-ray studies of the stomach and duodenum will usually show an ulcer crater or scarring in the proximal portion of the duodenum (duodenal bulb). Endoscopic examination of the duodenum will confirm the diagnosis in problem cases.

Treatment. Effective medical treatment involves drastic reduction of acid secretion through intensive antacid therapy (as frequently as every hour) or the use of histamine (H_2) receptor blockers, such as cimetidine, ranitidine or famotidine, given for a period of 6 to 8 weeks. Agents more potent than the H_2 blockers such as omeprazole (an inhibitor of the proton pump H^+K^+-ATPase) and various prostaglandin analogs are undergoing clinical trials. The majority of duodenal ulcers heal with these measures. It is debatable whether reduction of smoking and abstinence from alcohol, coffee, and tea play a significant role in the reduction of acid secretion.

An alternative therapy to acid reduction is sucralfate (a complex of sulfated sucrose and aluminum hydroxide). This adheres to proteinaceous exudate at the ulcer site and forms a protective coating that shields the ulcer from acid, pepsin, and bile salts. It may also exert a cytoprotective effect mediated by prostaglandins. High healing rates have been obtained in controlled trials. Surgical therapy is indicated for the small percentage of patients who develop complications, listed in order of frequency:

Complications

Bleeding. Bleeding occurs in 10% to 15% of patients with duodenal or gastric ulcers. Surgical treatment is indicated for severe, persistent, or recurrent bleeding. The decision for surgical therapy depends on such factors as the patient's age, general health, length of ulcer symptoms, and presence or history of other ulcer complications (see Chapter 24). Mortality for a single bleeding episode is 5% to 10%.

Perforation. Perforation occurs in 6% to 11% of patients with duodenal ulcer and in 2% to 5% of patients with gastric ulcer. An ulcer may perforate the duodenal wall, releasing caustic duodenal contents into the peritoneal cavity. Severe peritonitis with a boardlike abdomen and shock results, requiring emergency closure of the perforation or a definitive ulcer operation in selected patients who are in good condition and have slight peritoneal contamination. Mortality of perforation ranges from 7% to 26%, depending on the patient's age and the presence or absence of associated diseases.

Obstruction. Gastric outlet obstruction occurs in 5% of patients with duodenal or gastric ulcers and is especially common with pyloric channel ulcers. Chronic duodenal ulcers may cause gastric outlet obstruction from edema and spasm or cause severe scarring, with symptoms of nausea, vomiting, weight loss, and metabolic alkalosis. Obstruction causes stasis and excites the antral phase to increase gastric secretion. A vicious cycle results, which often must be interrupted by surgical correction. Mortality is 5% to 15% for duodenal ulcer and somewhat higher for gastric ulcer.

Intractability. Intractability used to be the major indication for surgery. Currently with effective medical therapy few patients need surgery for this indication. Operation is reserved for those who cannot comply with the medical regimen or have severe side effects from the medications.

In general, duodenal ulcers need not be removed. If the conditions causing duodenal ulcers are corrected by the surgical procedure, the ulcers will heal. Theoretically the ideal surgical treatment for duodenal ulcer is division of the vagus nerves (vagotomy) to control the vagal-antral phase plus antrectomy (distal gastric resection) to control the antral phase. Since vagotomy alone interferes with gastric emptying and leads to stasis, with nausea, vomiting, weight loss, and recurrent ulceration, antrectomy or some drainage procedure must complement it.

Three operations improve gastric emptying: Pyloroplasty (longitudinal division of the pyloric muscle with transverse closure) widens the gastroduodenal junction (Fig. 23-2, *A*). Gastrojejunostomy (anastomosis of the stomach to the jejunum) provides an alternative opening from stomach into small bowel (Fig. 23-2, *B*). Gastroduodenostomy (anastomosis of stomach to duodenum, the Jaboulay procedure) bypasses the pylorus. None of these emptying procedures sacrifices any of the stomach; its reservoir capacity remains unaltered.

Vagotomy combined with antrectomy or one of the emptying procedures has largely replaced the older surgical operations for duodenal ulcers, which involved removal of large portions (up to 80%) of the stomach (Fig. 23-2, *C* and *D*). The newer procedures are as effective but safer and technically easier to perform than extensive gastric resections, which may produce undesirable side effects in 25% of patients (dumping syndrome, chronic weight loss, diarrhea, malabsorption, anemia, metabolic bone disease, bilious vomiting, alkaline reflux gastritis, and an increased incidence of gastric cancer). These complications are much less frequent after vagotomy with antrectomy or drainage.

In the standard type of vagotomy, or truncal vagotomy (Fig. 23-2, *A* and *B*), the nerve trunks are divided as they lie on the lower esophagus. Not only is the acid-secreting area denervated, but also the antrum, pylorus, liver, gallbladder, pancreas, and other organs. Side effects of the vagotomy (diarrhea, increased incidence of gallstones) and of antrectomy or drainage

Table 23-1. Approximate Average Values of Volume and Acidity in 12 hour Collection of Gastric Juice for Conditions Listed

	12-hour nocturnal aspiration of stomach	
	mEq of HCl	*Volume of secretion (ml)*
Normal	20	200
Duodenal ulcer	60	500
Gastric ulcer	12	150
Zollinger-Ellison syndrome	100 or more	1000 or more
Gastric cancer	8	100

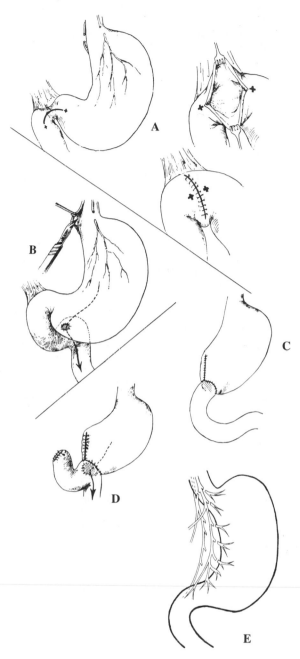

Fig. 23-2. Surgical treatment of peptic ulcer. **A,** Vagal nerve division and pyloroplasty. **B,** Vagal nerve division and gastrojejunostomy—arrow shows new exit for gastric contents. **C,** Billroth I partial gastric resection—stomach is anastomosed to duodenum. **D,** Billroth II partial gastric resection—duodenal stump is closed and stomach is anastomosed to jejunum. **E,** Highly selective vagotomy. Notice preservation of fibers supplying antrum and pylorus.

(mostly dumping and alkaline reflux gastritis) have led to the introduction of highly selective vagotomy (HSV), or parietal cell vagotomy (Fig. 23-2, *E*), in which branches to the lower esophagus and upper stomach are divided, denervating the parietal cells only. Because the antrum and pylorus remain innervated, the stomach empties normally and surgical

drainage is unnecessary. Although HSV reduces the usual side effects of vagotomy, it is complicated by a higher incidence of recurrent ulcers than is seen with the other types of vagotomy. This occurs in 11% to 25% of patients followed from 5 to 12 years after operation.

Recurrence. Depending on the type of operation, recurrent or stomal ulcerations may occur in 1% to 15% of patients. Recurrences usually indicate incomplete vagotomy or inadequate drainage. Other causes include insufficient resection of the acid-bearing portion of the stomach, retention of antral mucosa, hyperparathyroidism, or the Zollinger-Ellison syndrome. Diagnosis of stomal ulceration is based on the history, barium studies, and endoscopy. Complications of stomal ulcers include obstruction, hemorrhage, perforation, and gastrojejunocolic fistula. Some recurrent ulcers heal after treatment with cimetidine or ranitidine. Those that occur after incomplete vagotomy respond well to transthoracic vagotomy. Sluggish gastric drainage, detected by barium studies, often necessitates refashioning the gastric outlet.

Chronic Gastric Ulcer.

Incidence. Clinically, gastric ulcer is three to four times less common than duodenal ulcer. It occurs more frequently in middle aged and elderly persons and about equally in men and women.

Cause. About 80% of gastric ulcers appear in stomachs that secrete normal or smaller amounts of acid. Evidence points to a defective mucosal barrier and back-diffusion of acid (from stomach lumen into the mucosa) as the immediate cause. A defective pyloric sphincter allows bile reflux into the stomach where it disrupts the vital mucosal barrier; the resulting chronic gastritis precedes most gastric ulcers.

The other 20% of gastric ulcers usually occur just inside the pylorus or are associated with duodenal ulcers near it, causing pylorospasm or obstruction. These ulcers, arising in a hyperacidic environment, belong in the duodenal ulcer group.

Several drugs may disrupt the mucosal cell barrier or the protective mucus. Aspirin, phenylbutazone, indomethacin, reserpine, and steroids are the chief offenders, in addition to the antiarthritis drugs ibuprofen, tolmetin, and naproxen. Nonsteroidal antiflammatory drug (NSAID) gastropathy is usually antral or prepyloric disease which ranges from simple erythema, through diffuse erosions with or without microbleeding, to frank gastric ulcers. It usually occurs in older women and shows a poorer response to cimetidine therapy than does classic peptic ulcer disease.

Clinical features. The clinical picture of gastric ulcer simulates that of duodenal ulcer. Gastric ulcers tend to occur in patients who are older and of lower social status than those with duodenal ulcers. The pain localizes more often to the left upper quadrant and sometimes is provoked by food or hot or cold liquids. Gastric ulcers are more worrisome than duodenal ulcers because about 5% are malignant; duodenal ulcers are virtually never malignant (Table 23-2).

Laboratory examination. Overnight collections of gastric secretions show a decrease in both volume and concentration of acid in gastric ulcer as compared to duodenal ulcer (Table 23-1). Barium x-ray studies often show an ulcer crater in the stomach (Figs. 23-3 and 23-4). Gastroscopy with multiple biopsies or gastric washings with careful cytologic studies helps to exclude cancer.

Treatment. The same conservative treatment is tried for gastric ulcer as for duodenal ulcer. During the period of therapy, aspirin and other barrier-breaking drugs must be stopped. Because gastric ulcers may be malignant, the physician must recommend operation if the ulcer fails to heal after 8 weeks of treatment. About 15% of benign gastric ulcers fail to respond satisfactorily to medical treatment and must ultimately be treated surgically. Indications for surgery are failure to heal, suspicion of malignancy, recurrence, persistent bleeding, perforation, and obstruction. This last complication rarely occurs except with pyloric channel ulcers.

Removal of the distal half of the stomach gives excellent results for gastric ulcer. (The antrum is, of course, removed in this procedure.) A Billroth I reconstruction is preferred, since it reduces the risk of bile gastritis, iron deficiency, and afferent loop syndrome. The recurrence rate is negligible.

In patients with pyloric channel ulcers or combined gastric and duodenal ulcers surgical treatment is the same as for duodenal ulcers.

Acute Gastric Mucosal Ulcers (AGM Ulcers or Stress Ulcers).

Cause. AGM ulcers arise in critically ill patients after varied insults including shock, burns, sepsis, operations, and drugs. *Ischemia* and a *damaged mucosal barrier* are the common denominators underlying these superficial erosions. Almost all patients in severe shock show AGM ulcers. Ischemia disrupts the vital mucosal barrier; adynamic ileus, with reflux of bile, adds to the mucosal damage. Gastric acid diffuses through the impaired mucosa, and ulcers—often multiple—result.

Clinical features. Upper gastrointestinal bleeding that develops in a critically ill patient with no prior his-

Table 23-2. Comparison of Duodenal and Gastric Ulcers

	Duodenal Ulcer	*Gastric Ulcer*
Cause	Increased acid secretion, increased gastrin, defect in acid disposal	Abnormal pyloric sphincter-bile reflux gastritis, increased back diffusion of hydrogen ion
Location	Duodenum	Stomach
Age	Younger (30 to 50 years)	Somewhat older
Sex	Male:female, 7:1	Male:female, 1:1
Incidence	1% to 20%	1% to 5%
Symptoms	Much the same	
Malignancy	Rare	5%
Free HCl (12 hour night secretion)	60 mEq (average)	12 mEq (average)
Medical treatment	Excellent (successful in over 90%)	Poor (successful in 50%)
Surgical treatment	Vagotomy and antrectomy or emptying procedure, parietal cell vagotomy	Removal of the ulcer with limited partial gastrectomy

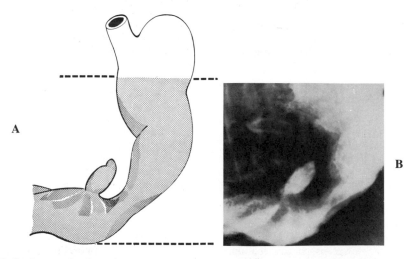

Fig. 23-3. Benign gastric ulcer. **A,** Diagram of x-ray findings. **B,** Upper G.I. series showing gastric folds radiating away from ulcer and sharp margins that are not elevated.

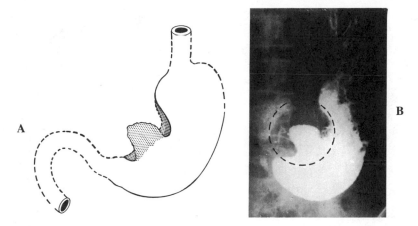

Fig. 23-4. Malignant gastric ulcer. **A,** Diagram of x-ray findings. **B,** Upper G.I. series showing no radiating folds and heaped-up ulcer margins.

tory of peptic ulceration should indicate AGM ulcers. Because of clots within the stomach and the superficial nature of AGM erosions, diagnostic barium studies often fail to detect them. Gastroscopy and celiac arteriography help to localize the bleeding site or sites.

Treatment. Prevention is probably the most important measure. The physician should anticipate these ulcers in any critically ill patient. Continuous nasogastric suction with instillation of antacids helps neutralize gastric acidity. Cimetidine is a useful adjunct because it reduces the need to give large amounts of antacids, which can cause undesirable side effects. Sucralfate is at least as effective as antacids or cimetidine, is cheaper, and has less risk of gram-negative nosocomial pneumonia caused by retrograde colonization of the pharynx from the stomach, which occurs with the use of agents that elevate gastric pH.

However, these measures alone do not give adequate protection. Concurrent treatment of shock, sepsis, and other conditions will relieve gastric ischemia.

If a patient presents with bleeding AGM ulcers, treatment consists of blood volume replacement, gastric lavage, and neutralization of gastric acid. If hemorrhage persists or recurs, bleeding points may be controlled by transendoscopic laser photocoagulation using the neodymium-YAG laser. Alternatively, arteriography may be used to localize the bleeding site, and in suitable cases, selective infusion of Pitressin into the left gastric artery may induce spasm and thrombosis of the bleeding vessel. The associated decrease in mucosal perfusion does not cause further ulceration if the gastric contents are kept alkalinized during this treatment. If these conservative means fail, most surgeons rely on vagotomy and pyloroplasty (and oversewing the bleeding sites) to stop the bleeding. Severe hemorrhage sometimes demands total or nearly total gastrectomy.

Peptic Ulcers From Other Causes
Zollinger-Ellison Syndrome

A rare syndrome of recurrent, severe ulcer disease, the Zollinger-Ellison syndrome emphasizes the impor-

tance of gastrin in gastric secretion; it explains the frustrating phenomenon of recurrent ulceration in some patients who have had adequate previous treatment.

The cause is a gastrin-secreting non-β islet cell tumor of the pancreas (Fig. 23-5). Gastric secretion is enormous (the 12 hour volume is over 1,000 ml, and free HCl, is over 100 mEq). Serum gastrin levels in these patients average over 600 pg/ml (normal: 200 pg/ml). Also, the basal acid secretion is high, usually 60% or more of maximal acid output (after stimulation with betazole [Histalog]). Approximately 23% of tumors occur in the duodenum or in extrapancreatic, extraintestinal locations. Approximately 25% of gastrinomas are associated with the multiple endocrine adenopathy (MEA) I syndrome (see below).

Until recently the only effective treatment was a total gastrectomy that removed the target organ. Approximately 20% of patients can be cured by surgical excision of pancreatic or extrapancreatic gastrinomas. In most cases this is not possible because the tumors are frequently multiple and microscopic in size or are malignant and have already metastasized.

Cimetidine or ranitidine effectively controls the hyperacidity and symptoms and must be given indefinitely. Because of the prodigious doses needed to control symptoms, some surgeons add highly selective vagotomy to the treatment with the aim of reducing drug dosage and side effects. Because of effective control of hyperacidity, patients may survive for many years. They seldom die of complications of ulcer disease but from metastases of the slowly growing but malignant gastrinomas.

Hyperparathyroidism

Because hypercalcemia increases gastric secretion, patients with hyperparathyroidism develop a higher than normal incidence of duodenal ulcers. These usually fail to respond to medical therapy but subside with treatment of the hyperparathyroidism.

Multiple Endocrine Adenopathy

Two main syndromes involving adenomas of endocrine glands have been described: MEA I (parathyroid,

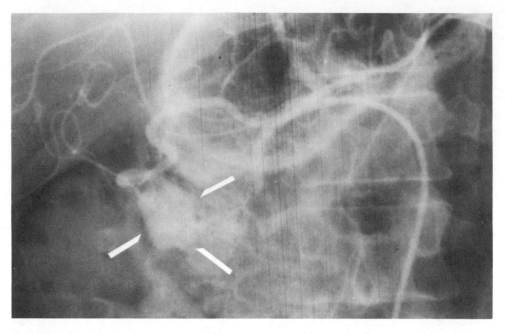

Fig. 23-5. Angiogram demonstrating 2.5 cm solitary tumor in head of pancreas. Fasting serum gastrin was 4,300 pg/ml.

pituitary, and pancreas) and MEA II (parathyroid, adrenal medulla, and thyroid C-cells). Both entities are associated with peptic ulcers, probably because of hyperfunctioning parathyroid (parathormone) and pancreatic (gastrin) tissues.

GASTRIC CANCER

Stomach cancer currently makes up 3% of malignancies in the population of the United States. Although the incidence is decreasing for unknown reasons, about 25,000 new cases of gastric cancer occur each year.

Carcinoma of the Stomach

Pathology. The varieties of gastric carcinoma are carcinoma in situ (rare), superficial spreading carcinoma (rare), ulcerative (28%), fungating or polypoid (23%), infiltrative (13%), and advanced (33%). Linitis plastica (leather bottle stomach), a diffuse form of the infiltrative variety, has a poor prognosis. The gross appearance of these tumors correlates poorly with their histology.

In decreasing order of frequency the sites most often involved are the pylorus and prepyloric region (about half of all cases), the body of the stomach, and the area of the cardia.

There are two basic histologic types—intestinal and diffuse. The former, usually well-differentiated and often accompanied by intestinal metaplasia, has a better prognosis. The latter, less well-differentiated and infrequently accompanied by intestinal metaplasia, has a poorer prognosis.

Spread. Regional lymph node metastases are present in 90% of cases at autopsy and in 70% of surgical specimens. Metastases commonly involve nodes along the greater and lesser curvatures and around the

pylorus, celiac axis, and porta hepatis. Cancers in the upper stomach also spread to splenic hilar and peripancreatic nodes. Rarely, cancer cells invade the left supraclavicular nodes (Virchow's nodes), presumably through the thoracic duct.

Microscopic metastases may extend submucosally and subserosally for surprising distances. Gastric cancer often invades the pancreas, liver, and transverse colon. Hematogenous spread occurs most frequently to the liver and lungs. Tumor cells may shed and grow on peritoneal surfaces as multiple implants and may cause massive ascites. Deposits on the pelvic floor are known as Blumer's shelf and on the ovary as Krukenberg's tumor.

Staging. The following system of clinical staging helps in treatment and prognosis:

Stage I. Cancer confined to stomach
  A. Cancer confined to mucosa
  B. Cancer extending to but not through serosa
  C. Cancer extending through serosa with or without invasion of adjacent structures
Stage II. Diffuse involvement of gastric wall (linitis plastica) or involvement of regional lymph nodes
Stage III. Involvement of regional nodes remote from the tumor or on both gastric curvatures
Stage IV. Distant metastases

This system gives a reasonably accurate idea of prognosis; stage IA has an excellent prognosis, stage IV, a dismal one.

Clinical characteristics. Specific or early symptoms are notoriously lacking in cancer of the stomach. Epigastric pain, weight loss, anorexia, vomiting, fatigue, and anemia occur insidiously and are often ignored. Dysphagia occurs with lesions in the cardia. A mass is palpable in one third of patients. Hepatomegaly raises suspicion of liver metastases. Males outnumber females about 3 to 1. Diseases that may precede and predispose to cancer of the stomach include pernicious anemia (achlorhydria), gastric polyps, and chronic atrophic gastritis.

Diagnosis. Cancer of the stomach is suspected from x-ray evidence, gastroscopy findings including biopsy, and cytologic evidence of malignant cells in the gastric aspirate.

Treatment. Surgical excision of the lesion and involved nodes is the only treatment of definite value. Radiation therapy offers little help.

Prognosis. If all tumor can be removed, with no spread beyond the stomach, up to 50% of patients live 5 years; however, because of the lack of early symptoms, the rich lymphatic supply, and the aggressiveness of these tumors, less than 10% of all patients with gastric carcinoma survive 5 years.

Gastric cancer is common in Japan, where extensive screening programs ensure that approximately one third of cases are diagnosed at an early stage and 5-year survival exceeds 90%.

Lymphomas of the Stomach

Lymphomas constitute about 5% of gastric neoplasms. They occur primarily in the stomach or as manifestations of a generalized process. Grossly they appear as mucosal thickenings, multiple nodules, or a single polypoid growth. Since lymphomas are radiosensitive and gastric carcinoma is not, biopsy of gastric tumors for specific diagnosis is often indicated even when the lesions appear far advanced. Treatment consists of radical resection followed by postoperative radiotherapy. Chemotherapy may be needed in patients with extensive lesions.

Sarcomas of the Stomach

The most common gastric sarcoma is leiomyosarcoma, which represents about 1% of gastric malignancies. It responds best to excision.

MISCELLANEOUS CONDITIONS OF STOMACH AND DUODENUM
Gastric Polyps

Polyps of the stomach are rare. Usually single, they may number in the hundreds. Most polyps, especially multiple lesions, are hyperplastic, not neoplastic, and do not become malignant. Adenomatous polyps are the usual type of neoplastic polyp. Malignancy potential increases with the size of the polyps. Those greater than 2 cm are likely to be malignant and should be removed either endoscopically or surgically.

Multiple benign polyposis (Peutz-Jeghers syndrome), an inherited syndrome, may involve the stomach as well as other parts of the gastrointestinal tract. It is associated with melanin spots on the lips and buccal mucosa. Conservative treatment usually is indicated.

Duodenal Diverticula

Duodenal diverticula are outpouchings in the duodenum. Although common, they usually cause no symptoms and should be left alone unless they are a suspected cause of bleeding or inflammation, both of which are rare complications.

Gastritis

Acute gastritis may occur after dietary indiscretion such as ingestion of a large amount of alcohol. It also may complicate use of NSAIDs. *Atrophic gastritis,* associated with hypochlorhydria or achlorhydria, may cause malabsorption of vitamin B_{12}. The thinned atrophic mucosa is clearly visible during gastroscopy. Enlarged rugal folds, often present in the Zollinger-Ellison syndrome, indicate *hypertrophic gastritis.* After operations that destroy or bypass the pylorus, duodenal contents sometimes reflux into the stomach causing alkaline *reflux gastritis,* with epigastric pain, anemia, and weight loss. Although usually responsive to medical therapy, this condition, if it becomes intractable, may necessitate surgery to divert duodenal contents away from the stomach.

Mallory-Weiss Syndrome

Mallory-Weiss syndrome is an uncommon complication of severe vomiting that results in a laceration through the mucosa of the esophagogastric junction. Surgical suture of the laceration is sometimes necessary to stop bleeding.

Dumping Syndrome

Dumping occurs to some extent in about 10% to 20% of patients who have gastric operations involving pyloric bypass or destruction. This syndrome features two types of symptoms, gastrointestinal and hemodynamic. Gastrointestinal symptoms include nausea, vomiting, abdominal pain (fullness, cramps), and diarrhea. Hemodynamic symptoms are weakness, fatigue, palpitations, sweating, pallor, and sensation of warmth. These symptoms begin within 30 minutes after a meal; they usually last less than 60 minutes and their intensity varies widely.

Although the precise cause remains unknown, the basic trigger seems to be rapid distension of the jejunum from hyperosmolar fluid rushing (or dumping) into it. Investigators are less certain about the hemodynamic aspects of dumping. Older theories cite the importance of hypovolemia from plasma elements pouring into the jejunum in response to the sudden hyperosmolar load. Newer theories, focused on chemical mediators released from the distended mucosa, have implicated both serotonin and bradykinin.

Treatment consists of a high-protein–low-carbohydrate diet, recumbency after meals, and withholding fluids during meals. Symptoms improve with time as patients adjust to their postgastrectomy state; less than 5% of patients have protracted dumping. Thus operative treatment should be reserved for patients with severe and chronic symptoms. Interposition of a short reversed segment of jejunum between the gastric remnant and the small bowel helps to slow the rush of fluid into the jejunum.

Foreign Bodies

Children and mental incompetents may swallow an astonishing variety of foreign bodies (Fig. 23-6). Most pass through the gastrointestinal tract in 3 to 4 days without symptoms or complications. *Trichobezoars* are hair balls that accumulate in the stomach from chronic hair ingestion. *Phytobezoars* are accretions of indigestible food fibers. Gastrectomy, particularly when accompanied by vagotomy (poor gastric drainage; Fig. 23-7), improper mastication, and high cellulose diets, favors their formation. Cellulase or other enzymes may break up the mass.

Gastric Operations for Morbid Obesity

Morbid obesity is a condition in which a person is at least 100 pounds overweight or whose weight exceeds twice the ideal weight. It affects 7% of females and 5% of males in the United States. Most likely causes are a genetic predisposition and excessive intake of food arising from overactive appetite centers in the midbrain. It is refractory to medical treatment. Complications include adult-onset diabetes, hypertension, ischemic heart disease, cerebrovascular accidents, varicose veins, restrictive lung disease, hernia, osteoarthritis, accidents, sleep apnea, and gallstones. Death rates are 11 times greater than in the nonobese.

The aim of surgery is to reduce daily intake of food to less than 800 calories until weight reduction is achieved and to prevent the complications of morbid obesity. All gastric operations are designed to create a small proximal gastric pouch (capacity 50 ml) that

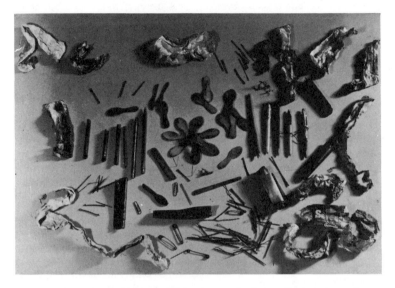

Fig. 23-6. Foreign bodies removed from stomach of mentally defective patient.

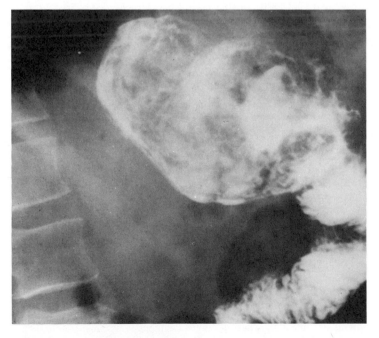

Fig. 23-7. Large filling defect in stomach on barium meal study caused by phytobezoar that developed following vagotomy and Billroth I partial gastrectomy.

empties slowly through a small opening (not greater than 1 cm). Eating brings on a feeling of early satiety. Gastric bypass consists in constructing a small gastric pouch that drains into a loop of jejunum. Disadvantages are high operative morbidity, stomal ulcers in 5% of patients, and uncertainty as to future problems associated with bypass of most of the stomach and duodenum. The more popular operation is gastroplasty in which two rows of staples form a small (50 ml) pouch with a 1 cm outlet in the upper stomach. Various measures are used to reinforce the outlet, since a cause of failure in the past has been gradual dilation of the pouch and the outlet permitting egress of excessive quantities of food. These operations achieve 50% loss of excess weight in 75% of patients treated. Postoperative complications include gastric leaks, outlet stenosis, wound infections, and (rarely) vitamin deficiencies.

24

Gastrointestinal Hemorrhage

Nathaniel J. Soper
Robert T. Soper

Recognition
Initial Management
Upper Gastrointestinal Hemorrhage
Lower Gastrointestinal Bleeding

Massive hemorrhage from the gastrointestinal (GI) tract continues to represent a major diagnostic and therapeutic challenge that enlists the cooperative efforts of surgeon, endoscopist, and radiologist. Regardless of the apparent magnitude of the bleeding, GI hemorrhage is an ominous manifestation that deserves thorough evaluation. Despite improved methods of diagnosis and increasingly sophisticated intensive care, mortality from severe GI hemorrhage is still approximately 10%, which represents little decline over the past 30 years. Massive bleeding more commonly arises from the upper GI tract, yet its diagnosis and treatment may be even more challenging when it occurs from a colonic source. Goals to be achieved in the individual patient include recognition of GI hemorrhage, hemodynamic stabilization (resuscitation), cessation of bleeding by the safest technique possible, and prevention of recurrent hemorrhage.

RECOGNITION

GI bleeding may be either occult or manifested by obvious efflux of blood. If gross blood is not apparent, a chemical test for occult blood (e.g., Hemoccult) can be performed, which will detect between 10 and 50 ml of blood entering the gastrointestinal tract per 24 hours. False-positive results may be caused by vitamin C ingestion or dietary hemoglobin or myoglobin, but not by iron ingestion. Hematemesis, hematochezia, or melena is present unless the rate of GI bleeding is minimal. Vomiting of bright red or dark blood indicates that the source of bleeding lies proximal to the ligament of Treitz. The characteristic coffee-grounds nature of "changed" blood is due to the conversion of hemoglobin to methemoglobin by gastric acid. Melena (black, tarry stool) is usually due to bleeding from a source in the proximal GI tract; however, hematin (the black pigment produced by oxidation of heme) can be seen in the stool when the bleeding point is as far distal as the cecum, if transit time is prolonged. Melena can be produced by as little as 100 ml of blood in the stomach and can persist for up to 5 days after bleeding has ceased.

INITIAL MANAGEMENT

Having confirmed the presence of acute or recent bleeding from the GI tract, the physician must acertain whether the hemorrhage is ongoing, gauge its magnitude, and begin resuscitation. A patient with evidence of acute GI bleeding should be treated as though he or she were exsanguinating until it is proven otherwise. Generally, this entails admitting the patient to the intensive care unit and obtaining surgical consultation.

The volume and rate of blood loss must be determined with a fair degree of accuracy since therapy will have to be instituted immediately in the patient with massive bleeding. The triad of hematemesis, hematochezia, and hypovolemia indicates massive GI bleeding and requires urgent treatment (discussed later in this chapter). Signs and symptoms of hypovolemia, including weakness, pallor, sweating, dizziness, tachycardia, and extreme thirst, signify massive bleeding. A large-bore nasogastric tube should be passed immediately to evacuate the stomach and measure the rate of blood loss. A catheter should be placed in the bladder to monitor hourly urine output. Patients who are hemodynamically unstable may require continuous monitoring of central venous and arterial pressures to optimize resuscitative efforts. If the rate of bleeding slows, as measured by vital signs, hematocrit determinations, the number and character of stools, and the volume of nasogastric aspirate, a more exhaustive diagnostic workup can be instituted. In all patients, blood should be drawn for type and cross match, coagulation studies, and blood chemistries. Elevation of blood urea nitrogen (BUN) can be seen with upper GI bleeding due to absorption of a large protein load and to reduced renal perfusion. In patients with slow GI bleeding, serial hematocrit determinations are probably the most reliable indicator of the rate of blood loss.

The location and the specific lesion that is producing the bleeding should be ascertained as soon as possible in the patient with massive hemorrhage. Most patients with brisk upper GI bleeding have hematemesis, so the distinction between lower and upper GI bleeding is made by history. When hematemesis has not occurred in the presence of massive hematochezia, aspiration of clear bile from the stomach usually indicates a source of bleeding below the ligament of Treitz. Endoscopy or angiography is usually necessary to determine the precise source of hemorrhage.

The general condition of the patient should be assessed as quickly as possible because the so-called poor-risk patient will require a more precise diagnostic and therapeutic approach than the good-risk patient, who has no cardiovascular or other systemic disease.

For the purpose of clarity, in this chapter we will deal first with upper GI bleeding and then with lower GI bleeding and will emphasize general principles rather than attempting either to deal thoroughly with the basic disease processes or to outline a complex formula to manage GI hemorrhage.

UPPER GI HEMORRHAGE

Massive upper GI hemorrhage produces signs of acute hypovolemia following closely on the heels of both hematemesis and hematochezia. For all practical purposes, this type of bleeding is distributed among peptic ulceration, gastritis, and ruptured esophageal varices, bleeding ulcer being approximately twice as common as either of the other two.

Unusual causes of massive upper GI hemorrhage are worthy of brief mention so that they will not be forgotten in the haste of the moment. Oronasopharyngeal bleeding may be suspected if the patient appears to be swallowing blood; bleeding can be quite massive but usually stops with direct tamponade. Hematobilia can be diagnosed only by angiography, endoscopy, or choledochotomy but should be suspected when there are symptoms and signs of hepatobiliary disease or a history of blunt hepatic trauma. The possibility of an aortoduodenal fistula should be considered in any patient with an aortic prosthesis. The Mallory-Weiss syndrome (emesis-induced hemorrhage from a mucosal tear at the gastroesophageal junction) and angiodysplastic lesions are most commonly diagnosed at gastroesophagoscopy. Bleeding disorders should be considered in all cases, and an accurate history, inspection for cutaneous bleeding, and laboratory bleeding studies should be carried out (see Chap. 4).

General Considerations of Diagnosis and Management

After admitting the patient to the hospital and initiating the above steps for assessing the status of the circulatory system and the magnitude of the bleed, a history should be taken and physical examination performed. Of the commonly encountered causes of upper GI bleeding, only portal hypertension with esophageal varices is associated with characteristic physical findings. However, over half of cirrhotic patients who bleed from an upper GI site do so from nonvariceal lesions. Historic features of note include previous bleeding episodes, heartburn or dyspepsia, ulcer-type pain, alcohol abuse, ingestion of salicylates or nonsteroidal antiinflammatory drugs (NSAIDs), and emesis or prolonged retching preceding the onset of hemorrhage. Despite a thorough history and physical examination, experienced clinicians can correctly diagnose the source of upper GI hemorrhage in only half of the cases.

After placing large-bore (14-gauge or larger) intravenous catheters, a No 36 Fr Ewald tube is passed into the stomach for lavage with large volumes of saline. The temperature of the lavage fluid probably is not important; in fact, ice-cold saline lavage may be injurious to the gastric mucosa. Gastric lavage performs several functions: the rate of hemorrhage is monitored, blood clots are evacuated, and hemostasis may be augmented. Bleeding ceases during gastric lavage about 90% of the time. When active hemorrhage stops, the Ewald tube may be replaced with a standard (16 Fr) nasogastric tube.

Although it was never proven to be of benefit, empiric therapy with histamine H_2-receptor antagonists is usually begun at this time. Preliminary data suggest that intravenous somatostatin may produce cessation of nonvariceal bleeding, but this therapy is considered experimental at the present time.

The most important diagnostic maneuver in the patient with massive upper GI bleeding is endoscopy, preferably with a flexible fiberoptic esophagogastroscope. Endoscopy should be performed within 12 to 24 hours of admission. If bleeding is present during the examination, its source and magnitude can be determined simultaneously, and in some cases control can also be attempted. For example, if bleeding esophageal varices are encountered, not only is the diagnosis made with certainty but definitive therapy can be administered by injection of sclerosing agents. In the presence of somewhat localized gastritis, angiodysplasia, or bleeding peptic ulcer, the endoscopist can attempt control of hemorrhage by using electrocautery, neodymium-YAG laser, or heater probe application through the endoscope. It should be emphasized that these proce-

dures have the potential hazard of perforation if applied inappropriately.

Once diagnosis is established, subsequent management is instituted, as shown schematically in Fig. 24-1. It is unusual for pulsatile hemorrhage from the gastroduodenal or left gastric artery to stop with gastric lavage; in that situation the patient will require urgent surgical intervention. On the contrary, bleeding from minor or small vessels often justifies a period of further medical management. Initially, saline lavage is continued, but intensive therapy with antacids or H_2 blockers may be more important. Gastric pH should be measured hourly by aspiration through the nasogastric tube. The antacid regimen is adjusted to achieve a neutral pH.

Although the flexible fiberoptic endoscope has substantially increased the diagnostic accuracy of bleeding lesions of the esophagus, stomach, and duodenum, ultimate outcome for the individual patient has not been affected significantly. Selective visceral angiography provides added dimensions to both diagnosis and ther-

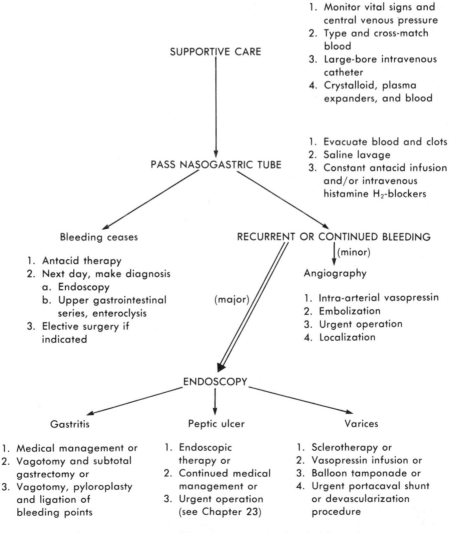

Fig. 24-1. Management of massive upper gastrointestinal hemorrhage.

apy. If bleeding persists and the definitive diagnosis is not made endoscopically, or if the diagnosis is made and the patient is a poor operative risk, emergency angiography should be carried out. The skilled angiographer can selectively cannulate the left gastric artery, infuse vasopressin, and frequently stop the bleeding of hemorrhagic gastritis; he can cannulate the gastroduodenal artery and infuse either preformed blood clot or vasopressin to stop duodenal ulcer bleeding, and he can cannulate the superior mesenteric artery and infuse vasopressin to lower portal pressure and stop variceal bleeding.

Peptic Ulceration

The cause of 40 to 50 percent of all cases of massive upper GI bleeding is peptic ulcer, nearly equally distributed between gastric and duodenal ulcer. When hemorrhage occurs from a peptic ulcer, whether the source is in the stomach or the duodenum, the immediate aim is to control the bleeding. The diagnosis is often suggested by history, unless bleeding is occurring for the first time as the symptom of an acute stress ulcer. Physical examination and laboratory studies are usually of little help.

If the bleeding stops as a result of gastric lavage or if bleeding has stopped before admission to the hospital so that a nasogastric tube aspirate yields only old or changed blood, gastroscopy may be deferred and angiography will not be helpful. The patient should be managed with gastric suction to decompress the stomach and gastric pH neutralization, as outlined previously. Most patients should undergo elective esophagogastroduodenoscopy, but an upper GI contrast radiographic study may be safely performed if bleeding has not recurred for 12 hours. If bleeding recurs, emergency endoscopy, with or without subsequent angiography, should be carried out to identify the precise source of bleeding.

Once the diagnosis of peptic ulcer is made by any of these measures, it is treated medically, endoscopically, or operatively, depending on the previous history of bleeding, pain, and chronicity. Emergency operation is indicated for patients whose estimated blood loss exceeds 2500 ml in the first 24 hours or 1500 ml in the second 24 hours, or for those whose bleeding recurs while they are hospitalized; using these criteria, approximately 25% of patients bleeding from a peptic ulcer require emergency surgery. The choice of operation (discussed in Chap. 23), is designed to reduce gastric acidity and prevent recurrence of peptic ulcer disease.

Esophageal Varices

The diagnosis of bleeding from a ruptured varix is suggested in the patient with upper GI hemorrhage who has a history of chronic alcoholism or liver disease. Frequently the patient is in a precomatose state, and physical examination reveals mild jaundice, ascites, and muscle wasting. Definitive diagnosis of variceal hemorrhage is made by esophagoscopy. A barium swallow that will outline the extent of the varices is more useful when the patient is not bleeding (Fig. 24-2). Patients with portal hypertension may bleed from hemorrhagic gastritis or peptic ulcer disease rather than from varices; endoscopy will establish the diagnosis.

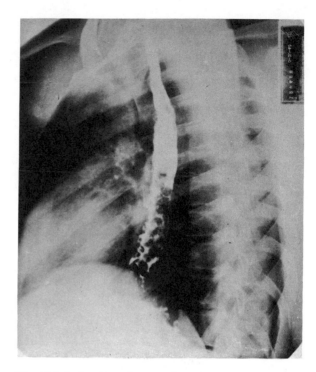

Fig. 24-2. Barium in esophagus outlining large esophageal varices.

Emergency management of the patient with bleeding varices is directed toward stopping the hemorrhage as soon as possible. In addition to the deleterious effects of blood loss and shock common to all patients with upper GI bleeding, hepatic encephalopathy may also ensue because of the large amount of ammonia released by the bacterial action on intraluminal blood. Therefore, coincident with attempts to control the hemorrhage, efforts should be made not only to rid the gastrointestinal tract of blood by vigorous catharsis but also to impede its breakdown. This latter goal can be achieved by administration of either poorly absorbed antibiotics, such as neomycin, that reduce the bacterial flora of the colon, or unabsorbed sugar, such as lactulose, that decreases ammonia production by interfering with bacterial metabolism.

Massive variceal bleeding usually will not stop with gastric lavage alone, necessitating additional nonoperative measures. Pharmacologic control of bleeding varices has been widely reported using infusion of vasopressin (Pitressin), which lowers portal pressure by reducing splanchnic blood flow. Although early experience dictated intraarterial infusion through the superior mesenteric artery, it has been demonstrated clearly that simple intravenous administration is as effective and eliminates the need for a skilled angiographer. Pitressin is administered as a 20-unit bolus followed by continuous infusion of 0.2 to 0.4 units/minute. This approach has been successful in at least temporarily halting variceal hemorrhage in approximately 70% of patients.

Endoscopic sclerosis of bleeding varices is an alternative method of managing the acute bleeding. Although sclerotherapy is easier to accomplish in non-bleeding patients, with practice it can be performed in the active bleeder by most endoscopists with a success rate of approximately 75%. Several courses of therapy may be needed to obliterate the entire variceal network, during which time rebleeding can occur. Nevertheless, repeat procedures are usually tolerated well by the patient, so this form of therapy has become the procedure of choice in many medical centers.

If these measures fail to arrest the variceal hemorrhage, an attempt at balloon tamponade is warranted. Triple-lumen tubes (Fig. 24-3) can be used to compress the bleeding veins by inflating the gastric and esophageal balloons. The use of these tubes is attended by a significant risk of complications such as ischemia of the gastroesophageal junction, perforation of the esophagus, or massive aspiration. Nevertheless, balloon tamponade may be a life-saving maneuver if other nonoperative measures do not control variceal bleeding. The combination of all of these nonoperative techniques results in cessation of the hemorrhage in 85% to 90% of patients.

Surgical approaches to acute variceal hemorrhage include portasystemic shunting, esophagogastric devascularization procedures as described by Sugiura in Japan, simple esophageal transection with the end-to-end anastomosis (EEA) stapler, and transesophageal variceal ligation. Both emergency portacaval shunting and variceal ligation have high mortality (approaching 50% in patients with poor liver function) thus reducing their

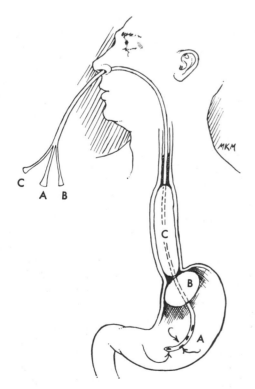

Fig. 24-3. Sengstaken-Blakemore tube. Triple-lumen tube: *A*, gastric suction; *B*, balloon in gastric fundus; *C*, balloon in lower esophagus. Tube is passed into stomach, inflated gastric balloon is snugged up to esophageal junction, and esophageal balloon is then inflated to compress varices.

usefulness. Because only limited experience has been reported for use of the various devascularization procedures in the typical poor-risk cirrhosis patient, these techniques cannot yet be recommended as procedures of choice.

Long-term management of patients with bleeding varices after control has been achieved through nonoperative measures remains controversial. Elective portasystemic shunts in good-risk patients carry low mortality and have a negligible rebleeding rate, but are complicated in many patients by the late development of encephalopathy. Distal splenorenal shunts control variceal bleeding equally well (5% failure rate) and are followed less frequently by encephalopathy than shunts that totally divert portal venous flow away from the liver. Esophagogastric devascularization is a difficult and potentially dangerous operation that should only be attempted by those with experience. On the other hand, sclerotherapy may be repeated as needed, does not further compromise function of the diseased liver, and is safe, making it a highly attractive alternative to the various surgical alternatives.

Gastritis

Massive hemorrhage from erosive gastritis was once a common cause of upper GI bleeding in critically ill patients. In recent years, the routine use of prophylactic acid-reducing medical therapy has diminished the incidence of this entity. Bleeding from stress gastritis is most frequently encountered in patients with extensive burns, trauma, or sepsis. In fact, the development of hemorrhagic gastritis in a postoperative patient should alert the physician to the possibility of an occult source of sepsis. In other patients with bleeding gastritis, the history may reveal ingestion of substances that are toxic to gastric mucosa such as aspirin, indomethacin, steroids, or alcohol. Diagnosis is made exclusively with gastroscopy and more often than not reveals diffuse disease that precludes both endoscopic coagulation and limited gastric resection.

The initial management of hemorrhagic gastritis should be nonoperative because the majority of patients stop bleeding spontaneously. Medical management is similar to that for peptic ulcer and includes evacuation of gastric blood clots, saline lavage, sedation, and blood replacement. Early neutralization of gastric acidity with intensive antacid therapy adjusted according to hourly gastric pH values is of utmost importance. The histamine-receptor antagonists cimetidine and ranitidine have been helpful in this respect, though alone they may not be adequate in the face of severe bleeding and therefore should be used in concert with topical antacids. As with variceal hemorrhage, administration of vasopressin may also be helpful in controlling difficult cases. This drug may be administered intravenously or through selective cannulation of the left gastric artery at the time of angiography.

Surgical intervention often is not necessary—fortunately, because the appropriate operation for hemorrhagic gastritis is controversial. Near total gastrectomy enjoys the lowest rebleeding rate but is a major undertaking that is not without complications. Vagotomy and pyloroplasty with oversewing of individual bleeding points through a large gastrotomy is tolerated better by the extremely sick patient but is accompanied by a greater probability of recurrent hemorrhage. Individualization is the best policy. For example, a surgeon might select the latter procedure for patients who can best tolerate a rebleed should it occur and, paradoxically, reserve gastric resection for those least able to endure a second operation.

Other Causes of Upper GI Hemorrhage

Aberrant blood vessels, tumor undergoing necrosis, aortoduodenal fistulas, and lesions of the small intestine including vascular malformations and Meckel's diverticulum are managed with operations that are applicable to the particular lesion. Recurrent slow bleeding from chronic peptic ulcer disease is managed according to the principles outlined in Chapter 23.

LOWER GI BLEEDING

Rarely is colonic bleeding massive and life threatening; more commonly it is slow and intermixed with stool. Persistence of chronic rectal bleeding warrants an immediate and thorough investigative work-up to establish its cause. In this situation the bleeding is not the problem, but its cause can be serious and life threatening.

Massive Colonic Bleeding

It must be emphasized at the outset that upper GI sources of bleeding should be eliminated as possibilities in the patient with massive rectal bleeding. Aspiration of clear bile from the stomach for all practical purposes establishes the locus of bleeding as being at least below the ligament of Treitz.

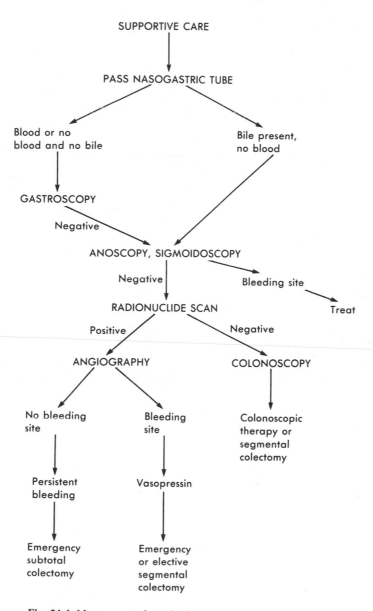

Fig. 24-4. Management of massive lower gastrointestinal hemorrhage.

History is not usually as helpful as it is in upper GI bleeding, and the physical examination may be equally unrevealing. The most common causes of massive lower GI bleeding are angiodysplasia of the right side of the colon and diverticula, and these should be highly suspect, especially in the older patient. Numerous other conditions, however, can often produce brisk rectal bleeding such as internal hemorrhoids, an ulcerating colonic neoplasm, colonic ischemia, ulcerative colitis, solitary ulcer, and, in rare instances, superficial erosions of the colon, or Crohn's colitis.

As with upper GI bleeding, appropriate screening tests should be performed and plasma expanders followed by blood transfusions should be instituted immediately while diagnostic measures are undertaken. A general plan for management of massive lower GI hemorrhage is outlined in Fig. 24-4. Anoscopy and sigmoidoscopy with adequate facilities to aspirate blood should be undertaken as soon as possible. If a bleeding lesion is detected in the anorectum, it should be treated appropriately. If the bleeding arises above the end of the sigmoidoscope and is persistent but not exsanguinating, the patient is evaluated by radionuclide scanning using technetium–99m–labelled red blood cells. This test may detect bleeding that exceeds the rate of 0.5 ml/min and may assist with localization of the lesion. If the radionuclide scan is positive, selective arteriography should be carried out immediately. Injection of contrast material into the inferior mesenteric artery followed by the superior mesenteric artery frequently identifies the source of bleeding. When the bleeding point is identified and is localized to either the left or the right colon, continuous intraarterial infusion of vasopressin is begun. Success with this technique has eliminated the need for urgent laparotomy and colon resection in many patients. If bleeding is not controlled or if it recurs, limited resection of the appropriate segment of bowel can be carried out.

Angiography is rarely, if ever, positive when the radionuclide scan is unrevealing. Therefore, if the bleeding scan is negative, colonoscopy should be performed after rapid cleansing of the colonic lumen with saline-polyethylene glycol (Golytely). A bleeding site will be discovered in about two thirds of such cases, and some lesions (e.g., angiodysplasias) can be treated by electrocoagulation or laser.

Operation is necessary for hemorrhage that persists or recurs despite conservative therapy. In most instances, the bleeding site will have been localized and a segmental colon resection can be performed. Intraoperative attempts at localization generally have been disappointing; therefore, every effort should be made to identify the source of hemorrhage preoperatively. When such information is lacking and intraoperative examination of the gut is unrevealing, the colon, small intestine, and stomach can be examined endoscopically during the procedure. If all localizing efforts fail, total abdominal colectomy with either ileorectal anastomosis or end ileostomy may be the only recourse. Today the mortality rate from lower GI hemorrhage is about 10%.

Chronic Lower GI Bleeding

Slow and recurrent or persistent colonic bleeding is suggested by a history of blood passed rectally in a patient with chronic anemia. Bright red rectal blood indicates a point of origin within the anus or rectum, especially when it coats the stool. Anal fissures, hemorrhoids, and low-lying carcinomas are the most likely sources of this type of slow rectal bleeding. Tarry material or dark blood intermixed with stool suggests the origin to be in the right colon or small bowel. Bloody diarrhea mixed with mucus suggests ulcerative colitis, granulomatous enterocolitis, or amebic colitis. The diagnostic work-up is performed with dispatch but not as an emergency. Careful rectal examination, anoscopy, and sigmoidoscopy should be carried out when the patient is first seen. These procedures will confirm the diagnosis of numerous conditions, including hemorrhoids, fissures, ulcerative colitis, and about three fifths of the colonic neoplasms. The next diagnostic maneuver should be a barium enema, usually with air contrast. This procedure will confirm the diagnosis of colonic diverticulosis, neoplasms above the reach of the sigmoidoscope, chronic ulcerative colitis, and colonic polyps.

If these procedures fail to reveal the source of the bleeding, colonoscopy should be carried out. When performed by an experienced operator, diagnostic colonoscopy carries little morbidity; furthermore, transcolonoscopic therapy of certain lesions (removal of polyps, laser coagulation of angiodysplastic vessels) may be performed.

25

Small Intestine

Robert T. Soper
Siroos S. Shirazi

Anatomy
Physiology
Surgical Diseases of the Small Intestine

The small intestine is the longest segment of the gastrointestinal tract, extending from the pyloric sphincter to the ileocecal sphincter, or valve. Curiously enough, although the small bowel is operated on frequently (resection, bypass, decompression, lysis of adhesions, placement of indwelling catheters for suction or feeding purposes), few of these operations are done *on* the small bowel for diseases that originate *within* the small bowel. Thus, duodenal ulcer is caused by acid-peptic factors originating within the stomach with the major effect on the duodenum; mesenteric vascular occlusion infarcts and perforates the small bowel but originates primarily as a vascular lesion; small bowel obstruction is most commonly caused by extrinsic factors (hernias, adhesions) not of primary origin from the small bowel itself. Numerically, few surgical diseases arise primarily *within* the small intestine itself.

ANATOMY

The small intestine measures 7 to 8 m in the adult and a surprisingly long 200 cm in the newborn infant. Its subdivisions (duodenum, jejunum, and ileum) are continuous, and only the duodenojejunal junction is marked clearly (by the ligament of Treitz).

The duodenum begins at the pylorus, measures roughly 25 cm in length, and is largely retroperitoneal. It receives the contents of the stomach proximally, and the bile and pancreatic enzymes in the concave mesenteric surface of its second portion, which is occasioned by embryonic rotation. It can be mobilized partially by the *Kocher maneuver,* which divides the peritoneal attachments to its convex surface. The juxtaposition of large vessels, pancreas, and vital duct structures makes surgical manipulations of the duodenum hazardous and necessitates removal of the distal stomach, common bile duct, and pancreatic head if the duodenum must be resected. (See discussion of Whipple's procedure, Chapter 19.)

In contrast, the jejunum and ileum are suspended freely in the peritoneal cavity by the dorsal mesentery and are, therefore, easy to inspect, manipulate, and resect at laparotomy. The jejunum encompasses the proximal 40% of the bowel from the ligament of Treitz to the ileocolic valve, and the ileum makes up the remainder. The junction between the two is not clearly defined. In general, the jejunum has a larger lumen, thicker walls, larger and more numerous transverse mucosal folds *(valvulae conniventes),* and a better blood supply delivered through fewer vascular arcades than the ileum.

Arterial blood to the small intestine is supplied entirely from the superior mesenteric artery and largely through end arteries. There is little collateral blood flow to the small bowel (in striking contrast to the stomach and colon); therefore, vascular occlusion is more likely to produce bowel infarction.

Venous blood from the small bowel carries fluid end products of digestion to the liver through the portal vein. The small bowel lymphatics, or *lacteals,* travel in the mesentery and collect retroperitoneally into the *cisterna chyli;* they transport products of fat digestion (chyle) into the systemic venous system through the thoracic duct.

The nerve supply to the small bowel is entirely from the autonomic nervous system. The efferent nerves ensure coordinated aboral peristaltic waves to carry intestinal contents downstream during digestion. The sensory afferents localize and discriminate pain of small bowel origin very poorly as a dull, vague aching in the epigastrium or periumbilical area of the abdomen.

The wall of the small intestine is composed of four layers: The inner mucosa is composed of simple columnar epithelium with innumerable intestinal glands (the absorptive surface being increased enormously by the presence of villi) plus the mucosal folds known as the *valvulae conniventes.* The submucosa consists of fibrous and supporting tissue and is richly supplied by the intrinsic vascular and nervous elements of the intestine. The outer longitudinal and inner circular muscle layers contribute the peristalsis necessary to propel intestinal material downstream. The outer serosa is visceral peritoneum, which, in its pristine state, allows free motion of the intestine, provides an impermeable barrier to the passage of bacteria to the peritoneal cavity, and adds considerably to the suture-holding qualities of the bowel wall.

PHYSIOLOGY

During intrauterine life, the intestine functions as an integral part of normal amniotic fluid circulation. Amniotic fluid is swallowed by the fetus, and a portion is absorbed, utilized, and then excreted as urine back into the amniotic fluid. Interruption of this cycle at any stage results in retention of abnormal amounts of amniotic fluid, a condition known as *polyhydramnios.* Fifty percent of babies born of mothers with polyhydramnios will have major congenital anomalies that interfere with this circulatory system, including hydrocephalus, anen-

cephaly, myelomeningocele, upper gastrointestinal tract obstruction, and congenital hydronephrosis.

In postnatal life the small intestine has digestive and absorptive functions. In the adult, 8 to 10 L of digestive secretion is produced daily in the oral cavity, stomach, small bowel, pancreas, and liver to aid enzymatic breakdown of ingested food to molecules small enough to be absorbed. The small bowel adds somewhat to the digestive secretions and propels the succus entericus downstream in an orderly and relatively slow manner. After digestion has been completed, the mucosal surface of the small intestine absorbs water, electrolytes, and the basic breakdown products of the food. Fat travels through the lacteals and lymphatic ducts to the superior vena cava, and the bulk of the remaining products is conveyed to the liver through the portal venous system for further metabolic alteration. Normally up to 98% of the liquid volume of the succus entericus is absorbed, largely from the lower portion of the small intestine.

Resection or bypass of up to 50% of the small intestine is generally followed by an initial period of diarrhea and weight loss but is compatible with perfectly normal subsequent growth and development, regardless of age at the time of operation. Chronic diarrhea, anemia, osteomalacia, and varying degrees of malnutrition, at least temporarily, occur after loss of more than half of the small intestine.

SURGICAL DISEASES OF THE SMALL INTESTINE

The majority of operations performed on the small bowel are done because of peptic ulcers, intestinal obstruction (including those of congenital origin), or as a necessary part of operations primarily on the colon; these entities are discussed in their own specific chapters and are not considered further here. The remainder of this chapter is devoted to the small fraction of surgical diseases that arise primarily within the small intestine.

Neoplasms

The small intestine is singularly free of neoplasms, both benign and malignant, as compared with the esophagus, stomach, and colon. The reasons for this discrepancy are unknown. Small intestine lesions represent well under 5% of all primary neoplasms of the gastrointestinal tract. Benign tumors include polyps, villous adenomas, myomas, leiomyomas, fibromas, lipomas, and aberrant gastric or pancreatic tissue. They commonly are asymptomatic and are found incidentally at autopsy or laparotomy. They become symptomatic by ulcerating the overlying mucosa with bleeding or by acting as the leading point for small bowel intussusception; the larger tumors may obstruct the lumen. Diagnosis is made at laparotomy, but occasionally the tumors show as filling defects in the barium column during small bowel x-ray examination (Fig. 25-1). Duodenal lesions can now be viewed by the flexible fiberoptic endoscope, allowing precise preoperative biopsy diagnosis (Fig. 25-2). Lesions of the jejunum and ileum require laparotomy for diagnostic confirmation and surgical excision.

The *Peutz-Jeghers syndrome* is the association of

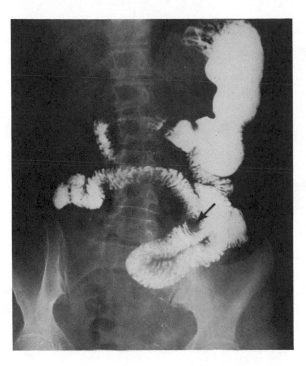

Fig. 25-1. Small bowel polyp designated by arrow.

intestinal polyps with melanin spots on the mucosa of the lips, mouth, and anus. The disorder is inherited, usually as an autosomal-dominant trait, but occasionally as a spontaneous mutation. The polyps are generally localized to the small intestine and number from one to five; occasionally they are more numerous and are located within the stomach or colon. Malignant degeneration is extremely unusual with the Peutz-Jeghers type of polyp, and surgical treatment is undertaken only when the polyps produce symptoms.

The most common malignant neoplasm of the small intestine is the *adenocarcinoma*, about one half of which are primary within the duodenum. Bleeding and obstruction are the most common signs and often occur late in the evolution after metastasis has already occurred. *Lymphosarcomas* are the next most common variety, generally occurring in children and young adults and often in association with widespread disease.

The signs of small bowel malignancy in roughly descending order of frequency are intestinal obstruction, gastrointestinal tract bleeding, an abdominal mass, and perforation. Diagnosis is made at laparotomy, but plain and barium contrast studies of the intestine may be helpful. Treatment is wide surgical resection of the involved bowel and its draining lymphatic pathways when possible and if distant metastasis has not already occurred. X-ray therapy is useful in additional treatment of lymphomas. Local resection or bypass occasionally palliates incurable neoplasms. The overall 5-year survival rate is from 10% to 15%, the prognosis for lymphosarcoma being materially better than that for primary small bowel adenocarcinoma.

Carcinoid tumors (Fig. 25-3) arise from argentaffin cells near the base of the intestinal glands. They are most commonly found in the appendix and small intes-

tine, respectively; however, they can arise anywhere in the gastrointestinal tract, and pulmonary carcinoids have occasionally been reported. Carcinoid tumors are yellow or gray; the cells have a columnar arrangement and stain with chromic acid to allow a specific histologic diagnosis.

Carcinoid tumors may be benign or malignant, probably related more to the time at which they are discovered than to any inherent difference in malignant potential. This supposition is supported by the observation that although 60% of carcinoid tumors arise within the appendix, they are never malignant in this location; they probably produce early obstruction of the very small appendiceal lumen that initiates signs of appendicitis leading to prompt surgical excision and cure. On the other extreme, carcinoid tumors arising in the small intestine are almost always malignant by the time of discovery. The larger lumen of the intestine allows years of undetected growth to occur before symptoms are produced and surgical treatment is carried out. Metastasis occurs through the portal venous system to the liver.

The *carcinoid syndrome* is seen only when malignant carcinoids have *metastasized* widely to the liver or other extraportal sites such as the lungs; it is present in about 25% of reported malignant carcinoids. The clinical features of the *carcinoid syndrome* are periodic attacks of (1) colicky abdominal pain with diarrhea and weight loss, (2) flushing of the face, neck, and torso, and (3) asthmatic wheezing. Late in the course of the carcinoid syndrome, pulmonic or tricuspid valvular stenosis develops gradually, leading to cardiac failure and death.

Argentaffin cells normally produce minute amounts of hydroxytryptophan (as an intermediate in the biosynthesis of serotonin), which is believed to play a role in hemostasis and maintenance of smooth muscle tone in blood vessels and intestine. Carcinoid tumors synthesize enormous amounts of serotonin which, however, is altered and "detoxified" by the liver so long as the venous drainage goes into the portal system. However, large hepatic or extraportal metastases secrete serotonin directly into systemic blood to induce the smooth muscle contractions responsible for the characteristic signs and symptoms previously related. The reason for the periodicity of attacks is unknown. Diagnostic confirmation is provided by demonstration of excessive levels of serotonin (5-hydroxytryptamine, or 5-HT) in the serum or its degradation products (5-hydroxyindoleacetic acid, or 5-HIAA) in the urine. Serotonin is also excreted by the lungs into expired air, explaining why valvular disease is limited selectively to the valves on the right side of the heart.

Malignant carcinoids are the exception to the rule that metastases of incurable primary intestinal neoplasms should not be resected. Malignant carcinoids grow slowly, and removal of portions of the metastases may provide gratifyingly long relief from the distressing and ultimately serious (or fatal) effects of hyperserotoninemia.

Trauma

The small intestine is damaged by both *penetrating* and *nonpenetrating* abdominal trauma, often in associ-

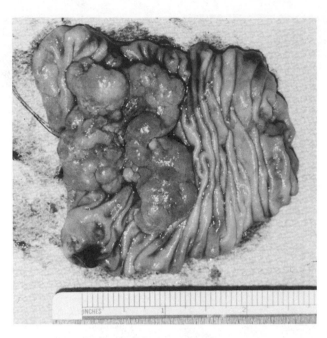

Fig. 25-2. Benign villous adenoma resected from third portion of duodenum; seen preoperatively by fiberoptic endoscopy.

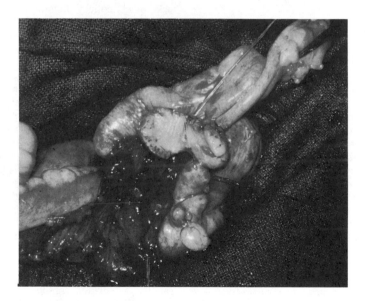

Fig. 25-3. Carcinoid tumor at base of appendix. Probe *(upper white line)* points to yellow-white tumor, which has been sectioned. Appendix is retracted toward upper right of field.

ation with other visceral injuries. The penetrating missile may perforate intestine or produce mesenteric vascular injury, ranging from a minor hematoma confined to the mesentery to massive hemorrhage into the free peritoneal cavity with shock and serious compromise to the blood supply of the involved segment of intestine. Plain supine and decubitus abdominal radiographs will often show free air and will locate the missile if it has been retained in the body to help map out its path. Laparotomy is almost always indicated with a painstaking and orderly inspection of the entire peritoneal cavity for injury. The missile need not be removed, but damage to the viscera must be repaired. Minute or sharply demarcated puncture wounds of small intestine may be turned in, but large or ragged lacerations and severely contused or devascularized bowel require resection and anastomosis. Mesenteric bleeding must be controlled by pressure or ligature. Because of the chemically irritating and septic content of the small intestine, the peritoneal cavity should be lavaged and suctioned, and appropriate antibiotics administered postoperatively if spillage has occurred.

The mortality for nonpenetrating abdominal trauma is approximately three times that for penetrating injuries, probably because there are less compelling indications for exploratory laparotomy in the former. The intestine ranks fourth behind the spleen, kidneys, and liver in frequency of damage by nonpenetrating abdominal trauma. The jejunum and ileum are relatively mobile and tend to slide away and escape injury from a nonpenetrating blow, though sudden dislocation may indeed lacerate the small bowel mesentery. The duodenum and duodenojejunal junction are anchored retroperitoneally and cannot escape, resulting in a much higher incidence of injury. This is especially true for the fourth part of the duodenum, trapped between the wounding blow anteriorly and the rigid second lumbar vertebra posteriorly. Intramural hematoma and laceration are the common duodenal injuries incurred in this manner. If the duodenum is lacerated beneath its peritoneal cover, extravasation of duodenal contents occurs retroperitoneally.

Intramural *duodenal hematomas* produce symptoms by obstructing the lumen, which may take several hours or even days to complete. Diagnosis is suggested by narrowing of the lumen and a "coil spring" appearance of the duodenal mucosa on upper gastrointestinal barium studies. Surgical treatment consists in evacuating the hematoma through a serosal incision, careful inspection for a break in the mucosa, and drainage. Operative therapy is indicated only if 5 to 7 days of intravenous fluids and nasogastric suction fail to relieve the obstruction.

The diagnosis of retroperitoneal laceration of the duodenum may be extremely difficult to establish, though the abdominal plain film often shows obliteration of the right kidney profile and small bubbles of gas above the kidney. In view of the subtle clinical signs and the disastrous results of untreated duodenal laceration, any patient with a nonpenetrating abdominal injury must be hospitalized and observed very closely. Diagnostic laparotomy should be carried out if the patient's condition does not improve promptly. The laparotomy is not complete without Kocher's manuever to allow inspection of the retroperitoneal duodenum and exploration of the lesser sac for associated pancreatic injury. Duodenal lacerations are closed, and the area is generously drained.

People involved in automobile accidents while wearing abdominal seat belts suffer a peculiar type of subtle injury to the abdomen that deserves special mention. Rapid deceleration whips the upper part of the torso forward, and if the seat belt is above the bony pelvic girdle (where it generally is), it momentarily traps the viscera against the vertebral column and imposes many different shearing and compression injuries to gut and mesentery. The abdominal injuries most commonly seen are mesenteric hematoma, devascularization of bowel, severe damage leading to rupture of the bowel wall, and delayed ecchymosis and hemorrhage of the abdominal wall in a beltlike pattern. Symptoms are likely to be slow in onset and often are overshadowed by other injuries. Any automobile accident victim who bears the ecchymotic imprint of a seat belt injury on the abdomen and who develops late abdominal pain, distension, paralytic ileus, or slow return

of gastrointestinal function is a prime candidate for serious visceral injury. Repeated abdominal examinations, x-ray examinations, and paracenteses are often helpful in confirming this diagnosis, but laparotomy often must be the final arbiter.

Infections

None of the primary infections of the small intestine or its mesentery is treated primarily by surgical means, but often the symptoms produced by them mimic surgically treated diseases (appendicitis) or are complications often seen in hospitalized patients (pseudomembranous enterocolitis).

Acute Gastroenteritis

Acute gastroenteritis is generally caused by food poisoning or virus infections, and in North America it is less commonly caused by dysentery *(Shigella, Salmonella)* or paratyphoid infection, and very rarely by typhoid fever. Profuse vomiting and diarrhea are associated with colicky abdominal pain, diffuse abdominal tenderness, and hyperactive bowel sounds. Attention to these features on physical examination will in most cases adequately distinguish gastroenteritis from appendicitis. The temperature is often elevated, but tachycardia is not seen until the late stages of the disorder when the patient becomes dehydrated. Stool culture and serum agglutination tests are helpful in the diagnosis, and leukopenia is a characteristic finding with both typhoid and viral infections.

Primary Intestinal Tuberculosis

Primary intestinal tuberculosis is extremely rare in countries that have eliminated bovine tuberculosis and controlled human pulmonary tuberculous infection. Intestinal tuberculosis involves the distal small bowel and cecum with a granulomatous mass and is best treated by chemotherapy; obstructive complications of the tuberculous mass may require surgical bypass.

Tuberculous Peritonitis

Tuberculous peritonitis is a bland form of peritonitis that is self-limiting in its course; it is characterized by yellowish deposits on the mesenteric surface that are composed of typical tubercles. The diagnosis is confirmed by biopsy of one of the tubercles. Intestinal tuberculosis is often the source of peritoneal involvement, though hematogenous spread may be responsible.

Mesenteric Lymphadenitis

Mesenteric lymphadenitis is a hyperplastic enlargement of mesenteric lymph nodes, generally seen only in children and young adults, which produces pain difficult to distinguish from that of appendicitis. It is probably caused by a viral enteritis (adenovirus) with secondary mesenteric lymph node involvement. The clinical picture is characterized by central and right lower quadrant abdominal pain in a mildly febrile child who commonly has evidence of pharyngitis or tonsilitis. Abdominal tenderness is maximal in the right lower abdominal quadrant or right paraumbilical area without sharp localization or signs of peritoneal irritation. The enlarged nodes can be palpated as irregular, tender nodules if the patient is adequately relaxed. Treatment is supportive, and the patient is observed for signs of supervening appendicitis. Exploratory laparotomy is indicated when appendicitis cannot be ruled out, at which time prophylactic appendectomy is recommended to avoid subsequent confusion should the disease recur.

Acute Necrotizing Enterocolitis

Acute necrotizing enterocolitis (pseudomembranous enterocolitis) (Fig. 25-4) is a fulminating infection of the small bowel or colon that is sometimes caused by an overgrowth of staphylococci but may also occur in the absence of any cultured pathogen. The clinical settings favoring the development of acute enterocolitis are chronic low-grade intestinal obstruction (children with Hirschsprung's disease) or treatment with broad-spectrum antibiotics that upsets the balance of the intestinal flora to allow overgrowth of bacteria in the gastrointestinal tract. There is widespread denudation of the intestinal mucosa, especially in the small bowel, with edema and inflammation of the wall and pooling of large amounts of fluid within the bowel lumen.

Acute enterocolitis is characterized by the sudden onset of profuse diarrhea containing desquamated mucosa and blood that is associated with a high fever, tachycardia, nausea and vomiting, abdominal pain, and tenderness. Dehydration, electrolyte imbalance, and hypovolemic shock quickly occur from the massive amounts of fluid entrapped in the bowel lumen, which may not become evident as diarrhea for several hours because of an adynamic ileus. Hypovolemic and septic shock is the most common cause of death.

Treatment must be heroic, with rapid replacement of fluids, electrolytes, and blood. Nasogastric suction is begun, and cleansing enemas are given to expel the fluid retained within the bowel lumen. Antibiotics to which staphylococci are sensitive (penicillinase-resistant penicillin, vancomycin) should be given if stool smear and culture suggest an overgrowth of staphylococci. Steroids and fecal enemas are sometimes helpful. When present, chronic intestinal obstruction should be relieved as soon as possible.

Granulomatous (Transmural) Enterocolitis

The term *granulomatous (transmural) enterocolitis* includes regional enteritis, regional ileitis, regional ileocolitis, and Crohn's disease. It is preferable to the older terms, Crohn's disease and regional enteritis, because a granulomatous reaction is the most characteristic microscopic feature of the disorder, and it can indeed involve all layers of any or all portions of the intestine. It was first described in 1932 by Crohn and his associates as a specific entity distinct from tuberculous enteritis and other less specific infectious disorders of the intestine.

Granulomatous enterocolitis is an uncommon disease that affects principally young adults. It is rare among blacks and has an equal sex incidence. The cause of the disease is unknown, though allergic, infectious, and autoimmune factors have been suggested as contributing factors.

Granulomatous (transmural) enterocolitis either originates in, or is totally confined to, the distal ileum in the majority of cases. It commonly spreads proximally and occasionally distally to the colon. During the latter stages it often has multiple sites of involvement with uninvolved "skip areas" intervening. In early phases the bowel mucosa ulcerates and the wall becomes grossly thickened, erythematous, and edematous, with thickening of the adjacent mesentery and rubbery enlargement of the mesenteric lymph nodes. At this stage the outstanding histologic features are mucosal ulceration, submucosal lymphoid hyperplasia, and transmural lymphangiectasis, infiltrates of inflammatory cells and eosinophils, sclerosing lymphangitis, and granulomas without caseation. Involvement of all layers of the bowel wall justifies the descriptive term *transmural* and, when this peculiar disease attacks primarily the colon, serves to distinguish it from the primarily mucosal inflammation of chronic ulcerative colitis.

If limited to the ileum, the early stages of acute granulomatous enterocolitis often mimic appendicitis and are distinguished only at laparotomy. If the cecal base is not involved, prophylactic appendectomy may safely be performed at this time, along with confirma-

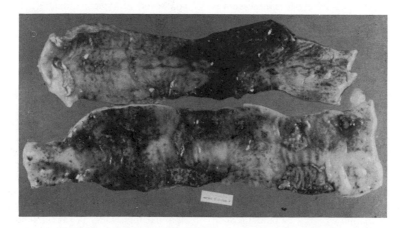

Fig. 25-4. Acute necrotizing enterocolitis. Notice hemorrhage, edema, superficial ulceration, and exudation of mucosa.

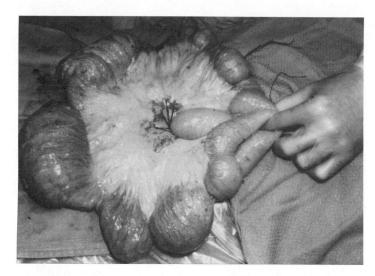

Fig. 25-5. Operative photograph of ileum extensively involved with granulomatous enteritis; note the multiple narrow areas (strictures) separated by less involved bowel (skip areas).

tory biopsy of a mesenteric lymph node. Approximately 50% of such patients will have spontaneous subsidence of the small bowel inflammation, with lengthy periods of remission.

In later stages of the disease, the edema and erythema of the involved bowel wall are replaced by fibrous tissue with rigidity, contracture, and narrowing of the lumen (Fig. 25-5). A moderately tender mass can usually be palpated at this stage, which is clinically manifested by periodic bouts of crampy abdominal discomfort and diarrhea associated with weight loss and anemia caused by occult blood loss in the stool. Fever and leukocytosis parallel the activity of the disease, and for unknown reasons perianal abscesses and fistulas are common.

The later stages of transmural enterocolitis are characterized by abscess formation and inflammatory involvement of adjacent viscera leading to both external and internal fistulas. The viscera more commonly involved in these fistulas are small bowel, bladder, and sigmoid colon, with varying symptoms related to the fistulas. The signs and symptoms of chronic low-grade intestinal obstruction (caused by the extreme narrowing of the lumen) are often superimposed.

The course of granulomatous enterocolitis is characterized by chronicity and periods of remissions and exacerbations. Generally speaking, the younger the patient and the more acute the onset, the more guarded the prognosis must be in terms of later recurrences and complications.

The diagnosis of transmural enterocolitis is generally confirmed by barium x-ray examination. The early radiographic signs include a modest degree of narrowing of the lumen associated with flattening and a raggedness of the mucosal pattern with puddling of barium. Later stages show extreme narrowing of the lumen, referred to as the *string sign* (Fig. 25-6), with dilation of the proximal loops according to the degree of intestinal obstruction present. Occasionally fistulas

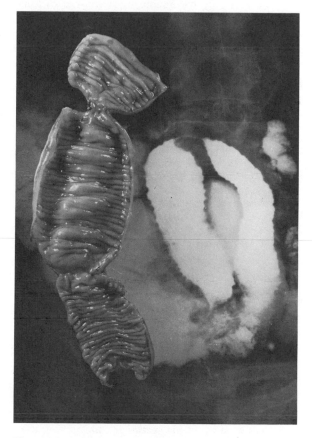

Fig. 25-6. Granulomatous enterocolitis (regional ileitis). "String sign" and uninvolved "skip areas" illustrated in distal ileum superimposed on barium study.

or extravasation of barium into abscess cavities is seen. Barium enema with retrograde filling of the distal ileum occasionally is helpful in the diagnosis of transmural ileitis.

Treatment of granulomatous enterocolitis is non-operative until and unless complications occur. Indications for operative treatment are the development of intestinal obstruction, fistulas, intra-abdominal abscesses, and hemorrhage, or if the patient's general well-being is severely compromised by chronic malnutrition, anemia, pain, and debility. Malignant degeneration rarely occurs. In a large series of cases, over one half will ultimately require surgical intervention.

Specific treatment for granulomatous enterocolitis is nonexistent. Evaluation of different forms of therapy is difficult because of the unpredictable and remitting course of the disease. Corticosteroids or ACTH, a nutritious low-residue diet, supplements of vitamins and iron, ingestion of nonabsorbed sulfonamides (Azulfidine), rest, and symptomatic treatment for diarrhea are all employed in the nonoperative treatment of granulomatous enterocolitis. Operative treatment is directed to the specific complication or indication for surgery, including resection of the involved intestine. Recurrence of the disease in previously uninvolved bowel can be expected in fully one fourth to one third of patients who are followed for many years after surgical treatment. Repeated resections and bypass procedures are fraught with nutritional and metabolic disturbances in themselves, thus warranting intensification of nonoperative treatment and avoidance of operative therapy when possible.

Vascular Diseases
Superior Mesenteric Vascular Occlusion

Occlusion of the superior mesenteric artery and vein may occur singly or together, because of a host of disparate influences. Trauma, stagnation of flow, compression, a state of hypercoagulability, and atheromatous plaques favor thrombosis. Occlusion also may occur from emboli originating within the left side of the heart, generally associated with auricular fibrillation. Rarely is the superior mesenteric vein alone thrombosed, but venous thrombosis predictably occurs after occlusion of the arterial inflow. The inferior mesenteric vessels are rarely involved.

Occlusion of the superior mesenteric vessels produces vascular compromise of that segment of small intestine distal to the point of occlusion; the more proximal the occlusion, the longer the segment of bowel that will be involved. Primary venous occlusion is associated with a "wet gangrene" type of reaction with noticeable hemorrhage and edema of the involved bowel and an effusion of sanguineous fluid from its surface. Arterial occlusion produces initial blanching of the intestine with venous stagnation subsequently inducing a blue-red discoloration. The intestine becomes slightly distended and hypotonic because of paralytic ileus that, with continued ischemia, progresses to perforation and peritonitis. Bowel infarction is generally limited to the jejunum, ileum, and right colon, even when the superior mesenteric artery is occluded at its junction with the aorta, because of collateral arterial blood flow to duodenum and colon.

Clinically, acute occlusion of the superior mesenteric vessels is characterized by rapid onset of abdominal tenderness and distension associated with vomiting, shock, and later the passage of blood-tinged stool. Signs of peritoneal irritation ensue as transudation of fluid and bacteria into the peritoneal cavity occurs.

Prime candidates are the very elderly with advanced generalized arteriosclerosis, patients who have thrombocytosis (postsplenectomy) or are recuperating from operations on the aorta or portal vein, and patients with recent fibrillation (often associated with mitral stenosis).

Physical examination reveals a distended abdomen with dullness to percussion and generalized tenderness, often with guarding and rebound. Bowel sounds are absent and rectal digital examination may reveal bloody stool. Often a vague central abdominal mass is palpable. Plain flat and decubitus x-ray studies of the abdomen are not very helpful in the diagnosis.

Diagnosis and treatment are made at early laparotomy after nasogastric suction and rapidly administered supportive treatment in the form of intravenous fluids, electrolytes, blood, and antibiotics. Thrombectomy, embolectomy, endarterectomy, and arterial bypass are indicated if frank necrosis has not occurred, but generally the surgeon's efforts are limited to resection of frankly necrotic intestine. Prognosis is poor unless the infarcted segment is short or the occlusion can be corrected before bowel necrosis occurs.

Abdominal angina and *postprandial intestinal angina* are terms used to describe a clinical syndrome associated with gradually developing superior mesenteric artery insufficiency generally caused by atheromatous plaques. Intestinal ischemia follows the stimulus to intestinal secretion and activity provoked by ingestion of a large meal. Retrograde aortic angiography demonstrates narrowing at the takeoff of the superior mesenteric artery from the abdominal aorta. Direct arterial reconstructive surgery relieves symptoms and may avert the later development of total occlusion.

Superior Mesenteric Artery Syndrome

The superior mesenteric artery syndrome is characterized by obstruction of the distal duodenum where it is compressed by the superior mesenteric artery against the unyielding second lumbar vertebral body posteriorly. The obstruction may be acute or chronic and intermittent. Epigastric distension and bilious vomiting parallel the degree and acuteness of the duodenal compression. Diagnosis is suggested by a very carefully performed barium upper gastrointestinal tract series demonstrating a dilated stomach and duodenum with abrupt narrowing at the point where the duodenum crosses under the vessel. Normal small bowel is seen distal to this point. Differentiation from other types of duodenal obstructions (intrinsic stenotic membrane) is made at the time of laparotomy, and the obstruction is bypassed by a side-to-side duodenojejunal anastomosis.

Diverticula
Meckel's Diverticulum

Meckel's diverticulum (Fig. 25-7) is the most common type of small bowel diverticulum, occurring in 2% of the general population. It represents a persistence of

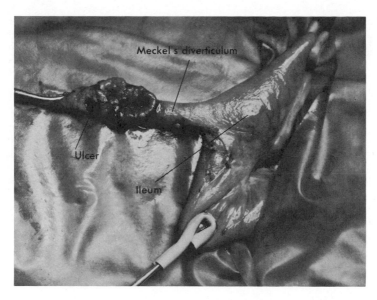

Fig. 25-7. Meckel's diverticulum with bleeding peptic ulcer perforation.

the atavistic structure known as the vitellointestinal tract (omphalomesenteric duct), which connects the distal ileum to the yolk sac early in embryonic life. The vitellointestinal tract normally obliterates and disappears entirely by the seventh week of gestation. Persistence of the entire tract is rare but is manifested early in life by drainage of ileal content at the umbilicus. Diagnosis is confirmed by injection of the fistula with radiopaque material to show a connection with the distal ileum. If the lumen of the retained tract is obliterated, the anomaly appears as a fibrous cord between the ileum and the umbilicus; the diagnosis is made incidentally at laparotomy or when small bowel obstruction occurs because of external compression by the fibrous cord.

The most common remnant of the vitellointestinal tract is persistence of its proximal end, known as Meckel's diverticulum. It is represented by a blind diverticulum situated on the antimesenteric border of ileum, which in the adult is located about 2 feet proximal to the ileocecal valve. The majority of these common types are asymptomatic and are discovered incidentally at autopsy or laparotomy.

The symptoms of Meckel's diverticulum are produced by peptic ulceration, intussusception, or diverticulitis. About 50% of the symptomatic diverticula (and about 15% of all Meckel's diverticula) contain ectopic gastric mucosa that secretes hydrochloric acid directly on unprotected adjacent ileal mucosa. Peptic ulceration occurs with pain, bleeding, inflammation, or sometimes perforation. Dark red to tarry blood passed rectally is the most common complaint prompting surgical consultation. The diverticulum may become inverted into the lumen of the ileum to provide the leading point of an ileoileal intussusception, with ultimate symptoms of intestinal obstruction and currant jelly type bloody stools. Most Meckel's diverticula are wide necked and drain readily, but occasionally the neck is narrow with

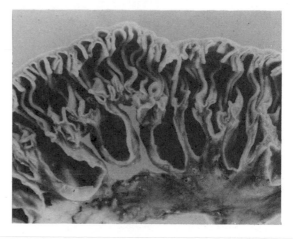

Fig. 25-8. Photograph of resected segment of small bowel. Numerous diverticula that arise from its mesenteric surface are visible in this opened specimen.

poor drainage of intestinal material producing primary diverticulitis.

The diagnosis of Meckel's diverticulum is virtually impossible by barium contrast x-ray examination. Abdominal scan after infusion of technetium-99m may show a hot spot of uptake in Meckel's diverticulum, provided that it contains functioning ectopic gastric mucosa. Asymptomatic Meckel's diverticula are discovered incidentally at exploratory laparotomy carried out for other purposes, and the symptomatic ones are found at laparotomy undertaken for symptoms produced by the various complications. Appendicitis is the most common presumptive diagnosis when pain, inflammation, and perforation are the symptoms. Treatment is complete surgical excision.

Other Small Bowel Diverticula

Diverticula of the small bowel unrelated to the vitellointestinal tract remnant usually arise from the mesenteric surface and are much more common in the duodenum than in the jejunum or ileum. Duodenal diverticula are said to be present in 6% of patients who have upper gastrointestinal tract barium studies performed, but they are present in about 20% of cadavers at autopsy. Duodenal diverticula commonly arise at or near the ampulla of Vater, are generally single, and are rarely symptomatic. They must be distinguished clinically from other, much more common, symptom-producing lesions of the pancreas, stomach, and biliary tract. Jejunal and ileal diverticula are likely to be multiple (Fig. 25-8). Large diverticula may cause diarrhea, weight loss, and malabsorption-like states attributed to stagnation of contents producing inflammation, infection, and ulceration. Small bowel diverticula are diagnosed from barium x-ray studies as sacculations that readily fill with barium.

Symptomatic diverticula of the jejunum and ileum are uncommon, but they are treated surgically with ease by resection of the involved segment of the bowel. Duodenal diverticula are more frequent, less commonly symptomatic, and dangerous to approach surgically because of the relative inaccessibility of the duodenum. Resection or inversion of duodenal diverticula must be done with infinite care and meticulous dissection, protecting the common bile duct by cannulation when necessary. For these reasons, conservatism is the rule in the treatment of duodenal diverticula.

26

Large Intestine

George E. Block
Richard D. Liechty

Diagnostic Studies
Inflammatory Diseases
Neoplasms
Trauma

Diseases of the colon range from congenital malformations to degenerative processes. They include developmental defects (aganglionosis, Hirschsprung's disease), trauma, inflammation (specific or nonspecific), neoplasia, and degeneration of colonic musculature or vasculature.

Of all the organs in the body, none harbors a more septic internal environment. Proper surgical management of colonic disease demands an understanding of this milieu and the diseases that arise within it.

DIAGNOSTIC STUDIES

Sigmoidoscopy

No physical examination of an adult is complete without a sigmoidoscopic examination. Although flexible instrumentation has added a vital new dimension to this procedure, the rigid sigmoidoscope remains an excellent diagnostic tool. Inexpensive and easy to use, this instrument allows visualization of tumors, and sites of inflammation or trauma. The patient assumes the Sims, jackknife, or knee-chest position, usually after being prepared with a prepackaged enema. The examiner advances the scope under direct vision as far as possible without discomfort. He then slowly and methodically withdraws it, circumferentially scanning the entire bowel wall. Unfortunately, the rigid instrument often fails to pass through a sharp bend at about 15 to 17 cm.

Because it can easily pass through the normal rectosigmoid curvatures, the flexible sigmoidoscope overcomes this barrier and extends the viewer's range to the full length of the sigmoid colon. It also allows biopsy or removal of lesions.

Colonoscopy

Colonoscopy, with instruments ranging up to 200 cm, allows scanning of the entire colon, biopsy of large lesions, and removal of small ones. This examination requires careful bowel preparation and technical expertise. It carries a greater risk of complications (bleeding, perforation) than sigmoidoscopy. Colonoscopy finds its greatest application in detection and follow-up of cancers, polyps, and inflammatory disorders.

Radiography

Diagnostic radiographic examinations include plain films that can indicate obstruction, ileus, or perforation. The cornerstone of radiographic evaluation, the barium enema, outlines most polypoid or constricting lesions, especially when barium is followed by air insufflation (double-contrast technique). Radiographic

techniques for locating colonic bleeding sites are discussed in Chapter 24.

Colonic bypass procedures. Colostomies divert the fecal stream through the abdominal wall and away from areas of the distal colon that are *obstructed, perforated, severely traumatized, infected* (diverticulitis), or the site of *difficult, tenuous anastomoses*. Notice that in all these conditions *perforation* or *erosion* exists or threatens. Perforation of the colon engenders *continued contamination*, which may result in generalized peritonitis and death. Colostomies are not done if resection and primary anastomosis of the lesion can be performed safely. Three main options in designing colostomies are available (Fig. 26-1 and Table 26-1).

Loop colostomy. Loop colostomies are technically simple procedures in which a segment of colon (usually transverse colon) is brought out through a small inci-

Table 26-1. Comparison of Types of Colostomies

Type	Advantages	Disadvantages
Loop (proximal to lesion)	Sterile procedure; rapid and simple; easy closure	Fecal "spillover"; large cumbersome stoma; in perforations, feces in distal limb may continue peritoneal soilage; more stages to surgical treatment
Divided limb (proximal to lesion)	No fecal "spillover"; small stoma, easily cared for	Contaminated field; later colostomy closure is more difficult; technically more difficult; in perforations, feces in distal limb may continue peritoneal soilage; more stages to surgical treatment
Exteriorization of lesion itself	Well adapted to perforations (no fear of continued fecal contamination); double-barreled colostomies simplify closure; removed lesions allow histologic diagnosis; fewer operations required	Technically often difficult; limited to mobile areas of colon; cancer operations are often compromised; double-barreled stoma is clumsy

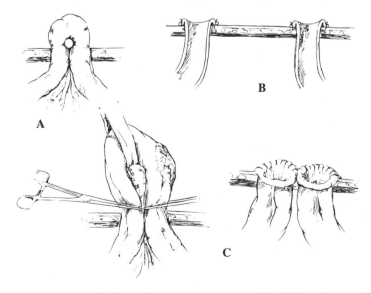

Fig. 26-1. Types of colostomies. **A,** Loop colostomy unopened. **B,** Divided limb colostomy. **C,** Exteriorization of diseased portion of colon; *on left,* segment of colon with tumor is brought out through abdominal wall incision—specimen is removed above clamps; *on right,* clamps are later removed—colon ends sutured to skin.

sion in the abdominal wall (Fig. 26-1, *A*). A small rod or tube under the loop supports it until healing takes place. If the proximal portion is distended with gas, aspiration with a needle or a small rubber catheter will immediately decompress it. This is essentially a sterile procedure since the bowel lumen is not entered until the wound is closed. The exteriorized loop may be opened and "matured" by suturing the mucosa of the bowel to the skin at the termination of the operative procedure. Although subsequent "spillover" may result, excessive gas pressure in the distal limb is immediately and permanently relieved. Loop colostomies should be considered temporary, with anticipated closure at a later date. Loop colostomy closure is technically simple.

Divided limb colostomy. Divided limb colostomies (Fig. 26-1, *B*) prevent "spillover" of fecal material, but since the colon must be divided, some operative contamination invariably results. With careful technique, however, contamination is minimized. The divided bowel ends are exteriorized through separate incisions. Divided limb colostomies require more dissection than loop colostomies, but the resultant proximal stoma is smaller, more esthetic, and easier to fit with a colostomy appliance. Divided limb colostomies are preferred when permanent fecal diversion is desired.

Exteriorization. Exteriorization is often the safest and most rapid method of fecal diversion. However, it requires an adequate length of mesentery (natural or tailored) and implies a second operation to close the resultant stomas. Exteriorization is best used for perforation but may be adapted to obstructing or perforated colon cancers if the surgeon meticulously dissects the entire lymph node–bearing colonic mesentery (Fig. 26-1, *C*).

INFLAMMATORY DISEASES
Appendicitis

For a full description of appendicitis, see Chapter 39. Some of the features associated with adult appendicitis are mentioned briefly here.

Although appendicitis chiefly afflicts the young, no age is immune. The basic initiating factor in most adult appendicitis is *obstruction* secondary to a fecalith (Fig. 26-2), impacted within the appendiceal lumen. Obstruction of the left colon from carcinoma has been cited as a precipitating factor in adult appendicitis, presumably because of increased intraluminal pressure in the colon. Perforation of the appendix is less common in adults than in children. (It is most common below 2 years of age.) In the aged patient the response to appendicitis may be deceptively mild. In some older patients, for example, the white blood cell count and temperature remain normal with acute suppurative appendicitis; however, pain and tenderness are remarkably constant factors in appendicitis, regardless of the age. In the adult patient a fistula occurring after appendectomy should always be suggestive of distal colonic obstruction, usually from a neoplasm or an inflammation. The obstruction must be relieved before the fistula will close.

A perforated carcinoma of the cecum or terminal ileitis (Crohn's disease) often mimics acute appendicitis.

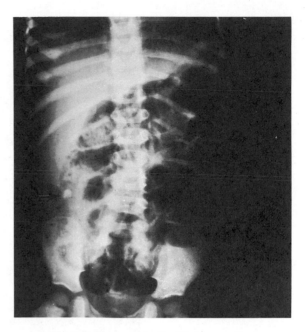

Fig. 26-2. Arrow marks fecalith in appendix.

Diverticulosis and Diverticulitis

Incidence. Diverticulosis occurs in about one third of all adults. (This incidence increases with age.) About one sixth of all persons with diverticulosis develop symptoms of diverticulitis. Operation is required for the *complications* of the disease (perforation, obstruction, hemorrhage, fistula, and abscess).

Site. Diverticulosis has a predilection for the sigmoid and distal descending colon (about 80% of patients); (Fig. 26-3). The reason for this relationship is not clear (firmer feces and increased pressure in the sigmoid loop may be important). Diverticula are usually acquired and appear where blood vessels penetrate the colon wall. Since vessels normally course through the bowel wall in the mesenteric border and beneath appendices epiploicae, diverticula most commonly appear in these areas, though no part of the bowel wall is immune. Diverticula rarely occur in the rectum.

Epidemiology. Diverticulosis chiefly afflicts developed societies. Lack of dietary roughage may play a leading role in causation. Other probable factors include aging, obesity, genetic trait, and chronic constipation.

Pathology. Although the area of diverticulitis is usually less than 10 inches in length, it may extend to include the entire colon. Obstruction of the neck of the diverticulum (by feces or barium) initiates diverticulitis. Inflammation and consequent edema in the bowel wall may constrict adjacent diverticula, inducing "secondary diverticulitis." This process may continue as a chain reaction limited only by the extent of diverticulosis. Massive *lower* gastrointestinal bleeding (the most common cause is diverticulosis) results from anatomical proximity of the diverticulum and the blood vessel that accompanies it through the bowel wall.

The inflammatory process causes some degree of bowel narrowing and may progress to complete bowel

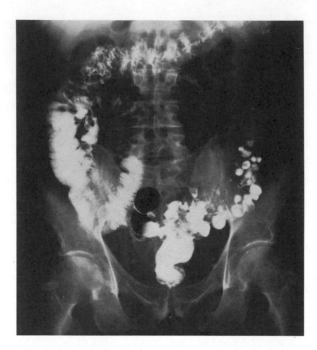

Fig. 26-3. Sigmoid diverticulitis. Globular collections of barium within diverticula.

obstruction that mimics carcinoma. Abscesses, fistulization to adjacent structures, or perforation often complicate the course of diverticulitis. Pericolitis and edema of the mesentery invariably accompany the inflammation. Muscular hypertrophy of the bowel wall usually coexists with these findings. Most evidence points to this hypertrophy as being associated with the inflammation and not a primary cause of the diverticula.

Clinical course. Clinical signs and symptoms vary with the pathologic stages and complications that have been described. Left lower quadrant pain, fever, and altered bowel habits (small-caliber stools or diarrhea) are common. Symptoms of pyuria (frequency, dysuria, urgency) are caused by the inflammatory mass impinging on the urinary bladder or forming a fistula into the bladder. A mass is sometimes palpable in the left lower quadrant or on pelvic or rectal examination.

Barium enema examination may show normal mucosa in the typically funnel-shaped constricted area, but this seldom, if ever, absolutely rules out carcinoma. (Some sigmoid cancers may also cause pain, fever, and a mass.) Sigmoidoscopy is of little help in the diagnosis of diverticulitis and the differential between an obstructing cancer and obstructing diverticulitis may be made by elective colonoscopy. Diverticulitis usually runs an intermittent course of remissions and exacerbations over periods of months or years, but we have seen acute perforation with *no* previous warning signs or symptoms.

Treatment. Medical treatment includes bed rest, broad-spectrum antibiotics appropriate to aerobic or anaerobic organisms, nasogastric suction, and sedation. This regimen may produce subsidence of the acute attack, and bulk-forming laxatives and bulky diets may prevent further attacks of the disease. Should recurrent

attacks or complications arise (perforation, hemorrhage, fistula, obstruction, abscess), operation is indicated. Resection and primary anastomosis are the treatment of choice for those patients undergoing elective operation after meticulous preparation of the bowel. With obstruction or perforation, *exteriorization-resection* is the treatment of choice. In some cases with severe inflammation, exteriorization or primary resection is not possible, and in these cases a three-stage operative treatment is elected: (1) The obstruction is relieved by a *proximal colostomy.* (2) After the inflammation subsides (3 to 6 months), the *diseased segment is resected* and the colon ends are anastomosed. (3) After subsequent healing of the anastomosis (in 4 weeks), the *colostomy is closed* as the final stage.

When operation is indicated for massive hemorrhage, the offending segment is resected or exteriorized. In some persons who require emergency operation for massive hemorrhage, the site of hemorrhage is not identified. In these patients the site of hemorrhage may occasionally be disclosed by selective angiography of the inferior mesenteric artery. In this rare situation the affected site alone may be resected. If the site of massive hemorrhage is not disclosed, an abdominal colectomy with ileoproctostomy is recommended for these patients.

Mucosal (Ulcerative) Colitis

Idiopathic ulcerative colitis, or mucosal colitis, is an inflammatory disease of unknown cause that is confined to the colon and rectum and usually affects the entire large bowel, with the most pronounced disease in the distal portion. The idiopathic inflammation may be a consequence of abnormal responsiveness of the patient to his internal or external enviroment, exposure to a foreign agent, or both. Exogenous agents such as polysaccharides, specific bacteria, and bacterial products have been suggested, but not identified, as the cause of the disease. Similarly, vascular, neurogenic, lymphatic, and degenerative abnormalities have also been suggested as a cause of colitis. Up to now, no specific entity has been universally accepted as the cause of ulcerative colitis.

Pathology (Figs. 26-4 and 26-5). The pathological findings, most noticeable in the mucosa, feature inflammatory cells, ulcerated areas, and many small microscopic crypt abscesses. The submucosa is edematous with evidence of fibrosis. The seromuscular layer shows significantly little abnormal reaction, except in areas of perforation or abscess formation. The pathologic findings vary with the clinical course. In the fulminant variety little mucosa remains and the outer colonic layers are edematous and infiltrated by inflammatory cells. In the chronic form the colon is contracted, and the mesentery is fibrotic (Fig. 26-6), shortened, and edematous. Ulcerations may coalesce leaving islands of intact or proliferated mucosa known as pseudopolyps.

In the majority of patients the rectum is involved with or without retrograde involvement of the remainder of the colon. The so-called "backwash" ileitis is a nonspecific inflammation undoubtedly attributable to the propinquity of the terminal ileum to the inflamed colon. In this entity no specific mucosal lesion is found, and it is a reversible phenomenon.

Cancer of the colon develops in 4% to 6% of patients with chronic ulcerative colitis. Certain subsets of colitis patients are identified as being particularly cancer prone: patients with pancolitis, patients whose colitis occurred during adolescence or earlier, and patients whose disease has been present 10 years or longer. If all three of these factors are operative, the lifetime cancer risk exceeds 40%. Patients who are likely to develop a colon cancer associated with colitis may be identified by certain cytologic changes or by random biopsies of the colonic mucosa. The appearance of dysplasia or carcinoma in situ is indicative of the tendency to colitic cancer. Patients with cancer of the colon arising in ulcerative colitis have the same prognosis as their noncolitic counterparts.

Clinical course. Ulcerative colitis can occur from early childhood to late life, but it is characteristically a disease of the second and third decades. It may be fulminant or chronic with exacerbations and remissions occurring over a period of years. In the fulminant presentation a bloody diarrhea with concomitant protein and blood loss characterize the disease, as well as fever, abdominal cramps, distension, and electrolyte loss. A particularly virulent form of ulcerative colitis occurs as *toxic megacolon*. In this entity there is transmural progression of the disease with destruction of the myenteric plexus; the colon passively dilates from swallowed and fermented gas. Radiographs of the abdomen will reveal an immensely dilated colon with asymmetric ulcers shown in relief. Toxic megacolon is

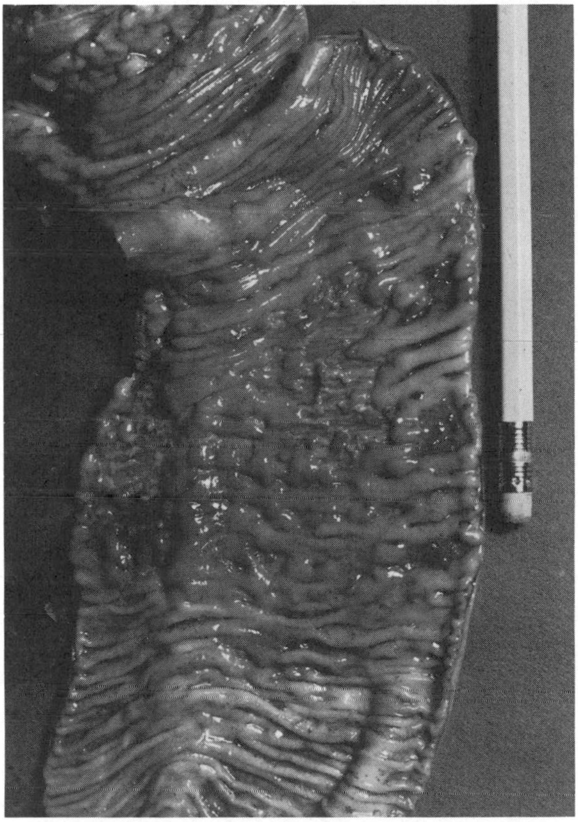

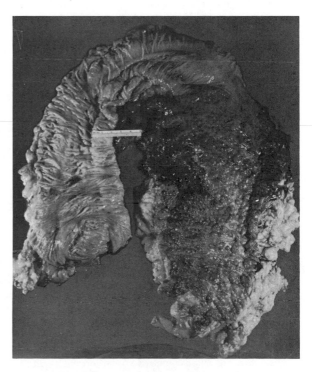

Fig. 26-4. Ulcerative colitis. Notice shallow ulcers oriented longitudinally and areas of edematous mucosa.

Fig. 26-5. Ulcerative colitis. There is diffuse involvement of half of specimen and pronounced pseudopolyposis.

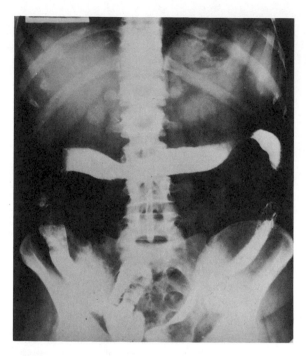

Fig. 26-6. Ulcerative colitis. Barium enema shows contraction, foreshortening, ragged mucosa, and loss of haustral markings.

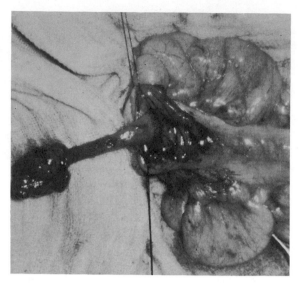

Fig. 26-7. Adenomatous polyp of colon on long stalk.

usually associated with severe constitutional manifestations of the disease subsequent to blood, protein, and electrolyte deficiencies and local septic complications.

Abnormalities of other organs, such as uveitis, arthritis, stomatitis, cirrhosis, and biliary duct fibrosis, accompany many chronic cases of mucosal colitis. The precise cause and relationship of these associated ailments remain obscure, but metastatic sepsis has been implicated in a number of these entities. The diagnosis of mucosal colitis is confirmed by the clinical course, the appearance of the mucosa on sigmoidoscopy, biopsy of the rectal mucosa, and the absence of specific pathogens on culture and biopsy.

Treatment. Medical treatment is successful in the majority of cases with ulcerative colitis, but 30% of patients with ulcerative colitis eventually require operation. Medical treatment includes sedation, repletion of specific deficiencies, bowel rest, and antiinflammatory agents such as sulfasalazine (Azulfidine) and corticosteroids. Operation is indicated for toxic megacolon, severe hemorrhage, perforation, fistula or abscess formation, failure of medical treatment, relapsing chronic colitis, or when cancer is suspected or present. The treatment of ulcerative colitis is total proctocolectomy in one or two stages with the establishment of a permanent ileostomy. Various attempts at preservation of the rectum for eventual anastomosis have failed.

In selected persons, however, preservation of the rectal musculature with total excision of the rectal mucosa allowing an anastomosis of the terminal ileum to the anus through a muscular cuff of the rectum has achieved a varying degree of success for voluntary def-

ecation. These patients have from five to 20 stools per day. An ileal pouch is usually constructed proximal to the ileoanal anastomosis. This procedure, the endorectal pullthrough procedure, is not indicated when operation is done on an emergency basis for such entities as hemorrhage, fulminant colitis, or toxic megacolon.

Another attempt to avoid a noncontrolled stoma is the so-called continent ileostomy, or Kock ileostomy. In this procedure a prestomal pouch is constructed intraabdominally and the patient defecates by irrigating the pouch through the stoma and its nipple valve several times per day. This procedure found wide initial acceptance, but its failure rate (reoperation in over 30% of the cases) has dimmed enthusiasm.

Transmural Colitis (Granulomatous Colitis, Crohn's Disease)

Transmural colitis (see Chap. 25) involves the colon in up to 50% of all cases previously believed to be exclusively mucosal colitis. Patients with transmural colitis have much the same symptoms as those with mucosal colitis—diarrhea, abdominal cramps, and fever. We cannot differentiate between the two diseases from symptoms, but we can get help from clinical findings as outlined in Table 26-2.

The symptoms of mucosal and transmural colitis are identical; the medical treatment is also the same. Why should we bother to distinguish them? Because a precise diagnosis helps the clinician to anticipate complications, including cancer, plan the operation, and justify radical procedures (total colectomy and ileostomy) when necessary.

Diagnosis. Ulcerative colitis is associated with bloody stools, rectal involvement, episodes of toxic megacolon, and the occasional development of cancer (Table 26-2). Perianal and internal fistulas are commonly associated with Crohn's colitis, whereas carcinoma is rare. When performing an emergency operation, the surgeon often lacks preoperative information to make an accurate diagnosis. Even postoperatively

Table 26-2. Comparison of Ulcerative Colitis and Crohn's Colitis

Diagnostic Features	Ulcerative Colitis	Crohn's Colitis
Distribution	Continuous with rectum	Often discontinuous (segmental)
Rectum	Almost always involved	Often normal
Internal fistulas	Rare	Frequent
Strictures	Uncommon: suggests carcinoma	Frequent
Mucosa	Shallow ulceration may have pseudopolyps	Longitudinal fissures, cobblestone appearance
Symmetry	Symmetric	Asymmetric (one wall involvement)
Terminal ileum	Normal	Usually involved
Megacolon	Frequent	Less common
Colon perforation	Common	Infrequent
Operative findings		
Serositis	Absent	Common
Inflammatory masses	Rare	Frequent
Enlarged mesenteric lymph nodes	Infrequent	Usual
Anal lesions	Nonspecific	Common with granulomas present

definite diagnosis will not be established in approximately 5% of patients. The appearance of the colon at the time of operation is helpful. If the diagnosis is not apparent, the surgeon must make every effort to preserve the rectum at the initial operation unless there is overwhelming rectal involvement.

Treatment. Ulcerative colitis responds to medical treatment in two thirds to three fourths of the patients. Crohn's colitis is less likely to respond to medical treatment. Crohn's colitis infrequently develops into toxic megacolon. Although cancer has been reported in Crohn's colitis, it is extremely rare, and strictures may be considered benign. Similar strictures in ulcerative colitis must be considered as a carcinoma until proved otherwise.

Total colectomy and permanent ileostomy cure the patient with ulcerative colitis. A similar operation for Crohn's colitis will eventually result in recurrences in the neoileum in 10% to 16% of the patients, usually depending on the extent of initial small bowel disease.

Specific Infections

Pseudomembranous Colitis

Pseudomembranous colitis is discussed in Chapter 25.

Amebiasis

Amebiasis of the colon is unusual in the United States except in inmates in mental institutions. Amebic infiltrates have a predilection for the rectum and cecum. They may mimic carcinoma, or a diffuse amebic colitis may be confused with ulcerative colitis. Sigmoidoscopic examination with biopsy specimens and stool cultures usually confirms the diagnosis. Emetine and other antiamebic drugs control most cases. Complications such as the development of toxic megacolon or perforation with peritonitis or abscess formation necessitate operation.

Tuberculosis

Tuberculosis of the colon is almost always associated with pulmonary tuberculosis. A primary form, probably of bovine origin, seldom arises in our country. The typical granulomatous nature of tuberculosis involves, in the large bowel, chiefly the cecum and right colon. Although the diagnosis can be suspected preoperatively, it is seldom confirmed except at operation. When obstruction occurs, resection of the involved portion of the large bowel may be necessary. Antituberculosis drugs must be used to control the systemic infection.

Bacillary Infections

Bacillary infections may be confused clinically with chronic ulcerative colitis. The sigmoidoscopic findings are also similar, but bacterial culture establishes the diagnosis of bacillary dysentery.

An overgrowth of *Clostridium difficile* after administration of many of the common antibiotics may result in pseudomembranous enterocolitis or colitis. This diagnosis may be established by serologic detection of the offending organism, which is best treated by cessation of the inducing antibiotic and the substitution of oral vancomycin or metronidazole.

Actinomycosis

Actinomyces bovis is a rare cause of human intestinal disease, though it is a relatively common inhabitant of the gastrointestinal tract. Biopsy, cultures, or hanging-drop preparations usually reveal the diagnosis. Persistent (and confusing) abdominal wall fistulas may occur, sometimes months after an operation. Treatment with new penicillin preparations has been gratifying.

NEOPLASMS

Adenomatous polyps and adenocarcinoma are the most common tumors of the colorectum. Although polyps may bleed and occasionally cause bowel obstruction, their overwhelming significance resides in the possibility of associated malignancy.

Polyps

Polyps are sessile or pedunculated (Fig. 26-7). About 70% arise within range of the sigmoidoscope, and most of the others are visible through the colonoscope. Barium studies, especially double-contrast studies, outline most polyps in the upper colon (Fig. 26-8 and Table 26-3). Five chief types of polyps are seen: tubular, villous, juvenile, hereditary familial, and those associated with the Peutz-Jeghers syndrome.

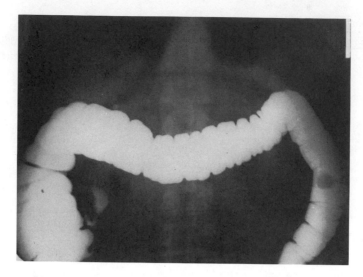

Fig. 26-8. Polyp of colon shows as filling defect on barium enema.

Table 26-3. Comparison of Polyps of the Large Bowel

Type	Frequency	Site	Malignancy	Treatment
Tubular	Most common polyp; 10% of all adults; increases with age	Rectosigmoid 70%	Premalignant	Endoscopy and biopsy excision; excise larger upper colonic polyps
Villous	Relatively common in the aged	Rectosigmoid 80%	About 25% malignant Increases with size	Total biopsy; radical operation if malignant
Juvenile	Common in first decade; rare in adults	Chiefly rectum	Never	Excise only for bleeding, intussusception, diagnosis
Hereditary familial	Very rare	Scattered	100%	Total or near-total colectomy
Peutz-Jeghers	Very rare	Chiefly small bowel	Never(?)	Excise for bleeding or obstruction

Pseudopolyps

Pseudopolyps are discussed above in the section on mucosal, or ulcerative, colitis.

Adenomatous Polyps

Tubular adenomatous polyps (polypoid adenomas, pedunculated polyps) are without question the most common polyps.

Age. Tubular polyps reach a peak incidence during the eighth decade. Before 20 years of age they are nonexistent (except for genetic multiple polyposis). Tubular polyps are more common in males than in females.

Site. About 70% of tubular polyps arise in the rectosigmoid area. A similar occurrence for carcinomas is suggestive of a causal relationship between adenomatous polyps and colorectal carcinoma.

Incidence. The incidence of tubular polyps varies with age. Clinical studies indicate that about 10% of patients over 40 have rectosigmoid polyps. Autopsy studies indicate a much higher incidence (20% to 50%). Multiple polyps (2 to 10) occur in about 30% of all patients with polyps.

Malignant potential. The potential for malignancy is the most important factor concerning polyps. Advocates for the malignant potential of polyps cite as corroborative evidence the striking parallelism between polyps and cancer in location, age and sex incidence, frequent association of polyps and cancer, the absolute 100% incidence of cancer with familial polyposis, and the occasional finding of an invasive cancer arising in an adenomatous polyp.

At the present time the evidence is overwhelming that tubular adenomatous polyps and villous adenomatous polyps are premalignant. Wide-based polyps and large polyps (greater than 2 cm in diameter) are often sites of occult malignancy and should be totally excised for whole-mount examination.

Treatment. *Sigmoidoscopic removal* of polyps is usually safe and is accomplished simply. Wide-based rectal polyps are removed by transanal excision (after sphincter dilation) and direct suture closure.

Colonoscopy has added a dramatic new dimension to upper colonic polypectomy (or biopsy). Experienced colonoscopists can reach the cecum in about 90% of all patients, and they can successfully visualize (and biopsy or excise) an even larger percentage of polyps in the distal colon. By preempting laparotomy, colonoscopy has made polypectomy safer for many patients and allowed biopsies of wide-based polyps that help select those lesions that require laparotomy and excision.

Celiotomy and polypectomy. Polyps that defy visualization and excision by sigmoidoscopy or colonoscopy necessitate celiotomy and polypectomy. Multiple polyps throughout the colon require abdominal colectomy with ileosigmoid or ileorectal anastomosis, as indicated. The premalignant potential of adenomatous polyps demands an aggressive course of removal.

Laparotomy and polypectomy. The student should realize that repeated diagnostic barium enema studies and endoscopy are time consuming, costly, and uncomfortable. For patients who accept repeated examinations reluctantly or diffidently, laparotomy may prove to be the most prudent plan.

Villous Adenomas

Villous adenomas (villous papilloma, villous tumor, papillary adenoma, and true papilloma) are velvety, broad-based tumors that may grow to encircle the bowel. About 80% reside in the rectum. In contrast to cancer, which they resemble, they are usually soft and pliable, so soft, in fact, that they can be missed by digital examination of the rectum.

Malignant potential. Although some surgeons look upon villous adenomas as malignant tumors per se, only about one fifth are actually malignant. The percentage increases with the size of the tumor, so that tumors of 5 cm or more may be considered to always harbor an occult carcinoma.

Treatment. Most villous adenomas occur in older persons, occur in the rectum, and have broad bases (therefore small biopsy specimens are inconclusive). Combined abdominoperineal resection, which would be required for most of these rectal lesions if malignant, carries an imposing mortality in aged patients. Therefore *total biopsy* of the tumor with frozen-section diagnosis of several cross sections of the tumor helps greatly in determining whether radical resection is necessary. If the lesion is benign, nothing more need be done: if it is malignant, a cancer operation is performed. In some critical-risk patients, focal cancer has been treated by such local resections alone—or cauterization—in deference to the forbidding mortality of radical operations.

In no instance has malignant recurrence occurred after total biopsy of benign tumors in our experience. In rare instances severe fluid and electrolyte problems have been caused by the copious diarrhea (mucorrhea) that these patients so frequently exhibit. Potassium loss is especially high. Large tumors can be removed by spreading the sphincters and direct excision. Coccygectomy and posterior proctotomy help to expose lesions high in the rectum.

Juvenile Polyps

Juvenile polyps are hamartomas, not true neoplasms. Grossly they are smooth, round, and cherry red and exude mucus when cut across; microscopically they are characterized by mucoid cystic spaces with a large amount of interstitial fibrous tissue. Generally single, they occur most frequently in the first decade of life and tend to disappear spontaneously. Because of bleeding they may be a persistent nuisance. They rarely induce intussusception, and *malignancy never occurs* in juvenile polyps. Biopsy excision to control bleeding or to differentiate familial polyposis should be the extent of treatment. The polyps in a patient with multiple or scattered polyps almost invariably share a single histologic pattern; thus, if the physician can prove micro-

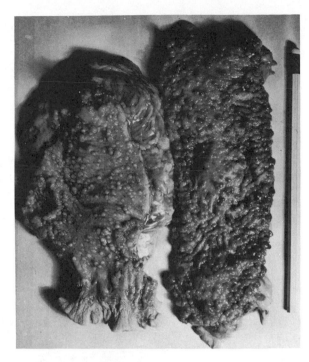

Fig. 26-9. Multiple polyposis of colon.

scopically that one accessible polyp is of the juvenile variety, he need not remove any others unless they are symptomatic.

Familial Polyposis

Familial polyps will become malignant in 100% of the instances. This rare inheritable trait is autosomal dominant and may be transmitted by either parent (Fig. 26-9). The polyps rarely appear before adolescence, and in some instances they appear sporadically because of a mutant gene.

Treatment. Either total removal of the rectum and colon with ileostomy or total colectomy with preservation of the rectum (an ileoproctostomy) must be performed. If there are fewer than 20 polyps in the rectum, some consider an ileorectal anastomosis "safe." The experience of several centers does not bear this out, however, and it is advisable to remove all rectal mucosa. The endorectal pullthrough operation is ideal for patients with familial polyposis, as it preserves the voluntary sphincter and excises all the premalignant mucosa.

After the physician diagnoses familial polyposis, it is necessary to examine all other members of the family who might carry the inheritable trait.

Peutz-Jeghers Syndrome

Peutz-Jeghers syndrome is discussed in Chapter 25.

Adenocarcinoma

Adenocarcinoma of the colon and rectum rivals lung cancer as the most common killing cancer in humans.

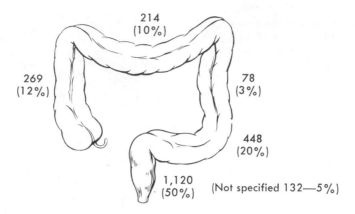

Fig. 26-10. Sites of 2,261 colorectal cancers at University of Iowa Hospitals, 1940 to 1960.

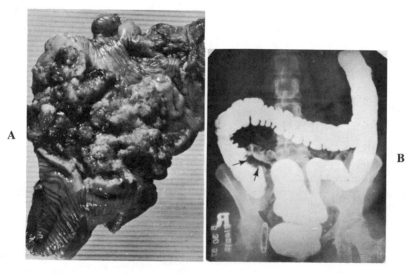

Fig. 26-11. A, Polypoid, ulcerating carcinoma of cecum. Distal ileum at left. **B,** Barium enema with arrows marking filling defect of cecal carcinoma.

About 60% of these tumors lie within range of the sigmoidoscope; now that the colonoscope can reach the remaining 40%, diagnostic efficiency should improve (Fig. 26-10).

Epidemiology. Mortality for colorectal cancer is high in North America, western Europe, Australia, and Israel and in patients with ulcerative colitis or familial polyposis. Colorectal cancer is uncommon in Asia and Africa. Burkitt hypothesizes that low-fiber, high-sugar diets induce colon and rectal cancers.

Age. The relative incidence of colorectal cancer increases with age; 90% appear in patients past 40 years of age. Under 30 years of age, familial polyposis and ulcerative colitis often coexist. The prognosis for youthful patients (mostly mucoid carcinoma) is poor.

Symptoms. Alteration in bowel habits, blood in or with the stools, obstruction, and anemia keynote the symptoms. *Anemia* is most common with right-sided colon lesions because the tumors are characteristically polypoid, and the ileal contents that bathe these tumors are caustic (Fig. 26-11, *A*). An unexplained iron-deficiency anemia in an adult over the age of 40 must be considered to be a gastrointestinal neoplasm until proved otherwise. *Obstruction* predominates in left-sided colon lesions because of a narrower lumen, firmer feces, and a characteristic annular lesion at this location (Fig. 26-12, *A*).

Diagnosis. *Physical signs* are often scant. Masses are sometimes palpable, most often by rectal examination, and stools usually show blood, sometimes grossly but most often in the occult form. Endoscopy greatly aids early diagnosis.

The adoption of the Hemoccult examination for occult blood in the stool has added greatly to the early diagnosis of carcinoma of the colon. For this the patient merely abstains from meat for 3 days and sends to his physician paper folders containing minute specimens of stool. A "positive" report for occult blood is then followed up by appropriate examination. It has been gratifying to see the patient and physician response to this easy and inexpensive examination, and it has resulted in the detection of many early carcinomas and polyps.

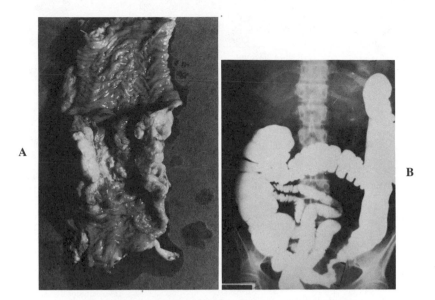

Fig. 26-12. A, Annular, constricting carcinoma of sigmoid colon. **B,** Barium enema outlining "apple core" defect of sigmoid carcinoma shown in **A.**

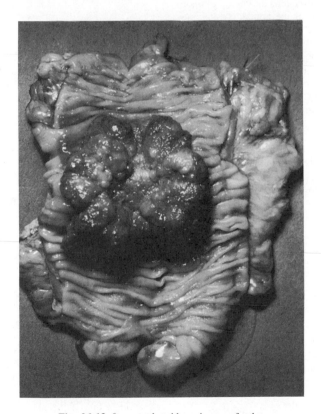

Fig. 26-13. Large polypoid carcinoma of colon.

Barium enema examination and colonoscopy help detect colonic cancers above the reach of the sigmoidoscope (Figs. 26-11, *B*, and 26-12, *B*).

Differential diagnosis. Since large polyps that resemble carcinomas should be removed (Fig. 26-13),

they present few diagnostic problems. Distinguishing diverticulitis from cancer, usually in the sigmoid colon, is the major diagnostic problem. Even at laparotomy some cases defy diagnosis until the specimen is opened. (Cancers always involve mucosa; diverticulitis

Table 26-4. Operations for Colorectal Carcinoma

Tumor Site	Operation	Anastomosis or Colostomy
Cecum, ascending colon	Right colectomy	Ileum to midtransverse colon
Hepatic flexure	Right and transverse colectomy	Ileum to midtransverse or left transverse colon
Transverse colon	Right, transverse, and upper left colectomy	Ileum to upper descending colon
Splenic flexure	Right, transverse, and upper left colectomy	Terminal ileum to descending colon
Descending colon, sigmoid colon	Left colectomy	Left transverse colon to rectosigmoid
Rectum	Left lower colectomy with low anastomosis or anal anastomosis; abdominoperineal resection	Descending colon to rectal stump; terminal sigmoid colostomy

causes mucosal edema.) Since diverticulosis and cancer of the colon may coexist, barium studies seldom exclude carcinoma absolutely. Colonoscopy often will. If, however, the diagnosis remains in question, the surgeon must assume the worst and perform an appropriate cancer operation. This will obviously cure the complication of the diverticulitis and give the greatest chance for cure of any cancer.

Tuberculosis and other infections and benign tumors (lipoma, fibroma, mucocele of the appendix, endometriosis) are on rare occasions mistaken for carcinoma of the colorectum. In all such cases, biopsy diagnosis must exclude colorectal cancer.

Metastases. Metastases from large bowel cancers spread in a number of ways: intramurally, lymphatically, through the veins, by implantation in the bowel lumen (often by the surgeon at the time of resection), by direct extension, and transperitoneally. Two factors that influence the prognosis of a colorectal lesion are the depth of penetration of the bowel wall by the tumor and the presence or absence of regional lymph node metastases. Several classifications are used to describe colorectal cancers. These are as follows:

Dukes' Classification	Extent of Disease	5-Year Survival (%)
A	Confined to bowel wall	80-90
B	Extension into pericolic tissues; nodes—negative	50
C	Involving adjacent structures; nodes—positive	20

Astler-Coller Classification	Extent of Disease
A	Confined to mucosa
B1	Extension into the muscularis propria; nodes negative
B2	Penetration of the muscularis propria; nodes negative
C1	Extension to the muscularis propria; nodes positive
C2	Penetration of the muscularis propria; nodes positive

TNM Classification	Extent of Disease
T1	Mucosal or submucosal involvement
T2	Involvement of the muscular wall
T3	Involvement of all layers of the colon with extension to immediately adjacent structures
T4	Fistula present
T5	Tumor is spread by direct extension beyond the immediately adjacent organs or tissues
N0	Regional nodes not involved
N1	Regional nodes involved
M0	No known distant metastases
M1	Distant metastases present

T designates primary tumor, N designates lymph nodes, and M designates distal metastases. Example: A modified Duke's B2 would be under the TMN classification T2 N0 M0. Survival is inversely proportional to extent of disease by any staging method.

Treatment. The aim of treatment of colorectal cancer is to remove the cancer with its areas of local extension and areas of lymphatic spread (Table 26-4). During these procedures, early ligation of the venous return and ligation of the bowel above and below the tumor have been advocated to help prevent operative dissemination of cancer cells. Up to now neither laboratory nor clinical proof indicates that either of these two maneuvers substantially decreases local or systemic recurrences.

Operations are designed to remove the lymph node–bearing tissue, contiguous bowel, and any adjacent organs involved by the tumor such as small bowel, bladder, and uterus.

Major colonic resections are preceded by a thorough cleansing of the bowel by a clear liquid diet, a laxative, and enemas. An attractive alternative to this is the oral administration of large amounts (5 to 7 liters) of a balanced saline solution containing potassium before operation for patients whose tumor is not obstructing the gut. Obviously, patients with congestive heart failure are not candidates for such massive fluid administration. For healthier patients this has proved to be an excellent and rapid method of mechanical cleansing. Most surgeons use some type of preoperative antibiotics to reduce the concentration and total number of gut organisms. The prophylactic antibiotics may be administered orally or systemically. If systemic antibiotics are adopted, no more than two postoperative doses are necessary, but the preoperative dose must be given early enough so that adequate blood and tissue levels are present at the time of incision. Whether or not systemic or oral antibiotics are utilized, all surgeons agree that a thorough mechanical cleansing is the most important factor in the preoperative preparation of the colon.

Prognosis. Results vary with age, extent of tumor, pathologic type of tumor, location of tumor, the presence or absence of involved nodes, associated diseases (ulcerative colitis or familial polyposis), and the operative procedure. A summation of the prognostic importance of these factors follows, highlighted (as in many other cancers) by the presence or absence of involved lymph nodes: Without positive lymph nodes, the 5 year survival is about 80%; with positive lymph nodes, the 5 year survival is about 60%. In *all* cases the 5 year survival is more than 50%. Transverse colon cancers have a poor prognosis. Men and blacks show a poorer prognosis in all age groups. Large bowel cancers in young people (under 40 years) have a poor prognosis. Cancers that originate *above* the peritoneal reflection have a better prognosis than those that originate *below* the peritoneal reflection. Obstructing and perforating cancers of the colon have a poor prognosis. If the colon is not removed in *familial polyposis*, almost all patients develop cancer by 50 years of age. Radiation therapy decreases pain in many advanced cases, but neither radiation nor chemotherapy increases survival.

TRAUMA

Trauma to the large bowel may be *penetrating* or *blunt*. *Penetrating* wounds may occur from *outside* (knife wounds, missile wounds) or *inside* from objects inserted into the rectum (thermometers, sigmoidoscopes, enemas) or swallowed (safety pins, toothpicks, fishbones). *Blunt trauma* is most common from automobile accidents in civilian life and from blast injuries in combat military personnel. Improperly worn seat belts (that ride too high) can themselves induce intraabdominal injury.

Diagnosis. The extent of *penetrating* wounds from the outside is usually indeterminant from examination of the wound. Probing small abdominal wall wounds is misleading, since contraction of the musculofascial layers overrides and obscures the original tract. Most penetrating abdominal injuries demand immediate laparotomy.

In all instances of abdominal trauma two serious threats arise: *bleeding* and *perforation*. If sufficient blood is lost (1000 to 1500 ml), shock occurs. The bleeding vessel must be ligated. With losses of lesser amounts of blood, the findings are more subtle. In these instances, paracentesis or peritoneal lavage (500 to 1000 ml. of balanced salt solution through a peritoneal dialysis catheter, then evacuated by placing the bottle on the floor) gives the most accurate information. Blood (above 100,000 RBC/mm^3), bile, bacteria, or amylase indicates intraperitoneal disease.

Perforation is suggested by abdominal pain and tenderness (acute abdomen, discussed in Chapter 21). The diagnosis of perforation of a hollow viscus is not always easy, since trauma to the abdominal wall may induce both pain and tenderness in the wall itself.

Plain and upright films of the abdomen are helpful, since free peritoneal air is diagnostic of perforation of a hollow viscus. Negative films for free air, however, do *not* rule out perforation since small amounts of free air may be overlooked. Thus frequent, repetitive examinations, abdominal films, and peritoneal lavage form the core of successful management of the patient with possible colon damage.

Treatment. When intraperitoneal hemorrhage or perforation is diagnosed, operative treatment must be immediate. In perforation the elapsed time since the injury determines treatment. When the patient arrives soon (within 4 to 6 hours) after the wound and peritoneal soilage is limited, simple closure of the wound may suffice. When the patient arrives late and peritoneal soilage is extensive, exteriorization of the damaged bowel segment (when possible) or a diverting colostomy when exteriorization is technically difficult are the treatments of choice. In penetrating wounds of the abdominal wall, when uncertainty exists concerning intraperitoneal damage, watchful waiting and diagnostic laparotomy are the two main therapeutic options. Laparotomy is, of course, the most certain plan, but under battlefield conditions or with multiple-person injuries in civilian practice, the physician must sort out the patients who require operation from those he can keep under observation. In battle wounds, high-velocity missiles may damage a wide area around the wound because of shock waves. Adequate debridement of the bowel wall before closure helps prevent necrosis.

27

Intestinal Obstruction

Greg Van Stiegmann

Intestinal obstruction is defined as an interference in the normal movement of the bowel contents through the intestinal tract. Two main types of obstruction occur: (1) mechanical obstruction, which arises from structural lesions (adhesive bands, stones, tumors, etc.) that block the bowel lumen, and (2) *paralytic ileus,* which arises from a failure of the neuromuscular propulsive action of the bowel wall. The distinction between these types is vitally important because mechanical obstruction, if unrelieved, may progress to strangulation (shutting off of the blood supply to the obstructed segment) or *perforation*. Both complications pose a serious threat to life. Paralytic ileus, on the other hand, rarely threatens life and is treated conservatively with gastrointestinal decompression and correction of the factors causing the bowel wall paralysis.

Simple obstruction, in contrast to *strangulation obstruction,* occurs when the blood supply to the obstructed bowel is adequate. *Vascular obstruction* occurs when an impedance to the arterial flow or venous return sets the stage for bowel infarction. In *partial obstruction* the signs and symptoms of bowel obstruction occur, but some passage of bowel contents continues.

MECHANICAL OBSTRUCTION
Site of Mechanical Obstruction

The small bowel is about 20 feet long, and the large bowel is 5 feet long. This 4 to 1 ratio parallels the ratio of mechanical obstructions that occur in the small and large bowel; 80% occur in the small bowel, and only 20% involve the large bowel. The student can recall the relative incidence favoring small bowel obstruction by this helpful question: Given a certain amount of traffic, will more accidents occur along a 20-mile two-lane curving highway or along a 5-mile four-lane straighter highway?

Etiology

The "big three" causes of adult mechanical intestinal obstruction are hernias (incarcerated or strangulated), adhesions, and tumors (Fig. 27-1). Hernias and adhesions together account for about 70% of all bowel obstruction. Tumors cause about 15% of all intestinal obstruction, but they are, by far, the most common cause of *large bowel obstruction*. Intussusception, volvulus, obturation (fecal impactions, gallstone ileus), inflammatory lesions, and vascular obstruction are the remaining causes of adult intestinal obstruction. Intestinal obstruction in the child, limited primarily to congenital defects and intussusception, is discussed in Chapter 39.

Hernias

The various sites of hernias (including incisions) should be inspected and palpated carefully (see Fig. 27-1, *C*). Hernias in obese people are often difficult to detect through fatty tissue. Richter's hernias (a knuckle of bowel in the defect) may be deceptively small. If a hernia becomes tense, tender, and nonreducible, the surgeon must assume that it is strangulated. He should operate immediately reducing it surgically and resecting any necrotic bowel.

Adhesions

The incidence of intestinal obstruction caused by adhesions appears to be increasing (see Fig. 27-1, *A* and *B*). *Lower abdominal incisions* are more likely to produce adhesive obstruction than *upper abdominal incisions* because the omentum shields the small intestine from the incision in the upper abdomen. About 15% of obstructions caused by adhesions are strangulating. *Closed loop* obstructions, in which a portion of bowel is closed at both ends, threaten perforation from increasing gas pressure (from putrefaction) within the bowel lumen. Early operative release of the obstructing bands can prevent these complications.

Tumors

Neoplasms of the *small bowel* (carcinoma, carcinoid, lymphoma, and benign tumors) are rare causes of obstruction. In contrast, neoplasms cause most obstructions of the colon (see Fig. 27-1, *D*) (diverticulitis is next in incidence). Left colon lesions may cause tremendous dilation of the proximal colon when the ileocecal valve is competent. Because the proximal colon wall is thinned from dilation and the bowel cannot be prepared preoperatively, decompressive colostomy or cecostomy usually must precede resection of the tumor. In certain cases the obstructing tumor, with bowel and mesentery, can be exteriorized and removed (obstruction resection; see Chap. 26).

Intussusception

Intussusception, common in children (Chap. 39), is rare in adults. Polypoid tumors often "lead" the adult intussusception (Fig. 27-2, *A*). Because of these mechanical lesions underlying adult intussusception, we never attempt hydrostatic reduction as in children but immediately explore and resect the involved bowel.

Volvulus

Volvulus is twisting of a portion of the gastrointestinal tract on its mesentery. The blood supply is always threatened, if not completely occluded, in this situation (see Fig. 27-2, *B*).

Sigmoid volvulus (Fig. 27-3) is the most common type of volvulus because the sigmoid mesentery is long and redundant. In eastern European and some Asian countries sigmoid volvulus is one of the most common causes of bowel obstruction. The high-cellulose diet in

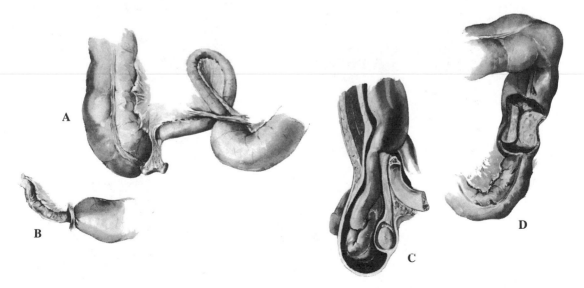

Fig. 27-1. The three leading causes of intestinal obstruction—adhesions, hernias, and tumors. Adhesions causing bowel obstruction. **A,** Fibrous band causing obstruction and volvulus about band. **B,** Fibrous band obstructing segment of small bowel. Notice proximal dilatation. **C,** Inguinal hernia with loop of obstructed small bowel. Notice that obstruction occurs at internal inguinal ring. **D,** Cancer of colon causing bowel obstruction.

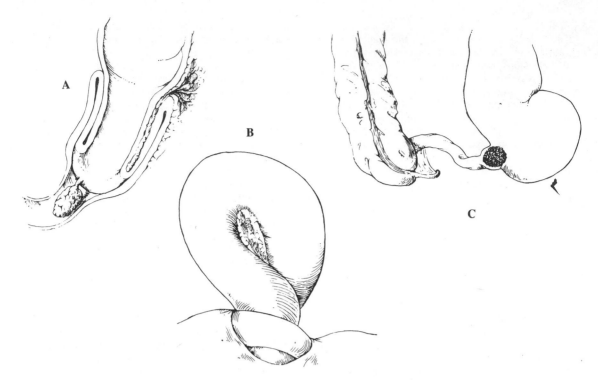

Fig. 27-2. A, Polyp of bowel "leading" an intussusception. **B,** Volvulus of bowel. **C,** Gallstone ileus. Large gallstone obstructing distal ileum.

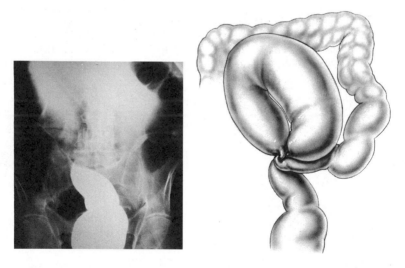

Fig. 27-3. Sigmoid volvulus. Roentgenogram shows large fluid-filled mass and typical bird-beak deformity outlined by barium in distal sigmoid colon. Diagram shows twist.

these areas may be an etiologic factor. In western areas sigmoid volvulus usually occurs in older, debilitated patients. Barium enema will often outline the twist. Sigmoidoscopy with insertion of a soft rubber rectal tube usually effects decompression amidst a rush of gas and liquid feces. Operative treatment (detorsion or sigmoid resection) is utilized for recurrence, strangulation, or failure of decompression by a rectal tube.

Cecal volvus (Fig. 27-4) occurs when the cecal mesentery is long, allowing the cecum free movement within the peritoneal cavity. The twisted cecum, containing gas usually (and paradoxically), appears in the left upper abdomen on x-ray examination. Barium enema confirms cecal volvulus and differentiates the contained gas from air within the stomach.

Volvulus of the stomach is rare. It is usually associated with paraesophageal hernias. *Small intestinal volvulus* almost invariably results from adhesions. Adhe-

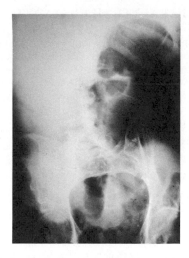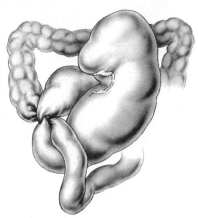

Fig. 27-4. Cecal volvulus. Notice dilated, gas-filled cecum in left upper quadrant on roentgenogram. Diagram shows twist.

sions pathologically join two portions of the small bowel that form the base of the loop. Volvulus results from a twisting of this loop about the base. *Midgut volvulus,* which occurs almost exclusively in children, involves an abnormality in the embryonic rotation and return of the developing intestine (see Chap. 39).

Obturation

Obturation results when materials *within* the gut occlude the lumen. *Fecal impaction* and *gallstone ileus* (see Fig. 27-2, *C*) are the most common causes of intraluminal obstruction in more advanced countries. Parasitic infections (chiefly *Ascaris lumbricoides,* which may produce a ball of worms) cause intestinal obstruction in underdeveloped areas. Bezoars of various types are common in mentally defective patients.

Inflammatory Causes

Tuberculosis, regional enteritis, ulcerative colitis, and amebiasis are the more common causes of intestinal obstruction associated with inflammation. The diagnosis, usually obscure, depends on biopsy and culture specimens.

Vascular Obstruction

Vascular obstruction is the reverse, pathologically, of *strangulation obstruction; primary* blood vessel blockage precedes and causes bowel obstruction (see Chap. 25).

The final clinical picture is identical to that in strangulation obstruction. The early stages of vascular obstruction feature extreme abdominal pain that comes on abruptly (with crescendos) before becoming steady, vomiting, and diarrhea. Many patients, perhaps one third, give a prior history of crampy pains after meals.

The diagnosis of vascular obstruction is difficult, especially in older patients, in whom it occurs frequently. The onset may be deceptively subtle with minimal symptoms. In younger patients the onset is frequently sudden and confusing. A thorough knowledge of the patient and of the possible antecedent causative fac-

tors gives the physician the best opportunity to make this diagnosis.

Embolism (cardiac or arteriosclerotic), *increased venous pressure* (abdominal tumor, cirrhosis, congestive heart failure), *hypercoagulability* (polycythemia, some cancers), or *vascular diseases* (collagen diseases, vasospastic diseases, prolonged infections, or trauma) should be considered in the differential diagnosis. Arteriograms will often pinpoint the obstructed artery. Immediate operation, with embolectomy when possible, and bowel resection (often massive) are the only therapeutic options. In older patients the mortality is extremely high.

Clinical Features

Symptoms. Pain, obstipation, distension, and vomiting are the characteristic symptoms in intestinal obstruction.

Pain is typically crampy and intermittent, resulting from forceful contraction of the bowel wall musculature attempting to push fluid and gas past the obstruction. Continuous pain usually signifies strangulation or perforation. Vomiting temporarily relieves the pain from upper gastrointestinal obstructions as bowel distension is ameliorated. In colon obstruction the crampy pains occur at longer intervals than with small bowel obstruction.

Because intestinal obstruction may be only partial or intermittent, *obstipation* is not absolutely necessary to make the diagnosis of intestinal obstruction. Gas or feces in the bowel segment distal to the obstruction may pass in small amounts, especially in response to enemas. However, complete obstruction usually produces eventual failure to pass either gas or feces.

Distension, to some degree, always accompanies obstruction. In high (proximal small bowel) obstruction, distension is minimal. In lower obstructions, distension is massive because of the greater amount of bowel that is filled with gas and liquid.

In higher obstruction *vomiting* ocurs as an early symptom because the upper small bowel receives bile and pancreatic and gastric juice (in addition to its own secretions) and is poorly absorptive. In obstructing lesions of the low ileum or colon *feculent vomiting* results from stagnation and bacterial putrefaction and strongly suggests the low site of obstruction. In obstruction of the colon with a competent ileocecal valve, vomiting seldom occurs as a "back-up" phenomenon, but it does result on a reflex basis.

Laboratory Diagnosis

X-ray examination. Plain films of the abdomen taken with the patient in the upright (or decubitus) and supine positions are the most important aids in the diagnosis of intestinal obstruction. Small intestinal gas and fluid levels in the adult patient invariably indicate mechanical intestinal obstruction (Fig. 27-5). This pattern usually appears within 12 hours of the onset of symptoms. Air fluid levels throughout both large and small bowel indicate adynamic (paralytic) ileus.

Plain films of the abdomen may also show free air in the peritoneal cavity (from perforation of a hollow viscus), calculi in the biliary or renal areas, fecaliths, tumors, or radiopaque foreign bodies. Barium enemas help to localize the area of colon obstruction. In suspected cases of obstruction, radiologists use oral barium cautiously because of the threat of inspissation of the barium above the obstruction.

Blood studies. Elevations in the hemoglobin and hematocrit commonly indicate dehydration and hemoconcentration. The white blood count is usually elevated, with a shift to the left, especially with strangulation obstruction.

Urinalysis. A high specific gravity and ketonuria indicate a common complication of intestinal obstruction: dehydration and fluid sequestration. Adynamic ileus may be caused by *diabetic acidosis* or *primary renal disease*. Glycosuria or proteinuria (with abnormal cellular elements in the urine) should always indicate the possibility of these diseases.

Blood chemistry. Amylase may be slightly elevated in intestinal obstruction. Usually, electrolyte determinations guide preoperative fluid replacement (see Chap. 3).

PARALYTIC ILEUS (ADYNAMIC ILEUS, NEUROGENIC ILEUS)

In evolutionary terms *paralytic ileus* is a protective mechanism that "splints" the gastrointestinal tract after abdominal injury. It prevents the muscular contractions of the gastrointestinal tract from continuously pouring out noxious bowel contents into the peritoneal cavity after a hollow viscus is perforated, thus allowing the perforation to seal.

Etiology

Four general causative mechanisms for paralytic ileus are as follows:

Direct peritoneal irritation from any source: acute cholecystitis, pancreatitis, appendicitis, perforation of a hollow viscus, or any abdominal operation (this is the commonest cause).
Extraperitoneal irritation: pneumonitis, hemorrhage, fractured ribs or spine, trauma to retroperitoneal nerves, renal lesions, etc.
Systemic imbalances: infections, electrolyte imbalance, shock, myxedema, Addison's disease, uremia, diabetes, or porphyria.
Neurogenic disorders: spinal cord lesions, severe strokes, or central nervous system trauma.

Bowel sounds are absent, and gas appears scattered throughout the gastrointestinal tract (Fig. 27-6). Nasogastric suction, correction of the mechanisms causing the paralytic ileus, and parenteral fluid replacement are the cornerstones of treatment.

Colonic ileus (Ogilvie's syndrome) is commonly seen in association with other diseases and may complicate the postoperative course of patients who have undergone other abdominal operations. Massive colonic dilation, particularly of the cecum, is typical and may lead to perforation. Diagnosis of this condition can be made by abdominal plain films or Gastrografin enema if mechanical obstruction is suspected. Initial treatment involves nasogastric intubation and correction of any fluid or electrolyte imbalances. Colonscopic decompression should be undertaken if the diameter of the cecum approaches or exceeds 12 cm. Such

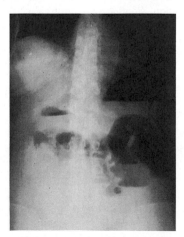
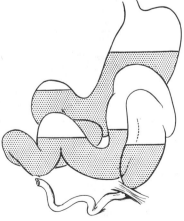

Fig. 27-5. Mechanical bowel obstruction. Localized air-fluid levels seen on upright film of abdomen. Diagram shows dilated proximal bowel and stomach, air-fluid levels, and adhesive band causing obstruction.

treatment is successful in about 75% of patients. Alternatively, operative tube cecostomy may be performed.

DIFFERENTIAL DIAGNOSIS
Simple Versus Strangulation Obstruction

Since strangulation obstruction requires immediate operative treatment, the physican must constantly look for these five diagnostic features: when intermittent, colicky pain becomes steady and unrelenting; when abdominal tenderness (and rebound) become evident; when a mass becomes palpable; when the temperature and pulse increase; and when laboratory studies suggest acute inflammation. In brief, the "warm" abdomen changes dramatically to the hot abdomen when strangulation of the bowel occurs. Diagnostic laparotomy is a certain method for determining strangulation obstruction in the difficult diagnostic case.

Mechanical Obstruction Versus Paralytic Ileus

In *paralytic ileus* an obvious cause of the ileus is usually evident, such as acute peritonitis from appendicitis, pancreatitis, cholecystitis, gastroenteritis, abdominal surgery, pneumonitis, or trauma (Figs. 27-5 and 27-6). The abdomen is silent. When the cause of the ileus is not associated with peritonitis, the abdomen is painless and nontender. The radiograph of paralytic ileus shows gas distributed evenly throughout the large and small bowel (Fig. 27-6). Radiographs of the abdomen are not infallible, however. Because any condition that causes peritonitis also causes some degree of paralytic ileus, these abdominal disorders mimic strangulation obstruction. The abdominal films are usually the only objective method, other than a diagnostic laparotomy, for differentiating paralytic ileus (associated with peritonitis) from strangulation obstruction (Table 27-1).

Small Bowel Versus Large Bowel Obstruction

Differentiating colon from small bowel obstruction depends on radiographic evidence, either plain abdominal films or barium enema demonstration of an obstructing lesion of the colon. Differentiation is important so that the patient (and the family) can be prepared for a colostomy, if it is necessary. Clinical localization, though less accurate, is also possible. Obstruction in an older patient with no hernia or history or previous abdominal operations and with distension and no vomiting, usually indicates carcinoma of the large bowel. Sharp frequent abdominal cramps, severe vomiting, and early fluid and electrolyte imbalance are suggestive of small bowel obstruction.

PATHOPHYSIOLOGY

Simple intestinal obstruction causes death, if untreated, because of two factors: *distension* of the bowel proximal to the obstruction and *dehydration*.

Distension

Distention of the proximal bowel constantly threatens ischemia of the involved bowel wall. Violent contractions of the proximal bowel wall attempting to force bowel contents past the obstruction ultimately cause edema of the bowel wall. An edematous bowel wall loses some of its absorptive capacity while secretions (and edema fluid) increase. Anxiety, pain, and nausea cause increased aerophagia (air is mostly nitrogen, which is poorly absorbed). Thus intraluminal pressure (both gas and fluid) builds up to the point where it compresses the small vessels in the bowel wall, and eventually it exceeds the capillary perfusion pressure. Consequent ischemia causes further edema and results in bowel wall necrosis, perforation, and peritonitis. As this final phase approaches, the edematous, stretched, and thinned bowel wall loses its power to contract. The

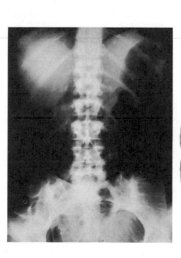
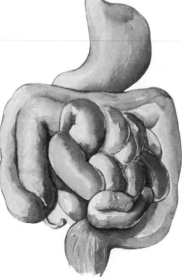

Fig. 27-6. Paralytic ileus. Upright film of abdomen shows dilated small and large intestine. Gas is scattered diffusely throughout intestinal tract. Diagram shows diffuse intestinal dilatation.

Table 27-1. Comparison of Paralytic Ileus and Mechanical Obstruction

	Paralytic Ileus	Mechanical Obstruction
Cause	Peritoneal irritation Extraperitoneal irritation Neurogenic disorders Metabolic disorders	Hernia Adhesions Tumors Volvulus Intussusception Obturation Inflammation
Site	Entire bowel is dilated	Dilatation proximal to obstruction
Clinical findings	Distension, vomiting, obstipation; silent abdomen; abdomen may or may not be tender	Crampy pain, distension, vomiting, obstipation, hyperactive bowel sounds at first; later bowel may be silent
X-ray findings	Gas throughout (Fig. 27-6)	Gas and fluid proximal to obstruction No gas distal to obstruction (Fig. 27-5)
Treatment	Conservative with treatment of the cause of the ileus	Operative release or bypass of the obstruction
Prognosis	Usually good after correction of cause; strangulation and perforation are rarely a threat	Strangulation or perforation constant threat until obstruction relieved

patient no longer complains of cramping pains, and the abdomen is forebodingly silent. Thus every case of simple obstruction will ultimately become "self-strangulating" obstruction if proximal bowel distension is not relieved.

Dehydration

Dehydration occurs rapidly because oral intake is impossible and water and electrolytes are lost by vomiting, increased net secretions from the gastrointestinal tract (because the reabsorptive power of the mucosa is impaired), and edema of the bowel wall with transudation into the peritoneal cavity.

As strangulation approaches, bacteria and their toxins escape into the peritoneal cavity, causing edema of the parietal peritoneum, venous thrombosis with more anoxia, and eventually endotoxic shock. When strangulation precipitates the bacterial phase of intestinal obstruction, all the lethal effects of diffuse peritonitis are suddenly superimposed on an already critically ill patient. The mortality is understandably high.

TREATMENT OF MECHANICAL BOWEL OBSTRUCTION

The treatment of bowel obstruction is keyed to the pathophysiologic developments, but in *reverse order*. *Dehydration* and *proximal bowel distension* initiated by the obstruction must be treated first, and the obstruction is relieved subsequently.

Dehydration

Severe dehydration poses the serious threat of hypovolemia and shock, which threat is heightened by the vasodilator effect of anesthetics, which causes further decrease in circulating blood volume. Thus replacement of these abnormal fluid losses is a vital first step in the treatment of bowel obstruction. In estimating the amount of replacement fluids, the physician must realize that obstructed patients lose fluids from increased net secretions into the bowel lumen, transudation, edema (bowel wall, mesentery), and vomiting. When signs of shock appear in advanced stages of bowel ob-

struction in the adult, the patient has lost at least 5 or 6 L of fluid.

Proximal Bowel Distension

Intestinal intubation with suction to remove accumulated gas and fluid keynotes the treatment of bowel distension. Surgeons use nasogstric tubes, long intestinal tubes, or tubes inserted directly (at laparotomy) to decompress the distended gastrointestinal tract.

Nasogastric-Tube Versus Long-Tube Decompression

In proximal small bowel obstruction nasogastric suction is adequate to relieve intestinal distension. In lower obstructions many surgeons cite the advantage of the long intestinal tube, which more completely decompresses the dilated loops of bowel, thus decreasing pressure on the stretched and edematous bowel wall. Subsequent operative correction of the obstruction is aided by the flattened, decompressed small bowel. Several long and trying hours may be required to pass a long tube into the lower small bowel, so other surgeons favor nasogastric intubation with immediate operative decompression and removal of the obstruction.

Intestinal Intubation as Definitive Treatment

In a minority of instances long-tube decompression may relieve intestinal obstructions completely (usually those caused by adhesions). This treatment requires several days of suction and intravenous feedings (and immobility) to be certain that the obstruction is relieved. During this treatment, the threat of recurrent obstruction constantly plagues both surgeon and patient. Because of the hardship and uncertainty of this treatment, most surgeons lack enthusiasm for the conservative treatment of mechanical bowel obstruction.

Removal of the Obstruction—Operative Treatment

The final goal in treating mechanical bowel obstruction is removal of the obstruction. Strangulating or potentially strangulating lesions (hernia, volvulus, intussusception in older patients, and complete obstruction because of adhesions or closed-loop obstructions) demand emergent operative treatment. With partial or early obstructions, the surgeon has valuable time for diagnostic studies.

SMALL BOWEL OBSTRUCTIONS

Since most small bowel obstructions are extrinsic, the surgeon can easily lyse adhesions or reduce hernias. If the small bowel is necrotic, he can safely resect it, since the small bowel is relatively sterile. Bypass operations (enteroenterostomies or enterocolostomies) are useful in complicated situations such as multiple dense adhesions in critically ill patients. To prevent recurrent obstructions, some surgeons pass a long tube with an inflatable balloon (Baker tube) into the proximal jejunum and manipulate it to the cecum. It serves as an internal stent to allow adhesions to form without sharp kinking of the small bowel.

LARGE BOWEL OBSTRUCTIONS

The majority of large bowel obstructions (in contrast to those of the small bowel) are caused by intrinsic lesions (cancer or diverticulitis). Most obstructions of the colon occur in the sigmoid area because this is the most common site for both cancers and diverticulitis, and the sigmoid lumen is smaller and the feces more solid than in the more proximal colon.

Closed Loop Obstructions

Because the ileocecal valve is competent in about 50% to 60% of all people, closed loop obstructions constitute a similar percentage of all large bowel obstructions. Radiographs of the abdomen show gross dilation of the colon between the one-way cecal valve and the obstructing lesion. Immediate operative decompression key-notes the treatment. Foolish reliance on long-tube decompression of the small bowel may cause a deadly delay. Mounting gas pressure from putrefaction within the closed loop will eventually burst through the thinned bowel wall (usually the cecum) contaminating the peritoneal cavity with toxic bowel content.

Incompetent Ileocecal Valve Obstruction

When the ileocecal valve permits regurgitation, the distal obstruction differs very little clinically from a low small bowel obstruction. Barium study of the distal colon will usually detect the colonic site of obstruction.

Large Bowel Decompression

Because the large bowel teems with bacteria and the weakened colon wall holds sutures poorly, primary anastomosis is always hazardous (Chap. 26). (Infection jeopardizes any anatomosis.) Proximal colostomy is a safe and simple procedure, decompressing the bowel and totally bypassing gas and feces through the abdominal wall. Cecostomy differs from colostomy in providing only a vent through the abdominal wall; it does not provide a bypass for all cecal contents.

In certain cases when sufficient mesentery provides adequate mobility, the colon lesions may be exteriorized and removed (obstructive resection). The proximal and distal portions of the colon remain above the skin and may subsequently be reunited.

28

Anorectum

Richard D. Liechty

Anatomy
Physiology
Examination
Diseases of the Anorectum

In terms of physical agony (from painful anorectal disorders) or mental anguish (from concern with bowel function or cancer) the anorectum assumes an importance that belies its insignificant anatomic status (e.g., hemorrhoids are one of the commonest of all human ailments). The pain from one small, thrombosed, external hemorrhoid can completely overwhelm an otherwise healthy person. In our cancer-conscious generation, fresh blood on the toilet paper or a lump appearing at the anus sends patients trembling to their physicians, even though both signs often result from simple hemorrhoids. The anorectum, the site of a variety of disorders (both simple and complex), is an area of understandable patient concern.

ANATOMY

Pertinent anatomic points are shown in Figs. 28-1 and 28-2: The anatomic *key* to the anorectum is the *pectinate line*. Above it pain sensation is absent, blood drains to the portal and caval systems, and lymph drains along the superior rectal vessels or lateral to the obturator or iliac nodes. *Below* the pectinate line, pain is notably present, blood drains to the inferior vena cava, and lymph drains to the inguinal nodes. *Anal glands* empty into anal crypts at the pectinate line. When obstructed or infected, these glands become the source of abscesses and fistulas.

PHYSIOLOGY

When the rectosigmoid colon distends with feces, autonomic nerve impulses stimulate the colon to contract involuntarily, forcing the feces toward the anus. Voluntary relaxation of the tonically contracted puborectalis and external sphincter muscles permits this passage.

Chronic or injudicious use of laxatives thwarts this

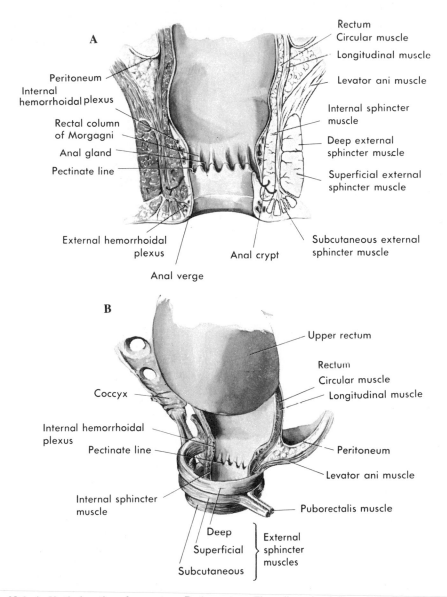

A, Peritoneum
Internal hemorrhoidal plexus
Rectal column of Morgagni
Anal gland
Pectinate line

Rectum
Circular muscle
Longitudinal muscle
Levator ani muscle
Internal sphincter muscle
Deep external sphincter muscle
Superficial external sphincter muscle

External hemorrhoidal plexus
Anal crypt
Subcutaneous external sphincter muscle

Anal verge

B, Coccyx
Internal hemorrhoidal plexus
Pectinate line
Internal sphincter muscle

Upper rectum
Rectum
Circular muscle
Longitudinal muscle
Peritoneum
Levator ani muscle
Puborectalis muscle

Deep
Superficial
Subcutaneous

External sphincter muscles

Fig. 28-1. A, Vertical section of anorectum. **B,** Anorectum. Three-dimensional diagram showing relationship of external sphincter to internal sphincter; notice that superficial portion of external sphincter inserts into both coccyx and pubis.

remarkably efficient mechanism by stimulating the colon when the rectum is not distended with feces. This process, repeated many times, results in temporary loss of the natural response. Thus habitual laxative (or enema) use becomes physiologically disrupting in the vain effort to "regulate" (or coerce) bowel movements.

When laxatives liquefy the stool, another disruption occurs. Normal stools (the consistency and shape of bananas) gently compress the anal canal, "milking" the anal glands and crypts. Chronically liquid stools lack this milking effect. Thus liquid stools bathe the crypts and glands with bacteria; chronic cryptitis and anal gland infection result. The increased frequency of anal disease in patients who practice chronic self-purgation is, we are convinced, more than coincidental.

Regular bowel movements are the result of balanced diet, exercise, adequate fluid intake, and heed to nature's demands. Laxatives and enemas for constipation in an otherwise healthy person should be condemned for what they are—nostrums.

EXAMINATION

In no other area of the body is a physical examination more important than in the anus and rectum. For complete examination, three important elements are good illumination, proper positioning, and patient cooperation.

Inspection of the perianal area can yield much information. Excoriations from scratching (in pruritus), fissures, external fistulas, external hemorrhoids, abscesses, and occasionally tumors can be seen.

Digital examination of the rectum should be an inte-

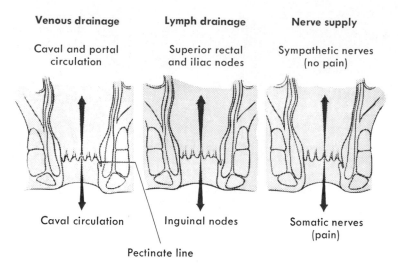

Venous drainage

Caval and portal circulation

Caval circulation

Pectinate line

Lymph drainage

Superior rectal and iliac nodes

Inguinal nodes

Nerve supply

Sympathetic nerves (no pain)

Somatic nerves (pain)

Fig. 28-2. Pectinate line marks important differences in nerve supply, venous drainage, and lymph drainage.

gral part of all physical examinations except when pre-empted by pain (anal fissure). In this situation the digital examination is performed with anesthesia or is deferred until acute inflammation subsides. Sphincter tone, prostate size, point tenderness, extrinsic or intrinsic rectal masses, pelvic hernias, or a "rectal shelf" (tumor deposits in the cul-de-sac) is noted. Remember that *many malignant large bowel tumors can be palpated by rectal examination.* A specimen of stool from the examining finger is immediately available for testing for occult blood.

Anoscopy is carried out simply and without prior enemas. The diseases of the anorectum that can be observed or palpated are discussed below. (Sigmoidoscopy is discussed in Chapt. 26.)

DISEASES OF THE ANORECTUM
Hemorrhoids

Internal hemorrhoids are dilated veins of the superior and middle rectal plexuses that occur above the dentate line and underlie mucosa. *External hemorrhoids* are dilated inferior rectal veins that lie below the dentate line and are covered by squamous epithelium. Factors that increase pressure in these venous systems are theoretically responsible for development of hemorrhoids. The common ones are constipation, straining at stool, hereditary varicose tendencies, pregnancy, prolonged upright position, abdominal or pelvic tumors, and portal hypertension. Chronic anal infection from colitis and ileitis, or chronic laxative use may also dilate the vein walls by causing chronic cryptitis and anal vein phlebitis with consequent dilation.

Bleeding, protrusion, dull pain, and *pruritus* (in any combination) characterize uncomplicated hemorrhoids. Thrombosis or acute prolapse (with edema or ulceration) is exquisitely painful. Toxic symptoms may accompany acute episodes.

The diagnosis is usually obvious from inspection, but diagnostic efforts must *always* include barium studies and sigmoidoscopy to rule out other large bowel disease. Many patients with colon cancer have had

hemorrhoidectomies *shortly before* the cancer was diagnosed.

Treatment. The three common indications for hemorrhoidectomy are *pain, prolapse,* and *bleeding.* Since most adults eventually develop hemorrhoids, excision is advised only when symptoms warrant the risk and inconvenience.

Treatment of an acutely thrombosed external hemorrhoid is incision and evacuation of the painful clot, followed by warm sitz baths. Small internal hemorrhoids may be injected with a sclerosing solution with good success. This promotes microthrombi formation and ultimate fibrosis of the hemorrhoid. Sodium morrhuate and 5% phenol in oil are commonly used solutions for injection. Rubber band ligation of internal hemorrhoids is now the preferred treatment.

Larger external hemorrhoids and internal hemorrhoids, that are symptomatic are sometimes excised. All methods of hemorrhoid removal have the same goal: complete removal of the hemorhoids with preservation of an intact, functional anus.

After hemorrhoidectomy an important problem is pain control. Pain followed by perianal muscle spasm induces many postoperative complications, such as urinary retention, constipation, fecal impaction, and pulmonary difficulties caused by immobilization. Pain is alleviated by warm, moist packs, adequate analgesia, sitz baths, and maintenance of a soft stool. Gentle daily digital dilation for several days promotes normal healing and discourages stenosis.

Anal Fissure

Anal fissures are slitlike ulcers in the anal mucosa. They are, of course, always infected. The commonest causes are (1) trauma, usually from passage of hard stools, (2) cryptitis, in which the anal crypts become inflamed and subsequently develop a mucosal break that extends distally, and (3) ulceration of mucosa over a thrombosed hemorrhoid. Spasms of the anal sphincters help sustain anal fissures by decreasing blood flow.

These fissures occur most frequently in the posterior

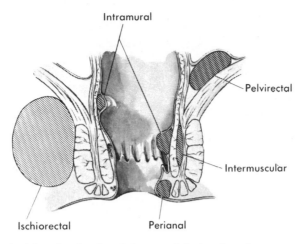

Intramural

Pelvirectal

Intermuscular

Ischiorectal   Perianal

Fig. 28-3. Location of pelvirectal and perirectal abscesses. Infections in anal crypts are usual source.

midline. A "sentinel tag," a small projection of skin, usually lies just below and marks the fissure.

Severe pain on defecation and blood-streaked stools characterize anal fissures. The anus is, of course, very sensitive to digital examination.

Anal fissures are treated conservatively by scrupulous anal hygiene, hot sitz baths, and stool softeners. If the fissure fails to heal within 3 weeks, *sphincter dilation* (under anesthesia), *fissurectomy*, and *partial sectioning* of the *internal sphincter* or the *external sphincter* (subcutaneous portion) are the operative options. These procedures used alone or in combination are advocated with varying degrees of enthusiasm. They have in common relaxation of the sphincter mechanism. We prefer partial division of the internal sphincter. With sphincter muscle spasm relieved, stool passage is easier, which aids healing. Complicated fissures occasionally progress to abscesses, fistulas, or anal stenosis.

Anorectal Abscesses and Fistulas

Since fistulas are the result of perianal abscesses, these diseases are discussed together. *Perianal abscesses* almost invariably result from infected anal glands that erode into underlying tissues. Chronic use of purgatives, regional enteritis, and ulcerative colitis have liquid stools in common as a probable causative factor. Uncommon infections (actinomycosis, tuberculosis, other fungal diseases), pelvic inflammatory disease, prostatitis, and cancer may rarely be associated.

Fig. 28-3 shows the common locations of these abscesses. Opinions vary as to frequency of occurrence in various anatomic sites. The ischiorectal abscess is probably the most common.

Early symptoms of dull rectal aching and mild systemic complaints progress to severe, throbbing perianal pain with fever, chills, and malaise. A fluctuant, "pointing" area is not always apparent because of the thick perianal skin. Redness, tenderness, and generalized bulging are the usual findings. Prompt incision and drainage *without* waiting for fluctuation (as in other subcutaneous infections) can prevent serious extensions. We have seen mutilating extensions that involved thighs, scrotum, and even the abdominal wall.

Because of severe pain, general or regional anesthesia is preferable, but some surgeons drain perirectal abscesses under local anesthesia.

Supralevator abscesses. Supralevator abscesses are uncommon. Anal gland infections and pelvic or intraperitoneal infections engender these abscesses.

Intramural abscesses. Intramural abscesses cause little discomfort since the bowel wall has no pain sensation. They are drained through a sigmoidoscope. Pelvirectal abscesses are drained through the skin. Drains are always brought out through external incisions.

Perirectal fistulas. After drainage, most perirectal abscesses eventually heal with no sequelae, but those that fail to heal primarily evolve into fistulas. The external opening may close temporarily only to reopen when pus accumulates in the tract, and eventually the tract becomes lined with epithelium. Multiple openings ("pepper pot anus") complicate some cases. Extensions to the urinary tract, perineal area, thighs, or bone may occasionally occur.

Usually the fistulous tract follows a variable course, but a few general rules are available for simplification: The primary or internal opening is usually found in one of the anal crypts. Most lie at one side or the other of the posterior midline. If the cutaneous opening is anterior to a *transverse* line drawn through the anus, the internal opening is on a radial line directly into the anorectum. If the cutaneous opening is posterior to the line, the internal opening will probably be in the posterior midline (Fig. 28-4, *A*).

Symptoms are usually confined to intermittent swelling, drainage, pruritus, and varying discomfort. The history of an abscess is of obvious help in the diagnosis.

The cutaneous opening is characteristically a slightly raised, gray-pink papule of granulation tissue. In time scarring along the tract becomes palpable. A probe can sometimes be passed through the fistula to the pectinate line. This is ordinarily not painful. Common courses of anal fistulas are shown in Fig. 28-4, *B*.

Simple, early fistulas are incised with saucerization (excision of the overhanging margins) of the tract. In severely scarred fistulas, excision of the tract, leaving

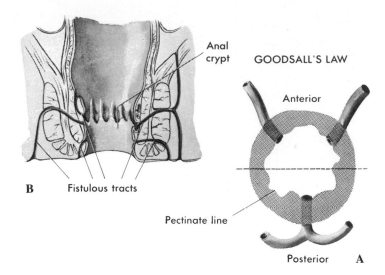

Fig. 28-4. A, Anorectal fistulas. Location of external fistulous opening is key to position of internal opening. **B,** Common courses of anorectal fistulas tracts. Internal (primary) opening is almost always in crypt; fistulas are usually single and involve only portions of sphincter muscles; multiple fistulas or fistulas that involve all external sphincter muscles are less common.

the skin open, is the best method of removal. In either case the internal opening must be obliterated or the fistula will recur. If the fistula follows a course that necessitates cutting of the sphincter, the incision must traverse the muscle fibers perpendicularly and *at only one level*; none of the muscle should be removed.

If the fistula is the result of carcinoma, tuberculosis, Crohn's disease, or mucosal colitis, the primary disease must of course receive treatment priority. Most surgeons are extremely reluctant to perform anorectal operations on patients with mucosal colitis or Crohn's disease because of local recurrence with failure of wound healing.

Pruritus Ani

Pruritus ani, intense itching of the perianal area, is a symptom, not a disease. Common and frequently dibilitating, it offers a constant therapeutic challenge. A busy general practitioner will see numerous patients every month with this complaint.

A classification of etiologic factors is listed below:

Surgical
  Hemorrhoids
  Fissures
  Fistulas
  Prolapse
  Cryptitis
  Neoplasm
Nonsurgical
  Local
    Dermatitis, bacteria, fungal, contact
    Pinworms
    Antibiotic irritation
Systemic
  Jaundice
  Diabetes
  Psoriasis
  Syphilis
  Seborrheic dermatitis
  Leukemia
Idiopathic
  Including psychophysiologic

With such a broad spectrum of causes, the necessity for cultures and other pertinent laboratory tests is obvious.

Treatment. Underlying anatomic factors are treated surgically (fissures, fistulas, hemorrhoids, or neoplasm). Similarly, in systemic conditions such as diabetes or jaundice or with local irritants and infestations such as antibiotics or pinworms the offending cause is specifically treated. "Smothering" symptoms with local treatments (for specific disorders) is unacceptable.

Even after extensive search the cause of pruritus ani often remains elusive. Idiopathic pruritus accounts for approximately half of the patients seen. The single common denominator in all patients with this complaint is feces being excreted through the anus and thus perianal fecal irritation. Immaculate perianal hygiene alone will often relieve the itching. The perianal area should be washed with water and dried with cotton or a soft cotton cloth. Cornstarch applications help to keep the area dry. Hydrocortisone ointment, 1%, is nonspecific but usually helpful. Many patients suffer from anxiety states.

Subcutaneous alcohol injections, radiation therapy, and presacral neurectomy are heroic treatments reserved for a few patients with truly intractable pruritus ani.

Prolapse of the Rectum

The three types of rectal prolapse (Fig. 28-5) are: mucosal prolapse, rectal intussusception, and true prolapse.

Mucosal prolapse (see Fig. 28-5, *B*) occurs with an intact sphincter and involves extrusion through the anus of *rectal mucosa* only. The remainder of the wall is not involved. It becomes symptomatic because of irritation, and occasionally ulceration, of the prolapsed tissue. Soiling results from mucosal secretions. This condition is common in infancy (theoretically because of the lack of sacral curvature) and in the aged. Infant pro-

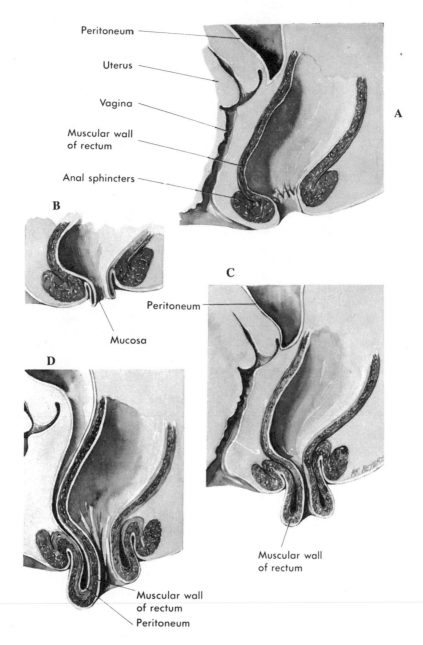

Fig. 28-5. Rectal prolapse. **A,** Normal. **B,** Mucosal prolapse most common type of prolapse; mucosa shows radial folds. **C,** Rectal intussusception; all layers of rectal wall prolapse—peritoneum does not. **D,** True prolapse; all layers of rectal wall prolapse; peritoneum descends as hernial sac anteriorly. Both C and D show concentric folds from accordion-like effect of mucosa that has not been depicted.

lapse almost invariably disappears by 5 years of age. In the adult, radial incisions, similar to hemorrhoidectomy incisions, result in scarring, which holds redundant mucosa in place.

Rectal intussusception (see Fig. 28-5, *C*) involves protrusion of the entire rectal wall without a peritoneal sac. It starts above the pectinate line. The palpable full-thickness wall in the prolapsed portion and *concentric* folds distinguish it from nucosal prolapse. A sulcus can be palpated along the periphery of the prolapsed part of the anal ring that is not present in true prolapse.

True prolapse (Fig. 28-5, *D*) occurs by herniation of the pelvic peritoneum through the pelvic diaphragm, the anterior rectal wall, and the anus. Anal sphincter tone is poor. True prolapse occurs mainly in infants, men in their twenties or thirties, and woman at any age. In men it probably represents a congenital weakness because the prostate and seminal vesicles lend adequate support anteriorly to prevent herniation.

Several operations have been devised for correction of intussusception and true prolapse, and, as is usually the case when several operations are used for a particular condition, all leave something to be desired. The operations that give the best results utilize obliteration

Table 28-1. Venereal Diseases

Type	Cause	Diagnosis	Treatment
Lymphogranuloma venereum	Virus	Frei test; biopsy	Noneffective
Condylomata acuminata	Virus	Biopsy; multiple warts	Podophyllin (25%) electrocautery
Syphilis	Spirochetes	Biopsy; dark-field examination	Penicillin Other antibiotics
Gonorrhea	Bacteria	Smear; intracellular diplococci	Penicillin

of the peritoneal sac, shortening and fixation of the rectosigmoid colon, and approximation of the levator ani muscles.

Specific infections

Specific infections of the anorectum are uncommon yet must be remembered when sinus tracts, ulcers, or tumors appear that defy the usual categorization or treatment. The venereal diseases listed in Table 28-1 may be the offenders in such instances.

Anorectal Tumors

Basal cell carcinomas and *melanoma* of the anus are curiosities treated by wide excision (as in other parts of the body) with or without preoperative irradiation. *Epidermoid carcinoma* of the anus occurs in the elderly, is associated with chronic infection (an excellent reason for biopsy of chronic lesions), and metastasizes to pelvic and inguinal nodes. (Inguinal nodes are also involved with anal infections.) Radical abdominoperineal resection with resection of involved inguinal lymph nodes (or, in low, early lesions, conservative resection) appears to offer about the same 5-year survival as rectal adenocarcinoma.

Pilonidal Sinus

Although it does not arise from the anorectum, pilonidal disease often enters the differential diagnosis of anorectal diseases; it can mimic anorectal abscesses or fistulas.

As the name suggests, a nidus of hair is almost invariably found within these sinus tracts. Almost all the hairs enter the sinus *root end first*. Hair scales pointing away from the root end (like feathers on an arrow) apparently are driven inward by a rolling action between the buttocks. Hair *follicles* or other skin appendages are *never* found within the sinus walls. These lesions occur in the intergluteal region of young hirsute males, and less commonly in females. Pilonidal disease is common in young military personnel. It almost never occurs in person 45 years of age or older. An analogous pilonidal sinus of indriven hairs occasionally afflicts the hands of barbers.

Infection with rupture through the skin (which forms sinuses), chronicity, and recurrence keynote the problem. Simple incision and drainage of infected cysts and excision with open healing of chronic sinuses have evolved, since World War II, as the most prudent treatment. Excision with primary closure is preferrred by some surgeons.

III

Surgical Specialties

29

Thoracic and Pulmonary Surgery

John H. Lemmer, Jr.
Nicholas P. Rossi

The spectrum of general thoracic surgery ranges from rare congenital deformities of the chest wall to the operative management of the leading cause of cancer death today, lung cancer. Contained within the thorax are the pleura, lungs and airways, mediastinum, and esophagus, each of which may be affected by inflammatory, neoplastic, functional, or traumatic disorders that require surgical intervention. This chapter outlines the more common thoracic disorders encountered by thoracic surgeons, the indications for surgery, and the prognosis of these diseases.

CHEST WALL

Congenital Malformations of the Chest Wall

Pectus Excavatum

The most common congenital chest wall abnormality is pectus excavatum, a depression of the sternum (Figs. 29-1 and 29-2). In patients with this defect, the lower costal cartilages turn posteriorly to join the depressed sternum but the rest of the thoracic wall develops normally. With growth, the mediastinal structures are displaced to the left, and the deformity becomes asymmetric, the depression being angulated to the right side. This developmental abnormality is more common in boys than girls and tends to run in families. Although uncommon in the general population, pectus excavatum does occur with increased frequency in patients with Marfan's syndrome.

Although the mediastinal structures are displaced to the left, surprisingly, impairment of cardiopulmonary function is minimal and the great majority of patients

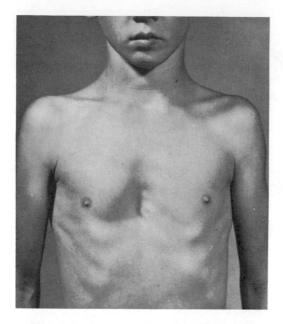

Fig. 29-1. Pectus excavatum, preoperative appearance.

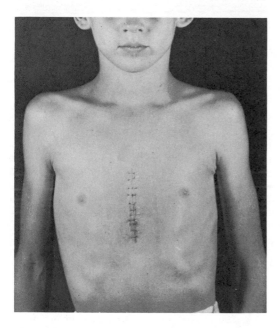

Fig. 29-2. Pectus excavatum, postoperative appearance.

are asymptomatic. Occasionally a patient with a severe deformity demonstrates significant physiologic changes (detected by pulmonary function studies and cardiac catheterization). Patients with mild and nonprogressive abnormalities may not require therapy, and the most frequent indication for surgical repair is to improve the cosmetic appearance of the chest and, as a result, the patient's self-image. There are several alternatives for surgical repair of pectus excavatum, but the most frequently performed techniques are based on that devised by M. M. Ravitch. In brief, this procedure in-

volves removing the deformed costal cartilages (subperichondrially), releasing the sternum from its xiphoid and intercostal bundle attachments, and lifting the sternum to a more anterior position (usually with the aid of an osteotomy). The risks of surgery for this condition are minimal, and the results are generally good.

Pectus carinatum (pigeon breast) is a protrusion deformity caused by anterior displacement and bulging of the sternum with associated deformity of the costal cartilages. Physiologic impairment is rare and most patients are asymptomatic. As in the case of pectus excavatum, operation is indicated most frequently for cosmetic reasons.

Neoplasms of the Chest Wall
General Considerations

Chest wall tumors are unusual lesions that account for less than 1% of all neoplasms. About one half of all thoracic wall tumors are benign, and the most common malignant tumor of the thoracic wall is metastasis from a distant primary site. Nearly all tumors arising in the sternum are malignant. Chest wall tumors in children are more likely to be malignant than those in adults. Most of these tumors present as painful masses and the various tumor types can have characteristic radiographic appearances. Excisional biopsy is nearly always indicated without prior needle biopsy to avoid problems with diagnostic accuracy (because of the small amount of tissue obtained by needle) and the potential for seeding the needle track with malignant cells. All chest wall tumors should be considered malignant until proved benign. If, at operation, the tumor is found to be malignant, wide excision of a margin of normal-looking tissue surrounding the tumor (often with a portion of the rib above and the rib below the lesion and complete removal of the involved rib) is performed. Significant chest wall defects can be reconstructed by the transposition of muscle flaps, such as the latissimus dorsi, or by the placement of prosthetic materials.

Benign Chest Wall Tumors

The most common benign chest wall tumor is fibrous dysplasia, which most often occurs on the posterior or lateral aspect of the involved rib. This lesion may be solitary or may be associated with fibrous dysplasia of the long bones and skull. The tumors usually are not painful. Resection is generally performed to rule out malignancy. Chondromas, the second most common chest wall tumor, are most frequently located anteriorly and should be completely excised to prevent local recurrence, progressive painful enlargement, and malignant degeneration. Eosinophilic granulomas are benign neoplasms that often occur as part of a collection of disorders of the reticuloendothelial system and may be associated with lesions in other bones (especially the skull) and with systemic symptoms.

Malignant Chest Wall Tumors

More than 50% of malignant chest wall tumors are chondrosarcomas. These tumors tend to occur in middle-aged persons, are most frequently anterior in location, and arise near the costochondral junction (Fig. 29-3). Because of their propensity to recur locally and to

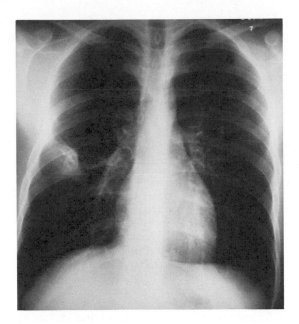

Fig. 29-3. Chondrosarcoma of rib.

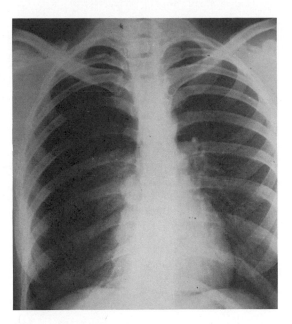

Fig. 29-4. Spontaneous right pneumothorax; lung about 60% collapsed by pleural air.

metastasize after several recurrences, radical resection en-bloc should be performed with chest wall reconstruction. Early complete removal may result in more than 70% 5-year survival in patients with this malignancy. Other less common primary chest wall malignant tumors include malignant fibrous histiocytomas, rhabdomyosarcomas, and osteogenic sarcomas. Solitary myelomas may occur in the rib but most frequently are associated with Bence-Jones proteins in the urine, abnormal plasma protein electrophoresis, and bone marrow involvement. If myeloma is suspected, limited incisional biopsy followed by radiation and systemic therapy is preferred to excisional biopsy.

THE PLEURAL SPACE

The pleural spaces normally contain only a thin film of serous fluid, which is the result of the negative pressure (-5 cm H_2O) present within each pleural space. The parietal and visceral pleural membranes possess a mesothelial cell layer that has absorptive abilities.

Thoracentesis and Tube Thoracostomy

Two procedures utilized commonly in the management of pleural space problems are thoracentesis and tube thoracostomy. Thoracentesis is simply needle aspiration of the pleural cavity. Under sterile conditions, with local anesthesia, a needle is introduced between ribs, the location of which is determined by the nature of the substance to be removed. To remove air in the pleural space (pneumothorax), the second or third intercostal space is appropriate. For the patient with pleural fluid to be drained, a lower intercostal space is commonly utilized. If the fluid is loculated or localized, radiographic examination of the chest or fluoroscopy should guide placement of the needle. Portions of the fluid should be sent for cytologic examination, bacterial culture, and antibiotic sensitivity, pH, protein content, glucose level, and other biochemical determinations.

Tube thoracostomy is the placement of a tube into the pleural space for removal of air and/or fluid to allow for full lung expansion. Performed aseptically with local anesthesia, placement of the tube is usually guided by radiographic studies demonstrating the location of the material to be drained. Conventional radiography, computed tomography (CT), fluoroscopy, and sonography may be utilized for this purpose. The chest tube often is attached to underwater seal suction drainage to aid in full expansion of the lung within the hemithorax.

Spontaneous Pneumothorax

Spontaneous introduction of air into the pleural space with varying degrees of lung collapse occurs as the result of lung bleb rupture. These thin-walled air spaces that can burst without warning are most frequently located at the apices of the lungs. Spontaneous pneumothorax occurs typically in tall, thin young men and is heralded by the acute onset of chest pain, tachypnea, and tachycardia. A chest film confirms the diagnosis (Fig. 29-4). Treatment depends upon the size of the pneumothorax. Occasionally, very small asymptomatic air collections may be observed with serial radiographs. Drainage by a chest tube (closed tube thoracostomy) is, however, most often required to obtain full lung expansion. This tube may be relatively small in diameter, since only air is being drained, and it is usually attached to underwater seal suction drainage at -20 cm H_2O. The tube is removed 24 hours after cessation of air leakage from the lung.

About one fifth of patients suffer recurrence, and one recurrence makes subsequent recurrences more likely. Thus, for patients with two or more episodes of spontaneous pneumothorax, surgery to create symphysis between the parietal and visceral pleura is recommended. The procedure involves thoracotomy, wedge resection of visible apical blebs, and mechanical abrasion of the pleural surfaces (pleurodesis; Fig. 29-5). This stimulates the formation of adhesions between the pleural membranes, thus preventing the possibility of future pneumothorax.

Tension Pneumothorax

The development of air under pressure in the pleural space is a surgical emergency. Tension pneumothorax occurs most frequently as a result of chest trauma or secondary to underlying lung disease such as emphysema. Air from the lung is forced into the pleural space by the act of respiration but cannot exit because of a flap-valve mechanism that prevents two-way flow. As more air accumulates, the pressure developed becomes greater than atmospheric pressure, causing collapse of the lung on that side. As even higher pressures develop, the mediastinal structures are pushed away from the affected side and impairment of cardiac function occurs, resulting in shock and, if untreated, death. Relief of the pressure by introducing a needle between the ribs into the pleural space can be life saving.

Pleural Effusions

Pleural effusions occur as the result of imbalance between pleural fluid formation and absorption. In general, pleural effusions are divided into two groups based on the character of the fluid. Transudative effusions have a lower protein content, lactate dehydrogenase level, and specific gravity than exudative effusions. Transudative effusions are commonly associated with conditions such as congestive heart failure, renal insufficiency, and liver cirrhosis, whereas exudative effusions occur in conjunction with infections, neoplasms, trauma, and connective tissue disorders.

Malignant pleural effusions are a special problem frequently encountered. Common primary sources are breast cancer, lung cancer, ovarian neoplasms, and lymphomas. Patients with this condition, although they suffer from incurable disease, often live for considerable periods of time and may have symptomatic dyspnea secondary to lung compression caused by the fluid. Repeat needle thoracentesis is often unsuccessful in the

long term, owing to rapid reaccumulation of fluid. Chemical pleurodesis can be accomplished by draining the fluid and instilling a pleural irritant such as tetracycline. This results in the formation of adhesions between the parietal and visceral pleural membranes and obliteration of the pleural space.

Hemothorax

Blood in the pleural space occurs most commonly as a result of trauma. Tube thoracostomy should be performed in all trauma patients suspected of having significant intrathoracic bleeding. This allows for drainage of the blood and monitoring of the bleeding rate. Most frequently, the bleeding is self-limiting, and emergency operation for control is not required. Continued profuse bleeding (over 300 ml/hour for 3 hours) is usually an indication for emergency operation. Chest tube drainage is usually sufficient treatment for traumatic hemothorax. In some cases, insufficient drainage and resorption of the blood clot occurs resulting in the formation of a chronic fibrous peel encasing and restricting the lung. In these patients, an elective thoracotomy and removal of the peel (decortication) may be required.

Empyema

Empyema is the presence of pus in the pleural cavity. It develops as a result of pneumonia, trauma, surgical operation, or, rarely, extension of infection from adjacent regions such as the neck. Diagnosis is based on evidence of systemic illness (fever, leukocytosis) and radiographic changes. Confirmation is made by needle aspiration of the infected fluid, portions of which should be sent for bacteriologic examination and culture and antibiotic sensitivity studies. Oil-based dye can be injected into the empyema cavity to provide details of its anatomic limits and to help plan treatment. Expeditious drainage of an empyema is the keystone of its treatment. The goal of surgery for empyemas is to obtain optimal drainage of the purulent fluid and to allow for full expansion of the lung to obliterate the empyema space. In some cases (particularly postpneumonic empyemas with thin fluid or empyemas in chil-

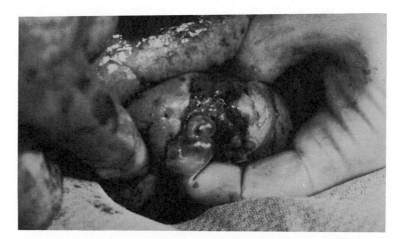

Fig. 29-5. Subpleural bleb, rupture of which produces spontaneous pneumothorax.

dren), tube thoracostomy drainage will be curative. For thick fluid and most postoperative empyemas, resection of a portion of rib at a dependent location and placement of a large-bore soft tube is advisable. For very large and chronic empyemas, other surgical options include empyemectomy, open flap (Eloesser) creation, and decortication. In general, although survival of treated empyema patients depends on the nature of their underlying illness and overall health, failure to provide early and adequate drainage of an empyema may lead to systemic sepsis and death.

Chylothorax

Chylothorax is the presence of chyle in the pleural space, which is most commonly caused by trauma, tumor, or previous operation. Conservative management with tube thoracostomy drainage and dietary manipulation (to decrease lymph flow in the thoracic duct) is often curative. The loss of chyle into the chest tube can be substantial (up to 1 L/day) and may result in serum protein depletion. In such patients, timely thoracotomy is recommended. At operation, the thoracic duct can be ligated at the diaphragm, which is usually curative and has no untoward sequelae. In patients who develop chylothorax "spontaneously" without previous trauma or operation, malignancy is often present, lymphoma being the most common.

Mesothelioma

Although the pleura is a frequent site for metastatic implants from distant malignancies, primary cancer of the pleura is uncommon. By far the most common primary pleural neoplasia is mesothelioma, which occurs in assocation with asbestos exposure. This exposure is usually quite remote, having occurred 15 to 30 years before the development of the tumor. Although benign localized mesotheliomas occur and may be cured by operative resection, most of these tumors are malignant and diffuse and beyond surgical cure. The prognosis for these patients is very grave.

THE LUNGS AND BRONCHI
Diagnostic and Preoperative Evaluation

Chest radiographic studies are essential to evaluate patients with pulmonary conditions who are being con-

sidered for surgical treatment. Conventional chest films are frequently supplemented by tomographic studies (either plain or computed), which can provide further information. CT provides a cross-sectional view of the thorax and, in particular, improves visualization of the lung hilum and mediastinum (Figs. 29-6 thru 29-8). Magnetic resonance imaging (MRI) is a newer technique that provides views of the thorax in sagittal and coronal section in addition to cross section (Figs. 29-9 and 29-10). When malignancy is suspected, needle aspiration of lesions to obtain tissue for cytologic examination can be performed under fluoroscopic or CT guidance. For further evaluation of conditions involving the bronchi, bronchography may be performed to provide better detail of endobronchial lesions and bronchial anatomy. This technique involves injection of viscid radiopaque material through a nasotracheal catheter into the bronchial system of one lung; radiographs are taken in various positions (Fig. 29-11). Close cooperation between the surgeon and the radiologist is essential for the proper preoperative evaluation of the patient with suspected surgical disease of the lung or respiratory passages.

Following appropriate radiographic studies, it is frequently advantageous to visualize the interior of the tra-

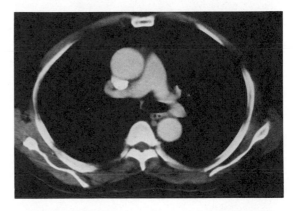

Fig. 29-7. CT of chest at level of pulmonary artery bifurcation.

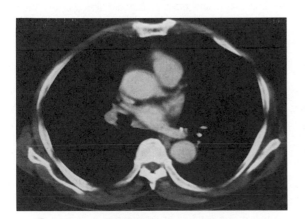

Fig. 29-6. CT of chest at level of left atrium.

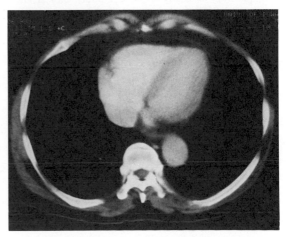

Fig. 29-8. CT of chest at level of left ventricle.

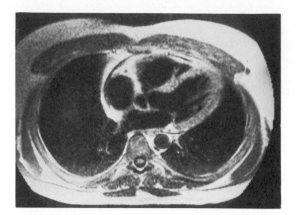

Fig. 29-9. MR image of chest, cross-sectional view.

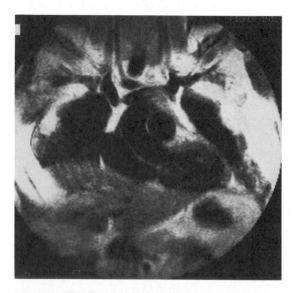

Fig. 29-10. MR image of chest, coronal view.

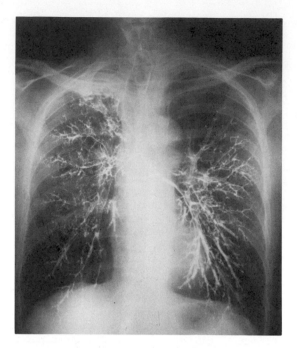

Fig. 29-11. Normal bronchogram.

chea and bronchi by bronchoscopy. Flexible fiberoptic bronchoscopy is easily conducted under topical anesthesia. The flexibility and small diameter of this instrument allows for manipulation into subsegmental bronchi, and biopsies of suspicious endobronchial lesions can be obtained through the bronchoscope. Indications for bronchoscopy include evaluation of radiographic abnormalities, hemoptysis, chronic cough, suspected foreign body in the airways, and suspected broncholithiasis. Rigid bronchoscopy entails the use of a larger-caliber, rigid lighted tube and is most often performed under general anesthesia. Ventilation of the patient is maintained through a separate port in the scope. This instrument allows the passage of larger biopsy forceps and suction catheters and is therefore most frequently used to evaluate severe active airway bleeding, mucus plugs, and foreign bodies. Tracheal strictures are best visualized through the rigid bronchoscope, and it is usually the instrument of choice for pediatric patients. Examination with the rigid bronchoscope is, however, limited, because only the segmental bronchi can be visualized by this technique.

Mediastinoscopy is a technique for obtaining biopsy of mediastinal lymph nodes. Mediastinoscopy requires general anesthesia and is performed by inserting a lighted scope through a small cervical incision in the suprasternal notch. The instrument is passed along the anterior surface of the trachea to the level of its bifurcation. Lymph nodes adjacent to the trachea, proximal left and right bronchi, and subcarinal area are visualized and biopsied. Anterior mediastinotomy is an extrapleural mediastinal exploration through the bed of the second or third costal cartilages. This form of open biopsy is especially useful to obtain specimens of enlarged lymph nodes in the left upper mediastinal region, a region not accessible by the mediastinoscope. Mediastinoscopy and mediastinotomy are nearly always diagnostic in sarcoidosis or lymphoma when adenopathy is present, and these techniques are also useful to detect mediastinal spread of bronchogenic carcinoma preoperatively.

Pulmonary function tests are an integral part of the preoperative assessment of the patient with disease of the lung or bronchi (Table 29-1). Many patients with lung disease have underlying pulmonary dysfunction, frequently as the result of chronic cigarette smoking. In patients who are to undergo resection of functioning pulmonary parenchyma (e.g., lobectomy or pneumonectomy) it is imperative to predict preoperatively whether the patient's postoperative pulmonary function status will be adequate for survival and nearly normal activity. Spirometric pulmonary function tests measure lung volumes and air-flow rates, whereas gas transport can be measured by diffusion capacity studies. There are two major patterns of dysfunction:

Table 29-1. Frequently Used Pulmonary Function Tests

Test	Definition	Normal	Remarks
Vital capacity (VC)	Volume of air exhaled by maximum voluntary effort after maximum inspiration	Depends on age, sex, and size (30-50 ml/kg body weight)	Reduced in restrictive disease, may be normal in obstructive disorders.
Forced expiratory volume in 1 second (FEV_1)	Amount of VC exhaled in 1 second	About 85% of VC is exhaled in 1 second	Reduced, especially in obstructive lung disease.
Maximal midexpiratory flow rate (MMFR or $FEF_{25-75\%}$)	Average flow rate during middle half of forced expiration	4.5-5.0 L/second	Reduced in obstructive disorders; less dependent on patient effort.
Maximum voluntary ventilation (MVV)	Amount of air moved during maximal breathing for 12 seconds	100 L/minute	Dependent on patient effort; reflects obstructive or neuromuscular disease.
Diffusing capacity (DL_{co})	Measure of carbon monoxide transfer across alveoli	Reported as percentage of predicted value based on known dependent factors	Nonspecific measure of pulmonary gas transfer.

Obstructive disorders are exemplified by emphysema (chronic obstructive lung disease). Patients have a low forced expiratory volume in 1 second (FEV_1) and maximum mid-expiratory flow rate (MMFR). Forced vital capacity (FVC) may be somewhat reduced or relatively normal.

Restrictive disorders are exemplified by pulmonary fibrosis. These patients have marked decrease in FVC-without evidence of air flow obstruction (FEV_1 relatively normal).

As a general rule, lobectomy is contraindicated for patients whose preoperative FEV_1 is less than 1.2 L, and pneumonectomy should not be performed in patients whose FEV_1 is less than 1.7 L. A postresection FEV_1 of at least 800 ml is generally required if a patient is to survive without being a "pulmonary cripple," although larger patients may require an even greater postoperative volume.

Equally important is the determination of arterial blood gases in the patient who is being considered for pulmonary resection. Measurements of resting arterial blood gases while the patient breathes room air are easily obtained and inexpensive and provide valuable information about the patient's ability to oxygenate and to ventilate. Hypoxia (low arterial O_2 tension) reflects the adequacy of delivery of unoxygenated blood to ventilating alveoli and the diffusion of O_2 across the alveolus. Since CO_2 is much more diffusable than O_2, severe hypoxemia can occur in the presence of a normal CO_2 level. Causes of hypoxemia reflect situations in which an uneven distribution of ventilation to alveolar blood flow is present. Examples are atelectasis (airway closure with normal perfusion), congenital heart conditions with right-to-left shunting (unoxygenated blood bypasses the lungs and mixes directly with arterial blood), and diffusion abnormalities (alveolar thickening).

Hypercarbia (high arterial CO_2 tension) reflects inadequate ventilation of alveoli that may be perfused normally. Inability to ventilate adequately may be due to large airway obstruction or failure of respiratory muscles.

Emphysema (chronic obstructive lung disease) is the most common chronic lung disorder in adults and is frequently present in patients who are undergoing evaluation for thoracic surgery. In this condition, chronic airway obstruction and alveolar destruction lead to both hypoxemia and hypercarbia, but it is the latter that is commonly the most severe. As a general rule, the presence preoperatively of resting (room air) arterial O_2 tension less than 50 torr or CO_2 tension greater than 45 torr indicates underlying lung disease so severe that pulmonary resection is contraindicated.

Congenital Malformations of the Lung and Bronchi
Congenital Lobar Emphysema

Congenital lobar emphysema is an important cause of respiratory distress in young infants and may be life threatening. Due to maldevelopment of bronchial cartilage of the involved lobe, air enters the lobe, but, upon expiration, the bronchus collapses and air remains trapped in the affected lobe. This ball-valve effect leads to progressive enlargement of the lobe and compression atelectasis of uninvolved lobes. The left upper, right upper, and middle lobes are the most frequent sites of congenital lobar emphysema. About one third of affected infants become symptomatic within the first month of life and the remainder within the first 6 months of life. Associated congenital heart defects are common. Examination reveals decreased breath sounds and hyperresonance on the side of the thorax containing the emphysematous lobe. Chest films show an enlarging air-filled cyst that compresses the other lobes and may cross the midline. Further diagnostic studies are not usually necessary, and resection of the involved lobe gives excellent results.

Cystic Adenomatoid Malformation

Cystic adenomatoid malformation is an unusual lesion that results from the failure of cartilaginous maturation with overgrowth of mesenchymal elements and the formation of cysts due to air trapping. In contrast to congenital lobar emphysema, multiple cysts are present, usually without associated heart defects. Respiratory distress is the most frequent presenting symptom, and chest films reveal multiple cystic structures and mediastinal shift to the opposite side of the chest. The left lower lobe is the most common site, although any lobe may be involved. Resection is usually curative.

Agenesis and Hypoplasia of the Lungs

Bilateral lung agenesis is inconsistent with life after birth; infants with unilateral lung agenesis survive and the clinical picture is variable. Although most of these infants present early with respiratory difficulties, some may not be discovered to have the disorder until later if sufficient functioning pulmonary parenchyma is present on the contralateral side. Upon examination, infants with this disorder demonstrate lack of breath sounds and dullness to percussion on the side of agenesis. Chest radiographs show a homogeneous density that can be confused with total lung atelectasis (such as would occur secondary to an obstructing foreign body). Pulmonary angiography, bronchography, and bronchoscopy are methods used to confirm the diagnosis. In congenital pulmonary hypoplasia the involved lung is underdeveloped, as are the corrersponding bronchus and artery. This condition is invariably present in infants with congenital diaphragmatic hernia. In this malformation, the presence of abdominal contents within the chest (via the hernia) in fetal life impairs lung development, and frequently it is the lung hypoplasia, rather than the hernia itself, that is most detrimental to the survival of the infant.

Bronchogenic Cysts

Bronchogenic cysts result from lung bud tissue that apparently becomes isolated during development and is not connected normally to the bronchial tree. Although they represent a congenital abnormality of the lung, the cysts are most commonly mediastinal in location and account for 10% of mediastinal masses in children. They are usually near (but do not communicate with) the tracheal bifurcation and main bronchi. Most often the cysts are single, but they may be multiloculated. They are lined by respiratory epithelium, and the walls often contain smooth muscle and cartilage. As mucus collects within the cyst, gradual enlargement occurs. Many patients with bronchogenic cysts are entirely asymptomatic, and the cyst is discovered on routine chest

films (Fig. 29-12). Other patients may become symptomatic due to bronchial obstruction (causing wheezing, painful cough, atelectasis) or infection of the cyst. CT is useful to determine the anatomic location and limits of the mass (Fig. 29-13). Excision should be performed.

Arteriovenous Fistulas

Congenital connections between a pulmonary artery and vein occur occasionally. The shunting of unoxygenated pulmonary blood directly to the pulmonary vein without passing through the alveolus (a right-to-left shunt) leads to hypoxemia, the degree of which is determined by the number and size of the fistulas. Multiple fistulas may be present in patients with hereditary hemorrhagic telangiectasia (Rendu-Osler-Weber syndrome), but only about one half of patients with arteriovenous fistulas have this disorder. Because of the chronic right-to-left shunt, patients with arteriovenous fistulas develop clubbing, cyanosis, and polycythemia. Occasional patients may present with hemoptysis. Evaluation includes chest radiography and CT, arterial blood gas analysis, echocardiography, and pulmonary arteriography. Surgical resection of isolated fistulas is indicated. For patients with multiple small fistulas this may be impractical,and radiographic techniques (miniballoon occlusion) can be of value. Untreated, these patients are subject to the complications of chronic polycythemia, including cerebrovascular accident.

Pulmonary Sequestration

Sequestration, another congenital maldevelopment of the lung, may occur in two forms—intralobar and extralobar. In both forms, the abnormal lung mass is composed of nonfunctioning pulmonary tissue with no direct communication to the airways, and the arterial blood supply is from the aorta. Intralobar sequestra-

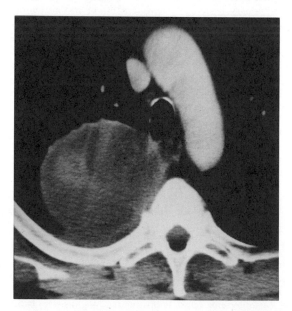

Fig. 29-13. CT of bronchogenic cyst (same patient as in Fig. 29-12).

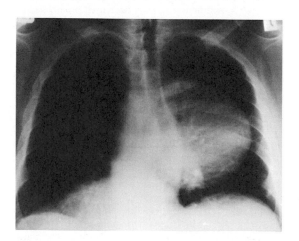

Fig. 29-12. Huge bronchogenic cyst found on routine chest film in asymptomatic patient.

tions occur most commonly in the left lung, and the blood supply is most often from a single large branch of the aorta; venous drainage is into the pulmonary veins. On chest radiography the intralobar sequestration is usually cystic, frequently with an air-fluid level. Symptoms develop from recurring infection; lobectomy is generally indicated and provides cure.

In contrast, the extralobar form is a separate mass of nonfunctioning pulmonary tissue contained within its own pleural envelopment. These are also more common on the left and are usually nonaerated. The blood supply to extralobar sequestration is usually by way of multiple small aortic branches, and the venous drainage is into the azygos or hemiazygos vein (instead of pulmonary vein). Frequently, connections to the gastrointestinal tract (especially esophagus) are present. Associated congenital abnormalities are rare. Most often the extralobar form of sequestration causes no symptoms and is found on routine chest radiography. Resection is indicated to confirm the diagnonsis.

In both forms, the anatomy of the arterial supply to the sequestration is of surgical importance (Fig. 29-14). Failure to recognize the aortic origin of the feeding vessel(s) can lead to inadvertent transection of the vessel(s) and severe hemorrhage at operation.

Lung Abscess

Lung abscess is a destructive, suppurative process in the lungs caused by microorganisms. The infection is often polymicrobic and the abscess forms as the result of lung necrosis. Unlike bronchiectasis, which follows anatomic segments of the lung, the destructive process of lung abscess may cross segmental lines. The incidence of lung abscess has decreased dramatically over the past 50 years owing to the development of antibiotics. With improved culture techniques, the important role of anaerobic bacteria has become evident.

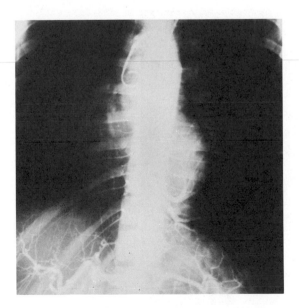

Fig. 29-14. Arteriogram demonstrating aortic branches to pulmonary sequestration.

Several underlying causes must be considered:

Aspiration of ingested material. This occurs especially in patients who have been unconscious (alcoholics, epileptics, patients with central nervous system diseases) or patients with esophageal disease causing regurgitation. The location of the abscess generally corresponds to the most dependent pulmonary segment at the time of aspiration. If the patient is supine at the time of aspiration, abscesses most commonly occur in the posterior segment of the right upper lobe or the superior segment of the lower lobes. Aspiration is the most common cause of lung abscess in recent published reports.

Bronchial obstruction. An abscess may develop distal to an obstruction that prevents clearance of the bronchial tree. Causes include endobronchial carcinoma, bronchial stenosis, and foreign body.

Pneumonia. The type of organism causing the pneumonia determines the pattern of resulting abscesses. *Klebsiella,* formerly a major cause of lung abscesses, produces multilocular cavities. *Staphylococcus,* the most common cause of abscess in infants and children, produces a necrotizing bronchopneumonia leading to multiple abscesses. Pneumonia-associated abscesses occur particularly in immunosuppressed and pediatric patients.

Abscess developing in a structural abnormality. Pulmonary abnormalities such as intralobar sequestration, cystic adenomatoid malformations, lung infarction, or necrotic tumor tend to become infected and form abscesses.

Blood-borne infection. Septic pulmonary emboli or blood-borne bacteria from a distant infection can lodge in the lung and lead to abscess formation.

Clinical symptoms due to lung abscess include those of systemic illness (fever, chills, malaise) and those resulting from the inflammation in the lung (cough, hemoptysis, foul-smelling sputum, pleuritic chest pain). Radiographic examination of the chest usually confirms the presence of a lung abscess, although the cavity may not be evident in studies performed early in the course of the illness. When formed, the cavity possesses an air-fluid level and has a relatively thick wall (Fig. 29-15). Evaluation begins with sputum analysis with bacterial culture and antibiotic sensitivity testing. Bronchoscopy should be performed in all cases to exclude the presence of obstructing lesions.

Surgery is rarely indicated for lung abscesses. The majority of patients can be treated successfully with systemic antibiotics, postural drainage, and chest physiotherapy. Aspiration of the abscess contents through the bronchoscope is useful and may be repeated periodically to drain the cavity and hasten resolution. While these measures may have to be carried out for a period of months before there is radiographic evidence of resolution of the abscess, they are nearly always successful and surgery is avoided; however, in some instances surgical excision of the abscess is necessary. The indications for resection include the presence of carcinoma, massive hemoptysis, significant bronchial stenosis, the presence of a congenital cyst, and failure of the cavity to respond to medical management in 8 to 12 weeks. Lobectomy is usually the operation of choice.

Bronchiectasis

Bronchiectasis is a chronic suppurative disease of lung segments characterized by bronchial dilation and surrounding inflammation. Bacterial infection of the bronchial wall and adjacent lung leads to airway destruction and enlargement. The smaller bronchi become obliterated, and the larger proximal bronchi undergo dilation during the healing, fibrotic phase of the inflammatory process. The cause of this disorder is often obscure, but it is usually an acquired condition thought to be secondary to chronic bronchitis and peribronchial pneumonitis. In children, bronchiectasis is commonly associated with aspiration of foreign bodies, chronic upper and lower respiratory tract infections, and cystic fibrosis of the pancreas. It also occurs in the rare triad of Kartagener's syndrome (bronchiectasis, situs inversus, and sinusitis). Once a common clinical disease and cause of premature death, bronchiectasis has become rare since the development of effective antibiotic therapy.

Affected patients have a history of recurrent respiratory infections, often in conjunction with sinusitis. Fever, morning cough, production of foul-smelling sputum, hemoptysis, and chest pain occur, particularly during acute exacerbations. Chest films may not be diagnostic. Bronchoscopy should be performed to rule out obstructing lesions or foreign bodies and to obtain sputum samples for bacterial culture. Bronchography, which also documents the extent and location of the disease, is the most important diagnostic examination. Bronchiectasis usually affects the lower lobes, and bronchography will demonstrate bronchial dilation, usually in a pattern corresponding to the anatomic segments of the lobe (Fig. 29-16). Complications of the disease are hemorrhage, empyema, and metastatic spread of the infection (brain abscess).

Treatment of bronchiectasis consists of rest, adequate nutrition, antibiotics, and postural drainage. In many cases the bronchiectatic changes are reversible and respond well to these measures. Operative removal of segments involved with irreversible disease is carried out during a quiescent phase in selected patients who have adequate pulmonary function.

Pulmonary Tuberculosis

In 1900, tuberculosis was the most common single cause of death in the United States. Surgery of the chest evolved around operations devised to treat pulmo-

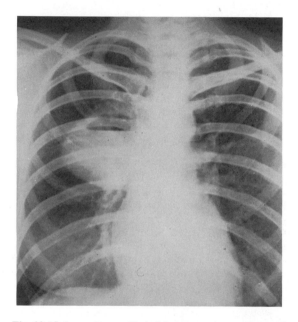

Fig. 29-15. Lung abscess. Underlying cause was carcinoma of lung.

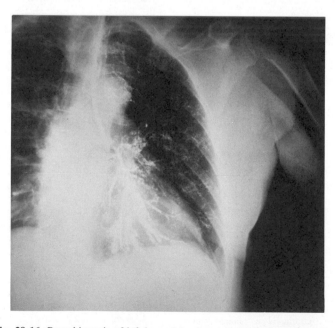

Fig. 29-16. Bronchiectasis of left lower lobe demonstrated by bronchography.

nary tuberculosis. With advances in tuberculosis chemotherapy and improved living conditions, control of this disease has become a reality. Surgical procedures for pulmonary tuberculosis are performed rarely now, but the disease has not disappeared. In fact, with increasing numbers of immunocompromised patients and an increasing incidence of infections caused by primary drug-resistant mycobacteria and atypical mycobacteria, complete eradication of this condition is not expected in the near future.

Initial inhalation of *Mycobacterium tuberculosis* most often leads to the formation of a primary complex called the Ghon complex, consisting of a primary tubercle in the lung and enlarged hilar lymph nodes that also harbor the organism. At this point the patient with normal immune system reactivity will have a positive purified protein derivative (PPD) skin test. The development of hypersensitivity is followed by caseous necrosis and fibrosis and calcification of the tubercle. In some patients, especially those who are immunosuppressed, this primary infection may progress to pneumonia, endobronchial disease, or miliary spread. Most instances of clinical pulmonary tuberculosis are the result of postprimary infection, usually from reactivation of the primary lesion. This most commonly progresses from a pneumonic infiltrate to a cavitary lesion with bronchial communication, which may lead to endobronchial and systemic spread. The diagnosis of pulmonary mycobacterial disease requires isolation of the organism from sputum or tissue.

Treatment of pulmonary tuberculosis is primarily medical. The most common drugs utilized today are ioniazid, rifampin, streptomycin, and ethambutol, which are usually utilized in combinations of two or three for periods of 6 to 9 months. Close monitoring of the patient is required because of serious drug side effects.

Surgery is recommended for patients who fail to respond to medical treatment or develop complications that require operative intervention. Prior to the development of effective antituberculous chemotherapy, various surgical procedures were employed. Surgically induced pneumothorax, phrenic nerve paralysis, placement of foreign material between the parietal pleura and chest wall (plombage), and thoracoplasty were forms of "collapse" therapy used to effect pulmonary collapse. For reasons that are unclear, these procedures did lead to the remission of pulmonary tuberculosis in some patients, but they are no longer used for this purpose. Today, surgical treatment for tuberculosis generally involves resection (lobectomy) for patients with persistently positive sputum following multidrug therapy, persistent cavitary disease, massive hemoptysis, destroyed lung, severe lower lobe bronchiectasis, bronchopleural fistula, and suspicion of carcinoma. Preoperative bronchoscopy is important to rule out the presence of endobronchial involvement, which would lead to poor healing of the transected airway. Because of the success of antituberculous chemotherapy, surgery for this disease is rarely required today.

Atypical mycobacteria *(M. kansasii, M. intracellulare)* tend to be resistant to chemotherapy; localized *M. intracellulare* disease may require excisional therapy, whereas *M. kansasii* can usually be cured with prolonged multidrug treatment.

Although it is no longer the "white plague" of previous generations, pulmonary mycobacterial disease is not expected to disappear entirely. It is being seen with increasing frequency in patients who are immunosuppressed for the treatment of medical conditions (transplant patients) and in those suffering from acquired immunodeficiency syndrome (AIDS).

Pulmonary Actinomycetic and Mycetic Infections

Actinomyces israelii and *Nocardia asteroides* are two organisms classified as bacteria that are associated with chronic pulmonary infection. Actinomycosis may occur as a cervicofacial, abdominal, or thoracic infection. The region of involvement is characterized by chronic suppuration, proliferative granulomatous inflammation, and "sulfur granule" formation. When the lungs are involved, extension through the chest wall may occur. Treatment is antibiotic therapy (penicillin, tetracycline), and surgery is usually required only for abscess drainage or excision of chest wall disease. Nocardiosis occurs mainly in immunosuppressed patients. The organism has a propensity for chest wall and subcutaneous tissue involvement and may also form "sulfur granules." When found in the sputum or biopsy specimen of a patient with altered resistance, *Nocardia* should be considered a pathogen. Central nervous system involvement occurs frequently. Treatment is medical (sulfadiazine), and surgery is reserved for diagnostic excision, empyema, and excision of sinus and chest wall abscesses.

Candida, Cryptococcus, and *Aspergillus* are three fungi with worldwide distribution. Candidiasis is often an opportunistic infection associated with broad-spectrum antibiotic therapy. *Cryptococcus* is a cause of pulmonary granulomas, granulomatous pneumonia, and other forms of pulmonary involvement; surgery is usually necessary to diagnose the origin of a cryptococcal pulmonary nodule. *Aspergillus* is another opportunistic fungus that causes various forms of pulmonary infection. Invasive or disseminated disease is most common in the immunosuppressed patient. Saprophytic infection can occur when the organism takes up residence in a preexisting pulmonary cavity, leading to the development of a fungus ball, or aspergilloma. Generally, these cavitary fungus balls should be excised as they are associated with a high incidence of serious hemoptysis.

Histoplasmosis, coccidioidomycosis, and blastomycosis are three forms of pulmonary fungal disease that have individually distinct geographic distributions. Details of their distribution, manifestations, and treatment are found in Table 29-2.

Benign Tumors of the Lung

Truly benign neoplasms of the lung are much less common than the malignant variety. Hamartomas, the most common benign lung tumors, are composed of tissue elements normally found in the lung (cartilage, cuboidal and ciliated epithelium, and muscle fibers) but arranged in an abnormal fashion. These tumors present most commonly as an asymptomatic, round, well-circumscribed nodule on chest films and often have a characteristic, "popcorn," pattern of calcification suggesting their identity. Most commonly discovered by

Table 29-2. Fungous Diseases of the Lungs

Disease	Agent	Endemic Geographic Distribution	Transmission	Roentgenographic Findings	Clinical Findings and Symptoms	Treatment
Actinomycosis	*Actinomyces bovis*	Worldwide	Aspiration from mouth to lower respiratory tract	Dense, progressive infiltrates; abscess	Chronic cough, purulent sputum, low-grade fever, weight loss	Penicillin, tetracycline, drainage or resection of abscesses and chest wall extension
Nocardiosis	*Nocardia asteroides*	Worldwide	Saprophytes in soil; opportunistic disease	Pneumonia or infiltrate process; cavitation; nodular lesion	Nonspecific, may have chest wall or nervous system involvement	Sulfonamides, excision of involved chest wall, drainage of abscesses or empyemas
Candidiasis	*Candida albicans*	Worldwide	Invasion under conditions of reduced resistance or prolonged antibiotic or steroid therapy	Pneumonia or miliary spread	Those of severe bronchopneumonia	Amphotericin B
Cryptococcosis	*Cryptococcus neoformans*	Worldwide; soil especially contaminated by pigeon excreta	Lung principal port of entry; occurs especially in debilitated or immunosuppressed patients	Solitary or multiple nodules, pneumonitis, mediastinal adenopathy; cavitation rare	Usually subclinical; may cause meningitis	Amphotericin B, resection of localized pulmonary disease
Aspergillosis	*Aspergillus*	Worldwide	May be saprophyte in normal sputum; usually found in sick patients with lymphoma, carcinoma, tuberculosis, or immunosuppression	Pneumonic abscess, intracavitary fungus ball	Bronchitis; acute or chronic pneumonia, allergic form, hemorrhage a serious threat	Amphotericin B; resection of fungus ball
Histoplasmosis	*Histoplasma capsulatum*	Most common in Mississippi River Basin area	From soil contaminated by excreta of birds, bats, and rodents	Variable pneumonia; dense infiltrates, miliary patterns, nodular lesions, sclerosing mediastinitis	Primary infection is transient; mediastinitis may cause superior vena cava obstruction; protean symptoms in disseminated form	Amphotericin B; resection of single nodules performed at times to exclude lung carcinoma
Coccidioidomycosis	*Coccidioides immitis*	Southwestern United States	Airborne, highly infectious but not contagious; can be passed on by fomites	Variable; thin-walled cavity, solitary lesion; infiltrates; pneumonitis, pleural effusion, adenopathy	Primary infection "flu-like," most asymptomatic, small number with hematogenous spread	Amphotericin B, but not for most cases that are self-limited; surgery for persistent cavities
North American blastomycosis	*Blastomyces dermatitidis*	Mississippi Valley, southeastern United States	Inhalation of spores, not contagious, common in persons in contact with soil	Variable; usually dense pneumonitis or infiltration; may resemble lung cancer	Skin lesions, symptoms similar to tubercular cough, nonspecific symptoms	Amphotericin B, 2-hydroxystilbamidine, resection usually not required except for cavitary lesions

routine radiographic studies, the peak incidence occurs in the sixth decade of life. Because they are located within the pulmonary parenchyma and not endobronchially, most hamartomas are asymptomatic. Resection is almost always indicated to exclude malignant lesions, which are more common in this age group.

Other truly benign tumors of the lung and bronchi include lipomas, nodular amyloidosis, leiomyomas, and hemangiomas. Rarely, benign intrapulmonary lymph nodes mimic the appearance of a neoplasm on chest radiographs.

Bronchial Adenomas

Bronchial adenomas are a group of tumors with relatively low malignant potential, but they are not truly benign. Most common in this group are bronchial carcinoids. These endobronchial tumors arise from neuroendocrine (Kulchitsky's) cells of the bronchial mucosa. They can occur as a component of the multiple endocrine neoplasia (MEN) syndrome but usually do not give rise to the carcinoid syndrome unless they are metastatic. The other major group of bronchial adenomas are the endobronchial tumors of salivary gland origin (adenoid cystic carcinomas and mucoepidermoid adenomas).

Most patients with bronchial adenomas present with symptoms of partial bronchial obstruction, most commonly cough and hemoptysis. Owing to recurrent infection distal to the obstructing lesion, symptoms such as fever and chills may occur. The tumor may be difficult to visualize on normal chest films but often is demonstrated by CT. Bronchoscopy is indicated in all patients with chronic cough, and careful biopsy (because of the risk of hemorrhage from vascular tumors) provides the diagnosis. Most commonly, bronchial adenomas are found in a mainstem or lobar bronchus. Surgical excision is indicated. Although they are called adenomas, these tumors have been known to metastasize and cause death.

Cancer of the Lung

In the United States cancer of the lung is the leading cause of death due to malignancy in both men and women. Clearly caused by cigarette smoking, other environmental factors such as asbestos and uranium exposure are also important contributing causes. Except for the small-cell (oat-cell) type of lung cancer, surgical extirpation is the treatment of choice. At the time of diagnosis, however, many patients have disease that is too extensive or widely metastatic for potential surgical cure, and some patients have underlying pulmonary disease too severe to allow for survival following pulmonary resection. The role of the thoracic surgeon in the management of lung cancer is to evaluate patients with respect to these considerations and to offer potential surgical cure to the greatest number of patients with the disease while avoiding unnecessary operations for those with no hope of surgical cure and avoiding pulmonary resection in those who have no reasonable chance of surviving the procedure.

Lung cancers are divided into two major groups on the basis of cell type: non–small cell lung cancers have the potential for surgical cure unless specific contraindications, such as extensive local disease (invasion of mediastinal structures) or metastases outside of the affected hemithorax, are present. In contrast, small cell carcinoma is almost never curable by surgery. The great majority of these tumors present with widespread metastases and are best treated nonsurgically by radiation and chemotherapy.

There are three major types of non–small cell carcinoma: *Squamous cell carcinoma* is most closely associated with cigarette abuse. This neoplasm tends to occur in the larger (central) airways and to spread by regional lymph node metastasis. The results of surgery for this cell type tend to be better than for the others, although

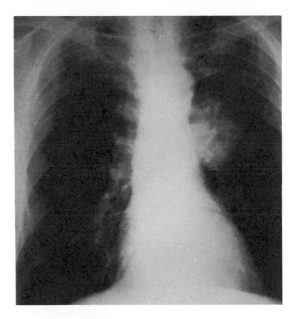

Fig. 29-17. Carcinoma of lung; left hilar mass.

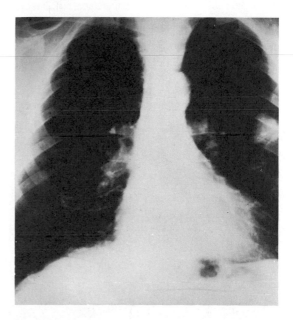

Fig. 29-18. Carcinoma of lung; nodule in left midlung field.

this difference may be slight and is highly dependent upon the stage of the disease. *Adenocarcinoma* tends to arise more peripherally in the lung and to spread more rapidly by both vascular and lymphatic routes. The relative incidence of this cell type appears to be increasing. *Large cell carcinoma* also commonly arises peripherally in the lung, may grow to be quite large, and tends to metastasize later than adenocarcinoma.

Small cell carcinoma is a tumor that tends to occur centrally and spread quickly to regional lymph nodes and distant sites (brain, bone, liver). Approximately 20% to 25% of all lung cancers are of this cell type. The great majority of patients with this disease have other organ involvement at the time of diagnosis, so surgery is not indicated. Although the initial response to chemotherapy and radiation may be quite good, small cell carcinoma usually recurs. Overall survival with this form of lung cancer is decidedly poorer than for the non–small cell types.

The clinical presentation of the patient with lung cancer depends on the site and extent of the disease. Asymptomatic patients may be found to have a single pulmonary mass on routine chest films, while other patients with more extensive disease may present with weight loss and weakness (Figs. 29-17 and 29-18). Endobronchial tumors frequently cause cough, hemoptysis, and recurrent or unresolving pneumonia. Extrapulmonary manifestations include clubbing, Cushing's syndrome, hypercalcemia, carcinomatous neuropathy, and osteoarthropathy. The diagnosis may be confirmed by sputum cytology (especially if cough or hemoptysis is present), bronchoscopy with biopsy, and needle biopsy. For patients with a single, new, enlarging, peripheral pulmonary nodule (coin lesion) and adequate pulmonary function, the procedure of choice is often thoracotomy both to establish the diagnosis (by frozen section) and to perform definitive therapeutic resection if the nodule is malignant.

Preoperative assessment of patients with non–small cell lung cancer is of great importance and has two goals: to determine the potential resectability of the lesion and to determine whether the patient's cardiopulmonary status is adequate for surgery and survival following the removal of functioning lung tissue. Patients are not helped by an operation that fails to remove all known tumor completely (there is no proved advantage to tumor debulking for lung cancer) nor by one in which all tumor is removed but the patient is chronically ventilator dependent because of postoperative respiratory insufficiency due to inadequate remaining functional lung.

Computed tomography (CT) is frequently employed preoperatively to delineate the anatomic limits of the tumor and to determine the presence or absence of mediastinal adenopathy. Tumors with extensive mediastinal invasion are usually unresectable (Fig. 29-19). The presence of enlarged lymph nodes on CT does not mean, however, that the nodes contain metastatic cancer, as lymph node enlargement secondary to inflammation is common. If information about the lymph node status is crucial to decisions concerning operability, then biopsy of the CT–identified nodes can often be performed by mediastinoscopy or anterior mediastinotomy without subjecting the patient to thoracotomy.

Certain contraindications to surgical resection of lung cancer have evolved with experience (see box below). They are associated with extremely poor cure rates and patients with these conditions should not be subjected to the risk and pain of thoracotomy. Note that old age alone is not a contraindication, and pulmonary resection can be performed in the otherwise healthy elderly patient with early lung cancer, with relatively low morbidity and mortality and good long-term survival. The operability of patients with biopsy-positive mediastinal lymph node metastases is a controversial subject. In some institutions, involvement of the mediastinal lymph nodes is considered a sign of inoperability. In others, involvement of accessible mediastinal lymph nodes does not preclude surgery, and mediastinal lymph node dissection is performed at the time of operation. Patients with contralateral hilar or contralateral mediastinal node involvement are clearly incurable by surgery. The presence of positive lymph nodes at the hilum of the lung in which the cancer has arisen is not a contraindication to resection, and these nodes are removed at the time of lobectomy or pneumonectomy.

The amount of lung removed at operation depends on several factors. Large central tumors with mainstem bronchus involvement require pneumonectomy, whereas more peripheral tumors may be removed by lobectomy if they do not cross the intrapulmonary fis-

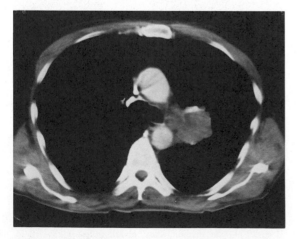

Fig. 29-19. Carcinoma of lung invading mediastinum.

Contraindications to Pulmonary Resection for Lung Cancer

Prohibitive pulmonary function tests (FEV_1 <1.7 for pneumonectomy; FEV_1 <1.2 for lobectomy)
Prohibitive arterial blood gases (pCO_2 >45 torr; pO_2 <50 torr on room air)
Distant metastasis
Involvement of trachea or contralateral mainstream bronchus with carcinoma
Superior vena cava obstruction
Malignant cells in pleural effusion
Recurrent laryngeal nerve paralysis from carcinoma
Histology showing small-cell carcinoma

sure. Occasional small peripheral tumors may be excised by segmentectomy or wedge resection, especially in patients with borderline pulmonary function. By removing less pulmonary tissue, the risk of postoperative respiratory insufficiency is lessened, but the adequacy of these limited resections as cancer operations has not been proved conclusively.

Pulmonary resection is performed through a thoracotomy incision, usually with the patient in the lateral decubitus position. It is frequently helpful to utilize a double-lumen endotracheal tube, which permits selective ventilation of the unoperated lung, thereby improving exposure for the surgeon. Control of the pulmonary artery and vein (or their branches) is of prime importance and, at times, can be difficult owing to the friability of these vessels. Surgical stapling devices are frequently employed to provide permanent occlusion of the bronchus to be transected. Careful exploration of the lymph node–bearing regions is routinely performed, and all nodes are removed, carefully labeled, and submitted for histologic examination. These include the intralobar, lobar, and hilar nodes and those in mediastinal sites (paratracheal, subcarinal, paraesophageal, pulmonary ligament, and paraaortic). After resection, chest tubes are introduced through small separate incisions and attached to underwater sealed drainage (except for pneumonectomy patients, in whom no chest tube is used). Following lobectomy or wedge resection, full expansion of the remaining lung is important to obliterate the resulting space as completely as possible. Following pneumonectomy, fluid gradually collects in the hemithorax and is slowly replaced by fibrous and gelatinous material.

Lung cancers are staged according to the TNM system based on tumor characteristics (size and location), node involvement (hilar or mediastinal), and the presence or absence of distant metastases. In an abbreviated form, the stages of lung cancer are:

Stage I: Tumors removed by at least 2.0 cm from the carina without direct extension into the mediastinum or chest wall. No lymph node involvement.

Stage II: Tumors with stage I characteristics with metastasis to parabronchial or ipsilateral hilar region lymph nodes only.

Stage III: Tumors with direct extension into the chest wall, diaphragm, mediastinum, or great vessels. Metastasis to mediastinal, subcarinal, or contralateral lymph nodes. Any malignant effusion.

Stage IV: Any distant metastasis.

Adjuvant therapy for surgically treated patients with non–small cell carcinoma is controversial. In general, there is currently no role for chemotherapy in patients who have undergone removal of all visible tumor (including lymph node dissection), although experimental protocols are under way to investigate the efficacy of such treatment and this recommendation may change based on the results of these studies. Radiation therapy is frequently recommended to patients who are found at surgery to have tumor-positive mediastinal lymph nodes, narrow surgical margins, or chest wall extension of tumor. While the rate of local recurrence is decreased by postoperative radiation therapy, an increase in the long-term patient survival rate has not been clearly demonstrated at this time.

One unique form of lung cancer is the superior sulcus (Pancoast's) tumor (see box). These neoplasms arise at the apex of the lung and involve chest wall, brachial plexus, and sympathetic ganglia. The patient presents with shoulder and arm pain, muscle weakness in the affected hand, and Horner's syndrome. For this particular tumor (which may be of any non–small cell type), preoperative radiation therapy to the primary lesion appears to have significant value. Resection may require removal of a portion of the brachial plexus (with resultant deficits in the affected arm) but, when no mediastinal lymph node metastases are present, the survival rate may be surprisingly high for this locally extensive neoplasm.

Complications of pulmonary resection for lung cancer include those common to other surgical procedures—wound infection, myocardial infarction, pulmonary embolus. In addition, specific complications that may occur are atrial arrhythmias (particularly after pneumonectomy), bronchial stump disruption, empyema, and chronic post-thoracotomy incision pain. The overall 30-day operative mortality for patients undergoing pneumonectomy is about 6%, for lobectomy 3%, and for wedge excision 1.5%.

The long-term results of surgical treatment of non–small-cell lung cancer are only fair. About 50% to 60% of patients with stage I disease survive 5 years after operation. Only approximately 25% of those with stage II tumors and about 10% of those with stage III tumors live that long. Because of the high rate of tumor recurrence and the significant incidence of second primary lung cancer, careful long-term follow-up with regular chest x-ray examination is required for patients who have undergone lung cancer resection.

Tumors of the Trachea

Although it is presumably subjected to the same carcinogenic influences as the bronchi, the trachea is rarely involved with cancer. Squamous cell carcinoma is the most common cell type. Patients present with stridor, cough, hemoptysis, and dyspnea. The diagnosis of tracheal cancer is made by bronchoscopy, while CT can help determine the extent of the tumor. Surgical excision of approximately 5.0 cm of the tracheal length can be performed, and primary anastomosis can be achieved. The long-term survival rate for patients with tracheal cancer is low, although certain cell types (carcinoid and mucoepidermoid) are associated with better results.

Features of Pancoast's (Superior Sulcus) Tumor

Carcinoma in superior sulcus of lung
Shoulder and arm pain (T1–C8 distribution)
Muscular atrophy of involved arm
Horner's syndrome (due to involvement of sympathetic chain and stellate ganglion)
Treat with preoperative radiation
Relatively good survival if lymph nodes are not involved

Metastatic Disease to the Lung

The lungs are a common site for the development of blood-borne metastases from other primary malignancies. Common primary tumors include head and neck, colorectal, breast, uterine, urinary tract, and male genital tract carcinomas and various soft-tissue and skeletal sarcomas. In selected patients, surgical resection of isolated pulmonary metastases can offer improved long-term survival. For this to be successful, complete control of the primary tumor must be achieved, and the planned resection procedure must encompass all the known metastatic disease. In terms of long-term patient survival, the results of the removal of a single pulmonary metastasis are much better than those for the excision of two or more metastases. While lobectomy may be required to remove a metastatic lesion deep within the lung in general, pneumonectomy should not be performed for metastatic disease. The 5-year survival of patients undergoing such procedures can be 25% to 50% depending largely on the source of the primary tumor.

Middle Lobe Syndrome

Middle lobe syndrome refers to intermittent or chronic collapse of the middle lobe of the right lung. The cause is obscure and variously attributed to extrinsic pressure from lymph nodes surrounding the middle lobe bronchus or to its acute angle of entry into the main bronchus. Tuberculosis is one of the known causes of lymph node enlargement leading to this syndrome, but often no specific infective agent is found.

The predominant symptoms are cough, chest pain, hemoptysis, and fever. Recurrent pneumonia in the middle lobe is a common presentation. Characteristically, radiographic examination of the chest shows a triangular density best seen on the lateral projection, which represents the atelectatic middle lobe (Fig. 29-20). Bronchoscopy should always be performed to rule out the presence of tumor and foreign body. Bronchography is useful to delineate the bronchial anatomy. Most patients with middle lobe syndrome can be managed medically with antibiotics, postural drainage, and bronchodilators. If these are not successful, resection of the middle lobe may be required. Middle lobectomy in this situation can be a difficult procedure because of inflammation surrounding the bronchus. Resected specimens may reveal congenital bronchial stenosis, cysts, specific infections, chronic nonspecific pneumonia, and granulomatous disease.

THE MEDIASTINUM

The mediastinum is that portion of the thorax bounded superiorly by the thoracic inlet, inferiorly by the diaphragm, and laterally by the pleural reflections. Contained within this space are the thymus, heart, aorta, pericardium, trachea and lung hila, esophagus, thoracic duct, nerves, and lymph nodes. The space has been divided into compartments to aid in the discussion of pathologic conditions that occur therein. One common system separates the mediastinum into anterosuperior, middle, and posterior divisions (Fig. 29-21). Diseases of the mediastinum reflect both inflammatory and neoplastic causes.

Mediastinitis

Mediastinitis is uncommon and can be acute or chronic. Acute mediastinitis may result from direct contamination (following surgery or trauma) or as an extension of inflammation in neighboring or contained structures (neck, lungs, esophagus). Patients with acute mediastinitis are typically quite toxic, with a wet cough and fever. Air may develop in the mediastinum or overlying subcutaneous tissues. A common cause is esophageal rupture, which can follow esophagoscopy or occur spontaneously (Boerhaave's syndrome). Treatment is early surgical drainage with appropriate antibiotic coverage.

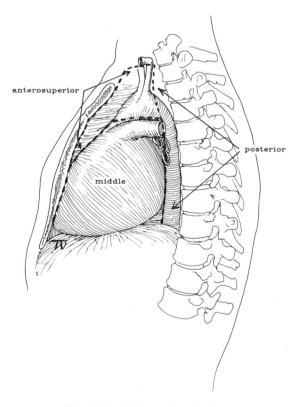

Fig. 29-21. Divisions of mediastinum.

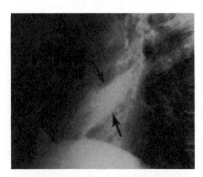

Fig. 29-20. Middle lobe syndrome. Triangular density of collapsed middle lobe is best seen between arrows on lateral chest film.

Chronic mediastinitis is insidious in onset and results from granulomatous infection, although specific organisms frequently are not identified. In the United States, *Histoplasma* is the most commonly cultured organism causing chronic mediastinitis. Chronic inflammation and lymph node enlargement can lead to mediastinal fibrosis and obstruction of the superior vena cava. Surgery for this condition usually is not required, although bypass procedures for the superior vena cava obstruction syndrome may be indicated in selected patients.

Mediastinal Tumors

In general, mediastinal tumors produce symptoms by compressing mediastinal structures; dysphagia and stridor are common presenting complaints. Evaluation includes chest films, CT examination, and, on occasion, barium swallow and bronchoscopy. Mediastinal tumors in children are more likely to be symptomatic and malignant than those in adults. In both groups, asymptomatic lesions are more likely to be benign.

Anterosuperior Mediastinal Tumors

Thymus tumors are the most common tumors of the anterosuperior mediastinum and are the most common primary adult mediastinal tumors (Figs. 29-22 and 29-23). The tumors may be benign thymomas, malignant thymomas, thymic cysts, or thymic hyperplasia. Thymic tumors occur in association with several clinical syndromes: myasthenia gravis, red blood cell aplasia, hypogammaglobulinemia, and Cushing's syndrome. Thymomas may be malignant or benign, and determination of this depends on the presence or absence of invasion of local structures rather than on histologic criteria. While resection of benign thymomas is curative, patients with clinically evident malignant thymomas have only 40% 5-year survivals and may benefit from

postoperative radiation therapy. The relationship between the thymus gland and myasthenia gravis has long been recognized. Forty percent of all patients with thymomas suffer from myasthenia gravis, and about 10% of all patients with myasthenia gravis have thymomas. Patients with myasthenia gravis suffer weakness and fatigue of voluntary muscles due to abnormal neuromuscular transmissions at the synaptic level. Medical treatment involves anticholinesterase inhibitors and corticosteroids. Plasmapheresis produces temporary improvement in the patient's muscle weakness symptoms. For reasons that are not entirely clear, removal of the thymus (whether or not a thymoma is present) can be very beneficial to patients with myasthenia gravis. Although reported response rates vary, about 35% of myasthenia gravis patients undergo remission following thymectomy, while another 50% show significant improvement in their symptoms. The results for patients found to have thymomas are less salutary. Current indications for thymectomy in myasthenia gravis patients are suspicion of the presence of a thymoma or generalized symptoms not well controlled with medical therapy. Remission or improvement in symptoms does not occur immediately after thymectomy and may not be evident for months. Thymectomy may be performed through a cervical or a sternotomy incision. Many thoracic surgeons prefer sternotomy because the exposure is better and removal of all thymic tissue is judged to be more complete. Preoperative plasmapheresis helps to prevent postoperative respiratory insufficiency secondary to ventilatory muscle weakness.

Lymphomas. Lymphomas may appear within the mediastinum (in the anterosuperior or middle division) as a part of disseminated disease or as localized primary disease. The majority of patients with mediastinal lymphoma have symptoms of compression, often with fever, weight loss, and pruritus. The goal of surgery for the patient with suspected lymphoma is to obtain adequate tissue for accurate histologic analysis. Generally, needle aspiration is inadequate, and a limited invasive procedure (mediastinoscopy or anterior mediastinotomy) is required. The treatment of choice is radiation therapy. Chemotherapy is added if disseminated disease is present.

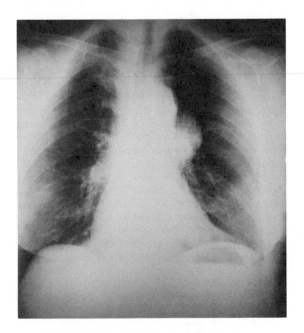

Fig. 29-22. Chest film demonstrating thymoma.

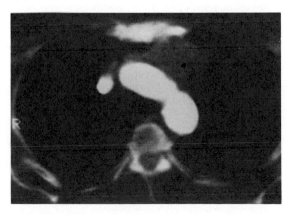

Fig. 29-23. CT of chest demonstrating thymoma between aorta and sternum.

Teratodermoid tumors. There are three major types of teratodermoid tumors: epidermoid cyst, dermoid cyst, and teratoma. In all three types, elements of more than one germinal layer are present, and teratomas contain elements of all three germinal layers. These tumors are usually asymptomatic, but rupture into the pleura, pericardium, or bronchus may occur. Radiographic examination is diagnostic if cartilage, bone, or teeth is seen in a tumor in the anterior mediastinum. Malignant teratomas may occur, and removal is always indicated.

Intrathoracic goiters. Intrathoracic goiters occur as extensions of cervical goiters. Most affected patients suffer stridor, dyspnea, or dysphagia, and the symptoms may be positional. Most patients are euthyroid and some may have no palpable neck mass on examination. Plain radiographs show a lobulated shadow high in the anterior mediastinum with displacement of the trachea. CT studies demonstrate the cervical origin of the mass and allow for examination of the remainder of the mediastinum. Resection of the intrathoracic thyroid tissue is recommended to relieve symptoms or to prevent the future development of stridor. Furthermore, occasional resected substernal goiters are found to harbor carcinoma (which may be occult). The operation can usually be accomplished adequately through a cervical incision.

Miscellaneous anterosuperior mediastinal tumors. Various other tumors may occur within the anterosuperior mediastinum including lymphangioma, hemangioma, lipoma, thyroid adenoma, and parathyroid adenoma.

Middle Mediastinal Tumors

Mesothelial cysts. Mesothelial cysts are relatively common in the middle mediastinum. Most are found closely applied to the pericardium and are called pericardial, or "spring water," cysts because of the clear fluid they contain. These arise from a portion of the pleuroperitoneal membrane that is pinched-off during the formation of the diaphragm. They are present close to the cardiophrenic angle and contain fluid similar to pericardial fluid. These cysts are always benign and usually asymptomatic. Needle aspiration is sufficient therapy, but excision is often recommended to confirm the diagnosis and rule out malignant tumors.

Bronchogenic cysts. Bronchogenic cysts also occur in the middle mediastinum. Since the tumors are derived from lung tissue, they are discussed above, under "Congenital Malformation of the Lungs and Bronchi."

Lymphomas. Lymphomas, both Hodgkin's and non-Hodgkin's type, are commonly found within the middle mediastinum. These tumors are discussed above, under "Anterior Mediastinal Tumors."

Posterior Mediastinal Tumors

Neurogenic tumors. Tumors of neural origin are by far the most common tumors of the posterior mediastinum. They are usually benign, and the major histologic types are neurofibroma, neurilemmoma, malignant schwannoma, ganglioneuroma, neuroblastoma, paraganglioma, and pheochromocytoma.

These tumors are commonly asymptomatic and are discovered on incidental radiographic examination of the chest. Widening of the involved intercostal space or enlargement of the intervertebral foramen may be evident. Symptoms may be due to pressure on adjacent structures or secondary to hormonal activity of certain tumors. Elevated urinary levels of vanillylmandelic acid occur with ganglioneuromas and neuroblastomas, symptoms of which include diarrhea, abdominal distention, hypertension, flushing, and sweating. Pheochromocytomas are hormonally active tumors associated with elevated urinary catecholamine levels and episodic hypertension. Neurofibromas are seen in association with von Recklinghausen's disease. They frequently arise at the intervertebral foramen, and there may be intraspinal extension of tumor. It is generally recommended that patients with tumors at this location undergo CT or myelography of the spine to determine whether intraspinal extension is present. Failure to realize this anatomic extension of the tumor can lead to intraspinal bleeding and spinal cord damage at the time of surgery.

Neuroblastomas are malignant sympathetic nervous system tumors that occur in children and are associated with catecholamine production. This interesting tumor has shown the ability to undergo transformation into benign ganglioneuroma or to regress without treatment, but the majority are highly malignant.

Neurogenic tumors of the posterior mediastinum are excised through posterolateral thoracotomy incisions. Patients with malignant lesions often receive postoperative radiation, and in some instances chemotherapy may be indicated.

Enteric cysts. Also known as duplication cysts, enteric cysts arise embryonically from that portion of the foregut from which the gastrointestinal tract develops. Commonly, they are smooth walled, the wall having a histologic resemblance to esophagus, stomach, or small intestine. They frequently occur closely applied to the esophagus and may cause symptoms due to esophageal obstruction. Resection is indicated to prevent bleeding, perforation, and compression symptoms.

DISORDERS OF THE ESOPHAGUS
Diagnostic Measures

Evaluation of symptoms suggestive of esophageal disease usually begins with a barium swallow. This easily performed radiographic study is very useful for diagnosing obstructive lesions and suggesting the presence of motor dysfunction. Confirmation of the presence of pathologic gastroesophageal reflux is not, however, made reliably with this examination. For further evaluation of the abnormalities demonstrated by the esophagogram, esophagoscopy frequently is performed with either flexible fiberoptic or rigid endoscope. Flexible esophagoscopy has the advantages of increased patient comfort (performed under topical anesthesia) and the ability to visualize the stomach and duodenum. Small biopsies of mucosal abnormalities may be obtained through the endoscope. Rigid esophagoscopy, best performed using general anesthesia, allows the operator to obtain biopsy specimens, remove foreign bodies, and perform dilation of the esophagus under direct vision; however, the stomach cannot be visualized with the rigid esophagoscope. For the evaluation of most common esophageal disorders, flexible esophagoscopy is usually the endoscopic technique of choice. Complications of esophagoscopy include aspiration and perforation of the esophagus.

Esophageal function tests are utilized frequently to evaluate possible motor disorders and to document significant gastroesophageal reflux. Esophageal manometry utilizes a multiport catheter attached to pressure transducers that record the pressure changes at various levels of the esophagus at rest and with swallowing. Abnormal esophageal peristalsis, muscle spasm, and abnormalities of the gastroesophageal sphincter can thus be documented. Techniques to measure distal esophageal pH are widely used to document gastroesophageal reflux. The acid reflux test involves instillation of 250 ml of 0.1 N hydrochloric acid into the stomach and placement of the peroral pH probe 5 cm above the gastroesophageal junction. Reflux of the acid into the esophagus (with pH lowering) indicates a positive result. Twenty-four-hour esophageal pH monitoring can also be accomplished, and frequent episodes of low distal esophageal pH are diagnostic of significant reflux.

Gastroesophageal Reflux and Esophageal Stricture

The esophageal mucosa is very susceptible to injury from gastric juice. Reflux of acid from the stomach into the distal esophagus leads to esophagitis with the potential for ulcer formation. Chronic esophagitis leads to fibrosis of the esophageal wall and subsequent stricture formation. Most commonly, reflux esophagitis is associated with the presence of a sliding hiatal hernia in which the gastroesophageal junction and a portion of the stomach are actually supradiaphragmatic. Sliding hiatal hernias are, however, relatively common, and most are not associated with significant gastroesophageal reflux. Patients with esophagitis complain of heartburn and suffer regurgitation of bitter-tasting material into the mouth. These symptoms are usually worse when the patient is supine and after meals. The diagnosis is suggested by barium swallow and confirmed by esophagoscopy (visualizing distal esophagitis) and pH monitoring tests. When stricture has developed, the patient's chief complaint is usually dysphagia, and a barium swallow reveals the site of esophageal narrowing. Esophagoscopy with biopsy should be performed to rule out malignant causes of esophageal obstruction.

The initial treatment of gastroesophageal reflux should be conservative. Antacids, avoidance of the supine position (elevating the head of the patient's bed 6 inches), not going to bed directly after meals, and eliminating certain foods (caffeine, alcohol, chocolate, and nicotine) and practices known to lower gastroesophageal junction pressure will ameliorate many patients' symptoms. Drugs to reduce gastric acid production (cimetidine) may be of value in selected patients.

The indications for antireflux surgery include failure of medical management, ulcerative esophagitis, stricture, recurrent aspiration, and bleeding. Various procedures have been devised to prevent gastroesophageal reflux, and the one commonly performed today in the United States is the Nissen fundoplication. Esophageal strictures usually may be dilated successfully at the time of antireflux operation. Severe nondilatable strictures may require removal of the esophagus and replacement with another conduit such as stomach or colon.

Paraesophageal Hernia

Paraesophageal hernias represent the situation in which the gastroesophageal junction maintains its normal subdiaphragmatic location but the stomach herniates through a defect in the diaphragm close to the gastroesophageal junction. This situation is very uncommon but represents a clear-cut danger to the patient. Bleeding, strangulation, or infarction of the intrathoracic portion of the stomach may occur and may be fatal. Although frequently asymptomatic, paraesophageal hernias should be repaired surgically.

Motor Disease of the Esophagus

The two major motor disorders of the esophagus are achalasia and diffuse esophageal spasm. Achalasia is an intrinsic disorder of the esophagus characterized by failure of the lower esophageal sphincter mechanism to relax with swallowing. The esophagus gradually hypertrophies, dilates, becomes tortuous, and loses effective peristalsis. The etiology is unknown but degeneration of Auerbach's plexus may be an underlying mechanism. The classical symptom triad is dysphagia, regurgitation, and weight loss; pain is not a prominent complaint. A significant number of patients with achalasia develop pulmonary complications secondary to aspiration, and the incidence of esophageal carcinoma in achalasia patients is approximately 10 times that of patients without the disorder. Barium swallow is diagnostic, showing concentric or sigmoid dilation of the esophagus with abrupt narrowing at its entrance to the stomach ("bird-beak" gastroesophageal junction; Fig. 29-24). Achalasia may be treated by pneumatic balloon dilation of the gastroesophageal junction or by surgi-

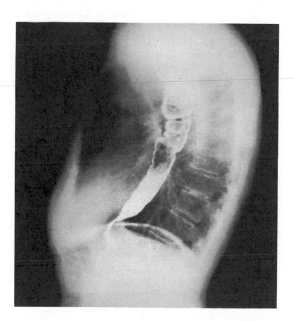

Fig. 29-24. Barium swallow of achalasia. Dilation and tortuosity of esophagus and narrowing of esophagogastric junction is demonstrated.

cally splitting the thickened constricting musculature at the esophagogastric junction (modified Heller myotomy operation). Pneumatic dilation may require several repeat procedures but gives satisfactory results in approximatley 65% of patients. The modified Heller operation may be performed with low morbidity and mortality and produces satisfactory results in 85% of patients, many of whom have failed previous pneumatic dilation.

Diffuse esophageal spasm is a disorder characterized by simultaneous high-pressure contraction waves in the distal two thirds of the esophagus with lack of propulsion in that region. Patients with this disorder suffer dysphagia and substernal pain, which may at times be confused with angina pectoris. The diagnosis is confirmed by barium swallow and manometric studies. In severe cases, a long esophageal myotomy is performed, but the results of this operation are not as successful as surgery performed for achalasia.

Esophageal Diverticula

Diverticula of the esophagus are of two major types; traction and pulsion. Traction diverticula occur in the midesophagus secondary to neighboring lymph node inflammation, causing traction on the wall of the esophagus and creating outpouchings. These are true diverticula in that they contain all coats of the esophageal wall. Pulsion diverticula are false diverticula— outpouchings of esophageal mucosa that herniate between the muscle fibers. Pulsion diverticula occur secondary to esophageal motor dysfunction distal to the site of the diverticulum. Increased motor tone causes locally high intraluminal pressure and forces the mucosa outward between the muscle layers to form the diverticulum. Pulsion diverticula most commonly occur in the cervical esophagus (Zenker's diverticulum) and just above the gastroesophageal junction (epiphrenic diverticulum). Zenker's diverticula are outpouchings of the esophagus in the neck just above the cricopharyngeal muscle. Dysfunction of the cricopharyngeus is characterized by failure to relax, creating a high-pressure zone above the muscular ring that causes herniation of the esophageal mucosa. Occurring most commonly in older patients, Zenker's diverticula cause choking, aspiration, and coughing. Surgery to correct the condition involves splitting the cricopharyngeal muscle and removal of the diverticulum if it is large. Epiphrenic diverticula are pulsion diverticula that occur just above the diaphragm and are also usually associated with motility abnormalities. Myotomy of the muscle fibers below the hernia sac is indicated, with excision of large diverticula.

Benign Tumors of the Esophagus

Benign tumors of the esophagus are rare. The most common type is leiomyoma. These extramucosal tumors produce smooth deformity of the esophageal lumen and their appearance on barium swallow is characteristic. They are usually found in the middle and lower thirds of the esophagus. Dysphagia is the predominant symptom. Enucleation via thoracotomy is curative.

Malignant Tumors of the Esophagus

Cancer of the esophagus is a disappointing disease to treat because of the advanced stage at which it usu-

ally presents and the low cure rate. Predisposing factors include alcohol abuse, tobacco abuse, Barrett's esophagus (transformation of esophageal mucosa from squamous to glandular type), previous caustic burns, and achalasia. The majority of esophageal carcinomas are squamous cell carcinomas, although adenocarcinoma predominates in the distal one third of the esophagus. The onset of the disease is insidious, and severe (more than 75%) obstruction of the esophageal lumen usually is present before dysphagia develops. Weight loss, malaise, and general weakness often are also present at the time of diagnosis. Barium swallow will reveal the obstructing lesion, and endoscopic biopsy confirms its identity (Fig. 29-25). The treatment of esophageal carcinoma depends largely on the stage of the disease. Clearly unresectable large tumors involving other intrathoracic structures are generally treated by radiation therapy and may require placement of a plastic tube through the remaining lumen to maintain patency. Cure rates with these techniques are low and complications are frequent. Surgery for esophageal carcinoma may be performed by various techniques, and the approach depends on the site of the tumor in the esophagus. Upper third lesions are often treated by radiation because the cure rate is extremely low after resection, which usually requires laryngectomy and complicated plastic reconstruction. Middle and lower third lesions may be resected for cure or palliation. Replacement of the resected esophagus by advancing the stomach into the chest or replacement with colon (maintaining its blood supply) are frequently performed procedures. Middle third tumors are approached through a right thoracotomy, whereas lower third lesions are best exposed by a left thoracotomy. Esophagectomy without thoracotomy may be performed through a combined transabdominal and cervical approach, the mobilized stomach being advanced into the neck where it is anasto-

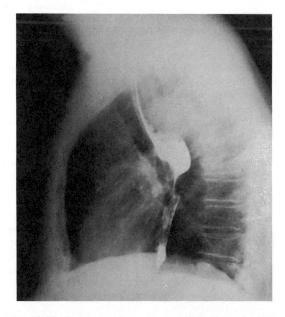

Fig. 29-25. Barium swallow showing carcinoma of middle third of esophagus producing abrupt narrowing of dye column.

mosed to the cervical esophagus. Unfortunately, despite the variety of potential management methods, cancer of the esophagus has a very poor prognosis, and the great majority of patients die within 2 years of diagnosis.

TRAUMA TO THE CHEST

Next to cardiovascular disease and cancer, trauma is the third leading cause of death for men and the fifth leading cause of death for women of all ages in the United States. Accidents are the leading cause of death for all people ages 1 to 34 years. Urban violence and automobile accidents are in large measure responsible. Trauma to the chest is estimated to be the chief cause of 25% of deaths from auto accidents, and 50% of accident patients who die have significant chest trauma. The sequence of evaluation of the chest trauma patient depends upon the location and nature of the injury. After initial airway control and maintenance of ventilation and circulation, chest films should be obtained. Further studies such as barium swallow, arteriography, or bronchoscopy may be indicated based on the history of the injury and the clues provided by the chest studies.

Chest Wall and Lung Injuries

While an uncomplicated rib fracture requires no specific therapy other than pain control, multiple rib fractures produce an unstable segment of chest wall that moves paradoxically inward upon inspiration and balloons outward during expiration (flail chest). This injury is commonly sustained when the chest hits the automobile steering wheel (Fig. 29-26). While chest wall instability does have some adverse affects on the mechanics of ventilation, it is usually the severe contusion of the underlying lung, which often leads to respiratory failure, that may be fatal. Interstitial and intraalveolar hemorrhage associated with contusive injury to the lung results in pronounced ventilation and perfusion abnormalities so that the oxygenated blood passes through the lung without proper gas exchange (physiologic shunt). This results in systemic hypoxemia. Splinting of the cough mechanism owing to pain and chest wall instability prevents adequate clearing of the airway and may result in secondary pneumonia. Treatment of severe cases requires endotracheal intubation, mechanical ventilation (often with positive end-expiratory pressure), and careful fluid management. Surgical stabilization of the chest wall is rarely required.

Pneumothorax and Hemothorax

Traumatic pneumothorax and hemothorax should always be suspected in patients who have suffered penetrating or blunt trauma to the chest. Broken rib edges can lacerate the lung and cause entry of air and blood into the pleural space. If air or blood accumulates rapidly, the mediastinum is shifted toward the uninvolved side and that lung may be compressed (tension pneumothorax or hemothorax). Twisting or compression of the vena cava limits venous return to the heart; cardiac output falls and circulatory shock results. Treatment is needle aspiration of the pleural space followed by tube thoracostomy. If persistent massive bleeding becomes evident, emergent thoracotomy is indicated for control. When a large amount of blood has collected in the pleural space and is not effectively removed by chest

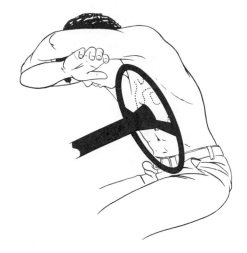

Fig. 29-26. Steering wheel injury to chest. Injury to chest wall may result in rib fractures and flail chest. Contusion of underlying heart and lungs causes reduced cardiac output and arterial hypoxemia. Rupture of thoracic aorta may also result.

tubes, elective thoracotomy and removal of the hematoma may be indicated to prevent lung entrapment.

An open pneumothorax is caused by penetrating trauma or avulsion injury that results in loss of chest wall continuity. This allows equalization of the intrathoracic and extrathoracic pressures. With breathing, air moves in and out of the hole in the chest wall, reducing the patient's tidal volume and leading to hypoxemia and hypercarbia. Management is insertion of a chest tube and placement of a sterile occlusive dressing over the "sucking" chest wound. Definitive treatment requires operative closure of the chest wall hole.

Rupture of a Major Airway

Most major airway ruptures are produced by blunt trauma that tears the large airway structures, producing severe air leaks. Dyspnea, cough, hemoptysis, tension pneumothorax, and subcutaneous emphysema promptly develop, which immediately place the patient in grave jeopardy. Bronchoscopy is utilized to confirm diagnosis. Early thoracotomy and repair should be performed, since bronchial stenosis, infection, and a destroyed lung might otherwise result.

Cardiac Trauma

Cardiac trauma may be classified as penetrating or nonpenetrating. Penetrating injuries to the heart are made by a sharp object or missile. If the patient survives the immediate penetrating injury to the heart, cardiac tamponade often develops. A relatively small amount of blood within the closed pericardial space is sufficient to interfere with cardiac filling, thereby reducing cardiac output. The patient is restless and has air hunger. Heart tones are distant, and there may be a pericardial friction rub; blood pressure is reduced and pulse pressure is narrow. Venous pressure is elevated and neck veins are distended. Chest radiographs show a normal-sized heart, and the electrocardiogram (ECG) is helpful in diagnosis only when there is coronary artery injury.

Immediate treatment is pericardiocentesis. A needle is passed into the pericardial space (under ECG monitoring) to remove accumulated blood. A large-bore needle connected to the ECG is inserted along the sternum at the left sternocostal angle and directed cephalad and posteriorly toward the heart at a 45-degree angle to the sternum. As the needle passes through the chest wall to the pericardial sac, the ECG reading is similar to lead V_2. If the needle contacts myocardium, a current of injury or multiple premature ventricular contractions will be noted on the ECG. The needle is then withdrawn slightly and the contents of the pericardial sac are aspirated. If the blood pressure improves and central venous pressure falls after pericardiocentesis, the patient may be observed and monitored closely. Should signs of cardiac tamponade return, immediate operation is indicated to remove blood from the pericardial sac and repair the myocardial injury. Because of its anterior position the right ventricle is lacerated more frequently in penetrating wounds of the heart. Simple suture closure that avoids injury to neighboring coronary arteries is the usual method of treatment.

Nonpenetrating injury of the myocardium caused by blunt trauma to the chest wall is probably more frequent than is clinically recognized. Steering wheel injury in an automobile accident and other forms of trauma to the anterior chest wall produce this injury, the physiologic consequences of which are cardiac arrhythmias and reduced cardiac output, which are directly related to the amount of contused myocardium. Despite these two complications, it is remarkable that patients often survive severe trauma to the heart. The diagnosis of cardiac contusion is difficult because ECG and serum myocardial enzyme patterns are nonspecific, although radioisotope techniques involving technetium-labeled phosphate complexes may be useful in demonstrating injured myocardium. Treatment of this condition is similar to that for myocardial infarction and involves rhythm monitoring, with aggressive treatment of arrhythmias, and inotropic agents to support cardiac output while the myocardium heals.

Aortic Injuries

Eighty-five percent of patients with thoracic aortic injuries die at the time of injury, commonly caused by collision between the anterior chest and the steering wheel or dashboard. The most common site of aortic rupture is in the proximal descending aorta, just beyond the origin of the left subclavian artery. The next most common site is the ascending aorta just above the aortic valve. These transverse tears may be partial or may involve the entire circumference; the aorta is held together by a thin adventitia layer in those who survive. The diagnosis is frequently missed because it is not considered. Radiographic examination of the chest shows widening of the mediastinum, and angiography confirms the diagnosis. Other suggestive signs are cervical hematoma, tracheal deviation, hemothorax, asymmetry of the radial pulses, and a paralyzed left vocal cord. Immediate repair should be performed. For ascending aortic tears, total cardiopulmonary bypass is required, but injuries to the more common site can often be performed without bypass or with modified forms of left heart bypass.

Ruptured Diaphragm

Blunt trauma and crushing injuries are the usual cause of a ruptured diaphragm. Diaphragmatic rupture most commonly occurs on the left side adjacent to the esophageal hiatus, but injury to every part of the diaphragm has been described. The symptoms are nonspecific and if there is no evidence of external trauma, the diagnosis can be missed. Progressive cardiorespiratory distress is observed as more and more viscera enter the chest and collapse the lung, push the mediastinal structures to the opposite side, and impede venous return to the heart and expansion of the lung. Signs suggestive of ruptured diaphragm are bowel sounds heard in the chest and difficulty passing a nasogastric tube. A chest film is extremely valuable in diagnosis, especially a lateral view showing bowel loops in the chest. Patients should undergo reduction of the viscera and closure of the diaphragmatic tear. Repair of acute rupture is most commonly performed through an abdominal incision. Diaphragmatic rupture is not always recognized at the time of injury and these patients may present to the surgeon later, often after the diagnosis has been made on the basis of an abnormal chest film. For these patients, repair through a thoracotomy is usually preferred owing to the presence of adhesions between the viscera and chest wall, which are more easily managed through this incision.

Esophageal Lacerations and Ruptures

Lacerations of the esophagus, usually caused by instrumentation or by penetrating objects, occur most frequently in the upper third. As a general rule, any cervical wound penetrating the platysma should be explored surgically. Penetrating injuries to the neck often require evaluation by barium swallow, esophagoscopy, and arteriography to exclude injuries to the esophagus, airway, and neck vessels. Cervical esophageal tears are repaired through a neck incision and drains are placed.

Ingestion of caustics may produce variable amounts of injury to the esophagus. Most commonly, there is evidence of mucosal burns in the mouth and pharynx, and early endoscopy is usually indicated to determine the extent of esophageal involvement. Management is variable, depending on the degree of tissue damage present.

Injuries of the thoracic esophagus from blunt trauma are rare, and the trauma need not be severe to cause disruption. Penetrating esophageal injuries are accompanied frequently by injuries to the heart and great vessels. In all such cases, repair of the injuries should be carried out as soon as possible. Instrumentation injuries are most common in the cervical esophagus, just above the cricopharyngeus muscle. Distal esophageal perforation is the second most common site of instrumentation injury. If recognized early, repair may be performed successfully, but those perforations diagnosed more than 6 hours after the injury have a high rate of complications and mortality.

Spontaneous rupture of the esophagus (Boerhaave's disease) occurs usually after large meals and strenuous vomiting. On occasion it is seen after lifting, seizures, and childbirth. Early surgical repair is indicated.

Perforations and lacerations of the esophagus usually cause dysphagia, vomiting, and subcutaneous emphysema. Movement and inspiration aggravate the pain. The presence of air bubbles, an air-fluid level, or widening of the mediastinum on x-ray examination is suggestive of esophageal injury. Pleural effusion (which will potentially become an empyema) frequently accompanies esophageal trauma. Recognition is based on radiographic studies. Water-base contrast material (Hypaque) is utilized because it is less irritat-ing to the mediastinum should extraesophageal extravasation occur.

Foreign Bodies

Foreign bodies in the chest are not in themselves an indication for emergency removal unless associated with potential infection or lodged near important vascular or other intrathoracic structures.

30

Cardiac Surgery

Congenital Heart Disease

Flavian M. Lupinetti
Douglas M. Behrendt

GENERAL CONSIDERATIONS

Proper treatment of patients with congenital heart disease begins with accurate diagnosis. In most cases this requires cardiac catheterization and contrast studies, although echocardiography is becoming increasingly reliable. Since many patients requiring surgical treatment of congenital heart defects are neonates, thorough preoperative preparation is essential.

Adequate ventilation and oxygenation should be confirmed. Intubation and mechanical ventilation may be required. Intravenous access should be provided and hypovolemia corrected appropriately. Metabolic acidosis is a frequent consequence of congestive failure in congenital heart disease and must be treated vigorously. Since neonates have difficulty with thermal autoregulation, temperature should be monitored continuously and external warming used as needed.

In more elective cases, many of these considerations are less critical. One should nonetheless insist on a thorough preoperative evaluation to ensure optimal surgical results. In particular, children must be evaluated for intercurrent infections, which generally are sufficient reason to delay elective procedures.

ABNORMALITIES OF THE AORTIC ARCH

The great arteries and their major branches are derived from six pairs of embryonic aortic arches. The third aortic arch forms most of the common and internal carotid arteries. The left fourth arch forms part of the definitive aortic arch, while the right fourth arch forms the proximal right subclavian artery. The right sixth aortic arch develops into the right pulmonary artery. The distal part of the left sixth arch persists as the ductus arteriosus. The greatest portions of the remaining aortic arches regress.

Patent Ductus Arteriosus

After birth, stimulated by the increase in blood oxygen tension and the fall in pulmonary artery pressure, the ductus arteriosus normally closes. A persistent patent ductus arteriosus (PDA; Fig. 30-1) produces excessive pulmonary blood flow and may result in congestive heart failure. Premature infants are particularly likely to have a patent ductus. These patients may exhibit tachycardia, tachypnea, poor feeding and growth, or even respiratory distress requiring mechanical ventilation. Administration of indomethacin is sometimes effective in closing the ductus, but often surgical closure is required. Term infants and older children with a patent ductus are typically less severely affected, although they too may display symptoms of congestive failure. When the shunt is large, examination of the heart reveals a hyperactive precordium and a continuous, harsh murmur that varies in intensity (the "machinery" murmur) audible in the upper left chest and back.

Operation should be considered for all patients with PDA. In early life, the primary reason for operative treatment is the relief of left ventricular volume overload and the prevention of failure. While failure may occur in an older child or even an occasional adult with a large patent ductus, the possibility of endocarditis constitutes the usual indication for operation in the patient with a small ductus. Operative closure of the ductus is accomplished via left thoracotomy. The ductus is dissected from between the aorta and the pulmonary artery. It is then ligated with multiple sutures, or it may be divided. Operative mortality should approach zero, and morbidity is quite low.

Coarctation of the Aorta

Coarctation of the aorta (see Fig. 30-1) is a narrowing of the aorta, most commonly in the vicinity of the left subclavian artery and the ligamentum arteriosum, the remnant left by a closed ductus arteriosus. It has been hypothesized that the presence of some ductus-derived tissue in the aorta causes narrowing to occur when this tissue undergoes the same involution displayed by the normally closing ductus. Coarctation may cause profound congestive failure in small infants. It may cause no symptoms in older children and may be discovered during a diagnostic evaluation for hypertension. Physical examination demonstrates diminished lower extremity pulses and a marked difference in blood pressures between the arms and legs.

Coarctation should be corrected to avoid the long-term consequences of hypertension and congestive failure that are likely in the absence of operative intervention. There are several accepted operations for coarctation. Excision of the coarct segment with end-to-end anastomosis was the first approach employed. Because of concern about problems such as growth of the anastomosis, other procedures have evolved. These include the use of the subclavian artery as a patch to enlarge the aorta and the use of a synthetic graft to patch open the

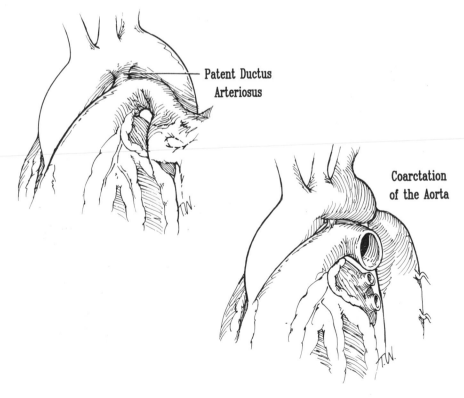

Patent Ductus
Arteriosus

Coarctation
of the Aorta

Fig. 30-1. Aortic arch anomalies: *left;* Patent ductus arteriosus; *right;* coarctation of the aorta.

narrowed segment. A small percentage of all of these repairs are complicated by recurrent coarctation, and reoperation is sometimes required. The probability of curing the hypertension is greatest when operation is performed early in life and quite small when operation is performed in adults.

Vascular Rings

Anomalies of the aortic arch and its major branches that encircle the trachea or esophagus are referred to as vascular rings. The anatomy of a vascular ring may include a double aortic arch, anomalous origin of a subclavian artery, a ligamentum arteriosum arising from a right aortic arch, or other abnormalities. Vascular rings produce esophageal obstruction and dysphagia or tracheal obstruction and dyspnea, stridor, chronic cough, and recurrent pulmonary infections. The diagnosis is made by barium swallow, and arteriography is rarely needed. All patients who have symptoms from vascular rings should undergo operation. Surgical treatment requires division of part of the ring and thorough dissection of the vessels from the other mediastinal structures.

Interrupted Aortic Arch

Interrupted aortic arch is a rare condition characterized by complete separation of the aorta at a point along the transverse arch. In most cases the distal aorta is perfused by a PDA. When the ductus begins to close perfusion to the lower portion of the body falls to dangerously low levels, and profound acidosis, renal failure, and heart failure develop. Operative approaches to this problem include direct anastomosis of the inter-rupted ends and graft interposition; both approaches are associated with extremely high operative mortality.

ABNORMALITIES OF THE ATRIAL AND VENTRICULAR SEPTA

The interatrial septum develops from two embryonically separate structures. The septum primum arises from a depression in the common atrium formed by the expansion of the atrium around the truncus arteriosus. The septum primum extends from the roof of the atrium toward the endocardial cushions in the atrioventricular canal. The remaining opening between the right and left sides is the ostium primum. Before this opening is sealed, perforations appear in the septum primum and coalesce into the ostium secundum. The continued expansion of the right atrium incorporates the primitive sinus horn of the superior vena cava. This incorporation results in the infolding of a second ridge of atrium, the septum secundum. The septum secundum does not completely partition the atrium; instead it overlaps with the septum primum, leaving an oblique pathway, the foramen ovale, between the right and left atria. After birth, the fall in pulmonary vascular resistance results in a relatively higher left atrial pressure, closing and usually sealing the foramen ovale.

Atrial Septal Defect

Atrial septal defect (ASD, Fig. 30-2) results from an abnormality of the embryonic sequence described above. Inadequate development of the septum secundum results in the ostium secundum type of ASD. There are several morphologic variants of this defect, not including the probe-patent foramen ovale, which

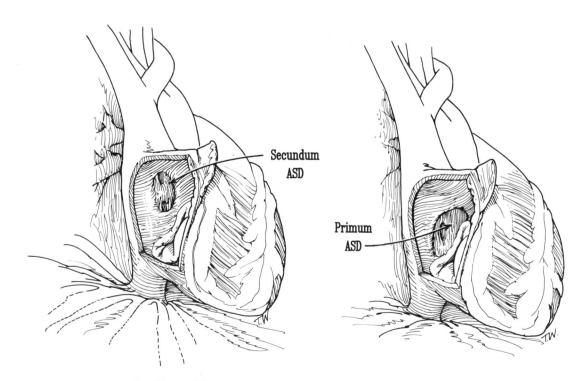

Fig. 30-2. Atrial Septal defects: *left;* secundum ASD; *right;* primum ASD

occurs in many asymptomatic individuals. The ostium primum ASD is related to a defect in formation of the septum primum and the endocardial cushions and represents the less severe end of the spectrum of complete atrioventricular canal.

The clinical manifestations of ASD are determined by the relative amount of left-to-right shunting of blood across the defect. This is typically expressed as the Q_P/Q_S, or the ratio of pulmonary to systemic blood flow. The Q_P/Q_S is determined not so much by the size of the ASD as by the relative compliance of the left and right ventricles. A Q_P/Q_S of less than 1.5 usually does not cause symptoms, nor does it require surgical intervention in many cases. At higher ratios, especially over 2.0, the eventual development of symptoms such as progressive heart failure or arrhythmias becomes more probable.

It is fortunate that many patients with ASD are diagnosed in childhood on routine physical examination by the detection of a murmur before the onset of symptoms. When not discovered and treated early, ASD may produce dyspnea on exertion, easy fatigability, palpitations, and, eventually, pulmonary hypertension and congestive failure. Rarely, a paradoxical embolus, a systemic arterial embolus resulting from a venous thrombus, may be the first presentation.

Physical findings of an ASD are attributable to the increased pulmonary blood flow. They include a parasternal lift, a systolic flow murmur near the upper left sternal border, and fixed splitting of the second heart sound. The chest film typically demonstrates an enlarged heart and an increase in the pulmonary vasculature. The diagnosis is confirmed by cardiac catheterization, which shows an increase in oxygen saturation of the atrial blood over that in the venae cavae.

Operation is indicated for any patient with symptoms or in asymptomatic patients with a Q_P/Q_S exceeding 1.5 to 2.0. Operation is performed using cardiopulmonary bypass. The right atrium is opened and the defect is visualized. Closure is accomplished with simple suturing of the defect or with a patch of pericardium or synthetic material. Operative mortality should approach zero, and long-term results are excellent.

Ventricular Septal Defect

The membranous portion of the interventricular septum develops partly from the endocardial cushions and partly from the conotruncal ridges of the embryonic great arteries. The muscular portion of the septum is formed by fusion of the medial walls of the ventricles as they expand and dilate. A developmental abnormality of this process results in a ventricular septal defect (VSD, Fig. 30-3), the commonest of all serious congenital heart defects.

VSDs are classified by their location. Muscular VSDs are located in the muscular portion of the septum and are frequently multiple. This is the type of VSD most likely to undergo spontaneous closure. Perimembranous VSDs, which are found adjacent to the tricuspid anulus near the anteroseptal commissure, are the type that most commonly require operative closure. Less common types of VSD are the supracristal type, immediately inferior to the pulmonary valve, and the atrioventricular canal type, located posteriorly in the inlet portion of the right ventricular wall, inferior to the septal leaflet of the tricuspid valve.

Of all VSDs present at birth, most close spontaneously within the first year of life. VSDs still present at age 5 or 6 years rarely close. The physiologic consequences of this condition are determined primarily by

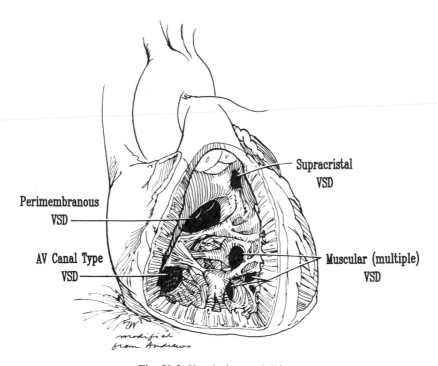

Fig. 30-3. Ventricular septal defects.

the size of the defect. Very large defects can cause severe failure in the early months of life. Infants with large VSDs exhibit tachypnea and poor feeding and have an active precordium with a harsh, pansystolic murmur. Moderate to large defects may be tolerated for several months, but typically growth retardation is a problem. Delayed treatment of large VSDs may prevent the normal maturational changes in the pulmonary arteries and lead to irreversible pulmonary hypertension. Older children with smaller VSDs may have symptoms ranging from mild to severe fatigue. These children may be diagnosed by the characteristic loud, pansystolic murmur, biventricular lift, and chest film that shows increased pulmonary markings.

Operation is indicated for patients with VSDs and severe symptoms at any age. In very small patients with complex or multiple defects, pulmonary artery banding protects against pulmonary hypertension and relieves symptoms while allowing the child to grow until definitive surgery can be performed. The definitive procedure consits of closure of the defect, usually with a prosthetic patch. Large VSDs should be closed before age 2 years if possible, since the risk of pulmonary vascular disease increases after this age. Patients with long-standing severe pulmonary hypertension leading to increased pulmonary vascular resistance are not likely to benefit from closure of the defect and, in fact, can be made more seriously ill. The results of operating on all other patients with VSDs are quite good. Mortality is limited almost exclusively to patients with severe cardiac failure in the preoperative period. The most common operative complication is injury to the conduction system; avoiding this problem requires intimate knowledge of the anatomy of the His bundle and its branches.

Arterioventricular Canal Defect

The embryonic endocardial cushions contribute to the formation of the atrioventricular valves as well as the interatrial and interventricular septa. Abnormalities in the development of these structures give rise to a variety of endocardial cushion, or atrioventricular canal (AVC), defects. The spectrum of these defects spans the primum ASD (above); the complete AVC, with large atrial and ventricular defects and a common atrioventricular valve; and a number of intermediate forms.

Patients with complete AVC generally present within the first year of life with severe and progressive cardiac failure. Physical findings include increased precordial activity, systolic murmur, and fixed splitting of the second heart sound. Increased pulmonary vascularity and cardiomegaly are typical radiographic findings.

Less complete forms of AVC may not cause symptoms for many years. For these patients operation should be performed to avoid long-term sequelae as in ASD. Patients with complete AVC often require operation early in the first year of life because of progressive failure. The incidence of pulmonary vascular disease increases markedly during infancy; thus, operation should be considered before 6 months of age in most cases to prevent irreversible changes.

Surgical treatment of complete AVC requires repair of both ASDs and VSDs. It is interesting that the atrioventricular valve is functionally competent in most cases, and it is important for the surgeon to preserve this competence at operation. Operative mortality for partial forms of AVC is essentially that of ASD repair. The risk of death after operation for complete AVC is much higher. In the absence of preexisting pulmonary vascular disease and mitral valve regurgitation, long-term results of operation are good, although many patients are left with some mitral valve incompetence.

AORTIC STENOSIS

Congenital aortic stenosis (CAS) most commonly involves the aortic valve itself. The valve is usually bicuspid, although stenosis of tricuspid valves occurs as well. Least common is the valve with an eccentric orifice, the so-called unicuspid valve. In all forms, the cusps are fused and the leaflets tend to be thickened. CAS can also occur from a narrowing in the aorta above the valve (supravalvular aortic stenosis) or from an obstruction in the left ventricular outflow tract below the valve (subvalvular stenosis). The latter is more common, and may be characterized by a discrete diaphragm below a structurally normal aortic valve or by an elongated, irregular tunnellike muscular obstruction.

Like acquired aortic stenosis, CAS is compensated for by an increase in intraventricular work to maintain peripheral pressure. Severe valvular stenosis in infants produces symptoms of congestive failure, including tachycardia, tachypnea, fatigue, diaphoresis, and poor weight gain. Patients who have milder stenosis may develop symptoms only when growth occurs and cardiac output increases. Dyspnea on exertion and fatigue predominate, but angina and syncope occur as well. Sudden death occurs in a certain percentage of patients with CAS but is rare in patients with few or no symptoms. Other congenital heart defects, most notably coarctation, ventricular septal defect, and patent ductus, may coexist with CAS and should be evaluated by catheterization or echocardiogram.

Nevertheless, some neonates with critical valvular aortic stenosis may require emergency operation. Operative mortality in the neonatal age group is as high as 50%. Older patients should be considered for operation when they manifest appropriate symptoms or when they are found to have a sufficiently high transvalvular gradient (>75 torr) at catheterization. Operation requires careful division of the fused commissures. Care must be taken to provide the maximum amount of valve opening without creating aortic insufficiency. The results of operation beyond the first year of life are good, although the valve remains abnormal and a pressure gradient may persist. As many as half of these patients will require reoperation later in life for recurrent stenosis.

Subvalvar CAS of the diaphragmatic type rarely requires operation in the very early years. Operative mortality is quite low in older children, and excision of the membrane is essentially curative. The tunnel form of subvalvar stenosis sometimes is treated by extensive excision of the muscular obstruction, often with poor results. An extracardiac conduit can at times be used to bypass the obstruction. Supravalvular CAS requires enlargement of the aortic root with a pericardial patch. This operation has low mortality and good long-term results.

CAS may be associated with an extremely small left ventricle (hypoplastic left heart syndrome) and/or congenital mitral stenosis. These entities have a dire prognosis, although some good palliative results have been achieved employing certain innovative operations. Recent successes with cardiac transplantation in neonates offer another option that may prove worthwhile.

PULMONARY VALVULAR STENOSIS

Pulmonary valvular stenosis (PVS) is characterized by fusion of the commissures of a valvular apparatus that otherwise appears grossly normal. Pulmonary valvular dysplasia refers to the small percentage of these valves that have abnormally thickened and noncompliant cusps without commissural fusion. This discussion will be limited to those cases of PVS that occur with an intact ventricular septum. One of the main consequences of PVS is right ventricular hypertrophy; this may include hypertrophy of the muscular component of the outflow tract as well, exacerbating the stenosis. Some patients with PVS have a hypoplastic right ventricle.

Patients with PVS of the most severe degree present in the neonatal period with congestive heart failure. When there is a concomitant ASD, cyanosis may also be prominent because of right-to-left shunting. Lesser degrees of stenosis may be manifest later in infancy with similar but milder symptoms. The mildest form may be diagnosed because of an asymptomatic murmur, or because of failure symptoms that gradually develop over many years. Physical findings include a loud systolic murmur and the absence of the pulmonary component of the second heart sound.

Neonates with critical PVS or those with atresia of the pulmonary valve and a hypoplastic right ventricle benefit from a systemic-pulmonary artery shunt, such as a Blalock-Taussig procedure, in addition to a direct approach to the valvular stenosis. In this instance, some surgeons have performed a closed valvotomy (i.e., one that does not require cardiopulmonary bypass). This may be accomplished by enlarging the valve opening using instruments inserted through a purse-string suture in the right ventricle or pulmonary artery, or by inflow occlusion and sharp division of the commissures. In older patients who are better able to tolerate an open heart procedure, the pulmonary artery is opened, the valve is visualized, and the commissures are incised. Operative results are good in all but the youngest and most severely ill patients. More experience is being acquired in balloon valvotomy for nonoperative relief of this condition. Early results with the procedure are encouraging.

TETRALOGY OF FALLOT

The right and left ventricular outflow tracts and the proximal portions of the great arteries develop from the ascending portion of the primitive heart loop, the bulbus cordis. The midportion of the bulbus is called the conus cordis and forms the outflow tracts; the distal portion, the truncus arteriosus, forms the proximal aorta and pulmonary artery. In the truncus two truncal ridges appear, enlarge, and fuse, dividing the truncus into an aortic and a pulmonary side. As the truncus grows, these two channels spiral around each other. If the conotruncal septum is displaced anteriorly, there are significant anatomic derangements. First, there is a large defect of the perimembranous ventricular septum. Second, there is narrowing of the outflow portion of the right ventricle, or infundibular stenosis. Third, unequal division of the truncus by the truncal ridges leads to the aorta arising over the ventricular defect from both ventricles. These are three of the defects that comprise tetralogy of Fallot (TOF, Fig. 30-4). The fourth component is right ventricular hypertrophy, a consequence of the elevated right ventricular pressures.

The degree of infundibular stenosis is great enough to prevent adequate pulmonary artery blood flow. Furthermore, the large VSD ensures that there are equal pressures in the right and left ventricles, and therefore right-to-left shunting occurs. The shunting of unoxygenated blood into the systemic arterial circulation produces cyanosis. Most patients with TOF are not notice-

Tetralogy of Fallot

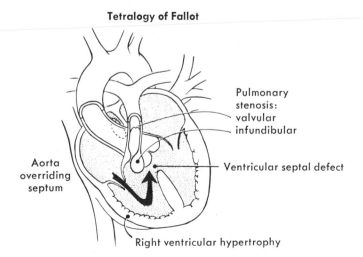

Fig. 30-4. Four defects of tetralogy of Fallot. Decreased pulmonary blood flow and direct ejection of right ventricle to aorta (right-to-left shunt) cause arterial hypoxia.

ably cyanotic at birth, presumably because the ductus arteriosus is patent and provides more nearly adequate pulmonary flow. In the occasional patient who maintains patency of the ductus, operative intervention may not be necessary for several years. Most patients, however, become quite symptomatic early in life. Exercise tolerance is limited, and any activity that increases pulmonary vascular resistance, notably crying, elicits marked cyanosis. Severe paroxysms of hyperpnea and cyanosis, so-called tet spells, are probably related to spasm of the infundibulum in response to endogenous catecholamines. As the child grows older, he or she assumes the characteristic squatting position when fatigued. Polycythemia is another compensatory mechanism in TOF patients; a hematocrit of 60% or more is not uncommon.

Untreated, most patients with TOF die before age 10 and only the rare patient lives beyond age 40. The degree of infundibular stenosis is the primary determinant of the natural history of this condition. Surgical approaches to the treatment of TOF can be divided into palliative and reparative operations.

Palliative operations are those that increase the quantity of pulmonary blood flow without correcting the fundamental cardiac anomaly (Fig. 30-5). The oldest and most commonly employed palliative procedure is the Blalock-Taussig shunt, an anastomosis of the subclavian artery to the pulmonary artery. A common modification of this operation employs prosthetic material to shunt blood from the subclavian or innominate artery to the pulmonary artery. Other palliative procedures include the Waterston shunt (ascending aorta to right pulmonary artery) and the Potts shunt (descending aorta to left pulmonary artery). In neonates and infants, many surgeons prefer to use one of these palliative operations to stabilize the patient and allow for further growth and development. Definitive repair is reserved for later in life.

Other surgeons prefer definitive repair of TOF at the time of diagnosis, regardless of the patient's age or condition. Whenever it is done, definitive operation for TOF consists of closing the ventricular defect and relieving the infundibular stenosis. A prosthetic patch is invariably required to close the ventricular defect be-

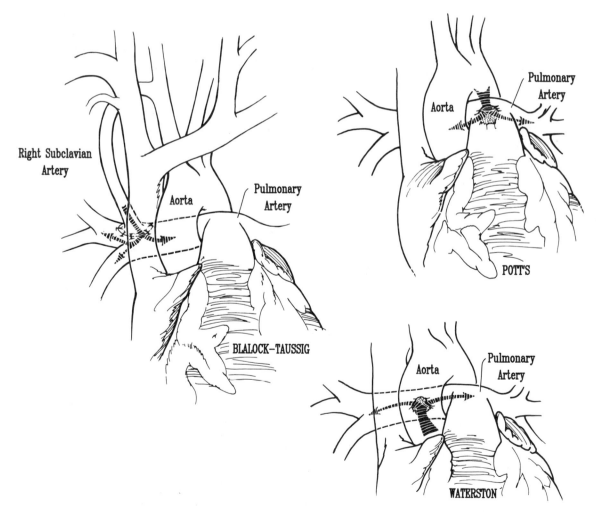

Fig. 30-5. Palliative operations for inadequate pulmonary blood flow. *Left;* Blalock-Taussig shunt; *above right;* Potts' shunt; *below right,* Waterston's shunt.

cause of its large size. Enlargement of the right ventricular outflow tract requires resecting some of the hypertrophied muscle and correcting the PVS when this is present. The valve may be relatively normal, moderately stenotic, or severely dysplastic. Appropriate division or excision of the valve leaflets is performed, and often a patch of pericardium or prosthetic material is needed to enlarge the outflow tract, valve ring, and proximal pulmonary artery. Much of the morbidity and mortality of operations to correct TOF are attributable to the incision into the right ventricle, which is often essential to achieve satisfactory relief of infundibular stenosis.

TRANSPOSITION OF THE GREAT ARTERIES

Like TOF, transposition of the great arteries (TGA, Fig 30-6) results from abnormal development of the conotruncus. In TGA the truncal ridges fail to spiral and instead fuse along a straight line. This causes the right ventricle to eject into the aorta and the left to eject into the pulmonary artery. This establishes two circulations in parallel, instead of in series, and would be uniformly lethal without some shunt connecting them. Most frequently, this is a patent foramen ovale but there may be a VSD or PDA. These patients are cyanotic from birth and usually have life-threatening problems when the PDA closes if the foramen ovale does not allow adequate mixing.

At the time of catheterization for diagnosis of TGA, there is an opportunity for palliation of this condition. A balloon septostomy, first described by Rashkind, can be used to enlarge the foramen ovale and thereby improve mixing of the two venous circulations. The Blalock-Hanlon operation is a palliative surgical procedure that does not require cardiopulmonary bypass. This procedure creates an atrial septal defect by excision of a piece of atrial septum within a vascular clamp placed across the interatrial groove.

Definitive repair of TGA can be carried out at the atrial, ventricular, or arterial level. Atrial level repairs baffle the returning venous blood to the "wrong" ventricles, which in turn remain connected to the "wrong" arteries, thus properly directing the course of the blood. Two popular atrial repairs are the Mustard procedure, which employs pericardium to construct the baffle, and the Senning procedure, in which the baffle is composed mainly of atrial wall. The Rastelli repair is performed at the ventricular level and requires the presence or the creation of a large VSD through which the left ventricular blood can be directed into the aorta by a patch. The right ventricle is then connected to the pulmonary artery by an extracardiac valved conduit. The Rastelli repair is generally reserved for patients with significant obstruction to left ventricular outflow into the pulmonary artery. Arterial level repairs involve switching the great arteries so that each is anastomosed to its proper ventricle. Since this requires switching the coronary arteries as well, the operation is technically demanding. The operative mortality for these operations is low at centers with extensive experience with TGA. Patients who survive the surgery can be expected to have excellent long-term results with any of these approaches.

Congenitally corrected TGA is characterized by transposition of the arteries as well as atrioventricular discordance (the right atrium connected to the left ventricle and vice versa). Thus the two circulations are in series and functioning normally. However, most patients with this condition have other abnormalities, such as VSD, PVS, or tricuspid (systemic) valve insufficiency, that require operative intervention.

DOUBLE-OUTLET RIGHT VENTRICLE

Double-outlet right ventricle (DORV) may be considered a variant of transposition. In DORV both great arteries arise more than 50% over the right ventricle, and a large VSD is almost always present. The clinical manifestations and natural history of DORV are highly variable and dependent on the degree of arterial obstruction that may exist and upon the size and location of the ventricular defect. The operative approach to this problem must be highly individualized to the particular anatomy. Usually the left ventricle can be connected to the aorta with an interventricular baffle, but sometimes operations similar to those used for TGA must be employed. The operative mortality in DORV is high, although specific sub-sets of patients with favorable anatomy can be expected to have good operative and long-term results.

TRUNCUS ARTERIOSUS

Failure of the truncus ridges to form and fuse leaves a single common artery, a persistent truncus arteriosus (PTA), arising from both ventricles. A ventricular septal defect is invariably present as well. The pulmonary arteries arise from a variable location along the common truncus. The truncal valve may consist of two to four cusps, which are frequently dysplastic and may be associated with valvular stenosis or insufficiency. Both of these latter conditions adversely affect survival.

Clinical manifestations of PTA include tachypnea, tachycardia, and an active precordium with continuous murmur and thrill. These are often present within the first few weeks of life, although a rare patient may not present for several months. The few patients who survive childhood without treatment for this condition de-

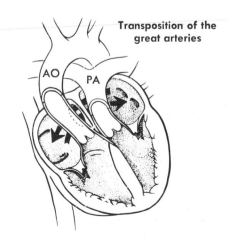

Transposition of the great arteries

AO PA

Fig. 30-6. Transposition of the great arteries. Position of great vessels reversed. Defect in atrial or ventricular septum allows mixing of systemic and pulmonary circulation.

velop profound changes of pulmonary hypertension and generally succumb in early adulthood.

Operation is indicated for most patients with PTA as soon as possible after the diagnosis is established. At operation the ventricular defect is closed with a patch that directs left ventricular flow into the truncus. The pulmonary arteries are detached from the truncus and must be connected to the right ventricle. A valved aortic allograft makes an excellent conduit to interpose between the right ventricle and the pulmonary arteries. The operative mortality is quite high, at least in part because of the poor clinical status of these patients in the preoperative period.

ANOMALIES OF PULMONARY VENOUS CONNECTION

Partial anomalous pulmonary venous connection (PAPVC) is commonly associated with the sinus venosus type ASD. In PAPVC the pulmonary vein from one or more lobes of the lung connects to the superior or inferior vena cava, azygous vein, coronary sinus, or right atrium. In the usual case the right upper lobe vein drains into the superior vena cava. The pathophysiology, clinical manifestations, and natural history of PAPVC are essentially the same as those of ASD. The indications for operation are also the same. In the presence of a PAPVC involving only one lung lobe with a Q_P/Q_S less than 1.5, operation is probably not indicated. With greater degrees of left-to-right shunting, operation should be performed. In most cases, surgical treatment requires closing the atrial defect with a large patch that also serves to baffle the pulmonary vein back into the left atrium.

Total anomalous pulmonary venous connection (TAPVC) is characterized by the absence of any direct communication between the pulmonary veins and the left atrium. In most cases the pulmonary veins have a common confluence. This confluence drains into a vertical vein that empties into the superior vena cava (supracardiac connection), directly into the coronary sinus (cardiac connection), or into a descending vein that drains into the hepatic veins or inferior vena cava (infracardiac connection). Multiple levels of connection may also occur.

Some degree of interatrial shunting is obligatory to maintain life beyond a few days. The severity of symptoms depends on the highly variable degree of pulmonary venous obstruction that is present. Greater obstruction produces profound pulmonary congestion, with cyanosis, tachypnea, and congestive failure. With lesser obstruction, 1 to 2 years may elapse before the onset of dyspnea, fatigue, poor weight gain, and cyanosis.

Operation is indicated in all patients. The goal of the operation is to create an anastomosis between the confluence of the pulmonary veins and the left atrium, close the ASD, and ligate the anomalous connection. This may require moving the interatrial septum to the right to accommodate the new anastomosis. Operative mortality for this operation is high when the patient's preoperative status is poor. Patients who survive the operation should be expected to have excellent long-term results.

PULMONARY ATRESIA

In typical patients with pulmonary atresia with intact ventricular septum, a fibrous membrane occupies the site of the pulmonary valve, the right ventricular outflow tract may be atretic, the tricuspid anulus is small, and the right ventricle, although present, is hypoplastic. Infants are cyanotic from birth and develop more intense cyanosis when the ductus arteriosus closes. Operation should be carried out immediately after the diagnosis is established. A shunting procedure such as the Blalock-Taussig shunt must be performed to provide pulmonary blood flow. A pulmonary valvotomy must be performed as well to allow blood to flow through the right ventricle, which is thereby stimulated to grow. These two procedures may be carried out either at the same operation or in stages. Operative mortality is high, the need for repeat palliative operations is also high, and the success of definitive operations is extremely limited. Best results are obtained in those rare patients who exhibit some degree of right ventricular growth following the initial palliative operations and who have a nearly normal-sized tricuspid anulus. The patient whose right ventricles does not grow may be a candidate for the Fontan operation (see below).

Tricuspid Atresia

In tricuspid atresia (TA) there is a failure to form a direct connection between the right atrium and right ventricle. Instead, there is an ASD, a fairly normal left atrium, mitral valve, and left ventricle, and typically a large VSD leading to a small right ventricle and a pulmonary artery of normal size.

Cyanosis is present from birth and may be progressive. In patients with small ventricular defects and pulmonary artery obstruction, inadequate pulmonary flow usually prevents the child from surviving infancy, and a shunt may be required.

Definitive surgical treatment of TA is based on the operations devised by Fontan and Kreutzer. Fontan's original procedure consisted of an anastomosis of the superior vena cava to the right pulmonary artery and placement of a valved conduit between the right atrium and left pulmonary artery. The ventricular and atrial defects were closed. Various modifications of this operation include direct anastomosis of the right atrium to the pulmonary artery and the use of valved or nonvalved conduits to connect the right atrium to the right ventricle or pulmonary artery. In all of these operations, the pulmonary circulation depends on venous pressure exceeding pulmonary artery pressure. Before considering patients for this type of procedure, it must be determined that all factors that would impede pulmonary perfusion are absent. In particular, patients are not candidates for Fontan-type operations if they have elevated pulmonary vascular resistance, small-caliber pulmonary arteries, atrial fibrillation, or left ventricular dysfunction.

UNIVENTRICULAR HEART

A variety of cardiac anomalies are most easily considered under the general heading of univentricular heart (UH). The anatomic features of the ventricle may be more consistent with those of a left ventricle (smooth walled) or a right ventricle (trabeculated) and there may be a rudimentary outflow chamber of the opposite morphology. Single ventricles of indeterminate morphology are also encountered. A variety of atrioventricular valve malformations may be expected as well. The great arteries may be normally related or transposed, and subarterial stenosis is common.

Clinical manifestations vary with the degree of pulmonary obstruction. Although some cyanosis is almost always present shortly after birth, some patients with good perfusion of the pulmonary bed survive for many years. When there is excessive pulmonary flow, pulmonary artery banding is usually performed initially.

When there is reduced pulmonary blood flow and severe cyanosis, a shunt is performed for palliation. At a later stage definitive operations, which include septation of the single ventricle into two pumping chambers and modifications of the Fontan operation, may be attempted. Operative survival for both the palliative and reparative operations is poor except in certain ideal patients.

CORONARY ARTERY ANOMALIES

Numerous variations of normal coronary artery anatomy that are of no hemodynamic consequence may be encountered in the hearts of otherwise healthy patients. Other coronary anomalies are secondary to some other cardiac defect. Examples of such abnormalities include variations in coronary origin and course in TGA and TOF. Although these anomalies have no intrinsic clinical significance, they may create difficulties in the operative correction of the underlying defect.

The most common clinically important coronary artery anomaly is the origin of a coronary from the pulmonary artery. The left coronary artery is far more frequently involved in this defect than is the right. The pathophysiology of this condition depends on the extent of collaterals between the right and left coronaries. After birth, when pulmonary artery pressure falls, there is shunting of blood from the right coronary into the left and then into the pulmonary artery, in essence an arteriovenous fistula. The pressure in the small coronary arteries is low when the collaterals are small and myocardial perfusion is inadequate. These patients present within the first several months of life with symptoms of angina as well as those of congestive failure due to ischemic myocardial dysfunction and mitral regurgitation.

Arteriographic demonstration of this anomalous origin of a coronary artery should be followed by prompt operation. Three surgical approaches have been employed. The first approach, simple ligation of the anomalous vessel at its origin, is a relatively easy operation and may be successful when there are extensive collaterals, usually in the older patient. Coronary bypass, using the saphenous vein or subclavian artery, is another option, but patency rates of these minute anastamoses are low. Excellent results have been obtained in some infants with inadequate collaterals by establishing a direct connection between the aorta and left coronary artery, either by direct reimplantation or by a tunnel created within the pulmonary artery.

The second most common major anomaly of the coronary arteries is coronary arteriovenous fistula. In these cases, the coronary arises from the aorta and connects with the right atrium, right ventricle, pulmonary artery, coronary sinus, or superior vena cava. Patients may present at any age and are frequently discovered during evaluation of an asymptomatic murmur. As with other left-to-right shunts, symptoms of congestive failure predominate when the fistula is large, although angina may be encountered as well. Operative treatment consists of obliterating the fistulous connection. This may be difficult, as there may be multiple fistulas. Successful operation is curative, and operative mortality should approach zero.

Acquired Heart Disease

Flavian M. Lupinetti,
Nicholas P. Rossi

PRINCIPLES OF CARDIAC SURGERY

Safe and effective cardiac operations begin with a careful preoperative evaluation of the patient. The surgeon must become intimately familiar with the patient's clinical history and physical examination. Appropriate radiographic and catheterization data must be reviewed for proper planning of the surgery. Thorough evaluation of related organ systems including the lungs, kidneys, and peripheral arteries must be carried out, and consideration must be given to any hematologic, endocrine, or neurologic abnormalities.

Monitoring devices used during heart surgery include an arterial line, for measurement of systemic pressure and convenient blood gas measurement; a Swan-Ganz catheter, for determination of central venous, pulmonary artery, and pulmonary capillary wedge pressures, and cardiac output; and a continuous electrocardiogram (ECG). An indwelling urinary catheter and nasal and rectal temperature probes are inserted as well.

Cardiopulmonary bypass (Fig. 30-7) refers to the use of a mechanical pump and oxygenating device to supply oxygenated blood to the body while the heart is emptied. This permits operation on the heart with good visibility and a quiet field. Cannulas are inserted into the right atrium or the venae cavae to return venous blood to the oxygenator using gravity flow. The oxygenator allows diffusion of carbon dioxide from the blood in a passive manner. Oxygen is taken up by the blood either by bubbling oxygen directly through the blood or by permitting it to pass into the blood across a semipermeable membrane. The oxygenated blood then

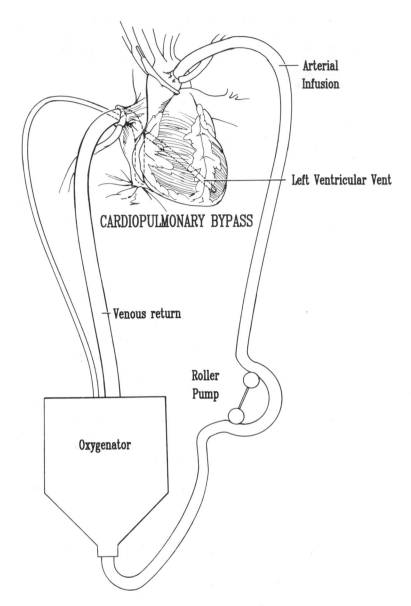

Fig. 30-7. Cardiopulmonary bypass. Blood is drained from the right atrium by gravity. It is oxygenated and then propelled into the aorta. A left ventricular vent helps to keep the heart empty.

passes through a roller-type or a centrifugal pump that drives it through a cannula inserted in the patient's aorta (the femoral artery is used in certain circumstances). This provides almost complete emptying of the heart; some other sources of blood return, notably the coronary sinus and bronchial circulation, require removal by means of a vent that may be placed in the left ventricle (via the pulmonary vein or apex insertion), pulmonary artery, or aorta.

Complete arrest of the heart requires clamping the aorta proximal to the arterial perfusion cannula. This establishes *global ischemia* and produces cardiac arrest. During global ischemia, aerobic metabolism is stopped, while adenosine triphosphate (ATP) stores are progressively depleted. Excessive depletion of the heart's energy stores results in the inability of myocardial cells to

control ionic gradients and cell volume. Ultimately calcium accumulation by the cells leads to further depletion of high-energy phosphates. Excessive calcium accumulation binds myosin and actin molecules into a tight *rigor complex*. An irreversible stage of injury occurs when the heart becomes firmly contracted, a state referred to as *ischemic contracture,* or "stone heart."

Myocardial injury can be avoided during global ischemia by modifying the conditions of arrest. Probably the most important component of myocardial protection is hypothermia. With every 10° C decrease in temperature, the oxygen demands of the myocardium fall by half. Hypothermia is ensured with systemic cooling of the patient by means of a heat exchanger on the cardiopulmonary bypass system, topical cold solution, and administration of cold *cardioplegia.*

Cardioplegic solutions arrest the heart in diastole and abolish its electrical and mechanical activity. Potassium is most commonly used to provide this rapid and complete arrest. Cardioplegic solutions should be slightly hyperosmolar, to prevent cardiac edema, and may require readministration during long periods of arrest. Other components of cardioplegic solution advocated by some investigators include blood, oxygen, calcium channel blockers, and substrates for cellular metabolism. The efficacy of these additives is not established.

Postoperatively, the patient is monitored with the same devices and the same degree of care used during the operation. Cardiac output is assessed clinically by examining peripheral pulses and skin temperature and color and by monitoring urine output and acid-base status; it is also measured directly with the thermodilution catheter. Arterial blood pressure should be followed closely and maintained in a normal range. It is possible, however, to have a satisfactory blood pressure due to peripheral vasoconstriction, and this can be a misleading measurement in the patient with poor perfusion. Central venous pressure and pulmonary capillary wedge pressure are useful indices of volume status, but they must be evaluated appropriately in the context of the patient's overall status and complicating factors. Cardiac rate and rhythm are monitored continuously.

Insufficient cardiac output should be addressed by understanding the etiology. Hypovolemia is common after open heart surgery and should be treated with blood or electrolyte fluid, depending on the patient's hematocrit and hemoglobin concentration. In patients with low output who appear to have adequate fluid volumes, inotropic agents, such as epinephrine, norepinephrine, isoproterenol, dopamine, or dobutamine, may be helpful. Low cardiac output with elevated peripheral vascular resistance may be treated by afterload reduction with agents such as nitroprusside or nitroglycerin.

Blood pressure management also may require administration of the drugs mentioned above. Cardiac rate disorders are often easily managed using temporary pacing wires placed on the atrial and ventricles in the operating room. Other rhythm disturbances may necessitate the use of a variety of antiarrhythmics.

ISCHEMIC HEART DISEASE

Ischemic heart disease is a condition that results when the myocardium does not receive enough oxygen and substrate to maintain its normal physiologic activities. In Western society, this is a common consequence of *coronary artery disease.* The two conditions are not synonymous, however. Coronary artery disease is thought to develop mainly as a result of accumulation of plasma lipids from the blood into the arterial intima. When the coronary artery is narrowed by greater than 50% of its diameter (75% of its cross-sectional area) there is a graded reduction in blood flow. Although the percentage of vessel stenosis compared to adjacent, presumably undiseased, artery is the most commonly used method of expressing the degree of coronary artery obstruction, this is a crude and inexact assessment of the physiologic consequences of coronary artery disease.

Ischemia occurs when the balance between myocardial oxygen demand and myocardial oxygen supply is not maintained. Oxygen demand is determined by myocardial wall tension, a function of systolic pressure and volume; the contractile state of the heart; and heart rate. Myocardial oxygen supply is determined by oxygen content of the arterial blood, ability of the myocardial cells to extract oxygen, endocardial-epicardial distribution of blood flow, and perfusion pressure across the coronary circulation, which is equal to the difference in the mean pressures of the aorta and right atrium.

Evaluating the patient with ischemic heart disease requires consideration of a number of prognostic factors in addition to *coronary anatomy* as demonstrated by angiography. It is also essential to consider *left ventricular function.* Left ventricular function can be determined clinically, based on the patient's symptoms and physical exam; it can also be determined quantitatively, using contrast or radionuclide ventriculography. *Objective evidence of ischemia* is yet another important consideration in evaluation of ischemic heart disease. This is often supplied by electrocardiographic monitoring of the patient during exercise. Because *recent history* is of considerable importance, the patient should be questioned carefully about recent changes in the nature, pattern, or intensity of the symptoms.

All indications to perform coronary bypass surgery can be grouped under one of two broader objectives: *relief of symptoms* or *preservation of myocardium.* Extension of life expectancy cannot be predicted for most patients undergoing coronary bypass. Some subsets of patients, notably those with greater than 50% diameter stenosis of the left main coronary artery, those with unstable angina, and those with three-vessel disease and poor ventricular function, do appear to live significantly longer with operative as opposed to nonoperative management. Most patients undergoing coronary bypass do so because of chest pain that is not sufficiently controlled by medication to permit a level of exertion that the individual finds acceptable.

Operative treatment of ischemic heart disease requires bypass of all coronary lesions that are thought to be both hemodynamically significant and surgically accessible (Fig. 30-8). Most bypasses are constructed with a length of greater saphenous vein, although lesser saphenous veins and basilic or cephalic arm veins are sometimes required. The grafts are interposed between the ascending aorta and the coronary artery beyond the most distal stenosis. Increasing use is being made of the internal mammary artery (IMA) as a bypass conduit. This artery may be used either as a graft in situ, remaining attached proximally to the subclavian artery, or as a free graft, with the proximal end anastomosed to the aorta, as with vein grafts. Synthetic grafts are rarely used for coronary bypass because of their low long-term patency rates.

Operative mortality following coronary artery bypass is very low in patients with stable angina and good ventricular function. Mortality increases with progressive hemodynamic instability and poor ventricular function. The optimal criteria for emergency operation for patients with evolving or recently completed infarction have not been defined.

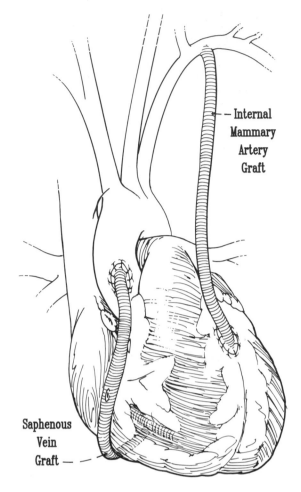

Internal Mammary Artery Graft

Saphenous Vein Graft —

Fig. 30-8. Coronary artery bypass. An internal mammary artery has been anastamosed to the left anterior descending coronary artery. A saphenous vein has been used to bypass the right coronary artery.

Long-term results of coronary bypass depend upon long-term graft patency. It is because of superior late patency that internal mammary arteries (90% patency at 10 years after bypass) are favored in addition to or instead of saphenous vein grafts (75% patency at 10 years). Late graft patency appears to be superior in patients who take aspirin on a continuing basis postoperatively and may be better in patients who comply with restrictions on diet and smoking.

Reoperation for disease affecting previous bypass grafts or vessels not diseased at the initial operation remains an option for patients with recurrent ischemic heart disease. While the operative risk is somewhat higher, the same prognostic analysis used in patients undergoing their first bypass surgery should be applied. The operative indications are essentially the same.

Complications of ischemic heart disease that may require operative treatment include ventricular aneurysm, acquired VSD, and mitral regurgitation. All usually result from transmural myocardial infarction. A ventricular aneurysm may produce congestive heart failure by impairing normal mechanical ejection. Pa-

tients with large aneurysms and failure symptoms often benefit from aneurysmectomy. Some aneurysms are associated with ventricular tachyarrhythmias that fail to respond to medical management and therefore require an operative approach. Acquired VSDs produce fulminant congestive failure. In most cases prompt operative closure of the defect is indicated to provide the patient with the best chance for survival. Postinfarction mitral regurgitation is dealt with as is mitral regurgitation from other causes (see below).

VALVULAR HEART DISEASE

Mitral stenosis, either in isolation or combined with mitral regurgitation, is usually a consequence of rheumatic heart disease. As the incidence of rheumatic fever has declined in North America and Western Europe, the incidence of mitral stenosis similarly has fallen. Mitral stenosis is a progressive disorder that produces pulmonary congestion, atrial enlargement leading to atrial fibrillation, systemic emboli, and congestive failure. Many patients who undergo operation can be treated by mitral valvotomy, which relieves the obstruction without the deleterious sequelae of prosthetic valves. Valve replacement is carried out when valvotomy is not possible.

Mitral regurgitation may result from ischemic heart disease, degenerative diseases (Barlow's syndrome, fibroelastic deficiency), or endocarditis. Incompetence of the mitral valve allows the left ventricle to eject a portion of its volume into the low-pressure left atrium. A fall in cardiac output and systemic pressure does not occur, however, because the left ventricular end-diastolic volume increases. At least for a time, this maintains an adequate forward flow, but the chamber dilation aggravates the mitral regurgitation, and eventually congestive failure results. Performed early, operation may consist of mitral valve repair, the techniques of which have been recently popularized by Carpentier and others. Mitral valve replacement is required in cases that come to operation later in the course, and is the procedure most commonly used by cardiac surgeons today.

It is unusual these days to discover *aortic stenosis* secondary to rheumatic heart disease. Most aortic stenosis is now encountered in patients with congenitally bicuspid valves that have undergone degenerative calcification or in elderly patients whose aortic valves have undergone senile calcific changes. Aortic stenosis increases myocardial oxygen and substrate demands, stimulates left ventricular hypertrophy, diminishes cardiac output, and may lead to serious arrhythmias. The cardinal symptoms of aortic stenosis—angina, syncope, and congestive failure—are indications for operation. Regardless of symptoms, individuals with a transvalvular gradient ≥50 torr should also be considered for operation. Reconstructive procedures for acquired aortic stenosis are not well established; valve replacement is the treatment of choice.

Aortic insufficiency is degenerative in etiology. Long-standing aortic insufficiency results in the left ventricle undergoing sometimes massive hypertrophy and dilation, the so-called *cor bovinum.* Quantitative operative criteria for this condition are less well defined than for other forms of valvular dysfunction. It is clear that development of symptoms, predominantly dyspnea on exertion, is an indication for valve replacement.

Tricuspid valve disease rarely requires operative intervention. It may occur in the presence of severe mitral stenosis, either because of tricuspid valve involvement with the rheumatic process or secondary to pulmonary hypertension and right ventricular dysfunction. Tricuspid insufficiency may be encountered due to endocarditis, especially among patients with a history of intravenous drug abuse. Many patients with tricuspid valve insufficiency can be treated with valve repair or anulus plication, although valve replacement remains an option.

Bacterial endocarditis may affect any heart valve, although the mitral and aortic valves are most commonly involved. Preexisting valve lesions predispose to this condition. Endocarditis responds in most patients to appropriate antibiotic therapy. Subsequent operation, employing the usual criteria, may be required at a later time, after the valve has been "sterilized." Earlier operative intervention is required if the patient has endocarditis due to a fungus or an antibiotic-resistant bacterium, if the valvular involvement causes severe congestive failure, or if there are infected embolic complications. Surprisingly, valve replacement may be performed in this setting with a low incidence of prosthetic valve infection. This is probably due to the high velocity of blood flow across the valves.

Prostheses available for use when valve replacement is indicated can be conveniently divided into the categories of mechanical valves, bioprostheses, and human allografts (homografts). Examples of each are shown in Fig. 30-9.

Mechanical valves in use today are composed of a ball in a cage or one or two tilting disks held in place by struts. These valves are very durable and have a low incidence of structural defects. The primary disadvantage of mechanical valves is the need for careful anticoagulation; thus, these valves are inappropriate for patients with bleeding disorders and those who cannot comply with a strict medical regimen.

Bioprostheses, on the other hand, do not always require anticoagulation. These valves are obtained from the aortic valve of the pig or are constructed from bovine pericardium. Both types of bioprostheses are fixed in glutaraldehyde to render them biologically inert and provide better structural stability. Disadvantages of bioprostheses include degeneration, which appears inevitable in valves implanted for many years, and their tendency to undergo rapid calcification in pediatric patients.

Homografts provide many of the advantages of both mechanical and bioprosthetic valves. Structurally, they are quite stable and do not require anticoagulation. Furthermore, they do not appear to be subject to rejection and have a very low incidence of infection. At present they are used to replace only the aortic valve. The technique of homograft insertion is more demanding than that for other valves.

DISORDERS OF CARDIAC RHYTHM

The most common rhythm disturbances that require operative intervention are the bradycardias, most of which are a result of *heart block* or *sinoatrial node dysfunction*. Both conditions may be congenital, acquired, or iatrogenic.

Heart block is characterized by normal sinus node function with a failure of normal conduction to the ventricles. First-degree heart block rarely causes symptoms, whereas second-degree block may result in symptomatic bradycardia, and complete, or third-degree, heart block frequently produces symptoms. The most common serious manifestation of complete block is the Stokes-Adams attack, which produces syncope.

Sinus node abnormalities may be produced by failure of the sinoatrial cells to undergo spontaneous depolarization at the normal rate or by failure of normal conduction between the sinoatrial and atrioventricular

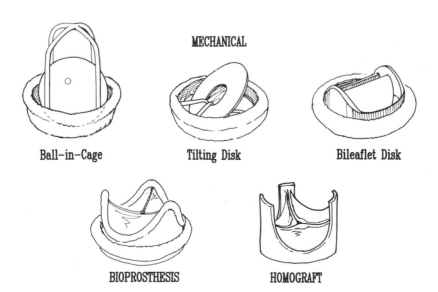

MECHANICAL

Ball-in-Cage   Tilting Disk   Bileaflet Disk

BIOPROSTHESIS   HOMOGRAFT

Fig. 30-9. Prosthetic valves used for cardiac valve replacement.

nodes. Again, syncope is the most common clinical manifestation.

Symptomatic bradycardia is an unambiguous indication for pacemaker insertion. Other indications are more complex and controversial. The selection criteria for the type of pacemaker employed are evolving as pacing technology advances. Many patients are well served with simple pacemakers that only maintain a constant rate of ventricular depolarization. Newer devices permit more elaborate pacing of both the atria and the ventricles, with coordination of all chambers. These more recent pacemakers may be particularly beneficial to patients with low cardiac output.

Pacemaking leads are usually inserted through the subclavian vein and directed under fluoroscopic control into the right atrium or ventricle (Fig. 30-10). A transthoracic approach with application of the leads to the epicardium is preferred for children, whose veins are not able to accommodate the leads. The generator is placed in a subcutaneous pocket that should be easily accessible for later replacement as the battery deteriorates.

Tachyarrhythmias have recently become amenable to surgical intervention. They may be conveniently divided into *supraventricular* and *ventricular* tachycardias.

The most common supraventricular tachycardia requiring operative treatment is the Wolff-Parkinson-White syndrome (WPW), in which the electrical impulse from the atria to the ventricles is conducted along an abnormal pathway, the bundle of Kent. This impulse is not delayed as is the normal depolarization in the atrioventricular node. This allows for the rapid conduction of atrial tachycardias, such as atrial fibrillation, to the ventricles. Alternatively, the Kent bundle may conduct retrograde from the ventricle to the atrium, thereby creating a circus movement.

WPW does not always produce symptoms and therefore need not require operative intervention in all cases. However, in patients with symptomatic or life-threatening tachycardias secondary to WPW, strong consideration should be given to surgical division of the Kent bundle. This operation has very little risk and a high rate of complete cure. Thus it may be favored even for patients who can be successfully managed with antiarrhythmic drugs as an alternative to a lifetime of medication.

Ventricular tachycardias (VT) are a frequent complication of ischemic heart disease. Most patients can be adequately managed for these arrhythmias with medication. Some patients have recurrent episodes of life-threatening VT despite optimal medical management. In these patients surgical ablation of the arrhythmogenic focus has gained increasing acceptance. Crucial to the success of surgical treatment of VT are careful preoperative and intraoperative electrophysiologic mapping studies to determine the site of origin of the arrhythmia. Various methods of ablating the focus have been employed including excision, cryoablation, and isolation. All have proved more successful than nondirected approaches such as coronary bypass alone or unguided aneurysmectomy.

Since these ablative techniques require cardiopulmonary bypass, they may be prohibitively dangerous in

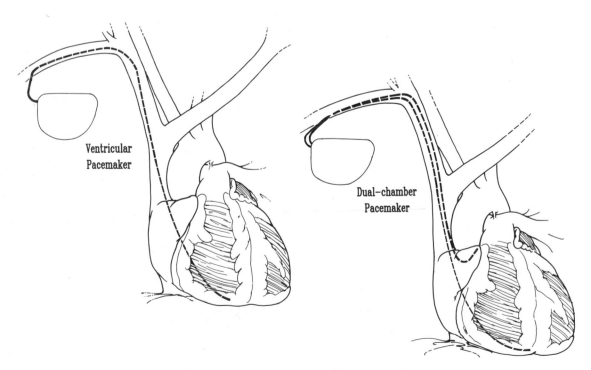

Fig. 30-10. Pacemakers. *Left;* Single-chamber pacemaker used for ventricular pacing; *right;* dual-chamber pacemaker coordinating atrial and ventricular depolarization.

some patients with very poor ventricular function. This group of patients may benefit from implantation of an automatic defibrillator-cardioverter. This device is capable of sensing a ventricular tachycardia and applying countershock to terminate it.

PERICARDIAL DISEASE

The pericardium is a flask-shaped sac that surrounds the heart and origins of the great arteries and veins. Fluid is formed by the visceral pericardium and resorbed by lymphatics in the parietal pericardium. About 50 ml of fluid is present in the average adult pericardial space. The pericardium provides anatomic fixation for the heart and acts as a barrier to infection and tumor. It also reduces friction between the heart and other organs and distributes hydrostatic forces among the cardiac chambers. Persons with congenital absence of the pericardium generally have no adverse clinical consequences.

Pericardial tamponade results from excessive fluid occupying the pericardial space. As little as 50 ml of additional fluid may be sufficient to produce tamponade in the acute situation, such as following trauma. Much larger volumes are required to cause tamponade when they accumulate over a longer period of time. Examples of these more chronic forms of tamponade include malignant effusions and uremic pericarditis.

Tamponade should be suspected in the appropriate clinical setting when there is evidence of elevated venous pressure with low systemic blood pressure. *Pulsus paradoxus* is a decline in systolic pressure of more than 10 torr on inspiration and is a strong indicator of tamponade. Other aids to diagnosis include measurement of central venous pressure and pulmonary capillary wedge pressure and echocardiography.

Emergent treatment of tamponade consists of pericardiocentesis by a percutaneous technique. When this is successful, the patient's clinical appearance improves rapidly. Continued drainage may be provided using an indwelling catheter. If percutaneous aspiration is unsuccessful or if fluid reaccumulates, operative drainage should be performed.

Pericarditis results from multiple etiologies, including bacterial and fungal infection, uremia, trauma, radiotherapy, rheumatologic conditions, and various medications. *Chronic constrictive pericarditis* represents the end stage of an inflammatory process resulting in a thickened, leathery pericardium that limits cardiac filling. Operation requires extensive resection of the pericardium to allow the heart chambers to distend normally. Bleeding from this operation is frequently heavy, and cardiopulmonary bypass should be available.

CARDIAC TRAUMA

Penetrating injuries to the heart are best treated by prompt transport of the patient to the operating room, median sternotomy, and control of the bleeding site with manual compression. Definitive control may be provided by large mattress sutures over felt pledgets. Emergency room thoracotomy is appropriate only when the patient's condition is deteriorating so rapidly that it seems impossible to delay even a few minutes. Even in these cases, removal of a small amount of fluid from the pericardium by needle puncture may allow transport to the operating room for exploration under optimal conditions.

Blunt cardiac trauma may result in very serious injuries, such as cardiac rupture, ventricular septal rupture, or valvular rupture. A more common manifestation of blunt injury is myocardial contusion. Diagnosis of myocardial contusion is often attempted on the basis of electrocardiographic findings and cardiac enzymes. Both of these methods are relatively insensitive and nonspecific. Radionuclide scanning is a much more specific method of diagnosing contusion, but is positive only in cases of transmural injury. Echocardiography is useful in detecting areas of diminished ventricular wall motion. While this method cannot distinguish old infarct from recent contusion, it provides information about the functional status of the myocardium that may be quite useful in managing the patient's care.

CARDIAC NEOPLASMS

Three out of four cardiac neoplasms are benign, myxomas being the most common benign tumor in adults and rhabdomyomas the most common in children. Myxomas are most frequently in the left atrium but may be encountered in any chamber. They may produce symptoms of dyspnea, congestive failure, emboli, and atrial arrhythmias that mimic mitral valve disease. The diagnosis may be established by echocardiogram or contrast studies, and operation should be carried out promptly to avoid embolic complications. The surgical procedure consists of complete excision of the myxoma, including its base, with a small margin of normal tissue. This wide resection is necessary to prevent recurrence.

Of malignant cardiac neoplasms, metastatic tumors are more frequently encountered than are primary malignancies. Lung cancer is the malignancy that most commonly metastasizes to the heart and pericardium. Angiosarcoma is the most common primary cardiac malignancy. Cardiac malignancies, primary or metastatic, tend to be rapidly progressive and only rarely amenable to excision. Radiation and chemotherapy may provide some palliation.

CARDIAC TRANSPLANTATION

Cardiac transplantation has become an increasingly successful treatment for patients with end-stage heart disease. Criteria for transplant have become somewhat broader as results have improved, and factors such as patient age are less likely to exclude a patient from consideration for this procedure. Candidates for heart transplant must be free of infection. Furthermore, pulmonary vascular resistance must be acceptably low to prevent acute right ventricular failure of the donor heart. Insulin-dependent diabetes and recent pulmonary embolus remain contraindications.

A potential donor must be unequivocally brain dead and have had no episodes of profound hypotension, cardiac ischemia by ECG or cardiac enzymes, or sepsis. The donor and recipient must be ABO blood type compatible, and the body weights should be within 10% of each other. Since most donor hearts come from

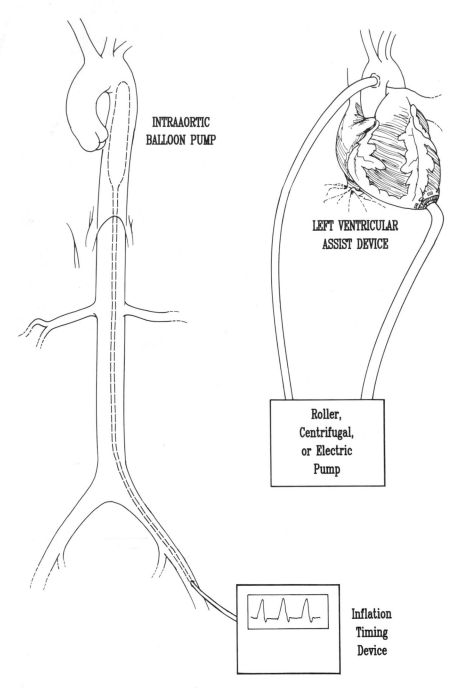

INTRAAORTIC
BALLOON PUMP

LEFT VENTRICULAR
ASSIST DEVICE

Roller,
Centrifugal,
or Electric
Pump

Inflation
Timing
Device

Fig. 30-11. Mechanical assist devices for treatment of low cardiac output. *Left;* Intraaortic balloon pump; *right;* left ventricular assist device.

locations remote from the recipient, consideration must be given to the transport time involved and the acceptable length of cold ischemic time that the donor organ can tolerate.

Close coordination between the harvesting and the transplanting teams is essential for best results. The recipient is placed on cardiopulmonary bypass as the donor organ is being retrieved. The recipient's heart is excised leaving as much atrial tissue, aorta, and pulmo-

nary artery as possible. Anastomosis of the atria is performed first, followed by that of the pulmonary artery and aorta.

Postoperative care is similar to that for other cardiac surgery with the exception of immunosuppressive therapy. Cyclosporine A is the cornerstone of treatment; prednisone and antithymocyte globulin are important as well. The use of azathioprine is controversial. Prevention of rejection requires routine endocardial biopsies to assess histologic evidence of leukocyte infiltration and muscle necrosis.

Heart-lung transplantation is being evaluated in some centers as an option for patients in whom cardiac transplantation alone is not an option. Most candidates for cardiopulmonary transplant have severe pulmonary hypertension. The criteria for this procedure are more rigid than those for cardiac transplant. Major problems that remain include the ability to preserve the delicate lung tissues during the operation and the detection of rejection postoperatively. Isolated lung transplantation has been performed successfully but remains an investigative modality at present.

COMPLICATIONS OF CARDIAC SURGERY

Severe hemorrhage is a common complication of cardiac surgery, in large part because cardiopulmonary bypass requires massive doses of heparin and causes consumption of platelets and clotting factors. The risk of hemorrhage can be minimized in the operating room by achieving careful surgical hemostasis and adequately reversing the heparin with protamine. Patients who develop postoperative bleeding should have clotting factors replaced by administration of fresh frozen plasma as indicated by the patient's prothrombin time. A prolonged partial thromboplastin time may indicate the presence of excessive circulating heparin and constitutes an indication for additional protamine. Platelets may be useful regardless of the actual platelet count, as platelet function may be abnormal despite adequate numbers of platelets. Fibrinolysis, determined by fibrinogen measurement, may necessitate administration of additional fibrinogen in the form of cryoprecipitate. When these measures are inadequate to stem the bleeding, operative reexploration may be required.

Reexploration may also be required because of cardiac tamponade resulting from accumulation of blood and clot around the heart. Tamponade is usually preventable by large-bore tube drainage of the mediastinum at the operation but should be suspected in patients with large blood losses and declining cardiac output and blood pressure. Delayed tamponade may occur days or even months after operation and may require percutaneous or open drainage.

Infections are a rare but serious complication of cardiac surgery. Even superficial wound infections must be treated aggressively with antibiotics and appropriate wound management. Sternal infections and mediastinitis are life-threatening problems that typically require operative débridement and reconstruction.

Renal failure following cardiac surgery is most likely in patients who had some degree of renal impairment preoperatively. Related factors are hypotension before, during, or after operation; lengthy cardiopulmonary bypass; and hemoglobinemia. Maintaining adequate renal perfusion is the best prevention for this problem. Dopamine is useful in achieving this goal by both improving cardiac output and stimulating renal artery dilation. Diuretics may also be helpful in maintaining urine flow. Dialysis may be indicated in the patient with established renal failure.

Neurologic complications may result from inadequate cerebral perfusion during bypass; this is best avoided by maintenance of adequate arterial pressure during the operation. Emboli, either air or particulate matter, are other sources of neurologic sequelae.

A number of poorly understood clinical constellations are grouped under the heading of postperfusion syndromes. These may be characterized by chest pain, fever, malaise, and pericardial friction rub. Some cases appear to be related to cytomegalovirus and others to the development of high titers of antimyocardial antibodies. Most cases have no clear etiology, however. Treatment consists of supportive care and antiinflammatory drugs.

Very low cardiac output may develop at any time in the perioperative period. Perhaps the most dramatic example is the patient with cardiac dysfunction so severe that he cannot be weaned from cardiopulmonary bypass despite adequate blood volume and maximum inotropic support.

In this setting, the intraaortic balloon (Fig. 30-11) counterpulsation device may be life saving. The balloon is synchronized with the patient's ECG to inflate during diastole, thereby reducing afterload and diminishing the work of the heart. This allows support of the circulation until the heart is able to recover from injury. A more recent aid in this situation is the ventricular assist device (VAD, Fig 30-11), which can be used to assume the total function of the left or right ventricle, or both. Both the intraaortic balloon and the VAD are used primarily for hearts that are expected to recover function. The VAD has also been used in patients awaiting cardiac transplant who have such profound heart failure that death is considered imminent. It has been successful in some cases as a "bridge to transplant."

The concept of a total artificial heart has occupied investigators for many years but has only recently been put into practice. The artificial heart has proved capable of maintaining adequate total body perfusion, but has been plagued by thromboembolic complications that thus far preclude wide use.

31

Vascular Surgery: Peripheral Arteries

Howard P. Greisler

William H. Baker

Diagnosis
Types of Arterial Disease
Occlusive Disease
Other Percutaneous Modalities
Inflammatory and Miscellaneous Arterial
Diseases

The four basic phenomena (obstruction, erosion, perforation, and a mass) that are so important in other surgical diseases are frequently and often dramatically evidenced in diseases of the arteries. Obstruction from arteriosclerosis is one of the most common of all vascular ailments. Aneurysms may erode or appear as pulsating masses. Perforation of a major artery may result dramatically from degenerative arterial diseases or trauma. In addition, there are a variety of rarer but interesting vascular syndromes.

DIAGNOSIS

The most important facet of the vascular examination remains the history and physical examination. Despite the recent development of various new laboratory and radiographic diagnostic modalities, arterial disease and its clinical significance are best evaluated at the bedside by the examining physician. The other tests (Table 31-1), however, are very useful in quantitating the suspected disease, localizing and otherwise characterizing arterial lesions, and often planning surgical procedures. Plain radiographs may demonstrate arterial calcification (Fig. 31-1). Although this finding demonstrates the presence of arterial disease, it is not informative regarding arterial patency and it has an excessive incidence of false-negative results. An enlarged artery demonstrated by ultrasound or computed tomography (CT) is more accurate for the diagnosis of aneurysm.

In the noninvasive vascular laboratory, physiologic data are collected by Doppler ultrasound and plethysmographic techniques, and anatomic information is col-

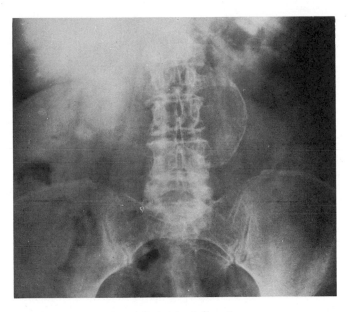

Fig. 31-1. Calcified abdominal aortic aneurysm.

Table 31-1. Diagnostic Aids in Arterial Disease

Diagnostic Method	Technique	Results
Plain x-ray studies	Conventional radiography	Shows calcification in vessels or aneurysm (Fig. 31-1)
Ultrasound velocity detector (Doppler)	Listen over the arterial tree to detect flow characteristics	Locates altered flow characteristics; can be used with a blood pressure cuff to accurately measure the arterial pressure at different levels of the extremity
Plethysmography	Gauge placed around extremity; cup placed on eyeball	Additive to Doppler
Ultrasound examination	Noninvasive scan of abdominal aorta or other arterial segment	Can measure accurately the size of aneurysms
Computed tomography	Computer-assisted radiographic scan	As with ultrasound, accurately quantitates aneurysm size
Intravenous digital subtraction angiography	Intravenous dye injection with computer-assisted arterial imaging after subtracting background from radiograph	Shows arterial intraluminal contour, often less defined than standard arteriography
Arteriography	Injection of contrast dye in artery	Shows intraluminal contour and abnormalities of flow (Fig. 31-7)

lected by other ultrasound studies. Ultrasonic waves are reflected by moving red blood cells. The reflected energy may be made audible or recorded on hard copy. The presence of a Doppler signal indicates that flow is present, and analysis of that signal may indicate reduced or abnormal flow. The Doppler signal can be detected in all major arteries in the extremities. When used in concert with ordinary blood pressure cuffs, the pressure in different segments of the arterial tree can be determined and the segment containing a significant obstruction to flow can often be localized. Analysis of the pitch of the Doppler signal and of the contour of the wave generated by the arterial pulse is often useful for further definition of the extent of the obstruction to flow. Doppler signals can be similarly detected in the extracranial carotid arteries. The response of the Doppler-detected supraorbital arterial flow to certain compressive maneuvers is an important part of the cerebrovascular examination. Analysis of the sound frequency (in Hertz; Hz) of the Doppler signals from the common, internal, and external carotid arteries is useful in determining the degree of obstructive flow in these vessels. Because of their noninvasive quality, such studies are especially useful when the course of arterial disease is followed over time. In addition, a sterile Doppler probe may be used in the operating room to verify patency of a vascular anastomosis and to help assess the immediate effect of a vascular procedure.

Plethysmography measures volume changes. Various-sized sensors are available to measure changes in the volume of the finger, arm, toe, calf, thigh, or penis with the cardiac cycle to quantitate flow or, when used with blood pressure cuffs, to measure pressure. Specially designed suction cups are used with either an air- or fluid-filled system to measure eyeball-volume changes as a reflection of the flow through the internal carotid and ophthalmic arteries.

Contrast angiography most precisely identifies the anatomy of occlusive arterial disease. Newer iodinated agents are relatively risk free, and sophisticated catheter techniques make virtually every artery in the body available for study. Although this invasive technique is uncomfortable, even the cerebrovascular examination has only 1% morbidity and mortality. Computerized digital subtraction angiography (DSA) is currently used clinically as a screening test in high-risk patients and perhaps as a substitute for conventional arteriography in assessment of certain lesions. Intraarterial DSA may supplement standard arteriography to more fully visualize arterial segments that are not well seen primarily because proximal arterial stenosis limits the distal flow of dye. Radionuclide angiography is also of value in

assessment of arterial anatomy in patients with a strong history of dye allergy, though the resolution of this technique does not yet rival that of conventional angiography. Magnetic resonance imaging (MRI) can be used to assess aneurysm size, although currently images are less clear than those of CT.

TYPES OF ARTERIAL DISEASE

Congenital Lesions

Congenital arteriovenous fistulas occur as café-au-lait spots, cirsoid aneurysms, or racemose connections between major arteries and veins. Even though the subcutaneous lesions may be disfiguring, nonoperative therapy is usually indicated initially, since they may disappear spontaneously or regress in size. Excision or irradiation is indicated if venous lakes or multiple arteriovenous fistulas enlarge or produce changes in cardiovascular dynamics. If they are localized, excellent palliation may be afforded by the occlusion of major "feeder vessels" surgically or by emobolization. However if there is widespread involvement, amputation is indicated (Fig. 31-2).

Arterial Injuries

Both blunt and penetrating trauma can result in any of three major types of injuries to blood vessels; laceration (incision), perforation (ice-pick injury, needle injury after arteriography or cardiac catheterization), or contusion (Fig. 31-3). After complete transection of an artery the ends retract and contract to assist in hemostasis. After partial transection this retraction is impossible and hemorrhage is often greater than with complete transection. Contusion of an artery may injure the intima and promote local thrombosis. Blunt trauma may similarly result in internal disruption followed by thrombosis or false aneurysm formation.

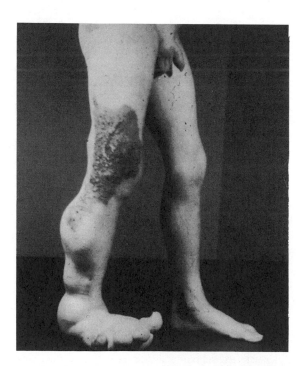

Fig. 31-2. Multiple arteriovenous fistulas in right leg associated with hemolymphangioma. Partial amputation was required.

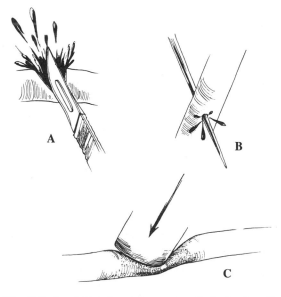

Fig. 31-3. Arterial injuries. **A,** Laceration. **B,** Perforation. **C,** Contusion. *Note:* Partial lacerations usually result in brisk bleeding because severed ends cannot retract. Complete transections permit severed ends to retract; spasm and thrombosis often limit bleeding.

These lesions are usually obvious on examination. However, occasionally even a complete transection is difficult to detect if hemorrhage is arrested by tamponade within a fascial compartment and distal pulses are present because of collateralization. Arterial injury threatens life or limb if not corrected promptly. Consequently, if there is any question, emergency arteriography is indicated if time permits; otherwise emergency operative control may be required. Hemorrhage must be controlled, blood loss replaced, and in most cases the artery reconstructed. Autogenous tissue (vein grafts, arterial grafts, arterioplasties) is preferred over a synthetic prosthesis because of the threat of infection. An infected graft produces septic emboli, thrombosis, or disruption of the graft with the threat of false aneurysm or exsanguination. The physician should never attribute peripheral ischemia after injury to "arterial spasm"; such patients should have either immediate arteriography for diagnosis or emergency exploration for treatment of a suspected arterial injury.

Delayed complications of arterial injury include arterial occlusion with intermittent claudication, rest pain or limb loss, false aneurysm (Fig. 31-4), or traumatic arteriovenous fistulas. False aneurysms have a predilection for sudden expansion and rupture with massive hemorrhage and can often be detected by palpation and auscultation. Traumatic arteriovenous fistulas may become manifest as congestive heart failure (the fistula increases venous return, dilating the cardiac chambers and producing high-output cardiac failure), pulsating veins, or typical bruits, heard over the involved vessels. Resection or ligation of the fistula often with reconstruction of the vascular system is the reparative procedure of choice. Smaller arteriovenous fistulas may

be obliterated by percutaneous transcatheter embolization of autogenous clot or other materials into the fistula to occlude the communication.

Arterial Emboli

Acute arterial occlusion is most commonly caused either by embolization of thrombus or atherosclerotic plaques from more proximally in the cardiovascular system or from thrombosis in situ of previously diseased arteries. Most arterial emboli arise from within the heart. Atrial fibrillation, aortic and mitral valvular disease, recent myocardial infarction with a mural thrombus, or rarely myxomas of the heart are antecedent causes. Another less common source is arteriosclerotic plaques that break off from more proximal arterial walls and embolize. The common sites of embolic obstruction are at the bifurcations of the major vessels: popliteal, femoral, iliac, aortic, and occasionally brachial, carotid, or mesenteric arteries. The lower extremities are the site of approximately 80% of embolic occlusions.

Peripheral arterial emboli appear as an abrupt onset of ischemia. The classical "five Ps" of acute arterial occlusion are pain, pallor, pulselessness, paresthesias, and paralysis. The sudden onset of ischemic pain allows the majority of patients to accurately recount the precise timing of the occlusion. Paresthesias and paralysis are suggestive of imminent limb nonviability and indicate ischemia severe enough to cause nerve or muscle damage. Despite prompt, excellent treatment, morbidity and mortality in this group will be increased because of neuromuscular ischemia, which eventually becomes irreversible.

When the diagnosis of an arterial embolus is made,

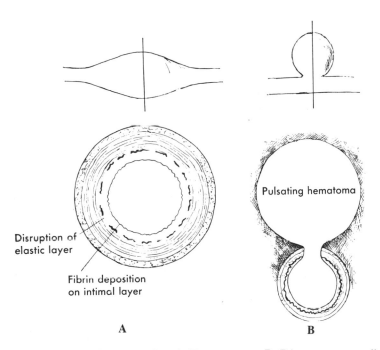

Fig. 31-4. Types of aneurysms in cross section. **A,** True aneurysm. **B,** False aneurysm usually caused by trauma; pulsating hematoma results; intimal layer grows into aneurysm that is covered by clot and later by fibrous tissue.

intravenous heparin is administered immediately (usually in the emergency room). This will not dissolve the embolus but will prevent propagation of the thrombus in the involved vessels. While localization of the occluding embolus is generally made by history and physical examination, the coexistence of long studies, atherosclerotic occlusive disease may make preoperative arteriography advisable. Such evaluation is not justified if imminent limb loss is suspected. Embolectomy is performed as soon as possible, preferably within hours. The balloon catheter technique of embolectomy accomplished through a peripheral artery (e.g., removal of an aortic saddle embolus through the femoral arteries) can be done under general, regional, or even local anesthesia. Although delayed embolectomy (duration of occlusion greater than 12 hours) is sometimes successful, it is fraught with lower success rates and with increased mortality in patients with nonviable limbs. The source of the emboli is treated to prevent recurrent embolization (i.e., anticoagulants, valvuloplasty, valve replacement, ventricular aneurysmectomy, or cardioversion). Occlusion of arteriosclerotic vessels may require combining embolectomy with endarterectomy or bypass grafting.

The sudden restoration of blood flow to the acutely ischemic limb in cases of advanced or relatively long-standing acute ischemia may result in swelling within the fascial compartments of the involved extremity. Such increased intracompartmental pressure can secondarily cause arterial insufficiency through extrinsic compression. Suspicion of a developing compartment syndrome, based either on physical examination or the measurement of intracompartmental pressures, is an indication for surgical fasciotomy to open the compartment and decrease the pressure.

In patients with acute occlusions from thrombus, an alternative therapy is intraarterial infusion of fibrinolytic agents. However, this treatment is also best performed in the immediate postocclusion period. Thrombolytic therapy must be combined with surgery or transluminal angioplasty in patients with atherosclerotic or other underlying arterial pathology. Because of the longer time required to reestablish arterial patency, it should not be used in patients threatened with imminent limb loss.

Aneurysms

Aneurysms are localized dilations of arteries. They may be true (containing all three layers of the arterial wall) or false (containing only adventitia and sometimes media; Table 31-2 and Fig. 31-4). Most aneurysms are atherosclerotic in origin, but a few result from trauma or infection.

The gross pathologic condition of aneurysms includes degenerative dilation with deposition of fibrin and clot within the lumen. Microscopically the tunica intima is thickened with fatty deposits and calcifications and the tunica media is disrupted (see Fig. 31-4). Many patients (60% to 70%) are unaware of the pulsating mass unless it occurs in a superficial location, such as the extremities.

Most aneurysms are discovered while still asymptomatic; however with progression they may rupture, thrombose, embolize, or erode into adjacent structures. The diagnosis of aneurysm is usually made by discerning plapation or by plain radiographs that show calcification within the wall of the aneurysm (Fig. 31-1). Accurate measurement of the dimensions of the aneurysm is best accomplished with either ultrasound scanning or CT. Arteriography is not mandatory unless the proximal and distal extent of the aneurysmal dilation must be known before operation (thoracic aortic aneurysm and aneurysms believed to involve the renal arteries) or the distal arterial tree is of questionable quality (femoral and popliteal aneurysms). Although even small aortic aneurysms can rupture, the risk of rupture increases with the size of the aneurysm. Rupture of an aortic aneurysm is fatal in the majority of cases. Ruptures occur usually into the retroperitoneum or occasionally into the overlying duodenum (aortoduodenal fistula) or inferior vena cava (aortocaval fistula). Most aortic aneurysms are asymptomatic, but since their rupture is such a threat to life, the treatment of choice is surgical excision of relatively large aneurysms (5 cm or greater) and replacement with a synthetic prosthesis (Fig. 31-5). All extremity aneurysms should be treated surgically because of the risk of thrombosis, distal embolization, or both. Popliteal and femoral aneurysms are frequently bilateral and/or coincident with aortic and other aneurysms. Because the thoracic and suprarenal aorta supply organs that do not tolerate prolonged an-

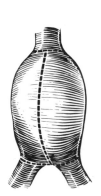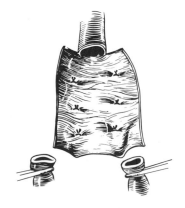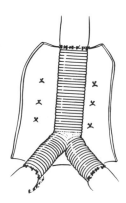

Fig. 31-5. Abdominal aortic aneurysm is incised after proximal and distal control is obtained. Bleeding lumbar arteries are controlled from within aneurysm. Anterior wall of aneurysm is resected, but posterior wall is left intact. Vascular integrity is reestablished with Dacron graft.

oxia (spinal cord, kidneys), aneurysms in these areas may require temporary bypass (with the pump oxygenator, atriofemoral bypass, or tube shunts) during repairs.

Occlusive Disease
Lower Extremities

Atherosclerosis is the almost universal cause of chronic occlusive disease of the legs. The characteristic pathologic features of atherosclerosis are intimal thickening and degeneration. Loss of the endothelial surface with lipid and calcium deposits in the intima and smooth muscle cell proliferation are followed by progressive obstruction, which may be partial (stenosis) or complete (occlusion).

Clinically atherosclerosis is characterized by slowly progressive arterial insufficiency. It occurs most commonly in older men but affects both sexes and sometimes emerges as early as the third decade of life. It is common in diabetics, in whom it affects both the larger, surgically accessible arteries and the smaller arteries of the foot and leg.

History. Pain is the most common symptom of arteriosclerosis obliterans. Intermittent claudication, a specific symptom of arterial insufficiency, is a cramping pain in muscles that occurs after a period of exercise and is relieved by a few minutes of rest. This pain is repetitive with precisely the same amount of exercise. Accumulation of acid waste products from anoxic muscle probably causes the pain. Calf claudication means that the obstruction is at or proximal to the popliteal artery, whereas hip or buttock claudication indicates aortoiliac disease. Aortoiliac atherosclerosis may produce not only claudication but also impotence (Leriche's syndrome; Fig. 31-6).

Pain at rest in the foot occurs from inadequate perfusion in the horizontal position (i.e., sleeping) in the patient with severe occlusive arterial disease. Pain at

Table 31-2. Aneurysms

Location	Cause	Relative Incidence	Treatment	Prognosis
Thoracic aorta	Arteriosclerotic, infection, trauma	Occasional	Medical or surgical (depending on anatomical site and patient)	Fair
Abdominal aorta	Arteriosclerotic	Frequent	Resection	Good
Femoral and popliteal	Arteriosclerotic, trauma, infection	Occasional	Resection or exclusion bypass graft	Good
Carotid	Arteriosclerotic	Rare	Resection	Good
Upper extremities	Trauma, arteriosclerotic, infection	Rare	Resection	Good
Splenic	Arteriosclerotic	Occasional	Resection if symptomatic or in females under 40 years	Good
Renal	Arteriosclerotic	Occasional	Aneurysm resection or nephrectomy, sometimes nonoperative	Good

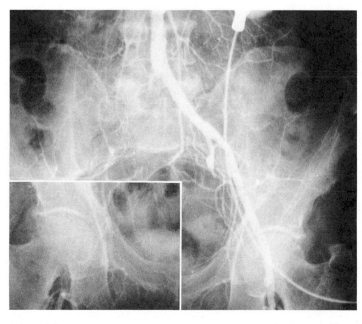

Fig. 31-6. Occlusion of right common and external iliac artery. Collateral flow from left internal iliac system supplies right profunda femoris artery through obturator and gluteal branches of right internal iliac artery.

rest is often alleviated when the foot is placed in a dependent position and must be differentiated from calf cramps from other causes.

Nonoperatively treated patients who have claudication uncommonly come to amputation, whereas patients exhibiting ischemic pain at rest have more advanced disease and, unless treated, face a major amputation.

Physical examination. Careful evaluation of the pulses is the most important part of examining a patient with peripheral artery disease. The pulse (arterial pressure) is directly related to the inflow of blood and inversely related to the resistance to flow. Diminished, absent, or asymmetric pulses often pinpoint the exact site of arterial obstruction. Auscultation of the pulses may demonstrate a bruit denoting turbulent flow past a stenotic lesion or through an arteriovenous fistula.

Chronic occlusive disease is characterized by cool, atrophic, shiny skin, absent hair and thickened toenails. A later, more grave, sign is ulceration of the distal extremity. Inadequate perfusion is suggested by slow capillary and venous refilling times. The skin blanches with pressure and the color returns slowly after releasing pressure. In acute obstructions the affected extremity appears suddenly and persistently cadaveric because of the absence of collateralization. Elevation of the ischemic extremity produces pallor, and dependency produces cyanosis. This results from the following chain of events: elevation lowers the perfusion pressure, producing pallor; local anoxia and metabolic acidosis result; capillary dilation occurs, causing slowing of an already inadequate blood flow and cyanosis with dependency.

The presence of leg complaints, diminished pulses, and deformed, arthritic joints makes a diagnosis difficult. In other patients typical complaints of intermittent claudication will be combined with satisfactory pulses. It is imperative that the physician exercise the problem patient to produce symptoms and reexamine him at that time. Exercise in a patient with symptomatic arterial insufficiency leads to a preferential perfusion of the exercising muscle bed at the expense of the more distal arterial beds resulting in a further diminution of distal pulses. Is the pain really calf pain or is it joint pain? Have the pulses changed? Are the bruits louder? Is the symptomatic foot paler? Many difficult problems can be solved in the astute clinician's office.

Vascular laboratory examination. A normal patient has the same systolic blood pressure in the arm and ankle (ankle/arm $\cong$ 1). A reduction in this ratio indicates arterial disease; the more extensive the occlusive disease, the lower the ankle-to-arm ratio. Segmental pressures obtained with either the Doppler technique or plethysmography or analysis of pulse wave velocity contours are used to localize the level(s) of disease. Any abnormalities can be exaggerated with stress (treadmill, inflow occlusion) testing, which decreases pressures and wave amplitudes in the ischemic extremity.

Arteriography. Contrast angiography is required, not to diagnose the level of obstruction (this is done on physical examination and in the vascular laboratory examination) but to aid in planning surgical intervention. All methods give excellent details and have low morbidity. Translumbar aortography is always associated with some bleeding, but transfusion is rarely necessary. Thrombotic and embolic complications are more common after the transfemoral approach. Bleeding after the transaxillary approach may occasionally lead to brachial plexus injury from compression unless the hematoma is recognized promptly and drained. DSA following intraarterial dye injection can often enhance the visualization of the smaller more distal arteries, which occasionally may not be seen adequately with conventional angiography.

Extracranial Cerebrovascular Disease

Although arteriosclerosis may involve any neck vessel, typically it causes a localized stenosis at the origin of the internal carotid artery. Symptoms arising from this lesion may result from embolization of atherosclerotic debris or platelet emboli distally, or from low flow past the lesion. In younger female patients fibromuscular dysplasia may involve a major portion of the extracranial internal carotid artery. Microscopically in this lesion the media is alternately thinned (areas of an-

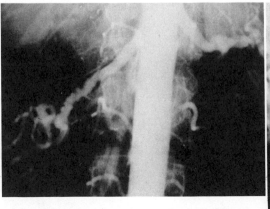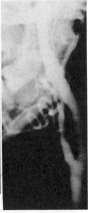

Fig. 31-7. These arteriograms represent fibromuscular dysplasia. Notice "chain of lakes" present in right renal artery and septa present in carotid artery.

eurysmal dilation) and thickened (areas of stenosis), producing a "chain of lakes" arteriographically (Fig. 31-7); this is the same picture seen in similar renal artery lesions. Fibromuscular dysplasia is frequently associated with intracranial aneurysms.

Patients with cerebrovascular disease may be grouped into at least three categories of neurologic insult. A *transient ischemic attack* (TIA) is a neurologic deficit that lasts less than 24 hours; a *reversible ischemic neurologic deficit* (RIND) lasts longer than 24 hours but neurologic recovery is complete within 1 week; and a permanent neurologic deficit, either an acute or chronic stroke, may occur. Amaurosis fugax is a transient blackening of the visceral field, often described as a window shade being pulled down and then up, resulting from embolization of the ipsilateral carotid artery. Cholesterol emboli called Hollenhorst plaques often can be seen on ophthalmic examination.

The patient's neurologic complaints and findings can be further categorized as follows:

Hemispheric
    Contralateral motor and sensory
    Ipsilateral visual symptoms—amaurosis fugax
    Dysphasias
Vertebrobasilar
    Vertigo (true)
    Ataxia
    Diplopia
    Bilateral visual aberrations
    Shifting paresis or paresthesias
    Drop attacks
    Dysarthrias
    Syncope
Nonspecific
    Dizziness
    Light-headedness
    Decreased mentation
    Headache
    Confusion
    Personality change
    Tinnitis
    Decreased visual acuity
    Seizures

Occlusive disease of the subclavian artery proximal to the vertebral artery can lead to the subclavian steal syndrome. Classically exercise of one arm leads to a reversal or exacerbation of reversed flow in the ipsilateral vertebral artery as blood from the circle of Willis and contralateral vertebral artery is redirected from the brain to the ischemic arm, producing neurologic symptoms. Upper extremity claudication may also occur.

On physical examination diminished carotid or subclavian pulses with overlying bruits may be found. It is important to differentiate these more distal carotid bruits from murmurs transmitted to the neck from aortic valvular disease. The blood pressure in each arm must also be compared.

Vascular laboratory examination. Periorbital Doppler examination detecting flow in the supraorbital artery should normally be unaffected by superficial temporal or facial artery compression and be reduced by common carotid artery compression. An abnormal examination indicates collateral blood flow secondary to stenosis (at least 75%) of the internal carotid artery. A carotid phonoangiogram (CPA) is a pictorial display of the neck bruit. Oculoplethysmography (OPG) compares the volume expansion of each eyeball. The globe on the side of a carotid stenosis expands at a slower rate than the contralateral globe supplied by normal arteries. The Gee modification of the OPG measures ophthalmic artery pressure indirectly. Frequency analysis of Doppler-detected carotid velocity aids in quantitating the degree of stenosis. The greater the stenosis, the faster the blood flows and the higher the pitch at the site of stenosis. Real-time B-mode ultrasound can provide anatomic information noninvasively. Duplex scanning combines frequency analysis with B-mode ultrasound imaging. The extent of noninvasive testing and its exact interplay with contrast studies has not been definitely decided and varies between institutions.

Arteriography and treatment modalities. Transfemoral cerebral angiography is preferred over direct carotid punctures. The extracranial and intracranial arteries must be visualized from the aortic arch for diagnosis of all lesions and formulation of a comprehensive treatment plan that may include anticoagulation therapy, surgery on the extracranial carotid or vertebral arteries, or extracranial-intracranial bypass. Most patients with acute strokes are not candidates for immediate operation, in contrast to patients with transient ischemic attacks. Patients who are asymptomatic but have a severe stenosis and access to a reliable surgeon are now frequently being treated surgically to lessen the chance of stroke. Stenosis in the internal carotid artery is typically suited for endarterectomy. The details of the operative procedure (use of an internal shunt, patch angioplasty, and hypercapnia or hypocapnia) remain controversial, but the reported results are excellent with a variety of techniques (combined mortality and morbidity of 1% to 3%).

Visceral Arterial Stenosis

Atherosclerotic stenosis of any or all of the visceral arteries (celiac axis, superior mesenteric artery, inferior mesenteric artery) may cause symptoms, as may external compression (by the median arcuate ligament). See Chapters 27 and 25 and Table 31-3 for clinical details.

Renal Artery Stenosis

Renal artery stenosis is becoming more commonly recognized as a cause of arterial hypertension. In patients in their fifth to seventh decades, atherosclerosis is the most common cause, but in younger women fibromuscular dysplasia is more common. Rarely, renal artery aneurysms cause hypertension.

On physical examination an abdominal bruit is heard in a hypertensive patient. Intravenous pyelography reveals a small kidney with delayed function. Renal vein renin is elevated on the affected side and often suppressed on the contralateral side. Split renal function studies show a diminished urine volume and sodium concentration with increased creatinine concentration from the involved kidney. The arteriogram reveals the nature and extent of the lesion.

Surgical treatment is directed toward the removal or bypass of the responsible lesion. More rarely nephrectomy is required for removal of a Goldblatt kidney. Percutaneous passage of a balloon catheter for dilation of the responsible stenosis is an alternative therapy in

Table 31-3. Chronic Occlusive Disease

Site	Clinical Findings	Diagnosis	Treatment	Comment
Aortoiliac	Men, fifth to seventh decade, pain, intermittent claudication, impotence	Decreased or absent femoral and distal pulses, bruits over stenotic arteries; aortography shows diseased areas	Thromboendarterectomy, bypass graft, sympathectomy, amputation	Results good if outflow adequate
Femoral	Men, fifth to seventh decade, intermittent claudication, skin changes	Decreased or absent distal pulses, evidence of ischemia in foot or leg	Bypass graft, patch angioplasty, sympathectomy, amputation	Results good if outflow adequate
Renal	Hypertension, males and females	Bruit over abdomen, renal arteriogram, intravenous pyelogram—small kidney with delayed function, differential renal function, renal vein renin assay	Bypass graft, endarterectomy, patch angioplasty, nephrectomy	Good results if case selection is strict, saves kidney function
Cerebrovascular	Hemispheric vertebrobasilar, nonspecific	Carotid pulse decrease, bruit over carotid, arteriography shows stenosis or ulceration	Endarterectomy	Good results
Celiomesenteric	Visceral angina: pain after eating, weight loss, diarrhea (constipation), abdominal bruit, infarction	Angiography, difficult diagnosis in acute occlusion	Bypass graft, endarterectomy, bowel resection	Good results if done before infarction
Upper extremities	Claudication, skin changes, sensory disturbances	Absent pulses, bruit over involved vessel, arteriogram	Endarterectomy, bypass vein graft, resection of first rib, cervical sympathectomy, amputation	Fair

some cases and has its best results in fibromuscular hyperplasia. Indications for surgical therapy or percutaneous transluminal angioplasty are uncontrollable hypertension and preservation of deteriorating renal function.

Treatment of Occlusive Arterial Disease

There are three levels of treatment in vascular disease: maintenance of life, maintenance of limb form, and maintenance or restoration of limb function. The vascular surgeon often resects an abdominal aortic aneurysm in a poor-risk patient, since this is a life-threatening lesion. A reconstructive procedure is indicated in less than ideal situations if limb loss is imminent. Operations designed to alleviate intermittent claudication alone must be accomplished by low-risk surgery.

Direct reparative arterial surgery is possible for localized segments of occlusive disease in medium to large arteries. When arterial disease is diffuse or involves small arteries, the only treatment options are nonoperative therapy, sympathectomy, and amputation.

Reconstructive arterial surgery. Reconstructive arterial surgery depends on the following fundamentals: An accessible lesion is responsible for the patient's symptoms or is life or limb threatening. There is adequate inflow and outflow of the proposed reconstructed segment (a superficial femoral artery stenosis is not bypassed with significant aortoiliac obstructive disease). Finally, the choice of operation must be tailored to the patient (a subcutaneous axillofemoral artery bypass is done in an extremely poor-risk patient). There are several methods of arterial revascularization.

Endarterectomy. The diseased intima is dissected from the media by the open (Fig. 31-8) or closed (loop endarterectomy) method. This is applicable in the aor-

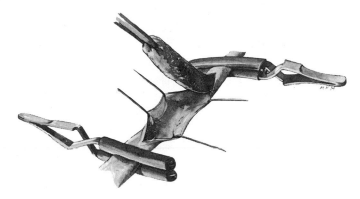

Fig. 31-8. Endarterectomy.

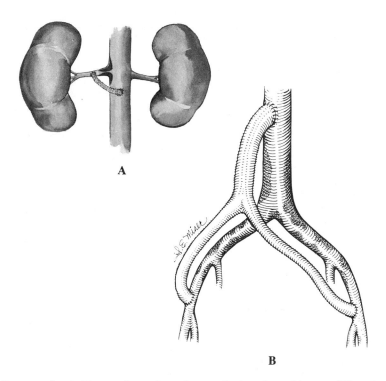

A

B

Fig. 31-9. Bypass grafts. **A,** Bypass of stenotic renal artery. **B,** Aortofemoral bypass of iliac atherosclerosis.

toiliac system, the proximal profunda femoris artery (profundoplasty, which is often done along with a patch angioplasty), and carotid bifurcation and visceral arteries, but this method has met with high recurrence rates in the superficial femoral and more distal arteries of the lower extremities.

Bypass graft. A graft (either a prosthesis or autogenous tissue) shunts blood around the diseased segment (Fig. 31-9). Dacron and polytetrafluoroethylene (PTFE) aortofemoral bypass grafts have largely supplanted endarterectomy as the treatment of choice for aortoiliac atherosclerosis. Excellent long-term results are expected even in patients with a distal superficial femoral artery stenosis, provided that the deep femoral artery is patent. Reversed autogenous vein or saphenous vein *in situ* after valve obliteration are the preferred grafting

techniques in femoral-popliteal-tibial disease, but synthetic material can be used in patients who lack suitable or available veins.

Replacement grafts. The diseased arterial segment is resected and replaced by a prosthesis or autogenous tissue (usually vein but sometimes another artery). This technique is performed less frequently than bypass grafting. It is not free of complication, however, including embolization, plaque dissection with subsequent thrombosis, and arterial laceration and rupture.

Patch graft (angioplasty). Either autogenous tissue or prosthetic material is used to enlarge stenotic arteries (Fig. 31-10).

Percutaneous transluminal angioplasty. In this technique a balloon-tipped catheter is percutaneously passed under fluoroscopic control to a stenotic arterial

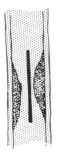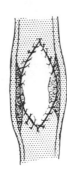

Fig. 31-10. Vein patch graft.

segment, and the balloon is inflated to dilate the vessel lumen. This method has produced good early success rates in short stenosis of the renal, aortoiliac, and femoral arteries and less success more distally in the lower extremities. It provides an alternative to open surgical intervention for patients with suitable highly localized obstructive disease, particularly those considered to be poor anesthesia risks.

Other percutaneous modalities. A number of fluoroscopically guided percutaneously introduced techniques are currently under evaluation. These include several laser techniques designed to vaporize plaque, atherectomy catheters to shave plaques, and aspiration catheters. The long-term results and morbidities are of these modalities remain controversial.

Nonoperative treatment of ischemic lower extremity. If the arteriosclerosis is diffuse, direct surgical correction is impossible. Nonoperative treatment involves the following:

1. Stop smoking!
2. Avoid trauma: corns and calluses should not be cut.
3. Avoid pressure by using soft mattresses and adequate-sized shoes.
4. Carefully wash and dry the feet every day and apply a bland ointment.
5. Exercise daily and frequently to tolerance to develop collateral circulation optimally.
6. We believe that vasodilator drugs have little value in generalized arteriosclerosis. (Theoretically, they dilate only pliable arteries and any pliable small arteries in ischemic beds are already vasodilated from high levels of tissue carbon dioxide.)
7. Ulcers are cleaned by sharp débridement and intermittent saline soaks, and skin grafts, if possible.
8. Local medications are contraindicated, since the ischemic skin is sensitive to chemical agents; antibiotic ointments are used only against specific organisms resistant to other treatment.
9. Pentoxifylline (Trental) and other agents used to increase red blood cell deformability have met with limited success in increasing the walking distance of patients with occasional claudication and may be tried.

Sympathectomy. Destruction of the sympathetic ganglia in the lumbar chain may dilate small and medium-sized arteries. If sufficient collateral arterial supply exists around obstructed arterial segments, sympathectomy may somewhat improve a marginal blood supply, primarily to the skin. The duration of its effectiveness and its value in improving the blood supply to the muscles are controversial. Usually at least one of the first lumbar ganglia is preserved in males to prevent impotence. Plethysmography and skin temperatures before and after sympathetic nerve block may help predict the efficacy of sympathectomy, but a negative result does not necessarily rule out a positive clinical result. Sympathectomy is less commonly of value in diabetics in whom auto-sympathectomy is commonplace. Sympathectomy alone will rarely heal large ulcerations or alleviate rest pain and is seldom recommended in modern practice.

Amputation. Gangrene, advancing infection, recalcitrant ulceration and unremitting pain at rest necessitate amputation. Amputation is a last resort after all nonoperative and direct attempts to treat ischemia have failed. The level of amputation depends on a blood supply sufficient to heal the incision. Despite an absent popliteal pulse, a below-knee stump can often thrive on collateral circulation. The adequacy of blood supply to the proposed level of amputation is estimated by physical examination and by vascular laboratory examination. If pressure is below 50 torr at the ankle, local digital or forefoot amputations are usually doomed to failure. Excellent results with below-knee amputations and early physical rehabilitation on prostheses are being obtained by use of plaster dressings postoperatively.

The effects of amputation need not be disastrous. With a proper prosthesis the patient may reenter society in a productive role. It is the surgeon's duty to encourage this goal.

Inflammatory and Miscellaneous Arterial Diseases
Buerger's Disease

Buerger's disease is an inflammatory disease of unknown cause that involves both arteries and veins. Also known as thromboangiitis obliterans, it was previously frequently diagnosed. However, newer diagnostic modalities have shown that its true incidence is quite low. It usually occurs in young men (onset 20 to 35 years) and involves small and medium-sized arteries in the lower extremities (posterior tibial, anterior tibial). Arteries in the forearm may also be involved. Besides sex and age, tobacco is the only other important associated factor.

Pathologically the arteries show an early panarteritis with chronic inflammatory cells and a relatively diffuse scattering of multinucleated giant cells. The internal elastic lamina remains intact. Fibrosis of the entire artery with small discontinuous recanalized channels occurs in late stages.

Clinical examination. Lower extremity pain from inflammation and ischemia, with appearance of small segments of migratory superficial phlebitis, keynotes the symptoms. Migrating phlebitis (with no other cause) is suggestive of Buerger's disease. Raynaud's phenomenon is common. Arteriography usually shows sharply demarcated obstruction of involved arteries, with the remaining arteries appearing surprisingly normal.

The course of this disease is variable. In some it smolders for years with minor sequelae. In contrast, we have been forced to amputate the lower extremity in a 19-year-old man after less than 6 months of symptoms.

Treatment. Abstinence from tobacco is probably the most important factor. Bed rest with protection of the extremity is the only other available treatment measure. Antibiotics are used only to treat secondary infections. Sympathectomy may delay or prevent amputation after subsidence of the acute process. Because of its distal nature, direct surgical revascularization procedures are often impossible but must be considered. Amputation is done only after all other treatment has failed.

Angiospastic diseases

The blood flow to surface areas of the body constantly fluctuates in response to tissue demands, temperature variations, and emotions. Vasomotor control is greater in the hands and feet, and these areas consequently reflect, most noticeably, abnormalities in vasomotor response. With exaggerated response the skin becomes white (with spasm), cyanotic (from anoxic capillary dilatation), and then intensely red (from reactive hyperemia) before becoming normal.

Raynaud's phenomenon, an intermittent, cold-induced peripheral ischemia, generally involves the upper extremities. It may become chronic with eventual loss of tissue. The phenomenon is associated with the following numerous conditions, with symptoms fluctuating with progression of the underlying disease:

Obliterative arterial disease
    Arteriosclerosis
    Buerger's disease
    Arterial emboli
Trauma
    After injury or operation
    Occupational
        Pneumatic hammer operators
        Pianists, typists
Neurogenic
    Thoracic outlet syndromes
    Primary neurologic diseases
Hematologic diseases
    Cold agglutinins
    Cryoglobulins
    Hemoglobinopathies (such as sickle cell anemia)
    Polycythemia
Systemic diseases
    Scleroderma
    Systemic lupus erythematosus
    Polyarteritis nodosa
    Rheumatoid arthritis
    Malignant disease
Drugs
    Ergots
    Heavy metals

If no underlying conditions causing Raynaud's phenomenon become evident, a diagnosis of Raynaud's disease is made. These patients, usually females less than 40 years old, develop numbness or burning pain in the fingers and hands with the typical color changes on exposure to cold. These changes are bilateral, and tissue loss is limited.

A modified Allen's test helps in the diagnosis of vascular disease distal to the wrist. Pressure is maintained over the radial and ulnar arteries by the examiner while the patient clenches his fist to empty blood from the hand. Release of either artery should produce a rapidly spreading erythema of the dependent hand and fingers, thereby demonstrating patency of that artery. Release of an occluded (radial or ulnar) artery will not produce erythema. If a distal or palmar artery is diseased, the portion of the hand it supplies will become erythematous later than the rest of the hand. This test and Doppler examination of the radial, ulnar, and digital arteries and the palmar arch help differentiate occlusive from vasospastic abnormalities

The diagnosis of Raynaud's disease is made clinically. Arteriography is not indicated unless the physical examination indicates major proximal artery disease. All efforts are made to diagnose an underlying condition.

Treatment includes avoiding cold and wearing warm clothing. Vasodilators and pharmacologic sympathectomy are occasionally beneficial. Surgical sympathectomy is reserved for patients with tissue necrosis but is usually only temporarily helpful. Calcium channel-blocking agents including nifedipine have been promising and are the agents of first choice.

Vasculogenic Impotence

Impotence has numerous vasculogenic, neurogenic, and psychogenic causes, and it has long been recognized as a symptom of aortoiliac occlusive disease (Leriche's syndrome). Newer diagnostic modalities have identified many cases secondary to disease within the hypogastric arteries and its branches supplying the penis. The diagnosis of vasculogenic impotence rests on noninvasive penile plethysmography and Doppler ultrasound penile artery pressures along with arteriography. Other psychogenic and neurogenic causes must be carefully considered. Direct arterial reconstructive procedures on selected patients are currently producing good results.

Erythromelalgia

Erythromelalgia is a rare condition of unknown cause. Clinically the patient complains of a red, warm, painful area on the lower extremities precipitated by excess heat and dependency. Sympathectomy is contraindicated in these patients.

Thoracic Outlet Syndrome

The thoracic outlet syndrome is a clinical syndrome of pain in the arm and numbness and sometimes coldness in the hand, secondary to compression of the neurovascular bundle as it leaves the chest. The most frequent symptom patterns refer to ulnar or median nerve involvement, but vascular compression often accompanies the brachial plexus compression. The neurovascular bundles is entrapped between a cervical rib and the first rib, the scalenus anticus muscle and the first rib, or the clavicle and the first rib. Clinically, hyperabduction of the shoulders (military position) or tensing the scalenus anticus muscle (Adson maneuver) will diminish the radial pulse. This clinical test will be abnorml in at least half the population without thoracic outlet syndrome. Nerve compression, either at the vertebral bodies or distal to the shoulder (i.e., carpal tunnel syndrome) must be differentiated. Treatment is surgical removal (either transaxillary, transpleural, or transcervical) of the first rib beneath the neurovascular bundle. The surgeon must be aware that a poststenotic dilation (aneurysm) may harbor thrombus leading to distal embolization. If present, this is repaired in order to ensure a successful therapeutic effort.

Arteritis

Although Buerger's disease is the most widely discussed inflammation of the arteries, there are numerous other causes of arteritis, as listed below:

Infective
    Pyogenic arteritis
    Fungal arteritis
    Tuberculous arteritis
    Mycotic aneurysm
    Syphilitic arteritis
Noninfective
    Systemic lupus erythematosus
    Polyarteritis nodosa
    Rheumatoid arthritis
    Pulseless disease (Takayasu's arteritis)
    Necrotizing arteritis after coarctation repair
    Buerger's disease

Specific infections are caused by direct bacterial invasion (i.e., from the retroperitoneal lymph nodes into the aorta), infection occurring after trauma or surgery, and septic emboli.

The causes of noninfective arteritis are many. Most are manifestations of a collagen vascular disease. The necrotizing arteritis that occasionally complicates successful repair of an aortic coarctation is allegedly secondary to mechanical stretching of the artery. Giant cell (temporal) arteritis causes headaches and visual disturbances. Physical examination discloses a tender, enlarged superficial temporal artery. Pulseless disease (Takayasu's disease, aortic arch syndrome) occurs in young women. Symptoms and findings depend on which arteries of the aortic arch are involved. Occasionally branches of abdominal aorta may be involved. Pathologically, the artery is thickened, with panarteritis, degeneration of the elastic fibers, and round cell infiltrations in all layers.

Specific infective arteritis responds to appropriate antibiotic, determined by cultures. Surgical therapy is reserved for resistant cases, complications, and mycotic aneurysms. Autogenous tissue is employed rather than synthetic material. Treatment (usually steroids) of a noninfective arteritis is directed toward the underlying disease. Steroids have also successfully ameliorated pulseless disease and temporal arteritis. Reserpine improves the necrotizing arteritis that sometimes occurs after repair of aortic coarctation.

32

Vascular Surgery: Peripheral Veins

William H. Baker
Howard P. Greisler
Robert T. Soper

Anatomy
Deep Venous Thrombosis (DVT)
Superficial Thrombophlebitis
Varicose Veins
Postphlebitis Syndrome
Pulmonary Embolism
Specific Large Vein Thrombosis
Lymphedema

Veins return blood to the heart from the vast capillary system, and in contrast to their arterial counterparts, flow rates are low and intermittent. Physiologically the veins return blood to the right side of the heart so that the cardiac output of the right and left ventricles is equal. Pathologic venous conditions, however, rarely interfere significantly with the filling pressure of the right heart but clinically cause increased venous pressure distal to the point of the pathologic entity. Increased peripheral venous pressure increases the egress of fluid out of the capillary bed causing clinical edema and poor nutrition of the limb. Additionally, emboli within the venous system may travel through the right side of the heart to the pulmonary tree and be associated with sudden death. This chapter deals with the prevention, recognition, and treatment of these problems.

ANATOMY

Since most venous surgical diseases involve the lower extremities, the discussion of venous anatomy is limited to these members. The normal venous drainage of the lower extremity includes a *superficial* network of veins traveling in the subcutaneous areolar tissue above the deep fascia of the leg and the *deep* venous system, which lies among the muscle groups in the lower extremity deep to the fascia.

Normally the superficial veins carry approximately 10% of the venous return from the legs, with deep veins carrying the rest. These two systems are interconnected segmentally by perforating or communicating channels, flow normally being from superficial to deep.

The normal direction of flow in both the superficial and deep venous systems is always from peripheral to central and from higher pressure to lower pressure areas.

The propulsive force generated by the left ventricles is mostly dissipated through the arterial and capillary systems, leaving inadequate pressure in the distal veins to overcome gravity in returning blood to the heart in the standing position. This problem is normally overcome by the milking action of the muscles, which generates flow in the deep system in the legs, and by humoral and sympathetic stimuli as well. There are several unidirectional bicuspid valves in both the superficial and deep set of veins as well as in the communicating (perforating) veins. When competent, the valves prevent retrograde flow with its resultant elevation of tissue pressure distally (Fig. 32-1, *A*).

The *greater* and *lesser saphenous veins* form the superficial set of veins of the lower extremity. The greater saphenous vein arises at the dorsal venous arch of the foot and ascends anterior to the medial malleolus, passing anteromedially up the thigh to empty into the deep venous system (the *common femoral vein*) in the groin via a fascial aperture known as the *fossa ovalis*. The greater saphenous system drains blood from the skin and subcutaneous tissues of the entire circumference of the thigh and the medial and anterior aspect of the leg and foot. The other component of the superficial saphenous system (the lesser saphenous vein) begins behind the external malleolus and ascends posterolaterally in the calf to empty into the deep system (the popliteal vein) in the upper portion of the popliteal space. The physiologically more important set of deep veins are often paired with and run along the like-named arteries.

DEEP VENOUS THROMBOSIS (DVT)

Thrombosis of the deep veins of the lower extremity is a debilitating, sometimes lethal, entity. Phlebothrombosis, an older descriptive term, implies less inflammation than thrombophlebitis, but this differentiation is moot. In general, stasis in the veins of the calf or stasis behind any valve cusp leads to thrombus formation, which then propagates proximally into the tibial,

popliteal, or larger veins. Virchow's triad of stasis, endothelial injury, and hypercoagulability is still considered central in the pathogenesis of DVT, platelets in sluggish blood adhering to subendothelial tissue. Initially the thrombus is almost free floating, but it soon attaches to the adjacent vein wall. The thrombus often propagates proximally until the next major tributary where blood flow increases. If vein wall and coagulation conditions permit, the thrombus may continue to propagate and occlude the tributary as well. If a portion of the thrombus becomes detached, pulmonary embolism is the result. Pulmonary emboli from the tibial veins are small enough to be well tolerated by most patients, but thrombus from the popliteal or large veins may produce sudden right-sided heart failure and death. Eventually the DVT may be cleared by the body's thrombolysins, but scarred valves or obstructed, fibrotic veins are often sequelae. DVT is associated with reduced blood flow and inactivity as in the postoperative state, obesity, age greater than 60 years, malignancy, trauma, elevated estrogen levels secondary to birth control pills or pregnancy, ulcerative colitis, and a previous history of DVT and varicose veins.

Signs and Symptoms

The classical patient with acute DVT has calf tenderness and edema. Dorsiflexion of the foot (Homans' or dorsiflexion sign) produces calf pain, and a palpable cord may be present in the popliteal space. As the thrombus progresses proximally and venous obstruction is increased, the entire lower extremity becomes painful, edematous, and pale (phlegmasia alba dolens).

With further progression and arterial compromise from tissue compression, the limb takes on a bluish hue (phlegmasia cerulea dolens). Massive thrombosis leading to venous gangrene is, fortunately, rare (Fig. 32-2).

These classical findings are present in approximately 50% of patients. That is, at least half of the patients with some element of DVT are entirely asymptomatic, whereas half of the patients with calf pain or swelling may not have DVT. Prophylactic treatment is therefore advocated in high-risk patients. However, any patient suspected of having DVT requires a more elaborate work-up before long-term, potentially dangerous anticoagulation is prescribed.

The differential diagnosis of DVT includes superfi-

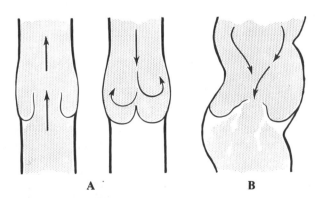

Fig. 32-1. A, Competent vein opens to allow forward blood flow but closes snugly to prevent retrograde flow. **B,** Imcompetent vein valve cusps cannot close; retrograde flow of blood results.

cial thrombophlebitis; ailments of the knee and in particular ruptured Baker's cysts; spontaneous or trauma-related rupture of the muscles of the calf (especially the plantaris muscles), which produces sudden pain in the calf and is followed some days later by ecchymosis of the calf; acute arterial occlusion that may produce pain and blanching, but swelling is rare and of course the absence of pulses should be an excellent clue; and edema from any cause (i.e., congestive heart failure, etc.).

Diagnosis

When carefully performed, noninvasive laboratory studies can allow accurate diagnosis of acute iliofemoral vein thrombosis in greater than 90% of affected patients. *Doppler ultrasound* detects flow in the major veins. When one is listening over any vein, compression distally in the extremity should produce a proximal rush of blood past the probe. Proximal compression should obliterate the flow unless there are incompetent valves between the compressing hand and the listening probe. Release of the proximal compression produces a release augmentation of flow beneath the probe. These maneuvers can be used to test the venous sounds at the ankle, behind the knee, in the midthigh, and over the common femoral vein in the groin. Although the accuracy of the test varies, 90% accuracy can be expected in good laboratories. These results have been duplicated, but not bettered, with duplex scanning.

A *plethysmograph* measures volume (i.e., a gauge placed around the calf measures the volume of the calf). When a blood pressure cuff placed proximally is inflated to between arterial and venous pressures, the calf plethysmograph records a volume increase (venous capacitance). When the cuff is suddenly deflated, blood flows from the calf and the calf volume is thereby reduced. The rate of volume change is calculated in terms of venous outflow. The overall results parallel those of the Doppler ultrasound, both tests being less accurate in diagnosing DVT of the calf than in finding more proximal disease.

^{125}I-labeled fibrinogen is injected intravenously, and both legs are scanned hours and days later. Since active ongoing thrombosis incorporates fibrinogen at the site of thrombosis, any increase in radioactivity indicates that thrombosis is occurring. This test is extremely accurate for diagnosing small, less clinically important calf vein thrombosis but is less accurate for the upper thigh and pelvis because of background radiation from the bones and bladder. We do not use the test to diagnose acute DVT because there is a waiting period (hours and sometimes days) between injection and the appearance of results. This is an excellent tool for studying the pathophysiology of DVT, prospectively monitoring high-risk patients, assessing therapeutic measures, and differentiating acute and chronic venous disease.

Isotope venography requires injection of an isotope into the dorsum of the foot and observation of its course up the leg with a scanning device. It is not accurate in the diagnosis of calf vein thrombosis, but it allows reliable diagnosis of thrombosis of the veins of the thigh and pelvis.

Contrast venography is the "gold standard" of venous diagnosis. Iodinated contrast material is injected into a foot vein with the patient in reverse Trendelenburg's position. All the veins of the deep and superficial system should become visualized. When the contrast medium reaches the groin, the legs are quickly elevated to fill the veins of the pelvis. A partially occluding thrombus will be outlined by the contrast material (Fig. 32-3), whereas no contrast medium will be seen in totally occluded veins (i.e., only collateral channels will be visualized).

A patient suspected of having DVT should have this diagnosis confirmed by one of the previously mentioned tests (Table 32-1). If the testing procedures are necessarily delayed, treatment is started immediately to prevent the complications of pulmonary embolism. However, diagnostic confirmation is always obtained before treatment is continued on a long-term basis to avoid anticoagulating patients who have complaints from other causes. If one of the noninvasive tests is nondiagnostic or does not correlate well with the clinical picture, contrast venography is obtained.

Treatment

The treatment of DVT is anticoagulation. An initial dose of between 5,000 and 10,000 units of heparin is given intravenously followed by 1,000 to 2,000 units hourly on a continuous basis using an infusion pump. The exact dose of heparin is that which maintains the partial thromboplastin time (PTT) between 60 and 80 seconds. Either the activated partial thromboplastin time (APTT) or the activated coagulation time (ACT) can be used to monitor heparin dosage. Continuous intravenous heparin has an advantage over intermittent heparin in that there are no wide swings of the measured clotting times, so bleeding complications are kept at a minimum. Intermittent subcutaneous heparin does

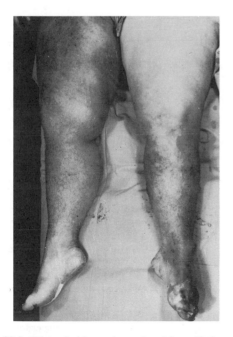

Fig. 32-2. Bilateral phlegmasia cerulea dolens. Notice swelling and mottling of both legs and necrosis of skin of left foot.

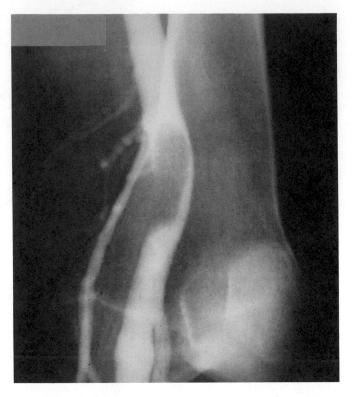

Fig. 32-3. Contrast venogram showing popliteal vein thrombosis.

Table 32-1. Diagnosis of DVT

| | Sensitivity | | |
Method	Calf	Thigh	Pelvis
History and physical examination	±	±	±
Doppler ultrasound	±	+	+
Plethysmograph	±	+	+
^{125}I fibrinogen scan	+	±	−
Radionuclide venogram	−	+	+
Contrast venogram	+	+	+

not ordinarily achieve adequate levels of anticoagulation, and intramuscular heparin may produce significant bleeding complications. The heparin itself is not considered to be a thrombolytic agent, but it protects against the propagation of thrombus, thus reducing the risk from pulmonary embolism. The patient usually requires bed rest for as long as the leg is symptomatic. Ambulation is then cautiously begun with the leg supported in elastic bandages or stockings.

Warfarin (Coumadin) is overlapped with heparin for 5 to 7 days and continued for 3 to 6 months to protect against late pulmonary embolism. Thrombolytic therapy more promptly eliminates clot and, theoretically, preserves functioning valves. This advantage has not been clinically obvious and is balanced by bleeding complications. Thrombolytic therapy may yet assume a greater role if tissue plasminogen activator (TPA) is shown to be less dangerous yet effective.

Surgical extraction of venous thrombi is rarely performed. This operation is reserved for patients who have threatened limb loss and who do not respond immediately to heparin therapy. Past published series have shown that the incidence of rethrombosis is high and, in addition, the late results of surgery are not superior.

Interruption of the inferior vena cava (IVC) to prevent pulmonary embolism is indicated in the patient who has recurrent pulmonary embolism on therapy or who has an absolute contraindication to anticoagulation (recent gastrointestinal or intracranial hemorrhage). The preferred method is the transjugular or the transfemoral insertion of the Greenfield filter into the infrarenal inferior vena cava using local anesthesia and fluoroscopic control. These filters have an excellent long-term patency rate compared to older devices and have been used in the suprarenal IVC in patients with infrarenal thrombus. The IVC also may be approached surgically via the retroperitoneal or transperitoneal approach. The transperitoneal approach has the advantage of allowing ligation of the left ovarian vein in female

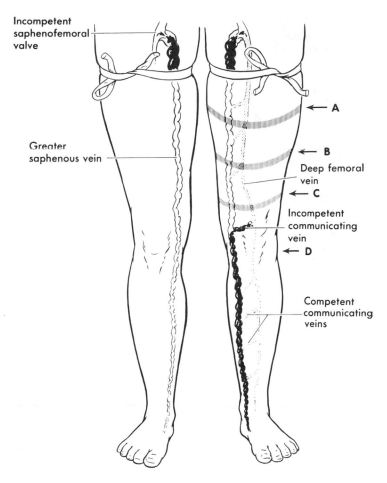

Incompetent
saphenofemoral
valve

← A

← B

Deep femoral
vein

← C

Incompetent
communicating
vein

← D

Greater
saphenous vein

Competent
communicating
veins

Fig. 32-4. Modified Trendelenburg (tourniquet) test for varicose veins. Tourniquet on the patient's *right* leg prevents filling of varicosed greater saphenous vein distally, proving competency of all communicating valves and incompetency of saphenofemoral valve. One patient's *left* leg, incompetent communicating vein valve at knee allows filling of greater saphenous vein distal to this point, but tourniquet at points *A, B,* or *C* would not alter findings. However, had second tourniquet been placed at point *D,* greater saphenous vein would have filled only from knee down to this level.

patients. The IVC ligature is placed directly beneath the renal veins so that there is no cul-de-sac in which a thrombus may form between the ligature and the renal veins.

Prophylaxis

Prevention of DVT is indicated in hospitalized patients who have at least one risk factor. Early postoperative ambulation reduces stasis. Elastic stockings increase femoral vein flow velocity, but their clinical value is debated. Intermittent calf compression devices, with or without support stockings, not only reduce stasis but appear to activate the fibrinolytic system. Low-dose heparin administered subcutaneously (5,000 units/12 hours) has been shown to reduce DVT pulmonary embolism and death in general surgical patients. This effect is based on heparin's ability to activate antithrombin III, an effect not detected by the PTT. Low-dose heparin combined with ergotamine, which decreases venous capacitance (and increases velocity flow), is also effective. Low-dose heparin is not as ef-

fective as low-dose coumadin in orthopedic patients. Most reports minimize the effect of prophylactic drugs on operative bleeding. If prophylaxis is not undertaken in high-risk patients, they should at least be closely monitored for DVT with noninvasive studies to avoid the grave complications of pulmonary emboli.

SUPERFICIAL THROMBOPHLEBITIS

Thrombosis and inflammation involving the superficial veins immediately underneath the skin is a very troublesome, but not medically serious, disorder in most patients. Pulmonary embolism and leg ulceration from isolated superficial thrombophlebitis are distinctly unusual. The involved vein is tender, has overlying erythema, and may form a palpable cord. Lymphangitis mimics superficial thrombophlebitis, but the patient's temperature is usually elevated and a site of distal infection is evident.

Superficial thrombophlebitis may be associated with DVT; thus these patients are noninvasively evaluated to rule out DVT. Treatment is symptomatic and consists of bed rest, heat, and analgesics, including aspirin. Phenylbutazone is reserved for refractory patients. In recurrent or resistant cases, heparin, warfarin (Coumadin) anticoagulation, or surgical excision and ligation of the involved veins may be indicated. If the thrombophlebitis is septic in origin (associated with prolonged intravenous cannulation, etc.), excision of the infected vein is required.

VARICOSE VEINS

Primary varicosities form without any evidence of prior DVT. A specific cause in these patients is often difficult to pinpoint, but about 40% have a family history of varicose veins, often with onset early in adult life. Varicose veins have a pronounced female preponderance (2 or 3 to 1), presumably related to the smooth muscle–relaxing effect of female sex hormones manifest by cyclic dilation of veins and increase in tissue fluids premenstrually. Commonly, pregnancy is associated with the onset of worsening of varicose veins. Perhaps the upright position of *Homo sapiens* is important.

Patients with *secondary* varicosities have had a prior episode of DVT, which either has destroyed valvular competency or has created venous obstruction. Incompetent deep veins lead to a reflux of blood pedally with the resultant dilation of distal veins, which itself causes valvular incompetence, setting up a vicious cycle. Patients with primary and secondary varicosities are differentiated by history, by the previously mentioned noninvasive tests, and by the Trendelenburg test (Figs. 32-4 and 32-5). With the leg elevated and the veins emptied, digital pressure or a tourniquet is placed over the saphenofemoral junction. The leg is quickly placed in the dependent position. No filling of the varicosities is seen if the communicating or perforating veins are competent. Rapid filling of the varicosities with the tourniquet in place indicates incompetent perforating veins (secondary varicosities). Release of the tourniquet leads to retrograde filling of the saphenous vein in patients with an incompetent saphenofemoral function (primary varicosities). Any patient whose varicosities are filled through incompetent perforators is assumed to have had previous deep vein disease.

Clinical Features

The most common reason women bring their varicose veins to the attention of the physician is purely cosmetic. Occasionally, however, the varicose veins cause a dull nagging ache or discomfort in the calves and ankles, that is exacerbated by prolonged standing or a day of activity. This sensation of heaviness and fullness is not usually associated with significant ankle edema. Excessive bleeding may occur if these superficial veins are traumatized.

Treatment

The treatment for most varicosities is expectant. Some patients feel much better wearing elastic stockings and should be encouraged to do so. Sheer support hose, though not ideally compressive, are usually preferred for cosmetic reasons. There are some patients, however, who wish to have the varices excised. Ligation and stripping of primary varicosities can be expected to give an excellent cosmetic and functional result. The patient with secondary varicosities may initially be improved, but the varicosities and symptoms are likely to recur because of the deep vein disease; thus stockings are recommended for this group of patients. Sclerotherapy is usually reserved for small varicosities that involve veins other than those of the greater or lesser saphenous system. Although this treatment is very popular on the European continent and in England it is less frequently employed in the United States. Sclerotherapy with 23% saline is used to treat smaller spider, or sunburst, varicosities.

POSTPHLEBITIS SYNDROME

The patient with postphlebitis syndrome and superficial varicosities (Fig. 32-6) should be recognized as having a complication of extensive DVT and not a complication of varicose veins. A patient with an ankle ulcer rarely has isolated varicosities but almost always has valvular incompetence or occlusion of the deep veins of the legs.

The hallmark of treatment is effective external compression. Most patients do not wrap an elastic bandage evenly, and in addition the bandage may become dis-

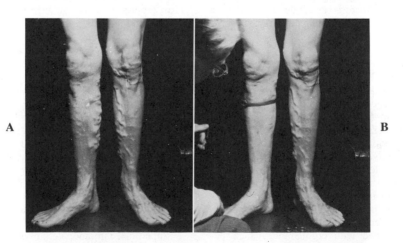

Fig. 32-5. A, Bilateral greater saphenous varicosities; veins fill promptly on standing. **B,** Vein does not fill distal to tourniquet; communicating vein valves are competent below this point.

lodged several times during the day. A fitted elastic stocking is applied on arising. The patient should not stand or sit for prolonged periods; activity that encourages the pumping action of the soleus muscle (walking) is prescribed. Resting with legs elevated several times daily is advised. Some patients find that the swelling goes down spontaneously at night, but others require elevation of the foot of the bed. Most importantly the patient should have excellent skin care and avoid irritation to the skin. Any skin breakdown along the medial aspect of the ankle, regardless of the cause, should be treated promptly.

Skin ulcers are managed initially by bed rest to reduce the edema and dressing changes to clean the ulcer. Sometimes antibiotics are necessary to combat deep infection. Once edema and infection have been controlled, a medicated compressive dressing is applied and changed as required, usually weekly. These dressings have the advantages of being bacteriostatic, maintaining a constant pressure over the leg and thus assisting in venous hemodynamics, and keeping the patient's irritating hands away from the ulcer. Some patients wear them for many months before the ulcer finally heals, but during this time, they maintain an active lifestyle.

Patients may also be hospitalized to have the ulcer excised surgically and skin grafted. This treatment has the advantage of healing the ulcer in a relatively short period of time (weeks) but has the disadvantage of requiring an expensive hospitalization.

Although some surgeons advocate it, extensive excision of ulcers with ligation of perforating veins and excision of all superficial varicosities is infrequently carried out. This method of treatment does not treat the cause of the patient's problem, namely, deep venous incompetence. Despite this extensive operation, compressive stockings are still required on a lifetime basis.

New methods of surgical therapy for selected patients with chronic venous insufficiency are being used in some centers. Patients with isolated unilateral ileofemoral venous thromboses can benefit from anastomosis of the distal end of the divided contralateral greater saphenous vein to the deep venous system on the affected side (femorofemoral venous cross-over graft). Patients with incompetent valves in the deep veins occasionally benefit from transplantation of a segment of brachial or greater saphenous vein containing a competent valve into the deep venous system. However, the selection of suitable candidates for these operative procedures must be scrupulous, and the benefits are apparently short lived.

PULMONARY EMBOLISM

Each year approximately 400,000 patients suffer fatal pulmonary embolism, the most dreaded complication of DVT. Minor pulmonary emboli may go undetected and estimates of the true incidence are as high as 25 patients per 100 hospital admissions, 5 of whom die. The pathophysiology reflects pulmonary hypertension and bronchoconstriction. The clinical diagnosis at times is difficult to make, and a high index of suspicion is required. The common symptoms of pulmonary embolism are dyspnea, cough, apprehension, chest pain, sweating, and syncope. The most reliable physical finding is tachypnea followed by rales, accentuated pulmonary second sound, tachycardia, and fever. An accentuated S_3 and S_4 gallop sound may be present in more massive pulmonary emboli.

The so-called classic signs of pleural friction rub and hemoptysis reflect pulmonary infarction and are present in less than 25% of cases. The white blood cell count is most often below 15,000, and the so-called di-

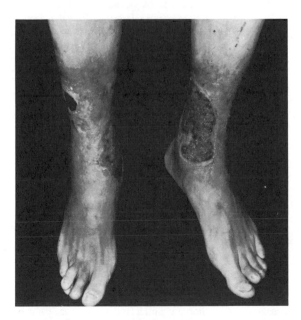

Fig. 32-6. Stasis dermatitis with skin ulcers. Although this patient may have secondary varicosities, ulcers are attributable to old deep venous disease.

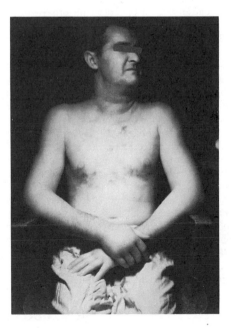

Fig. 32-7. Superior vena caval syndrome—dilated veins on chest wall, swelling of neck and upper extremities caused by lung cancer obstructing vena cava.

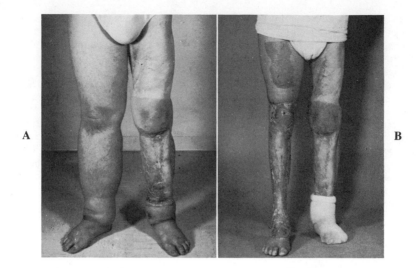

Fig. 32-8. A, Lymphedema praecox in 21-year-old patient; left leg was treated surgically 10 years before; right leg developed recent edema. **B,** Same patient 3 weeks after surgical treatment of right leg.

agnostic triad of elevated (LDH) and serum bilirubin with a normal serum glutamic oxaloacetic transaminase (SGOT) is seldom found. The chest film is normal early, but in severe and late pulmonary embolism, pulmonary consolidation, effusion, and a high diaphragm on the side of the embolus are common findings. The electrocardiogram (ECG) may show some right-sided heart strain, but more commonly the tracing remains unchanged.

Occluding pulmonary emboli cause hypoperfusion and, by necessity, hypoxemia. A PO_2 greater than 90 torr virtually rules out pulmonary embolism. Patients should be evaluated noninvasively for the presence of DVT because 95% of patients with proved pulmonary emboli will have demonstrable DVT. Other emboli may derive from the pelvic veins. A ventilation-perfusion lung scan should show a diminished perfusion in the area of pulmonary embolism with normal ventilation. Later, as the lung consolidates, ventilation may also be decreased. In equivocal cases a pulmonary angiogram is performed. The contrast material will either outline partially occluding thrombi or show decreased perfusion in certain areas.

The treatment of established pulmonary embolism is intravenous heparin. If repeated embolism occurs or there is a contraindication to anticoagulation, interruption of the inferior vena cava, as outlined previously, should be performed. Pulmonary embolectomy is performed on patients with massive pulmonary embolism with refractory hypotension. Thrombolytic therapy is considered in massive pulmonary embolus as an alternative to pulmonary embolectomy. Although less invasive, this method is slower in its effect and may produce hemorrhages and immunologic complications.

SPECIFIC LARGE VEIN THROMBOSIS

Acute occlusion or thrombosis of any major vein produces a syndrome of signs and symptoms specific to the vein, the region drained by it, and the adequacy of collateral venous circulation. Two recognized clinical syndromes are associated with obstruction of the superior vena cava and the axillary (subclavian) vein, respectively.

Acute superior vena caval obstruction occurs with extrinsic compression of the vein by tumor or enlarged lymph nodes or by thrombosis associated with direct trauma, infection, or long-term indwelling catheters (Fig. 32-7). Clinically, the superior vena caval syndrome consists of a plethora or cyanosis of the skin of the head and neck associated with varying degrees of venous distension and edema of the upper torso and extremities. This is attended by headache, vertigo, tinnitus, epistaxis, and sometimes fainting. Elevated upper extremity venous pressure and delayed arm-to-lung circulation times support the diagnosis; venography confirms the level and length of obstruction. Treatment is directed at the cause of the original obstruction, including surgical resection of the extrinsically compressing tumor or nodes, heparin anticoagulation, or thrombolytic therapy. Rarely, the obstruction is bypassed by use of a vein graft.

Acute axillary (subclavian) vein thrombosis, often termed "effort thrombosis," is seen in younger men who strenuously use their upper extremities in sports or occupation, particularly in activities requiring frequent and violent abduction of the arm on the shoulder. Progressive trauma to the vein probably initiates the thrombosis, which then propagates to totally occlude the vessel. If the venous collaterals are poor at this point, insidious swelling and cyanosis of the upper extremity occur with distension of the superficial veins. Elevated venous pressure, delayed arm-to-lung circulation times, and venography again are useful in diagnosis. Anticoagulation is indicated acutely; mechanical causes such as thoracic outlet syndrome, cervical rib, and lymph node enlargement must be sought and appropriately treated.

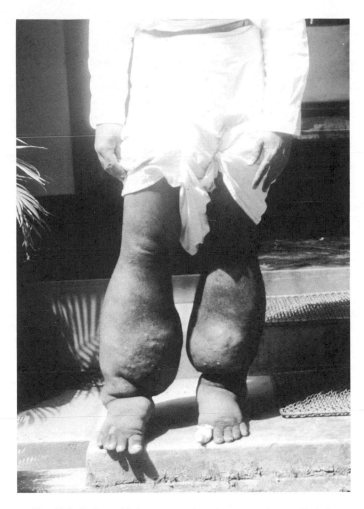

Fig. 32-9. Patient with lower extremity edema secondary to filariasis.

Thrombolytic therapy and venous thrombectomy have been used successfully in effort thrombosis.

LYMPHEDEMA

The remarkable appearance of lymphedema (excessive lymph in the tissue spaces) caused Caesar's lesions to coin the term *elephantiasis* to describe the afflicted lower limbs of their North African opponents, whose lymphatics were obstructed by filariasis.

Primary lymphedema occurs early in life as a result of developmental defects of the lymphatics of a specific site. It may be hereditary or simple (nonhereditary). More frequently the lower limbs and less frequently the upper limbs, genitals, or facial features are affected. Under the microscope the diseased tissue shows any of three patterns: aplasia, hypoplasia, or dilation and tortuosity of the lymphatics. Injected vital dyes diffuse randomly through the subcutaneous tissues and are not picked up by the defective lymphatic system. *Congenital* (primary) *lymphedema* (10%) is obvious at birth. (Milroy's disease is congenital lymphedema limited to one or both lower limbs and characterized by permanence, steady progress, increasing severity, and ab-

sence of constitutional symptoms.) *Lymphedema praecox* (71%) has the characteristics of congenital lymphedema except that it becomes obvious in patients 10 to 30 years old (Fig. 32-8). (The rare cause of primary lymphedema arising in later years is the *forme tardive*, 19%.)

Secondary lymphedema characteristically occurs later in life and results from obstruction, destruction, or overload of the lymphatics from any of a number of causes, such as (1) repeated lymphangitis or chronic bacterial (commonly streptococcal) infections, (2) neoplastic invasion of lymphatics, (3) filariasis (Fig. 32-9), (4) extensive fibrosis and scarring from radiation, burns, or other trauma, and (5) repeated allergic reactions. Lymphedema of the lower limbs beginning after 40 years of age should raise suspicions of intrapelvic carcinoma in women, or carcinoma of the prostate in men, or lymphoma. Lymphedema of the upper limb after radical mastectomy may signal the presence of lymphatic metastases of breast carcinoma, but more frequently it results merely from fibrosis, thrombosis, and localized infections in the postoperative period. A rare malignancy, *lymphangiosarcoma*, appears in a chronically lymphedematous arm (Stewart-Treves syndrome) or leg decades after the onset of the lymphedema.

Unlike venous edema, lymphedema rarely causes brown (hemosiderin) discoloration or ulceration.

Diagnosis and Treatment

The diagnosis is usually made on clinical grounds. Deep venous obstruction is ruled out in most patients by a noninvasive test. In patients whose history of lymphedema is relatively short, CT of the pelvis helps to rule out obstructive malignancies. Lymphangiography is not required to make the diagnosis, so this examination is usually not obtained.

Patients with secondary lymphedema require treatment of their infection or neoplasm. All patients require well-fitted elastic support garments (30 to 50 torr pressure). In addition, intermittent compression devices have been successfully used. The patient must elevate the extremity periodically, exercise to tolerance, and protect the skin from injury. Long-term prophylactic antibiotic treatment may be required to prevent repeated episodes of acute lymphangitis.

Lymphedema uncontrolled by these measures may be relieved by direct surgical attack (Fig. 32-8, *B*). The defective lymphatics, and therefore the lymphedema, are chiefly limited to the tissues lying between the superficial 1/50 inch of skin (epidermis has no lymphatics,

uppermost dermis has very few) and the lymphatics superficial to the deep fascia.

In severe, long-standing cases the afflicted skin, often including the investing fascia, is completely excised, and split-thickness skin grafts are placed directly on the investing fasciae or muscles. The grafts may be cut from the excised specimen or from unaffected areas.

A currently popular surgical approach is to supply an escape route for the trapped lymph with a pedicle. One pedicle consists of skin and subcutaneous tissue from the affected leg, which is denuded of its epidermis. The denuded skin is passed through a long incision in the deep fascia and is attached intimately to the underlying muscles, which always have normal lymphatics. The lymph exits from the skin across this bridge to the muscle (Noel Thompson procedure). A novel pedicle consists of omentum tunneled subcutaneously from the abdominal cavity to the limb; lymph is returned from the limb to the abdominal cavity.

Other surgical approaches have included lymphaticovenous anastomoses and direct microvascular lymphatic reconstructions. However, the long-term success of surgical therapy in relieving lymphedema is not encouraging, and these methods should be applied only to carefully selected patients.

33

Orthopedic Surgery

Reginald R. Cooper

Orthopedics encompasses the investigation, preservation, and restoration of form and function of the musculoskeletal system and related structures. Orthopedists employ medical, surgical, and physical methods of treatment.

Numerous conditions affect the musculoskeletal system, but I will discuss only the ones most commonly seen in clinical practice. These disorders can be categorized according to etiology as follows:

Congenital and developmental
Infectious and inflammatory
Traumatic
Metabolic
Neoplastic
Neuromuscular
Degenerative
Mechanical and postural
Idiopathic

Some disorders involve only one region, but others are not so restricted.

ORTHOPEDIC EVALUATION OF A PATIENT

Medical, emotional, social, and economic factors influence the patient with an orthopedic disorder. The astute physician considers each of these in its proper perspective. The patient who seeks the advice of an orthopedist usually complains of one or more of the following: something feels wrong (pain, numbness, tenderness), something looks wrong (deformity, limp, bump), or something moves wrong (limp, weakness, stiffness, instability).

If the disorder is localized, complaints often remain in the involved part; however, pain can be referred to a remote site (e.g., knee pain from hip disease). A lesion that irritates a peripheral nerve produces pain in the area supplied by the nerve (e.g., pain in the lower extremity from a herniated lumbar intervertebral disk). In the back and extremities, protective muscle contraction frequently produces symptoms at a distance from the disease.

With the doctor's guidance, the patient must relate a pertinent, integrated, chronologic history of all complaints. Important questions about pain include the following: What are the circumstances surrounding its onset? What is its progression? Was the onset associated with injury? Was it sudden or gradual? Was this the first episode? Has the pain been continuous? Is it sharp or dull, superficial or deep? What relieves it? What makes it worse? Does it interfere with function or sleep? A similar chronology must be documented for complaints other than pain.

A normal opposite part serves as a valuable standard for comparison during examination of a patient with a musculoskeletal problem. Depending on the involved region, the physician can modify the following physical examination outline:

Joints
  Inspection: In what position is the joint held? Is this normal? What is the joint contour? Is it swollen? Is the overlying skin normal? Are there discolorations, venous distension, cuts, scars?
  Palpation: Is there tenderness? Does it feel hot or cold? Is there excessive joint fluid? Is a fluid wave ballotable? Is the synovium thickened? Are all the ligaments intact? Is there unstable, abnormal motion?
  Range of motion:
    Active: Is motion produced by the patient limited? If so, why? Is there pain, muscle spasm, contracture (fixed, spasm), bony block? In what direction is the limitation? Record range of motion in degrees.
    Passive: Can you move the joint through a greater range than the patient can? If so, is muscle torn, paralyzed, or reflexly inhibited? Record range of motion in degrees.
Muscles
  Does each one contract?
  What is its strength?
    Grade 5, normal, 100%—range of motion against full resistance
    Grade 4, good, 75%—range of motion against some resistance
    Grade 3, fair, 50%—range of motion against gravity
    Grade 2, poor, 25%—range of motion with gravity eliminated
    Grade 1, trace, 10%—slight contraction, no motion
    Grade 0—no contraction
  Is there measurable atrophy or enlargement?
  Compare limb circumference with the opposite side.
    Find the same level on two sides by measuring from a *fixed* part to a given site. *Example:* To find thigh circumference, measure 6 or 7 inches proximally to the tibial tubercle (a fixed part), not from the patella (a movable part).
  Does the tendon glide freely? Is it tender? Is it intact?
  Are there masses in muscle or tendon?
Bone
  Is the integrity maintained (stability, crepitus [grating of bone fragments on each other])?
  Is it obviously deformed (angulated, curved)?
  Is it of normal size (length, width)?
  Is it in proper relation to other bones?
  Is it tender?
  Is the overlying skin normal?

Are any masses present? If so, notice type, location, size, consistency, fixed or free, pulsatile, bruit, transillumination.
Neurologic examination
  Motor, sensory, reflexes
Vasculature
  Skin changes of vascular insufficiency, pulses, veins, masses, bruit
Function
  Put the part through voluntary motions of everyday activities
  Gait: Is it normal? If not, what abnormal components are present (short-leg limp, hip abductor weakness—lurch to involved side, hip dislocation, waddle)?

Radiographic studies are usually necessary, if not mandatory, for complete evaluation of a complaint related to the musculoskeletal system. Comparable views of the opposite normal side sometimes aid in making a diagnosis.

REGIONAL ORTHOPEDICS
Neck (Table 33-1)
Torticollis (Wryneck, Congenital Muscular Torticollis)

A fibrotic, contracted sternocleidomastoid muscle tilts the head to the ipsilateral side and turns the face to the contralateral side (Fig. 33-1). The cause remains unknown. Theories include birth trauma, muscle fibrosis, and abnormal muscular development. Many involved babies were breech presentations. About 3 weeks after birth, the parents find a lump in the child's sternocleidomastoid muscle. The mass disappears in a few weeks, and some of these infants develop torticollis later. Some afflicted children had no noticeable mass. Asymmetry of face and skull bones accompanies torticollis.

The parents should stretch the tight muscle gently each day. They should position the bottle and toys so that the baby turns to them in a way that stretches the tight sternocleidomastoid muscle. Many cases correct spontaneously and do not develop into wryneck. Severe persistent deformity at 2 or 3 years of age warrants excision of a segment of the contracted muscle. Much of the asymmetry disappears with subsequent face and head growth.

Any of the following can produce torticollis: hemivertebra and other cervical spine abnormalities, visual disturbances in which the patient tilts the head to see

Table 33-1. Disorders of the Neck

Age	Disorder	Cause
Birth to 2 years	Torticollis	Developmental
4-8 years	Acute wryneck	Traumatic or inflammatory
Adult	Stiff neck	Inflammatory(?)
	Degenerative joint disease (cervical-spine arthritis, degenerative disk disease, cervical spondylosis)	Degenerative
	Acute sprain	Traumatic

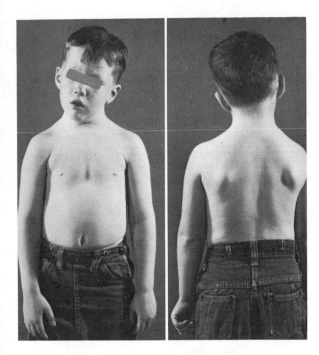

Fig. 33-1. Congenital torticollis. Head tilts to side to fibrotic sternocleidomastoid muscle, and face turns to opposite side.

better, or acute cervical lymphadenopathy that causes the patient to tilt the head to relieve pain.

Acute Wryneck

Children develop acute wryneck because of inflammation and cervical lymphadenopathy associated with acute pharyngitis or because of rotatory subluxation of the cervical spine. A history of acute onset differentiates either from congenital muscular torticollis.

At times during acute pharyngitis, hyperemia and inflammation around cervical spine ligaments allow rotatory subluxation of cervical spine facets. Treatment consists of appropriate therapy of the primary disorder, head halter traction to realign facets, and postreduction immobilization for 2 to 3 weeks in a cervical collar.

Occasionally a child suddenly twists the neck, hears a click, experiences sharp neck pain, and locks in a twisted position. An open-mouth radiograph of the first and second cervical vertebrae (C1-C2) demonstrates a subluxated facet of C1 on C2. Head halter traction with the spine neutral or slightly flexed reduces the subluxation. The child should wear a collar or brace for 3 weeks.

Stiff Neck

A person who has slept with the neck twisted or who has been in cold air often complains of a stiff neck. He or she holds the head rigidly inclined to the involved side and complains of sore, tender neck muscles. Neck motion produces pain. The cause is unknown. Some believe that an inflammatory myositis produces stiff neck. With heat, analgesics, rest, and support by a collar or traction, symptoms usually subside in 3 to 10 days. Transcutaneous electrical nerve stimulation (TENS) may be of value.

Degenerative Joint Disease (Cervical Spine Arthritis, Degenerative Disk Disease, Cervical Spondylosis)

In degenerative joint disease, intervertebral disks and cervical facets degenerate. Spurs of bone and inflammation adjacent to disks, intervertebral body joints, and facets impinge on cervical nerve roots at one or more levels. At times, degeneration occurs after trauma, but it can arise spontaneously. Symptoms vary from mild to severe. Frequently, pain radiates from the neck to the head or upper extremities. Pain and paresthesias can follow a nerve root distribution. Persistent nerve root irritation causes reflex sympathetic nerve stimulation with blurred vision, loss of balance, and headaches. Often, the patient inclines the head away from the painful side to get temporary relief. Neck motion decreases. Pressure over spinous tips and longitudinal compression of the spine produce pain. Reflexes and sensation decrease. Radiographic examinations help localize the level(s) of disk narrowing and spur formation (Fig. 33-2).

Periods of rest, pillows designed to support the cervical spine in neutral position or extension, moist heat, salicylates, intermittent head halter traction (7 pounds for 15 minutes, 3 times a day), and night head halter traction often relieve symptoms. If conservative measures fail, the patient may need surgery. Depending on the severity and location of the disorder, surgeons can remove the disk, enlarge the foramina, or fuse the cervical spine.

Cervical disk herniation can produce motor loss, decreased reflexes, and sensory loss that follows a definite nerve root pattern. Myelograms help confirm the diagnosis and localize the level.

Acute Sprain

Cervical sprains concern the legal profession about as much as they concern the medical profession. The occupant of an automobile struck from the rear often sustains neck injury. Some patients have immediate neck pain, but others have none for 12 to 36 hours. Patients complain of diffuse pain over the posterior surface of the neck and head. Protective muscle contraction decreases neck motion in an attempt to prevent pain. At times, patients develop sore muscles, stiff neck, severe pain, vertigo, nausea, headache, and paresthesias. Symptoms tend to be intermittent and frequently persist for months but subside eventually in most instances.

Interspinous ligaments and neck and shoulder muscles are tender. Cervical spine motion decreases. Decreased sensation in the upper extremities usually does not follow a well-defined nerve distribution and varies from examination to examination. Definite, severe, and persistent neurologic signs suggest more than ligament or muscle damage. Radiographs are usually normal but *must be taken* to rule out fracture and dislocation.

Analgesics, heat, rest, massage, and mild head halter traction for 2 to 10 days often relieve acute symptoms. If so, the patient should gradually increase neck motion as symptoms decrease. The use of a neck support may be necessary in some instances. TENS may help. Many patients with persistent symptoms have pending lawsuits. Physicians often speculate about the relation of symptoms to insurance settlements.

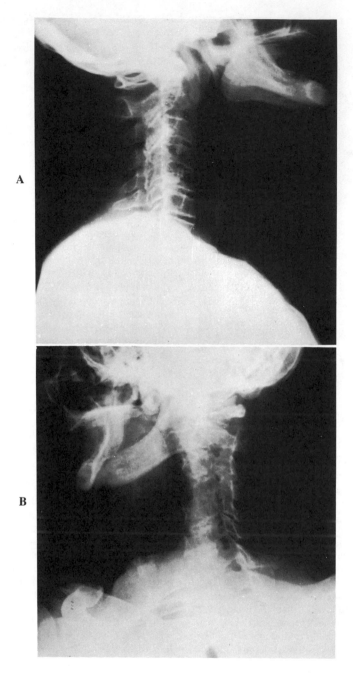

Fig. 33-2. Degenerative joint disease of cervical spine. **A,** Lateral view. Normal cervical curve is gone, and C4-C5 disk space is narrow. **B,** Oblique view. Degenerative spurs have narrowed intervertebral foramina.

Shoulder (Table 33-2)

Fractured Clavicle

The clavicle is the bone most frequently fractured during delivery. It begins ossification before other long bones, and the shoulders are the widest part of a newborn's body. When an examiner attempts to elicit a Moro reflex, the baby with a fractured clavicle does not move the arm on the involved side (pseudoparalysis). Brachial plexus injury, fracture of the humerus, and dislocated shoulder produce a similar sign.

No reduction is necessary. Strapping the baby's arm to the chest for 7 to 10 days relieves discomfort. A lump of callus appears within a few days and disappears during the ensuing weeks, and full function returns.

Brachial Palsy (Obstetric Palsy)

Mechanical stretch of the brachial plexus during delivery paralyzes various muscles of the upper extremity and produces loss of sensation in the distribution of involved nerves. Nerves may remain intact but stretched or they may rupture completely. The infant does not move the involved arm or forearm. Signs depend on the anatomic location of the lesion. In the common up-

Table 33-2. Disorders of the Shoulder

Age	Disorder	Cause
Birth to 2 years	Fractured clavicle	Traumatic
	Brachial palsy (obstetric palsy)	Traumatic
2-4 years	Pulled shoulder	Traumatic
Adult	Rotator cuff degeneration (acute bursitis, noncalcific or calcific; rotator cuff disease)	Degenerative
	Frozen shoulder (adhesive pericapsulitis)	Degenerative
	Acute rupture of the rotator cuff	Traumatic and degenerative
	Snapping scapula	Inflammatory(?) Degenerative(?)

per arm type of Erb-Duchenne (caused by downward traction of the shoulder), an injury of C5-C6 nerve roots paralyzes deltoid, supraspinatus, infraspinatus, and biceps muscles. The arm adducts and internally rotates, and the forearm pronates. In the lower arm paralysis of Klumpke (caused by upward traction with the arm overhead), an injury of C8 and T1 paralyzes intrinsic muscles of the hand or the long finger flexors, or both. In the whole-arm type, various combinations of paralyses lead to severe dysfunction.

During the months after birth, the infant usually improves but seldom recovers completely. Prognosis is best in the upper arm type. Treatment soon after birth prevents contractures. Each day the child's shoulder should be moved passively into abduction and external rotation and the forearm into supination. In older cases release of contractures, transfer of tendons, and osteotomies might improve function.

Pulled Shoulder

Occasionally a parent grabs a child by the hand and pulls him or her onto a curb or in a given direction. The infant has immediate pain and refuses to move the arm. The shoulder is tender. If roentgenograms reveal no fracture, the child probably has a partial tear of the shoulder capsule and bleeding into the joint. Resting the part for a few days by strapping the arm to the body relieves symptoms. If left to his or her own devices, with pain as a guide, the child will regain motion in the arm. No physical therapy is needed.

Rotator Cuff Degeneration (Acute Bursitis, Noncalcific or Calcific; Rotator Cuff Disease)

The rotator cuff, composed of the supraspinatus, infraspinatus, teres minor, and subscapularis muscles, holds the head of the humerus downward and medially against the glenoid, thereby producing a stable fulcrum for arm abduction. The floor of the subdeltoid (subacromial) bursa covers the superior surface of the rotator cuff, and a disorder of one involves the other. Frequently cuff degeneration of unknown cause produces pain and limits shoulder motion. The supraspinatus usually degenerates near its insertion into the greater tuberosity of the humerus. If the degenerated area and

surrounding repair tissue extend to the external surface of the tendon, subacromial bursitis develops. If the degenerated tendon calcifies, this calcium can rupture into the bursa. Degeneration can partially rupture the rotator cuff. Symptoms vary with the following syndromes.

Acute degeneration and bursitis. With acute degeneration, the patient notices sudden, sharp, severe pain in the subacromial region. Pain radiates down the arm. Shoulder motion, especially abduction and external rotation, decreases. Examination discloses point tenderness over the greater tuberosity, and active and passive motions produce pain. As the greater tuberosity passes beneath the acromion during abduction from 30 to 80 degrees, the patient experiences the most severe pain (painful arc syndrome). Radiographic studies either reveal no abnormality or show calcification in the tendon or bursa.

The patient should rest and use analgesics and hot packs to relieve pain. Oral analgesics and antiinflammatory drugs or local injection of an anesthetic or steroids into the bursa often helps. Pain should decrease in 48 to 72 hours. If it does not, the physician might wish to aspirate calcium or remove it by operative incision. When pain subsides, the patient must begin shoulder circumduction, abduction, and external rotation to prevent a frozen shoulder (see below).

Chronic degeneration and bursitis. With or without a previous acute episode, the patient with rotator cuff disease complains of intermittent aching in the shoulder, tenderness over the cuff insertion, and pain on motion. If the cuff ruptures, shoulder abduction weakens. Patients with chronic and recurrent rotator cuff disease should use heat and analgesics to relieve pain. Between acute episodes, they should initiate active range-of-motion exercises. If calcium produces a mechanical obstruction to motion, it should be excised.

Tenosynovitis of the long head of the biceps. Tenosynovitis produces symptoms much the same as those of acute rotator cuff tendinitis except that tenderness is over the biceps groove. Supination of the forearm against resistance produces shoulder pain. Conservative treatment is the same as in acute bursitis. If the process continues and motion gradually decreases, the patient might need surgical release of the long head of the biceps.

Frozen Shoulder (Adhesive Pericapsulitis)

Adhesions form in the gliding planes about the shoulder after trauma, shoulder disease, or any disorder that limits shoulder motion. Patients, usually 40 to 60 years old, complain of severe pain. Motion decreases greatly. Radiographs usually disclose no abnormalities. Occasionally they show signs of previous shoulder disease. Heat and active circumduction exercises help restore shoulder function. On rare occasions, if the range of motion is not improving, manipulation under anesthesia may be necessary. This disorder tends to subside in 12 to 18 months, and motion increases.

Acute Rupture of the Rotator Cuff

A force applied during lifting or during a fall can rupture a normal rotator cuff or a previously degenerated one. With a complete tear, the patient experiences severe pain, feels a sharp snap, and loses active abduction and external rotation of the shoulder. If the arm is

Table 33-3. Disorders of the Elbow

Age	Disorder	Cause
2-4 years	Pulled elbow (nurse-maid's elbow)	Traumatic
Adult	Tennis elbow (lateral humeral epicondylitis tendinitis)	Degenerative, traumatic

Table 33-4. Disorders of the Hand

Age	Disorder	Cause
Birth to 2 years	Syndactyly	Congenital and developmental
	Polydactyly	Congenital and developmental
	Congenital bands	Congenital and developmental
Adult	Dupuytren's contracture	Idiopathic
	de Quervain's disease	Developmental, inflammatory
	Trigger finger	Developmental, inflammatory

Table 33-5. Disorders of the Spine

Age	Disorder	Cause
Birth to 2 years	Spina bifida and meningomyelocele	Congenital and developmental
2-4 years	Scoliosis	Idiopathic, infantile, congenital
4-8 years	Scoliosis	Idiopathic and paralytic
8-14 years	Scoliosis	Idiopathic and paralytic
	Juvenile round back (vertebral epiphysitis, Scheuermann's disease)	Developmental—osteochondritis, epiphysitis (?)
Adult	Spondylolysis and spondylolisthesis	Developmental defect; traumatic (?)
	Acute back sprain	Traumatic
	Intervertebral disk degeneration, herniation, and spinal stenosis	Degenerative
	Coccygodynia	Traumatic (?), unknown(?)

passively elevated above the head, the patient might be able to hold it there by use of the deltoid muscle. Immediate surgical repair of a complete tear produces a good chance for recovery of function. Partial tear is common. The patient complains of mild pain and moves the shoulder to a limited extent. With symptomatic treatment, the patient regains function.

Snapping Scapula

The patient complains of grating, snapping, or pain as the scapula rotates over the chest wall. Persons in certain occupations have difficulty working. Although a subscapular exostosis can produce symptoms, snapping is usually caused by poor posture, an abnormally formed scapula, subscapular bursitis, or inflammation in fascial planes. The physician should obtain radiographs to rule out lesions of the scapula. Usually attempts to correct poor posture, injection of tender areas with local anesthesia, and exercises to strengthen the scapular muscles relieve symptoms.

Elbow (Table 33-3)

Pulled Elbow (Nursemaid's Elbow)

The history of a child with a pulled elbow is similar to that of one with a pulled shoulder. Pulled elbow is more common. The child holds the forearm pronated and the elbow flexed 30 to 40 degrees. Radiographs are normal. In this disorder the radial head probably subluxates through the annular ligament. In a child over 6 years of age the larger radial head does not subluxate. If the doctor quickly manipulates the child's forearm into supination and extension, a click occurs as the radial head reduces. To prevent recurrent subluxation, the physician should splint the forearm in supination and extension for 7 to 10 days. The patient then initiates motion. No physical therapy is needed.

Tennis Elbow (Lateral Humeral Epicondylitis, Tendinitis)

The patient with tennis elbow complains of pain over the lateral humeral epicondyle. This often occurs after injury or activities wherein the forearm repeatedly supinates and extends (a backhand in tennis). The cause of symptoms is debatable. Some attributable complaints to a disrupted common extensor origin at or immediately distal to the lateral humeral epincondyle. Others believe that the radiohumeral bursa beneath the common extensor origin becomes irritated. In any case, the lateral humeral epicondyle is tender. The patient complains of pain during attempts at forearm supination or wrist extension against resistance. Warm, moist packs, rest, analgesics, and injections of local anesthetic and occasionally steroids usually relieve symptoms. Some patients have recurrence that again responds to conservative therapy. In these instances exercises to strengthen the wrist extensors may be of value. Some obtain relief with a strap around the forearm over the tender point. In 5% to 10% of the cases, persistent symptoms warrant surgical exploration and excision of the degenerated and torn extensor tendon.

Hand

The age for and cause of disorders of the hand are given in Table 33-4 and are discussed in Chapter 34.

Spine (Table 33-5)

Spina Bifida and Meningomyelocele

In spina bifida, a developmental disorder, one or more vertebral arches fail to fuse in the posterior midline. At times the incomplete neural arch allows the contents of the spinal canal to herniate. Spina bifida occurs in about one of every 1000 births. It most frequently involves lumbar and sacral vertebrae but can affect others. In many children with meningomyelocele, extensive defects lead to death at birth or soon thereafter. Within the last few years medical teams

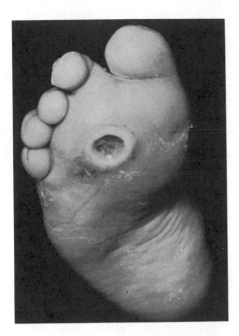

Fig. 33-3. Chronic foot ulcer in patient with spina bifida and meningomyelocele.

have improved prospects for increasing the life span of these children.

The several types of spina bifida depend on the anatomic defect. In spina bifida occulta the neural arch is defective but neural contents do not herniate, or at least not enough to cause neurologic symptoms. In some instances the overlying skin is pigmented, indented, or hairy. Later in life some of these children gradually develop incomplete paralysis, sensory loss, weakened intrinsic foot muscles, cock-up toes, and pes cavus. In spina bifida with meningocele one or more layers of the meninges herniate through the neural arch defect. In spina bifida with meningomyelocele the hernial sac contains meninges, cerebrospinal fluid, spinal cord, or nerve roots. Frequently these children have extensive paralysis, sensory loss, lack of bowel and bladder control, and associated hydrocephalus.

Symptoms and signs in spina bifida are produced by the protruding mass, neurologic loss, and resulting deformities. Frequently the skin over the hernia sac ulcerates and becomes infected. Meningitis follows. Neurologic defects vary with extent and location of the lesion. Sensory loss and skin ulcers are common (Fig. 33-3). Paralyzed muscles are usually flaccid. Deformities depend on the level of nerve root involvement. Many children have hip flexion contractures, dislocated hips, knee contractures, and pes equinovarus.

The complex treatment of the child with spina bifida is best done by a team that includes parents, pediatrician, neurosurgeon, orthopedic surgeon, urologist, orthotist, physical therapist, and social worker. The neurosurgeon closes the hernia sac and treats hydrocephalus. Urologists prevent and treat urinary tract infections and provide proper emptying of the urinary collecting system. Orthopedic surgeons prevent and correct deformities by physical therapy, manipulation, splints, braces, and surgery. Therapists help in gait training and instruct the child in self-care. The child needs nursing care to prevent ulcers. Parents must understand the magnitude of the problem and be willing to help with therapeutic programs.

Scoliosis

Lateral curvature of the spine can result from neuromuscular disorders (polio, muscular dystrophy, spinal cord tumor, neurofibromatosis), congenital defects (wedge vertebra or failed segmentation), or any disorder that produces muscle spasm (disk herniation); however, most cases of idiopathic scoliosis develop during rapid spine growth at adolescence.

Idiopathic scoliosis is more frequent in girls 8 to 14 years of age and often consists of one main thoracic or lumbar curve and one or two compensatory curves. In thoracic curves the spine and chest not only deviate laterally but also rotate. The chest protrudes anteriorly on the concave side of the curve and posteriorly on the convex side of the curve to produce hunchback. In lumbar curves the hip and pelvis on the side of the concavity appear prominent.

Patients with scoliosis usually have no symptoms. The patient or the parents notice the curve, the high shoulder, or the prominent thorax or hip. The physician must rule out all known causes of scoliosis before classifying it as idiopathic. Spinal radiographic studies (Fig. 33-4) with the patient standing up and lying down and bending to each side indicate the amount of curve flexibility. From these, the orthopedist measures the angle of the curve. If it is over 20 or 30 degrees, treatment should start at once. If it is not, the physician might observe the patient carefully to see whether the curve increases. If radiography 3 months later show an increased curve, the patient needs treatment. In general, the thoracic curves progress rapidly, especially if the patient is young. After spine growth stops, curves progress slowly if at all.

A Milwaukee brace or another type distracts the head from the pelvis and applies corrective lateral and rotatory forces to the spine by means of pads against the ribs. The orthopedist must check the brace frequently to be sure that it fits well. As the curve corrects and as the child grows, the orthotist must adjust and lengthen the brace. Some curves, if treated early by the brace, improve greatly or correct almost completely. If a curve progresses despite a brace or if a severe curve remains, the orthopedic surgeon can correct the curve and fuse the spine with or without internal fixation by rods. Even then, pseudoarthrosis may develop. This break in the fusion may produce no pain but might allow progression of the curve and necessitate refusion.

Juvenile Round Back (Vertebral Epiphysitis, Scheuermann's Disease)

Occasionally the secondary ring epiphyses and the upper and lower margins of vertebral bodies ossify poorly. Boys between 12 and 16 years of age develop epiphysitis more often than girls. Thoracic vertebrae are most commonly involved. Anterior vertebral body growth is decreased. The patient at times has mild backache. Thoracic kyphosis increases, producing a round back and stooped shoulders. X-ray examination discloses an irregular upper and lower vertebral surface and anterior wedging of the vertebral body (Fig. 33-5).

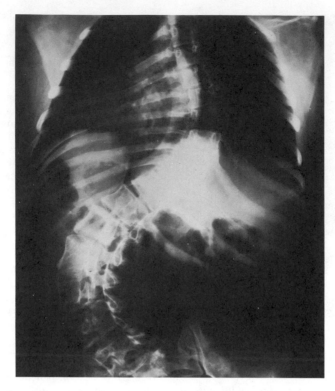

Fig. 33-4. Postpoliomyelitis scoliosis with right thoracic and left lumbar curve. Notice rotation of vertebral bodies.

The patient should limit activity to the point where he or she is free of pain. In the case of rapid progression of dorsal kyphosis, a Milwaukee brace helps prevent and correct deformity. The disorder is self-limiting. Spine fusion is indicated in severe deformity.

Spondylosis and Spondylolisthesis

In spondylolysis the pars interarticularis of the neural arch is defective and the posterior portion of the arch has no bony continuity with the remainder of the vertebra. In spondylolisthesis the neural arch is defective, and one vertebral body slides forward upon another (usually L5 or S1; Fig. 33-6). The defect may be congenital, but the actual slip tends to occur between 6 and 12 years of age. Once established, the slip usually does not progress; however, the intervertebral disk degenerates sooner than normal at the involved site. Spondylolisthesis is usually not so painful unless the disk degenerates. The patient might then have low back pain with radiation into the posterior aspect of the lower extremities. The patient must be taught to lift properly. He or she should stoop so that the spine does not bend but the hips and knees do. The patient builds up abdominal muscles by sit-up exercises with the hips and knees flexed. If pain persists, spinal fusion becomes necessary.

Acute Back Sprain

Acute flexion during a fall or while lifting frequently tears ligaments, fascia, and muscles of the low back. Patients experience sudden, sharp pain. On ex-

amination, muscle spasm and tenderness are found. Spine motion decreases. Radiographs may reveal no abnormalities. Rest, heat, and protection against extremes of motion relieve symptoms in 1 or 2 weeks.

After a sudden twist or bend, the spine at times locks in one position. Patients have severe pain. Based on the theory that facets lock in a subluxated position, doctors have called this a facet syndrome. Radiographic studies commonly show asymmetry of lumbosacral facets. Bed rest and sedation relieve acute symptoms.

Intervertebral Disk Degeneration and Herniation and Spinal Stenosis

Because of its ability to retain fluid and its intradiskal tension, the intervertebral disk gives the spine both flexibility and stability. With age intervertebral disks lose their elasticity and ability to retain fluid. Some disks then consist of nonelastic connective tissue, and others have clefts. Whether degeneration represents a variation of normal aging or is a disease is debatable. Disk degeneration often produces spine instability in the involved segment. This places abnormal stresses on ligamentous structures and spinal facet joints. In an attempt to repair and stabilize the spine, the body produces bone spurs. The inflammatory process often involves nerve roots. Frequently the patient complains of back pain and pain radiating into the thigh along the sciatic nerve. Pain is usually mild and intermittent for several months. Lifting, bending, and twisting increase pain, and rest relieves it. In some, pain starts in the low

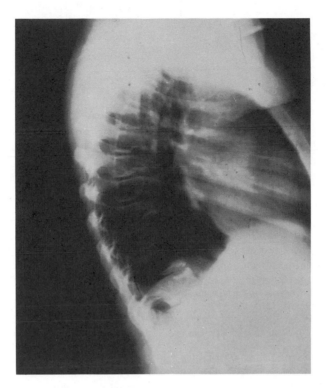

Fig. 33-5. Scheuermann's disease. Dorsal kyphosis is increased, vertebral bodies are wedged anteriorly, and epiphyseal rings are irregularly ossified.

back and later radiates into one lower extremity. Motion of the involved segment of the spine decreases. The doctor sees this best by viewing the patient from the side as the patient bends forward. Normally, motion starts at the neck and continues smoothly until the entire spine forms a continuous curve. In a patient with disk degeneration, involved segments remain flat. Hyperextension causes discomfort. Pressure over the spinous tip at the involved site produces pain. If the patient then hyperextends the back by lifting the head and shoulders off the table and pressure produces less pain, this is a positive instability test that helps localize the level of degeneration. The straight leg–raising test is positive when it reproduces radiating pain or back pain. Reflex, sensory, and motor activity vary from patient to patient. Radiographs often reveal a narrowed interspace and degenerative changes, most often at L5-S1 or L4-L5. Flexion and extension lateral views of the spine at times show sliding of one vertebral body on the other or tilting open of a disk space anteriorly on hyperextension.

During the acute stage of pain, bed rest usually relieves symptoms. The patient must then use the back properly. He or she should avoid bending, lift only by bending the knees, and avoid soft chairs and beds that allow the spine to sag. In the early stages of treatment, a low back brace reminds the patient of the proper position for the spine. Later, the patient should start progressive resistance exercises (sit-ups with hips and knees flexed) to build up the abdominal muscles and spine flexors. Most patients improve with this therapy.

If the anulus tears, the nucleus pulposus can herni-

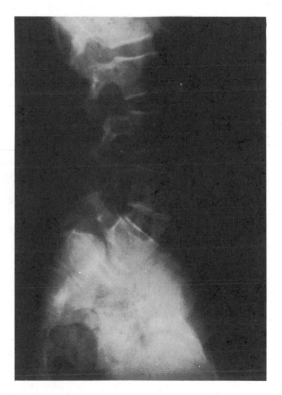

Fig. 33-6. Spondylolisthesis. L5 has slipped anteriorly on S1. Neural arch is defective.

Table 33-6. Disorders of the Hip

Age	Disorder	Cause
Birth to 2 years	Congenital dislocation	Developmental
4-8 years	Legg-Calvé-Perthes disease (coxa plana)	Metabolic (?)
	Synovitis	Viral (?)
8-14 years	Slipped capital femoral epiphysis	Metabolic (?)
Adult	Snapping hip	Anatomical variation

ate and press on a nerve root. This causes radiating pain and often interferes with reflex, motor, and sensory function in the lower extremity. The patient usually gives a history much like that of a patient with a degenerated disk. In many instances the most recent episode is severe and unrelenting. On physical examination, the physician often finds changes similar to those in a person with degenerative disk disease. In addition, the patient's reflexes decrease (ankle or knee jerk), muscles lose strength (toe extensors), and sensation in the L5 or S1 dermatome decreases.

Bed rest and medication for relief of pain lead to improvement in most patients, who are then treated as outlined for disk degeneration. Some patients need surgical removal of the intervertebral disk if they fail to improve in 3 or 4 weeks on a conservative therapeutic regime, or if their neurologic loss progresses. The physician should do a myelogram if he or she is not sure of the level of herniation or if there is a question about the diagnosis. After disk removal, some surgeons fuse the involved level of the spine. Others do not. After surgery, the doctor should treat the patient as one with a degenerated disk until the intervertebral region stabilizes. Spinal fusion is probably indicated if the patient has a defect such as spondylolisthesis. Recently proteolytic enzymes have been injected into intervertebral disks for treatment of acute disk symptoms.

Spinal stenosis, a narrow spinal canal, results from disk degeneration, osteophytes, or spondylolisthesis. In addition to the other symptoms of disk degeneration, this produces pain and paresthesias in the legs during walking (neurogenic claudication). Decompression of the spinal canal and foramina may be necessary.

Coccygodynia

Women develop a painful tailbone more often than men do. Some give a history of an acute injury to the coccyx. In others trauma seems to play no role. Sitting and motion of the coccyx increase the pain. The physician must rule out psychoneurosis, spine disease (bone tumors), and spinal cord and nerve lesions with pain referred to the coccyx. Rectal examination is mandatory. X-ray examination helps rule out bone lesions. Rest and heat often relieve acute coccygodynia. The patient is instructed to sit on a soft pillow or ring. Excision of the coccyx is rarely warranted since most patients continue to have pain despite surgery.

Hip (Table 33-6)
Congenital Dislocation

The physician must diagnose congenital dislocation of the hip soon after an infant is born. If the physician does not, he or she often commits the child to a life of disability. Hip joint capsule relaxation and acetabular dysplasia of unknown cause produce congenital dislocation of the hip. Girls are affected seven times more often than boys are. The disorder is at times familial. The doctor should warn parents of an affected child to have all subsequent children examined carefully. The degree of involvement varies from mild dysplasia (shallow acetabulum) to complete dislocation. In some babies the hip is dislocated before birth. In others the femoral head slips out of the acetabulum after birth. For clinical purposes, the disorder is classified as a dysplastic hip, subluxation, or dislocation.

The doctor examining a newborn must look for signs of hip dislocation. The most common reliable sign is a slight jerk and snap as the femoral head slides

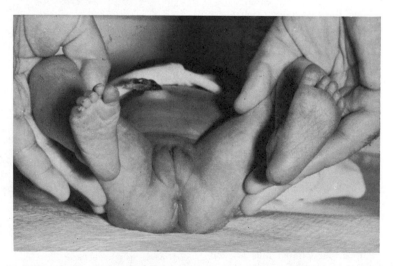

Fig. 33-7. Ortolani's test for congenital dislocation of hip. Examiner's thumb pushes posteriorly on baby's knee while examiner's fingers lift greater trochanter anteriorly and push medially to snap femoral head into acetabulum.

in and out of the acetabulum (Ortolani's sign). This is produced when the thighs, in flexion and slight abduction, are alternately pushed posteriorly and pulled anteriorly (Fig. 33-7). Other signs include limited abduction while the hip is flexed, posterior and lateral displacement of the greater trochanter, an extra fold or asymmetric gluteal folds, and telescoping (abnormal cephalocaudad motion of the femur with push and pull). If diagnosis and treatment are delayed until the child walks, she waddles. The involved leg is shorter. When the patient stands on the involved extremity, the pelvis drops toward the opposite side (positive Trendelenburg test).

Initial x-ray examination often reveals only lateral displacement of the proximal femur. Later films (Fig. 33-8) show a shallow, sloping acetabular roof, a laterally displaced proximal femur (if the acetabular region is divided into quadrants by a line passing through the triradiate cartilage of both acetabulums and a line dropped from the superior acetabular edge, the femoral head should lie in the lower inner quadrant), a delay in ossification of the femoral head, a break in Shenton's line (the normal continuous arch formed by a line drawn along the inferior border of the femoral neck and head and continued along the superior border of the obturator foramen), and an acetabular angle over 30 degrees (the acetabular angle is formed by one horizontal line that goes through the triradiate cartilages and another that goes from the superior acetabular edge to the triradiate cartilage on the involved side).

A child who remains undiagnosed has abnormal hip mechanics and develops early degenerative changes in the hip. To prevent crippling sequelae, the doctor must diagnose and treat congenital hip dislocation soon after birth. With the appropriate treatment, results are gratifying.

Treatment in the newborn depends on the degree of hip involvement. If the patient has a mild dysplastic hip, the mother should keep the child's legs abducted by pillows designed for this purpose. If the femoral head is well centered, a dysplastic acetabulum deepens and develops as the child grows. If the femoral head is subluxated or dislocated, the orthopedist can do a gentle, manipulative reduction after a few days of skin traction. Tight hip adductors might necessitate a subcutaneous adductor tenotomy. A plaster cast then holds the child's hips reduced. After this, the patient wears a brace to hold the hips in place. As the acetabulum deepens, the brace is gradually worn less, but it is worn at night for several years. If closed reduction is impossible, operative measures are needed. The doctor must follow a child with congenital dislocation during the growth years to be sure that the hip does not displace again.

Legg-Calvé-Perthes Disease (Coxa Plana)

Avascular necrosis of the femoral head of unknown cause is more common in boys 4 to 9 years of age than in girls. Biopsy of the epiphyseal plate shows derangement of chondrocytes and clefts in the cartilage. These probably interfere with blood vessels passing through the periphery of the epiphyseal plate and supplying the femoral head.

The child first complains of mild pain in the medial aspect of the knee and thigh or in the anterior part of

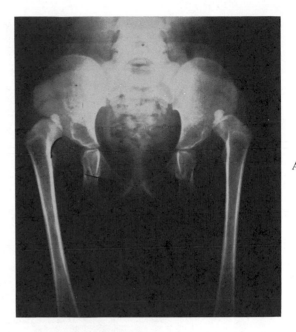

A

Fig. 33-8. Bilateral congenital dislocation of hips. **A,** Notice shallow, sloping acetabular roofs, superior lateral displacement of femoral heads, and broken Shenton's line.

Continued.

the hip. The parents notice a limp. On examination, the physician finds limited motion of the child's hip. Abduction and internal rotation decrease greatly. The child complains of tenderness and pain on motion. Muscle spasm is frequently severe. In early stages of the disorder radiographic examination shows a distended joint capsule and slight flattening of the femoral head. Later the femoral metaphysis widens, and the epiphyseal plate becomes irregular. The necrotic portion of the femoral head is radiopaque as compared to surrounding bone that has undergone disuse atrophy (Fig. 33-9). If the child bears weight, the femoral head collapses, widens, and leads to joint incongruity that can produce degenerative joint disease.

Treatment does not always restore a normal hip joint. Early treatment includes rest or traction with the thighs in abduction to relieve the pain of muscle spasm and acute synovitis and to center the femoral head in the acetabulum. The child walks with crutches or a brace to limit weight bearing on the involved extremity until the new bone replaces necrotic bone. After this, the child gradually increases the amount of weight bearing. A differential diagnosis in Legg-Calvé-Perthes disease should include tuberculosis, rheumatoid arthritis, and idiopathic synovitis.

Synovitis

Occasionally children complain of hip or knee pain and limp to protect the involved extremity. The history is noncontributory. Hip motion decreases. The child holds the hip flexed, externally rotated, and abducted. Pressure over the hip anteriorly produces discomfort. The doctor must do laboratory and radiographic studies to rule out pyogenic arthritis, osteomyelitis, and rheumatoid arthritis. By exclusion, he or she diagnoses idiopathic synovitis, treats the child by rest with traction,

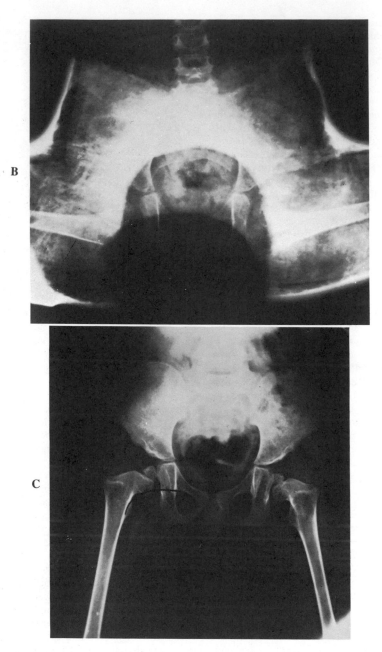

Fig. 33-8, cont'd. B, Roentgenogram through plaster after traction, adductor tenotomy, and closed reduction. **C,** Roentgenogram 8 months later. Femoral heads are centered in acetabulum, and Shenton's line is unbroken.

bed, or crutches, and follows the patient at frequent intervals. If, in fact, the child has idiopathic synovitis, he or she improves in 2 or 3 weeks and has no residual difficulty.

Slipped Capital Femoral Epiphysis

Slipping of the capital femoral epiphysis is usually a gradually progressive displacement of the femoral neck anteriorly and superiorly in relation to the femoral head. The cause is unknown, but the disorder involves epiphyseal plate cells. The changes in the cartilage cells of the plate are similar to those in Legg-Calvé-Perthes disease. Slipped epiphysis develops be-

tween 10 and 16 years of age. The patient complains of discomfort in the knee, thigh, or hip. Discomfort, though mild and intermittent at first, usually persists and becomes more pronounced. The parents notice that the child limps. Slipped epiphysis commonly affects one of two types of childrern. The child is either overweight and physically and sexually immature, or he is tall and thin. In the latter instance he has recently grown rapidly.

The patient holds the involved hip externally rotated and adducted. He or she complains of pain on motion and limits internal rotation and abduction as compared to the normal side. Characteristically the leg goes into

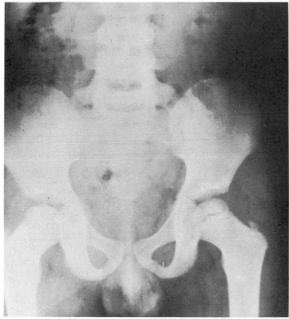

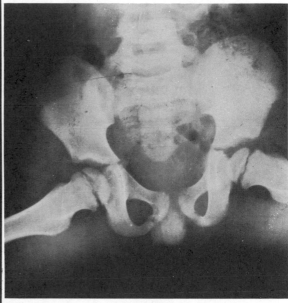

A

B

Fig. 33-9. Legg-Calvé-Perthes disease. **A** and **B,** Anteroposterior and lateral roentgenograms a few weeks after child limped and complained of mild right hip discomfort; right femoral head is somewhat irregular and smaller than left. *Continued.*

Table 33-7. Disorders of the Knee

Age	Disorder	Cause
Birth to 2 years	Bowlegs (genu varum)	Developmental or metabolic
	Knock-knees (genu valgum)	Developmental
	Congenital pseudarthrosis of the tibia	Developmental (?)
8-14 years	Osgood-Schlatter disease	Traumatic (?)
	Recurrent dislocation of the patella	Developmental
	Osteochondritis dissecans	Traumatic (?)
Adult	Baker's cyst (popliteal cyst)	Developmental or inflammatory
	Bursitis	Bursal inflammation
	Chondromalacia	Degenerative(?)

external rotation on flexion of the hip with the knee flexed. Often anteroposterior radiographic studies show slight widening of the epiphyseal plate and metaphysis, but lateral views reveal anterior displacement of the femoral neck (Fig. 33-10). This varies from minimal displacement to complete separation of the femoral head from the femoral neck.

To prevent further displacement and serious hip disability, the child should bear no weight. A patient with a mild displacement should have the epiphysis fixed to the femoral neck by means of threaded pins. He or she then uses crutches until the femoral head unites by bone to the femoral neck. In a person with pronounced displacement, the physician applies skin or skeletal traction to the limb over a period of several days to ab-

duct and internally rotate the leg in a manner that reduces displacement to the point where the head can be fixed to the femoral neck by pins. Vigorous manipulative reduction damages the blood supply to the femoral head and produces aseptic necrosis.

A few children with slipped capital femoral epiphysis develop one of the following complications: acute arthritis of the hip, chondrolysis, residual joint incongruity, or aseptic necrosis. These can produce a degenerative joint that later needs reconstructive surgery.

Snapping Hip

Flexion, abduction, or internal rotation of the hip produces an audible, palpable, or visible snap located over the greater trochanter of the femur. A thickened band of fascia snaps over the trochanter. Differential diagnosis includes loose bodies in the hip or subluxation. In case of a fascial band, pain is usually not severe enough to warrant treatment. Rest and antiinflammatory drugs may give relief.

Knee (Table 33-7)
Bowlegs (Genu Varum)

Bowlegs are most often a variation of normal, but the doctor must be sure that the child does not have rickets or an epiphyseal plate disorder.

Most newborns have bowlegs. This physiologic bowing persists for several years, but the majority correct spontaneously with growth. A few severe and persistent bowlegs need treatment with a long-leg brace designed to apply pressure laterally at the knee and medially over the thigh and lower leg. Even fewer persist to the point of needing osteotomy to correct the bowing.

In this country bowlegs caused by vitamin D–

Text continued on p. 333.

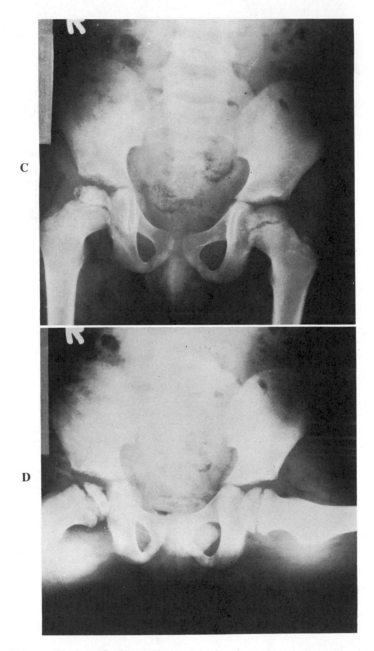

Fig. 33-9, cont'd. C and **D,** Six months later, the flat, dense, necrotic femoral head is obvious.

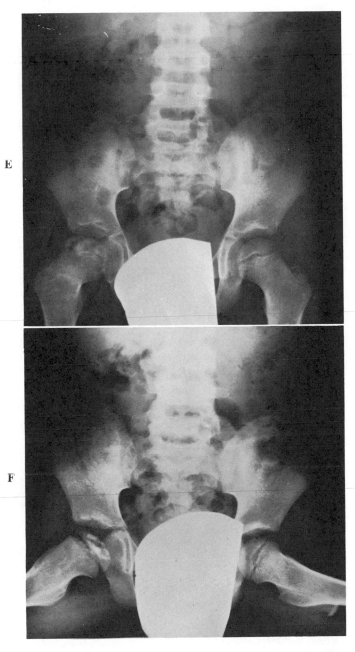

Fig. 33-9, cont'd. E and **F,** In another 6 months, new bone is replacing dense, dead bone; femoral head is still flat, and metaphysis is wide.   *Continued.*

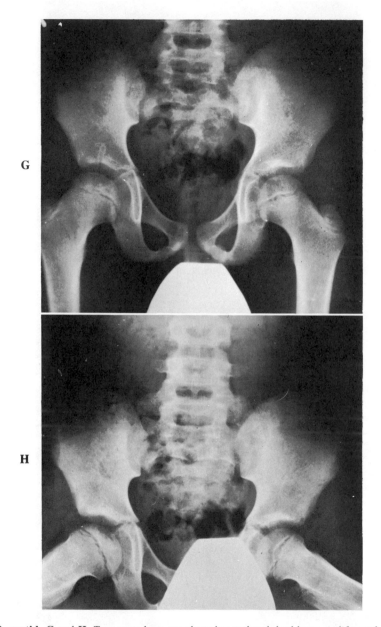

Fig. 33-9, cont'd. G and **H,** Two years later, new bone has replaced dead bone, and femoral head has only mild residual flattening.

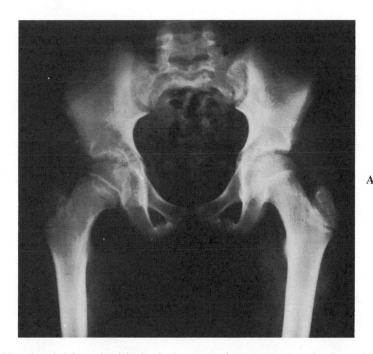

Fig. 33-10. Slipped capital femoral epiphysis. **A,** Anteroposterior roentgenogram showing early slip of right femoral epiphysis; epiphyseal plate is widened, and femoral neck is displaced superiorly and anteriorly in relation to femoral head. *Continued.*

deficient rickets are infrequent. An occasional patient with vitamin D–resistant rickets may develop bowlegs. Radiographs of a child with rickets show the widened epiphyseal plate and metaphysis wherein cartilage and bone matrix are produced but fail to mineralize. The physician must treat the primary disorder. Some of these children need osteotomies to straighten the legs.

Tibia vara (Blount's disease) produces bowlegs by delay in growth and irregular development of the medial and posterior portion of the epiphyseal plate of the proximal tibia. The deformity increases until the epiphyseal plate disturbance subsides. A child with severe deformity needs tibial osteotomy.

Knock-Knees (Genu Valgum)

Knock-knees are usually a variation of normal. Probably because of their wider pelvis, girls have knock-knees more frequently than boys do. Most children need no treatment. The legs straighten as the child grows. The physician must rule out an underlying bone disorder. A few children with severe knock-knees need a long-leg brace or an osteotomy.

Congenital Pseudarthrosis of the Tibia

The term *congenital pseudarthrosis* is a misnomer for this rare condition of unknown cause. Most children who develop this disorder are born with an intact tibia that is thin at the junction of its middle and distal thirds and bowed anteriorly (Fig. 33-11). Some of the children have manifestations of neurofibromatosis. The bone breaks soon after birth and resists healing. Surgeons have used numerous operative procedures, most with bone grafts, to try to obtain union of these defects.

Often pseudarthrosis remains and the leg is short and must be amputated. Recently, treatment with electric current shows some promise in obtaining union.

Osgood-Schlatter Disease

In Osgood-Schlatter disease, common in boys 10 to 15 years of age, the tibial tubercle becomes fragmented. The patient complains of a tender bump and has pain if he kneels or jumps. On examination, the physician finds a swollen, hard, tender tibial tubercle. Extension of the knee against resistance produces pain. Radiographs show a dense fragmented portion of bone separated from the underlying tibia (Fig. 33-12). This process is similar to "osteochondritis" in other areas. In most cases the fragment ossifies normally and complaints subside. The child should limit activity during the acute painful stage to relieve strain on the tibial tubercle. A cylinder cast alleviates severe pain. The child resumes activity as symptoms subside. In a few children the fragment does not heal, and a small separate dense piece of bone remains surrounded by fibrous connective tissue or a bursa, or both. These may remain symptomatic and necessitate removal of the fragment.

Recurrent Dislocation of the Patella

Recurrent dislocation of the patella is more likely to occur in girls 8 to 16 years of age than in boys. One or more of the following predisposing developmental defects cause this disorder: high-riding patella, knock-knees, flattened lateral femoral condyle, and lax medial patellar retinaculum. The patient reports that the leg gave way during vigorous physical activity while the knee was flexed. This produced severe knee pain, and the knee locked in flexion. Some astute observers tell

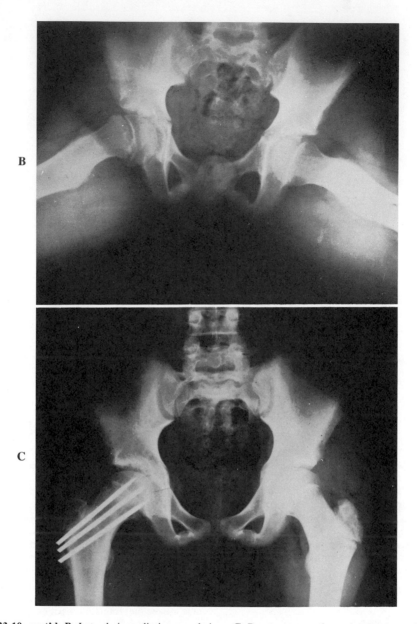

Fig. 33-10, cont'd. B, Lateral view; slip is more obvious. **C,** Roentgenogram 6 months after internal fixation.

the doctor that the kneecap slid to the outside of the knee, and the knee was swollen and tender for a week or so. Young girls with such a history often have subsequent episodes of subluxation wherein the kneecap slides over and back without locking in complete dislocation.

On examination, the physician often finds the patella higher than it should be, and it does not lock against the femur as it normally should when the knee is flexed 30 degrees. Radiographs often show no abnormalities, but they might disclose a high-riding patella, valgus knees, or an underdeveloped lateral femoral condyle. At times they show a chip fracture of the lateral femoral condyle produced by the patella sliding over it. A patient who has repeated episodes of patellar dislocation usually wants treatment. The older the pa-

tient, the smaller the likelihood of subsequent dislocation. The physician might advise girls 16 to 18 to wait and see if the frequency of dislocation decreases. In other instances he or she will advise surgical repair. The orthopedic surgeon reconstructs the extensor apparatus by transferring the patellar tendon insertion distally and medially on the tibia, reefing the medial patellar retinaculum, or releasing the lateral retinaculum, or all three. In some patients who have had multiple dislocations, patellar cartilage degenerates. In such cases the orthopedist might remove the patella and transfer the extensor apparatus to prevent it from dislocating.

Osteochondritis Dissecans

In osteochondritis dissecans of the distal femur an osteochondral fragment, usually on the lateral surface

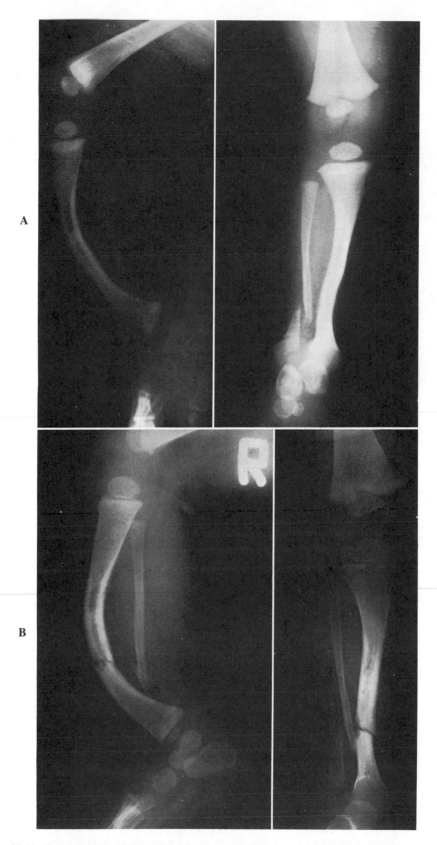

Fig. 33-11. Congenital "pseudarthrosis" of tibia. **A,** Lateral and anteroposterior roentgenograms soon after birth show anterior bowing of tibia and fractured fibula. **B,** Five months later tibia has broken.

of the medial femoral condyle, loses its blood supply and separates from the rest of the femur. No one knows the cause. The fragment can revascularize and be replaced by new bone but frequently detaches and becomes a "joint mouse." If the fragment is not detached, the patient usually complains of vague knee pain and

swelling made worse by activity. If the fragment becomes a loose body, the knee frequently locks and gives way. At times the patient feels loose bodies sliding about in the joint.

Radiographs show the fracture line with the overlying dense bone, if the fragment does, in fact, contain much bone (Fig. 33-13). Radiographs show a free fragment only if it contains bone or mineralized cartilage. The defect on the femoral condyle is often visible.

If the physician sees a patient with an intact fragment, he should advise no weight bearing and observe to see if the fragment revascularizes. If a free body produces symptoms, it should be removed.

Baker's Cyst (Popliteal Cyst)

Baker's cyst is not unusual in children. The cysts result from enlargement of the semimembranous bursa or the bursa beneath the medial head of the gastrocnemius muscle. Herniation of knee joint synovium through the posterior capsule of the knee also produces popliteal cysts. Symptoms consist in dull aching, swelling that fluctuates in size, and at times, constant pain. If the patient has severe symptoms, the surgeon can excise the bursa and close any defect in the posterior knee capsule.

Bursitis

Bursas, synovium-lined sacs located between tendons, muscles, and fascia in gliding areas, reduce friction. Adventitious bursas are produced by constant friction or repeated trauma. There are many bursas about the knee. They can be acutely or chronically inflamed, infected, or involved by a systemic disorder such as rheumatoid disease or gout. Pain is the most prominent symptom, and swelling and tenderness are the prominent signs. Treatment depends on the underlying cause.

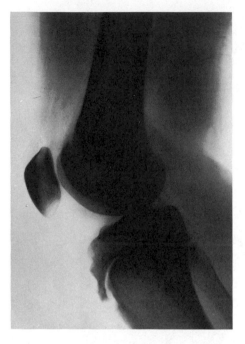

Fig. 33-12. Osgood-Schlatter disease. Tibial tubercle is irregular and fragmented. Small, dense piece of bone remains ununited.

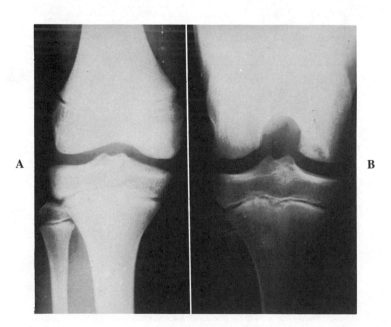

Fig. 33-13. Osteochondritis dissecans. **A,** Routine anteroposterior roentgenogram does not outline defect well. **B,** Anteroposterior roentgenogram with knee flexed shows fragment in its most common location of lateral surface of medial femoral condyle.

Any systemic disorder must be treated. Locally, trauma and irritants should be eliminated. Rest, hot packs, elevation, and compression help relieve symptoms. In noninfected cases bursas can be aspirated. To avoid infection, the physician must use extreme care. If aspiration is to be done, the skin must be prepared as for an open operation. One should not inject directly through the skin over the bursa; rather, the needle should start at a distance from the bursa in normal skin and subcutaneous tissue and enter the bursa from its deep surface. In this way infection is less likely to be introduced. Incision and drainage and antibiotics usually cure an acutely infected bursa. Excision of a chronically infected bursa might be necessary.

Chondromalacia

Chondromalacia, of unknown cause, consists of softening, yellow discoloration, fraying, and degeneration of the articular surface of the kneecap. Women 14 to 28 years of age frequently acquire chondromalacia. They complain of knee discomfort that is mild at first but later is severe. Activities such as stair climbing that produce forcible knee flexion increase the pain. The joint swells, and patellar compression produces pain and crepitus. Joint fluid increases, and patellar margins become tender. Radiographs often show no abnormalities. Straight leg-raising exercises to increase quadriceps strength and avoidance of strenuous activities that aggravate symptoms usually relieve discomfort. In some patients conservative treatment does not control symptoms. In these instances the surgeon might explore the knee joint and either skive (pare) the diseased cartilage or remove the patella. Arthroscopy might be used to carry out treatment.

Foot (Table 33-8)

Clubfoot

Congenital defects or neurologic disorders (myelodysplasia, cerebral palsy) produce clubfoot. The name of the most frequent congenital variety, talipes equinovarus, describes the position of the foot. The heel cord is tight, the ankle (talipes) is in plantar flexion (equinus), and the foot is inverted (varus, Fig. 33-14). The forefoot is adducted. Talipes equinovarus affects boys much more frequently than it does girls. In most instances no one knows the cause of clubfoot. The heel cord and the structures on the medial side of the foot contract. This pulls the calcaneus into plantar flexion, the navicular medial to the talus, and the cuboid medial to the os calcis. Children do not outgrow talipes equinovarus, and in fact the older they get, the more the foot bones become deformed. The orthopedist must institute treatment soon after birth while contracted soft tissues are more easily stretched. Long-leg casts are changed at 5- to 7-day intervals. Each cast produces a corrective force that slides the foot beneath the talus, thereby correcting forefoot adduction and inversion. The casts extend above the knee to prevent rotation of the cast. Some of the deformity corrects with each cast until the foot overcorrects except for the equinus. At this stage, subcutaneous section of the heel cord (Achilles tendon) corrects equinus immediately. After this, the child wears a cast in a corrected position for 5 weeks while the tendon heals. (Some physicians use

Table 33-8. Disorders of the Foot

Age	Disorder	Cause
Birth to 2 years	Clubfoot	Developmental
	Metatarsus adductus (metatarsus varus)	Developmental
	Calcaneovalgus	Developmental
	Congenital bands (constriction rings)	Developmental
	Toeing in	Developmental
	Toeing out	Developmental
	Flatfoot (pes planus)	Developmental
2-4 years	Köhler's disease	Osteochondritis
8-14 years	Sever's disease	Osteochondritis
	Freiberg's disease	Osteochondritis
Adult	Bunions (hallux valgus)	Developmental (?)
	Hallux rigidus	Arthritis (?), developmental (?)
	Metatarsalgia	?
	Corns	Traumatic
	Heel spur	Traumatic (?)
	Ingrown toenail	Traumatic (?)
	Digital neuroma (Morton's neuroma)	Traumatic (?), developmental
	Cockup toes and hammer toes	Congenital, neuromuscular, arthritic

casts to correct the equinus. Extreme caution is needed to avoid pressing up beneath the forefoot while the heel cord holds the os calcis in equinus. Such pressure "breaks" the foot and produces a rocker-bottom foot.) After correction of deformity, the infant should use night splints to hold the feet corrected until 5 to 7 years of age. Such treatment instituted soon after birth produces satisfactory results in 90% of cases. However, the foot tends to redeform until maturity. The doctor must stress this point to parents. Frequently, resistant, neglected, or recurrent clubfoot require surgery of soft tissues or bones of the foot. Such surgery may leave the foot more rigid than normal.

Metatarsus Adductus (Metatarsus Varus)

In the congenital disorder metatarsus adductus, the child's forefoot adducts (Fig. 33-15). On examination, the doctor might be able to passively correct the forefoot to neutral. If so, he or she advises the parents to hold the child's heel fixed in one hand and stretch the forefoot into a corrected position several times daily. If the infant is walking, he might also wear straight-last shoes. If the child's foot is too rigid to correct to neutral, a series of casts will produce gradual correction. This should be done between 3 and 6 months of age. The child wears straight-last shoes to keep the feet out of a deformed position.

Calcaneovalgus

Occasionally newborn babies' feet dorsiflex in front of the tibia and evert (valgus). In contrast to talipes equinovarus, these feet improve with time and need only gentle daily stretching. Calcaneovalgus must be differentiated from vertical talus, a rare disorder in which the foot is rigid and must be corrected surgically.

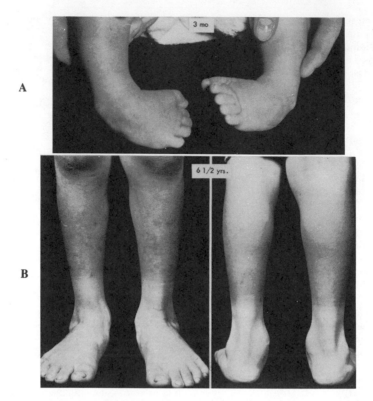

Fig. 33-14. Congenital talipes equinovarus. **A,** Feet at beginning of treatment when child was 3 months old. **B,** Feet at age 6½ after treatment with corrective casts and night splints.

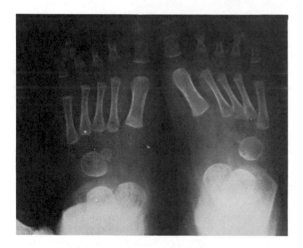

Fig. 33-15. Metatarsus adductus. Roentgenogram shows adduction of right forefoot.

Congenital Bands (Constriction Rings)

Tight fibrous connective tissue bands that surround a digit or extremity involve the skin and subcutaneous tissues and constrict underlying muscle and vessels (Fig. 33-16). Occasionally edema and vascular insufficiency distal to the band produce gangrene. These bands, once believed to be amniotic remnants, probably represent developmental defects. Frequently, the patient has associated congenital anomalies (syndactyly and polydactyly). The surgeon should excise the bands by multiple Z-plasties several weeks apart to avoid interruption of circulation to the extremities. Z-plasties prevent circumferential scarring with subsequent recontracture (see Chap. 40).

Toeing In

Parents frequently bring pigeon-toed children to the doctor. Usually toeing in results from one of three disorders: metatarsus adductus, internal tibial torsion, or medial femoral torsion or femoral neck anteversion. The physician often obtains a clue as to which of these is present by observing the child walk. He or she diagnoses metatarsus adductus when the forefoot adducts in relation to the hindfoot. If the child has no foot deformity and the kneecaps point straight ahead during gait, the problem is probably internal tibial torsion. Normally, the lateral malleolus is 15 to 20 degrees posterior to the medial malleolus. In internal tibial torsion this angle may decrease or reverse. If, on the other hand, the kneecaps point medially when the child walks, femoral torsion or anteversion of the femoral neck is likely. Sitting and sleeping with the feet turned in aggravates tibial and femoral torsion. As the child grows and sitting and sleeping positions change, femoral and tibial torsion usually correct. Although thousands of dollars are spent each year on shoe corrections, they probably do not influence toeing-in caused by bone torsion. The physician should follow the patient, and if the disorder is not correcting, the child should wear a night splint to hold the feet externally ro-

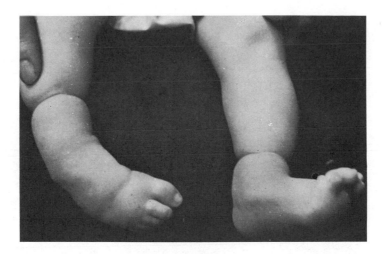

Fig. 33-16. Congenital bands (constriction rings) of both legs.
From Kenney, W.E., and Larson, C.B.: Orthopedics for general practitioner, St. Louis, 1957, The C.V. Mosby Co., p.27.)

tated. This splint consists of a metal bar fixed to the shoe soles in a manner that holds them rotated to the desired position. A few persons with severe residual torsion need corrective rotational osteotomy.

Toeing Out

Toeing out, too, is produced by intrinsic foot deformity, external tibial torsion, or external femoral torsion. A child just learning to walk frequently toes out to obtain a wider base for balance. External femoral or tibial torsion tends to correct with growth.

Flatfoot (Pes Planus)

The physician should exercise caution in diagnosing flatfoot in a child under 2 or 3 years of age. Before this age a fat pad in the foot obscures any arch that might be present. Flatfeet in children are either flexible or rigid. In the common, flexible type the arch flattens and heel goes into valgus during weight bearing. These correct when body weight is removed. These feet are not painful in childhood, and most of them correct as the child gets older and foot ligaments tighten. Even if a flexible flatfoot does not correct, the child has no functional handicap. Shoe corrections probably do nothing to help these feet. Medial heel wedges and arch pads keep shoes from running over and wearing out rapidly. These inexpensive corrections save the parents the cost of buying new shoes at frequent intervals.

Bone defects such as congenital fusion of tarsal bones (tarsal coalition) produce most rigid flatfeet. These feet are not passively correctable. If the child has foot and leg pain, an orthopedic surgeon should be consulted. Surgery might be necessary to relieve pain and deformity.

Köhler's Disease

Aseptic necrosis of the tarsal scaphoid usually affects children 6 to 11 years of age. Activity accentuates foot pain and rest relieves it. The physician finds tenderness in the medial side of the foot arch. Radiographic studies show a dense, narrow scaphoid. Limit-

ing the child's activity controls discomfort. Osteochondritis is self-limiting, and the scaphoid usually revascularizes.

Sever's Disease

A child 7 to 12 years of age with fragmented ossification of the os calcis apophysis complains of pain over the posterior aspect of the heel. The doctor finds tenderness in this area. Radiographs show a dense fragmented os calcis apophysis. Shoes that raise the heel and relieve pressure over the tender area and limitation of activity decrease symptoms. The disease is self-limiting.

Freiberg's Disease

Osteochondritis of the second metatarsal head affects girls 10 to 15 years of age more often than it does boys. Symptomatic treatment is instituted until the area revascularizes. Occasionally the articular surface of the metatarsophalangeal joint collapses, and pain continues. In such an instance excision of the metatarsal head or arthroplasty might be necessary.

Bunions (Hallux Valgus)

A painful bunion results when the great toe deviates laterally at the metatarsophalangeal joint (hallux valgus), the head of the first metatarsal bone becomes prominent medially, and a callus or bursa, or both, develop over the metatarsal head (Fig. 33-17). Congenital adduction of the first metatarsal bone or lax ligaments produce deviation of the great toe. Perhaps aggravated by some of the ridiculous shoes they tolerate, women develop bunions much more often than men. Some bunions produce slight discomfort. In such an instance shoes fitted to relieve pressure or cut out over the bunion relieve pain. The patient with severe pain often needs surgical correction including arthroplasty to remove overgrowth on the metatarsal head, decompression of the metatarsophalangeal joint, and correction of angulation between the great toe and first metatarsal bone.

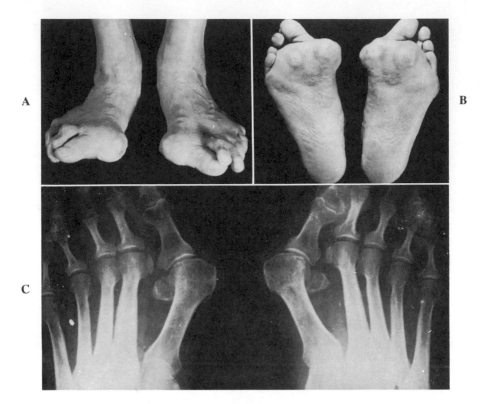

Fig. 33-17. Bunions. **A,** Dorsal view, showing lateral deviation (hallux valgus) of great toe and overlapping second toes. **B,** Plantar views showing callosities beneath prominent metatarsal heads. **C,** Roentgenogram showing bilateral hallux valgus.

Hallux Rigidus

In hallux rigidus the great toe fails to dorsiflex normally at the metatarsophalangeal joint. A bunion of long duration or any process that destroys the metatarsophalangeal joint can cause hallux rigidus. The patient who lacks dorsiflexion at the first metatarsophalangeal joint develops pain and walks in a protective manner to relieve this pain. Surgical treatment is by resection of the bunion and decompression of the metatarsophalangeal joint by removal of the proximal half of the proximal phalanx of the great toe.

Metatarsalgia

Pain beneath metatarsal heads is common. Weight bearing increases pain. Painful calluses develop over a prominent metatarsal head. Proper shoes and a pad in the shoes decrease pain. The pad must support weight in the region posterior to the metatarsal heads. Removal of a prominent metatarsal head beneath a persistent callus might be necessary.

Corns

Pressure on the skin against an underlying bony prominence produces corns that frequently become exquisitely painful. Treatment consists in the use of proper shoes, pads and cutouts to relieve pressure, and gentle trimming of the superficial dead skin. If conservative measures fail, the underlying bony spike can be removed.

Heel Spur

A heel spur per se is not a disease but is a manifestation of bone repair reaction at the site of degeneration of the plantar ligaments near the os calcis. The patient may give a history of a recent change from one type of shoe to another or of walking a long distance. The doctor should treat the heel spur with a pad cutout to relieve pressure. This disorder tends to repair itself after several months. In general, excision of the spur does not hasten repair time.

Ingrown Toenail

An abnormal shape of the great toenail, an infected area along the toenail, pressure from tight shoes or socks, and trimming the nail too close at its corners all contribute to ingrown toenail. The patient develops intermittent acute inflammation of soft tissues at the medial side of the great toenail (Fig. 33-18). During the acute stage, warm soaks, elevation, and antibiotics help control infection. After the acute episode, the patient should let the nail grow out, trim it straight across and not back at the corners, and avoid shoes and socks that cause pressure on the toe. At times elevating the nail edge and packing sterile cotton beneath it help the nail to grow out. If a deformed nail causes continued symptoms, the patient might want surgical treatment. The surgeon can remove the medial one third of the nail, curet the nail base, and suture the skin beneath the nail bed to close the defect and create a new nail groove. If

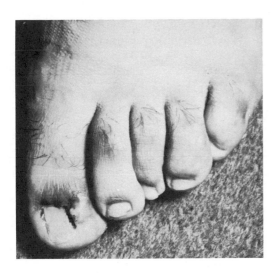

Fig. 33-18. Ingrown toenail. Soft tissues at lateral edge of great toenail are hypertrophied and infected.

this fails, he can remove the entire nail, nail bed, and distal portion of the phalanx.

Digital Neuroma (Morton's Neuroma)

The patient, usually a woman, with a neuroma of the common digital nerve to the contiguous sides of the third and fourth toe gives a classic history of episodes of severe, sharp, knifelike pain and paresthesias radiating into the adjacent sides of two toes. She removes the shoe and rubs the foot to relieve discomfort. Metatarsal pads may relieve pressure. If symptoms are severe enough, surgical excision of the neuroma may be necessary.

Cock-up Toes and Hammer Toes

Cock-up toes hyperextend at the metatarsophalangeal joints and flex at the proximal interphalangeal joints. A variety of disorders (congenital, neuromuscular, arthritic) cause them. Any muscle imbalance that produces relatively strong extrinsic toe extensors and weak intrinsic toe extensors might produce cock-up toes. These toes correct passively in contrast to hammer toes, which are fixed in their deformed position. Painful callosities develop over the proximal interphalangeal joints of hammer toes or cock-up toes. During the flexible stage, deformity is corrected when the muscle balance is restored through the use of intrinsoplasties—the restoration of intrinsic muscle function by transplantation of the extrinsic toe flexors into the extensor hood. If deformities are fixed, excision or fusion of the proximal interphalangeal joint relieves symptoms.

INFECTION

In osteomyelitis, an infection of bone, offending organisms migrate through the bloodstream from a remote soft-tissue infection to the bone (acute hematogenous osteomyelitis) or they invade bone directly through an open wound or extend from an adjacent infection. Pyogenic bacteria induce the majority of bone infections. *Mycobacterium tuberculosis, Treponema pallidum,* and fungi infect bone infrequently.

Acute Hematogenous Osteomyelitis

Acute hematogenous osteomyelitis is one of the few orthopedic emergencies. Bacteria invade the bloodstream from a boil, cellulitis, a sore throat, or a similar site. They travel to bone and lodge in the metaphysis where the bone blood flow is greatest but where the *rate* of flow is slow and capillaries are open. The bacteria provoke an inflammatory reaction, suppuration, bone erosion, and bone death. A piece of dead bone surrounded by pus or infected granulation tissue is a *sequestrum*. If phagocytosis, body defense mechanisms, and antibiotics do not destroy the bacteria, the abscess takes one or more of the following routes:

1. Pus extends into the medullary cavity of the bone, and its pressure compromises the blood flow in nutrient vessels that enter the endosteal surface of the cortex and supply its inner half to two thirds. Much of the bone shaft becomes sequestrated.
2. The abscess perforates the cortex, dissects beneath the periosteum, strips it from the bone, destroys the periosteal blood supply, and sequestrates the outer third of the cortex. Subperiosteal and endosteal new bone form around the sequestrums. This new bone is an *involucrum*. If the infection subsides, granulation tissue erodes the sequestrums and replaces them with new bone.
3. The infection perforates the periosteum and forms a soft tissue abscess.
4. Pus enters the adjacent joint, especially if the metaphysis is intracapsular as in the hip.
5. Although the epiphyseal plate acts as a barrier to infection, granulation tissue occasionally destroys it and alters growth.

Occasionally bacteria reenter the bloodstream, perpetuate septicemia, and establish metastatic foci in other sites including bone.

Acute hematogenous osteomyelitis usually affects children, boys more than girls, and most commonly attacks the upper tibia or the distal femur. The most common offending organism varies somewhat with the patient's age. In the child under 1 month of age, a gram-negative rod enters the bloodstream from an infected umbilicus and produces osteomyelitis. In the infant *Streptococcus* is common, but in the older child and adult *Staphylococcus* causes most bone infections.

In most instances the child has an infected cut, a boil, or a sore throat; 2 to 10 days later, he or she suddenly develops bone pain and loses function of the involved part. Generalized symptoms vary with the severity of the septicemia. If the organism is of low virulence or antibiotics have been used, the temperature often increases only slightly. At times, antibiotics suppress clinical symptoms while underlying bone destruction continues. In an infant with severe septicemia the temperature frequently rises to 104° or 105° F. The child is warm, dry, restless, and sometimes develops toxic myocarditis and pericarditis.

On examination, the physician finds heat, redness, and well-localized tenderness. By using a small object such as a pencil eraser to press on various parts of the bone, one can demonstrate circumscribed point tenderness in the infected portion of the bone. A fluctuant mass indicates subperiosteal or soft-tissue abscess. If the infection involves only bone, the child moves adjacent joints slowly without pain. Usually the sedimentation rate and white cell count rise, and the differential count shifts to the left. During septicemia, offending organisms can be grown from a blood culture.

The doctor *must* make the diagnosis clinically because during the first several days radiographic studies show nothing but soft tissue swelling. Only after 8 to 10 days do radiographs disclose periosteal new bone (Fig. 33-19). To avoid disastrous sequelae, the physician *must make the diagnosis before this,* while the infection remains confined in metaphyseal bone. The orthopedist should treat the child with acute hematogenous osteomyelitis by general supportive measures correct dehydration, restore an adequate hemoglobin level, start antibiotics, surgically drain bone abscesses, culture the pus, obtain sensitivities, and institute appropriate antibiotic treatment. The patient improves dramatically within a few hours. Postoperatively, rest with a cast or plaster splint prevents pathologic fracture until new bone replaces dead bone and areas of bone destruction. The patient takes antibiotics for 4 to 6 weeks after all symptoms and signs have disappeared. With this treatment, the child has the best chance to control the infection and avoid chronic osteomyelitis.

Chronic Osteomyelitis

Chronic osteomyelitis is difficult to cure. It follows one of several courses. Some patients develop intermittent acute exacerbations. In some the infection remains dormant only to flare up years later, whereas in others draining sinuses persist. After years of drainage, a few of these patients develop epidermoid carcinoma in sinus tracts.

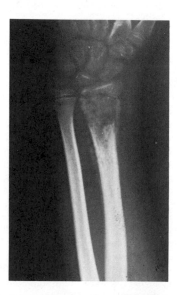

Fig. 33-19. Acute hematogenous osteomyelitis of radius 3 weeks after onset of symptoms. Infection has destroyed metaphyseal bone. Periosteal new bone is forming.

Unresorbed sequestrums and unobliterated cavities surrounded by sclerotic bone perpetuate chronic infection (Fig. 33-20). Patients with acute exacerbations need appropriate antibiotics and drainage of abscesses. In those with chronic draining areas, surgeons remove underlying diseased bone, collapse cavities, and use appropriate antibiotics in an attempt to close wounds.

Osteomyelitis Associated With Open Wounds

Open-wound osteomyelitis usually localizes and gives fewer generalized symptoms than acute hematogenous osteomyelitis does. Surgeons can prevent most of it by thoroughly débriding wounds and using antibiotics if indicated. A patient with this type of infection needs drainage of abscesses, removal of diseased bone and dead tissues, and antibiotics.

Acute Pyogenic Arthritis

Bacteria enter a joint from underlying osteomyelitis, from an open wound, or directly from the bloodstream. Infected synovium and purulent joint exudate interfere with proper nutrition of articular cartilage by synovial fluid. This, and perhaps proteolytic enzymes, destroys cartilage in the weight-bearing area. The infection extends to subchondral bone. Capsular and intraarticular adhesions combined with incongruous joint surfaces limit joint motion.

The patient with acute pyogenic arthritis develops acute joint pain. The joint swells, and the part loses function. Often generalized symptoms of infection prevail. On examination, the doctor finds a swollen joint with excessive joint fluid. Joint motion triggers pain.

Radiographs reveal a distended capsular outline. After several days, the joint space narrows. If uncontrolled, infection destroys bone. In many instances, at 8 to 10 days a focus of osteomyelitis becomes evident.

The physician confirms the diagnosis by aspirating purulent synovial fluid and finding bacteria on microscopic examination. The patient should have general supportive measures, much the same as in acute hematogenous osteomyelitis, surgical drainage of the joint and underlying bone infection, and appropriate antibiotics. To avoid permanent joint damage, *treatment must be started at once.*

Acute idiopathic synovitis of children presents one of the most confusing differential diagnostic problems. The child holds the joint, usually the hip, immobile, complains of tenderness, and cries with pain on motion. Usually there are no generalized symptoms. The patient often gives no history of prior infection; joint fluid contains no bacteria; radiographs show no abnormalities; and the condition subsides spontaneously with rest.

Cellulitis overlying the metaphysis of a child must be considered osteomyelitis until proved otherwise. The patient with cellulitis has fewer generalized symptoms, less pain, and more diffuse tenderness than one with osteomyelitis.

Acute rheumatic processes often begin gradually. The patient gives no history of prior infection. He or she has fewer generalized symptoms and no bone tenderness. The process involves many joints. The white blood count and sedimentation rate rise less than in patients with osteomyelitis.

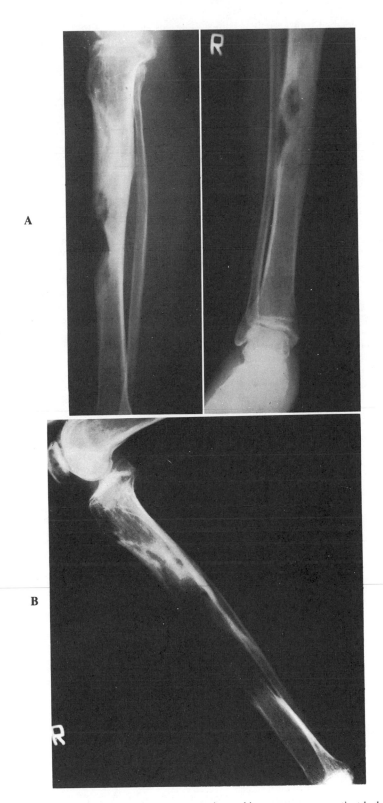

Fig. 33-20. Chronic osteomyelitis. **A,** Seventy years prior to this roentgenogram, patient had acute hematogenous osteomyelitis. Since then, recurrent chronic infection has drained intermittently. For 2 years, drainage had been continuous. Multiple lytic areas are surrounded by sclerotic bone. **B,** Eight months later, patient had increased drainage and pain and foul-smelling wound. Roentgenograms reveal extensive destruction from epidermoid carcinoma that developed in draining sinus.

At times neoplasm, especially Ewing's sarcoma, simulates an acute infection even to the extent of demonstrating heat and tenderness, generalized symptoms, fever, and sedimentation rate and white blood count elevation. X-ray studies usually reveal the bone involvement.

Tuberculosis

At times tuberculosis involves bone without entering a joint, but more often it infects both. The bacteria from a pulmonary lesion (less often from an enteric lesion) travel through the bloodstream to subarticular bone or synovium. Synovium proliferates with a tuberculous, granulomatous pannus that grows across and erodes beneath articular cartilage. The pannus from opposing joint surfaces bridges the joint with fibrous tissue that limits joint motion. Sometimes this ossifies and fuses the joint. The infection frequently destroys the joint capsule and forms a soft tissue abscess (cold abscess) of caseous material. This can penetrate skin and form sinuses that become secondarily infected with pyogenic organisms.

Bone tuberculosis often attacks the hip and spine of children. The patient notices gradual onset of pain, joint swelling, and loss of motion. Later, contractures ensue. Children with tuberculosis commonly perspire and cry at night. The temperature rises in the afternoon, and the white count increases. In early stages of the disease x-ray examination shows distension of capsular outlines and bone atrophy, especially of subchondral cortex. Later, marginal notching is visible. In advanced lesions bone and joint are destroyed.

Pulmonary tuberculosis and a positive skin test support the diagnosis. Isolation of bacteria by culture or guinea pig inoculation proves the diagnosis.

The doctor should treat the patient with general supportive measures, continue appropriate antituberculous drugs for 12 to 18 months, and immobilize the part by a cast, splint, or traction. When the patient is in good general condition, the orthopedist can excise localized lesions and attempt to restore function of the part, drain abscesses, excise advanced lesions, and fuse the involved joint.

TRAUMA
Fractures

A *fracture* is a break in continuity of bone or articular cartilage (Fig. 33-21).

Etiology

Fractures result from (1) a direct force at the site of fracture, or (2) an indirect force transmitted from a distance (e.g., fracture of the humerus from a fall on the outstretched hand).

Types

In *closed* fractures there is no communication between the external surface of the body and bone. In *open* fractures there is communication between the external surface of the body and bone through an open wound. A *pathological* fracture is usually produced by less force than that required to break a normal bone; the affected bone has been weakened by disease (infection, neoplasm, osteoporosis). In *avulsion* injuries a fragment of bone is pulled off by a ligament or tendon at its attachment. *Epiphyseal separation* is a break in the region of a child's epiphyseal plate (Fig. 33-22). Most involve subepiphyseal spongy bone, but some cross the epiphyseal plate or crush epiphyseal cells and result in subsequent growth disturbance (angulation or length discrepancy); (Fig. 33-23). In a *greenstick* fracture, one side of a child's bone "bends," and the other side breaks (Fig. 33-24). A *comminuted* fracture is one that has three or more fragments (Fig. 33-21).

Diagnosis

The physician should suspect a fracture in a patient who gives a history of injury and complains of pain, swelling, and loss of function. Displaced fragments

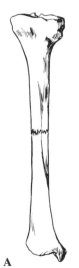 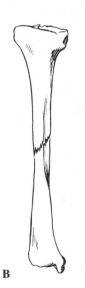 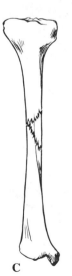 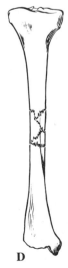

A   **B**   **C**   **D**

Fig. 33-21. Fracture configuration. **A,** Transverse. **B,** Oblique. **C,** Butterfly. **D,** Comminuted.

produce obvious deformity. Point tenderness at the fracture line is demonstrable, and gentle motion produces crepitus—one bone fragment grates on the other. Radiographic studies in at least two planes at right angles to each other are mandatory, and views of the opposite normal counterpart are valuable, especially in children where epiphyseal plates, nutrient arteries, and irregular ossification centers might be confused with a fracture.

Before treating a fracture, the physician must examine and record the neurovascular status of the extremity distal to the fracture plus *associated nerve, artery, ligament, or other soft tissue injuries.*

Treatment

By applying certain basic principles, the physician can treat the great majority of fractures satisfactorily, especially in children. Deviation from these principles frequently produces disastrous sequelae. Many fracture complications result from poorly indicated and improperly applied therapy, usually in the form of overtreatment with nuts, bolts, rods, and various pieces of hardware. Before treating a fracture, the physician must diagnose and treat associated injuries that threaten life and that demand priority (airway obstruction, hemorrhage, shock, perforated viscus).

Goals in treatment of fractures are to (1) prevent further damage, (2) gain satisfactory position of involved bones, (3) obtain union as rapidly as possible, (4) use the safest method, and (5) preserve or restore function of the involved part. Stages in fracture treatment are as follows.

First aid. Prevent further damage and relieve the patient's discomfort until institution of definitive therapy. The following two actions usually accomplish first aid of extremity injuries: Cover wounds with a pressure dressing of the cleanest bandage available to *prevent further contamination and control hemorrhage.* As a general rule, tourniquets are unnecessary and can be dangerous. *Immobilize the involved part* to relieve pain

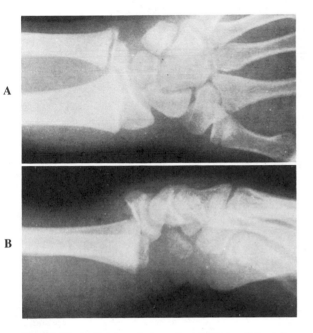

Fig. 33-22. A, Epiphyseal separation of distal radial epiphysis. Lateral view, **B,** shows triangular fragment of metaphysis that remained with dorsally displaced epiphysis.
(From Cooper, R.R.: J. Iowa Med. Soc. **54:**689,1964.)

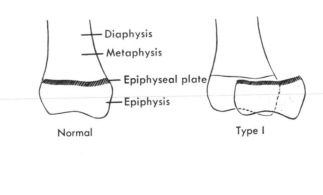

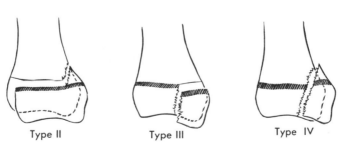

Fig. 33-23. Four types of epiphyseal fractures.

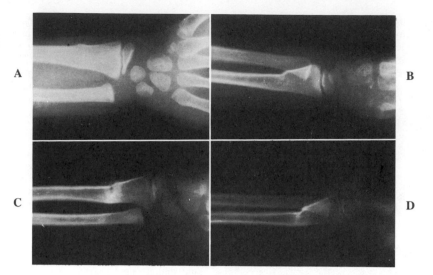

Fig. 33-24. Greenstick fracture. **A,** Anteroposterior view shows expanded cortex at site of fracture. **B,** Lateral view shows "buckle" of dorsal cortex of radius. **C,** Anteroposterior view after 3 weeks of treatment in long arm cast; repair has made fracture more obvious. **D,** Lateral view at 3 weeks. (From Cooper, R.R.: J. Iowa Med. Soc. **54:**689, 1964.)

and prevent further damage—penetration of nerves, arteries, and muscles by bone ends and penetration of skin, thereby converting a closed fracture to an open one. One can immobilize the part effectively with simple splints of magazines, pillows, boards, and strips of cloth.

Reduction. Place bone fragments in proper relationship to each other. Before this can be done, the doctor must relieve the patient's pain by:

1. Local injection of an anesthetic into the fracture hematoma. Two precautions are necessary: Strict sterile techniques must be used since a tract is established between a closed fracture and the body surface with the risk of subsequent infection. To obtain satisfactory anesthesia, the needle is inserted into the hematoma as evidenced by aspiration of blood
2. Regional anesthesia (axillary block, sciatic block, etc.)
3. General anesthesia; to minimize the risk of vomiting and aspiration, allow sufficient time to elapse after the patient eats or drinks (±6 hours)

Thoroughly and carefully débride (i.e., remove all-devitalized tissue and foreign bodies) all open wounds. Decide whether to close the skin, considering time since injury, amount of contamination, site of injury, and degree of tissue damage. Making this decision requires clinical judgment that comes only with experience. If an open wound accompanies a fracture, tetanus prophylaxis must be instituted, and prophylactic antibodies are warranted.

Three considerations in the reduction of a fracture are listed in order of importance as follows:

Alignment. Malalignment of a fracture resolves into two components (Fig. 33-25). *Rotatory malalignment:* Malposition of one fragment in relation to the other because of turning about an axis parallel to the long axis

of the bone is rotatory malalignment; (e.g., if a patient fractures his tibia and his toes point posteriorly, one may reasonably assume that rotatory malalignment exists). A fracture unites in a malrotated position and does not correct with time in either a child or an adult. *Angulation:* Malposition of one fragment in relation to another because of rotation about an axis at 90 degrees to the long axis of the bone is angulation (Fig. 33-26). In certain instances angulation is acceptable. In children growth corrects angulation in some locations depending on the child's age and the degree and direction of angulation. In general, the younger the child and the nearer the fracture to the end of a long bone, the more angulation is permissible, provided that the apex of the angle points in the direction of the plane of greatest motion of the adjacent joint (anteriorly or posteriorly in a fracture) near the knee. In no case should more than 25 degrees of angulation remain. Even in adults, in a bone buried deep in muscle, some angulation does not mean an unsatisfactory result.

Length restoration. In completely displaced fractures, fragments override because of muscle spasm. The physician must restore appropriate length. Anatomic reduction is not always necessary. In certain instances some overriding is not only acceptable but even desirable. In a child with a completely displaced long bone shaft fracture, 1 cm of overriding is acceptable with side-to-side union. After such a fracture, blood supply to the limb increases and causes increased growth of the involved extremity. In an adult, side-to-side union of a deeply buried bone is permissible. One should err on the side of overriding rather than distracting the fracture, since distraction predisposes to delayed union or nonunion.

Apposition. The amount of end-to-end contact of fragments ranks least important of the three factors, unless the fracture involves a joint surface or unless the bone is subcutaneous where the "stepoff" produced by

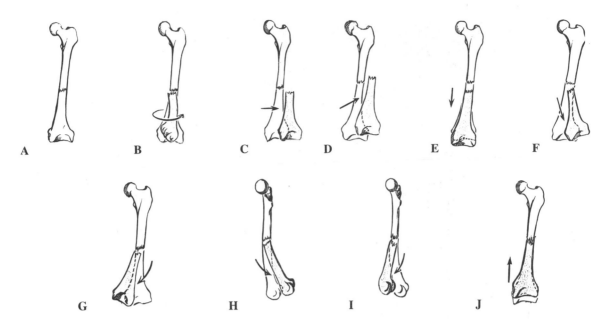

Fig. 33-25. Fracture deformities. **A,** No deformity. **B,** Rotation. **C,** Apposition loss. **D,** Overriding. **E,** Distraction. **F,** Angulation: valgus. **G,** Angulation: varus. **H,** Angulation: anterior apex. **I,** Angulation: posterior apex. **J,** Impaction.

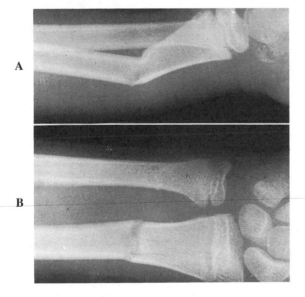

Fig. 33-26. Angulated fracture of distal third of child's forearm. Lateral view, **A,** shows angulation. Anteroposterior view, **B,** shows no loss of length or apposition.
(From Cooper, R.R.: J. Iowa Med. Soc. **54:**689, 1964.)

appositional loss would be cosmetically undesirable. Side-to-side union constitutes complete loss of cross-sectional apposition (Fig. 33-27).

When the preceding factors have been correlated, the fracture is reduced. In obtaining a reduction, the physician should always think in the following sequence:

"Can I manipulate the fracture and apply a plaster cast?"

If so, this is the best method yet devised for treatment of a fracture. If he cannot do this or if he knows from experience that he cannot, he should next think:

"Can I apply traction either to the skin, by attaching adherent tapes to the skin, or to the skeleton, by placing a pin through bone distal to the fracture?"

Traction is retained until fracture fragments adhere sufficiently to go without immobilization or to maintain position in a cast. Both methods of traction have advantages and disadvantages. Skin traction is easily applied and does not open a bone. In some patients the skin reacts to tape. The amount of traction and the length of time it can be maintained with skin tapes are limited. Skeletal traction is comfortable and tolerates more weight for a longer time than skin traction does. It can be applied under local anesthesia, but strict sterile technique and a threaded pin must be used to decrease the risk of infecting the bone.

A physician should use no other methods in treating children's fractures except for a few rare articular fractures and three common elbow fractures. Most fractures of the lateral condyle of the humerus require open reduction. Fractures of the medial epicondyle need open reduction if the bone fragment is entrapped in the elbow joint or the ulnar nerve is impinged. A few fractures of the radial neck cannot undergo closed reduction.

"Must I do an open reduction?"

Open reduction is appropriate only in instances in which the first two methods do not work. Fractures must have a blood supply in order to heal. Any open reduction destroys some vessels. Open reduction must definitely be indicated and should be performed only by

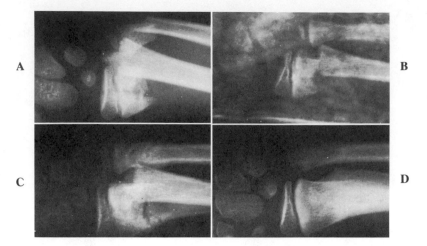

Fig. 33-27. Loss of apposition in fracture of distal third of child's forearm. **A,** Anteroposterior roentgenograms showing loss of apposition and length. **B,** With manipulative reduction, length is restored; 50% loss of apposition remains. **C,** Four weeks later, new bone has united fragments. **D,** Six months later, loss of apposition is being corrected by resorption of bone on medial side and bone deposition on lateral side. (From Cooper, R.R.: J. Iowa Med. Soc. **54:**689, 1964.)

one aware of all risks and who is technically competent to do open reductions.

Fixation. The fragments are held in reduction by plaster, traction, or in certain instances internal devices.

Immobilization. The fracture must be as free of motion as possible until the fracture unites as determined by clinical examination (lack of tenderness and motion) and x-ray examination (obliteration of the fracture line by new bone). Union usually occurs more rapidly in children than in adults.

Preserve or restore function to the involved part. The physician must constantly remember the goal of preservation or restoration of function. It is useless to obtain a perfectly united fracture if, in so doing, function is lost. Children restore function well if left to their own devices with pain as their guide to activity. Some adults need physical therapy to help restore function during and after fracture treatment. After an epiphyseal injury, the physician must follow the child to see if the bone becomes deformed.

Specific Fractures
Clavicle

Children and young adults frequently fracture the clavicle, usually by indirect force transmitted up the arm from a fall on the outstretched hand or through the acromion from a fall on the shoulder. Less frequently, a direct blow breaks the clavicle. After fracture, the weight of the upper extremity displaces the distal fragment caudad and the sternocleidomastoid displaces the proximal fragment cephalad (Fig. 33-28). Despite its subcutaneous location, the fractured clavicle usually fails to perforate the skin.

Children commonly sustain a greenstick fracture of the clavicle. In adults, brachial plexus, vessel, rib, and pulmonary injuries infrequently accompany clavicle fractures.

A figure-of-eight dressing relieves pain, lifts the di-

stal fragment, and pulls it posteriorly to appose the proximal fragment (Fig. 33-29). In children the dressing consists of a stockinette filled with padding. In adults plaster over padding effectively holds the clavicle.

Clavicle fractures nearly always unite, and excellent function returns even if moderate displacement remains. Anatomic reduction becomes a goal only if cosmesis is the primary concern.

Humerus

Usually a force transmitted upward through the hand and forearm fractures the humerus. Although shaft, lateral condyle, and medial epicondyle fractures and proximal epiphyseal separations are not uncommon in children, the bone breaks most often at the supracondylar level. In adults the shaft or surgical neck fractures most frequently.

Humerus fractures usually remain closed. Associated injuries include radial nerve injuries, either at the time of fracture or by entrapment in callus during healing. In adults arterial damage is uncommon. Brachial artery injury must always be considered during treatment of supracondylar fractures in children.

A supracondylar fracture of the humerus constitutes perhaps the most dangerous common fracture in a child's extremity. The distal fragment usually displaces posteriorly and proximally and compresses the brachial artery and median nerve between swollen soft tissues and the sharp distal end of the proximal fragment. Most children with this fracture should be hospitalized and the fracture reduced as soon as possible with skin traction applied to the forearm or with skeletal traction by a pin in the proximal ulna. The hand must be observed carefully and frequently for signs of neurovascular compression (pain, pallor, paresthesias, paralysis, lack of capillary refill, and disappearance of a radial pulse). Progression of any of these signs may necessitate surgical exploration of the brachial artery to prevent the dread complication of Volkmann's ischemic contrac-

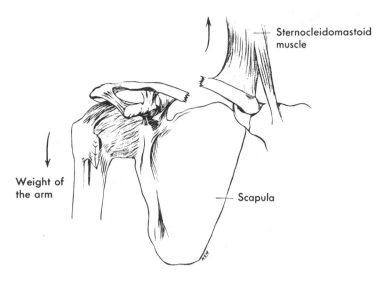

Fig. 33-28. Deforming forces in clavicular fractures.

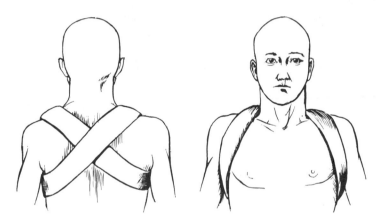

Fig. 33-29. Figure-of-eight splint dressing.

ture (see "Complications of fractures," below). After 5 to 10 days in traction, the elbow can be held safely in flexion during immobilization in a posterior splint or Velpeau dressing for 3 or 4 weeks.

Treatment of humeral shaft and surgical neck fractures usually is by a long-arm hanging cast. The latter acts as a weight on the arm to prevent overriding and to align fragments during healing. The hanging cast allows early shoulder joint motion, an important consideration in the elderly. Most humeral fractures unite readily. Radial nerve defects occurring at the time of fracture usually resolve. Late entrapment of the radial nerve by callus may require neurolysis.

A lateral humeral condyle fracture in a child extends into the articular surface. Usually, the common extensor muscle origin rotates the fragment 180 degrees so that the articular surface of the distal humerus contacts the fractured surface of the proximal fragment. These fractures fail to reduce by closed methods and if left alone become nonunited, with a subsequent progressive cubitus valgus deformity. This produces delayed ulnar nerve paralysis from stretching the ulnar nerve around

the increased valgus angle of the elbow. Appropriate treatment is by open reduction of the fragment and fixation with one or two pins in an anatomically reduced position. Care must be taken not to strip the common extensor origin from the fragment since this constitutes its only blood supply. After reduction, the child remains in a posterior splint or cast for 5 or 6 weeks, at which time the pins are removed.

A medial humeral epicondyle fracture in a child results when the common flexor muscle origin avulses the epicondyle. The fracture remains extraarticular. It requires open reduction if the fragment displaces and becomes entrapped in the joint or signs of ulnar nerve compression exist. Open reduction may also be indicated if there is noticeable displacement, since a fibrous union or a lack of union might weaken forearm muscles. The fragment is fixed to its original position either with sutures or a wire.

Forearm

Radial neck fractures in children ordinarily angulate only mildly and reduce by pressure applied directly over the radial head as the forearm is rotated into pronation and supination. Occasionally a radial neck fracture angulates nearly 90 degrees and fails to reduce by closed methods. In this instance open reduction and replacement of the radial head into the radial shaft become necessary. Postoperatively, the part is immobilized for 3 or 4 weeks until the fracture unites firmly.

Unlike children, adults frequently fracture the radial head. This at times is severely comminuted and, if left in place, produces degenerative changes in the radiohumeral joint. In adults an injured radial head can be safely excised.

Olecranon fractures in adults frequently result from a fall on the elbow with application of direct force to the proximal ulna. If the proximal fragment includes less than one third of the ulnar articular surface, the fragment may be excised and the triceps tendon attached to the remaining portion of the ulna. If the olecranon fragment is larger, it can be replaced and fixed to the ulnar shaft by means of an intramedullary screw or wires. Postoperatively, the elbow is immobilized in a posterior plaster splint for 3 to 6 weeks and then progressive active motion begins.

A direct blow or a fall on the outstretched hand may fracture the radius or ulna, or both. In children forearm fractures are commonly greenstick. In older children distal radial epiphyseal separations are not unusual. Older adults frequently fracture the distal 3 cm of the radius and the ulnar styloid (Colles' fracture). The mechanism of injury, a fall on the outstretched hand, displaces the distal fragment dorsally, proximally, and radially (Fig. 33-30). Surrounding tissues usually remain uninjured.

Local anesthesia affords satisfactory relief of pain for closed reduction of many forearm fractures in adults and children. After the fracture hematoma is injected, distraction accomplished by finger traps and a counterweight on the upper arm (Fig. 33-31) often corrects an-

gulation, overriding, and displacement. In children a long-arm cast then holds the fracture until it unites. In the older patient with Colles' fracture, a plaster cast from metacarpophalangeal joints to elbow for 3 to 4 weeks often suffices. This allows elbow, shoulder, and finger motion so necessary to avoid crippling stiffness of the arm and hand.

In adults with a radial and ulnar shaft fracture, closed reduction may be impossible, thereby necessitating open reduction and internal fixation.

Hand

See Chapter 34.

Vertebra

Vertebral fractures may be classified as vertebral body fractures, usually with anterior wedging and compression, and fractures that involve the neural arch, often with a shift of one vertebral body upon the other. The mechanism of injury in the first type is usually compression of the vertebral body, as in a fall from a height onto the legs or buttocks or from striking the top of the head as in diving into shallow water. The second type of fracture may also occur by these mechanisms but often follows severer rotational and displacement forces such as those produced in an automobile accident.

Vertebral fractures usually remain closed. Frequently spinal cord or nerve injuries accompany these fractures. Usually no external deformity is seen in vertebral fractures, though with great compression there may be visible angulation. Radiographs show anterior wedging of the vertebral body or fractures of the neural arch with displacement of one vertebral body on the other. Treatment is aimed at preventing spinal cord damage or further cord damage in patients who demonstrate initial neurologic deficit.

Fracture dislocations of the cervical spine require

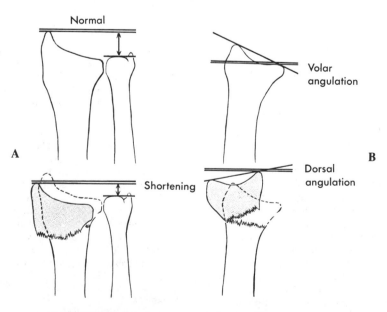

Fig. 33-30. Distal radial fracture. **A,** Anteroposterior. **B,** Lateral.

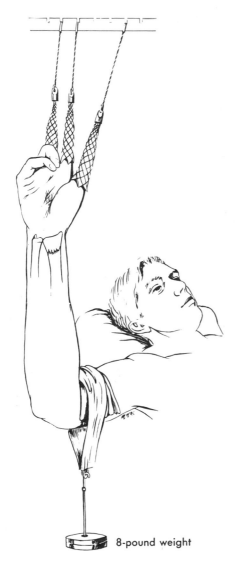

Fig. 33-31. Traction using finger traps and counterweight.

8-pound weight

reduction by tongs placed in the skull followed by further immobilization in plaster or by operative fusion of the involved vertebral bodies, or by both methods. Mild dorsal and lumbar compression fractures may be treated by bed rest with walking as soon as pain disappears. Residual deformities do not usually limit function, and late results often depend on the degree of spinal cord injury.

Fractures with spinal cord or nerve injury, especially if the loss progresses, require early neurosurgical or othopedic care.

Pelvis

Pelvic fractures result from direct trauma or from forces transmitted to the pelvis through the femur. Some fractures pass through weight-bearing portions of the pelvis, and some do not (Fig. 33-32). Pelvic fractures usually remain closed. Associated bladder, urethral, or rectal injuries must be suspected. Sacral

fractures may lacerate nerves that pass through sacral foramina. Displacement in pelvic fractures is often minimal. Displaced fractures in one part of the bony pelvic ring usually signify fractures through opposite portions of the ring. In some fractures the hemipelvis displaces craniad (Fig. 33-33). Treatment in this situation is traction through the corresponding leg to attempt restoration of alignment. Nondisplaced fractures warrant ambulation as early as symptoms permit.

Acetabular fractures that involve displacement with incongruity between the femoral head and the weight-bearing acetabular dome often require open reduction and fixation. These frequently result in subsequent degenerative joint changes and hip pain.

Other pelvic fractures usually produce no residual severe deformity. Appreciable displacement in women of childbearing age may make future vaginal delivery impossible.

Hip (Femoral Neck and Intertrochanteric)

Hip injuries usually occur from minor trauma in aged patients with osteoporosis. Pathological fractures from metastatic carcinoma often involve these locations. The deformity in both femoral neck and intertrochanteric fractures consists in shortening and external rotation of the extremity, a deformity usually obvious clinically and radiographically.

Treatment of femoral neck fractures consists in closed reduction by traction, internal rotation, and abduction of the limb followed by internal fixation with multiple threaded pins or a nail or screw through the femoral neck and head (Fig. 33-34). The femoral head is replaced by a prosthesis in selected cases. Intertrochanteric fractures are treated by closed reduction and internal fixation with a nail or screw and side plate (Fig. 33-34). Fixation permits patients to sit by 1 or 2 days postoperatively and walk in a walker or on crutches without bearing weight if they have sufficient strength. This prevents a multitude of complications (thrombophlebitis, pulmonary emboli, pneumonia, renal stones, pressure ulcers) that often lead to death.

Results in hip fractures leave much to be desired. Many elderly patients die during the first year after treatment. Intertrochanteric fractures usually heal, but nonunion with aseptic necrosis may follow femoral neck fractures. Replacement prostheses eliminate nonunion but introduce unique problems of their own.

Femoral Shaft

The injuring force to the femoral shaft may be a direct blow or transmission of stress upward through the foot and tibia. Most femoral shaft fractures remain closed. Considerable blood loss (up to 3 L) accompanies femoral shaft fractures. Varying degrees of muscle injury, especially to the quadriceps, may produce fibrosis with subsequent functional loss.

The clinical examination usually reveals shortening of the extremity and swelling of the thigh, both from the fracture hematoma and the shortened musculature. The fracture fragments almost always override, angulate, and rotate. Distraction because of excessive traction greatly increases chances of nonunion. A small amount of overriding is desirable, especially in the

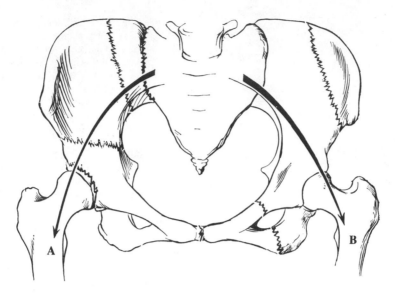

Fig. 33-32. Pelvic fractures. **A,** Fractures through weight-bearing line. **B,** Fractures not through weight-bearing line.

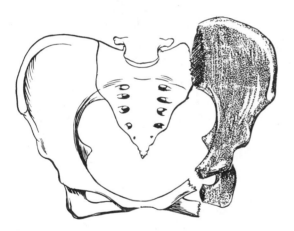

Fig. 33-33. Double vertical fracture of pelvis.

growing child, since the stimulus of increased blood supply to epiphyseal plates increases linear bone growth. Rotational deformities must be avoided, since even the child's growing bone will not correct rotational malalignments spontaneously.

Femoral shaft fractures in adults may be treated with 8 to 20 pounds of traction through a skeletal traction pin followed by the use of a cast brace. This is designed to permit knee motion and to take partial weight bearing through the fractured bone and partial weight bearing on the ischial tuberosity and through the soft tissues of the thigh. This method has the advantage of allowing healing to be stimulated by some forces being transmitted through the bone, and it allows earlier walking. In children skin traction often suffices. Toddlers may bear full weight with solid bony union in about 4 weeks. Certain femur shaft fractures in adults-can be treated by an intramedullary rod. This shortens hospitalization but adds risks of an operation.

Patella

Fracture of the patella includes two general types that often differ in mechanism of injury, associated damage to surrounding structures, and treatment.

Transverse fractures occur with violent sudden contraction of the quadriceps muscle (when one slips and attempts to prevent a fall). Less often, a direct blow produces a transverse fracture. The two fragments may be equal, or the fracture line can occur toward either pole of the patella, producing dissimilar fragments. If the fragments retain opposition, physical examination shows only mild local swelling and tenderness with pain on knee extension. Wide separation of the fragments produces a palpable sulcus. This also indicates medial and lateral tearing of the quadriceps expansion and the joint capsule.

If the fragments do not separate, treatment is by use of a posterior plaster splint or cylinder cast with graduated quadriceps exercise started at 2 to 3 weeks and with progressive weight bearing soon thereafter. Wide separation of fragments demands operative realignment, suture of the torn quadriceps expansion, and 6 to 10 weeks of plaster immobilization. Great disparity in fragment size justifies removal of the smaller one and repair of tendon or muscle attachments to the retained fragment.

Comminuted patellar fractures generally result from a direct blow. Associated lacerations of the joint capsule or quadriceps expansion are less severe; however, damage of the articular surfaces of femur and patella is frequently extensive. Treatment then is by patellectomy and suture of the patellar tendon to the quadriceps tendon. A plaster cast immobilizes the extremity in extension for 6 to 10 weeks.

Tibia

Tibial shaft fractures result from torsional force of from a direct blow (bumper fracture), and tibial plateau fractures result from a force transmitted up the tibia and

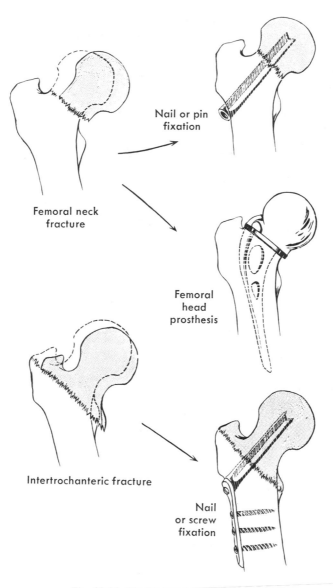

Nail or pin fixation

Femoral neck fracture

Femoral head prosthesis

Intertrochanteric fracture

Nail or screw fixation

Fig. 33-34. Hip fractures and their treatment.

to the femoral condyles (body weight). Bone fragments from the subcutaneous tibia frequently protrude through skin lacerations. Tibial fractures may injure the posterior tibial artery. Skin injuries often make it difficult to obtain soft tissue closure over open tibial fractures. Lateral displacement sufficient to cause overriding is uncommon in transverse fractures but common in oblique fractures. Rotational deformity must be suspected in displaced tibial fractures. Tibial plateau fractures angulate into varus or valgus.

Tibial shaft fractures can usually be treated by closed reduction and a long-leg plaster or by skeletal traction distal to the fracture until the fragments unite sufficiently to prevent displacement in a cast. Solid union may not occur for 3 to 8 months.

Tibial plateau fractures may be comminuted and require splinting with subsequent early motion, or they

may consist of one large fragment that can be openly reduced and fixed to the remaining tibia.

Ankle (Medial and Lateral Malleoli and Ankle Ligaments)

The medial malleolus (tibia), posterior malleolus (posterior lip of the distal articular surface of the tibia), and lateral malleolus (fibula) fracture alone and in various combinations. Ligament injuries may accompany one or more of these fractures and often demand as much or more attention than the fracture itself. The mechanism of injury is excessive movement of the mobile leg upon the fixed foot or of the mobile foot upon the fixed leg. The injuring force frequently externally rotates or abducts the foot, talus, and distal tibia and fibula. Certain combinations of forces produce characteristic fracture patterns. Ankle fractures remain closed unless a direct injury lacerates the skin or the injuring force dislocates the talus from the tibia with resulting skin loss or subsequent necrosis.

The deformity of a fracture dislocation of the ankle is obvious on inspection (gross loss of the relationship between the foot and leg). Without dislocation, the injury produces swelling and tenderness over the injured malleoli. Final distinction between bony and ligamentous injuries requires radiographic studies in the anterior, posterior, lateral, and oblique projections.

Adequate reduction demands reconstitution of the forklike configuration of the medial and lateral malleolus (closing the ankle mortise). Interposition of a flap of soft tissues (deltoid ligament) between the medial malleolus and talus may necessitate open reduction to restore normal congruity between the articular surfaces of the talus and tibia (Fig. 33-35). Many ankle fractures can be reduced closed and immobilized 6 to 8 weeks in a short-leg walking cast. More complicated fractures and fracture dislocations may require a long-leg cast and no weight bearing for varying periods or open reduction with ligament repair and internal fixation of the fracture.

The results of treatment are usually good if tibiotalar congruity is restored (the ankle mortise is closed) and ligamentous injuries are recognized and treated adequately. Delayed union or nonunion occasionally occurs in medial malleolar fractures.

Foot

Talus. Fractures often involve the neck of the talus and are frequently accompanied by ankle or subtalar dislocation. These fractures reduce with difficulty and may require surgical reduction. Because of the source of blood supply, aseptic necrosis of the body of the talus frequently develops and adds to morbidity and produces long-term complications.

Calcaneus. Fractures of the calcaneus usually occur during a fall from a height. These falls crush the bone and frequently extend into the subtalar joint. The foot becomes extremely swollen. Initial treatment is by rest, elevation, and compression. After swelling decreases, many fractures can be managed with a short leg-cast and weight bearing as tolerated. Several operations are designed to attempt reconstruction of various calcaneal fractures. After treatment, subtalar joint motion often remains decreased.

Metatarsus and phalanges. Metatarsal and phalangeal fractures usually require closed reduction and plaster immobilization for 3 to 4 weeks. Some, with great displacement, demand open reduction and internal fixation.

Complications of Fractures
Complications of Casts—Compartment Syndrome

Improperly applied plaster or subsequent swelling produces pressure of the cast against underlying soft

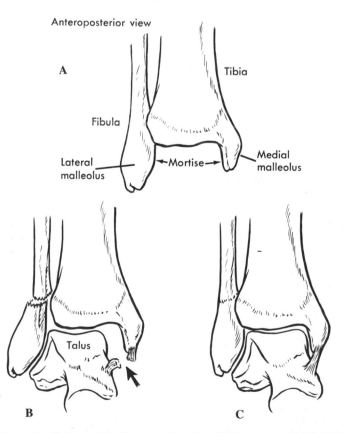

Fig. 33-35. Ankle mortise. **A,** Normal. **B,** Fracture of lateral malleolus and tear of deltoid ligament *(arrow)* opens mortise. **C,** Mortise closed with restored congruity of talus and tibia.

tissues over bone prominences. Skin circulation decreases, and necrosis results. In applying a cast the physician should expose the tips of the patient's toes or fingers in order to observe the parts for signs of neurovascular compression. Pressure from a tight cast or padding, or hemorrhage and swelling into a muscular compartment compromise circulation to the extremity. Persistent neurovascular interference invokes the dreaded compartment syndrome which, if ignored, leads to Volkmann's ischemic paralysis, especially after humeral supracondylar fractures and fractures or dislocations near the knee. In this syndrome circulation to muscle decreases, necrotic and fibrotic scar replaces muscles, and permanent contractures ensue (Fig. 33-36). Associated sensory loss further impairs function.

Because of these disastrous sequelae, the doctor must investigate and correct complaints of pain and numbness beneath a cast. Pain, pallor, swelling, discoloration, and lack of capillary refill indicate circulatory embarrassment. The doctor must treat a patient with any of these immediately by splitting the cast and the underlying padding, elevating the part, and observing the patient carefully to see if surgical exploration of the involved compartment is indicated. Intracompartmental pressure can be measured by insertion of a wick catheter. A persistent pressure of 35 to 40 mm H_2O is an indication to open the tight osteofascial compartment.

Malunion

If a fractured bone is improperly reduced or loses reduction as swelling decreases, the bone unites in an unsatisfactory position. To avoid this complication, the doctor must reduce the fracture properly and follow the patient to be certain that reduction is *maintained*. If a malunion is cosmetically or functionally unacceptable to the patient, an orthopedic surgeon can rebreak the bone (osteotomy) and restore satisfactory position.

Delayed Union

At times a bone fails to heal solidly after a reasonable period as determined by location of the fracture, type of fracture, and method of treatment. Continued adequate immobilization corrects most delayed unions.

Nonunion

Some bones fail to unite. Gross motion is generally demonstrable. X-ray examination reveals sclerosis of adjacent bone ends and obliteration of the medullary canal. Fibrous scar tissue or a false joint (pseudoarthrosis) fills the gap between bone ends. Bone grafting stimulates repair at these sites.

The causes of delayed union and nonunion are not always immediately apparent and usually include a combination of inadequate reduction, inadequate fixation, inadequate immobilization, severe trauma to soft parts, improper operative treatment, distraction of fragments, infection, and fracture location. The femoral neck, carpal scaphoid, and junction of the distal and middle thirds of the tibia unite slowly.

Shock

Bone is extremely vascular. At the time of fracture large volumes of blood escape from the circulating blood into soft tissues or externally through an open wound. Neurogenic shock from pain aggravates shock from blood loss. For the patient in shock, the physician must provide an adequate airway and oxygen, control hemorrhage and pain, and restore blood volume.

Fat Embolism

Patients who sustain massive trauma occasionally develop clinical signs and symptoms of fat embolism. This syndrome results from vascular impaction by fat, especially in lung, brain, and kidney. After massive trauma to long bones, marrow fat may contribute to intravascular aggregation of lipoproteins.

Classically, the patient begins to recover from the initial acute trauma and then regresses clinically. Regression occurs on the average of 24 hours after the acute injury and appears as an increase in pulse, temperature, and respiration. The patient becomes apprehensive, delirious, may eventually exhibit focal neurologic signs, convulse, and lapse into stupor and coma. Cyanosis may accompany these signs and symptoms.

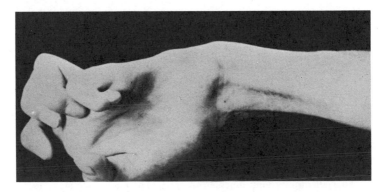

Fig. 33-36. Volkmann's ischemic contracture. Clawhand is rigid and useless.
(From Steindler, A.: The traumatic deformities and disabilities of the upper extremity, Springfield, Ill., 1956, Charles C Thomas, Publisher, p. 296.)

Frequently, petechiae appear with, or before the development of, other signs and symptoms, especially over the upper chest wall and in the conjunctivae. Chest films often reveal diffuse cloudlike densities in the lungs. Fat may be demonstrated in the urine of some patients. Blood gas studies are of critical importance in monitoring the status of a patient with fat emboli. Therapy must be instituted promptly if the patient's life is to be saved. Further manipulation of injured extremities should be avoided. The patient needs appropriate blood, fluid, and electrolyte replacement therapy and digitalis if cardiac failure develops. Blood gases serve as a guide to the need for and the use of oxygen therapy. The degree of pulmonary damage may necessitate positive pressure oxygen by means of tracheotomy and a respirator.

Some have advocated the use of steroids, alcohol, and heparin in management of fat embolism, but their status is more debatable than that of the critical need of oxygen by the patient with this syndrome.

Peripheral Nerve Injuries

At the time of fracture or during reduction, bone ends can injure nerves. Before attempting reduction, the physician must evaluate motor and sensory nerve function distal to the fracture and record these observations. Closed fractures occasionally contuse nerves. These usually recover fully. Immediate open exploration is not warranted. In open fractures with nerve injuries, the surgeon inspects the nerve at the time of wound débridement and, if it is severed, plans appropriate surgical repair.

Infection

Bacteria can enter bone from an open fracture or from implantation during surgery. (See discussion on treatment of osteomyelitis, above.)

Posttraumatic Degenerative Joint Disease

After articular fractures, incongruous joint surfaces can subsequently develop degenerative joint changes. At times the physician can minimize this by adequate apposition of fragments. If trauma is extensive, subsequent degenerative changes cannot be prevented. Patients with degenerative changes must be treated with appropriate measures depending on the severity of their symptoms. (See the discussion of degenerative joint disease, below.)

Acute Atrophy (Reflex Dystrophy, Postimmobilization Atrophy, Sudeck's Atrophy)

In certain patients, a part that remains immobile undergoes acute atrophy, including bone atrophy (Sudeck's atrophy). Patients who do not use portions of the extremity that are free of a cast develop atrophy more frequently than others. They complain of pain, motion decreases, edema develops, and the skin atrophies and becomes shiny. If the disorder progresses, contractures develop, adhesions limit joint function, and a useless part results. To prevent or treat this disorder, patients must use the part actively and institute range-of-motion exercises.

Aseptic Necrosis

When a fracture isolates bone from its blood supply, the bone dies. Necrosis most often develops after fracture of the femoral neck, carpal navicular, and neck of talus. Dead bone appears radiopaque in contrast to surrounding normal bone that atrophies from disuse. Dead bone is slowly destroyed by granulation tissue and replaced by new bone. If force is transmitted before repair is complete, the bone fractures in the zone of replacement at the junction of dead and new bone. Bone grafting hastens repair of necrotic areas and, by supporting bone, prevents collapse.

Joint Injuries
Sprains

A sprain is a tear in ligament and capsule fibers. Without proper treatment, ligaments heal in an elongated position with residual laxity that predisposes to further episodes of injury and the eventual need for surgical reconstruction. Sprains are classified clinically and treated as follows:

Mild (first degree). In the mild sprain, a few fibers separate. The region is tender, swollen, and bruised. The joint retains stability. The patient is treated with analgesics, rest, elevation, and cold packs for the first 12 to 24 hours, after which warm packs, a compression wrap or taping, and rest of the part for 7 to 10 days are in order.

Moderate (second degree). In the moderate sprain, several fibers tear. The patient complains of more tenderness and the part swells and becomes ecchymotic. On examination, the doctor notices some effusion and slight instability of the joint. Immobilization in a plaster cast for 3 to 6 weeks, depending on the joint involved, permits healing.

Severe (third degree). In the severe sprain, the ligaments disrupt completely, and the joint loses stability. An orthopedic surgeon should repair these ligaments.

Dislocations

During a dislocation, articular surfaces of opposing bones completely and persistently separate. During subluxation, opposing articular surfaces separate partially and temporarily. A dislocation damages joint capsule and ligaments. Prior to reduction of a dislocation, the physician should obtain radiographs for diagnostic and legal purposes. Fractures accompany many dislocations, and if a fracture is found after reduction, some might assume that the doctor produced it. Only if dislocation compromises vascular supply must reduction be done on an emergency basis before radiographs are obtained.

Before a dislocation is reduced, the patient needs proper anesthesia or analgesia. Complicated maneuvers are unnecessary to reduce most dislocations. Simple traction reduces many of them. Some must be reduced surgically.

The physician must obtain postreduction films to be sure that the dislocation is reduced. The part is immobilized for 3 to 6 weeks so that the ligaments heal properly. The patient restores function by using the part.

Torn ligaments that are not well protected heal in an elongated position with predisposition to recurrent dislocation that must often be treated by surgery.

Intraarticular Derangement

Knee joint menisci are particularly prone to injuries. Medial menisci tear 10 to 12 times more frequently than lateral menisci. The patient usually has the foot fixed and the knee partly flexed. He or she then forcibly rotates the body to the opposite side and feels sudden pain over the joint line. The joint *locks* (the knee will not fully extend or fully flex). An effusion develops over the next few hours. At times, traction unlocks the knee. Most meniscal tears do not heal but result in subsequent episodes of locking and giving way. Surgical removal of a torn meniscus alleviates these symptoms. Differential diagnosis includes osteochondral fractures and osteochondritis dissecans. During an os-

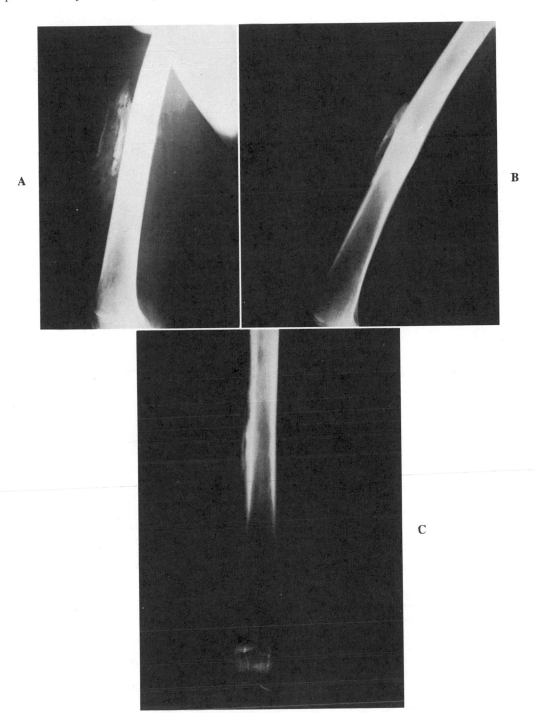

Fig. 33-37. Myositis ossificans. **A,** Roentgenogram of thigh 1 month after injury showing ossification in quadriceps muscle and beneath periosteum of femoral shaft. **B,** Twelve months later myositis ossificans is resorbing. **C,** Two and one-half years after injury, some periosteal bone remains.

Table 33-9. Benign Lesions Often Diagnosed as Malignancies

Lesion	Common Age (Years)	Sex Distri- bution	Common Location	Symptoms	Radiographic Appearance	Treatment
Osteocartilaginous exostosis: A cartilage-capped projection of bone; enchondral ossification at the cartilage-bone junction contin- ues until growth stops; develop- mental defect	6-10	Equal	Metaphysis, distal femur, proximal tibia	Mass; pain if: (1) bursa, (2) fracture, (3) nerve irrita- tion	Sessile or peduncu- lated bony prom- inence projects from the meta- physeal cortex (Fig. 33-38)	Less than 1% be- come malignant (chondrosarcoma from the carti- lage cap); re- move for pain, neurologic symp- toms, or rapid growth, espe- cially after the epiphyseal plates close
Metaphyseal fibrous defect: A devel- opmental defect that consists of fibrous connec- tive tissue, giant cells, and foam cells in the corti- cal and subcorti- cal bone	4-10	Equal	Metaphysis, distal femur, proximal tibia	None; incidental x-ray finding	Eccentric metaphy- seal lytic lesion surrounded by scalloped edge of reactive new bone (Fig. 33- 39)	*Do not* ascribe pain to them; find the true cause of limb pain in a child
Bone cyst: A jux- taepiphyseal cav- ity lined by a thin layer of con- nective tissue and filled with yellow serum	4-14	Males	Metaphysis, proxi- mal humerus, proximal femur	Pathological frac- ture	Metaphyseal central lytic and trabecu- lated cyst; the cortex expands on either side (Fig. 33-40)	Some heal after one or more frac- tures; others need treatment by curettage and bone grafting, preferably after 10 years of age
Osteoid osteoma: A reactive lesion consisting of a central nidus of osteoid and new bone in a fibrovascular stroma	10-25	Males	Femur and tibia	Severe pain, worse at night; relieved by aspirin	Lytic lesion less than 1 cm in di- ameter; a dense, central nidus sur- rounded by reac- tive new bone	Excision
Osteoblastoma: A reactive lesion similar to but larger than os- teoid osteoma	15-35	Equal	Vertebra, metacar- pus, femur	Pain that is less severe than in osteoid	Central lytic lesion over 1 cm in diameter sur- rounded by reac- tive new bone	Excision if possible

teochondral fracture, a piece of articular cartilage and subchondral bone breaks free from the underlying bone. In osteochondritis dissecans, common in teenag- ers, a piece of articular cartilage and underlying bone separates from the remainder of the bone. The bone fragments and dies. This disorder is usually located on the lateral surface of the medial femoral condyle. Fre- quently the fragment revascularizes and heals, but it sometimes drops into the joint. In either of these disor- ders a free fragment in the joint gives symptoms like those of a torn meniscus. Radiographs often reveal a defect in the femoral condyle where the fragment sepa- rated. If the fragment contains bone, a radiograph shows it. These free fragments should be removed.

Injuries of Muscles and Tendons

Excessive force produces separation of musculoten- dinous units at the junction of muscle and tendon,

through the tendon, or at the site of tendon insertion into bone. The patient notices immediate pain, swell- ing, ecchymosis, and loss of function. Soon after dis- ruption, the muscle or tendon should be restored surgi- cally, especially if it is an important functional unit. If treatment is neglected, many units regenerate suffi- ciently to give adequate function. If not, surgical re- construction is indicated.

Myositis Ossificans

A direct blow to a muscle causes intramuscular hemorrhage that usually resorbs but on occasion ossi- fies. Several days or even weeks after injury, the pa- tient notices a lump. The mass enlarges and becomes firm during the next 5 to 10 weeks. In some instances it is mildly tender and interferes with muscle function. Usually the mass then decreases in size and disappears after 6 to 8 months. Radiographs reveal increased ossi-

Table 33-9, cont'd.

Lesion	Common Age (Years)	Sex Distribution	Common Location	Symptoms	Radiographic Appearance	Treatment
Aneurysmal bone cyst: A reactive "blowout" of the cortex by a lesion composed of vascular lakes surrounded by fibrous connective tissue, foam cells, and giant cells	12-25	Females	Femoral metaphysis and vertebra	Pain and expanding mass	Lytic lesion with a "blowout" distension of the cortex; frequently a thin layer of periosteal new bone surrounds the cyst	Curettage and bone grafting
Enchondroma: A mass of hyaline cartilage within the confines of bone	10-50	Equal	Diaphysis, phalanx of hand, metacarpus, humerus, femur	Swelling, pain, fracture	Oval lytic area with "expanded" cortex, stippled calcifications	Curet and pack bone chips if fracture, rapid growth, or symptomatic; long bone enchondromas can become malignant (chondrosarcoma)
Fibrous dysplasia: A developmental error; certain regions of bone are replaced by a dense, fibrous connective tissue stroma from which trabeculae of new bone arise	5-25	Males	Diaphysis, ribs, femur, humerus	Incidental finding; fractures or deformity	Lytic, ground glass–appearing lesions; cortex expands and bones deform	Curet and pack if symptomatic
Giant cell tumor: A lesion of polyhedral stromal cells and many multinucleated giant cells within the confines of bone	20-50	Females	Epiphyseal, distal radius, distal femur, proximal tibia	Pain and mass	Central or eccentric epiphyseal destructive or trabeculated area surrounded by an expanded cortex	Excise if compatible with function of the part; if not, curet and graft; on recurrence, do wide local excision or amputation, since a strong potential for malignancy exists

fication while the mass grows (Fig. 33-37). The bone becomes mature and usually resorbs. In a few instances it remains. A thorough history helps differentiate myositis ossificans from a bone-forming tumor. Despite this, the doctor must observe the patient carefully. Excision of the mass soon after it develops leads to more hemorrhage and greater ossification. If after a year or 18 months the mass persists, the physician can safely excise it.

BENIGN BONE TUMORS

To diagnose bone tumors, the physician must use a correlative approach, integrating clinical facts, radiographic appearance, and histopathology, each in its proper perspective. Doing so is especially important in the diagnosis of a malignant tumor and perhaps even more important in prevention of misdiagnosis of malignancy in a benign lesion. Such an error would lead to

unwarranted, mutilating overtreatment. Table 33-9 describes in detail benign lesions that are frequently misdiagnosed as malignancies.

MALIGNANT BONE TUMORS
Tumors Primary in Bone

Malignant bone tumors produce the same symptoms regardless of their histologic type. Patients complain of pain, often mild and intermittent at first, but increasing to become severe and constant, especially at night. On examination the physician finds a mass, local tenderness, and warm skin with dilated subcutaneous veins. In more advanced cases generalized symptoms include weakness and weight loss. Anemia is common. If a patient's complaints are suggestive of a malignancy, the physician must make the diagnosis. This usually involves a biopsy. The orthopedist, radiologist, and pathologist must maintain close liaison to make the cor-

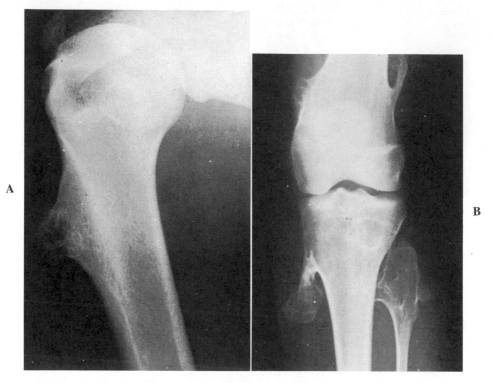

Fig. 33-38. Osteocartilaginous exostosis. **A,** Single exostosis of humeral shaft. **B,** Hereditary multiple exostoses.

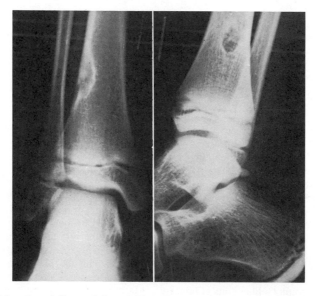

Fig. 33-39. Metaphyseal fibrous defect of tibia. Reactive new bone surrounds radiolucent defect.

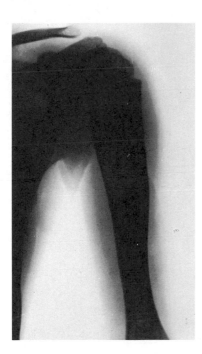

Fig. 33-40. Solitary bone cyst. Humeral metaphysis is expanded, and cortex is thin. Ridges of bone on cyst walls produce trabeculated appearance.

rect diagnosis and outline the plan of treatment. Table 33-10 gives the characteristics of malignant tumors primary in bone.

Tumors Metastatic to Bone

Carcinoma commonly spreads to bone. In extensive autopsy studies of patients dying from carcinomatosis, pathologists find bone metastases in as many as 70%. Metastases most frequently involve the vertebral column, pelvis, skull, humerus, and femur. They rarely spread to bones distal to the elbow and knee. Carcinomas of the prostate, breast, kidney, lung, and thyroid produce most bone metastases. Lesions can lyse bone (hypernephroma, thyroid), provoke an osteoblastic reaction (prostate), or be a mixture of the two (breast, lung).

Some metastases produce no symptoms. With others, the patient complains of pain and swelling. Frequently the involved bone fractures. At times the bone lesion causes symptoms before the primary tumor does. If in such a case the history, physical examintaion, and routine radiographs do not readily reveal the primary lesion, the orthopedist can biopsy a bone. This not only rules out a primary bone tumor, but in certain instances the histology of a metastatic lesion provides a clue to the primary site. Pathologic fracture through a metastatic tumor usually heals. Orthopedists treat these fractures with internal fixation so that the patient is free of pain and can be ambulatory. Depending on the type of tumor, its size, and its location, treatment of the bone lesion is by radiotherapy, chemotherapy, and hormone therapy, or a combination. The physician strives to prolong life and to make the patient as comfortable and functional as possible.

Secondary Invasion of Bone By Adjacent Soft Tissue Tumors

Fibrosarcoma, synovial sarcoma, neurosarcoma, liposarcoma, and hemangioendothelioma at times erode adjacent bone. They produce symptoms like those of a malignant bone tumor. Radiographs reveal the soft tissue mass and an underlying lytic defect in the outer surface of the bone cortex. At times the tumor destroys the entire cortex and invades the medullary canal. The physician uses the same diagnostic methods and treats the patient much the same as one with a primary malignant bone tumor.

NEUROMUSCULAR DISORDERS
Poliomyelitis

Poliomyelitis has disappeared as a major cause of neuromuscular disability in children. Vaccines have precipitously reduced the incidence of the disease. The poliovirus attacks brain stem motor nuclei and spinal cord anterior horn cells in a spotty distribution. The virus kills some cells and temporarily inactivates others. The localization and severity of muscle paralysis vary from person to person. If motor neurons recover, weakened muscles regain function. Many patients improve for 1 or 2 years after their acute attack of poliomyelitis; however, about 70% of muscle strength returns within 3 or 4 months.

Paralysis and deformity produce loss of function in poliomyelitis patients. Various factors result in deformity: muscle imbalance, decreased growth of a severely paralyzed extremity, and abnormal bone growth caused by irregular forces from muscle imbalance and gait disturbances.

Depending on the extent and location of postpoliomyelitis residuals, orthopedists treat patients with a variety of measures:

1. Bracing to:
   a. Support body weight
   b. Stabilize a joint—limit abnormal motion
   c. Counteract muscle imbalance—prevent a strong muscle from stretching a weak antagonist and deforming the part
   d. Assist a weak muscle—a spring-loaded brace
   e. Prevent deformity—distribute forces in muscle imbalance or gait disturbances
2. Tendon transfers—restore muscle balance by moving one or more strong musculotendon units to replace function in a paralyzed muscle group
3. Tendon lengthening—if a contracture develops
4. Arthrodesis (fusion)—to control a frail, unstable joint
5. Osteotomy—to correct bone deformities
6. Leg length equalizations—an extremity with loss of muscle function grows slower than normal; significant leg length discrepancy produces deformity and disordered gait mechanics, which strain the hips and spine and result in pain and further deformity.

Leg lengths are measured from the anterosuperior iliac spine to the tip of the medial malleolus. Ortho-

Table 33-10. Malignant Tumors Primary in Bone

Lesion	Age (Years)	Sex	Common Location	Radiographic Appearance	Treatment	Prognosis
Osteosarcoma: A connective tissue tumor composed of malignant stromal cells that have osteogenic potential as manifested by the ability to produce tumor osteoid and bone	10–25	Male	Metaphysis, distal femur, proximal tibia	Metaphyseal osteolytic or osteoblastic, or both; a triangle of subperiosteal reactive new bone, a sunburst appearance from striae of new bone, cortical destruction in a jagged manner (Fig. 33–41)	Amputation or disarticulation, chemotherapy	30% to 50% 5-year survival; tends to spread rapidly through the bloodstream
Juxtacortical sarcoma: An uncommon lesion that arises in relation to the periosteum or adjacent tissue; tends to form a deceptively benign-looking fibrous stroma from which tumor bone arises; some areas contain clumps of cartilage	30–40		Distal femoral metaphysis	A sclerotic, lobulated mass extending from the cortex; tends to invade the underlying bone	Wide, local excision or amputation	30% to 50% 5-year survival
Chondrosarcoma: A tumor of malignant cartilage cells; *primary,* a chondrosarcoma arising at the site of no known preexisting defect; *secondary,* a chondrosarcoma arising from an osteocartilaginous exostosis or enchondroma; microscopically, chondrosarcoma is difficult to differentiate from benign enchondroma; evidence for malignancy includes history, radiographic evidence of destruction, microscopic hypercellularity, plump nuclei, and double nuclei	30–50	Female	Diaphysis, ribs and pelvis, proximal femur and humerus	Mottled osseous destruction with fusiform expansion of the shaft; mottled calcification	Wide excision or amputation	40% to 60% 5-year survival; tends to spread locally and along veins; metastasizes through the bloodstream
Fibrosarcoma: A tumor composed of malignant stromal cells that produce a fibrous, nonossifying matrix	10–40	Male	Distal femur, proximal tibia	A lytic, destructive, non–bone producing defect	Amputation	20% to 30% 5-year survival
Ewing's tumor: A highly malignant round cell tumor probably derived from primitive reticular cells of the bone marrow	10–25	Male	Diaphysis of femur or tibia, pelvis	A lytic, destructive process, reactive periosteal new bone in layers and occasionally through reactive new bone much like osteogenic sarcoma	Irradiation, chemotherapy	30% to 40% 5-year survival
Reticulum cell sarcoma: A round cell tumor composed of reticulum cells of the bone marrow	20–40	Male	Pelvis, femur	A lytic, destructive lesion with little tendency to produce reactive new bone	Irradiation or amputation	60% 5-year survival
Multiple myeloma: A round cell tumor arising from primitive reticulum cells that have the capacity to differentiate into plasma cells	50–70	Male	Multiple sites, vertebra, skull, ribs, long bones	Multifocal lytic lesions without much tendency to reactive new bone; osteoporosis (Fig. 33–42)	Irradiation, chemotherapy	In many cases, eventually fatal

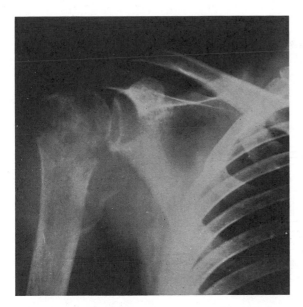

Fig. 33-41. Osteosarcoma of proximal humerus. Bone destruction is extensive. Thin layer of new bone outlines soft tissue extension of neoplasm. There is pathological fracture of neck humerus.

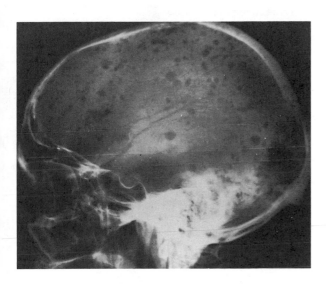

Fig. 33-42. Multiple myeloma. Roentgenogram shows multiple radiolucent lesions.

radiographs (films of both lower extremities against a centimeter scale); (Fig. 33-43) disclose the exact discrepancy. Orthopedic surgeons correct discrepancy in one of three ways:

1. Lengthen the short limb by osteotomy and gradual traction with extreme caution because of the distinct chance of neurovascular complications.
2. Stop growth of the normal limb. Charts based on studies of normal children show predicted growth from each epiphyseal plate at a given age. When a child with unequal leg lengths reaches an age where his expected leg growth

equals his length discrepancy, orthopedists arrest growth of the normal limb by curetting the epiphyseal plate or by placing staples across the plate. The shorter limb continues to grow, and leg lengths equalize.
3. Shorten the normal limb.

Cerebral Palsy

The term *cerebral palsy* denotes various syndromes that have in common nonprogressive neuromuscular dysfunction from brain damage. Causes are prenatal (fetal anoxia, German measles, developmental defects of the brain), associated with birth (prematurity and anoxia from drugs, prolonged labor), or postnatal (encephalitis).

Cerebral palsy is classified according to the type of neuromuscular dysfunction:

Spastic—stretch reflex, increased deep tendon reflexes, clonus
Athetoid—involuntary, writhing movements
Ataxia—poor coordination, nystagmus, adiadochokinesis
Rigidity—"lead pipe" resistance, absence of stretch reflex
Tremor—intention or nonintention tremor
Mixed—two or more of the above.

Cerebral palsy is also classified as to site involved: monoplegia (one limb), hemiplegia (one arm and one leg), paraplegia (both legs), triplegia (three limbs), and quadriplegia (all four limbs).

Many patients with muscular manifestations of cerebral palsy have associated defects of hearing, speech, and mentality. A team of physicians, physical therapists, occupational therapists, vocational counselors, speech therapists, and social workers should evaluate all aspects of the patient, establish realistic medical, social, and vocational goals based on motor and mental ability, and treat the patient with the proper modalities. *Physical therapy* aids in gait training, stretching tight muscles, sitting and standing balance, and muscle control. *Occupational therapy* teaches self-care. *Bracing* prevents deformity, prevents spasticity from stretching a weak or normal muscle, gives stability, helps control involuntary motion, and gives a solid base for walking. *Surgery* may be indicated to release or lengthen spastic muscle contractures. Neurectomy decreases spasticity. Arthrodesis stabilizes deformed and uncontrolled joints in functional positions. Tendon transfer restores muscle balance.

Myopathies and Neuropathies

In certain stages of their disease, some patients with muscular dystrophy or Charcot-Marie-Tooth disease and Friedreich's ataxia need orthopedic treatment. In early stages of a slowly progressive neuromuscular disorder, bracing relieves deformity and increases function. Tendon transfers and bone-stabilizing procedures are sometimes useful.

IDIOPATHIC DISORDERS
Rheumatoid Arthritis

Rheumatoid arthritis, one of the great cripplers, is part of a generalized disease that can involve almost

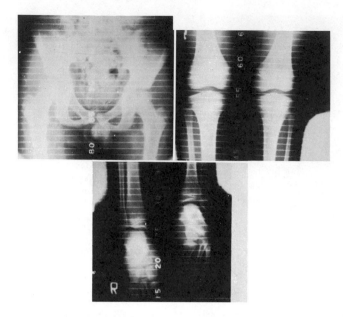

Fig. 33-43. Orthoroentgenograms showing that left leg is 6.5 cm. shorter than right.

any organ in the body. No one knows the cause of rheumatic disease, nor can its course be predicted in any individual. Rheumatoid arthritis attacks persons of all ages but is most common in women 25 to 40 years of age. Arthritis usually begins as a synovial inflammation in smaller joints, is migratory, and can involve any joint. Synovitis often subsides without residual damage. If the disease continues, inflamed synovium extends as a pannus across the joint, destroys cartilage, and erodes underlying bone. The joint loses stability and motion and becomes deformed.

The afflicted patient complains of pain, deformity, or loss of function. Early in the disease, radiographs reveal soft tissue swelling and marginal destruction of the joint. Later progressive disease narrows and destroys the joint.

Rheumatologists and orthopedic surgeons, working together, should manage the rheumatoid patient with medical and surgical therapy used at the proper time for optimal results. The rheumatologist initiates appropriate drug therapy. The orthopedist aids in treatment by splinting involved joints in a position that avoids undesirable contractures. He or she also directs the active exercise program and passive stretching of contractures. If a particular joint does not respond and synovitis and joint effusion persist, a synovectomy may prevent further joint destruction. After synovectomy, the synovium regrows and at times resists rheumatoid disease. At various stages of the disorder the surgeon might help the patient with one of several surgical procedures: release of tight muscles and fascia, transfer of muscles, arthroplasties (remolding of distorted joint surfaces with or without interposing metal or fascia over the reshaped bone surfaces), arthrodeses (fusion of painful and destroyed joints), and joint prostheses and total joint replacements (Fig. 33-44, *B*).

Degenerative Joint Disease

The term *degenerative joint disease* denotes changes wherein articular cartilage loses fluid, becomes less resilient, loses normal color, fragments, and thins. Weight-bearing portions of larger joints degenerate most often. The underlying bone contains cysts filled with fluid or granulation tissue. New bone production results in sclerosis of bone ends and spurs at joint margins. Free pieces of cartilage and bone frequently displace into the joint.

Degenerative joint disease can arise after processes that produce incongruity of opposing joint surfaces (infection, trauma) with resultant abnormal joint mechanics. In most instances, however, no one knows the cause. Some view degenerative joint disease as part of normal aging, and others believe that it is a disease. Degenerative changes in the knees, hips, and spine are common in persons over 65. A person with clinical and radiographic signs of degenerative joint disease is not necessarily symptomatic.

Patients often relieve joint stiffness and discomfort with rest, heat, antiinflammatory drugs, and analgesics. Severe pain and loss of function necessitate one of the following surgical measures: joint débridement (excision of loose bodies and rough areas on the joint surface); release of tight muscles, fascia, and joint capsule; arthroplasty (Fig. 33-44); arthrodesis; prosthetic replacement; or total joint replacement.

Paget's Disease (Osteitis Deformans)

Paget's disease, a disorder of unknown cause, usually affects men over 55 years of age. Bone is destroyed and produced in an irregular manner. Microscopic examination shows many fragments of bone fitted together in a mosaic with blue "cement lines" between the pieces. A fibrovascular stroma fills spaces

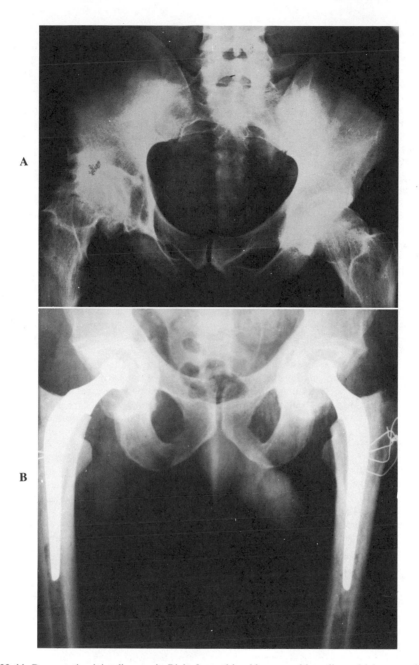

Fig. 33-44. Degenerative joint disease. **A,** Right femoral head has moved laterally, and joint space is narrow; notice osteophytic overgrowth of bone on inferior margin of femoral head and inferior acetabulum; acetabular cysts are surrounded by sclerotic bone. **B,** Recent method of treatment is total hip replacement with metal femoral component and polyethylene acetabulum.

between bone trabeculas. Paget's disease commonly affects the spine, pelvis, and proximal femurs. Radiographically, increased density from new bone production accentuates the major trabecular pattern. Bone destruction produces radiolucent areas. The involved bones often deform. At times patients with Paget's disease have aches and pains. Often, however, the physician discovers the disorder when he obtains radiographs for other reasons. Some patients obtain relief of dis-

comfort by the use of aspirin and other medications. They occasionally develop osteosarcoma superimposed on Paget's disease, and the doctor should follow them closely with this possibility in mind.

METABOLIC DISORDERS
Rickets

In rickets, a disorder of growing children, skeletal manifestations develop from a continued production of bone matrix and epiphyseal cartilage matrix that fails to mineralize properly. A deficiency of sunlight or vitamin D or a lack of response to vitamin D produces this lack of mineralization. In the absence of vitamin D the intestinal tract mucosa does not absorb calcium and phosphorus normally. In this country lack of vitamin D intake combined with lack of exposure to sunlight occurs only rarely and in lower economic groups. Patients with fat absorption disorders (celiac disease, sprue, and obstructive jaundice) lose vitamin D in the stool.

Children with rickets are restless and irritable. Their legs bow. The long bone metaphyses enlarge (trumpeting), the frontal and parietal bones protrude (craniotabes), costochondral junctions enlarge (rosary of rickets), the ribs sink in at the attachment of the diaphragm (Harrison's grooves), the pelvis collapses inward, and the spine curves. X-ray examination reveals a wide, cupped metaphysis, a wide, irregular epiphyseal plate, an irregular hazy zone of provisional calcification, and bowing of the long weight-bearing bones. Serum phosphorus decreases, serum calcium remains normal, and serum alkaline phosphatase increases. Urine calcium decreases, and phosphorus remains normal or increases.

Vitamin D–deficient children heal rickets in 3 or 4 weeks if they take 3000 to 6000 units of vitamin D daily. If they are positioned properly during the active stage of the disease, they will not deform soft bones. The surgeon corrects severe, persistent deformities by osteotomy.

Vitamin D–Resistant Rickets

In some children active rickets fails to respond to the usual doses of vitamin D. No one knows the exact cause of this disorder, which is often familial. An affected child often requires 10,000 to 1,000,000 units of vitamin D for treatment and 3000 to 500,000 units for maintenance. The physician should use 24-hour urine calcium studies to determine the correct dosage of vitamin D.

Renal Rickets

Patients who lose phosphorus or calcium because of renal defects frequently acquire rickets. Defective kidney tubules lose protein. If the glomeruli are defective, the patient frequently retains urea and sometimes becomes acidotic. The prognosis is not good in renal rickets. The physician must treat the associated defects.

Osteomalacia

Osteomalacia, the adult counterpart of rickets, is characterized by increased bone matrix and lack of mineralization. The bones soften and bend. In this country physicians rarely see this disorder on a vitamin D–deficiency basis. Steatorrhea or renal disease most frequently causes osteomalacia. Patients complain of weakness and deformity. Their bones fracture easily. Radiographs reveal a decrease in bone density, deformities, and Looser's zones (a fracture line surrounded by relatively dense bone). Serum and urine changes are similar to those in rickets. The physician must correct the underlying defect and use orthopedic measures to correct deformities.

Scurvy

Vitamin C deficiency is uncommon. Patients with scurvy do not produce normal connective tissue. Increased capillary fragility produces painful subperiosteal hemorrhage with resultant pseudoparalysis. Radiographs reveal osteoporosis produced by a lack of bone matrix. The zone of provisional calcification increases; a lytic zone (scorbutic band) crosses the metaphysis; a dense ring of bone surrounds the epiphysis; spurs form at metaphyseal edges; and periosteal new bone is produced. Occasionally an epiphysis separates from the metaphysis. Ascorbic acid, 100 to 120 mg daily, corrects this disorder.

Hyperparathyroidism (See Chapter 14)

Parathyroid hormone acts on kidney and bone to maintain normal serum calcium and phosphorus levels. Parathyroid adenoma or parathyroid hyperplasia produces hyperparathroidism most frequently in women 25 to 45 years of age. The following cause symptoms in hyperparathyroidism: increased serum calcium (lethargy, weakness, anorexia, constipation); bone destruction (pain or fractures), and calcium increase in the urine (renal stones, renal insufficiency).

Serum phosphorus decreases, serum calcium increases, and serum alkaline phosphatase increases. Urinary phosphorus and calcium increase. Radiographically, bones demineralize, the cortex thins, the lamina dura of the teeth disappears, subperiosteal bone of the midphalanx of the fingers is resorbed, and the outer table of the skull thins and becomes indistinct. "Brown tumors" composed of fibrous connective tissue, hemorrhage, and giant cells appear as bone cysts.

After the offending parathyroid glands has been removed, the surgeon must observe the patient carefully for postoperative tetany and must treat it promptly.

Osteoporosis

In a patient with osteoporosis, the total mass of bone matrix and mineral decreases. Osteoporosis can have a number of causes:

Disuse—normal stress is needed to prevent loss of bone mass
Endocrine disorders
    Cushing's disease—increased steroids and increased catabolism
    Postmenopausal—decreased stress and decreased sex hormones
    Hyperthyroidism
    Acromegaly
Scurvy
Protein deficiency caused by decreased intake or excessive loss
Multiple myeloma and carcinomatosis
Idiopathic, senile, or postmenopausal states

No one knows exactly why the bone mass decreases. Most patients remain in the idiopathic group. Osteoporosis is most common in women over 60 in whom diet, disuse, and endocrine changes probably play a role.

The patients complain of bone pain and tenderness. Vertebral bodies and femoral necks frequently break. Calcium, phosphorus, and alkaline phosphatase usually remain normal. Some patients are in negative nitrogen and calcium balance. X-ray studies disclose relatively radiolucent bone, thin cortices, and widened medullary canals. The vertebral bodies often collapse. Vertebral subchondral cortices curve, and vertebral bodies become biconcave.

Physicians diagnose idiopathic osteoporosis by excluding other disorders that have similar radiographic findings (osteomalacia, multiple myeloma, hyperparathyroidism, metastatic malignancies, Cushing's disease, and hyperthyroidism). Since one cannot determine the cause in most instances, treatment is difficult. The patient should consume at least one quart of milk and 70 g of protein each day. In addition to this regimen, some physicians add vitamin D, 5000 units a day for the first 3 months and then 1000 units a day. The patient remains as active as possible. Estrogens may be of value in certain patients. Some physicians use sodium fluoride to try to increase bone deposition. Physical therapy and spine supports sometimes provide symptomatic relief.

Gout

In gout, a metabolic disorder, the body produces excessive uric acid. Blood uric acid increases. Urate crystals form deposits (tophi) in joints and para-articular structures. These crystals destroy the joint surface and erode underlying bone. During an acute attack, patients complain of severe pain in a joint or bursa. Uricosuric agents alleviate symptoms during the acute episode. Patients then use drugs to maintain a decrease in the blood uric acid. In some patients with gout, orthopedists excise tophi and perform arthroplasties or arthrodeses on destroyed joints.

34

Hand Surgery

David W. Furnas
Adrian E. Flatt
Ivan M. Turpin

Man's hands have allowed him to put human thought into action, exerting control over his environment. Sensation in the hand (an organ containing one fourth of all pacinian [touch] corpuscles of the body) is the only sense among five in which man is clearly superior to animals. Pictures gained from earliest tactile and kinesthetic activities of the hand lay the groundwork for one's self-image and feelings of individuality. The hand also serves as a means of expression.

Thus afflictions of the hand are of great significance to the patient and his physician; moreover, they are very common: approximately one third of all industrial accidents and one third of injuries seen in the emergency departments of metropolitan hospitals involve the hand.

NORMAL ARCHITECTURE

Everyday use of the hand demands a structure that has stability and power combined with mobility, dexterity, and precision. Stability is furnished by the rigid central pillar of the hand (Fig. 34-1), formed by the firmly united carpal bones and the second and third metacarpal bones. Around this central pillar, in the manner of twin loading booms, rotate the two mobile units of the hand: the extremely mobile first metacarpal invested with thenar structures and the less mobile fourth and fifth metacarpals invested with hypothenar structures.

The digits with their two or three joints represent other highly mobile units. The metacarpophalangeal joints of the fingers have lateral mobility when they are extended, but lateral stability when they are flexed into grasp (where stability is required) because of the arrangement of their collateral ligaments (Fig. 34-2). All the interphalageneal joints have lateral stability throughout flexion and extension.

Three arches are formed by these units of the hand (Fig. 34-3): a proximal transverse arch, which is rigid, a distal transverse arch, which is flexible, and a longitudinal arch (the digital rays), which is rigid proximally and flexible distally.

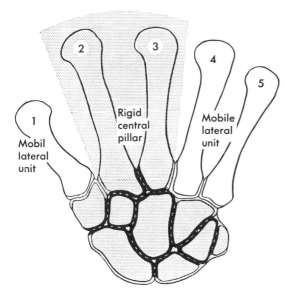

Fig. 34-1. Central pillar and lateral units of hand. Shafts of second and third metacarpals are firmly united to carpal bones, forming stable central pillar. Two lateral units of hand articulate freely with carpal bones and are mobile.

Power to the wrist and hand is supplied by five groups of muscles (Fig. 34-4): two extrinsic (muscle bellies in the forearm) and three intrinsic (muscle bellies in the hand). The muscles are innervated by three nerves: median, radial, and ulnar.

Extrinsic Muscle Groups

The flexor-pronator muscles pronate the hand and flex the wrist and digits. The flexor-pronator group (the three flexors of the wrist, the nine flexors of the digits, and the pronators teres and quadratus) is supplied by the median nerve (except for the ulnar half of the flexor digitorum profundus, which is supplied by the ulnar nerve). The extensor-supinator group supinates the hand and extends the wrist and digits. The extensor-supinator muscles (the three extensors of the wrist, the four common and two proper extensors of the fingers, the two extensors and the long abductor to the thumb, and the supinator) are supplied by the radial nerve.

Intrinsic Muscle Groups

The thenar muscles (short flexor, short abductor, and opposing muscles of the thumb) are supplied by the median nerve, and the hypothenar muscles (abductor, short flexor, and opposing muscles of the little finger) are supplied by the ulnar nerve. These two groups work together to cup the palm and to oppose the thumb to the fingers. The lumbricals, interossei, and adductor pollicis are supplied by the ulnar nerve (except for the first two lumbricals, which are median innervated). They furnish digital adduction-abduction movements, flexion at the metacarpophalangeal joints, and extension at the interphalangeal joints. (The extrinsic flexors are also able to flex the metacarpophalangeal joints, and the extrinsic extensors are also able to extend the interphalangeal joints.) The tendons of the intrinsic muscles in-

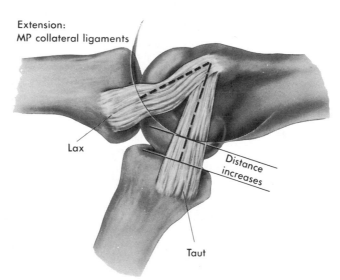

Fig. 34-2. Stability of metacarpophalangeal (MP) joints. In flexion, collateral ligaments are placed under tension because of eccentric profile and lateral bulges of metacarpal head; this prevents lateral motion of joints. In extension, ligaments are flaccid, and lateral movements are possible. Position of flexion is usually chosen when immobilizing this joint, to prevent shortening of ligament and deformity.

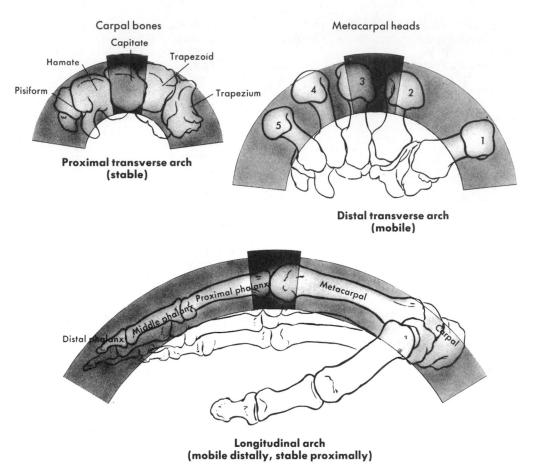

Fig. 34-3. Arches of hand. Stable, immobile proximal transverse arch is composed of firmly knit carpal bones. Mobile distal transverse arch is made up of metacarpal heads and intervening tissues. Longitudinal arches, which are extremely mobile distally and stable proximally, are made up of digital rays.

terweave with the tendons and aponeuroses of the extrinsic muscles, forming a coordinated network (Fig. 34-5). This system of motors, superbly linked with input from the eyes and the sensory organs of the hand, lends precision and dexterity to movements of the hand.

CLINICAL ASSESSMENT OF THE HAND
History

Intelligent assessment necessitates understanding the patient, including his personality, occupation, hobbies, and life expectations. Specific history relating to the hand should generate a clear understanding and documentation of the duration, nature, and onset of the complaint, as well as the patient's definition of his disability. Causes of hand disability arising proximally in the upper limb or higher, neurologically, should be routinely excluded.

Physical Examination

As a part of hand examination, consider the entire upper limb and a comparison of right and left sides at a minimum. Look at, feel, and move the hand to assess the five essential elements of function: cover, mobility, stability, sensibility, and circulation. Initially look for abnormal postures. These occur because of an imbalance of forces with loss, exaggeration, or disruption of normal arches. Common patterns of pathologic postures include claw deformity (intrinsic minus hand); (Fig. 34-6), dropped wrist and hand (Fig. 34-7), and intrinsic plus hand (Fig. 34-8). Assessing cover involves checking the skin for unstable scars or contractures and its color, temperature, and mobility as well. Active and passive mobility must be determined. During active motion, ask the patient to put his wrist through a full range of motion, to extend the wrist and fingers completely, and then to flex all the digits fully. The normal thumb can describe a cone, oppose, flex, and extend, as well as pinch and grasp (Fig. 34-9).

Active and passive motion must be compared and documented quantitatively, and any discrepancies between the two must be explained. Loss of passive motion is associated with a corresponding loss of active motion, but the converse does not hold. Before active motion can occur, any encumbrances of normal passive mobility such as joint, tendon, and skin contractures or

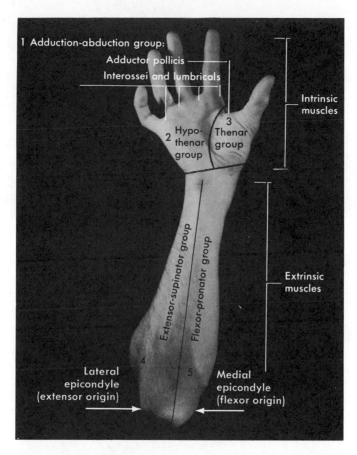

Fig. 34-4. Muscle power to hand. Three groups of intrinsic muscles: *1* and *2* supplied by *ulnar nerve* and *3* supplied by *median nerve*. Two groups of extrinsic muscles: *4* supplied by *radial nerve* and *5* supplied by median nerve and *ulnar half of flexor digitorum profundus* supplied by ulnar nerve.

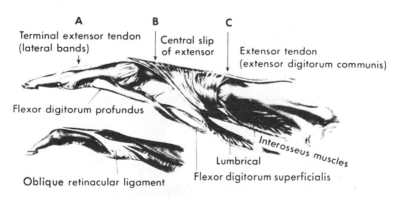

Fig. 34-5. Intrinsic and extrinsic networks for flexion and extension of fingers. Distal interphalangeal joint is flexed by *flexor digitorum profundus;* proximal interphalangeal joint is flexed by *flexor digitorum superficialis* (plus transmitted increment from *flexor digitorum profundus*); metacarpophalangeal joint is flexed by *interosseus muscles* through their direct osseous insertions and through their insertions into wings of dorsal aponeurosis. (This flexion force is augmented by transmitted increment from *flexor digitorum profundus* and *flexor digitorum superficialis.*) Distal interphalangeal joint is extended through insertion of lateral bands of dorsal aponeurosis, powered by extrinsic extensors and intrinsics (*interossei* and *lumbricals*) (either or both may act); proximal interphalangeal joint is extended by central slip of dorsal aponeurosis, powered in same way as distal phalanx; metacarpophalangeal joint is extended by extrinsic extensor tendons alone, acting through dorsal aponeurosis. *Oblique retinacular ligaments* assist in coordination of these movements. For injuries at levels *A, B,* and *C,* see Fig. 34-18.

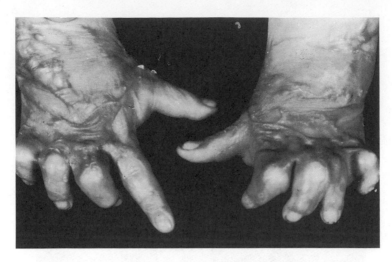

Fig. 34-6. *"Intrinsic-minus"* deformity or clawhand. Distal transverse arches are flattened. Metacarpophalangeal joints are hyperextended, proximal interphalangeal joints are hyperflexed (distal interphalangeal joints are sometimes flexed, sometimes hyperextended), thumb is held parallel to palm. Cause in this patient is scarring and skin destruction from scald of dorsum of hands, but in others paralysis of intrinsic muscles will result in same posture. (See Fig. 34-24.)

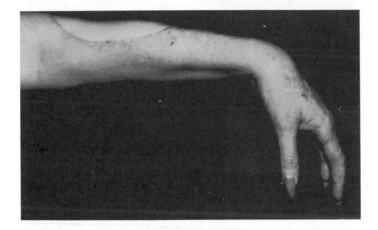

Fig. 34-7. *Wristdrop.* Ability to extend wrist against gravity is lost because of denervation of extensor-supinator group of muscles from resection of basal cell carcinoma of forearm that invaded *radial nerve*. Notice pale semicircle of skin, which is flap covering resected area.

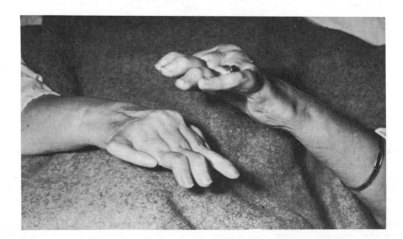

Fig. 34-8. *"Intrinsic-plus"* deformity. Arches are exaggerated. Metacarpophalangeal joints are flexed, and interphalangeal joints are in "swan-neck" position (proximal interphalangeal joint hyperextended [recurvatum], distal interphalangeal joint locked in flexion. Sometimes both interphalangeal joints are extended (accoucheur's hand).

(From Flatt, A.E.: The care of the rheumatoid hand, ed. 3, St. Louis, 1974, The C.V. Mosby Co.)

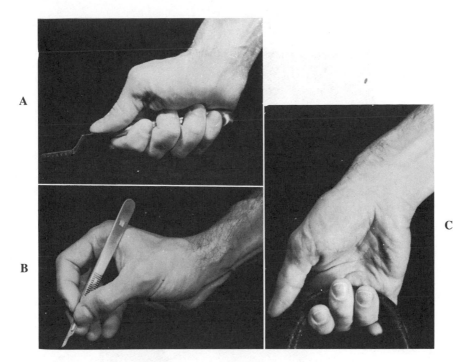

Fig. 34-9. A, Power grip. Object is clamped securely between flexed fingers and palm, counterpressure being applied by thumb. **B,** Precision grip (or "handling"). Object is pinched between flexor pads of opposing thumb and fingers. **C,** Hook grip. Only fingers are used, as a primitive hook.

adhesions must be eliminated. Stability requires normal functional integrity of the bones and joints of the hand. Disturbances of this integrity are particularly common after trauma, whether recent or remote, and in rheumatoid arthritis. Sensibility is determined by the usual pin and wisp of cotton, two-point discrimination (Fig. 34-10), a pickup test (Fig. 34-11), and stereognosis. Normally two points that are as close together as 2 to 4 mm can be distinguished with the tips and flexor surfaces of the digits, whereas on the dorsal skin two points closer than 10 to 12 mm are interpreted as one. Color and temperature are clues to adequacy of circulation. Normal perfusion requires adequacy of arterial supply, the capillary bed, and venous drainge. Loss of any of these three will compomise viability. Aberrations may be focal, as in an unstable scar or crushed skin, or involve the hand as a whole, as in combined radial and ulnar arterial injuries. Palpation of the pulses, Allen's test (Fig. 34-21), and examination with the Doppler flow detector are useful procedures. Injection with fluorescein and observation with Wood's light shows viable tissue.

Radiographic Examination

Radiography is an integral part of routine hand assessment. Careful examination will guide inquiry to an appropriate area. For example, the whole hand need not be examined if the terminal phalanx of the thumb has been injured, nor is it diagnostically accurate to assess the scaphoid without special scaphoid views. In short, requesting appropriate films reduces needless exposures.

PRINCIPLES OF MANAGEMENT OF HAND PROBLEMS

Restoration of grasp (both power and precision), fine tactile sense, dexterity, and normal appearance are the sometimes elusive goals of surgery of the hand. These are achieved by restoring cover and stability, mobility, sensibility, and circulation to the hand. Skin grafts and pedicles restore missing or contracted skin cover. Fracture fixation, bone grafts, and joint fusions may be required for bone and joint stability. Tendon repairs, grafts, or transfers restore transmission of power for active mobility. Loss of passive mobility is best managed conservatively. Motor nerve deficits may be corrected by nerve repairs, nerve grafts, or tendon transfers. Repairs or grafts of sensory nerves (or occasionally transferring sensory island flaps) may provide some restoration of functional sensibility. Finally, vascular repair may be essential.

Mobilization is a necessary element in managing accidental or surgical trauma. The hand reacts badly to prolonged immobilization, worse to swelling, and worst of all to both. Elevation and earliest feasible motion are immutable priorities.

CONGENITAL DEFORMITIES

Congenital deformities of the hand are relatively common and present a diverse array and range of disorders. Polydactyly, supernumerary digits, is the most common, occurring in 0.5% of live births. It is frequently bilateral and commonly the extra digit is the ulnarmost or radialmost of the hand.

Syndactyly (Fig. 34-12), failure of digits to separate

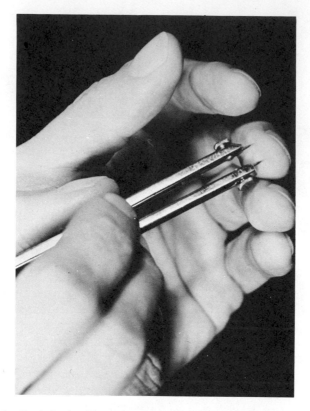

Fig. 34-10. *Two-point discrimination.* Two points are simultaneously pressed against skin; distance between points is varied to determine narrowest spread that can be distinguish as two separate points rather than one. Fingertips can usually distinguish two points spread as little as 2 to 4 mm. Proximal dorsal part of digit can only distinguish two points if spread is 10 mm. Two-point discrimination is one of the best means of detecting partial nerve injuries and in following nerve repairs.

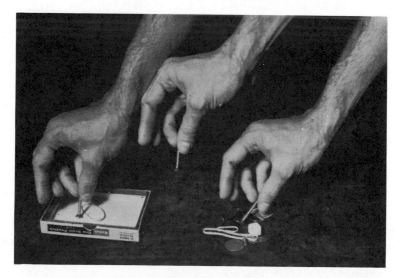

Fig. 34-11. *Moberg's "pickup" test.* Ask patient to pick up and place a number of small objects at top speed. This serves to reveal deficiencies in critical sensation and fine coordination that might be missed with cruder test. Incomplete return of median sensation indicated by patient's reference of ulnar-innervated ring finger.

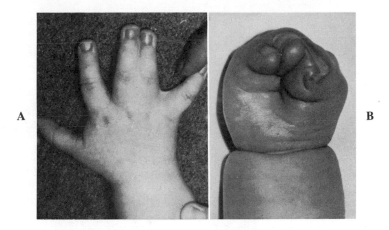

Fig. 34-12. Syndactyly. **A,** Simple syndactyly of ring and long fingers. **B,** Complex syndactyly causing mittenlike hand in patient with acrocephalosyndactyly, or Apert's syndrome.

from one another, is the second most common hand anomaly, occurring in 0.2% of live births. The long and ring fingers are the most commonly adherent, often bilaterally. Syndactyly ranges in complexity from a single slight obliterated web space to complete fusion of all the digits into a tight mitten.

Brachydactyly (shortened fingers), symphalangia (end-to-end fusion of phalangeal bones), ectrodactyly (absense of a part of one or more digits), and clinodactyly (lateral deviation of the fingers) are some of the less common congenital disorders.

In most instances the safest guiding principle is early referral to a surgeon with special interest in this field. Early operative treatment is mandatory if there is any distortion of growth or progression of deformity.

ACQUIRED DISORDERS
Traumatic (Table 34-1)
Laceration

Skin lacerations or wounds may be tidy or untidy. The tidy wound has clean incised margins that heal promptly after simple cleansing and closure. It is, however, essential to maintain a high index of suspicion of hidden problems. Severed tendons, nerves, arteries, and buried splinters of glass or metal can be present in the most innocent-looking wounds (Fig. 34-13). Untidy wounds are ragged, crushed, or torn at the margins and are more widely damaged in the depths. Missing or nonviable skin must be replaced. Dirt, foreign material, and devitalized tissue must be debrided. Complications of infection, excessive swelling, and necrosis are more likely to occur in an untidy wound.

No wound, tidy or untidy, should ever be considered for closure until the full extent of the injury is identified. If any uncertainty exists, formal exploration is mandatory.

Flexor tendon. The diagnosis of digital flexor tendon severance is confirmed by loss of the position of rest (Fig. 34-14) and the inability to perform the test for superficialis action (Fig. 34-15) or the test for profundus action (Fig. 34-16). If the patient performs

Table 34-1. Common Injuries of the Integument and Digits

Injury	Treatment	Injury	Treatment
Laceration	Cleansing, irrigation, and simple surgical closure	Partial amputation	Replace severed part if circulation appears adequate
Flaplike laceration	Suture into place if viable		Repair vessels microsurgically if needed
	If not viable, remove skin and close defect directly or with skin graft	Complete amputation	Microvascular replant if digit is important
Amputated skin	Defat the skin and replace as a skin graft, or		Closure with preservation of length
	take grafts from elsewhere	Crushed fingertip	Meticulous reassembly using magnification
Digital pulp	Cross finger flap, palmar flap, triangular island flaps, or skin graft	Avulsion of nail or nail bed	Trim nail and replace as a splint to wound; carefully repair nail bed
Degloving injury (skin peeled back from digit as if it were a glove, e.g., ring caught in machinery)	Repair injured vessels with vein grafts and close skin, or amputate ring finger or unimportant digit, or replace degloved skin with flap		Replace any missing areas of nail bed with split skin graft
		Subungual hematoma	Perforate overlying nail with heated paper clip or needle and evacuate hematoma

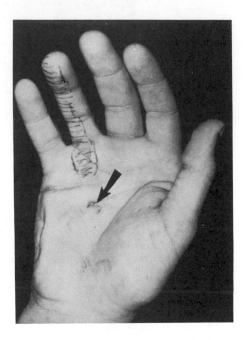

Fig. 34-13. "Tidy" injury of hand. This clean, penetrating wound of palm was caused by broken thermometer.Despite its innocuous appearance, examination revealed area of anesthesia (crosshatches in ink on ring finger), inability to abduct-adduct fingers, and positive Froment's sign (Fig. 34-20, *B*). Transection of motor branch of ulnar nerve, transection of part of sensory branch of ulnar nerve, transection of deep palmar arterial arch, and partial transection of flexor digitorum profundus tendon to ring finger were found at operation.

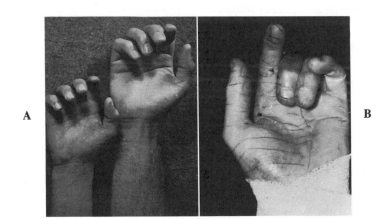

A   B

Fig. 34-14. *Position of rest.* **A,** Normal position of rest. With hand lying palm upward on flat surface, muscle tone of flexors causes slight flexion of thumb and orderly gradation of flexion of fingers, which increases from index to little finger. **B,** *Loss of position of rest.* Razor slash of flexor compartment of wrist has caused loss of position of rest of thumb and index finger because of complete severance of associated flexor tendons; small strand of intact profundus tendon prevents complete loss of position of rest in little finger; all sublimis tendons were divided, as median nerve and radial artery were; areas of sensory loss from transection of median nerve are crosshatched with inked lines; notice that *much of damage to wrist is readily assessed without removal of dressings.*
(**A,** From Flatt, A.E.: The care of minor hand injuries, ed. 4, St. Louis, 1979, The C.V. Mosby Co.)

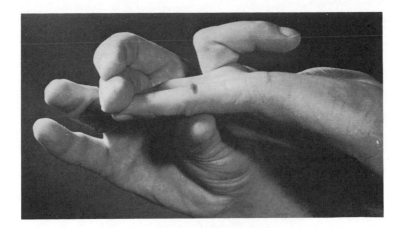

Fig. 34-15. Test for *flexor superficialis* action. Flexor digitorum profundus muscles and tendons form more or less solid sheet in forearm, dividing only quite distally into separate tendons that have little or no independence of action, i.e., the four tendons tend to act as one unit. Therefore, if three of the four digits are forcefully held in extension, flexor digitorum profundus to remaining digit is carried into extended position with its fellows and is unable to act as flexor. However, flexor digitorum superficialis, which has distinct and independent muscle belly for each of the four tendons, can still act as flexor; flexion takes place only at proximal interphalangeal joint, not at distal interphalangeal joint. Flexor digitorum superficialis to long finger shows normal function in photograph.
(From Flatt, A. E.: The care of minor hand injuries, ed. 4, St. Louis, 1979, The C.V. Mosby Co.)

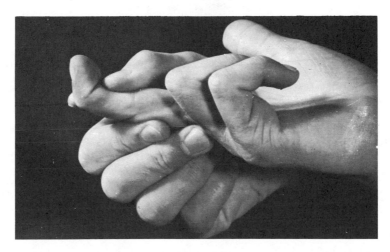

Fig. 34-16. Test for *flexor digitorum profundus* action. Finger is held forcefully in passive extension at metacarpophalangeal and proximal interphalangeal joints. Ability to flex distal interphalangeal joint indicates normal action of flexor digitorum profundus.
(From Flatt, A.E.: The care of minor hand injuries, ed. 4, St. Louis, 1979, The C.V. Mosby Co.)

these tests but shows pain and weakness, suspect partial division of the tendon.

The level of severance determines the therapeutic approach. Tendons divided distal to "no man's land" (where the flexor digitorum profundus and -superficialis cross through the fibrous digital sheath; Fig. 34-17) may have their proximal end advanced and sutured into the distal phalanx. Tendons severed proximally to no-man's land are anastomosed immediately with nonabsorbable suture material.

Flexor tendon injuries in no-man's-land yield noto-

riously poor results in anything but optimal circumstances. If divided tendons are sutured primarily, the exuberant fibroblastic outgrowth causes dense adherence between the tendon and sheath with loss of function. The best course of action for the primary physician is to clean the wound, close the skin, and send the patient promptly to an experienced hand surgeon. The surgeon may choose to perform immediate repair of one or both tendons. If the circumstances are less than ideal, the surgeon will postpone definitive surgery and instruct the patient in exercises to maintain joint sup-

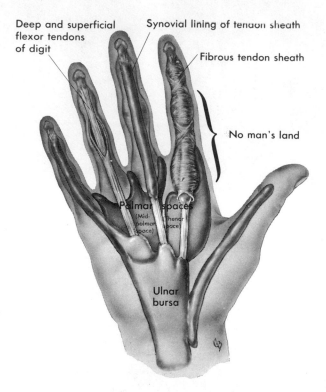

Fig. 34-17. *No man's land:* here the two flexor tendons of each finger of right hand are tightly enclosed in synovium-lined fibrous sheath made up of unyielding cruciate and annular ligaments; tendon anastomoses in this region tend to fail because of massive adherence to surrounding structures. *Palmar spaces:* these two fascial clefts are located behind digital flexor tendons; midpalmar space is separated from thenar space by septum that connects bursa or flexor tendons (ulnar bursa) to third metacarpal bone.

Table 34-2. Extensor Tendon Injuries

Entity	Mechanisms and level of severance	Treatment
Drop finger (Fig. 34-18, *D*; injury at level *C*, Fig. 34-5)	Laceration or rupture of extensor tendon on dorsum of hand or wrist or at metacarpophalangeal joint	Direct suture
Boutonnière deformity (develops several weeks after injury; Fig. 34-18, *B* and *C*; injury at level *B*, Fig. 34-5)	Laceration, rupture, or erosion of extensor tendon at proximal phalanx or proximal interphalangeal joint	Immobilization in extension with cast extending to forearm for 3 weeks; if chip fracture present, direct suture; late treatment requires complex operation
Mallet finger (or baseball finger) (Fig. 34-18, *A*; injury at level *A*, Fig. 34-5)	Avulsion or laceration of insertion of tendon into distal phalanx (fragment of distal phalanx frequently avulsed with tendon insertion)	Immobilize in plaster with distal interphalangeal joint in hyperextension and proximal interphalangeal joint in flexion; if wound is open, suture tendon ends and place intramedullary wire through distal interphalangeal joint

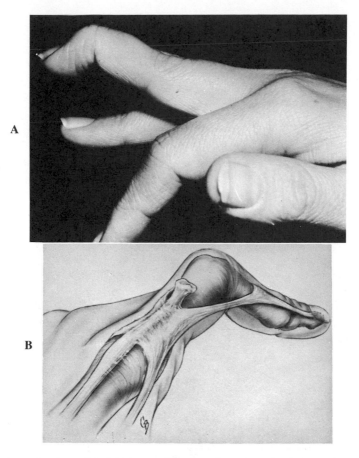

Fig. 34-18. A, *Mallet finger* (baseball finger): disruption of insertion of extensor tendon at distal phalanx. (Injury near level **A,** Fig. 34-5.) **B** and **C,** *Boutonnière deformity:* after disruption of central slip of the extensor tendon where it inserts on middle phalanx, lateral bands of extensor apparatus tend to migrate in palmar direction causing flexion of proximal interphalangeal joint and extension of distal interphalangeal joint. (Injury near level **B,** Fig. 34-5) **D,** *Drop finger:* long, ring, and little fingers cannot be extended against gravity (see level *C* of Fig. 34-5) because of tendon rupture at wrist; patient has rheumatoid disease and attrition of tendons on bony projection. (Injury proximal to level *C,* Fig. 34-5.)   *Continued.*

pleness. A silicon rubber rod may be placed to maintain a patent tendon sheath. When reaction to the initial jury has subsided sufficiently (weeks or months later), elective tendon grafting can be carried out.

In flexor tendon injuries of the wrist (Fig. 34-14, *B*) it is best to assume injuries to major nerves and arteries. If this is confirmed clinically, hemorrhage should be controlled by pressure and the patient should be transported to a surgeon competent to perform multiple nerve, artery, and tendon repairs. Circumstances such as transport over a distance may demand exploration and ligation of bleeders, irrigation of the wound, and closure of the skin. *Accurate repair* of tendons and nerves is more important than immediate repair.

Extensor tendon. The extensor tendons are flat, fine structures that are interwoven with tendons of the intrinsic muscles forming the intricate extensor aponeuroses. They do not hold sutures well, and surgical restoration is frequently difficult. Diagnostically, the most frequent error is overlooking closed injuries to this extensor apparatus. The most common closed extensor in-

juries (cited in Table 34-2) must be excluded when assessing a "sprained finger."

The boutonnière deformity (Fig. 34-18, *B*) is caused by loss of restraint of the lateral bands of the extensor mechanism. After the central slip has been divided, these lateral bands become attenuated and migrate volarward, allowing the proximal interphalangeal joint to protrude dorsally as if through a buttonhole. Extensor tendons are prone to attrition injuries. Drop fingers (Fig. 34-18, *D*) is seen in rheumatoid arthritis when slips of the extensor digitorum communis rupture because of tendon disease or erosion from a rough bony prominence at the level of the distal radius and ulna. Drummer's palsy, or drop thumb, is caused by rupture associated with avascular necrosis of the extensor pollicis longus near the lower end of the radius. Open disruption of an extensor tendon is treated by direct suture unless delay, contamination, or other circumstances contraindicate primary repair. Immobilization for 4 to 5 weeks is customary after suture of extensor tendons, whether open or closed.

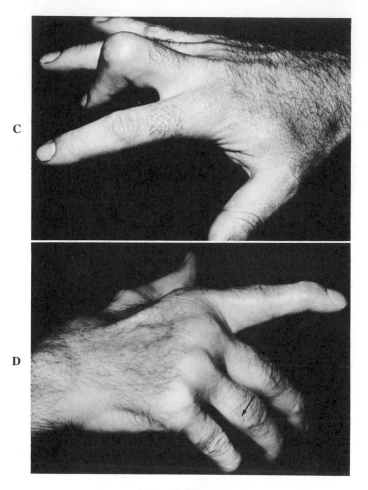

C

D

Fig. 34-18, cont'd.

Nerve injuries. Compulsive care must be taken to rule out nerve injuries in hand lacerations. For example, a child falling with outstretched hand onto broken glass must be assumed to have significant nerve injury. This assumption is essential because of the difficult and frustrating task of attempting accurate clinical asessment of a frightened, agitated child.

If the median nerve is divided (Fig. 34-14, *B*), the hand is "blinded" from loss of critical sensibility in the most important parts of the thumb and index, long, and ring fingers, and motor power is lost in the thenar muscles. Ulnar nerve transection cripples the greater part of the intrinsic musculature, depriving the hand of dexterity; it also numbs sensation to the ulnar side of the fourth and the entire fifth digit. Accurate testing of the motor and sensory branches of these nerves is mandatory in any hand injury. Even an inconspicuous nick can mark the entry point of glass or steel slivers that may have selectively divided a significant sensory or motor branch (Fig. 34-13).

In addition to the baseline assessment outlined earlier, the characteristic silky, dry texture is caused by disrupted sympathetic fibers that accompany sensory nerve injury. The most reliable tests for isolated motor function of the median nerve in the hand are the abductor brevis test and the opponens pollicis test (Fig. 34-19). For motor function of the ulnar nerve (Fig. 34-20, *A*) the most reliable test is adduction and abduction of the long finger. Froment's sign (Fig. 34-20, *B*) is useful in detection of paralysis of the adductor pollicis.

Distal nerve transections, transections of pure motor or sensory nerves, and nerve transections in children have the best prognosis after surgical repair. Immediate repair of cleanly cut nerve ends gives superior results to delayed repair. If a branch 1 mm or smaller in diameter is divided, it can be anastamosed accurately by use of an operating microscope or loupes.

Vessel injuries. The hand can usually survive with only one of its two major arteries intact and occasionally with neither. However, arterial anastomosis or grafts should be carried out if the blood supply is in question. Clinically, the Allen test (Fig. 34-21) is useful in determining patency of the radial or ulnar arteries. Operatively, viability is best assessed by bright red bleeding occurring at freshly cut edges of muscle or skin. If a tourniquet is used, one may assess viability by the "blush test" (i.e., noting the color that develops

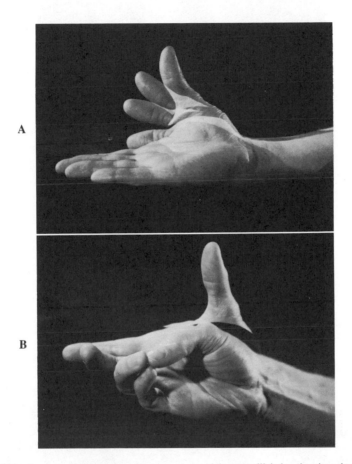

Fig. 34-19. Tests for motor function of median nerve. **A,** Abductor pollicis brevis raises thumb forward, perpendicular to plane of palm; ability to perform this movement against resistance is best single test of median nerve function. **B,** Opponens pollicis sweeps abducted thumb across palm so that flexor pad of thumb meets flexor pad of ring or little finger face-to-face and parallel.

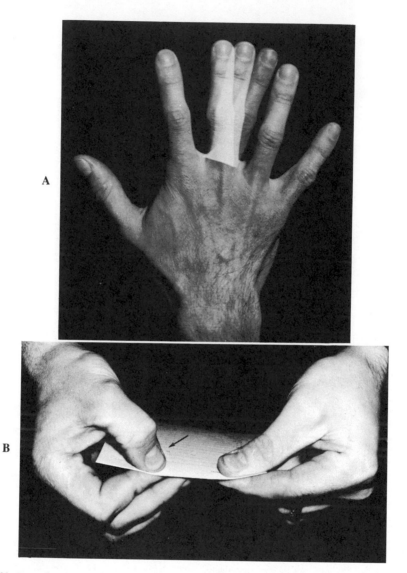

Fig. 34-20. Tests for motor function of ulnar nerve. **A,** Independent adduction-abduction of fingers, against resistance, and adduction of thumb with hand extended on flat surface demonstrates action of interossei and adductor-pollicis muscles, which are supplied by ulnar nerve; each muscle should be tested separately for localization of nerve damage. **B,** Froment's sign. Patient pinches piece of paper forcefully; examiner then pulls paper away, or patient pulls paper taut with both hands as if to tear it; to prevent paper from slipping away from weak adductor pollicis, patient must bring flexor pollicis longus into play causing flexion of interphalangeal joint of thumb; patient's right thumb shows Froment's sign because of transection of motor branch of ulnar nerve (same patient as shown in Fig. 34-13).

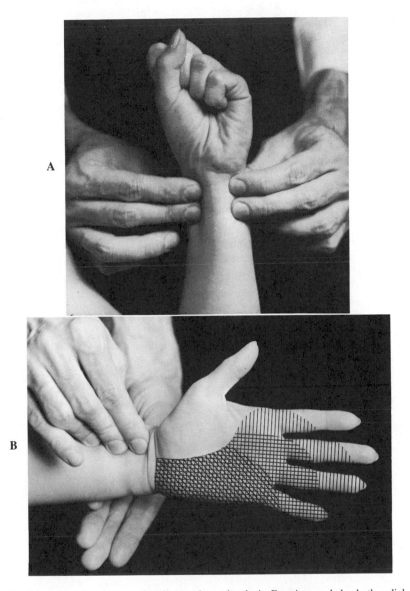

Fig. 34-21. Allen's test for patency of major arteries to hand. **A,** Examiner occludes both radial and ulnar arteries with his fingertips while patient holds his hand aloft and milks out any residual blood by repeatedly flexing digits into tight fist and extending them; hand is then lowered to dependent position, with arteries still occluded by digital pressure and digits extended. **B,** Artery in question is then released; rapid, bright, pink blush beginning near point of release signifies patent artery; slow or absent blush denotes occlusion or absence of artery. If blush does not occur after releasing one artery, remaining artery is released after pause of 1 to 2 minutes; patency of second artery is demonstrated by blush. Digital Allen's test uses same means for testing digital arteries.

in the questionable area after the tourniquet is released). The fluorescein test is useful.

Replantation. In the replantation of amputated digits the key to success is anastomosis of at least two veins and one artery. A specialty team using appropriate magnification and instruments can usually achieve a 90% or better survival rate (Fig. 34-22). Currently accepted indications for replantation include multiple digit amputations, thumb amputations, hand and palm amputations, and amputations in children. Single digits are replanted on a case-by-case basis, especially if distal to the flexor digitorum superficialis tendon insertion.

Fractures and dislocations

Fractures of the phalanges and metacarpals are the most common of all fractures. If accompanied by no deformity or displacement, they heal quickly with simple immobilization.

Deformity occurs when the fracture creates a disruption in the normal linkage system of the hand. The long bones of the hand constitute a delicate system of levers linked by mobile joints and controlled in space by the balanced pull of the flexor and extensor tendons. With disruption of a long bone a new "joint" is introduced into the system. Since no further controls have been added, the system buckles.

Deformity is tolerated very poorly in the hand, particularly in the proximal and middle phalanges and least of all in the joints. One must always look for rotational deformity, which is confirmed if the nail beds are not parallel or if the fingers tend to overlap in flexion (Fig. 34-23).

In treating deformity caused by fresh fractures one must be sure that reduction is obtained and maintained. If any uncertainty exists, open reduction and internal fixation are warranted.

Immobilization should be continued until there is clinical and radiographic evidence of union. For simple fractures 3 weeks often suffices; however, transverse fractures of phalangeal or metacarpal shafts often require 5 or 6 weeks. There is no justification for including the arm and shoulder in the immobilization. The

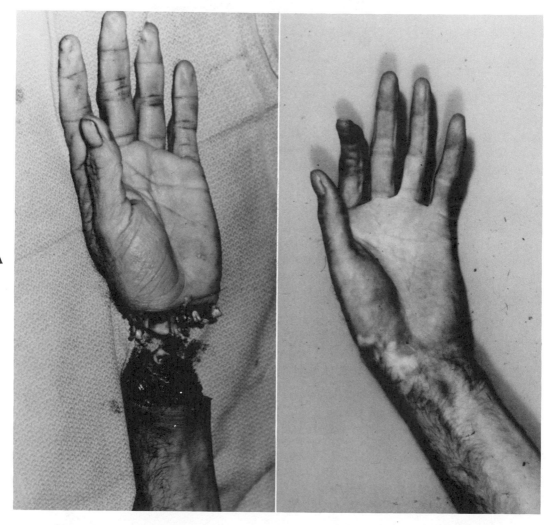

A

B

Fig. 34-22. A, Hand amputation. **B,** Successful replantation can usually be achieved in 90% of cases.

patient must faithfully exercise the remainder of the upper limb to prevent disuse atrophy.

Carpus. The most common carpal fracture is of the scaphoid. Classically a fall on the outstretched hand with tenderness in the anatomic snuffbox alerts the examiner to this injury. Even if radiographic findings are negative (including scaphoid views), immobilization is mandatory for at least 2 weeks and may be discontinued only if repeat films and clinical examination are negative at that time. It is essential to look very closely for evidence of displacement of scaphoid fractures, which may indicate concomitant soft tissue injury and

the necessity for open reduction and internal fixation. Furthermore, the possibility of avascular necrosis of the proximal pole of the scaphoid should be considered. It is wise to forewarn the patient of this possibility at the commencement of treatment. At times the scaphoid can heal very slowly and occasionally many months of immobilization are required to gain satisfactory union and function.

The lunate is the most commonly dislocated carpal bone. It usually dislocates in a *palmar* direction and may compress the median nerve in that position. Reduction can usually be accomplished by closed means

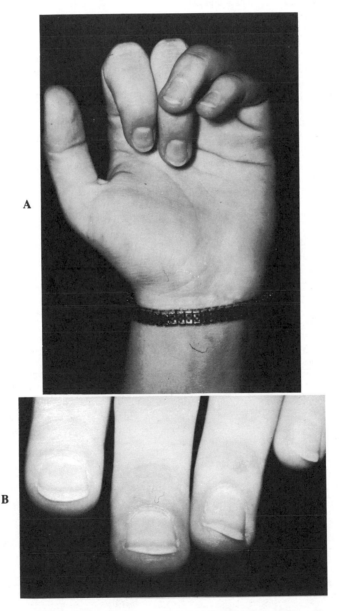

Fig. 34-23. "Scissoring" of fingers. **A,** Fingers overlap when flexed because of poor alignment and rotational malunion from fractures of index and ring proximal phalanges. **B,** Clue to malalignment is nonparallel fingernails.

but there is a risk of subsequent avascular necrosis. Follow-up radiographs are necessary to rule out this complication.

Metacarpus. Bennett's fracture-dislocation is a dislocation of the thumb carpometacarpal joint associated with a fracture of the metacarpal base extending into the joint, with resultant subluxation or disclocation. Skeletal fixation is generally required to maintain reduction.

The most common fracture of the remaining metacarpals is the "boxer's fracture" of the fifth metacarpal, commonly resulting from a fistfight. Fractures of the shaft of the long and ring metacarpals tend to be more stable than those of the border digits.

As a rule, dislocations of the metacarpophalangeal joints are easily reduced and maintained unless a phalangeal or metacarpal head is trapped in a "buttonhole" rent in the joint capsule. In the latter circumstance open reduction of the dislocation is required.

Phalanges. Displaced fractures of the proximal and middle phalanges of an articular surface often require open reduction and internal fixation. Displaced fractures of the distal phalanx are usually caused by crush injury and are adequately managed by simple immobilization after appropriate soft-tissue management. The fingernail should not be thoughtlessly discarded in these crush injuries, for it often serves as an excellent biological splint.

In a patient with a history of trauma and a swollen, tender digit but without any fracture on radiographs, exclusion of significant soft tissue injury is essential. The extensor apparatus and the collateral ligaments of either the interphalangeal or the metacarpophalangeal joints of the thumb are particularly prone to traumatic disruption.

Burns

Burns of the exposed and vulnerable dorsum of the hand most commonly result from open flames in adults or scalds in children. Suppleness and extensibility of the dorsal skin are destroyed by edema and inflammation and result in trouble-some scar tissue formation in deep second-degree and third-degree burns. The resultant claw deformity (Fig. 34-6) is extremely disabling. Therefore in burns of this depth assiduous physical therapy should begin as soon as possible. The joints should move through a full range of motion many times daily. Between exercise periods, plaster or dynamic splints will prevent clawing (Fig. 34-24). If these methods fail or are likely to, internal splinting with Kirschner wires immobilizing the proximal interphalangeal joints in slight flexion may be necessary.

Burns of the palmar surface are most often seen in children who have grasped hot objects. For deep second- and third-degree burns skin grafts may be required to prevent flexion deformities.

Electrical burns of the hand usually result from contact of the hand with a high-voltage conductor. Ongoing deep coagulation necrosis imposes an onerous and frustrating therapeutic burden and frequently neccessitates amputation. Arterial hemorrhage and gas gangrene are occasional complications.

Inflammatory Conditions
Septic (Fig. 34-25)

The dorsum of the hand with hair follicles and sweat and sebaceous glands acquires the same staphylococcal infections seen in the skin elsewhere on the body (folliculitis, carbuncles, furuncles, and subcutaneous abscesses). Simple streptococcal infections of either the dorsal or palmar aspect of the hand may lead to lymphangitis or lymphadenitis, which both respond promptly to appropriate antibiotics and local wound care. Mixed infections with anaerobic streptococci, bacteroids, or spirochetes (see Chap. 6) may be very destructive and demand aggressive systemic therapy (intravenous antibiotics) with complete and thorough débridement of the wound. A common source of these dangerous infections is human bite resulting from the collision of a closed fist with an open mouth.

Infections originating on the palmar surface or around the nail have distinct characteristics, which are listed in Table 34-3. When these infections are seen

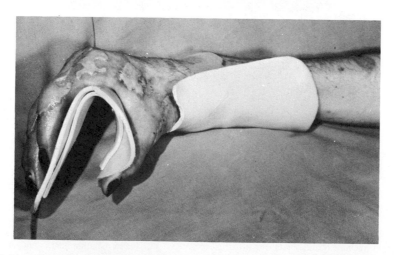

Fig. 34-24. "Anti-claw" splint placed on burned hand when at rest, to prevent claw deformity (see Fig. 34-6).
(From Furnas, D.W.: A bedside outline for the treatment of burns, Springfield, Ill., 1969, Charles C Thomas, Publisher.)

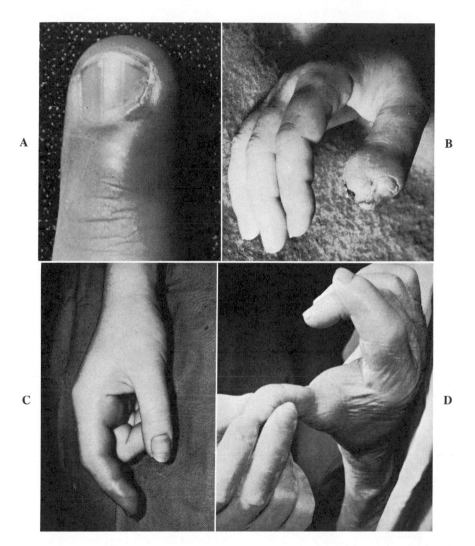

Fig. 34-25. Infections of hand. **A,** Acute paronychia. Infection tends to run around nail in surrounding subcuticular tissue; it may also tunnel beneath nail, forming subungual abscess. **B,** Felon. Pus is localized and tightly compressed within flexor pad or pulp space of tip of thumb. **C,** Tenosynovitis. Finger is (1) uniformly swollen, (2) slightly flexed, and (3) tender along tendon sheath, and (4) passive extension causes exquisite tenderness. **D,** Palmar space infection. Thenar space is swollen, tender, and distended with pus. (See Fig. 34-17.)

Table 34-3. Infections Originating on the Palmar Surface or Around the Nail

Entity	Findings	Cause	Site for Incision for Drainage of Pus	Complications
Paronychia (Fig. 34-25, A)	Inflammation of soft tissue around nail that tend to "run around" nail margin	Infection of torn hangnail or cuticle	Directly into pus collection	Subungual abscess
Subungual abscess	Pus collection under nail	Extension from other infections	Excision of proximal portion of nail	
Felon (Fig. 34-25, B)	Red, tensely swollen, extremely painful throbbing pulp space of distal phalanx; keeps patient awake	Minor puncture wound of fingertip	Lateral aspect of distal phalanx, cutting through fibrous septa	Necrosis and ostemyelitis of phalangeal bone caused by compression of arteries
Tendon sheath infection (Fig. 34-25, C)	Uniform swelling of finger; position of slight flexion of finger; exquisite pain on passive extension; maximum tenderness over tendon sheath area	Puncture wound or extension from other sites	Midlateral line of finger	Necrosis of flexor tendon; spread to palmar spaces or other bursae
Palmar space infections (Fig. 34-25, D; Fig. 34-17)	Tenderness and swelling of central and ulnar aspect of palm (midpalmar space) or of radial and thenar aspect of palm (thenar space)	Extension from tendon sheath infection; direct puncture wound	Skin crease incisions over most prominent area of swelling	Extensive damage to soft tissue of hand; extension to other spaces

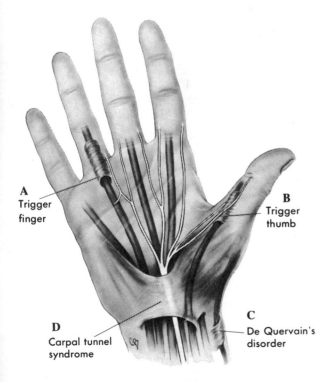

A
Trigger finger

B
Trigger thumb

D
Carpal tunnel syndrome

C
De Quervain's disorder

Fig. 34-26. Entrapment syndromes (right hand). **A,** Trigger finger caused by entrapment of digital flexor tendons in proximal portion of fibrous tendon sheath. **B,** Trigger thumb caused by entrapment of long flexor tendon to thumb. **C,** De Quervain's disorders or compression of abductor pollicis longus and extensor pollicis brevis tendon near radial styloid process. **D,** Carpal tunnel syndrome or compression of median nerve by transverse carpal ligament.

quite early in their course, they may be aborted by antibiotics, bed rest, elevation, and warm moist dressings to the hand. If the infection is not aborted, pus will collect and drainage is required.

In recent years the most common cause of hematogenous septic arthritis in the hand in patients under 40 is *Neisseria gonorrhoeae*. Culture of this organism is extremely difficult, and swabs should be taken routinely from the oropharynx, cervix or urethral meatus, anus, blood, and, if possible, the local site.

Nonseptic

Aseptic tenosynovitis is relatively common in the hand and wrist. De Quervain's disorder (Fig. 34-26) is caused by compression of the long abductor and short extensor tendons of the thumb in the fibrous sheath near the radial styloid process. It causes severe pain, particularly if adduction of the thumb is carried out while the wrist is held in ulnar deviation. Trigger finger or thumb results from stenosing tenosynovitis in the proximal portion of the fibrous flexor sheath and from nodule formation in the flexor tendon because of injury or rheumatoid disease. The tendon is trapped momentarily as it passes through the mouth of the sheath and then suddenly releases. Either flexion or extension may be blocked.

Treatment of these entrapment syndromes that fail to settle conservatively is surgical decompression by incision of the roof of the offending fibrous sheath.

Rheumatoid arthritis commonly occurs as an acute arthritis in the wrist or fingers. Multiple symmetrical small joint involvement, fluctuating clinical course, and appropriate laboratory studies serve to differentiate it from other forms of arthritis.

Degenerative Changes

Heberden's nodes are the most common form of degenerative change in the hand. They are present at the distal interphalangeal joint and reflect a local process of degenerative arthritis.

The carpometacarpal joint of the thumb is also commonly involved by degenerative processes and, as with Heberden's nodes, may relfect a systemic proclivity for osteoarthritis.

Carpal Tunnel Syndrome

The carpal tunnel syndrome, caused by compression of the median nerve in the flexor compartment of the wrist by the transverse carpal ligament, may occur as the result of diminution in the size of the canal (as with Colles' fracture) or of increase in the size of the contents (as with rheumatoid synovitis). Characteristically it results in pain in the hand and forearm, hyperesthesia and paresthesia of the three radial digits, and weakness and atrophy of the thenar muscles. Quite commonly the pain is experienced as far proximally as the shoulder. It is most common in middle-aged women and is frequently bilateral. Surgical decompression of the transverse metacarpal ligament (Fig. 34-26) usually gives results that are gratifying to surgeon and patient alike.

Tumors and Tumorlike Conditions
Dupuytren's Contracture

Dupuytren's contracture (Fig. 34-27) is a fibrous metaplasia (often bilateral) of the superficial palmar fascia that causes a characteristic flexion contracture in the subcutaneous layer of the palm. A hypertrophic fibrous nodule appears in the palm or finger (most commonly the ring finger) as is followed by the formation of thick, fibrous bands that may extend distally. These bands slowly shorten until extension of the metacarpophalangeal and proximal interphalangeal joints is prevented. The contracture is corrected by excision of the offending metaplastic tissue.

Benign

Ganglia, epidermal cysts, mucous cysts, xanthomas, lipomas, enchondromas, glomus tumors, and neurilemomas are benign tumors characteristically found in the hand (Fig. 34-28, *A* to *E*; Table 34-4).

Malignant

Squamous cell or epidermoid carcinoma (Fig. 34-29) is the most common malignant tumor of the hand.

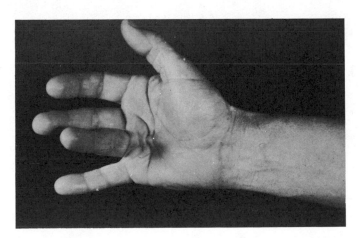

Fig. 34-27. Dupuytren's contracture. Band of hypertrophied and contracted superficial palmar fascia projects distally from nodule in palm; proximal interphalangeal joint of ring finger is forced into permanent flexion.

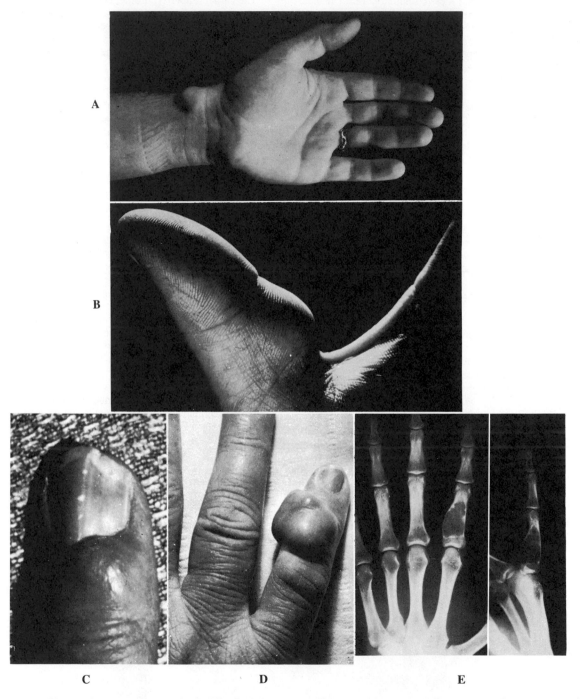

Fig. 34-28. Tumors of hand. **A,** Ganglia. **B,** Epidermal cyst. **C,** Mucus-retention cyst. **D,** Xanthoma. **E,** Enchondroma

Table 34-4. Benign Tumors of the Hand

Entity	Description	Comment	Treatment
Ganglia (Fig. 34-28, *A*)	Multilocular cyst growing from capsule of carpal joint (dorsum of wrist, snuffbox, or just proximal to thenar eminence) or volar aspect of metacarpophalangeal joint	Most common (approximately one third of tumors of the hand)	Excision using equipment for major hand surgery (aspiration of cyst, injection of cortisone occasionally effective); recurrences are seen after any type of treatment
Epidermal cyst or implantation cyst, inclusion cyst (Fig. 34-28, *B*)	Subcutaneous cyst filled with epithelial debris located on flexor surface of proximal phalanges or distal palm	Caused by bits of epidermis, stabbed into subcutaneous site by tools or sharp objects	Excision
Mucous cyst (myxomatous cyst, myxoid cyst, or synovial cyst; Fig. 34-28, *C*)	Translucent cyst embedded in thick, reddish skin just proximal to nail fold; frequently groove of nail in direct line with cyst	Filled with synovial fluid; usually communicates with distal interphalangeal joint	Excision of cyst and communication using magnification; avoid injury to extensor tendon
Xanthoma (benign giant cell tumor of tendon sheath; benign synovioma; Fig. 34-28, *D*)	Firm, irregular yellowish tumor growing from fibrous flexor tendon sheath	Multinucleated giant cells, synovial clefts, hemosiderin, foam cells seen on microscopic examination	Excision with equipment for major hand surgery
Lipoma	Soft, multinodular fatty mass	Frequently grow forward from middle palmar or thenar space displacing tendons and presenting as mass in palm	Excision with equipment for major hand surgery
Enchondroma (Fig. 34-28, *E*)	Cartilaginous pocket within bone or proximal phalanx (or other phalanges or metacarpal heads)	Usually asymptomatic, incidental finding on x-ray examination	None, unless symptoms of pathological fracture; then curettage and packing with bone chips
Glomus tumors (glomangioma or angioneuromyoma)	Tiny, very painful, reddish purple nodules frequently visible under fingernail, also seen in other sites	Growth of neuromyoarterial glomus, a heat-regulation arterial shunt	Excision
Neurilemmoma and neuroma	Painful, tender nodule along course of previously injured nerve; Tinel's sign (distal paresthesias elicited by percussion at site of neurilemoma	Most common in a digital nerve of thumb or index finger	If nerve is not functioning, excise neuroma and anastomose the nerve, or excise neuroma and bury stump of nerve in a recess where it will not be stimulated

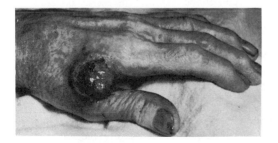

Fig. 34-29. Squamous carcinoma.

It usually develops from premalignant keratoses on the dorsum of the hand decades after chronic exposure to sunlight, ionizing radiation, or organic hydrocarbons or after long-standing chronic dermatologic disorders. Ingestion of arsenicals is associated with keratoses and carcinomas of the palmar surface of the hand. Growth is slow, malignancy is low grade, lymph node metastases occur in only about 5% to 15% of cases, and mortality is proportionately low. Wide excision of the lesion and repair of the defect by skin grafts or pedicles is the usual treatment. In far advanced cases, amputation, axillary lymphadenectomy, and perfusion of the limb with chemotherapeutic agents must be considered. Basal cell carcinoma is rare in the hand.

Malignant melanoma of the hand behaves essentially as malignant melanoma elsewhere on the body surface. Wide excision or amputation with or without regional lymphadenectomy or perfusion of chemotherapeutic agents is performed.

35

Neurologic Surgery

Hiro Nishioka

Neurologic surgery and other surgical specialties constitute areas of limited but essential fields of knowledge for the student. Although details of operative techniques and the complications of surgery are of concern principally to the practitioners of the specialties, the ability to recognize the need for surgical intervention, especially under emergency conditions, remains an indispensable part of every physician's armamentarium. Many uncomplicated neurosurgical conditions such as simple concussions and skull fractures can and should be managed by the primary care physician in a local setting. More complex problems may require specialized monitoring techniques or surgical intervention in a neurosurgical facility.

In considering neurosurgical problems, some basic working principles should be borne in mind. The specialized neurons of the central nervous system, once destroyed, are incapable of replacement. Furthermore, the pathways by which neurons are interconnected cannot be reestablished once severed or interrupted. A cell or its connections may be damaged by pressure, penetration by foreign objects, inflammation, invasion by neoplasm, or biochemical processes. Of these, pressure is the only factor that can be relieved surgically. Reparative surgery in the central nervous system is prophylactic only and is utilized to prevent additional damage by infection, hemorrhage, or trauma.

The degree of cellular or tract damage by pressure is proportional to the amount of pressure, the rapidity of pressure rise, and its duration. The most severe and permanent damage is produced by the sudden application of pressure, as in acute trauma. Pressure of lesser degrees can be tolerated without permanent damage if its rate of increase is slow (e.g., neoplasm). If surgical decompression is to be worthwhile, it must be performed before irreversible damage has occurred and it must be sufficiently extensive. The surgeon must occasionally sacrifice nerve tissue that appears grossly non-viable or even normal in the interest of preserving useful functioning tissue that appears capable of recovery.

The neurosurgical armamentarium also contains procedures for the planned focal destruction of tracts and nuclear elements and for electrical or chemical blockade of normal nerve pathways. These operations are utilized for the relief of intractable pain, involuntary movement and abnormal states of muscle tone.

The emphasis of this chapter will be the management of pressure-producing lesions. Descriptions of infrequently used or highly specialized techniques are omitted, so that the reader may concentrate on the commonly encountered neurosurgical problems.

SPECIAL DIAGNOSTIC STUDIES

Neurologic examination alone does not localize intraspinal or intracranial lesions accurately enough to allow the physician to proceed with operative treatment. Accurate delineation of the extent and location of the lesion prior to operation is desirable and requires the use of special investigative procedures.

Table 35-1 lists the common diagnostic studies utilized. Whenever possible, the specific tests that give the best chances of demonstrating a lesion should be chosen, based on the clinical impression of the location and type of pathosis expected. Although several tests might discover a tumor mass, one of them may provide information that is particularly useful to the operating surgeon (e.g., computed tomography [CT] or magnetic resonance imaging [MRI] may disclose and outline a tumor mass but an angiogram will show both the internal vascularity and the position of important vascular structures in the immediate vicinity of the tumor (Fig. 35-7). The routine use of a "battery" of tests is deplorable. All such tests are costly, and some carry significant risks of complications and even death. Therefore careful neurologic evaluation is essential to the efficient and safe investigation of the patient. The evaluation should consist of an accurate and detailed history of illness or injury, followed by a general physical and neurologic examination that should lead to a clinical diagnosis or impression specific enough to indicate the need

for one or more special investigations. General screening tests are, of course, never to be overlooked. Blood count, urinalysis, chest roentgenogram, and any other appropriate tests should be completed before special studies.

Electroencephalography, echoencephalography, radioisotope scanning, CT, and MRI are useful screening tests, since they can be performed without significant risk or discomfort to the patient. The information obtained by CT or MRI is often sufficient to proceed with surgical treatment; however, in many instances additional preoperative studies such as CT or MRI enhanced with contrast media, angiography, or positron-emission tomography (PET) may be desirable to obtain more specific information about a lesion's vascularity, its relation to the subarachnoid space, or its metabolic activity. The costly equipment required to perform all these tests is not available in many locales, so the choice of tests in smaller medical communities may be governed by the availability of diagnostic technology rather than by what may be the optimal test for a particular pathosis.

Considerable confusion exists in the minds of most students regarding the indications and contraindications for *lumbar puncture*. In the presence of a pressure-producing intracranial pathologic condition, lumbar puncture is potentially hazardous to the life of the patient. The withdrawal of spinal fluid from below, and particularly the leakage of fluid into the spinal epidural space after the needle has been removed, encourage herniation of the cerebellar tonsils and temporal lobe uncus, with resultant brainstem compression. Therefore lumbar puncture should be performed for specific indications only. Increased intracranial pressure is usually associated with clinically recognizable symptoms and signs such as vomiting and papilledema. There is no advantage in measuring the exact degree of abnormal pressure in the presence of such signs. The diagnosis of infections (meningitis, encephalitis) and of subarachnoid hemorrhage depends on the finding of the appropriate cells in the cerebrospinal fluid. Lumbar puncture is therefore indicated in all patients suspected of harboring the preceding, based on the clinical finding of

Text continued on p. 399.

Table 35-1. Diagnostic Studies Utilized Most Frequently

Diagnostic Test	Procedure	Information Obtained	Possible Complications	Lesions Best Demonstrated
Noninvasive Studies				
Electroencephalography	Application of electrodes to scalp and recording of cortical electrical activity	Abnormal wave forms and seizure discharges from areas irritated or compressed	None	Brain abscess, seizure focus
Echoencephalography (Fig. 35-1)	Transmission of ultrasonic waves coronally through the brain and recording echo at brain-fluid or brain-tumor interfaces (requires opening in bone, e.g., open fontanelle)	Ventricular size, neoplasms, or hematomas close to bony opening	None	Hydrocephalus, acute hematomas in infants

Table 35-1 continued.

Table 35-1. Diagnostic Studies Utilized Most Frequently—cont'd

Diagnostic Test	Procedure	Information Obtained	Possible Complications	Lesions Best Demonstrated
Computed tomography (Figs. 35-2, 35-3)	Radiographic tomography of head or spine with computed digital images based on x-ray attenuation of finite volumes (voxels) of tissue	Axial cross-sectional images of brain and spinal cord, outlines of ventricular system and subarachnoid space, showing lesions having tissue density different from normal structures	None	Hydrocephalus, intracranial hematomas, herniated lumbar disk, spinal stenosis and spondylosis, vertebral body fractures
Magnetic resonance imaging (Figs. 35-4, 35-5)	Tomography of head or spine in multiple planes, with computed digital images based on intensity of radiowave signals from tissue protons aligned by a strong magnetic field and perturbed by resonant frequency pulses	Same as CT scanning plus ability to image structures in multiple planes	None known, but study is hazardous if body harbors any ferrous metals (e.g., metal fragments in eyes, older aneurysm clips)	Hydrocephalus, neoplasms of brain and spinal cord, infarcts, demyelinating and inflammatory lesions, vascular malformations, herniated lumbar disk, central cervical disk, and spondylosis
Invasive Studies				
Lumbar puncture	Insertion of needle into lumbar subarachnoid space and withdrawal of fluid	Presence of abnormal amounts of cells and alterations in chemical contents of cerebrospinal fluid	Herniation of temporal uncus or cerebellar tonsils with compression of brainstem	Meningitis, subarachnoid hemorrhage, neoplastic seeding
Radioisotope scanning	Parenteral injection of radioactive isotope and observation of its flow through carotid and cerebral arteries, noting its tendency to localize in abnormal areas as determined by radioactive counts over neck and head	Relative rate and volume of flow through carotid and middle cerebral arteries; presence of neoplasms, vascular malformations, and abnormal brain tissues that take up more than normal amounts of isotope	Allergic reaction to isotope or its carrier	Unilateral carotid stenosis or occlusion, middle cerebral thrombosis, arteriovenous malformation, vascular neoplasms (e.g., meningiomas, metastases)
Contrast-enhanced computed tomography (Fig. 35-6)	Tomograms as above after parenteral injection of iodinated contrast media	Circle of Willis and major cerebral arteries, vascular patterns in and around mass lesions in addition to information from unenhanced CT	Allergic reactions to enhancing contrast material	Vascular neoplasms, arteriovenous malformations
Angiography (Fig. 35-7)	1. Injection of contrast into superior vena cava and visualization of cervical and intracranial vasculature by computed digital subtraction 2. Injection of contrast directly into carotid or vertebral arteries with rapid serial radiographic examinations	Opacification of cervical and cerebral blood vessels to show vascular abnormalities, or neovascularity and displacement by mass lesions	Thromboembolism with cerebral infarction, local hemorrhage, allergic reaction to contrast medium	Vascular anomalies (aneurysm, arteriovenous malformation) vascular neoplasms, especially meningiomas
Myelography (Fig. 35-8)	Lumbar, cervical, or cisternal puncture and injection of positive contrast medium	Outline of spinal subarachnoid space that may be distorted or blocked by mass lesions in the spinal canal	Spinal arachnoiditis, inflammatory reaction to contrast medium or contaminant	Tumors in the spinal canal, herniated intervertebral disk, avulsion of nerve roots

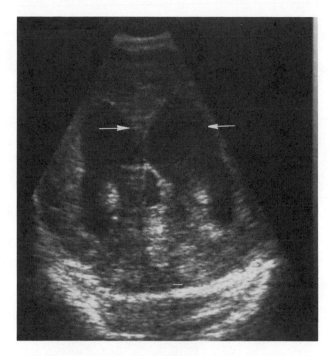

Fig. 35-1. Echoencephalogram (ultrasound study) through the anterior fontanelle of an infant, showing lateral ventricles *(arrows)* that are significantly larger than normal.

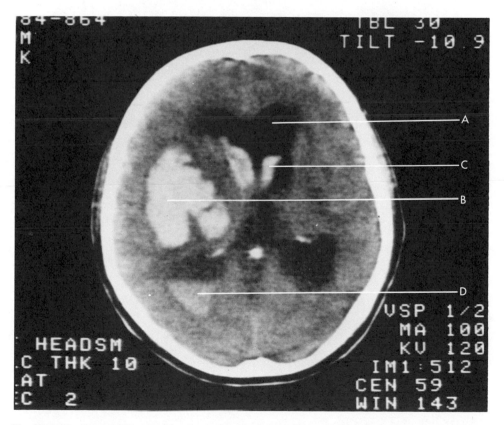

Fig. 35-2. Unenhanced CT scan of head at level of lateral ventricles. Skull appears as dense opaque outline; semisolid brain tissue as intermediate density; fluid in lateral ventricles, **A,** is least dense. Hemorrhage has occurred, **B,** into brain substance and into ventricles, **C.** With patient lying supine, some blood has settled into posterior horn of ventricle, **D.** These differentiations are made without injection of any radiopaque substances.

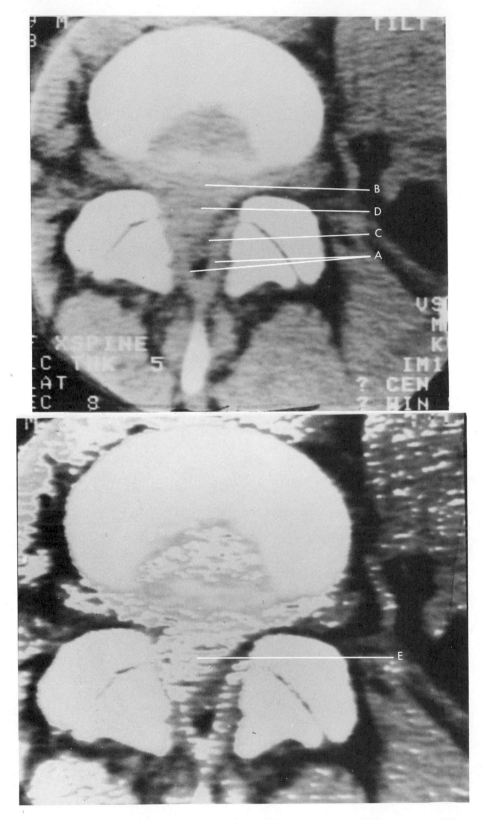

Fig. 35-3. Unenhanced CT scan of lumbar spine at level of L4-L5 disk. The spinal canal is bordered by ligamentum flavum, **A,** and the intervertebral disk, **B.** Roots of cauda equina, **C,** are greatly compressed by large fragment of herniated disk, **D,** occupying much of the canal. Differentiation of tissues can be accentuated by density-computed highlighting, **E,** without the need for injection of contrast media.

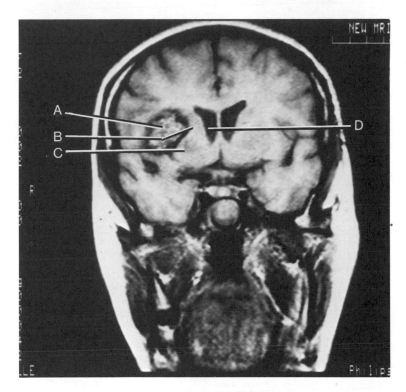

Fig. 35-4. Coronal MRI showing a clearly demarcated lesion **A** lying adjacent to the caudate nucleus **B** and putamen **C** but not displacing them or distorting the lateral ventricle **D** as would a neoplasm. The dark outer rim from hemosiderin and the reticulated center from large venous channels are chacteristic of a cavernous angioma.

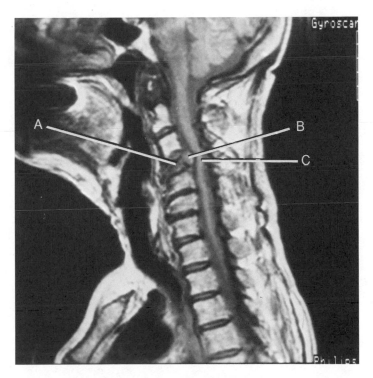

Fig. 35-5. MRI showing spinal cord compression by neoplasm. This sagittal image depicts the base of the brain, the entire cervical spine, and upper thoracic segments. Metastatic carcinoma has replaced the body of C4 **A,** causing it to collapse. The neoplasm is seen bulging posteriorly **B,** displacing and compressing the spinal cord **C** within its canal.

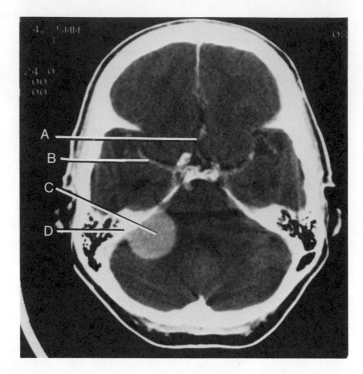

Fig. 35-6. CT following intravenous infusion of meglumine diatrizoate. The anterior **A** and middle **B** cerebral arteries are visualized by the contrast medium. This axial tomogram close to the skull base shows a rounded homogeneous tumor mass **C** attached by a broad base to the dura over the petrous portion of the temporal bone **D;** these characteristics are typical of a meningioma.

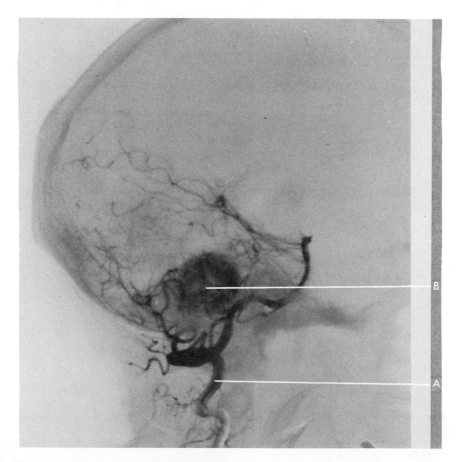

Fig. 35-7. Angiogram performed by injection of meglumine diatrizoate into vertebral artery, **A.** A highly vascularized tumor mass, **B,** lies in fourth ventricle. Lesion was a choroid plexus papilloma.

nuchal rigidity. That these same conditions are likely to be associated with increased intracranial pressure is apparent, but the possible risks of the procedure are outweighed by the necessity for deriving information that may be vital to the selection of proper treatment. In brain tumors the information obtained from lumbar puncture is usually not worth the hazards; in subdural hematoma the fluid may be entirely normal, misleading the clinician into a false sense of security. The Queckenstedt test (compression of the jugular veins) for all practical purposes, should *never* be performed when an intracranial pathosis is suspected, for the potential hazards of uncal or tonsillar herniation are acutely increased by that maneuver.

Lumbar puncture in intraspinal pathosis is worthwhile only if one suspects the presence of abnormal cells (inflammatory cells, neoplastic seeding, red cells from a spinal subarachnoid hemorrhage); the spinal indications are similar to those for intracranial pathosis. When a compressive lesion is present, lumbar puncture alone may yield supportive but nonspecific information, and, as with intracranial compressive lesions, a neurologic deficit can worsen following the puncture. Therefore, unless the facilities are available to proceed immediately with definitive myelography and surgical decompression, there is no advantage to performing a spinal puncture for intraspinal compressive lesions when MRI alone can provide a definitive diagnosis without risk or discomfort.

INCREASED INTRACRANIAL PRESSURE
Clinicopathologic correlations

The addition of fluid, blood, or neoplastic tissue to the normal contents of any body cavity may result in increase in the volume of that cavity, increase in the pressure within the cavity, or both. Adding to the contents of the cranial cavity results in an increase in the size of the head only in infants, whose cranial sutures are still open, but even then the increase can occur only slowly.

For practical purposes the cranial cavity may be regarded as a rigid box divided into two compartments, one above and one below the tentorium. Each has one principal outlet, the tentorial hiatus and the foramen magnum, respectively. Every increase in volume within these compartments is accompanied by a tendency for brain tissue to herniate through their outlets. The herniating tissue directly compresses and distorts the brainstem and is the primary cause of death from increased intracranial pressure.

Institution of treatment before irreversible damage has occurred depends on the recognition of danger signs indicating beginning or advancing herniation. The patient's responses to common environmental stimuli are the most reliable indicators of intracranial pressure. As pressure increases, the responses are progressively impaired in speed, accuracy, and propriety. Pupillary dilatation is always late in onset, occurring only in the presence of dangerous herniations. The "classic" alterations of vital signs (increasing blood pressure with slowing of the heart rate) may not occur until it is too late for effective treatment, if they occur at all.

Table 35-2 lists the progression of observable responses as intracranial pressure increases. Notice that the categorized responses for each stage are not abso-

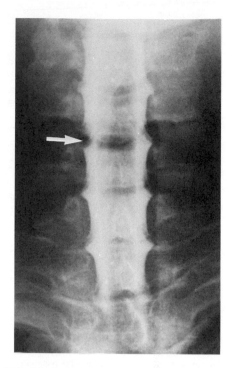

Fig. 35-8. Myelogram showing herniated cervical disk. The cervical canal is outlined by a column of contrast (Iopamidol), and nerve roots are seen exiting at each interspace. At C5-6 the root outline is indented and irregular *(arrow)*, indicating the presence of a small extradural mass, most commonly herniated disk fragments.

lute; these are general guidelines and are subject to some variation. Fig. 35-9 shows how a subdural hematoma distorts the brain and produces the neurologic signs of herniation. Dilatation of a pupil signifies herniation of the temporal uncus with compression of the oculomotor nerve. The nerve adjacent to the herniated uncus is usually affected first, resulting in dilatation of the pupil on the side of the lesion. Occasionally, however, the midbrain is shifted to the extent that the opposite oculomotor nerve is compressed against the edge of the tentorium resulting in pupillary dilatation on the side opposite the lesion.

Compression of the cerebral peduncle either directly by the herniating uncus or indirectly by shifting against the opposite tentorial edge results first in a *paresis* on the side opposite the primary lesion (since these fibers cross in the medulla at the decussation of the pyramids), commonly followed by a change in response to *extensor thrust* (decerebration). At this stage vasomotor and respiratory centers are easily compromised, so that cessation of respirations may occur at any moment.

The stage-by-stage progression to total decerebration and finally to complete flaccidity with no response to any stimulus may occur gradually over a period of hours or suddenly within a few seconds. Thus there is *no margin of safety after the onset of signs indicating midbrain compression.*

CONGENITAL MALFORMATIONS

A large variety of developmental abnormalities of the central and peripheral nervous system can occur,

Table 35-2. Clinical Changes with Progressive Brainstem Compression

Stage	Response to: Addressing Patient by Name	Patting or Shaking Patient's Shoulder	Pinching Tendon of Pectoralis Major	Relative Size	Reaction to Light
Normal	Looks at examiner, remains attentive	Looks at examiner, remains attentive	Removes pinching hand quickly and effectively, moves body away	Equal	Reactive
I	Opens eyes but tends to fall asleep while being spoken to	Open eyes and remains awake as long as stimulus is applied	Removes stimulus and moves away, but not as quickly as in "normal" stage	Equal	Reactive
II	No response	Little or no response	Sluggish and ineffectual attempts to remove stimulus, shrugs shoulders	Dilated on side of lesion*	Sluggish or no reaction
III	No response	No response	Extensor thrust (decerebrate posture) on side opposite the lesion*	Widely dilated on side of lesion	No reaction
IV	No response	No response or bilateral extensor thrusts	Bilateral extensor thrusts	Widely dilated bilaterally	No reaction
V	No response	No response	No response	Moderately dilated	No reaction

*Dilatation of the pupil and the appearance of extensor posturing occasionally occur first on the side opposite that listed in this table. For the anatomic explanation for this phenomenon, refer to text and to Fig. 35-9.

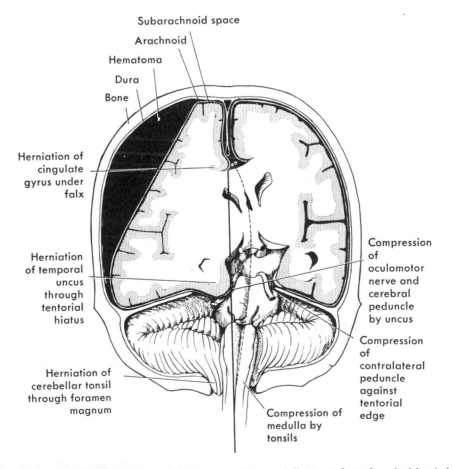

Fig. 35-9. Subdural hematoma. Although hematoma displaces and distorts surface of cerebral hemisphere, more serious and life-threatening changes are occurring in deeper structures at some distance from hematoma itself. These changes result in displacement and compression of vital centers within brainstem.

and many of them are compatible with survival of the infant and its development into a functional person. These malformations may occur singly, but all too frequently they are associated with anomalies of other body structures, so that careful assessment of all congenital abnormalities must be made before a reparative treatment program is proposed. Three common neurologic anomalies merit the attention of the student. These are spina bifida, hydrocephalus, and craniosynostosis.

Spina Bifida

Spina bifida occurs most frequently in the lumbar region but can occur at any level in the midline of the neuraxis, including the head (cranium bifidum). Failure of the neural tube to fuse posteriorly during the early weeks of embryonic life results in a bony defect through which intraspinal or intracranial contents may protrude. The defect may be minor and detectable only by radiographs, or it may manifest itself in the midline of the back by the presence of an overlying small tuft of hair (spina bifida occulta); in more severe abnormalities, the neural tube is incompletely covered by protective layers so that portions of the tube protrude beyond the normal cutaneous layers as a meningomyelocele (Fig. 35-10). Lumbar meningomyeloceles vary in their content of neural tissue, but almost all contain some elements of spinal cord or cauda equina, so they are frequently associated with some degree of paralysis. If no neural tissue is present in the sac or its walls, the lesion is called a meningocele.

Spina bifida occulta rarely requires any treatment, whereas most meningomyeloceles require surgical repair within the first 24 hours after birth of the child, in order to avert rupture or leakage of the sac with their attendant danger of meningitis. Surgical repair consists of excision of the sac with preservation and replacement of all salvageable neural tissue back into the floor of the dural canal. A plastic closure is then performed, beginning with a water-tight dural closure and then overlapping layers of paraspinous fascia over the dura to provide a reasonable thickness of protective soft tissue between neural tube and skin, for there will always be a significant posterior defect in the bony canal.

Hydrocephalus

Meningomyeloceles, regardless of location, are very often associated with the *Arnold-Chiari malformation*, (Fig. 35-11) a caudad displacement of the medulla and cerebellar tissue through the foramen magnum into the cervical canal. For reasons that have never been explained adequately, repair of the meningomyelocele is frequently followed by rapid enlargement of the head from obstructive hydrocephalus. The obstruction usually occurs at the aqueduct of Sylvius, which may have malformed as a series of semicontiguous channels rather than as a single tube, or may be simply too stenotic to accommodate the required flow of ventricular fluid. The enlargement of the lateral and third ventricles can be delineated easily by echoencephalography through an open fontanelle (Fig. 35-1), while CT and MRI studies can localize the point of obstruction with greater accuracy. Hydrocephalus may also occur as a late complication of neonatal intraventricular hemorrhage. Treatment consists of implanting a bypass or shunt from the enlarged ventricle to return its fluid to the systemic circulation directly, as in the ventriculovenous shunt (Fig. 35-12, *A*), or indirectly via the peritoneal cavity, where the fluid is absorbed back into the bloodstream (Fig. 35-12, *B*). Both methods incorporate calibrated unidirectional valve systems that allow fluid to leave the ventricles under controlled pressures and rates of flow while preventing reflux of blood or fluid into the ventricles. Many other methods of shunting the accumulated fluid have been devised, meeting with limited success and many complications; no single method has proven to be trouble free, so the infant with an implanted shunt must be followed into adulthood and any malfunctions, blockages, or infections of the shunt mechanism must be treated quickly and effectively. The successful long-term control of pressure usually results in useful survivals—children at least capable of being educated. On the other hand, inadequate control of pressure results in a child with very limited potential for mental development and with a monstrously large head.

Craniosynostosis

Craniosynostosis, or premature closure of the cranial sutures, is a curious condition that affects males

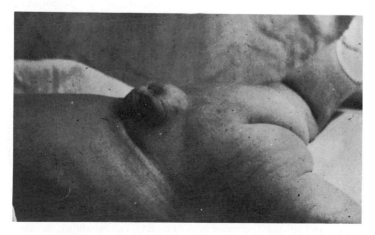

Fig. 35-10. Lumbar meningomyelocele. Lesion usually has wide base, so that closure of skin after excision of sac often requires extensive undermining and rotation of flaps.

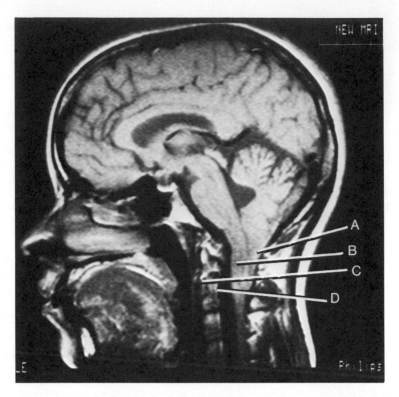

Fig. 35-11. The Arnold-Chiari malformation shown by midline sagittal MRI. A tongue of cerebellar tissue **A** along with an elongated and compressed medulla **B** extends downward through the foramen magnum into the spinal canal to the level of the atlas **C** and the odontoid process of the axis **D**.

six times more frequently than females. The abnormal shape of the head depends on which suture or sutures are prematurely fused. Closure of the sagittal suture prevents the skull from expanding laterally. This results in greater (compensatory) enlargement in the anteroposterior dimension so that the head becomes long and narrow (scaphocephaly). If the coronal suture fuses early, the skull cannot expand in the anteroposterior dimension, resulting in a short, wide configuration (brachycephaly). If all sutures close prematurely, the skull can expand only in an upward direction resulting in a "tower" shape (oxycephaly). In most cases treatment within the first 3 months of life is indicated to prevent mental retardation, blindness, and permanent disfigurement. Surgical correction may require only cutting out an artificial suture (linear craniectomy) or, in severely misshapen calvaria, may involve extensive repositioning and reconstruction of segments of the skull.

CRANIOCEREBRAL TRAUMA

The high incidence of head injuries in the general civilian population makes an adequate working knowledge of the problem essential to every physician. The pathologic condition that may result from trauma depends on the mechanism of injury, so this must be considered carefully in each patient. In this section the pathogenesis is considered along with the diagnosis and management of various types of patients. The management of the patient may be divided into four phases.

Phase 1
Assessment of the Type and Severity of Injury

The history of the traumatic event may provide valuable clues to the nature and areas injured. Unfortunately, patients are usually unable to provide this history because they are unconscious or because of amnesia generally associated with the injury. Therefore fragments of information from relatives, spectators, and police officers may have to be pieced together. Since head injury occurs frequently with injuries to other parts of the body, the physician must learn to evaluate quickly the relative severity of each and to determine which deserves priority in treatment. The force of a blow to the head is always transmitted in some degree to the cervical spine, so the possibility of a fracture or dislocation of the cervical spine accompanies every head injury. Respiratory and cardiovascular distress always take precedence over neurologic injury, for they are immediately life threatening and the resultant hypoxia enhances any damage to other tissues including those of the nervous system.

The type of injury may be classified according to the mechanism of trauma. It may be kinetic or static, nonpenetrating or penetrating. The kinetic injury results from the differential rates of motion between skull and brain tissues. Nonpenetrating kinetic injuries are by far the most common in civilian life. The stationary head may be struck, resulting in sudden movement of the cranium (acceleration), or the head in motion may strike a stationary object in such a way that motion of

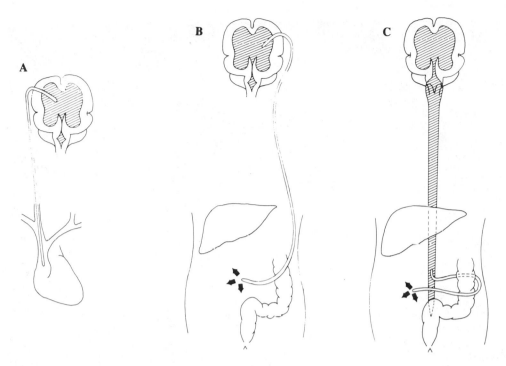

Fig. 35-12. Shunt procedures used most commonly for hydrocephalus. **A,** Ventriculocaval shunt. Fluid is shunted directly back into bloodstream through catheter inserted into jugular vein and threaded downward so that its tip lies in superior vena cava; one-way valve within system prevents reflux of blood upward from vena cava and controls pressure under which fluid drains out of ventricles. **B,** Ventriculoperitoneal shunt. Fluid is shunted into peritoneal cavity to be absorbed back into bloodstream. Catheter is threaded through subcutaneous tunnel over chest and upper abdominal wall to enter peritoneal cavity in lower quadrant. **C,** Lumbar peritoneal shunt. Fluid is shunted from lumbar subarachnoid space through subcutaneous tunnel around patient's flank. This procedure can be utilized only in a communicating hydrocephalus, i.e., when ventricular system communicates freely with spinal subarachnoid space. Any peritoneal shunt can be performed on patient's right or left side.

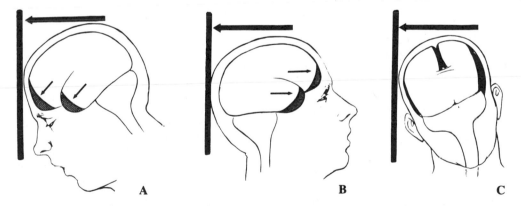

Fig. 35-13. Cortical contusion with relation to direction of head movement. **A,** Head moving forward and striking stationary surface—major injury found at tips of frontal and temporal poles. **B,** Head moving backward and striking stationary surface—major injury found in frontal and temporal lobes (contrecoup). **C,** Head moving laterally and striking stationary surface—major injury found on side opposite that which strikes surface (contrecoup); medial surfaces of hemispheres are also injured by impingement on relatively rigid falx.

the cranium is suddenly arrested (deceleration). The latter is more common and produces a more severe lesion. When movement is in a forward direction (Fig. 35-13, *A*), the major lesion is usually directly under the point of impact; when movement is in the lateral plane (Fig. 35-13, *C*), there is greater tendency for the maxi-

mal damage to occur on the side of the brain opposite the point of impact (contrecoup); (Fig. 35-14). Penetrating injuries are primarily static. In civilian life they are not uncommonly seen after a kick by a horse or after direct blows with small objects such as balls or hammers.

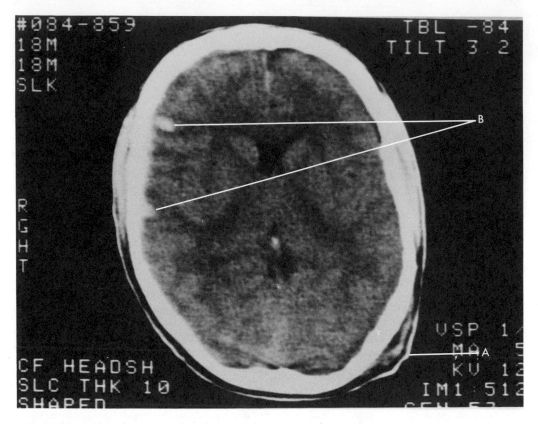

Fig. 35-14. CT scan showing contrecoup injury. Patient fell backwards, striking parieto-occipital region as indicated by swelling of scalp, **A.** Small intracerebral hemorrhages, **B,** are seen farthest from the point of impact on skull.

The *key* to the initial and subsequent neurologic evaluation of the head-injured patient is the assessment of the *level of responsiveness,* or *"consciousness."* This point cannot be overemphasized. Instability of vital signs is common immediately after head trauma, whereas localizing neurologic deficits may not become manifest until complications are far advanced. The rapidity, propriety, and accuracy of a patient's responses to verbal commands or to noxious stimulation wherever necessary must be observed carefully and recorded. The Glasgow coma scale (Fig. 35-15) offers a uniform assessment of basic cerebral functions after head injury and is used widely by medical and paramedical personnel. The patient's cerebral functioning level can be equated to a numerical value and plotted on a chart, so that significant changes in that value may be cause for specific treatment. Because alcoholic intoxication is associated so frequently with head injuries especially from vehicular accidents, the serum ethanol content must be taken into consideration in any assessment of cerebral responses.

The patient should be evaluated according to the *brain* injury as diagnosed by neurologic examination and the *bony* injury as diagnosed by physical and radiographic examinations.

Brain

Concussion	Hemispheres, brainstem
Contusion	or both
Laceration	

Bone

Closed fracture	Linear
Open fracture	Comminuted with or without
	depression of fragments

The severity of the brain injury does not correlate with the degree of skull damage. Therefore each component should be described, e.g., cerebral concussion with closed linear fracture, or cerebral laceration from open comminuted fracture with depression of fragments.

Concussion implies that the trauma has been sufficient to impair cerebral function temporarily, that there is no immediate structural damage, and hence that recovery may be expected. *Contusion* denotes a more severe injury, producing bruises or petechial hemorrhages in brain substance. Complete neurologic recovery can occur, but severe contusion may progress to infarction with permanent deficits or even death of the patient. *Laceration* denotes a break in the anatomic continuity of brain substance. It is usually associated with penetrating wounds (e.g., depressed fractures and bullet wounds), but it can occur in nonpenetrating injuries.

By far the most common type of head injury seen in practice is concussion with or without skull fracture. A blow to the head sends the victim into a state of unresponsiveness from which he cannot be aroused. Within seconds or minutes, he begins to move his extremities and then to open his eyes. He may be confused and disoriented for minutes or hours. During the first 6 to 12

Glasgow Coma Scale

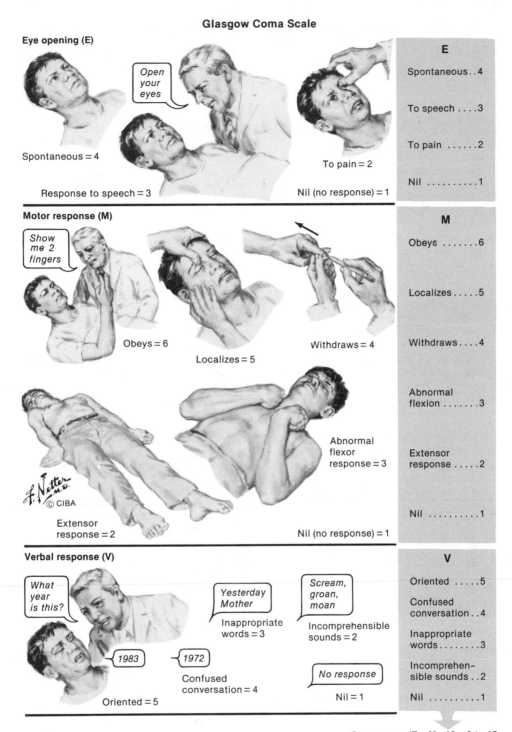

Coma score (E + M + V) = 3 to 15

Fig. 35-15. Glasgow coma scale.
(© 1983, CIBA Pharmaceutical Company, Division of CIBA-Geigy Corp., Ardsley, N.Y. Reprinted with permission from Clinical Symposia; illustrated by Dr. Frank H. Netter; all rights reserved.)

hours, there may be lethargy, nausea, and vomiting. Within 24 to 48 hours, he is lucid and oriented, with no neurologic deficit except for amnesia for the events just before or after the injury, or at both times. Headache and giddiness are common when ambulation is begun, except in young children, who complain very little of symptoms after 24 hours.

Since skull fractures without gross displacement will heal without specific treatment, they are not of therapeutic importance except in two instances. Fractures of the base of the skull with dural and arachnoid tearing resulting in *leakage of cerebrospinal fluid* (mixed with blood) from the ear or nostril may call for prophylaxis against meningitis. Cephalosporins are most satisfactory for this purpose. Fractures of the petrous temporal bone frequently cannot be seen in skull films, so that *diagnosis is based entirely on the finding of bloody spinal fluid otorrhea.* Fortunately this leakage from the ear almost invariably ceases spontaneously. Cerebrospinal fluid rhinorrhea, however, often persists, with its attendant threat of meningitis. In such cases intracranial repair of the meningeal laceration is necessary. *Depression of bone fragments* of such magnitude or in an area where functional cortex is compressed calls for immediate surgical elevation. In most instances the blow that produces such depression of bone also lacerates the scalp, so that there is danger of infection in sequestered bone fragments.

Performance of Ancillary Emergency Procedures

Establishment and maintenance of an unobstructed airway are the first and most important considerations. In the unconscious patient *endotracheal intubation* through the mouth or nostril provides an immediate and satisfactory route both for unobstructed breathing and for tracheal suctioning. When intubation is impossible because of local injuries or deformities, tracheostomy should be performed. These procedures are essential to the safe transport of the patient to a neurosurgical facility. *Replacement of blood loss* from scalp lacerations is not often necessary except in infants and children, whose blood loss may be sufficient to produce shock. Bleeding from the scalp edges can be controlled for short periods by tamponing, but if there is an extensive underlying fracture, bleeding from the *bone edges* may continue despite the application of pressure to the scalp. *Débridement* and *suture* of lacerations should be performed with adequate shaving and cleansing of the lacerated area and under good operating conditions. Too often, scalp lacerations are sutured roughly under the premise that the scar will be hidden by hair. Patients who may be expected to remain unresponsive for prolonged periods should have an *indwelling catheter* in the bladder. This will not only facilitate nursing care but will also allow accurate measurement of urinary output.

Summary of Phase 1

1. Record all available details of the history of injury and try to visualize how the body was injured.
2. General examination: define areas and extent of injuries and perform necessary emergency measures.
3. Record cerebral functional status:
   a. Level of responsiveness
   b. Memory and mentation
   c. Motor power in face and extremities
   d. Pupillary size and reactions
   e. Vital signs
4. Assign Glasgow Coma Scale rating on basis of above.
5. Obtain skull roentgenograms when the mechanism of injury or condition of the scalp suggests the possibility of a depressed fracture or of a temporal fracture that may cross the path of the middle meningeal artery
6. Obtain films of the cervical spine when the mechanism of injury indicates that the head was snapped suddenly forward or backward so as to fracture or dislocate the cervical vertebrae

Phase 2
Observation of Clinical Progress

The clinical course is observed to detect the development of complications. What are these complications, and what are their symptoms and signs? Four types should be under consideration at all times: *increased intracranial pressure, hemorrhage, infection,* and *convulsive seizures.*

Increased intracranial pressure after head injury may result from reactive cerebral edema or from the development of a localized hematoma in the epidural or subdural spaces, or within brain substance. Lethargy, vomiting, and dulling of responses are common to all cases regardless of the underlying pathosis, and localizing neurologic deficits are inconstant except in patients with intracerebral hematoma.

Cerebral edema begins immediately after injury and may continue to increase for 48 to 72 hours before beginning to subside. In relatively minor injuries it diminishes after 6 to 12 hours and requires no treatment. After severe cerebral contusions, edema and generalized infarction may convert the white matter into a pulpy mass.

Subdural hematoma is the most common of the complicating hematomas. The acute hematoma, which produces signs within 48 hours of injury, is usually caused by bleeding from a vein bridging between the superficial middle cerebral vein and the sphenoparietal sinus. Hence these hematomas are maximal in the *temporal region.* The clot may become organized and liquefy so that it becomes converted into a cystic cavity limited by a capsule and containing fluid having a much higher osmotic pressure than that of the adjacent cerebrospinal fluid. By osmosis through this semipermeable capsule or membrane, cerebrospinal fluid is imbibed, resulting in gradual expansion of the cavity. Symptoms may then appear after a delay of several weeks or months after injury (Fig. 35-16; chronic subdural hematoma). There may occur small subdural collections that cause no symptoms and require no treatment; they may resolve into thin scars and sometimes become calcified. An intermediate entity, the subacute hematoma, is recognized. Its definition is arbitrary, but generally it applies to hematomas that become clinically manifest between the third and fourteenth day after injury. An alternative explanation for the formation of chronic hematoma is tearing of the pacchionian granulations from their dural attachment resulting in the immediate leakage of cerebrospinal fluid and blood into the subdural space. This lesion is therefore maximal over the *convexity of the hemisphere.* After a lapse of about 3 months from the time of injury, the possibility of a clinically significant subdural hematoma is so small that, for practical purposes, it need not be entertained seriously in the differential diagnosis.

Epidural hematoma (Figs. 35-17 and 35-18) usually results from laceration of branches of the middle

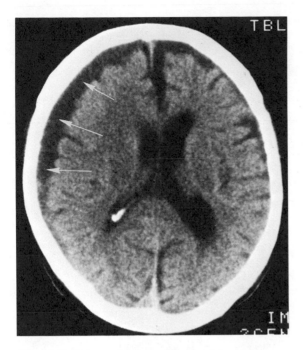

Fig. 35-16. CT scan showing a chronic subdural hematoma. The density of this fluid lesion *(arrows)* is much lower than brain tissue, but greater than that of ventricular fluid.

meningeal artery. Often a fracture line can be seen radiographically in the temporal region, crossing the grooves formed in the inner table of the skull by the artery. Because bleeding is arterial, the symptoms are usually rapid both in onset and in progression. This lesion is less common in the elderly because the dura becomes so adherent to the inner table with advancing age that the artery is tamponed effectively.

Intracerebral and intracerebellar hematomas form when bleeding occurs into bruised and edematous brain tissue. These "hematomas" are frequently a mixture of blood and necrotic white matter. Most are subclinical and are detected only by CT, but occasionally they are large enough to warrant surgical evacuation with concomitant débridement of nonviable adjacent brain tissue.

The appearance of signs of increased intracranial pressure varies with the lesion producing the pressure. Signs develop within the first 24 to 48 hours from cerebral contusion and edema and from epidural hematoma, whereas they tend to appear slightly later with intracerebral hematomas. Evidence of subdural hematoma may appear early or up to 3 months later, by which time the causative traumatic episode may have been forgotten. Since every head injury of any consequence is followed by some degree of increased pressure from reactive edema, one must establish a critical level at which point specific investigation and treatment are indicated. This level is generally reached *when the patient is no longer able to respond appropriately to verbal or non-noxious tactile stimuli.* If the patient has been incapable of such a response from the time of injury, it is appropriate, in the absence of localizing neurologic deficits, to await signs of progression.

The presence of hemiparesis is inconstant and unpredictable in patients with traumatic hematoma. Hemiparesis present immediately after injury is likely caused by cerebral contusion rather than by a compressing hematoma. The slow development of a mild hemiparesis is consistent with the presence of an extracerebral hematoma (epidural or subdural), whereas a dense hemiplegia, especially in an alert patient, is rarely produced by such a lesion. Subdural hematoma may arise with no paresis or with hemiparesis contralateral or ipsilateral to the hematoma. Hence the *neurologic picture of subdural hematoma is often confusing and nonspecific.*

Frequent recording of the vital signs—pulse, respirations, blood pressure, and temperature—is an integral part of the observation routine. Unfortunately the so-called classic alterations in the vital signs described under the section on increased intracranial pressure are so *frequently absent* in patients with proved intracranial hematomas that they cannot be relied on to occur. Intracranial pressure may not be assumed to be normal because vital signs are stable. Shock is never produced by increased intracranial pressure, except in the terminal stages. The development of shock demands a search for an extracranial source of blood loss.

Hemorrhage from the gastrointestinal tract not uncommonly accompanies severe head injuries, particularly with brainstem damage. The pathophysiology of this phenomenon is presumably the same as stress ulcers associated with burns and other major traumatic incidents. Bleeding may occur from a single acute ulcer or from multiple superficial erosions, and it may cause death by exsanguination. Whenever shock occurs during the clinical course of an unresponsive patient, gastrointestinal hemorrhage should be suspected. Subgaleal bleeding (cephalohematoma) in infants can be of sufficient magnitude to produce shock. In adults it is impossible to lose a sufficient quantity of blood intracranially or into the subgaleal space to produce shock from volume loss alone.

Infections involving the pulmonary and urinary tracts are frequently encountered in patients who remain unresponsive for prolonged periods of time. Tracheostomy is often indicated for adequate removal of tracheobronchial secretions. Prophylactic antibiotic therapy should be given in certain circumstances, particularly to elderly patients. *Meningitis* is a threat when an open fracture allows the leakage of cerebrospinal fluid outside the cranial cavity. Whenever there is bleeding from the ears, nose, mouth, or scalp, the blood should be examined for spinal fluid content. Blood containing cerebrospinal fluid is usually watery, forms a pale outer ring when dripped onto a gauze sponge, and does not clot. High fever and nuchal rigidity call for diagnostic lumbar puncture. Abscess formation produces pressure symptoms similar to that of hematoma, except that seizures and localizing paresis are much more common.

Convulsive seizures occur infrequently after head injury. They are much more likely to occur in infants and children under 10 years of age. The seizures may be focal or generalized (grand mal) and usually denote cerebral contusion. Except in infants, subdural hematoma is rarely associated with seizures before treatment.

Progressive facial nerve paralysis occasionally fol-

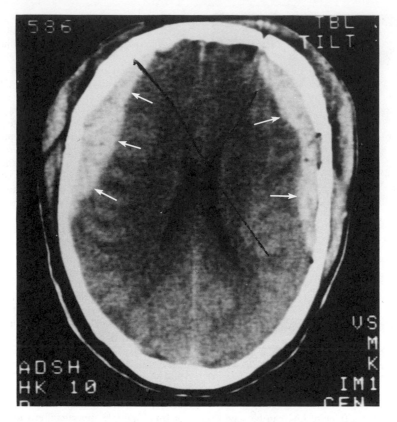

Fig. 35-17. CT scan showing bilateral extracerebral compressing hematomas, *arrows*. Acute hematomas are always of high density and are easily demonstrable by rapid scanning techniques.

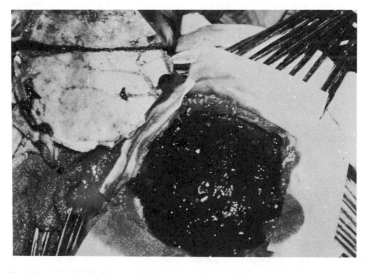

Fig. 35-18. Epidural hematoma. Reflected skull flap shows linear fracture crossing grooves formed by middle meningeal artery. Underlying hematoma is entirely solid clot, so that it could not have been drained through burr holes only.

lows basal skull fracture, and so it should be watched for in every patient with cerebrospinal fluid drainage from the ear. It begins 1 to 3 days after injury and may be partial and self-limited or may progress to total loss of facial nerve function.

Supportive Medical Care

Vomiting is common during the first 8 hours after head injury, so that oral intake should be withheld during that period. Clear fluids may be given thereafter if the patient desires them, and solid food after 24 to 48 hours depending on the severity of the injury. If parenteral fluids are required, the volume administered during the first 48 hours should be somewhat less than the normal daily requirements—1500 to 2000 ml for an average adult. Overhydration enhances cerebral edema. Feeding by nasogastric tube should be instituted if the patient is unable to swallow after 3 days.

To minimize the risk of gastrointestinal ulcers and hemorrhage, the gastric pH should be maintained above 5 with histamine (H_2) blockers such as cimetidine or famotidine. Seizures must be treated vigorously, as respiratory interruption accompanying convulsions adds the insult of hypoxia to an already injured brain. Phenytoin (Dilantin) should be given intravenously in doses sufficient to establish and maintain a therapeutic serum level; a loading dose of 1 g infused intravenously over a 10-minute period is appropriate for any adult. Individual seizures can be stopped by direct intravenous injections of diazepam (Valium). Both of these medications in their normal diluents are highly irritative to vein intima, frequently causing thrombophlebitis; therefore, these drugs should be injected into large veins or through central venous catheters rather than into the small peripheral veins of the wrist or hand.

Sedation should be avoided whenever possible, but the extremely restless, struggling, and vociferous patient should be quieted with small doses of chlorpromazine or other tranquilizing drugs rather than by the simple application of restraining bonds. Progressive facial nerve paralysis usually can be arrested by adrenal corticosteroids, but complete paralysis may require surgical decompression of the nerve within its canal.

Attention to the care of the eyes, oropharynx, and respiratory and urinary tracts is essential to the prevention of ulcerative and infectious complications. The program for such supportive care is the same as that required after any major operation or trauma.

Summary of Phase 2

1. Observe for
   a. Deterioration of cerebral functional status (decrease in the Glasgow Coma Scale rating)
   b. Specific signs of dangerously increased intracranial pressure
2. Treat any medically treatable complications such as gastrointestinal hemorrhage, convulsions, high fever.
3. Decide whether the patient's progress warrants continued care in a primary facility or indicates the need for more specialized observation at a neurosurgical facility

Phase 3
Performance of Special Diagnostic Tests

Acute traumatic intracranial hematomas are detected and delineated best by CT, which may also indicate the degree of cerebral swelling. Therefore optimal evaluation and management planning for any patient who does not regain consciousness fully and rapidly after a head injury should include immediate unenhanced CT studies. Certainly any patient whose level of responsiveness is reduced to or near the critical level discussed previously or who develops a neurologic deficit or fails to show satisfactory neurologic improvement should have such a study. Occasionally a subdural hematoma becomes exactly the same in density (isopycnic) as the adjacent brain, so that the interface between them is very difficult to define by unenhanced CT. In such instances, contrast enhancement or an MRI study may be necessary to confirm the presence of an extracerebral compressive mass.

Lumbar puncture is of no value except in the diagnosis of a complicating meningitis or gross subarachnoid hemorrhage. Subdural taps can be performed on infants, but only liquefied (chronic) hematomas can be aspirated through the small-bore needles used for such taps.

Phase 4
Nonsurgical Treatment

The goal of definitive treatment is to alleviate increased intracranial pressure. Although the removal of a significant hematoma is mandatory, that alone may be insufficient to accomplish this goal if there is severe cerebral swelling. Nonsurgical decompressive aids may then be necessary if the patient is to derive practical benefit from the removal of the primary lesion. These aids are to be used only if CT has ruled out the presence of a major hematoma; their indiscriminate use before definitive diagnostic testing not only may mask the signs of a lesion that demands surgical removal but also by reducing the tamponing effect of the brain adjacent to the hematoma, may *promote* further bleeding and expansion of the hematoma.

Two nonsurgical adjuvants are commonly utilized: infusion of dehydrating agents and administration of barbiturates in coma-inducing doses. Intravenously administered mannitol or urea usually produces considerable reduction of intracranial pressure. The degree and duration of this effect depends on the dosage and agent administered. When the effect has been exhausted, intracranial pressure tends to rise to a level even higher than that before the agent was given (rebound phenomenon). Hence the dose of mannitol or urea should be governed by intracranial pressure measurements monitored continuously by implanted sensors. Intravenous thiopental sodium given in high doses to induce and maintain a comatose state can also reduce intracranial pressure significantly; this technique is reserved for patients with prolonged, dangerous elevations of pressure that cannot be controlled by dehydrating agents. In patients whose respirations are inadequate to maintain at least a normal Pa_{CO_2} the intracranial pressure can be lowered by paralyzing spontaneous respiration with curariform drugs (pancuronium bromide) and then ventilating the patient into a hypocapnic state with a mechanical respirator. High-potency adrenal corticosteroids (e.g., dexamethasone) may reduce the degree of cerebral edema, but statistical studies have never proved that their use reduces the morbidity or mortality of head injuries. Their primary ability to reduce intracranial pressure is too delayed to be worthwhile in acute situations, but they do prolong the beneficial effects of dehydrating agents, and therefore their use as adjuvants to these agents is indicated. Because of the frequency of gastrointestinal hemorrhage in severe head injuries and the possible potentiation of this problem by adrenal corticosteroids, the prophylactic use of cimetidine is advisable. Furosemide increases the effect of mannitol but, used alone, has minimal effect on acutely elevated intracranial pressure.

Surgical Treatment

Surgical management consists of evacuation of hematomas, débridement of necrotic nonfunctional brain tissue, and extracerebral decompressive procedures. Chronic liquid hematomas can be drained through simple burr holes, whereas acute solid clots and necrotic brain require larger openings for effective removal. One can provide these by rongeuring the bone (craniectomy) or by removing a full bone flap. Additional decompression may be accomplished by the complete removal of large bone flaps and by sectioning of the tentorium to relieve direct pressure of the brainstem. The use of the latter procedures has largely been supplanted by the application of the nonsurgical adjuvants discussed previously.

In order for surgical treatment to be effective, one must choose an appropriate and adequate operation based on the history, clinical findings, and the characteristics of the lesion as delineated by CT or MRI. Hence the patient should be treated in a neurosurgical facility. Although in very rare circumstances a simple bur hole placed in the emergency room might provide life-saving decompression of an acute intracranial hematoma, it is much more likely that such an undertaking will be futile and will delay transporting the patient to a proper facility for more definitive treatment.

Of special interest in the postoperative care of patients with subacute and chronic subdural hematomas is the high incidence of convulsive seizures. The risk is sufficiently great to warrant routine use of anticonvulsant medications for 3 to 6 months after operation.

Prognosis After Head Injury

Although the threat of serious or fatal complications attends every head injury, no matter how trivial, some general prognostications may be applied to the majority of patients, depending on their neurologic findings immediately after injury. The capacity for neurologic recovery is profoundly influenced by the age of the patient. An infant or child suffering a concussion with loss of consciousness for not more than a few minutes will usually be asymptomatic within 48 hours. Young and middle-aged adults often complain of postural headache and giddiness for perhaps a week or more, whereas the elderly patient is often mentally confused for days and complains of symptoms for weeks. Severe brainstem injury with decerebrate responses may be completely reversible in the child and young adult, though several months are required for recovery. With such an injury, chances of fatality are quite high in middle-aged and even higher in elderly persons.

If epidural hematoma is diagnosed and treated in time, complete recovery usually occurs. However, the younger age of persons who typically sustain this complication contributes to the low mortality and morbidity. Acute subdural hematoma is fatal in the majority of cases, even with immediate operation. Gross cerebral contusion that accompanies most of these hematomas

contributes to high mortality. Chronic subdural hematomas can usually be treated satisfactorily, but the incidence of postoperative complications remains high.

Symptoms that cause varying degrees of prolonged or permanent disability may persist in many forms. The most obvious of these are motor deficits (e.g., hemiparesis and speech disturbances); however, there may be more subtle symptoms noticed by the patient and immediate family that are not easily recognized by the clinician. They include changes in affect and difficulties with cognition and concentration that can be quite disabling and may be attributed incorrectly to a posttraumatic neurosis. Psychometric testing may be necessary to prove organic brain dysfunction resulting from a head injury, particularly if the injury appears to have been mild.

SPINAL TRAUMA

Management of the spine-injured patient may be considered in the same four phases described for craniocerebral injuries. It is directed toward achieving the following goals: (1) relief of compression on the spinal cord and nerve roots; (2) prevention of additional trauma to neural elements until bone healing has taken place; (3) provision of conditions for bone healing that will result in permanent stability and satisfactory alignment.

Phase 1

Assessment of the Type and Severity of Injury

The mechanism of injury, resultant neurologic disability, and prognosis differ greatly depending on the level of injury. Table 35-3 lists the types of deficits with relation to the injured vertebral segments. Fracture-dislocations of the cervical spine (Figs. 35-19 and 35-20) usually result from acute hyperextension (e.g., a blow to the forehead or chin driving the head backward). Thus significant craniocerebral injury may be associated with any cervical spine injury, and *any injury to the head may be accompanied by damage to the cervical spine*. The thoracic and lumbar spine are more often damaged by hyperflexion.

As in craniocerebral trauma, the spinal injury is considered from two aspects, neurologic and vertebral:

Neurologic
    Concussion
    Contusion
    Compression   Spinal cord, nerve roots
    Hematomyelia
Vertebral
    Compression   Vertebral body
    Comminution

                   Spinous process (with or
                     without dislocation)
Linear fracture   Laminal arch (with or without dislocation)
                     Pedicle (with or without dislocation)

Dislocation without
    fracture

Description of the injury should include the level of the injury, assessment of major motor and sensory functions, and the bony lesion (e.g., complete paraplegia

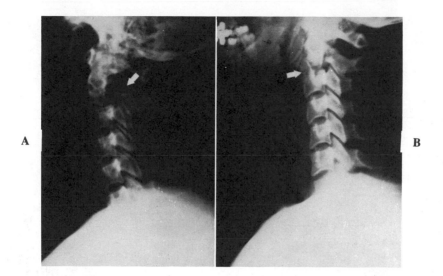

Fig. 35-19. Fracture-dislocation of C2 anteriorly on C3. **A,** Body of C2 is displaced anteriorly, and pedicles are fractured *(arrow)*. **B,** Dislocation has been reduced by traction and anterior interbody fusion performed with insertion of bone graft *(arrow)*.

Table 35-3. Clinical Picture After Injury to the Spinal Cord and Cauda Equina

Vertebral Segment	Neurologic Segment	Paralysis Resulting from Physiologic Transection	
		Partial Transection	Complete Transection
C1-C4	Spinal cord, cervical plexus level	Quadriparesis, becoming spastic*; Brown-Séquard syndrome	Instant or early death from respiratory failure
C5-T1	Spinal cord, brachial plexus level	Quadriparesis, becoming spastic; Brown-Séquard syndrome	Quadriplegia, becoming spastic
T2-T10	Dorsal spinal cord	Paraparesis, becoming spastic; Brown-Séquard syndrome	Paraplegia, becoming spastic
T11-L1	Conus medullaris	Flaccid or spastic paraparesis	Flaccid or spastic paraplegia
L2-S1	Cauda equina	Flaccid paraparesis	Flaccid paraplegia
Sacrococcygeal	Filum terminale	No deficit	No deficit

*Paresis or paralysis is always flaccid in the acute phase.

with motor and sensory loss to the T6 dermatome, fracture of pedicles of T5, with anterior dislocation of T5 on T6).

Concussion and contusion denote the same gross pathologic changes as in the brain. Hemorrhage into the substance of the cord may be petechial or localized into a hematoma (hematomyelia). Subdural and epidural hematomas sufficient to produce significant compression are so rare in the spinal canal that they are not of practical importance.

Unfortunately, the neurologic picture is frequently that of complete bilateral cord transection. There is usually a band of hyperesthesia at the dermatomal level of injury, with complete loss of all motor power and sensation, autonomic function (anhydrosis and paralytic ileus), and reflexes below this level. This is the picture of *spinal shock.* Autonomic activity returns in 48 to 72 hours and reflexes in 1 to 5 weeks. Paralysis of volun-

tary movement is permanent, but hyperactivity of reflexes often leads to severe spasms in paralyzed muscles. Lesser degrees of functional deficit are shown in Table 35-4.

Compression fractures of the vertebral body and linear fractures of laminae and spinous processes are generally not associated with neurologic deficits, for there is little displacement of the fracture fragments; however, very severe compressive forces may shatter the vertebral body, resulting in the "explosion fracture," in which fragments are displaced radially from the vertebral center, and those displaced posteriorly can compromise the spinal canal and compress the spinal cord (Fig. 35-21). Fractures of the pedicles are usually accompanied by dislocation, so nerve damage is common. Gross dislocations (Fig. 35-20) are still compatible with cord function if fractured laminal arches separate from the vertebral bodies so that the spinal canal is

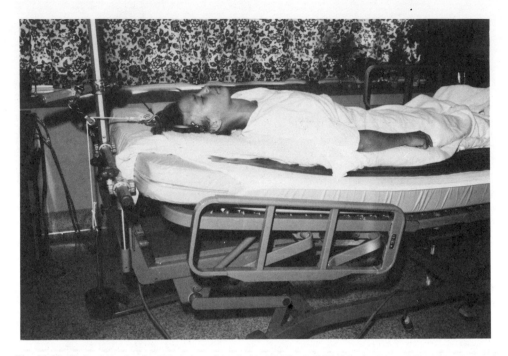

Fig. 35-20. Skeletal traction for dislocation of cervical spine. Gardner-Wells tongs *(arrow)* have been inserted into patient's skull, and traction has been applied by suspension of weights on pulley at head of bed. Position of head required to maintain vertebral alignment varies with individual features of dislocation. Patient is lying on automatic alternating pressure mattress, controlled by motor located at foot of bed.

Table 35-4. Clinical Syndromes of Partial Spinal Cord Damage

Portion of Cord Involved	Neurologic Picture
Central core	Severe paresis at level of injury only, with relatively intact motor and sensory functions below that level
Anterior half	Bilateral paresis and loss of pain and temperature sensation, with relative preservation of touch, position, vibration senses below level of injury
Lateral half	Ipsilateral paresis with contralateral loss of pain and temperature sensations below level of injury (Brown-Séquard syndrome)
Whole cord	Partial loss of all motor and sensory functions to approximately equal degree below level of injury

not narrowed beyond a critical dimension. Occasionally severe neurologic deficits can be present in the absence of any bone abnormality; a spontaneously reduced dislocation or acutely herniated disk should be suspected in such circumstances.

In assessing bony damage radiographically, the pa-tient should be moved as little as possible. The neck can be protected by sandbags or a collar, or the head and trunk can simply be strapped in a neutral position to stabilizing boards until the basic lateral roentgenograms of the spine have been taken to rule out dangerous malalignment of the vertebrae.

Performance of Emergency Procedures

Any dislocation of cervical vertebrae, with or without neurologic deficit, is treated and protected best by immobilization in skeletal traction (Fig. 35-20). Skull tongs of the Gardner-Wells type can be inserted quickly with minimal discomfort to the patient. Ideally, a traction halo (Fig. 35-23 A) can be applied initially, used to restore alignment, and then attached directly to a body jacket allowing the patient to be mobilized (Fig. 35-23 B). *Halter traction is unsatisfactory and can be dangerous to life in any patient with upper limb paralysis.* The halter may slip and asphyxiate, while the paretic patient may have insufficient strength to adjust or remove it. In most instances, proper alignment can be restored with traction alone. The traction is begun with 10 to 15 pounds, and weight is added successively as indicated by progress radiographs or fluoroscopic monitoring. Once the desired alignment has been obtained, it can usually be maintained with a comfortable traction level of 7 to 15 pounds.

Cervical dislocations above C6 associated with gross neurologic deficit may produce respiratory insufficiency from paresis of intercostal muscles and diaphragm. Tracheostomy plus the assistance of a mechanical respirator may be necessary.

Little can be done initially to restore the alignment

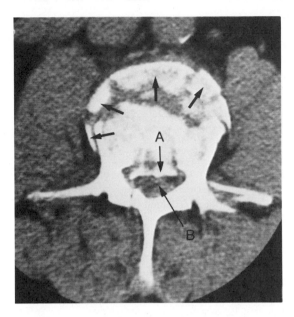

Fig. 35-21. CT showing compression/comminution ("explosion") fracture of vertebral body. Fragments have been displaced radially *(arrows)*, with the posterior fragment **A** encroaching significantly upon the central canal **B**, leaving only marginal space for the spinal cord.

after fracture-dislocation in the thoracic and lumbar vertebrae except by open operation. Since most of these fractures are the result of hyperflexion, the patient should be placed in bed on soft supports so that the spine is slightly extended. Pelvic traction is of no value.

If the patient is unable to urinate without leaving a significant residual, an indwelling catheter should be placed and drainage established.

Phase 2
Observation of Progress and Supportive Medical Care

The development of secondary compressive hematomas is so rare after spinal trauma that it is not the major consideration that it is after head injury; however, lack of neurologic improvement and certainly any progressive deterioration of function may be indications for surgical exploration and decompression.

Paralytic ileus constantly accompanies paralysis of the limbs, so oral intake should be withheld until there is evidence of return of good bowel activity. The normal daily requirement of fluids should be given parenterally.

Care of the skin is a major nursing problem in patients who are unable to change position in bed. Decubiti rapidly develop over the sacrum and heels. Use of revolving frame beds (e.g., Rotorest, Foster, Stryker)

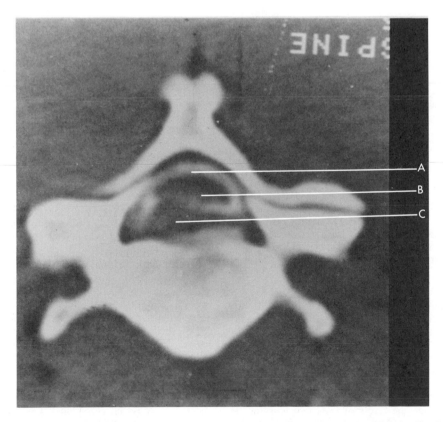

Fig. 35-22. High-resolution computerized tomogram showing compression of cervical cord by herniated disk. Subarachnoid space, **A,** is enhanced by intrathecal instillation of metrizamide. Spinal cord, **B,** is distorted and displaced posteriorly by large fragment of disk extruded into spinal canal, **C.**

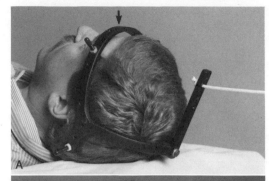

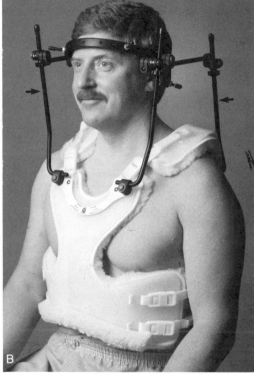

Fig. 35-23. A, Skeletal traction using a halo. The crown *(arrow)* is anchored securely to the skull by four pins inserted through the skin. Traction is applied via an upright bar bolted to the rear of the crown. **B,** When the patient is ready for ambulation, the traction bar is removed, and the crown is attached by upright struts *(arrows)* to a prefabricated body jacket. The crown and struts are of radiolucent and magnetically inert materials so that progress can be followed by radiography or MRI.

and of the alternating pressure mattress aid in the frequent redistribution of pressure on different areas of skin.

Phase 3
Special Diagnostic Procedures
Evaluation of the degree of pressure on the spinal cord or nerve roots is accomplished best by high-resolution CT through the levels of vertebral injury or the clinical levels of cord injury. Vertebral bodies are frequently comminuted, a fact that cannot be detected by normal radiographic techniques, and fracture fragments

may project posteriorly, impinging upon neural elements. Soft tissue projections such as acutely herniated disks can be demonstrated by MRI, myelography, or contrast-enhanced CT. It should be emphasized that the pathologic states revealed by these imaging techniques *do not always require surgical treatment.* The indications for surgical intervention must be determined by the clinician considering the patient's history, neurologic findings, and progress, and correlating them with the degree of neural compression visualized by the above imaging studies.

Phase 4
Nonsurgical Treatment
Contusion and laceration of the spinal cord are accompanied by reactive edema as in brain injuries. Therefore adrenal corticosteroids (dexamethasone) and dehydrating agents (mannitol) may be administered immediately to patients having neurologic evidence of spinal cord damage. Because the occurrence of clinically significant hematomas is rare, these nonsurgical adjuncts can be given by the first treating physician before transfer to a neurosurgical facility.

A fractured spine, like any fractured bone, requires approximately 6 weeks of immobilization to heal strongly. Unstable cervical fractures can be immobilized by skeletal traction until the patient has recovered from the immediate systemic effects of trauma. Thereafter, the patient can be ambulated with the fracture site immobilized by a halo apparatus (Fig. 35-23.) Early ambulation in this manner is particularly important in the elderly, for they are prone to develop systemic complications during any period of confinement. After the initial period of healing, a less restrictive support such as a plastic collar can be fitted. Periodic x-ray checks should be made to detect any subsequent dislocation. Lateral roentgenograms taken with the neck in flexion and then in extension are used to determine the degree of stability or instability. Thoracic and lumbar vertebral injuries require a minimum period of immobilization without weight bearing; thereafter, the patient can be ambulatory in a supportive brace or body cast. Usually the protective support must be worn for an additional 6 to 12 weeks.

Surgical Treatment
Having corrected to the degree possible by nonoperative measures any significant malalignment of the spine and having tended to the patient's sytemic needs, it remains for the physician to decide whether prolonged immobilization alone will produce satisfactory healing of both bone and nerve injuries or whether surgical intervention is desirable to improve the speed and completeness of recovery. Operative interbody fusion in cervical fracture-dislocations accomplishes (1) removal of a possibly herniated and compressing intervertebral disk, (2) much earlier mobilization and discharge from the hospital, and (3) a guarantee, barring complications, of achieving a permanently stable spine. The procedure may be undertaken as soon as the patient has recovered from the immediate constitutional effects of trauma, and ambulation may be begun within a few days of operation. Fracture of the odontoid process of the second cervical vertebra (C2) is treated by

halo immobilization for 8 to 10 weeks, whereas sublux- ation of C1 on C2 *without* odontoid fracture usually re- quires surgical stabilization. The posterior elements of the atlas and axis can be wired together for immediate protection, and the resultant C1–C2 relationship solid- ified using interlaminar strut grafts for a permanent fu- sion.

Anterior interbody fusion (Figs. 35-19 and 35-20) is applicable to all dislocations between C2 and T1. It is frequently necessary when there has been pronounced subluxation without major fracturing, for while a frac- ture reunites with strong new bone formation, inter- spinous ligamentous tears heal poorly and chronic in- stability is a common result. Simple compression frac- tures of the cervical vertebrae may heal satisfactorily in 6 to 8 weeks with an external supportive brace, but if the vertebral body has lost too much of its interior structure by shattering and compression, a late progres- sive gibbus (anterior angulation) may form (Fig. 35-24) and can result in myelopathy. In such cases, replace- ment of the damaged body with an iliac crest or rib strut graft bridging to normal bone will restore and maintain satisfactory alignment until a strong bony fu- sion has taken place.

In the thoracic and lumbar segments, decompression and interbody fusion by an anterolateral approach is feasible occasionally, but the posterior approach is more direct and satisfactory in the majority of cases. An effective decompression of the spinal cord and cauda equina can be accomplished with very limited re- moval of laminar arches; posteriorly protruding verte- bral body fragments can be repositioned anteriorly; the vertebrae can be aligned more precisely, and early sta- bility can be imparted by supportive devices such as Harrington rods (Fig. 35-25). Interlaminar fusions us- ing these devices can prevent late gibbus that in young patients, can progress years after the original injury.

Prognosis for Recovery After Spinal Injuries

The prognosis for neurologic recovery varies with the neurologic segment injured and the severity of the initial deficit. If there is immediate loss of all motor and sensory function below the level of injury, the chances for functional recovery are extremely small re- gardless of the promptness and type of tretment. Unfor- tunately, a high percentage of spinal injuries result in immediate functional cord transection with permanent loss of cord function. Any preservation of neurologic

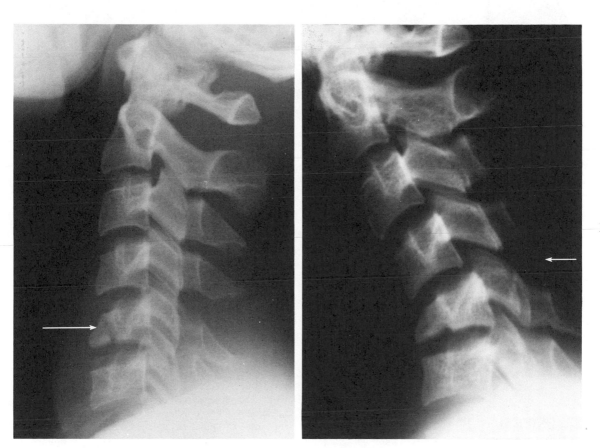

A   B

Fig. 35-24. Compression fracture with delayed angulation. The body of C5 was crushed in a diving accident, but normal alignment was restored and the patient ambulated with external support. Six weeks later, radio- graph **A** shows anterior angulation at C4-5 because of additional wedging of C5 vertebral body and rupture of the interspinous ligaments posteriorly. The central portion of C5 was resected **B** and a strut graft was used to bridge C4 to C6 *(arrow)* and restore satisfactory alignment. Once healed, C4, C5, and C6 become one solid block of bone.

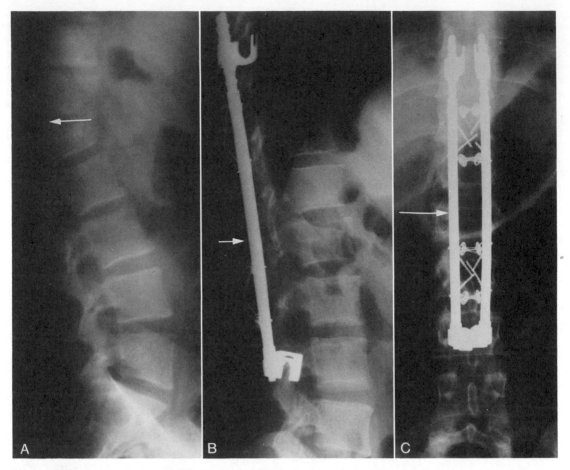

Fig. 35-25. Open reduction and posterior stabilization of T12-L1 fracture-gibbus. **A,** The body of L1 has been compressed and comminuted, causing an acute angulation at the thoracolumbar junction. **B** and **C,** Lateral and anteroposterior radiographs after operation show reduction of the angulation by Harrington rods *(arrows)* hooked above and below to the laminae and cross-wired through the base of the spinous processes to impart stability. Bone grafts are added to obtain permanent fusion of the posterior elements.

function alters the prognosis from one of almost complete hopelessness to one of possible, if partial, recovery. Complete recovery is rare with spinal cord injuries but occurs not infrequently when the cauda equina is the only area damaged. Death may ensue early or late as the result of pulmonary or urinary tract infection, especially after cervical cord transection.

The permanently paraplegic patient can usually be rehabilitated to an economically useful life. For some, crutch walking can be accomplished with external bracing of the legs, but for most the wheelchair is the only method of locomotion. The complete quadriplegic is usually a permanent invalid, incapable of gainful employment despite the availability of prosthetic aids.

PERIPHERAL NERVE INJURIES

Unlike the central nervous system pathways, the peripheral nerves are always capable of regrowth and reestablishment of neural connections after they have been traumatized or severed. The goal of surgical treatment is to provide the best possible conditions for the transected nerve to reestablish its connections with muscles and skin. Without the most optimal conditions, neuronal regrowth may be blocked, retarded, or disorganized and may result in incomplete or ineffective reinnervation.

Pathologic Changes After Injury

Trauma to peripheral nerve sufficient to produce clinically recognizable denervation may be accompanied by pathologic changes both proximal and distal to the site of injury. *Proximally* there is central chromatolysis *(axonal reaction)* in the cells of origin in the central nervous system; this is a temporary change and is reversible. *Distally* there is *wallerian degeneration,* which, once begun, is irreversible and continues until all axonal debris is removed. Within 4 to 6 days after the onset of wallerian degeneration, the nerve can no longer be made to conduct an electrical stimulus, so that direct stimulation of the nerve trunk through a needle electrode results in no contraction of the muscles that nerve normally innervates.

Axonal regrowth begins within 48 hours. If a proper pathway is available, regrowth proceeds at a rate of 1 to 1.5 mm/day until the target (muscle or skin) has been reached. If such a pathway is blocked, the axons curl back upon themselves, forming a heaped-up tangle of fibers called a *neuroma*. Although no recognizable degenerative changes occur in denervated skin, loss of tone and fiber size occurs in denervated muscle. The latter is most noticeable in the first 6 weeks after injury. If denervation is prolonged, the muscle becomes progressively replaced with fibrous tissue until it can no longer contract effectively even when stimulated directly. Thus, if effective reinnervation is to occur, the nerve must make contact with its muscle before too much fibrosis has occurred.

Using the foregoing principles, one can calculate the potential for effective treatment of most nerve injuries. Given a minimum neuronal regrowth of *1 mm per day* or *1 inch per month,* and considering that a muscle remaining denervated for more than 1 year may be extensively fibrosed, if a nerve is severed more than 1 foot proximal to its muscles, the potential for good functional motor recovery is poor. Furthermore, if, for example, a nerve is severed 9 inches proximal to its muscles but the lesion is neglected or goes undiagnosed for 6 months, a late anastomosis may not restore good function. Thus, although it may be prudent to delay exploration in cases in which the anatomic continuity of a nerve is believed to be preserved, *too long a delay may result in missing the opportunity for functional reinnervtion.* There are, of course, exceptions to these mathematical calculations, and so they may not be used as absolute criteria to determine whether surgery is indicated.

Management

The management of peripheal nerve injuries will be considered according to the three types of lesions encountered: stretching, compression and contusion, and laceration.

Stretch injuries affect principally the brachial plexus and, to a lesser extent, the sciatic nerve. A downward blow on the shoulder or falling and landing on the shoulder in such a way that it is forced downward put sudden tension on the roots and trunks of the brachial plexus. Axis cylinders may be ruptured, and the roots may be avulsed from the spinal cord. The result almost invariably is permanent loss of function. Management consists only in placing the limb in such a position that there will be minimal tension on the plexus (i.e., arm abducted 90 degrees and supported by an airplane splint). Myelography may be performed as soon as the patient can tolerate the maneuvers required without undue discomfort; extravasation of contrast medium at the site of an avulsed root is diagnostic. The lesion (Fig. 35-26) is untreatable. Posterior *dislocation of the hip* may result in stretching of the sciatic nerve over the head of the femur; other nerves may occasionally be stretched over the fractured ends of long bones. Surgical treatment of the stretch injury is most unsatisfactory because it is impossible to determine by gross inspection how long a segment of nerve has been damaged. Furthermore, such injuries in the brachial plexus and sciatic nerve at the hip are located so far proximal to denervaed muscles that even if regeneration occurs, it

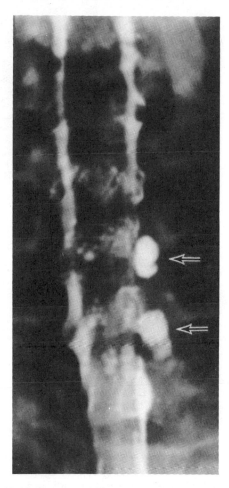

Fig. 35-26. Cervical myelogram showing extravasation of contrast media at site of avulsed C7 and C8 nerve roots *(arrows).*

cannot reinnervate muscles before extensive fibrosis has occurred.

Compression and contusion most commonly affect nerves that are relatively superficial and not protected by thick layers of muscle. The ulnar nerve at the elbow and the superficial peroneal nerve at the neck of the fibula are examples. Severe crushing trauma may injure any nerve trunk. There are three possible pathologic courses after peripheral nerve compression and contusion:

1. No wallerian degeneration—functional recovery within 2 to 6 weeks regardless of the distance from site of injury to denervated muscle or skin
2. Wallerian degeneration without significant internal fibrosis—regeneration and functional recovery after a delay consistent with the distance as calculated by distance from injury to muscle or skin ÷ rate of regrowth
3. Wallerian degeneration followed by significant internal fibrosis—formation of a neuroma-in-continuity (Fig. 35-27); partial reinnervation only, regardless of length of time elapsed

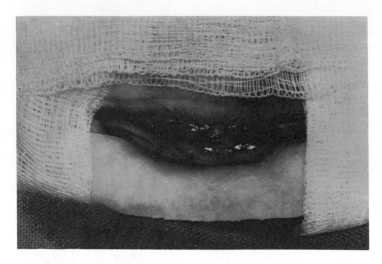

Fig. 35-27. Neuroma-in-continuity. Ulnar nerve in patient who fell on her elbow 6 months before operation and developed partial paralysis of interossei with preservation of all other ulnar nerve functions. Nerve is expanded to double its normal diameter by neuroma.

When there is no reason to suspect that a nerve has been severed (no penetrating wound, no fractured bone ends that might lacerate a nerve), management entails following the patient's course with frequent neurologic examination to determine whether regeneration is occurring. Paresthesias referred to the peripheral distribution of a nerve when the nerve is lightly percussed *(Tinel's sign)* indicate the most distal end of the regenerating nerve. If the sign can be elicited more than 2 inches beyond the point of injury, recovery will be likely to occur without surgical intervention. Electromyography is useful in detecting early reinnervation. If after 6 weeks there is no evidence of reinnervation or regeneration, exploration is indicated. If a significant neuroma is present with no electrical conduction distal to it, resection and anastomosis should be performed.

Laceration or transection of a peripheral nerve may be produced by penetrating foreign bodies or internally by the jagged ends of fractured long bones. Whenever such an injury occurs, neurologic function must be evaluated accurately and any deficit pointed out to the patient. The importance of the latter lies in the fact that surgical treatment of some kind is usually necessary in the treatment of associated injuries to bones, muscles, and tendons, so that a neurologic deficit that is not pointed out before such surgery may be blamed on the surgical procedure rather than on the injury. A clean field free of potential infection is a strict requirement for the anastomosis of a transected nerve. Most open wounds do not fulfill this requirement, and therefore emergency nerve repair is seldom indicated. Apposition of the lacerated ends with one or two sutures prevents their retraction and also facilitates identification at the time of definitive anastomosis. Such wounds should be debrided thoroughly and closed, and anastomosis should be delayed until clean healing has occurred. However, although it is prudent to wait whenever the sterility of a wound is in doubt, there is *equal disadvantage in waiting too long,* particularly when the site

of transection is nearly a foot proximal to denervated muscles, for reasons stated previously. Anastomosis can be performed by use of suture or various adhesives. Fresh cuts are made until healthy nerve ends are bared; the nerve trunk proximally and distally may be mobilized with its mesoneurium or transplanted in order to bring the ends together without tension. Marking the ends with radiopaque sutures through the epineurium provides a useful method of checking to see that they have not separated postoperatively (Fig. 35-28).

INTRACRANIAL NEOPLASMS

The morbidity and mortality potentials of an intracranial neoplasm differ from those of tumors elsewhere in the body. Local compression and invasion are as important to the prognosis as the histologic picture. Therefore anatomic localization of a tumor is all-important in the clinical diagnosis. A histologically benign tumor may inevitably be fatal if it is so located that surgical removal cannot be undertaken without undue risk of operative death or the production of an incapacitating neurologic deficit. The histologically malignant neoplasms spread infrequently within the subarachnoid space and very rarely outside the central nervous system. They cause death by invading or compressing vital centers.

The symptoms of intracranial neoplasms are of three types: *increased intracranial pressure*—headache, lethargy, vomiting; *local or neighboring compression and invasion*—paralysis and sensory loss; and local irritation—convulsive seizures.

Persistent headache, often accompanied by subtle changes in mental behavior and by vomiting, indicates abnormal pressure rather than common migraine or nervous tension headaches. The progressive onset of neurologic deficit distinguishes neoplasm from cerebrovascular accident with its sudden ictus. Convulsions, especially focal or jacksonian, beginning in adult life are suggestive of neoplasm rather than idiopathic epilepsy.

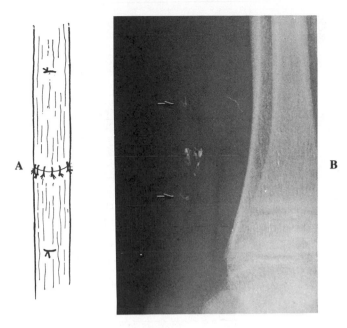

Fig. 35-28. Peripheral nerve anastomosis. **A,** Radiopaque suture is placed through the epineurium on each side of line of anastomosis. Postoperative roentgenogram, **B,** reveals these marking sutures to be approximately equidistant from anastomosis. Separation of nerve ends is diagnosed if marking sutures become separated.

Objective neurologic findings depend on the size, location, and rapidity of growth of the tumor. A slowly growing neoplasm, located at some distance from the sensorimotor cortex, may attain great size before producing recognizable neurologic signs other than those of generalized increased intracranial pressure. On the other hand, a small irritative lesion growing within the sensorimotor cortex may produce localized seizures and paresis long before there are any symptoms or signs of increased intracranial pressure.

Any of the foregoing symptoms coupled with any objective neurologic abnormality is sufficient to warrant investigation for brain tumor. In certain situations such investigations may be called for in the absence of any recognizable deficit. When it is reasonable to suspect the presence of a brain tumor, the most efficient and definitive diagnostic study one can order is MRI (Fig. 35-29). CT with intravenous contrast enhancement (Fig. 35-30) is available more widely and is nearly as reliable, but allergic reactions to iodinated contrast media are fairly common in patients who previously have undergone intravenous pyelography. Radioisotope and unenhanced CT are valuable when MRI is not available, but their diagnostic limitations must be kept in mind if such scans fail to reveal abnormalities in patients whose clinical findings strongly suggest the presence of a brain tumor.

A classification of more commonly encountered neoplasms is given below. For a detailed classification and description of all tumors, refer to textbooks of neuropathology. Only the clinical aspects of the common tumor are discussed here. Those tumors listed in the *plural* occur with varying histologic types and grades of differentiation.

Neuroepithelial
   Astrocytoma, grades I, II, III, and IV
   Ependymomas
   Oligodendrogliomas
   Medulloblastoma
   Pinealoma
   Papilloma of choroid plexus
   Paraphyseal (colloid) cyst
   Neurilemmoma
Mesodermal
   Meningiomas
   Hemangioblastoma
   Chordoma
Ectodermal
   Craniopharyngioma
   Pituitary adenomas
Congenital
   Epidermoid
   Dermoid

The age of the patient and the anatomic location of the lesion are of considerable importance in allowing prediction of the type of neoplasm. Infants and children under the age of 2 years rarely develop intracranial neoplasms. Up to the age of 15 years, tumors most often arise in the *cerebellum*. Of these, medulloblastoma and cystic astrocytoma comprise the majority. The highly malignant *medulloblastoma* occurs in the cerebellar vermis (disequilibrium) and blocks the outlets of the fourth ventricle (headache, vomiting from obstructive hydrocephalus). It frequently spreads in the subarachnoid space, producing secondary implants along the spinal neuraxis. Although it tends to infiltrate deeply in all directions, optimal treatment consists of surgical extirpation of as much tumor tissue as possible followed by irradiation of the entire brain and spinal

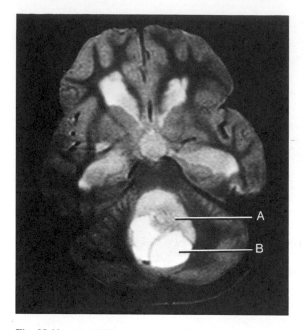

Fig. 35-29. Axial MRI showing cerebellar tumor in a child. In this T2-weighted image, ventricular fluid appears white as opposed to the T1-weighted image in Fig. 35-4. A large midline mass is present in the cerebellum having a solid cellular component **A,** and a large cystic component **B,** typical of cystic estrocytoma.

canal. Even though the neoplasm is highly radiosensitive, it cannot totally be eradicated, so survival is limited to 5 to 15 years.

The *cystic astrocytoma* occurs in the cerebellar hemisphere (limb ataxia) and later obstructs the fourth ventricle (headache, vomiting). The tumor consists of a large cyst containing xanthochromic fluid (Fig. 35-31) and a small nubbin of solid neoplasm. If this nubbin is resected completely, as it frequently can be, permanent cure results. Tumors of the cerebral hemisphere are less frequent in children, but when they occur, they are likely to be *ependymomas*. These tumors are moderately radiosensitive; therefore as much of the mass as possible is resected, followed by radiation therapy. Recurrence and death within 2 to 3 years are to be expected.

Of the remaining supratentorial tumors of children, *craniopharyngioma* deserves mention. This tumor, rising above the optic chiasm, is very often partially calcified, so that the combination of visual field defect, optic atrophy, and suprasellar calcium deposits provides an almost definitive diagnosis. The tumor can occur at any age, including the sixth decade or later, but does so most frequently before the age of 15. Complete curative surgical resection is possible in many instances, but the neurologic disability that may follow too radical an extirpation may be so disastrous that the surgeon may elect to stop short of total resection and treat small remnants by irradiation.

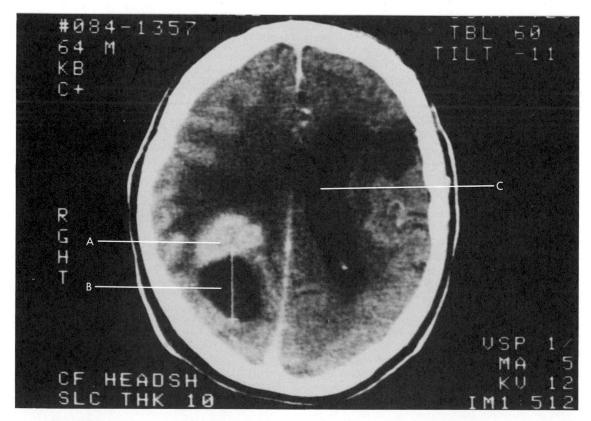

Fig. 35-30. Contrast-enhanced CT scan showing cystic astrocytoma in the parietal lobe. Solid portion of neoplasm, **A,** enhances densely with meglumine diatrizoate. Fluid within cyst, **B,** is slightly more dense than ventricular fluid, **C.**

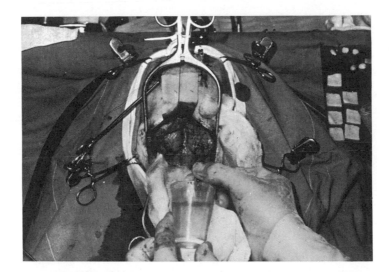

Fig. 35-31. Suboccipital craniectomy for cystic tumor of right cerebellar hemisphere. Cerebellar hemispheres are exposed, and their tonsils are seen herniated downward into cervical canal, right tonsil being larger than left. Cannula has been introduced into right hemisphere and about 25 ml. of fluid is drained off, resulting in collapse of hemisphere. Fluid is usually xanthochromic and often will clot on standing.

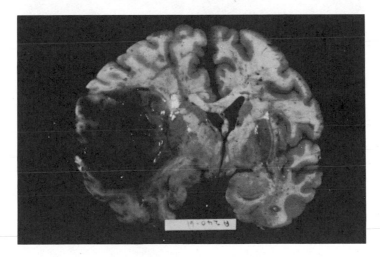

Fig. 35-32. Astrocytoma grade IV (glioblastoma multiforme). Tumor is often hemorrhagic. Its gross demarcation from surrounding brain tissue may appear fairly distinct at times, but microscopic examination will show invasion. Therefore, curative resection is not possible.

The 30- to 60-year age group produces the largest group of primary neoplasms, most of which are cerebral hemisphere malignancies with survival prognoses of less than 5 years. The *astrocytomas,* particularly the most malignant *glioblastoma* (Fig. 35-32), are the most frequently found lesions. They occur anywhere in the hemispheres, so the signs and symptoms depend on the anatomic location. If the neoplasm is located at the pole of a hemisphere, radical resection with lobectomy is the surgical procedure of choice. An entire frontal lobe anterior to the coronal suture can be excised without recognizable neurologic change if the opposite frontal lobe is normal; the anterior 5 cm of the temporal lobe can be excised without neurologic deficit if the opposite temporal lobe is normal; the occipital lobe can be excised without sensorimotor loss, but homonymous fields of vision will be lost. Since intrinsic neoplasms of the occipital lobe will likely destroy the visual area initially or inevitably, sacrificing that area in the interests of achieving maximum removal of tumor is usually justifiable. If the neoplasm is located deep in the hemisphere (e.g., in the thalamus) biopsy and limited resection of tumor is all that can be accomplished surgically; in such situations, locating and resecting the tumor is possible using a stereotactic guidance system coupled to CT or MRI. Only limited resection can be offered for neoplasms infiltrating the sensorimotor cortex, for any resection of tissue in that area is likely to result in additional undesirable paralysis. The neoplasms may infiltrate extensively (Fig. 35-33) and, when located near the midline, tend to cross to the opposite hemisphere via the corpus callosum; therefore recurrence

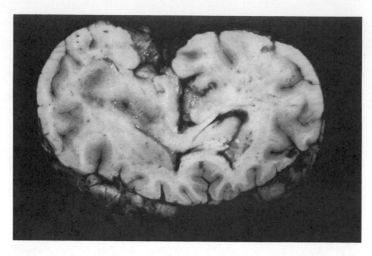

Fig. 35-33. Diffusely infiltrating frontal astrocytoma.Tumor blends imperceptibly with surrounding brain tissue and microscopically infiltrates brain. At operation, it is impossible to determine extent of tumor by gross inspection.

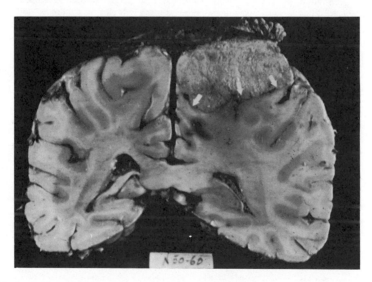

Fig. 35-34. Parasagittal meningioma. Tumor may arise from falx or from convexity and may invade superior longitudinal sinus. It does not invade brain tissue but slowly compresses it inferolaterally.

and eventual death of the patient are inevitable, even with the most radical resections.

Radiotherapy is considered appropriate for all gliomas, regardless of the extent of surgical resection. Although the more malignant neoplasms are the more radiosensitive, there is no accurate correlation between the grade of malignancy and the degree of radiosensitivity. The treatment is offered because the combination of surgical debulking followed by radiotherapy results in longer average survival than either treatment alone. Treatment can be accomplished either by externally focused irradiation or given internally by stereotactically implanted radioactive elements.

Chemotherapy with cytotoxic agents has resulted in some increases in postoperative survival, but like radiotherapy the effects are not accurately predictable and are still under extensive investigative study. In spite of

combined treatment of the malignant gliomas with these modes, survival remains a short 4 to 7 months for the glioblastomas, extending up to 1 to 2 years for the grade III astrocytomas, and up to 10 years for the gliomas of the lowest grades.

The most common benign tumor in adulthood is the *meningioma* (Figs. 35-34 and 35-35). A majority of meningiomas occur close to the midline, over the vault, or along the sphenoid wing. In the former position they are closely related to the superior longitudinal sinus and the falx cerebri, and they may invade the sinus or produce hyperostosis of the overlying bone. Some meningiomas erode through the bone and present as a mass under the scalp. Multiple meningiomas may occur as a manifestation of von Recklinghausen's disease. The tumors are readily diagnosed by CT. Focal or jacksonian seizures of months' or years' duration with a slowly de-

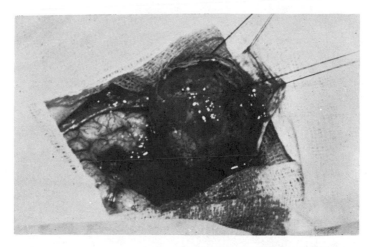

Fig. 35-35. Convexity meningioma. When tumor arises from convexity and has wide base, it can be removed from its bed in one piece, with it attached to dural flap. Since dura is invaded, flap to which tumor is attached is excised widely. Brain may then be covered with graft of tissue such as pericranium, or bone may simply be replaced over cortex.

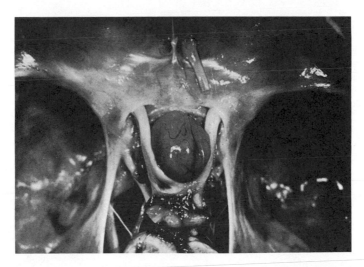

Fig. 35-36. Pituitary adenoma. Having ruptured through diaphragma sellae, tumor balloons upward between optic nerves, stretching them as well as optic chiasm to produce characteristic bitemporal hemianopsia.

veloping paresis are typical of this tumor. Total removal can usually be accomplished, but because many of these slow-growing neoplasms reach a large size before they produce symptoms (Fig. 35-4) extensive and permanent structural changes, which may result in significant postoperative morbidity, can occur preoperatively. Removal of large, long-standing meningiomas can be a difficult undertaking, but since these tumors are not generally considered to be radiosensitive, total extirpation is the only hope for permanent cure.

Neoplasms of the pituitary gland are common. They may be hormonally active, secreting prolactin (galactorrhea, infertility), ACTH (Cushing's syndrome), or growth hormone (gigantism, acromegaly). These neoplasms are usually small and contained within the sella turcica; they can be resected microsurgically by a nasal approach through the sphenoid sinus, or irradiated as a primary or postoperative treatment, if necessary. Pro-

lactin-secreting lesions can also be treated medically by use of bromocriptine mesylate. The hormonally inactive pituitary adenoma commonly grows upward out of the sella (Fig. 35-36), compressing the optic nerves and chiasm to produce a characteristic visual field defect (bitemporal hemianopsia) that is the hallmark of this neoplasm. When the tumor is small, it can be resected by the transsphenoidal route or treated by radiation; large tumors may require intracranial resection for adequate and precise decompression of the optic nerves.

Neurilemmomas arise most commonly from the auditory nerve but occasionally from the trigeminal and glossopharyngeal nerves. Tinnitus and slowly progressive hearing loss are the initial symptoms of the eighth nerve tumor; as the tumor enlarges and interferes with cerebellar function, ataxia is added to the symptom complex known as the cerebellopontine angle syndrome. Dysfunction of adjacent cranial nerves (trigem-

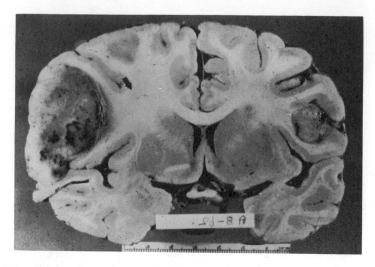

Fig. 35-37. Bilateral metastatic neoplasms. Multiplicity of metastases is unfortunate common characteristic. Lesions are grossly quite well demarcated in most instances. They often produce pronounced swelling of white matter. This patient had bronchogenic carcinoma.

inal and facial) is a late phenomenon, associated only with very large neoplasms. Removal of small tumors can be accomplished with preservation of some hearing; when large tumors must be removed it is not possible to save useful hearing, and facial motor function may be jeopardized, for the facial nerve is stretched and splayed over the dome of the neoplasm.

Above 50 years of age, the possibility of *metastatic carcinoma* must always be considered in the differential diagnosis of any expanding intracranial lesion. The metastases are frequently multiple (Fig. 35-37). In the male the most common source is the lung; in the female the breast is the usual source. A metastasis may become evident months or even years after the primary lesion has been removed; it may be solitary, particularly with hypernephroma, and surgical removal may extend life expectancy and has even resulted in apparent cures. Despite the ominous prognosis of metastatic carcinoma in the brain, one should not abandon hopes for worthwhile palliation. Surgical removal of any solitary intracranial metastasis may be worthwhile in selected cases, provided, of course, that there are no other known secondaries elsewhere in the body. In most instances a metastatic lesion excites considerable edema in the surrounding white matter. This edema can be overcome with high doses of dexamethasone and may result in dramatic symptomatic improvement. Hormone-dependent carcinomas of the breast and bowel carcinomas that have previously responded to chemotherapy may produce metastases that are sensitive to a combination of hormonal agents and cytotoxic chemicals. With a proper selection of modes of treatment, these unfortunate patients can be offered several months or even years of additional comfortable life. They should not be abandoned to die untreated simply because of the known presence of metastatic or recurrent malignant disease.

INTRASPINAL NEOPLASMS

Neoplasms within the spinal canal produce symptoms and signs by compression of the adjacent spinal cord or nerve roots and by obstruction of the blood supply to the cord. The patient complains of progressive weakness, clumsiness, or numbness of the extremities below the lesion. If a nerve root is involved, there may be pain radiating out into the dermatomal distribution of that root. In these respects the set of symptoms mimics that of vertebral spondylosis and herniated intervertebral disk. Spinal cord compression per se produces no pain, and loss of specific sensations often is not noticed by the patient.

Tumors involving the spinal cord almost invariably produce recognizable neurologic signs *bilaterally* by the time the patient is aware of any deficit. The small diameter of the cord makes it practically impossible for any mass lesion to produce compressive damage to one side only. Therefore, when the findings on examination are strictly unilateral, cord tumor is an unlikely diagnosis. The exact level of compression cannot be established reliably by clinical examination, for paresis and sensory loss do not necessarily extend up to the level of tumor (e.g., a tumor at C5 may produce paresis and sensory loss only to the T4 dermatomal segment). Only in the later stages, when function has been greatly impaired, does the neurologic level correlate with the anatomic site of the lesion.

Whenever the presence of a spinal cord tumor is suspected, MRI study of the appropriate segment of the spinal canal is indicated (Fig. 35-38). This diagnostic modality not only delineates whether the tumor is intradural and therefore a primary neoplasm, but also shows extradural neoplasms that infiltrate vertebrae and secondarily encroach on the spinal canal (Fig. 35-5). Clinical differentiation between the various types of tumors is difficult and not of practical value to the student. Early recognition of the presence of an intraspinal mass is important, for the sooner the mass is removed, the more rapid and complete will be the neurologic recovery. Operation performed after the patient has lost all cord function below the lesion stands little if any chance of producing worthwhile neurologic recovery.

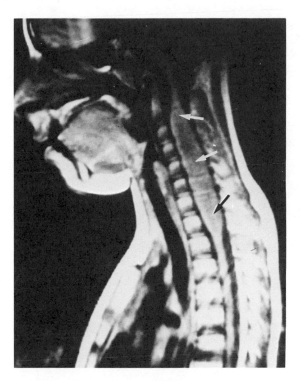

Fig. 35-38. Sagittal MRI showing intramedullary neoplasm. The cervical spinal cord is expanded from C2 to T1 by a cylindrical tumor mass *(arrows)*. This tumor was an astrocytoma; it was excised completely, without resultant neurologic deficit.

The common types of tumors are classified as follows:

Intradural
    Intramedullary
        Ependymoma
        Astrocytoma
    Extramedullary
        Primary
            Meningioma
            Neurofibroma
        Secondary
            Medulloblastoma (seeding from cerebellar tumor)
Extradural
    Primary
        Bone tumors
    Secondary
        Carcinomas (from prostate, lung, breast, gastrointestinal tract)
        Lymphoma
        Myeloma

Neoplasms within the cord substance (intramedullary) can be removed microsurgically. However, decompressive laminectomy followed by radiation may be the only treatment possible in some cases. The meningioma and neurofibroma can almost always be totally excised, with excellent neurologic results. Metastatic extradural neoplasms are seen more commonly than the aforementioned primary neoplasms. The history is usually short, with progression from apparently normal neurologic status to complete loss of all cord function within a few days. Such rapid progression indicates impairment of blood supply to the cord rather than compression as the principal feature and explains the overall lack of success of emergency decompression. Laminectomy with partial removal of tumor followed by radiation is offered in the hope of at least delaying progression to total paralysis.

INTRACRANIAL INFECTIONS

Infections within the central nervous system are generally chemotherapeutic rather than surgical problems. Two possibilities for surgical treatment exist, namely, evacuation of an abscess and prevention of reinfection. Abscesses are most frequently intracerebral, arising within the white matter by hematogenous spread from the lung or by contiguous spread through a tract from a paranasal sinus or the middle ear. The symptoms may be acute or chronic, characterized by headache, lethargy, vomiting, and paresis depending on the location of the lesion. Fever is often absent. Intracerebral abscesses are a common complication of acquired immunodeficiency syndrome (AIDS) and of cyanotic heart disease; in such cases, the lesions frequently are multiple or recurrent. Subdural abscess or empyema is next in frequency, arising almost invariably from a paranasal sinus or middle ear. Symptoms are acute and dramatic, with severe headache, convulsive seizures, and dense neurologic deficits. Epidural abscess also arises by direct extension from sinus or bone but is demonstrated less dramatically with pressure signs.

The presence of a focus of infection raises the possibility of abscess in the differential diagnosis of any mass intracranial lesion. It is obviously to the surgeon's advantage to be prepared for the finding of an abscess and to have given antibiotics appropriate to treat a known focus (or if the organism is unknown, a combination of penicillin and chloramphenicol) to establish adequate blood and tissue concentrations before intracranial surgery is undertaken. Subdural and epidural abscesses can usually be drained effectively through bur holes. Intracerebral abscesses, whenever encapsulated, are preferably resected completely. Postoperatively, the patient is treated with the same dosages of antibiotics as are used for active meningitis.

Concomitant with management of the abscess problem, any possible primary source for reinfection should be investigated. Meningitis without abscess formation also deserves such consideration if the responsible organism is other than *Meningococcus* or *Haemophilus influenzae*.

SPONTANEOUS INTRACRANIAL HEMORRHAGE

Intracranial bleeding in the absence of trauma may occur primarily into the brain substance (cerebral hemisphere, brainstem, or cerebellum) or into the subarachnoid space.

Intracerebral and intrapontine hemorrhages are most commonly seen in *hypertensive* patients in the 50- to 70-year age group. They are catastrophic in onset, with initial loss of consciousness and a severe lateralized neurologic deficit (e.g., hemiplegia). The hemorrhage usually occurs deep in the cerebral hemisphere near or in the internal capsule in the distribution of the lenticulostriate branches of the middle cerebral artery and frequently ruptures into the ventricular system

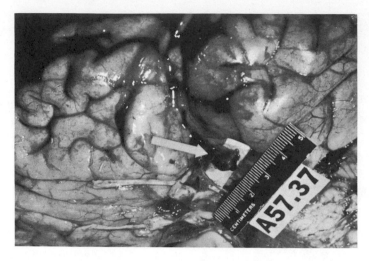

Fig. 35-39. Ruptured aneurysm, internal carotid artery. Aneurysm has ruptured at its neck *(arrow)*, producing fatal subarachnoid hemorrhage. Majority of aneurysmal ruptures occur at dome rather than at neck of sac.

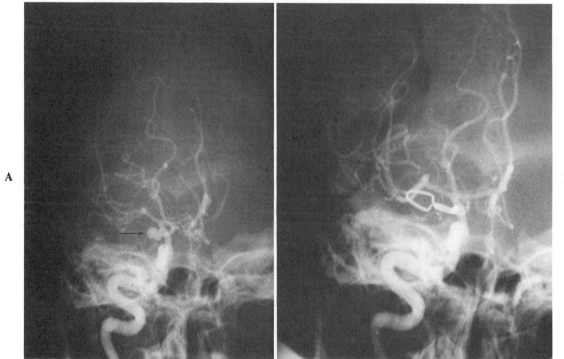

Fig. 35-40. Pre- and postoperative angiograms in patient with aneurysm of circle of Willis. **A,** Aneurysm *(arrow)* arises from right internal carotid artery at origin of posterior communicating artery. **B,** Postoperative angiogram shows neck of aneurysm occluded by metallic clip.

(Fig. 35-2). The immediate mortality is very high. Surgical treatment is directed toward preservation of viable functioning tissue by evacuation of hematomas and débridement of swollen and necrotic brain. Little benefit is derived from evacuating deep capsular hemorrhages because of their associated extensive destruction of functional structures, but more peripherally situated hematomas that have caused nondisabling paralysis can

be evacuated with little disturbance, so that the patient may recover much more rapidly and completely.

Subarachnoid hemorrhage is most often caused by a ruptured aneurysm of the circle of Willis (Figs. 35-39 and 35-40) and occurs maximally in the 40- to 60-year age group. The aneurysms develop gradually over many years, ballooning out of a relatively weak segment of a wall where an artery bifurcates or gives off a

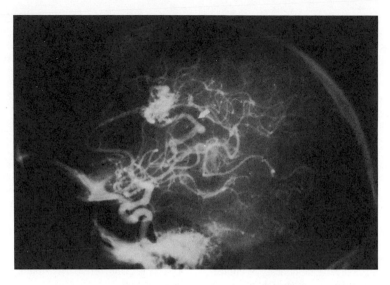

Fig. 35-41. Angiogram showing arteriovenous malformation. Lesion is fed principally by pericallosal artery. Rapid passage of contrast medium through malformation into venous system *(arrow)* is characteristic. Principal feeding and draining vessels depend on location of malformation.

branch; they enlarge but produce no symptoms until the wall of the sac becomes weak enough to rupture or the lesions become large enough to compress adjacent cranial nerves. The majority rupture before their maximum dimension reaches 1 cm. In over 20%, more than one aneurysm is present, but rarely does more than one aneurysm rupture at any given time. A hemorrhage can cause abrupt apnea and death; thus many victims never reach hospital. Of those who do, 12% to 15% die as a direct result of the initial hemorrhage and an additional 20% within 6 months die of rebleeding from the aneurysm. After 6 months, risk of rebleeding continues at an average rate of 2.2% per year for the next decade. This high risk of aneurysmal rebleeding and death is the indication for surgical treatment. Occlusion of the neck of the aneurysm sac by a spring clip (Fig. 35-40, *B*) is the most satisfactory and definitive operation; it is technically feasible in most aneurysms, but selection of the optimal time to perform the operation is very important to the overall outcome. Patients in good condition can be operated on within 3 days of their hemorrhage with low postoperative mortality and early protection against further bleeding, whereas those who are very ill from the effects of the subarachnoid hemorrhage may require a waiting period of 2 weeks or longer before definitive surgery can be performed with reasonable expectation of a satisfactory outcome. Hence it is essential that subarachnoid hemorrhage be recognized early (by the first physician who sees the patient), CT and angiographic studies be performed without delay, and that the patient be evaluated as a candidate for early surgical treatment. Aneurysms that, by their anatomic characteristics, do not lend themselves to clipping are sometimes treated by ligation of the carotid artery in the neck (if the aneurysm arises from the internal carotid artery in the cavernous sinus), by the external investment of the sac with gauze or plastics, or by filling the sac with fine wire or balloons to promote intraluminal thrombosis.

Subarachnoid and intraparenchymal hemorrhages occuring in the young (under 30) normotensive patient may result from *arteriovenous malformations* (Fig. 35-41). The malformations are present at birth but tend to enlarge slowly during life, opening up new vestigial channels into arteriovenous shunts that can sometimes significantly affect cardiac output. Hemorrhage occurs from the thin-walled veins that are too weak to contain blood under arterial pressure. Mortality from the first hemorrhage is low, but bleeding tends to recur over many years or even decades, and each succeeding hemorrhage adds to the mortality and morbidity. Therefore, surgical extirpation of the lesion is desirable whenever it is so located that operation does not carry too great a risk of producing a disabling neurologic deficit. To be effective the surgical resection must be complete, for any remaining arteriovenous shunts will expand over the years, opening up new abnormal channels of communication and giving rise to another malformation. Some of the larger and unresectable lesions can be obliterated satisfactorily by intraluminal embolization.

In approximately 19% of patients with proved subarachnoid hemorrhage, no cause can be established by all available diagnostic tests including repeated angiography. The prognosis for recovery and long-term survival for these patients is excellent and bears no relationship to the prognosis after bleeding from an aneurysm or arteriovenous malformation. No surgical treatment is necessary unless there is a localized hematoma of sufficient size to exert a dangerous mass effect.

CEREBROVASCULAR OCCLUSIVE DISEASE

The most common cause of cerebrovascular accident (stroke) is atheromatous occlusive disease. The internal carotid artery in the neck is the most common site of the stroke-producing atheromatous disease, whereas the vertebral artery in the neck and the intracranial vessels are less frequent sites. The age distribution of cerebrovascular disease closely parallels that of coronary artery disease, and the conditions often coexist in the same patient. Ischemia and infarction of the dependent cerebral hemisphere result in varying degrees of neurologic deficit that may be transient, temporary, or permanent.

The management of cerebral ischemia consists of angiography of the cervical and intracranial vessels for accurate diagnosis of the location and extent of arterial obstruction, followed by the restoration of vascular pathways by direct or indirect routes whenever feasible. However, if surgical treatment is to be effective, the diagnosis must be established and treatment completed before irreversible major cerebral damage has occurred. It is therefore important to recognize the signs and symptoms of an impending stroke. Clinically recognizable transient cerebral ischemia may precede a major infarction by several weeks or months. In cervical carotid artery disease, the cerebral hemisphere may suffer (with contralateral paresis, numbness, or clumsiness), or the retina may suffer (with ipsilateral loss of vision). In vertebrobasilar disease, brainstem symptoms occur (vertigo, incoordination, imbalance, or syncope). Such symptoms may be attributable to severe stenosis with inadequate blood flow through proximal vessels (Fig. 35-42) or to embolization of distal vessels from friable ulcerative atheromatous plaques occurring commonly at the origin of the internal carotid artery in the

neck (Fig. 35-43). Approximately 85% of patients with significantly stenotic or ulcerative carotid lesions have an audible bruit on auscultation over the neck vessels. Doppler evaluation and oculoplethysmography can provide an indication of the degree of stenosis, but angiography by either direct arterial injection or indirect venous injection with digital subtraction offer the only reliable assessment of the extent of arterial disease.

Carotid endarterectomy in patients with reversible neurologic symptoms caused by severe cervical carotid stenosis or ulceration produces excellent results in most cases, with a risk of surgical morbidity of 2% or less. The diseased segment of the artery is usually limited to the immediate area of the bifurcation of the common carotid artery, so that the distal limit of the atheromatous plaque in the internal carotid can easily be exposed. The intima and all underlying atheromatous tissue down to the adventitia of the artery can be excised, leaving a smooth and thin but adequately strong vessel. A venous patch graft occasionally is required to provide adequate lumen size. Not all patients, however, are candidates for the procedure. A completely occluded internal carotid artery rarely can be recanalized satisfactorily, and bypass anastomoses such as from the superficial temporal artery to the middle cerebral artery have failed to reduce statistically the incidence of stroke once the internal carotid artery has become completely occluded.

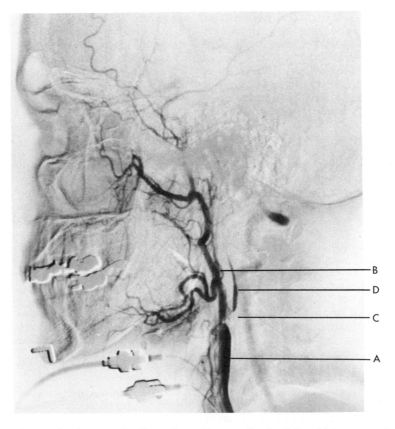

Fig. 35-42. Angiogram showing stenosis of internal carotid artery. Contrast injected into common carotid artery, **A,** passes readily up to external carotid artery, **B,** and its branches. Internal carotid artery, however, is so severely narrowed at its origin, **C,** that only wisp of contrast medium, **D,** has entered lumen.

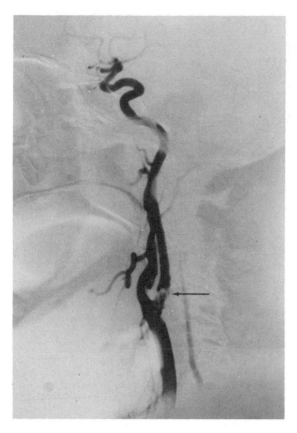

Fig. 35-43. Angiogram showing irregular, ulcerative atheromatous plaque at origin of internal carotid artery *(arrow)*. Such plaques are prone to fragmentation, with resultant embolization of intracranial vessels.

DEGENERATION AND HERNIATION OF INTERVERTEBRAL DISKS AND VERTEBRAL SPONDYLOSIS

Degeneration of the intervertebral disks is an aging process. It is essential for the student to have a sound understanding of the nature of disk degeneration as it relates to back disorders in general, for back disorders rank second only to the common cold as leading causes of absenteeism in the working population. An "abnormal" or "protruding" disk, as demonstrated by CT or MRI may not necessarily be the cause of the patient's presenting back symptoms, so treatment of that obvious abnormality may not achieve the satisfactory long-term resolution of that patient's disabling spine problems.

Herniation of an intervertebral disk into the spinal canal and degenerative changes in the disk and vertebral bodies resulting in spur formation (spondylosis) may cause compression and irritation of nerve roots and spinal cord. The former is a common condition affecting principally the 30- to 60-year age group, whereas symptomatic spondylosis is seen somewhat later in life (45 to 70 years). Although any vertebral segment may be involved in disk degeneration and vertebral spondylosis, there are definite levels of predilection, just as there are sites of predilection for atheromatous disease of the arteries. The fifth and sixth cervical and the third, fourth, and fifth lumbar intervertebral segments are the most frequently involved, whereas problems at other levels are rare in comparison. Spondylosis sufficient to produce *neurologic* symptoms occurs most commonly in the lower three cervical vertebrae (Fig. 35-45). Spondylotic spurs on the lumbar vertebrae may produce the symptoms and signs of nerve root compression; in the thoracic segments neurologic involvement is rare.

The symptoms of the two types of pathosis are clinically indistinguishable from each other. When nerve roots are involved, pain is the principal symptom, accompanied by variable degrees of sensory and motor impairment. The pain has the following characteristics: It is referred to the dermatomal distribution of the compressed nerve. It is aggravated by any maneuver that increases intraspinal cerebrospinal fluid pressure such as (a) coughing or sneezing, (b) straining at stool, and (c) compression of jugular veins (Naffziger's test). Cervical root pain is usually aggravated by extension of the neck. Lumbar and sacral root pain is aggravated by straight leg raising, which may be accentuated by forced dorsiflexion of the foot; occasionally, raising the contralateral leg may produce pain referred to the ipsilateral side. Spinal cord symptoms may be produced either by direct compression of the cord or compression of the incoming radicular arterial supply. The clinical picture is one of progressive spastic quadriparesis or paraparesis in rare thoracic disk herniations.

Distribution of symptoms and signs depends on the nerve roots compressed, as shown in Table 35-5. Because of individual variations in segmental innervation, the sensory pattern is much less reliable in the upper extremity than in the lower. In contrast, the motor pattern is less reliable in the lower extremity.

Management depends on the severity of symptoms and signs. Conservative measures, consisting of bed rest, traction (for cervical root pain), or immobilization, can be tried in all cases in which there is no disabling neurologic deficit. If symptoms are relieved satisfactorily, continued support of the involved area with a collar or brace may be the only treatment required. The presence of a definite neurologic deficit, particularly muscle weakness and atrophy, usually indicates surgical removal of the compressing lesion. Interference with bladder function by acute disk herniations requires immediate surgical treatment.

The diagnosis of lumbar disk herniation usually can be confirmed by unenhanced CT (Fig. 35-3) or by MRI (Fig. 35-44), but in some instances, myelography and postmyelographic CT are desirable prior to operative treatment. In special circumstances (e.g., patient in the first trimester of pregnancy) surgical treatment may have to be undertaken on the basis of neurologic findings alone. Wherever possible, however, radiographic confirmation is desirable, for segmental innervations can vary in individuals, and any lumbar nerve root can be compressed at either of two levels (e.g., the L5 root is compressed most often by a fairly medially herniated L4-L5 disk, but it can also be compressed by a far laterally herniated or a superiorly extruded L5-S1 disk).

Lateral cervical disk herniations are tiny lesions averaging 2 to 4 mm in diameter so myelography (Fig.

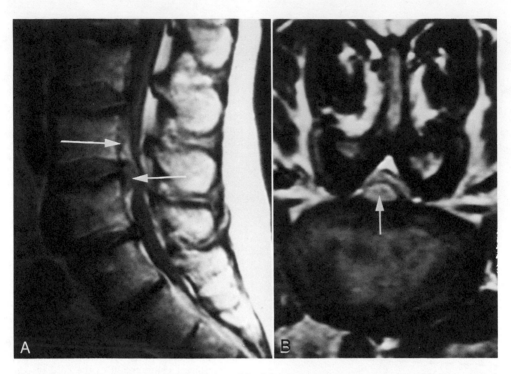

Fig. 35-44. A, Sagittal MRI showing herniation of the L3-4 disk. A large fragment of the disk has extruded out of the interspace *(arrows)* upward onto the body of L3 as well as caudad onto the body of L4, compressing the thecal sac severely. **B,** Axial MRI of same disk *(arrow)* shows how it has distorted the thecal sac.

Table 35-5. Common Neurologic Pictures With Herniated Disk and Vertebral Spondylosis

Distribution of Pain and Sensory Loss	Principal Motor Deficit	Reflex Diminution	Nerve Root Involved	Usual Intervertebral Disk Level*
Neck, shoulder, arm, radial side of hand, thumb, index finger	Biceps	Biceps	C6	C5-C6
Neck, shoulder, arm, index and middle fingers	Triceps	Triceps	C7	C6-C7
Neck, axilla, ulnar side of forearm and hand, ring and little fingers	Forearm/hand muscles	None	C8	C7-T1
Groin, anterolateral thigh, medial side of knee and upper calf	Quadriceps	Knee	L4	L3-L4
Back and hip, posterior thigh and calf, medial side of foot and medial two toes	Anterior tibial group	None	L5	L4-L5
Back and hip, posterior thigh and calf, lateral side of foot, lateral three toes	Gastrocnemius, soleus	Achilles	S1	L5-S1

*Far lateral disk herniation compresses the root above (i.e., lateral L4-L5 disk compresses L4 root). This phenomenon does not occur in the cervical spine.

35-8) or postmyelographic CT is necessary to confirm the diagnosis. On the other hand, midline cervical disk herniations that compress the spinal cord are demonstrated best by MRI. These considerations emphasize the need for careful clinical analysis of each disk problem to determine what is the most logical imaging study to perform for the given clinical situation.

Three modes of surgical treatment can be utilized for lumbar disk herniations. If the spinal canal is of adequate size and the disk protrusion is relatively small and still contained under the posterior longitudinal ligament, the intradiskal injection of the enzyme *chymopapain* may provide adequate root decompression and relief of symptoms. However, injection of this sub-

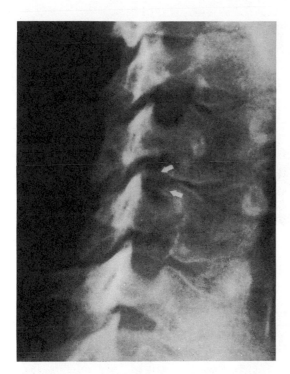

Fig. 35-45. Cervical spondylosis. Oblique view of cervical spine shows presence of osteophytic spurs *(arrows)* encroaching on an intervertebral foramen. Remainder of foramina are normal.

stance can produce anaphylactic reactions that can be fatal if not treated appropriately. Hence the procedure is performed under strictly controlled conditions. The degree of nucleolysis by chymopapain in the individual patient is unpredictable for it is not dose related; if it is too rapid and excessive, a dramatic loss of interspace height occurs, usually accompanied by disabling low back pain. Alternatively, given the same anatomic circumstances, intradiskal tension can be reduced by *percutaneous nucleotomy,* wherein a small cannula is introduced to the disk interspace percutaneously under fluoroscopic guidance; the nucleus pulposus is then morcellated and extracted piecemeal through the cannula. If the spinal canal is narrow or has become relatively stenotic by arthritic changes, or if the herniated disk fragment is very large or extruded into the epidural space, *open surgical diskectomy through a laminotomy* is the treatment of choice. This operation provides immediate relief of root pain in most cases.

Surgical treatment of the herniated lumbar disk remains a controversial problem, fraught with therapeutic failures from chronic disabling pain. Operation should be advised only after the most careful evaluation of the patient's neurologic, skeletal, and socioeconomic problems. Every patient must have a realistic expectation for long-term outcome, for at least 50% will experience some recurrences of low back problems in the years after operation as part of the natural history of disk disorders. Given such a suitably selected and well-prepared group of patients, more than 90% should be relieved of their symptoms to the extent that they can return to their normal work and physical activities.

Cervical root compression by herniated disk or spondylosis can be alleviated by removal of the herniated fragment through a hemilaminotomy and decompression of the root around a bone spur. When there is significant spur formation, the decompression can be accomplished better through an anterior interbody approach, and the interspace is fused with an iliac bone graft to prevent further spondylosis.

In contrast to the results of lumbar disk surgery, the above procedures for cervical disk herniation and spondylosis with nerve root pain produce highly satisfactory and permanent relief of symptoms with very few exceptions. However, when myelopathy results from spinal cord compression by a centrally herniated cervical disk or spondylosis, the reversal of neurologic deficit is frequently incomplete in spite of adequate anterior and/or posterior decompressions.

Stenosis of the entire spinal canal by bony thickening and overgrowth most commonly affects the lower lumbar segments. The clinical symptoms are numbness, heaviness, cramping, and weakness of the legs consistently brought on by exercise and can mimic *peripheral vascular insufficiency.* Therefore spinal canal stenosis should be considered in the differential diagnosis of claudicatory symptoms in the lower extremities. CT (Fig. 35-46) and myelography confirm the diagnosis, and a *generous* decompressive laminectomy provides excellent relief of symptoms.

PERIPHERAL AND CRANIAL NERVE COMPRESSION SYNDROMES

A variety of sensorimotor disturbances attributable to peripheral nerve compression, entrapment, or stretching have been identified. The more common anatomic sites of compression are as follows:

Median nerve at the carpal tunnel
Median nerve at the bicipital tendon
Ulnar nerve in the hypothenar eminence
Ulnar nerve at the elbow
Radial nerve in the forearm
Radial nerve in the spinal groove
Suprascapular nerve at the suprascapular foramen
Lateral femoral cutneous nerve at the inguinal ligament
Common peroneal nerve at the fibular neck

The most common of these, the carpal tunnel syndrome, is described in the preceding chapter. The ulnar nerve suffers with almost equal frequency, occasionally as a late complication of a deforming fracture at the elbow joint but more often because of entrapment of the nerve at its entrance to the fibromuscular septum just distal to the medial epicondyle of the humerus. Because most patients focus on the prominent sensory symptoms in the relatively unimportant fourth and fifth digits, one must not overlook the presence of a major disturbance of finger coordination—and therefore of hand function—caused by the loss of the ulnar-innervated interosseous and lumbrical muscles. Treatment consists in releasing the nerve from the compressing fascia and transposing it anterior to the epicondyle so that it is not stretched each time the elbow is flexed.

The lateral femoral cutaneous nerve is commonly compressed at its exit from the pelvis under the inguinal ligament, producing a characteristic pattern of burning dysesthesias and numbness of the anterolateral

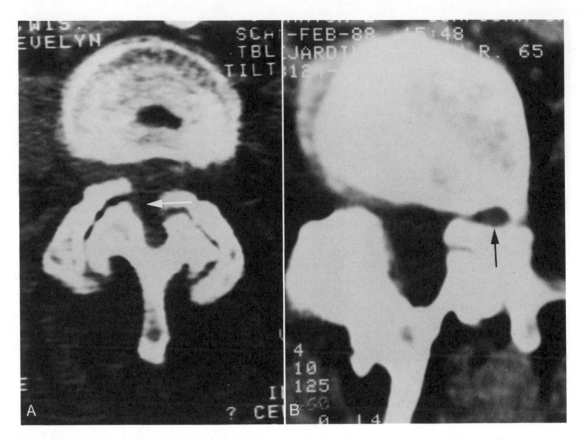

Fig. 35-46. CT showing spinal stenosis. **A,** The facet joints have hypertrophied and encroach medially, narrowing the central canal to a slitlike aperture *(arrow)* through which roots of the cauda equina must pass; the central stenosis causes bilateral numbness and claudicatory pains. **B,** The central canal is not significantly narrowed, but the lateral gutter *(arrow)* through which the nerve root courses toward its foramen of exit has become severely compromised; unilateral activity-related pain and paresthesias are the principal symptoms of this form of spinal stenosis.

thigh termed *meralgia paresthetica*. This and other less common but equally distressing nerve entrapment syndromes respond well to surgical decompression. Their possibility should always be borne in mind in the differential diagnosis of pain, numbness, paresthesias, and weakness in the extremities. *Electromyography* and *nerve conduction studies* are usually essential to confirm the diagnosis.

Trigeminal neuralgia (tic douloureux) is a relatively common condition characterized by lightning-like stabs of pain in the distribution of one or more branches of the trigeminal nerve. Occasionally the pain may follow the distribution of the *glossopharyngeal nerve (glossopharyngeal neuralgia)*. The condition occurs predominantly in the elderly and affects females more frequently than males. Attacks of pain can often be precipitated when one touches or rubs the area of skin involved ("trigger point"). In most instances the causative pathologic condition appears to be an abnormal arterial loop or a venous anomaly that presses on the nerve rootlets at their entry into or exit from the brainstem. Analgesics are of no value, for the pain is transitory. Carbamazepine is a very effective drug for tic pain, but untoward reactions occur frequently so that drug must be discontinued in a significant propor-

tion of patients. Alcohol injection of peripheral branches usually provides satisfactory relief, but the sensory loss obtained is not permanent, so the pain returns as the nerve regenerates. Intracranial sectioning of preganglionic fibers subserving the area of pain affords permanent pain relief but leaves an area of permanent numbness that can be distressing. Percutaneous radiofrequency coagulation of the trigeminal ganglion is also effective, with varying degrees of sensory loss, but the pain may recur. Decompression of either trigeminal or glossopharyngeal nerve at the root entry zone by rerouting or padding the compressing arterial loop or vein from the compressed nerve with an interposed sponge or muscle is usually effective and the most satisfactory, but there may be failures or recurrences because of irreversible demyelination of the chronically compressed nerves.

Hemifacial spasm (facial tic) is a motor nerve counterpart of trigeminal neuralgia, in which repetitive, involuntary twitching occurs in the muscles of one side of the face. The condition is frequently blamed on a nervous habit, but in reality it can be attributable to compression of the facial nerve intracranially by a redundant vessel loop just as in the case of the trigeminal and glossopharyngeal neuralgia. Surgical treatment is similar (i.e., moving the offending vessel away from the nerve or placing a muscle pad between the blood vessel and nerve, or doing both).

SURGICAL RELIEF OF PAIN AND DYSKINESIAS

Intractable pain caused by a lesion that cannot be eradicated can be alleviated by interrupting the pathways by which pain is mediated. That interruption can be accomplished physiologically by electrical blockade through transcutaneous electrical nerve stimulation (TENS), chemically by the injection of neurolytic agents such as alcohol and phenol, or surgically by the coagulation or transection of nerves and tracts. If management with combinations of analgesics, mood-altering drug therapy, and simple mechanical adjuncts such as TENS fail to control pain satisfactorily, procedures that leave permanent and irreversible sensory deficits can be considered. Spinothalamic tractotomy, performed at the C2 or T2 level by radiofrequency coagulation or open surgical transection destroys pain and thermal sensation below and contralateral to the operation. Posterior rhizotomy has limited applications because overlapping dermatomal segments makes adequate denervation difficult, and any significant deafferentation of an extremity renders it functionally useless from loss of proprioception. Although surgical deafferentation can render analgesic practically any painful area of the body, the procedures are intended primarily for clearly defined and severely painful syndromes such as those accompanying incurable malignancies and not for common pain problems that have no proveable cause. Once nerve pathways have been purposely destroyed, they can never be reestablished; the resulting sensory loss is permanent. Trigeminal root section performed for nonmalignant facial pain that is not typically trigeminal neuralgia will leave the patient with a permanent anesthetic face while the original pain for which the operation was performed may persist or recur despite the sensory loss. Rhizotomies, cordotomies, or other procedures performed for postherpetic neuralgia or for phantom limb pain fail too frequently to provide lasting relief of symptoms.

Section of anterior spinal roots *(anterior rhizotomy)* is a procedure reserved for the permanently paraplegic or quadriplegic in whom mass flexor reflexes result in painful spasms of the paralyzed extremities.

Stereotactically placed destructive lesions in the ventrolateral nucleus of the thalamus have, in selected cases, been effective in abolishing or reducing the tremor of Parkinson's disease. Patients under 60 years of age with unilateral tremor and without bradykinesia or pseudobulbar manifestations are the best candidates for the operation. The physiologic mechanism by which the tremor is stopped is unknown. The procedure has been tried with little success in the treatment of other disorders characterized by abnormal states of muscle tone and movement (dyskinesias).

36

Head and Neck Surgery

Charles J. Krause
Brian F. McCabe

Congenital Anomalies
Infections
Trauma
Neoplasms
Hearing Loss and Microsurgery of the Ear

A clear understanding of head and neck diseases is important for the general physician, since somewhere between 20% and 40% of all illnesses arise above the clavicles. Upper respiratory tract infections (nasal, sinal, aural, and pharyngeal) are by far the most common infections. A knowledge of these diseases is important for the specialist as well, because even the specialist must occasionally practice some general medicine. Furthermore, the specialist must not neglect disease in another organ system while treating that disease for which he is primarily trained. We must continuously dedicate ourselves to the welfare of the whole patient.

This chapter deals primarily with identification of otolaryngologic disease by pointing out the *nature* of the process. Principles of diagnosis are stressed, and treatment methods are described only so far as they are pertinent. The student is cautioned that treatment methods in this field change very rapidly.

CONGENITAL ANOMALIES
Congenital Anomalies with Respiratory Obstruction

Congenital abnormalities of the head and neck are important because they may affect vital processes such as respiration, deglutition, and nourishment. Some anomalies in this region impair the important modalities of communication. Of no small import are cosmetic defects imposed by congenital abnormalities of the head and neck. Function is the most important consideration, but appearance is also important. Here we do not speak of the gross abnormalities, such as anencephaly, cyclops deformity, and the other monstrous deformities that are for the most part incompatible with life. The minor abnormalities, such as prominent nose, outstanding ears, cleft lip, and hypognathia, though they do not necessarily compromise function, are major concerns to the patient as a person. The good physician bears in mind that in a person's physiognomy dwells the entity that that person calls "myself."

In this section we will consider chiefly entities that alter function and, therefore, demand early recognition and treatment.

Respiratory obstruction in the newborn is a problem of prime importance, and a thorough knowledge of its differential diagnosis is essential. The following is a list of some of the important causes:

Secretory obstruction (mucus or amniotic fluid)
Choanal atresia
Tracheoesophageal fistula
Congenital vascular ring
Laryngeal cyst and web
Congenital laryngeal stridor
Pierre-Robin syndrome
Treacher-Collins syndrome
Rhinomeningocele or encephalocele
Laryngomalacia and tracheomalacia
Laryngeal paralysis
Diaphragmatic hernia
Bronchial or pulmonary agenesis
Brain damage or agenesis, or both

Secretory obstruction of the nasal airways may result from retention of thick mucus or amniotic fluid in the perinatal period. The treatment consists of removal of the thick secretions using a flexible nasal suction device. This provides immediate improvement in the nasal airway, differentiating secretory obstruction from the other more serious causes discussed below.

Choanal atresia is obstruction of the posterior nares attributed to retention of the embryonic plate that separates the nasal chambers from the nasopharynx. The atresia may be unilateral or bilateral. Neonates afflicted with this abnormality do not breathe normally because *mouth breathing is not normal to the infant in the first 2 weeks of life*. Careful observation of the infant with bilateral choanal atresia reveals the following sequence of events: cyclic episodes of upper airway obstruction when the mouth is closed, associated with cyanosis and labored respiratory efforts that are dramatically relieved by crying. Air is freely exchanged during crying and the infant becomes pink and quiet, and closes his mouth. The cycle is then repeated. The infant cannot rest, and feedings are often aspirated because of the airway obstruction that this provokes. A true respiratory emergency exists. The diagnosis is made by inability to pass a catheter through the nasal chamber into the oropharynx. Radiocontrast studies confirm the diagnosis: lateral skull films show complete retention of dye instilled into the nasal chambers while the infant is supine. Treatment consists of tiding the infant over the 2-week period required for mouth breathing to be learned. Feedings are given by orogastric tube. A patent airway is obtained by whatever means proves most satisfactory: decubitus positioning, frequent suctioning, placement of an oropharyngeal airway; and occasionally a tracheostomy is required. The nasopharyngeal plate may be perforated with a blunt instrument or with a mastoid drill and operative microscope, but extreme care must be taken to avoid passing the instrument through the fragile and largely cartilaginous cervi-

cal vertebrae into the brainstem. Definitive operation for removal of the atresia plate transpalatally can be carried out as early as 1 year of age.

Tracheoesophageal fistulas are discussed in Chapter 39.

Congenital vascular ring is discussed in Chapter 30.

Laryngeal cysts and webs produce respiratory obstruction of the larynx and usually result in hoarseness. In the infant this is manifested as a husky or nonclear cry. Cysts may arise anywhere within the endolarynx or hypopharynx and are caused by malformations of mucous glands. Web formation occurs through incomplete separation of the true vocal cords. The cords are joined at the anterior commissure, much as fingers are connected in syndactylism. The laryngeal web is of minor consequence if it involves only the anterior commissure but is serious if it is nearly total with only a small airway at the posterior commissure. *Subglottic stenosis* is a less common condition of congenital narrowing of the airway at the level of the cricoid cartilage. Diagnosis is made by direct laryngoscopy. The treatment includes tracheotomy with excision of the stenotic area or expansion of the cricoid lumen through splitting it and interposing a cartilage graft. An indwelling stent for a period of several weeks is frequently necessary.

Congenital laryngeal stridor produces a clear, sharp inspiratory stridor on crying or straining. When the infant is breathing normally and quietly, the stridor is not present. Mild cyanosis is seen occasionally, but unconsciousness attributable to hypoxia does not occur. The lesion is caused by immaturity of the epiglottis ("infantile" or omega-shaped epiglottis), so that on sharp inspiration the aryepiglottic folds are drawn down into the glottic aperture, with consequent stridor. The stridor occurs *only on inspiration*. The condition is self-limiting. The child usually outgrows his symptoms during the second year of life, as the epiglottis gains maturity.

Pierre-Robin syndrome is one of the family of mandibulofacial dysplasias produced by anomalies of the first and second branchial arches. Respiratory obstruction of the oropharynx is immediate and alarming with the baby supine but is relieved in the prone position. The syndrome is recognizable at birth by simple observation of hypognathia, glossoptosis, cleft palate, and usually a cleft lip. The descriptive term *micrognathia* is used if there is no cleft palate. There is not room for the relatively large tongue in the patient's oropharynx because of the failure of anterior growth of the mandible. This must be differentiated from cretinism, in which the tongue is abnormally large and cannot be accommodated by the oral cavity of normal size. On inspection, the bulging floor of the mouth may resemble the tongue, but when this is pushed down, the tip of the tongue can be seen pointing up toward the hard palate, well back in the mouth. Although feeding may be difficult, airway obstruction is the most acute threat to life. Careful positioning is necessary for gravity to prolapse the dependent tongue away from the posterior pharyngeal wall to disobstruct the airway. An anterior tongue-tie with a base-of-tongue suture to the mandible may also hold the tongue forward to keep the airway clear. Tracheotomy may be necessary. Tube feedings

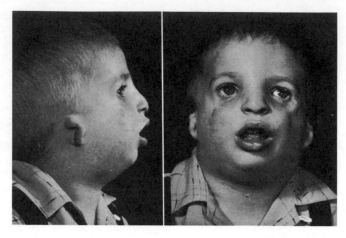

Fig. 36-1. Treacher-Collins syndrome, one of the congenital craniofacial dysplasias. "Bird shape" to face and eye and ear anomalies are striking. It is extremely important to place bone-conduction hearing aid on such patients by age 1 or 2, so that normal speech and intellectual development may occur.

are often required. Curiously, the airway problems improve with time. Other congenital anomalies are frequently present. Mortality is high, exceeding 20% in most series.

Treacher-Collins syndrome, another of the mandibulofacial dysplasias, is a striking developmental defect of the first and second branchial arches and the first branchial groove (Fig 36-1). Hypognathia and glossoptosis are present, as in the Pierre-Robin syndrome. In addition, an underformed maxilla produces the appearance of an abnormally prominent nose, outward and downward slanted eyes (sometimes called "antimongoloid"), a notched lower lid, bony atresia of both external auditory canals with severe conductive hearing loss, and small, low-set, deformed ears. The palate and the lip are usually intact. Early in life, the respiratory problem requires attention, but past infancy the mandible grows enough for adequate respiratory exchange without obstruction or stridor. In the second and third years of life, deafness is the greatest problem; the child needs a bone-conduction hearing aid to develop speech and learn at an adequate rate. The external auditory canal atresia is corrected surgically to improve hearing at about the time the child enters school; this should take precedence over cosmetic improvement of the external ears. These patients have such a characteristic appearance that they are sometimes called "bird people" (Fig. 36-1).

In *rhinomeningoceles* or *encephaloceles* cerebral contents herniate through an unformed cribriform plate or other portion of the floor of the anterior cranial fossa to produce masses in the nasal chamber of the newborn that may obstruct the airway. The appearance externally may be normal, or paranasal masses may pulsate. Rhinomeningoceles or encephaloceles are smooth, pale, and pulsate on close inspection. Radiographs reveal a bone defect in the floor of the anterior cranial fossa. Biopsy may be disastrous, of course, and must be avoided by awareness of this diagnostic possibility. Rhinomeningoceles are approached by anterior craniotomy, and the mass is retracted back into the cranial cavity and the defect is repaired.

Laryngomalacia and *tracheomalacia* are congenital defects in the ground substance of the airway cartilage, which cannot retain its shape on inspiration. The walls of the airway collapse in proportion to the degree of positive pressure created during expiration. The only treatment is tracheotomy when airway obstruction is severe. Congenital laryngeal stridor may be misdiagnosed as laryngomalacia and wrongly treated by tracheotomy.

Laryngeal paralysis may be unilateral or bilateral. If unilateral, the condition is asymptomatic, but if bilateral, severe inspiratory stridor is present at birth, and tracheotomy is mandatory. Bilateral laryngeal paralysis seldom occurs without associated neurologic disturbances, such as cerebral palsy. The diagnosis is made by direct laryngoscopy; the cords stay at or near the midline and do not abduct on inspiration.

Diaphragmatic hernia is discussed in Chapter 22, *pulmonary agenesis* in Chapter 29, and *central nervous system disturbances* in Chapter 35.

Congenital Anomalies Not Associated with Respiratory Obstruction

Branchial and *thyroglossal remnants* are discussed in Chapter 39.

A *cleft lip* or *cleft palate* (Fig. 36-2, *A)* is always alarming to the parents of the afflicted newborn, and they need reassurance that the child can develop almost normally in function and appearance with medical care that is properly timed and carried out. The appearance of the cleft lip or cleft palate is so varied as to defy description. It ranges all the way from a minor notch or slight alteration of the vermilion portion of the upper lip to complete clefts of both sides of the upper lip that extend into the floor of the nostrils and nasal chambers, completely back through the hard and soft palate. Restoration of the intact palate is as important for function as repair of the lip is for cosmetic appearance (Fig. 36-2, *B)*. Multiple operations, properly timed, are needed to avoid interference with proper growth of the middle third of the face. Dental anomalies, sometimes gross and bizarre, are invariably present. Speech and nourishment are difficult and require special help; cleft pal-

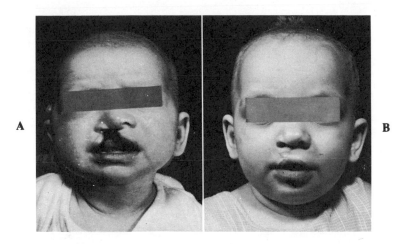

Fig. 36-2. Cleft palate and lip. **A,** Preoperative. **B,** Postoperative.

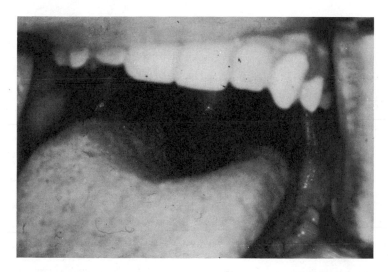

Fig. 36-3. Lingual thyroid, occurring at foramen cecum of tongue. Notice intact, unulcerated covering. Such lesions may be biopsied for diagnosis but should not be removed as a tumor, for this may be the only thyroid tissue patient has. [131]I scintiscan is simpler method of diagnosis.

ate adds vexing ear problems, such as repeated acute infections and chronic serous otitis media. Thus the modern care of cleft palate patients is a multidisciplinary effort of a highly specialized team. The cleft palate team includes an otolaryngologist, a plastic surgeon, an orthodontist, a prosthodontist, a speech therapist, a pediatrician, a pedodontist, an audiologist, a social worker, and a psychologist.

Lingual thyroid, a prominent mass overlain by normal mucosa (Fig. 36-3), is located at the junction of the middle and posterior thirds of the tongue. It is diagnosed by biopsy or scintiscan. Lingual thyroid should not be removed until it is proved that other thyroid tissue is present, unless thyroid replacement is given.

Protruding auricles (lop ears) result from failure of development of the anthelix, so that the rim of the ear stands outward from the skull (Fig. 36-4, *A)*. The ear is often cup shaped. Otoplasty will restore good contour if the patient is sensitive about the cosmetic deformity (Fig. 36-4, *B)*.

Pretragal cysts, or ganulomas, appear just anterior to the tragus of the ear and are caused by skin entrapped below the surface during development from hillocks of cartilage that form the outer ear. Incision and drainage are inadequate treatment; the entire skin-lined tract must be removed to effect a cure.

Floor-of-the-mouth cysts and tumors may be of many varieties. The *ranula* is the most common (Fig. 36-5). The *pseudoranula* is merely a blocked minor salivary gland in the floor of the mouth and is submucosal. The *true ranula* is an embryologic deformity of the sublingual glands and perhaps other glands, with fingerlike ramifications into the substance of the genioglossus muscles. Simple intraoral excision of the pseudoranula suffices. The true ranula generally requires an external approach for complete excision, though it may be managed satisfactorily by creation of a fistula of the ranula into the mouth. *Dermoid* and *epidermoid cysts* cannot be distinguished clinically. They are fusion-fault cysts, in which epithelial tissue is trapped between the

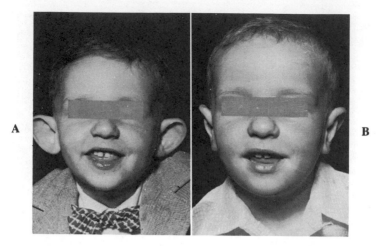

Fig. 36-4. Lop ears. **A,** Preoperative. **B,** Postoperative.

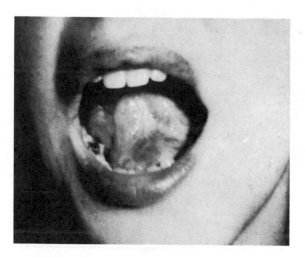

Fig. 36-5. Ranula, with intact epithelium over it. It is soft and cystic. Such lesions may be superficial in floor of mouth ("pseudoranula") or have deep extensions into diaphragm of floor of mouth and genioglossus muscles ("true" ranula).

joining mandibular arches. Differential diagnosis includes *minor salivary gland tumors, salivary gland calculi,* and *desmoid* or *desmoplastic tumors.*

INFECTIONS

Certain principles in the diagnosis and treatment of head and neck infections are important. Infections in this region are very common and may constitute as much as 20% of the family physician's office practice.

Despite their frequency, head and neck infections should not be taken lightly or dismissed with a superficial evaluation. The complications may be serious and life threatening (e.g., extension to bone or metastatic spread to other organ systems such as the kidney, heart, or joints). On the other hand, they hold no mystery to the alert physician who understands the specialized structures involved.

In the treatment of acute infections, full-dosage antibiotic therapy must be instituted early and maintained

for several days after symptoms have subsided. Whenever possible, cultures should be obtained before antibiotic therapy is instituted. Selection of a specific antibiotic will rest on what organism is suspected, a history of drug allergy, and the route of administration desired. Later it may be necessary to change the antibiotic when culture and sensitivity results are available. Acute abscesses, whether in the middle ear, neck, or another part of the body, must be afforded the time-honored principle of incision and drainage. Supportive measures are necessary, including aspirin for pain and fever, local wet or dry heat, bed rest, and increased fluid intake.

Chronic infections in this region, especially chronic sinusitis, mastoiditis (Fig. 36-6), and tonsillitis, are seldom amenable to antibiotic therapy alone. The treatment of chronic infections in this region is surgical. When bone is infected acutely, it is usually amenable to antibiotic therapy, but when chronic infection is present, the bone must be removed. This can usually be done without significant alteration of function or cosmetic deformity.

Viral

The *viral nose cold* is the most common infection of man. Little need be said about it except that antibiotics of any kind render the patient a disservice. The symptoms are well known, and the treatment is entirely supportive. The nose cold is generally said to be 3 days coming, 3 days present, and 3 days going. Any nose cold lasting longer than this is probably becoming complicated by suppurative infections of the nose, sinuses, or lower respiratory tract. *Adenopharyngoconjunctival (APC) fever* is a mildly epidemic viral infection of the nasopharynx that, after several days of sore throat, produces a nonsuppurative conjunctivitis of first one and then the other eye. *Infectious mononucleosis* is also a mildly epidemic disease of young people, often heralded by petechiae of the palate or buccal mucosa. The tonsils are usually involved in the nonsuppurative process. The tonsillitis may on occasion be extreme, with severe sore throat and necrotic slough of the surface of each tonsil. The diagnosis is made when two of the following are present: (1) posterior cervical adenopathy,

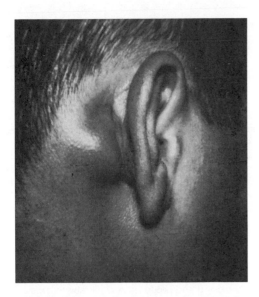

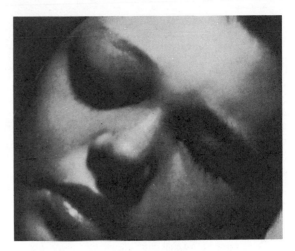

Fig. 36-7. Acute right frontal sinusitis that has perforated floor of sinus and produced an orbital abscess. Disease is now surgical. Differential diagnosis includes orbital cellulitis, cavernous sinus thrombosis or fistula, frontal or ethmoid neoplasm, and osteomyelitis.

Fig. 36-6. Acute mastoiditis. Swelling with pain and fluctuant mass in this region is most unlikely to be misdiagnosed. Incidence of acute mastoiditis has been very low in antibiotic era, but that of chronic mastoiditis is steadily rising. This patient has acute exacerbation of chronic mastoiditis. Disease chose to perforate mastoid cortex. If it had chosen rather the middle fossa plate (roof of mastoid) or inner ear, results could have been disastrous.

(2) a significant rise in the number of atypical "foamy" lymphocytes in peripheral blood, and (3) a positive heterophile agglutinin test in rising titer. The treatment is nonspecific but should include prolonged bed rest because of the possible complications of the disease, which include hepatitis and a prolonged postinfectious fatigue state.

Bacterial

Acute Suppurative Oropharyngitis, Nasopharyngitis, Laryngitis, and Tonsillitis

As with acute suppurative infections anywhere, acute infections of the oropharynx, nasopharynx, larynx, and tonsils result in fever, general malaise, pain in the affected organ, and altered function. The diagnosis is made when pus is observed over the greatly inflamed tissue. Antibiotic and supportive therapy is the treatment. A mirror is necessary in the diagnosis of all head and neck infections, or one may be led astray (e.g., the oropharynx of a patient with acute suppurative nasopharyngitis may be profusely inflamed but without pus visible on tongueblade examination, suggestive of a viral oropharyngitis). These infections are not communicable, though there are infections of this region that are (diphtheria and Vincent's infection). When the suppuration involves the larynx or trachea, modified voice rest must be a part of therapy to avoid the complication of speaker's nodule, vocal cord granuloma, or vocal polyp.

Paranasal Sinusitis

Clinically, the important forms of sinusitis are acute and chronic suppurative. Other forms of sinusitis exist (e.g., atrophic sinusitis, rhinoscleromatous sinusitis, and tuberculous sinusitis), but they are rare.

Acute suppurative sinusitis is accompanied by the usual signs of acute infection together with facial pain, usually over the involved sinus, and a purulent rhinorrhea (Fig. 36-7). The pain of sphenoiditis is either frontooccipital or bitemporal. The history is that of change of the watery nasal discharge to a suppurative one at the end of a viral nose cold. The diagnosis is not difficult to make on examination: there is pus at one of the sinus ostia within the nasal chamber. The edematous nasal mucosa is easily shrunk with a drop or spray of 1% to 3% ephedrine in normal saline solution, or with any of the commercial nose drops. The treatment is similar to that for any acute febrile infection, as described previously. Codeine may be necessary for relief of pain, and some benefit is afforded by antihistamines or similar agents to produce mucosal shrinkage, aid drainage, and diminish the mucoid element of the discharge.

Most acute suppurative sinus infections are never seen by the physician; they resolve spontaneously after a course of several weeks. But the *complications* of acute sinusitis always the bring the patient to the physician. The most common complication is that of chronicity, which is discussed later. Perhaps the second most common complication is *acute serous otitis media,* producing a stuffy ear, deafness, tinnitus, and autophony, of which the patient may complain bitterly without mentioning the nasal complaint. The sinusitis is then discovered as the cause during routine examination. More serious complications are *acute osteomyelitis, orbital abscess* (Fig. 36-7), *epidural, subdural, and brain abscess, cavernous sinus thrombosis,* and *acute empyema* of the sinus. All these complications are of major consequence, and each is accompanied by a specific set of symptoms that requires treatment by an appropriate specialist. They all produce external swelling and rapid deterioration of the general condition of the patient, which should immediately alert the physician.

Chronic suppurative sinusitis, however, is unaccompanied by facial pain, headache, or any signs of systemic infection, unless complicated. Let us dispel the widely prevalent notion that frontal (or frontal and occipital) headache plus a stuffy nose is equatable with chronic sinus disease. This set of symptoms generally signals tension headaches plus chronic vasomotor rhinitis. The diagnosis of chronic suppurative sinusitis is untenable if pus is not visible at one of the sinal ostia. This is true almost regardless of the x-ray findings, especially report of a "cloudy sinus." Perhaps the only diagnostic x-ray sign is that of an air-fluid level. The "cloudy sinus" frequently means nothing more than thickening of the lining—testimony of an old healed infection and scarification (Fig. 36-8, *A).*

The treatment of chronic suppurative sinusitis is surgical (the nasoantral window operation, or sinusectomy). Sinusectomy is accomplished transorally (antral region), intranasally (ethmoid or sphenoid sinus), or externally (for the frontal or frontoethmoid sinus). The *complications* of chronic sinusitis are of major importance, including those listed under acute sinusitis, plus one other, mucocele. *Mucocele* arises as a slowly enlarging cyst filled with mucus, or mucopus *(mucopyocele),* from the frontal sinus or a frontal ethmoid cell; it invades the surrounding sinuses and the orbit, often taking several years to produce proptosis and a downward and outward displacement of the eye (Fig. 36-8, *B).* A cystic mass is felt above the inner canthus of the eye. The treatment is always surgical removal.

The *role of allergy* in suppurative sinus disease deserves mention. There is no question that patients with allergic rhinitis are more predisposed to acute and chronic suppurative sinusitis than nonallergic patients. Identification of the underlying allergy directs treatment beyond that of the infection alone, which will not produce resolution of the basic disease. Allergic hyposensitization is then in order. An allergic component should be suspected whenever suppurative sinusitis fails to respond to the usual measures. Generally there is a family history of extrinsic allergy or a positive history of drug or food allergy in the patient, asthma in childhood, a labile nasal airway, perennial hay fever, or merely prolonged repetitive bouts of sneezing and epiphora. Pale, boggy, or violaceous nasal mucosa is often a clue, and the presence of allergic polyps (which resemble peeled grapes) is usually diagnostic. The treatment of allergic polyps is always surgical, but prior hyposensitization is carried out if allergies are found.

Infections of the Ear

External otitis, frequently mistermed otomycosis or "fungus of the ear canal," is a suppurative infection of the skin of the ear canal. In the *acute form* it is extremely painful and produces considerable edema of the skin. It does not produce deafness unless the canal is occluded by the edematous skin or exudate. Over half the reported cases are caused by *Pseudomonas aeruginosa,* and the remainder are caused by streptococci, staphylococci, or *Haemophilus influenzae.* Since it is an acute pyoderm, treatment is the administration of topical (not systemic) antibiotics. A cotton wick is placed deeply into the ear canal and kept soaked with Burow's solution or antibiotic-cortisone eardrops. The pain is relieved in 24 to 48 hours if the cotton wick extends the entire length of the ear canal. The wick is left in place for 1 to 3 days, after which drops are continued along with meticulous periodic cleaning of the ear canal until the infection has subsided.

The *chronic form of external otitis* may have a number of causes. The most frequent is atrophy of the ceru-

A 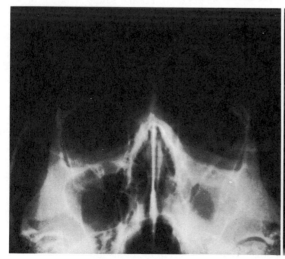 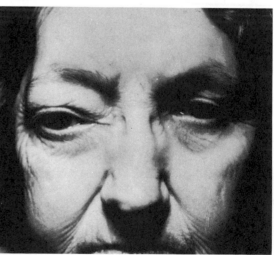 B

Fig. 36-8. A, Thickened lining of right maxillary antrum; this is not diagnostic of chronic sinusitis but may represent old healed disease. Only diagnostic radiographic sign of active sinusitis is air-fluid level. View roentgenograms you order; the good physician realizes that if roentgenogram is worth ordering, it is worth going to look at. **B,** Frontal mucocele; right eye is pushed down, out, and forward; cystic mass is palpable and easily visible above inner canthus of eye. This is one of complications of chronic suppurative sinusitis. Surgical intervention is indicated.

men glands resulting in a chronically dry, pruritic canal. Other causes are seborrheic dermatitis, eczematoid dermatitis, and the end result of an untreated acute external otitis. Repeated trauma to the canal is the usual result of the pruritus. Such trauma from a finger, cotton-tipped applicator, or pin propagates the infection. The treatment is avoidance of further trauma, careful cleaning by a physician, and long-term use of cortisone cream or ointment.

Acute suppurative otitis media is second in frequency to the nose cold. Few children escape it. It is also called *acute otitis media, middle ear abscess, acute ear, red ear,* and *bulging drum*. Signs and symptoms are those of an acute febrile infection with ear pain, which may be severe and protracted. Relief of the pain comes with either spontaneous drainage or the myringotomy knife. In the infant irritability and diarrhea may be the only symptoms; this has been termed "cholera infantum." The cause is the ascension of suppurative organisms from the nasopharynx (streptococci, pneumococci, *Haemophilus influenzae,* staphylococci, sometimes other organisms) through the eustachian tube or more probably through the peritubal lymphatics. It should be stressed here that not all "red ears" are acute suppurative middle ear infections. Distinction must be made from mere hyperemia of the membrane or tympanum, which can be caused by holding a struggling, crying child for otoscopy. Diagnosis is made by observation of a bulging, inflamed tympanic membrane or pus in the ear canal that has recently perforated the tympanic membrane. Bulging is recognized by a diminished or absent prominence of the short process of the malleus. The eardrum changes may be obscured by the thickening and desquamation that occur in the tympanic membrane in the medial portion of the canal with acute middle ear infection, requiring cleaning of the canal.

The treatment is by myringotomy (if the drum is bulging) and appropriate antibiotic therapy for at least 10 days. The following complications of an acute suppurative otitis media are probably more important than the disease itself:

Acute mastoiditis
Acute osteomyelitis of the temporal bone
Acute petrositis
Facial nerve paralysis
Chronic nonsuppurative otitis media
Chronic suppurative otitis media
Subperiosteal abscess
Acute suppurative labyrinthitis
Acute meningitis
Sigmoid sinus thrombus
Epidural abscess
Subdural abscess
Brain abscess (cerebellar or temporal lobe)

Each of these complications poses its own diagnostic and treatment problems. The most common complication of acute suppurative otitis media, *chronic non-suppurative otitis media,* is considered in the following paragraphs.

Chronic nonsuppurative otitis media is the most common cause of deafness in children and is conductive. It is of the magnitude of about 30 decibels (dB). The precise cause is not completely understood, though it follows eustachian tube obstruction and antibiotic-

treated acute suppurative otitis media. Mucus-secreting glands migrate from the eustachian tube epithelium into the middle ear mucosa and produce a thick, viscid, gluelike substance. The eardrum is gray, lusterless, retracted, and immobile. A synonym for the disease is *glue ear*. Treatment includes adenoidectomy, resolution of any suppurative disease of the upper respiratory tract, eustachian tube inflations by Valsalva maneuver or politzerization (forcible insufflation of the ear into the nasal chambers), elimination of inhalant allergies, antihistaminics, and, in refractory cases, temporary intubation of the tympanic membrane to give the middle ear a rest. In each case, myringotomy and aspiration of the gluelike material should accompany any other treatment.

Chronic nonsuppurative otitis media, with true secretion of mucus into the middle ear, should be differentiated from acute nonsuppurative otitis media, a transudation of thin amber fluid into the middle ear after acute eustachian tube obstruction. This is most commonly caused by a viral upper respiratory infection, with edema about the nasopharyngeal end of the tube. However, the physician must be aware that neoplasms of the nasopharynx usually produce middle ear effusion, and he must carefully examine the nasopharynx of each patient with middle ear effusion.

Chronic suppurative otitis media is another sequela of acute middle ear infection. It is essentially a nonresolution of the acute infection. This is always accompanied by perforation of the tympanic membrane and chronic, usually fetid, otorrhea. It is incumbent on the physician to distinguish a *safe* from a *dangerous* chronic suppurating ear. A "safe ear" seldom shortens anyone's life by one day; a "dangerous ear" produces the same complications that may occur after acute suppurative otitis media. The following criteria for this distinction demand careful consideration:

Character of the discharge
Site of the perforation
Presence of a cholesteatoma
Progressive unexplained hearing loss
Presence of bone destruction on inspection or radiographic examination
Presence of vascular pyogenic granulation tissue growing on bone
Positive reservoir sign
Positive fistula test

The *discharge* is suggestive of dangerous chronic osteomyelitis if it is highly fetid, the result of bone digestion by bacterial enzymes. Simple mucosal infection produces predominantly a mucoid discharge with no odor, or merely a musty odor from stasis and the action of saprophytic organisms.

Marginal perforation, including "attic" perforations or those in the pars flaccida, generally indicate a dangerous ear condition. Central perforations, or those in the pars tensa away from the annular region, generally indicate a nondangerous ear condition.

A *cholesteatoma (skin in the middle ear, where skin does not belong),* is virtually diagnostic of a dangerous ear condition. Once skin enters the middle ear space, it casts off layer upon layer of desquamated epithelium, which is surrounded by the thinned-out matrix. The matrix is the surrounding layer of living skin. The cholesteatoma invades and destroys bone by two processes: enzymatic digestion in the presence of vascular pyogenic granulation tissue, and pressure necrosis by a solid ball of cholesteatoma whose center is filled with desquamated keratin debris or "squame." The cholesteatoma may enlarge slowly over many years with no symptoms except the chronic otorrhea and perhaps *increasing deafness*. Then the cholesteatoma invades one of the many vital structures surrounding the middle ear, and catastrophe follows. These vital structures are the cochlea, the vestibular labyrinth, the sigmoid sinus, the jugular bulb, the dura of the cerebellum, the dura of the temporal lobe, and the subarachnoid space. Septic retrograde thrombosis of vessels may also be induced by chronic osteomyelitic bone. The cholesteatoma is recognized by its characteristic cheesy-white, flaky content. *The presence of bone destruction on either visual inspection or x-ray examination* indicates either a destructive osteomyelitic process or an expanding cholesteatoma. *Vascular pyogenic granulation tissue growing on bone* is diagnostic of chronic osteomyelitis. The *positive reservoir sign* is the re-formation of pus a few minutes after it has been thoroughly wiped away. A *positive fistula test* is conjugate deviation of the eyes to the opposite side on compression of the air in the external auditory canal, diagnostic of a fistula through the bone over a semicircular canal without actual suppurative invasion of the inner ear. It is then a matter of a few days to a few weeks before suppurative invasion takes place. When this occurs, sudden irrevocable total deafness follows, together with severe and prolonged vertigo and nystagmus. A labyrinthectomy is then necessary.

Only a few of these criteria may be present in a given patient, and no single test (except the positive fistula test in a chronic draining ear) is absolutely diagnostic of a dangerous ear. Thus it becomes a matter of meticulous observation, careful interpretation, and judgment to establish this. Recognition of the dangerous state is crucial *because the impending complication may be diagnosed in advance and prevented by surgical intervention*. Recognition is the physician's responsibility.

Fascial Space Abscesses

Peritonsillar abscess (quinsy) is the most common fascial space abscess. The organism is usually *Streptococcus* or *Staphylococcus,* and the cause is an acute or chronic tonsillitis. Pronounced edema of the tonsillar bed with fanning out of the anterior pillar over the swollen mass occurs. The uvula may be pushed across the midline. It is severely painful, causing sharp odynophagia and pain on opening the mouth. True trismus may be present. Incision and drainage is the treatment, along with antibiotic therapy. Distinction between peritonsillar abscess and peritonsillar cellulitis may be difficult. The cellulitis precedes the abscess, which takes at least 48 hours to form.

Retropharyngeal space abscesses are uncommon. They are generally seen in children, in whom an infected retropharyngeal lymph node gives rise to the infection. These nodes are usually absent in the adult. The diagnosis is made by a characteristic spongy or cystic feel to the posterior pharyngeal wall and widening of the retropharyngeal space on the lateral soft tissue radiograph of the neck. The collection of pus lies between the superior constrictor muscle and the prevertebral fascia. The treatment is incision and drainage.

Pharyngomaxillary space abscess (lateral or parapharyngeal space) is an abscess in the potential space between the fascia of the parotid gland and the internal pterygoid muscle laterally and the fascia of the superior constrictor muscle medially. In it are the carotid sheath structures and the styloid process with its muscle group. The abscess is recognized by medial displacement of the tonsil *and* lateral angle of the pharynx and brawny induration of the upper neck just below the angle of the mandible. However, bulging may be present in only one of these places. Trismus is pronounced. The treatment is external incision and drainage with antibiotic therapy.

A *masticator space abscess,* usually of dental origin, is an abscess under the periosteum of the mandible. Trismus is usually present. Ludwig's angina is a floor-of-the-mouth phlegmon and is also usually of dental origin. The patient frequently is a diabetic. The floor of the mouth is greatly swollen, and the tongue is pushed up and back, endangering the airway. Tracheotomy must be contemplated. Later, all the potential spaces of the floor of the mouth are involved, and the infection may spread down to the clavicular level. Wide incision and drainage is frequently necessary, though intensive antibiotic therapy early in the infection may suffice.

TRAUMA

Automobile accidents account for most severe maxillofacial trauma today. Although reduction and fixation of facial bone fractures may be delayed for as much as 14 days, a very careful evaluation of the patient must be carried out at the time of the injury. Other emergency conditions that require immediate attention may be developing such as airway obstruction, cervical vertebra fracture, long bone fracture, progressive intracranial or intraabdominal injury, or soft tissue lacerations.

Nose

The *nasal bone* is the most commonly *fractured* bone in the body. Even relatively minor nasal trauma may result in a fracture. When the patient is evaluated immediately after the trauma has occurred, the diagnosis may be obvious. Mobility of the nasal bones on palpation is diagnostic. X-ray studies may be misleading when old fractures have healed with scar tissue or when recent fractures are not demonstrated. Within a few hours after trauma the swelling about the nose may be extensive, making a clinical evaluation extremely difficult. In such a case, treatment may be delayed for as much as 7 days to allow the swelling to subside. Because of their intimacy, both nasal bones are usually fractured. After the nose is anesthetized, a blunt instrument may be placed beneath the nasal bone on the concave side and elevated outward. The other nasal bone is then moved medially into its proper position. This position is maintained with external splinting. When the nasal fracture is allowed to heal in a deviated position, a rhinoplasty is required later to restore normal nasal contour (Fig. 36-9).

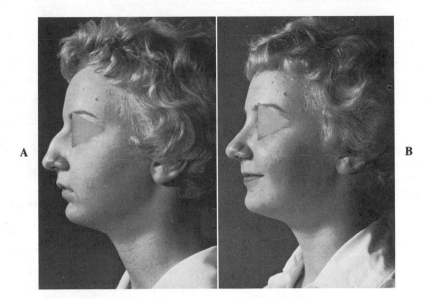

Fig. 36-9. Old nasal fracture. **A,** Unreduced. **B,** After rhinoplasty.

Fracture of the nasal septum sometimes occurs without nasal bone fracture. If the fractured septum is displaced significantly, it produces permanent airway obstruction. Fractures of the nasal septum are often difficult to reduce because the septum becomes dislocated off the maxillary crest. If the septum does not go easily back to the midline, nasal septal reconstruction (discussed on this page) may be required at the time of the acute fracture.

Another late sequela of untreated septal fracture is a *saddle deformity of the nose.* The middle third of the dorsum of the nose is supported by the nasal septum and not by the nasal bones. The support is lost by an inward fracture of the septum that may not be apparent immediately on external examination because a hematoma forms in its place, so that the nose retains roughly its former appearance. The "saddle" deformity becomes apparent after resolution of the hematoma and contraction of the resulting scar tissue. Correction of this deformity requires a bone or cartilage implant and rhinoplasty, a complicated procedure.

Deviation of the nasal septum may also be acquired by a differential growth pattern. Nasal septal spurs and bending of the nasal septum with encroachment of one nasal chamber are usually the result of unequal growth of the two sides of the septum. Deflection of the caudal (anteroinferior) edge of the septum into one nasal vestibule is usually traumatic. Septal deflections are important to the degree that they produce airway obstruction. Significant obstructions should be treated by nasal septal reconstruction. In this operation the mucoperiosteum and mucoperichondrium of each side of the septum are elevated and the deviated part of the cartilaginous septum is scored to allow it to straighten. Deviated bone is removed. These operations are relatively minor and often produce gratifying results. Deviated septa do not cause headaches, sinus disease, nervousness, weight loss, or the like.

Digital trauma to the nasal septum may eventually cause a septal perforation and today is its most common cause. Years ago, the most common cause was *syphilis.* A perforated nasal septum is not significant unless it produces annoying crusting and bleeding from perichondritis or chondritis at the edge of the perforation. This may be treated by covering the perforation with a silicone rubber prosthesis. Occasionally a septal perforation causes whistling in the airstream, when the perforation is of a critical size relative to the speed of the airstream. This may be resolved and the septal perforation closed with a special surgical procedure.

Epistaxis (Nosebleed)

Epistaxis is almost invariably a benign disease but frequently a trying one because it is frightening to the patient and difficult for the physician to treat. The single most common cause of epistaxis in the adult is *hypertension.* The most common season is the late fall, when the home heating plant is turned on and the humidity drops precipitously. This dries out the inspired air, cracking or splitting the delicate respiratory mucosa. In children *digital trauma* to the anterior area of the nose promotes this cracking, as crusts build up inside the nares. The usual location of the bleeding vessel is at the anteroinferior portion of the nasal septum, where a plexus of submucosal vessels is located (Kiesselbach's plexus) in *Little's area.* The plexus is formed by the confluence of the septal branch of the sphenopalatine artery, the anterior ethmoid artery, and the perforating branch of the anterior palatine artery. Such epistaxes are termed *anterior bleeders;* they account for nine out of ten nosebleeds.

The management of *posterior epistaxis* is sometimes difficult. In addition, the patients deserve a complete work-up in search of specific causes, such as hypertension, leukemia, neoplasms of the nasal chambers and paranasal sinuses, and hemorrhagic disorders.

The first step in the management of a patient with epistaxis is to locate the bleeding vessel. The important principles are threefold: *spot lighting, spot suction,* and *spot hemostasis.* Spot lighting requires a head mirror or a head light, because overhead operating room lighting or a flashlight is totally inadequate to the task. Spot suctioning apparatus (which will reach 25 torr negative pressure with a high flow) is available in every hospital emergency room. To this should be added a (Frazier type) suction tip, which has a finger cutoff valve. All clots are aspirated from the nasal chamber with the patient in a sitting or semi-Fowler's position, and the free-flowing source of blood is located.

Anterior septal bleeders may be managed, as a rule, by silver nitrate bead cautery. The silver nitrate bead must be placed directly over the opening in the bleeding vessel and held in position for 10 to 15 seconds. The patient is cautioned against straining and nose-blowing for several days. Occasionally petroleum jelly gauze packing is necessary. The use of topical vasoconstrictor agents such as epinephrine on a cotton tampon must be looked on as a temporary measure in the treatment of epistaxis.

Posterior epistaxis arises from either the ethmoid arteries (a part of the internal carotid system) or from the sphenopalatine arteries (a part of the external carotid system). In the former the bleeding will be from above the level of the middle turbinate and in the latter from below the level of the middle turbinate. This distinction is of vital importance should all local methods fail and vascular ligation be necessary.

Control of posterior epistaxis is usually possible by careful packing of ½-inch strip gauze impregnated with antibiotic ointment against the bleeding site. This packing is left in place for 4 or 5 days while the patient is hospitalized for observation. When the bleeding site is too far posterior to be controlled in this manner, a posterior pack of lamb's wool or Foley catheter balloon is added to the anterior pack. Recurrent or persistent severe epistaxis usually requires ligation of the internal maxillary artery or ethmoid artery, or both. Ligation of the internal maxillary artery is usually carried out following a transantral route, with removal of the anterior and posterior walls of the maxillary sinus to gain access to the artery.

Facial Bones

Fractures of the middle third of the face involving the maxilla have been conveniently classified by LeFort (Fig. 36-10). Type I is a fracture involving the alveolar ridges or palate, and the bodies of the maxillary bones are intact. Type II involves the medial portion of the middle third of the face, with the fracture line crossing the zygomaticomaxillary suture lines, so that grasping the incisor teeth allows motion of the entire middle third of the face and not just the palatal portion. Type III is termed a craniofacial separation, with the fracture line on almost a horizontal plane, separating the maxillary and zygomatic bones from the rest of the skull. *Proper treatment is very important because occlusion of the teeth is involved as well as cosmetic appearance.* Improper treatment results in malocclusion of varying types and degrees. If the molar teeth come together before the incisor teeth, biting through food with the front teeth is impossible. Arch bars are wired to the maxillary and mandibular teeth and then joined together with intermaxillary wires, so that the teeth are locked to-

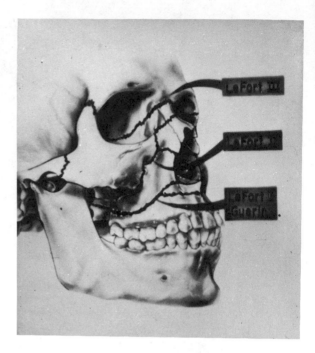

Fig. 36-10. Mid-third (maxillary) fractures of face tend to occur along certain lines and may be classified. LeFort classification is pictured here. LeFort III is craniofacial separation, LeFort II is pyramid-shaped fracture, and LeFort I is palatal separation.

gether in the natural occlusal relationship. The middle third of the face is stabilized when the arch bars are snugged up to the base of the skull with suspension wires circling the arches of the zygoma or passed subcutaneously through drill holes in the lateral orbital rims.

The supraorbital ridge, being very thick, is fractured only by a heavy blow. The infraorbital rim, however, is formed by thin bone and may be fractured by a relatively minor blow. A blow to the orbit may generate tremendous elevations of intraorbital pressure and result in a "blowing out" of the thin, bony orbital floor with herniation of orbital contents into the maxillary sinus below. Such an injury may result in enophthalmos, a depressed interpupillary line, and limitation of upward gaze in the affected eye (Fig. 36-11). Failure to recognize this fracture may result in permanent enophthalmos and diplopia. Treatment consists of retrieving the herniated tissue and restoring the integrity of the orbital floor.

Fractures of the zygoma occur from a direct blow high over the cheek. A crushing blow may fracture the arch of the zygoma to produce cosmetic deformity. The *tripodal fracture* involves the zygomaticofrontal suture, the zygomaticomaxillary suture, and the arch, resulting in a depression of the malar eminence. This fracture usually requires open reduction and fixation to assure a good cosmetic result.

Mandibular fractures are important for the same reason that maxillary fractures are important: faulty treatment will produce nutritionally crippling malocclusion. The most common types are *subcondylar,* which results in trismus; *ramus,* with displacement of the

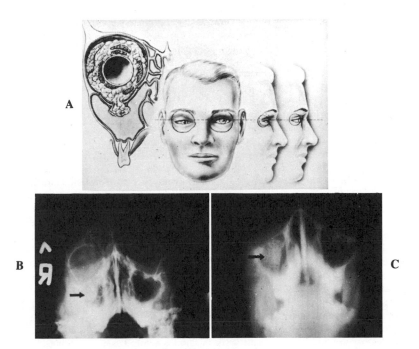

Fig. 36-11. Blowout fracture of orbit. Sharp blow to soft tissues of eye may fracture thin floor of orbit and allow orbital contents to drop into antrum. **A,** Eye is thus dropped, becomes enophthalmic, and upward-following gaze is lost. This is permanent unless recognized and treated. Water's view of sinuses can be very helpful, **B,** but sometimes laminagram, **C,** is necessary.

fracture ends produced by different muscle pulls exerted on the fragments; *body,* usually across the mental foramen; and *symphyseal.* Treatment is usually accomplished with simple closed reduction and stabilization with intermaxillary fixation. Occasionally, open reduction with fixation of the fragments is necessary.

Fractures of the frontal sinus are important to recognize in order to avoid the late sequelae of *cosmetic deformity, obstruction of the nasofrontal duct* (with ultimate production of a mucocele of the frontal sinus), and *cerebrospinal fluid leak* from a fracture tear of the posterior wall to which dura is firmly attached. An unrecognized cerebrospinal fluid leak may result in repeated episodes of meningitis, months or years apart. Open reduction is usually necessary.

Temporal Bone

Temporal bone fractures are the result of severe head injury, with the fracture line extending through the base of the skull, of which the temporal bone is a part. Hemorrhage from the ear canal or cerebrospinal fluid otorrhea is frequent, though not invariable. If there has not been a direct blow to the soft tissue over the mastoid, a bruise in this area is diagnostic (Battle's sign).

Temporal bone fractures are of two types. *Transverse temporal bone fractures* occur across the internal auditory canal and inner ear, producing immediate total deafness, labyrinthine vertigo and nystagmus, and frequently, facial nerve paralysis. *Longitudinal temporal bone fractures* cross the posterosuperior canal wall, middle ear, and eustachian tube, producing conductive deafness. A facial paralysis in this type is less common. Immediate facial nerve paralysis indicates sever-

ance of the nerve, which should be repaired as soon as the patient's general condition permits. A delayed facial nerve paralysis usually will resolve spontaneously.

Larynx

Laryngeal fractures are extremely important to recognize and treat early to avoid loss of the important faculties of speech and normal breathing. *In any patient with a neck injury, particularly an anterior blow to the neck, the symptoms of hoarseness or dyspnea demand immediate laryngoscopy.* Because progressive swelling continues for several hours after injury, airway symptoms that are very mild on admission to an emergency room may suddenly become severe and life threatening. Therefore, any patient with even mild airway symptoms must be carefully monitored for evidence of progression and treated with endotracheal intubation or tracheostomy should progression occur.

Within a week or 10 days of injury the diameters of the larynx can be reconstituted to restore normal speech and breathing. After this time, consequent scarring may require repeated operations on the larynx before the tracheotomy tube can be removed or may even sentence the patient to a permanent tracheostoma. The preceding points are extremely important and should be firmly in the mind of every physician attending an emergency room or treating acutely traumatized patients.

Frostbite

Cold injuries to the head and neck most frequently involve the external ear and the tip of the nose. The old maxim that a frozen member should be rubbed with snow is false. This only produces needless trauma to already damaged tissue. Cold, or frostbite, produces its injury by infarction and through cellular rupture by large ice crystals that form when tissue is slowly cooled below the crystallization point. Some tissue loss is then inevitable, but frequently this need be only the outer layers of the skin.

There is no uniformly successful method of treating frostbite, but it is generally agreed that the frozen tissue should be thawed reasonably rapidly. Further injury to the tissue should be avoided by immobility. Anticoagulation is not widely accepted. The skin should be protected against drying, fissuring, and the development of superficial infection by the application of petrolatum first, and later antibiotic ointments if necessary.

NEOPLASMS
Face

Basal cell carcinoma (rodent ulcer) is the most common neoplasm of the skin of the face. The lesion begins as a roughened area that ulcerates and fails to heal, classically above a line drawn from the tragus of the ear to the nasal ala. Farmers, because of their high exposure to actinic radiation, are prone to develop this lesion, as well as other skin neoplasms in exposed areas. Basal cell carcinomas rarely metastasize but continue to enlarge and destroy anything in their path until properly treated. The treatment is adequate excision, with closure of the excision site within skin lines to obtain optimal cosmetic results, especially for small lesions. When large basal cell carcinomas are excised, some type of skin flap is required for coverage. Excellent results are also obtainable by radiation therapy given in cancericidal doses, which usually means at least several weeks of daily treatments. Dermatologists frequently prefer to treat by electrodesiccation and curettage, or chemosurgery.

Epidermoid (squamous cell) carcinoma occurs anywhere on the face, including the lips, nose, lids, and external ear. Classically, the ulcerated lesion has a rolled, pearly border. The indurated border represents infiltration of adjacent normal tissue. In contrast to basal cell carcinoma, epidermoid carcinoma can metastasize. The nodes first involved are the submaxillary or submental nodes and then the deep cervical nodes, or the deep cervical nodes alone. Treatment is by adequate excision of the primary lesion, which must include 1 cm of normal tissue around its borders. Radiation therapy is also effective, but higher doses are necessary than in the basal cell carcinoma. When lymph nodes are involved, a radical neck dissection is necessary.

Carcinomas of the lids, lips, or external ear pose special problems in treatment and are best treated by a specialist. Where cartilage is immediately subjacent, as in the ear or nasal ala, special handling is required to prevent chondritis, whether treated surgically or by irradiation. Immediate reconstruction is necessary if the ear, eye, or nose is removed or is grossly deformed. Eyelid lesions must be managed with special care to avoid entropion, ectropion, and exposed cornea, which may lead to corneal damage and blindness. Lip lesions are treated by wedge resection or vermilionectomy. If the wedge is large, a plastic reconstructive procedure must be performed to supplant the tissue sacrificed so that a tight lip that limits speech and feeding does not ensue.

The *differential diagnosis* of facial skin cancer includes senile keratoses, seborrheic keratoses, nevi, and the keratoacanthoma. The last is an ulcerating reactive lesion of the skin that closely resembles cancer but is self-limiting.

Mouth and Oropharynx

Epidermoid (squamous cell) carcinoma is by far the most common neoplasm of the mouth and oropharynx. This lesion occurs most commonly in the tongue, floor of the mouth (Fig. 36-12), buccal mucosa, and tonsil but may involve the palate, alveolar ridges, mucosa of the jaws, uvula, and oropharyngeal walls. Treatment is simple excision to include an area 1 cm around the periphery or radiation therapy if the lesion is 2 cm. or smaller in size. A wedge resection is performed if the primary lesion involves the tongue. Tonsillar lesions are treated differently because of their propensity for early metastasis; small lesions are treated by irradia-

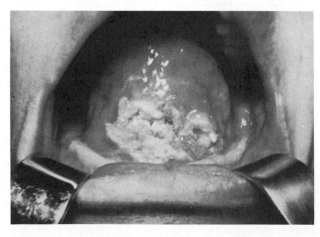

Fig. 36-12. Epidermoid carcinoma of floor of mouth. Notice its exophytic character and purulent membrane over entire ulcerated surface. Indurated lesions with ulceration anywhere in mouth demand biopsy.

tion, but those larger than 2 cm have usually metastasized and require neck dissection for cure. The involved cervical lymph nodes may be impalpable (subclinical metastases). Epidermoid carcinomas of the mouth and oropharynx that are larger than 2 cm in diameter require a large operation. Combination therapy is frequently used, including radiation therapy in a submaximal dose and surgical resection of the primary lesion with radical neck dissection in continuity. Resection of the primary lesion frequently requires partial mandibulectomy, partial glossectomy, or pharyngectomy. Reconstruction of the surgical defect is begun immediately to provide early functional and cosmetic rehabilitation. Five-year survival may approach 75% in small lesions located anteriorly in the mouth, whereas large lesions posteriorly with regional lymph nodes metastasis represent 25% or less 5-year survival.

Adenocarcinomas also occur in the mouth and oropharynx that are identical to those of the major salivary glands, because they arise in one of the many minor salivary glands in the region. They may be of many types. (See the discussion of salivary glands, below.) Thus mixed salivary gland tumors may occur on the palate, tonsillar pillars, or lateral angle of the pharynx. Treatment is always surgical because adenocarcinomas generally are not radiosensitive. The prognosis for these lesions is less favorable than for epidermoid carcinomas.

Connective tissue tumors are not unusual in this area. The most common are lymphomas that occur in tonsillar tissue. There may be connective tissue tumors of the bones of the jaws, such as osteogenic sarcoma, fibrosarcoma, and giant cell tumor. Muscle tumors such as rhabdomyosarcoma occur here, as well as neoplasms of other connective tissue elements (e.g., myxomas, fibromas, lipomas, and hemangiomas; (Fig. 36-13).

Tumors of dental origin appear as expansile lesions widening the alveolar ridge or the body of the mandi-

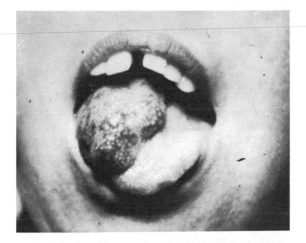

Fig. 36-13. Hemangioma of tongue. This lesion is common in upper digestive tract. Lesion is characteristically deep blue and empties and refills slowly on application and release of pressure. Varices on undersurface of tongue should be readily distinguishable from them and do not require treatment.

ble, or, less commonly, the upper jaw. The only common neoplasm of this type is the adamantinoma (ameloblastoma), a neoplasm of the enamel organ of the developing tooth. This benign tumor is cured by adequate simple excision. A dentigerous cyst is not a neoplasm, but it requires simple excision because it can be distinguished from an adamantinoma only by histologic examination.

Leukoplakia (white plaque) occurs wherever there is moist, stratified squamous, nonkeratinizing or respiratory epithelium. It appears as a thin, whitish plaque, most commonly in areas subject to chronic irritation, and can be identified in almost any denture-wearing patient. It is also very common on the buccal mucosa, lips, mucosa over the ascending ramus of the mandible, floor of the mouth, tongue and palate. It occasionally takes on a lacy pattern and may resemble lichen planus. Histologically, there may be any degree of abnormality from hyperkeratosis to invasive carcinoma. Not all leukoplakia requires treatment, but it must be observed periodically. If the lesion becomes thickened and palpable, this condition may indicate premalignant change, or if punctate ulceration occurs, excision must be carried out. If the area of leukoplakia is large, it may be excised in stages, or cryotherapy may be considered. Ordinarily, radiation therapy is not utilized unless there is evidence of malignant change.

The *differential diagnosis* of oral cancer includes the *epulides, chronic specific granulomas,* and *trauma* from ill-fitting dentures or jagged teeth. Giant cell epulis is not a neoplasm but a reactive phenomenon, found most frequently on the alveolar ridges. It is caused by trauma or great alterations in hormone levels, as in pregnancy. Chronic specific granulomas masquerading as neoplasms include *tuberculosis* (rare), *Vincent's angina, histoplasmosis* (Fig. 36-14), *actinomycosis, syphilis,* and *lethal midline granuloma* perforating the hard palate. The *brown hairy tongue* (Fig. 36-15), a peculiar biologic phenomenon that is poorly understood, should not be mistaken for a neoplasm. It is common in the chronically ill patient but also is seen in healthy persons. Brown hairy tongue is essentially hypertrophy of filiform papillae, with proliferating chromogen bacteria deeply embedded between the papillae. The treatment consists in repeatedly trimming the hypertrophied material with sharp dissection.

Early biopsy of lesions of the mouth and oropharynx is essential to cure. Once the lesion becomes larger than 1 cm, the cure rates drop precipitously. The prudent physician biopsies any suspicious lesion in this area. Practically no harm can be done, as functional or cosmetic losses from mouth or oropharyngeal biopsy are virtually negligible, but a positive biopsy of a small lesion will yield high dividends for the patient. A high index of suspicion is in order. The physician should never feel chagrined at a negative biopsy.

Nasopharynx

Cancer of the nasopharynx is common, especially in people of Oriental extraction. *Epidermoid carcinoma* and *lymphoepithelioma* of the nasopharynx are most insidious neoplasms, for in the majority of patients the first symptom is hearing loss from a middle ear effu-

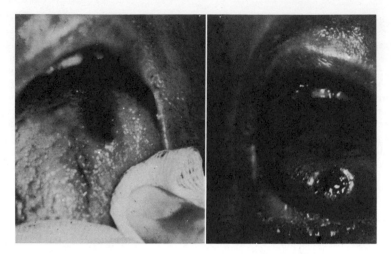

Fig. 36-14. Histoplasmosis of tongue. Notice sharp margination of ulceration and lack of exophytic response. This probably occurs by primary inoculation from chronic weed chewing. It is easy to confuse this or any other specific granuloma with malignancy.

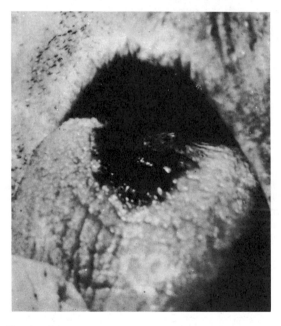

Fig. 36-15. Brown hairy tongue. This is not a disease per se but is often a great concern to patient. It is a frequent accompaniment of chronic disease state. Chromogen bacteria growing between greatly elongated filiform papillae produce picture. Treatment is by "tongue shave."

sion. Symptoms that may follow are a firm mass in the neck, odynophagia, epistaxis, or blood-streaked oral secretions. Any patient with a middle ear effusion or a hard mass in the neck must have a thorough examination of the nasopharynx before treatment is instituted. The treatment of primary nasopharyngeal carcinoma is radiation therapy. Once the primary tumor is controlled, neck dissection is performed if the cervical nodes are involved. Lymphoma may occur in this area

and liposarcoma and fibrosarcoma are rare neoplasms of the nasopharynx.

Benign tumors of the nasopharynx include the juvenile nasopharyngeal angiofibroma, a highly vascular tumor of young boys that is believed to arise in cartilaginous rests of sphenoid ossification centers. Its symptoms are nasal obstruction and epistaxis. The tumor can be diagnosed as a smooth blue-grey mass on mirror examination of the nasopharynx. The tumor contains a great many dilated blood spaces unlined with smooth muscle, and even biopsy may provoke profuse bleeding. Although it does not metastasize; it may erode the base of the skull. The treatment is by excision, usually with preoperative vascular embolization. The operation is extremely difficult and attended with much blood loss. *Craniopharyngioma* is a tumor arising from the embryonic Rathke's pouch. Most of these neoplasms are intracranial, but if the stalk of Rathke's pouch is persistent and becomes entrapped in the sphenoid bone, a sphenoid or nasopharyngeal tumor will result. This is also a benign tumor that is dangerous because of its position; an aid to diagnosis is calcification of the embryonic notochord. Chordomas occur most frequently in the body of the sphenoid bone and in the sacrum. Contents of the tumors are usually gelatinous; thus the tumor may be thought to be merely a cyst. However, unless the entire capsule is excised, it will recur.

Differential Diagnosis

The differential diagnosis of tumors in this area includes *chronic sphenoiditis, sphenoid mucocele, mucus-retention cyst of nasopharyngeal mucosa, Tornwaldt's bursa,* and *chronic adenoitis.*

Larynx and Hypopharynx

Epidermoid (squamous cell) carcinoma of the larynx afflicts men more commonly than women, in a ratio of about 10 to 1. One classification of neoplasms of the larynx is by location (1) glottic, including the entire true cord, (2) supraglottic, including the false vocal cord, aryepiglottic folds, epiglottis, and valleculae, and (3) subglottic, involving the conus elasticus and upper trachea. Cancer of the true cord has a good prognosis, ranking second only to epidermoid carcinoma of the skin in curability. The overall cure rate of carcinoma of the larynx is about 80%.

Carcinomas of the true cord are highly curable for two reasons: (1) symptoms (hoarseness, excessive throat clearing) annoy the patient enough to prompt an early visit to the physician, and (2) there is a paucity of lymphatics in the true cord so that metastases are rare. The 5-year cure rate of carcinomas of the true cord is between 80% and 90%. Treatment is by radiation therapy if cord mobility is unimpaired and the lesion extends to neither end of the cord; hemilaryngectomy is preferred if the lesion does extend to either end of the true cord. Because lesions of this area are so amenable to cure and so readily visible, *any patient with hoarseness of 2 weeks' duration or longer must have examination of the larynx.*

Larger glottic or supraglottic lesions without vocal cord fixation may be treated with a partial laryngectomy. These patients retain a serviceable voice and survival rates equal those of total laryngectomy. Even larger lesions require total laryngectomy and radical neck dissection. The patient must learn esophageal speech to gain full speech rehabilitation. Five-year survival is approximately 70%.

Epidermoid carcinoma of the laryngopharynx involves the lateral pharyngeal wall, posterior pharyngeal wall, or piriform sinus. Carcinomas that arise in the introitus of the esophagus are referred to as postcricoid lesions. These lesions are more common in women than in men. Dysphagia is the first symptom, and loss of laryngeal crepitus is the most important finding on examination. Laryngeal crepitus is that crackling sensation obtained when one pushes the larynx side to side over the cervical vertebrae. Barium swallow is indicated, and esophagoscopy confirms the diagnosis. The treatment is by partial or total laryngopharyngectomy and radical neck dissection followed by irradiation to 6000 rad. Five-year survival is approximately 50%.

Differential Diagnosis

Leukoplakia occurs on the true vocal cords and may be indistinguishable from carcinoma in situ or early invasive carcinoma. *Speaker's nodules* occur at the junction of the anterior and middle thirds of the vocal cords in patients who use their voices excessively. The nodules may be pinhead sized or polypoid and ulcerated, resembling a neoplasm. *Laryngocele* is a progressive enlargement of a noncommunicating portion of the laryngeal ventricle, producing a laryngeal cyst. Initially the laryngocele is internal, encroaching on the airway, and then it dissects up over the thyroid cartilage and externalizes as a neck mass. Laminagrams of the larynx are helpful in diagnosis of laryngocele. *Retention cysts* ordinarily present no problems in diagnosis because of their typical smooth, yellow-domed appearance. They are most common in the valleculae and on the aryepiglottic folds. The *chronic specific granulomas (syphilis, tuberculosis, actinomycosis,* and *lethal midline granu-*

loma) may present an identical appearance to cancer and require biopsy for distinction.

Nose and Paranasal Sinuses

Epidermoid (squamous cell) carcinoma is relatively rare in the nasal chamber but is common in the antrum and the ethmoid sinus. Unfortunately, the cure rate of this lesion is low because it does not produce significant symptoms until it has attained a large size. Ordinarily an antral carcinoma is not diagnosed or even suspected until it has eroded through one of its bony walls. Any of its walls may be eroded; the symptoms depend on which wall is involved. When the anterior wall is involved, the symptoms are fullness in the cheek, a mass, and numbness of the infraorbital region caused by infiltration of that nerve. Involvement of the inferior wall produces loosening or extrusion of teeth, widening of the alveolar ridge producing a poorly fitting denture, and a mass on the palate. Erosion of the medial wall produces blood-tinged nasal secretions and nasal airway obstruction. Erosion of the superior wall produces infraorbital nerve paresthesias and paralysis, proptosis, and interference with extraocular muscles. Bone destruction is present on appropriate computed tomographic examination. The treatment is a combination of radiation therapy and maxillectomy, which usually means sacrifice of that side of the hard palate. The patient can be rehabilitated in speech and chewing by the placement of an oral prosthesis that contains teeth.

Adenocystic carcinoma (adenoid cystic carcinoma, pseudoadenomatous basal cell carcinoma, cylindroma) is the most common adenocarinoma of the region. This may involve any of the paranasal sinuses or the nasal chamber. It is an extremely lethal neoplasm which tends to spread widely along nerves, and is somewhat sensitive to radiation therapy. These lesions are most commonly treated with surgical resection and postoperative irradiation. Other adenocarcinomas may occur here, arising in minor salivary glands, and the types are as listed in the discussion of salivary glands on this page.

Solitary myeloma of the respiratory tract (extramedullary myeloma) occurs in the ethmoid sinus or nasal chamber and produces symptoms of epistaxis and airway obstruction. It may exist as a solitary myeloma for many years, but frequently evidence of disseminated myeloma follows shortly. Treatment is excision or radiation therapy. Fibrosarcoma is another malignant connective tissue neoplasm that occasionally arises in this general area.

Olfactory neuroepithelioma (esthesioneuroblastoma) has been described only relatively recently. It is believed to arise from the neural elements of the olfactory epithelium. It is of relatively low-grade malignancy in most patients, though it may metastasize, and it is certainly malignant by position. There appears to be some radiosensitivity to this lesion. The treatment consists of wide surgical excision to include a craniotomy and resection of the cribriform plate.

Osteoma is the most common benign tumor of connective tissue origin that arises in the nasal and paranasal cavities. Osteoma usually involves the frontal sinus; it tends to grow slowly but may become very large. Excision must be carried out, especially if it arises adjacent to the nasofrontal duct or threatens to erode the inner wall of the sinus and the dura. *Ossifying fibroma* is one of the bony dysplasias that is not a true neoplasm but tends to act like one. The ethmoid sinus is the most common location, radiographic examination is diagnostic, and treatment is excision by external approach. *Giant cell tumor of bone* may affect any age group, is of generally low-grade malignancy, and may be treated either by surgical excision or by irradiation.

Differential Diagnosis

Chronic vestibulitis of the eczematoid variety is distinguished with difficulty from skin cancer of the nasal vestibule. When seen in a localized area of the nasal vestibule, or particularly when a brief trial of treatment fails, biopsy is mandatory. *Nasal polyposis* of the hyperplastic or allergic type should present no difficulty in distinction from cancer, since a nasal polyp has a striking resemblance to a peeled grape and the surface epithelium is always intact. Beefy red polyps associated with chronic sinusitis are a different matter, demanding prompt biopsy to rule out neoplasm. The presence of pus with inflammatory polyps does not exclude polypoid nasal malignancy because neoplasms of the nose alter nasal physiology and infection is the rule. *Nasal glioma,* representing heterotopic glial tissue, may be present anywhere in the nasal chamber and is overlain by normal skin or mucosa. *Meningocele* or *meningoencephalocele* should always be considered when a smooth nonulcerated mass is present in a nasal chamber. Pulsation of the mass is suggestive of meningocele and precludes biopsy. The chronic specific granulomas include *lethal midline granuloma, sarcoidosis, actinomycosis,* and *syphilis. Rhinoscleroma* and *rhinosporidiosis* are rare in this country.

Salivary Glands

Classification

Benign
  Mixed salivary gland tumor (pleomorphic adenoma)
  Benign mucoepidermoid tumor
  Adenoma
    Papillary cystadenoma lymphomatosum (Warthin's tumor)
    Serous cell adenoma
    Acidophilic cell adenoma
Malignant
  Epidermoid carcinoma (well- and poorly differentiated, including lymphoepithelioma)
  Mucoepidermoid carcinoma
  Adenocarcinoma
    Adenocystic carcinoma
    Acinic (serous) carcinoma
    Acidophilic (oxyphilic) cell carcinoma
    Unclassified salivary gland carcinoma

Connective tissue tumors also occur in salivary glands, though they are relatively rare. They include neurofibromas, fibromas, and neurofibrosarcomas. Salivary glands may also be the site of infiltration by lymphomas.

The physician should be aware of the relative frequency of malignant tumors found in various salivary glands. In the parotid gland approximately 25% of neo-

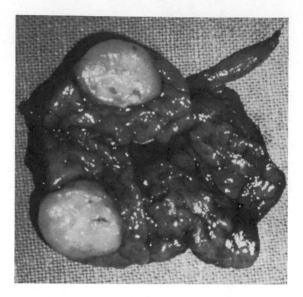

Fig. 36-16. Mixed salivary gland tumor involving submaxillary salivary gland. This particular neoplasm is much more common in parotid gland and may also occur in minor salivary glands of mouth and throat, particularly around palatine tonsil.

plasms are malignant; in the submandibular gland approximately 50% are malignant; and in the minor salivary glands approximately 70% are malignant.

About 60% of all salivary gland tumors are the so-called *mixed salivary gland tumor (pleomorphic adenoma),* which is almost always benign (Fig. 36-16). It acquired its name by virtue of an apparent mixture of two germ cell layers in its histologic pattern: nests, cords, and sheets of epithelial cells interspersed by a myxomatous stroma that sometimes condenses into pseudocartilage. It is characteristically a slowly growing, firm, freely mobile mass most commonly found in the tail of the parotid gland. When it is less than 2 cm in diameter, it may feel so mobile and superficial that the physician is tempted to remove it in the office. *This is always a mistake.* Adequate treatment for a mixed salivary gland tumor is lateral lobectomy. In our experience nothing short of this carries any assurance against recurrence. The mixed salivary gland tumor is notorious for its ability to produce seedling recurrences. This frequently happens when the tumor capsule is broken at the time of removal, or the tumor is simply shelled out.

Warthin's tumor is characteristically soft and almost cystic and occurs in the tail of the parotid gland, usually in old men. It may be bilateral. Simple excision effects a cure.

The distinction between a benign and a malignant salivary gland tumor is frequently a very difficult one. The surgeon is caught between Scylla and Charybdis: he or she does not want to biopsy a mass lest it be a mixed tumor and yet wants to go to the operating room prepared for whatever radical operation is necessary. Therefore it is wise to perform total parotidectomy for any parotid tumor. The only characteristic clinical fea-

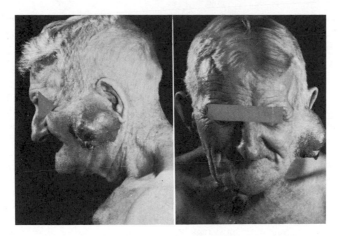

Fig. 36-17. Large, ulcerating adenocarcinoma of parotid gland.

ture of a malignant parotid tumor is a branch paralysis or total paralysis of the facial nerve. Benign tumors reach tremendous size without producing any paralysis of the facial nerve. Other characteristics of malignant tumors are fixation, pain, and tenderness (Fig. 36-17). However, benign tumors may be tender or painful as well, if recent hemorrhage into the tumor produces capsular stretch. If either one of these features is present, the surgeon should assume malignancy and make appropriate preparations. The facial nerve is not sacrificed at operation unless it is involved by tumor, in which event it is immediately grafted, using a sensory nerve as donor (Fig. 36-18).

Epidermoid carcinoma is the single most common malignant tumor to involve the salivary glands and is frequently metastatic from a skin tumor. The adenocarcinomas as a group more commonly arise in a salivary gland than epidermoid carcinoma. *Adenocystic carcinoma* is highly lethal, tending to metastasize early in regional lymphatics and to lung. *Mucoepidermoid carcinoma* is uncommon. Rarer still is *acidophilic cell adenocarcinoma,* which is believed to arise from ductal epithelium and is a tumor of old men. *Acinic cell adenocarcinoma* is the second most common of the adenocarcinoma group, occurring in females predominantly, and it tends to act more like a sarcoma than a carcinoma in that it metastasizes through the bloodstream.

Differential Diagnosis

Salivary gland calculi may mimic neoplasm by obstruction of salivary flow, but usually there is a clear history of fluctuation in the size of the gland. *Mikulicz's disease* and *Sjögren's syndrome* may resemble neoplasms, but they are diffuse diseases of the gland rather than localized; biopsy may be necessary to rule out cancer, and this is permissible in diffuse diseases of the salivary glands. A *high cervical lymph node* may be mistaken for a tumor in the tail of the parotid gland. If the mass can be brought out over the body or ramus of the mandible, it is a parotid gland mass rather than a cervical chain lymph node. A *hypertrophied masseter* or a *wing mandible* may be confused with a diseased parotid gland.

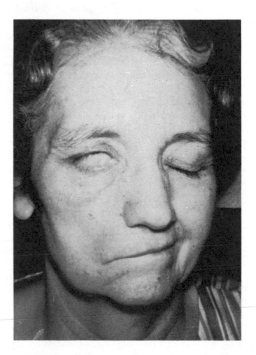

Fig. 36-18. Right complete peripheral facial paralysis with pronounced "Bell's phenomenon." This may be attributable to lesion anywhere along course of facial nerve trunk: internal auditory canal, middle ear, mastoid, or parotid gland. If cause is not determinable on complete work-up, diagnosis is Bell's palsy. This patient has just had parotid malignancy removed and facial nerve grafted. Facial motion will return in 9 to 12 months.

HEARING LOSSES AND MICROSURGERY OF THE EAR
Sensorineural Hearing Loss

Sensorineural deafness (sensory—hair cells of the organ of Cori; neural—eighth nerve or above this level in the central nervous system) is often called "nerve" deafness or perceptive deafness. It is the most common form of deafness. Here are some causes:

Congenital
Traumatic
Toxic
Vascular
Infection
Neoplasm
Ménière's disease
Degenerative

Congenital sensorineural deafness is usually very severe. As a rule it is bilateral, and so profound that the patient can hear only the loudest sounds and, of these, only low tones. Such a person will never develop normal speech and needs training in special schools throughout the early years. Congenital deafness may be attributable to Rh incompatibilities, birth trauma, virus infection in utero, malformation of the inner ears, or other causes. Mild forms of congenital deafness also occur.

Traumatic sensorineural deafness is of three kinds: noise-induced deafness, otic concussion, and transverse temporal bone fracture. The most common is *noise-induced deafness,* often called acoustic trauma, which results from an accumulation of the effects of intense sound over months or years. This is becoming more and more prevalent. It is manifest early as a selective 4906-hertz (Hz) dip on the audiogram, not impairing speech reception. *Otic concussion* produces a high-tone deafness and is the result of either cerebral concussion or the convergence of lines of force through the skull, which center on the temporal bone. *Transverse temporal bone fracture* (see above) causes total inner ear deafness.

Toxic deafness in the United States is generally caused by drugs, the most common of which are aspirin, streptomycin, and kanamycin. This is a direct effect of the drug on the hair cell.

Vascular deafness is the result of occlusion of the end artery to the labyrinth and produces total deafness together with loss of vestibular function. It is sometimes called "otic apoplexy."

Viral infection, the most common of which is the mumps virus, can cause deafness. Fortunately, this almost always spares one ear. It is quite common in children and may not be discovered until adult life or on a routine school audiometric program. Loss of hearing in one ear produces the inability to localize sound and the loss of stereo effect of hearing, preventing the person from separating one voice from another when there are multiple conversations in the room; this is sometimes called the "cocktail party effect" of binaural hearing. Bacterial infection from meningitis or from chronic mastoiditis can invade the inner ear and produce immediate total deafness and loss of vestibular function. Patients with severe sensorineural hearing loss may be candidates for a cochlear prosthesis (artificial ear).

Neoplasms that begin in the middle ear, the mastoid, or the auditory nerve produce deafness by growth and infiltration. Of these, the most common are acoustic neuroma, glomus jugulare tumor, and epidermoid carcinoma.

Ménière's disease is listed separately because we do not know whether it is caused by vascular, toxic, or metabolic factors. It is a pure hair cell deafness and as such is accompanied by a severe discrimination loss and *recruitment* (the abnormal growth of loudness in a deafened ear). The deafness fluctuates. The disease is characterized by tinnitus and vertigo, the spells lasting 20 minutes to many hours. The treatment is diuretics, vasodilators, and a low-sodium diet. Generally only one ear is affected. If treatment fails, destruction labyrinthotomy or vestibular nerve section may be necessary.

Degenerative sensorineural deafness is called *presbycusis.* It is the result of gradual loss of hair cells or first-order neurons, or both, because of the aging process. This strikes virtually all people and begins in the very high tones. It goes on all through life, but only in the middle-aged or older patient does it produce noticeable deafness by finally involving the upper and then the middle speech frequencies. Even a person 20 years of age does not have as extensive high-tone hearing as a younger person. There is no treatment for presbycusis. All the preceding causes of deafness tend to be additive to degenerative deafness, so that presbycusis may occur in such patients at an earlier age than otherwise.

Conductive Hearing Loss

A *conductive deafness* in any form of deafness that tends to prevent sound from reaching the sensorineural apparatus. There are many causes, the most common of which are the following:

Chronic nonsuppurative otitis media
Chronic suppurative otitis media
Canal problems, including congenital atresia and stenosis
Perforation of the tympanic membrane
Ossicular destruction or fixation, including otosclerosis
Trauma

Chronic nonsuppurative otitis media and *chronic suppurative otitis media* were discussed above. *Canal problems* that produce deafness do so by complete blockage of the canal. If even a very small passageway remains for air to reach the tympanic membrane, hearing is unaffected. Wax impactions and acute external otitis are the most common in this category. Other causes are osteomas of the canal, neoplasms of the skin of the canal, neoplasms about the ear such as neurofibromatosis, and congenital atresia, either occurring singly or as a part of a more general anomaly such as Treacher-Collins syndrome. A *perforation* of the tympanic membrane from unresolved middle ear infection or trauma produces conductive deafness by virtue of loss of the sound-gathering ability of the tympanic membrane. *Clinical otosclerosis* is a disease of young adults caused by ankylosis of the stapes by an overgrowth of spongiotic bone from the enchondral layer of the otic capsule. It is slowly progressive, and a history of repeated earaches or otorrhea is absent. There is usually a positive family history. It is slightly more common in females than in males. A normal tympanic membrane is compatible with this diagnosis. The deafness is frequently purely conductive, though there may be a mild to moderate sensorineural deafness superimposed. This form of deafness can usually be helped by an operation (Fig. 36-19). *Traumatic deafness* can be caused by bursting of the tympanic membrane that has failed to heal, a dislocation of the ossicles in the middle ear, or a temporal bone fracture of a longitudinal nature.

Hearing Testing

The *decibel* (dB) is the meaure used to describe degrees of hearing loss. It is important to note that the decibel is not a unit of measurement but a ratio. Hearing loss is expressed logarithmically, because the ear is able to work over a great expanse of energy input. The decibel is a logarithmic ratio between an observed sound pressure level and a reference level. For every increase in sound of 6 dB, sound pressure doubles.

The *audiogram* indicates hearing levels at thresholds over a frequency range of 125 to 8000 Hz. Across the ordinate of the audiogram, the threshold of hearing from 0 to 100 dB loss is indicated at that frequency. One also measures hearing thresholds at each of the speech frequencies (250, 500, 1000, 2000 Hz) by bone conduction, placing a transducer over the mastoid bone and stimulating the sensorineural receptor apparatus directly rather than through the ossicular chain and tympanic membrane.

With use of the audiometer, *discrimination testing* can be performed. This is a test of how clearly words are understood by the ear. The volume is raised 40 dB above the threshold of hearing, and the number of phonetically balanced words the patient can understand is recorded. The normal ear can understand at least 80%

of these words. When discrimination ability is definitely impaired, it indicates a sensory or a neural deafness. Conductive deafnesses do not impair word discrimination ability.

Tuning fork tests are important in the identification of hearing loss. The tuning forks most useful are the 512 and 1024 Hz and frequently the 256 and 2048 Hz. The *Rinne test* is performed by placing the stem of the fork sounded above threshold first over the mastoid bone just behind and above the external canal and then over the external canal an inch away from the ear. If bone conduction is louder than air conduction, the Rinne test is said to be negative, and if air conduction is louder than bone conduction, it is positive. A negative Rinne test is characteristic of conductive deafness. A positive Rinne test is compatible with normal hearing or sensorineural deafness. It is important to mask the opposite ear when there is a significant difference of hearing between the two ears, so that during bone conduction testing the sound is not perceived in the opposite, or better, ear. The *Weber test* is performed by placing the stem of the fork somewhere in the midline: the vertex, the forehead, or the upper incisor teeth. The fork will lateralize to the better ear in sensorineural deafness and to the deaf ear in conductive deafness. It is a rather sensitive test.

Tuning fork tests are supplemented by *whisper and speech tests* to determine the approximate level of deafness. The normal or very slightly deaf ear can perceive the lightest "residual air" whispered voice. Perception of a light whispered voice audible a few inches from the ear indicates hearing with 20 dB, a medium whispered voice tests at a 30 to 40 dB level, a low spoken

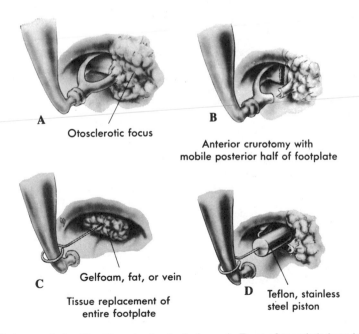

A Otosclerotic focus

B Anterior crurotomy with mobile posterior half of footplate

C Gelfoam, fat, or vein
Tissue replacement of entire footplate

D Teflon, stainless steel piston

Fig. 36-19. Various methods of handling otosclerotic deafness. **A,** Focus of spongiotic bone is visible at anterior portion of footplate binding stapes in oval window. **B,** Anterior crurotomy has been done. Footplate is fractured behind otosclerotic focus, and posterior assembly is mobile. **C,** Entire stapes has been removed; footplate is replaced with tissue graft or Gelfoam and crura with stainless steel wire; knot holding tissue graft is buried in it. **D,** Teflon piston secured by wire around incus replaces central portion of footplate.

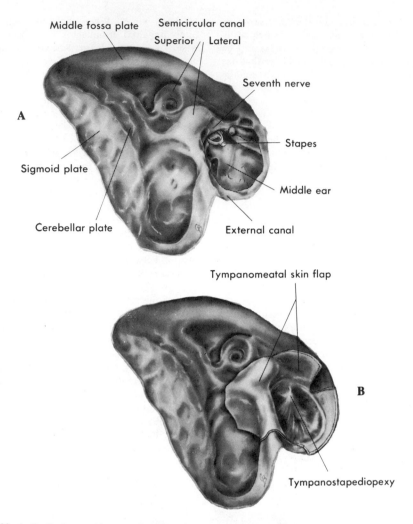

Middle fossa plate   Semicircular canal
Superior   Lateral

Seventh nerve

A

Stapes

Sigmoid plate

Middle ear

Cerebellar plate   External canal

Tympanomeatal skin flap

B

Tympanostapediopexy

Fig. 36-20. A, Radical mastoidectomy; here, one large common chamber is created, including mastoid bowl, middle ear, and external auditory canal; ossicles are removed except for stapes; this is essentially sculpturing of bony plates surrounding temporal bone and is reserved for advanced tympanomastoid disease. **B,** Modified radical mastoidectomy; if mesotympanum can be preserved, tympanic membrane is tilted inward to contact stapes and is held in this new position by reflection of tympanomeatal canal skin flap onto facial ridge and roof of cavity; this preserves hearing.

voice at a 50 to 60 dB level, and a medium spoken voice at the 70 to 80 dB level. If the ear cannot hear a loud voice or a shout with the other ear properly masked, it is said to be profoundly deaf.

A number of *special auditory tests* provide a relatively high degree of localization of the lesion (i.e., these special tests may tell us whether the deafness is hair cell, neural, or cortical in origin). Some of them are the short increment sensitivity index (SISI test), tone fatigue testing, brain-stem evoked response audiometry. There is also a wide variety of tests available for malingered deafness. There are even special tests available for objective evaluation of auditory acuity, not involving a judgment on the part of the patient. These include psychogalvanic skin response and evoked cortical potential recording using an analog computer.

Tinnitus Aurium

Tinnitus aurium means nothing more than ringing in the ears. This is a symptom and not a disease. Tinnitus of varying degrees is almost invariably associated with deafness, and it is present to the degree that the ear is deaf. Usually, the tinnitus will be at about the same frequency as the deafness, so that presbycusis or high-tone deafness produces a high-pitched ringing and conductive deafness produces a panfrequency or "white noise" ringing. Tinnitus may be subdivided into *subjective* and *objective*. Subjective tinnitus is that which the patient alone can hear, and the physician is unable to detect any sound using his stethoscope over the external canal or over the temporal region. Objective tinnitus is that which the physician can hear as well. Objective tinnitus always means that there is a physical basis for the tinnitus instead of a sensory or neural lesion.

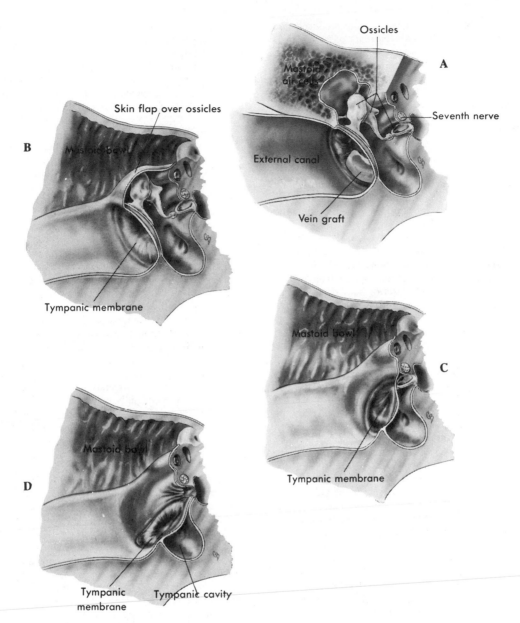

Fig. 36-21. A, Tympanoplasty type I. Notice that all structures are normal in the middle ear and mastoid, except for the perforation of tympanic membrane in its lower portion. Vein or fascia graft may be placed over perforation after careful removal of surrounding skin. More commonly, graft material is placed inside tympanic membrane. **B,** Tympanoplasty type II. Ossicular chain is preserved because it is free of disease. External auditory canal and mastoid bowl are one common chamber, from which middle ear is sealed. Normal hearing is obtainable with this operation. **C,** Tympanoplasty type III. Because of disease, malleus and incus were sacrificed, and tympanic membrane rests against head of stapes; otherwise it is same as tympanoplasty type II. Excellent hearing is attainable, because only lever ratio of ossicular chain is sacrificed and areal ratio (tympanic membrane to footplate) is maintained. This operation is same as modified radical mastoidectomy. **D,** Tympanoplasty type IV. Stapedial arch required sacrifice or was absent through disease. Footplate is left exposed to outside, and tympanic membrane is sealed against promontory. Round window (shaded area in center of hypotympanum) is thus joined with eustachian tube orifice as closed air-containing chamber. Because areal ratio is sacrified as well as lever ratio, normal hearing is not obtainable; the best level that is theoretically obtainable is 26 dB. below normal.

Examples of objective tinnitus are that produced by a cavernous sinus fistula, eddy currents of blood in the carotid system from an arteriosclerotic plaque, eustachian tube clicks, and tympanic muscle clicks from spasm of the tensor tympani muscle or stapedius muscle. The only treatment for tinnitus is detection of the underlying cause and its correction if possible.

Mastoidectomy

Mastoidectomy is performed for acute or chronic suppurative bone infection of the mastoid portion of the temporal bone (Fig. 36-6). The incidence of mastoidectomy for acute disease has dropped precipitously since antibiotics have been available, but at the same time, mastoidectomy done for chronic bone infection has risen.

A *simple mastoidectomy* is performed for acute osteomyelitis of the mastoid bone. The mastoid cortex and all air cells and diseased bone are removed. This usually means removal of the mastoid tip. The ossicles, tympanic membrane, and posterior bony canal wall are left intact. If the middle ear recovers, hearing is unaffected.

A *modified radical mastoidectomy* is performed for chronic suppurative mastoiditis and otitis media. The mastoid cortex is removed, and a meticulous removal of all mastoid air cells is done as the first step. The posterior canal wall is then removed, with the skin of the posterior and superior canal wall being preserved. The epitympanum is then exenterated of disease, and the incus and the head and neck of the malleus are removed. The tympanic membrane is reflected medially until it comes into contact with the head of the stapes, and the skin of the canal is used to line the mastoid cavity, sealing the middle ear from the remaining cavity. This operation joins the external canal and the mastoid cavity, making one large chamber. The cavity then heals by secondary intention, becoming lined with skin in a matter of weeks. Wax and skin debris must be removed from this cavity at twice yearly intervals, because it does not have the debris-removing characteristics of the normal ear canal. Excellent hearing may possibly occur after this operation. Theoretically only the lever ratio of the ossicular chain is sacrified, and thus it is possible to have as little as a 2 dB hearing loss (Fig. 36-20, *B*).

A *radical mastoidectomy* is the same as the modified operation except that portions of the middle ear and tympanic membrane are removed. The contents of the middle ear are exenterated, except for the stapes. Thus one large chamber is created, comprising the external canal, mastoid cavity, and middle ear, open for inspection the rest of the patient's life. The consequent hearing loss is, of course, severe: between 45 and 60 dB (Fig. 36-20, *A*).

Microsurgery of the Ear

Deafness is still man's most common physical impairment, despite the myriad ways modern man has found to maim and injure himself. Fortunately, a significant number of deafnesses are surgically correctable, especially those caused by defects in the tympanic membrane, ossicular chain, and stapedovestibular joint. Since that part of the tympanum containing the hearing mechanism is quite small (Fig. 36-21), these operations are done under magnification and are termed microsurgical operations. Some diseases causing deafness that may be helped by microsurgery are (1) tympanic perforation, (2) ossicular chain disruption with or without an intact tympanic membrane, (3) chronic suppurative otitis media (after mastoid disease is controlled), (4) certain varieties of chronic adhesive otitis media, (5) tympanosclerosis, and (6) otosclerosis.

These operations may be performed transmeatally or across the mastoid after mastoidectomy has been performed. The binocular operating microscope is used, which provides a coaxially lighted image of brilliant intensity, magnified from 6 to 40 times. Operations are done under general or local anesthesia. Where the tympanic membrane is intact, as in otosclerosis or tympanosclerosis, a skin flap is elevated from the posterior canal wall hinged on the posterior half of the tympanic membrane. Access to the tympanum is gained between the fibrocartilaginous annular ligament and the bony anulus of the tympanum. This renders the posterior half of the tympanum visible and, with it, almost all the conductive apparatus. A wide variety of special instruments is necessary for these operations. They are electrical and air turbine drills, chisels, needles, picks, hooks, knives, elevators, scissors, saws, suction tips, and various forceps. They are unique primarily in their diminutive size. Since these instruments are all handheld and not moved by micromanipulators, the surgeon's touch must be developed to an uncommon deftness. This usually takes several years of practice.

37

Urologic Surgery

Joseph D. Schmidt

Urology is that branch of medicine and surgery devoted to the study, diagnosis, and treatment of diseases and abnormalities of the urogenital tract of the male and the urinary tract of the female.

Urologists must work in close association with members of all other branches of medicine but particularly with internists and surgeons in the study and care of diseases of the adrenal gland, medical diseases of the kidney, and abdominal masses of all types.

The kidney is the most important organ of excretion. A clear understanding of the status of the urinary tract of every patient is essential to a complete evaluation of the patient's condition. Only by a complete history and general examination of the patient, analysis of the urine, estimation of renal function, and radiographic imaging of the urinary tract can the physician obtain an accurate knowledge of the patient's urologic status. Cystoscopy is often necessary to complete the urinary tract evaluation.

ANATOMY AND PHYSIOLOGY

The kidney has some endocrine functions that are related to the maintenance of blood pressure, hematopoiesis, and calcium metabolism, but its principal function is to form urine. This is the main pathway by which water, salts, nitrogenous wastes, and other products are excreted from the body, thereby helping to maintain the internal balance of these substances. The urine that is formed travels down through the calyces, renal pelves, and ureters to the bladder. In the adult, when about 400 ml has collected, the desire to urinate triggers contraction of bladder muscle, emptying the urine through the urethra. The kidneys, calyces, pelves, and ureters are normally duplicated, but there is normally only one bladder and urethra.

PATHOLOGY AND SYMPTOMATOLOGY

Diseases of the genitourinary tract conveniently fall into the following general classes: congenital anomalies, trauma, inflammations, neoplasms, and certain miscellaneous diseases. Since its excretory function links the genitourinary tract anatomically and physiologically to other organ systems, lesions involving the urinary tract may give rise to symptoms suggestive of lesions in organs outside the urinary tract. Moreover, since there is a direct communication and interrelationship between the functions of the various portions of the urinary tract, lesions in one portion may in turn produce disturbances of function in another portion. These two principles are extremely important to the understanding of urinary tract disease.

Thus disorders of this system not only may be multiple in distribution in the tract itself, but they may also be associated with or mimicked by lesions arising primarily in other organ systems. This is particularly true in *children* with congenital anomalies of the genitourinary tract. If an early diagnosis is to be made, a complete urologic survey must be made of children with unexplained symptoms or signs.

One should not infer from the preceding remarks that every person with a genitourinary disease should be subjected at the first visit to all the procedures necessary to evaluate the entire genitourinary system. This is not only unnecessary but in many instances may also be distinctly harmful; (e.g., in the presence of an acute inflammation of the urethra, prostate, or bladder, the instrumentation necessary to examine the urinary tract may be contraindicated). Only those examinations that accurately establish the location and nature of the disease needing immediate treatment are necessary. The more complicated diagnostic manipulations are deferred until the acute inflammatory findings subside or until the progress of the disease makes these examinations imperative.

Since *obstruction* and *infection* are complications common to most urinary tract lesions, the physician must determine the underlying problem.

THERAPY

Therapy, in general, consists of two phases after an accurate diagnosis has been established. The first phase is designed to relieve pain, dysuria, and frequency or signs of infection. The *sine qua non* is the *relief of obstruction* anywhere in the urinary tract, performed in the simplest way possible. In addition, antibiotics are given to control infection. With even this temporary relief of obstructive signs and symptoms, the patient's general condition will improve rapidly, and then one may proceed with the definitive phase of therapy.

The definitive phase is designed to cure, correct, or eradicate the causative lesion. This is done in such a way as not to disturb function but rather to restore it to as near physiologic normalcy as possible. Here again, adequate urine drainage is of paramount concern. All therapeutic efforts are aimed at restoring or maintaining normal renal function and urinary transport.

CLINICAL EXAMINATION
Approach

Patients may be shy about their complaints because of social taboos connected with the genitourinary tract.

It is especially important for the physician and nurse to assume a correct professional attitude toward them. Sympathy must be expressed and embarrassment avoided. They must be made to feel at ease. Deep human understanding and an intense feeling of responsibility on the part of the physician and nurse are mandatory qualities.

Remarks

The patient's history and chief complaint are important because they may point directly to some portion of the genitourinary tract, or they may indicate lesions elsewhere, but these extraurinary tract disturbances of function may be caused by impaired renal function. There may be no symptoms, and only a complete examination of the urinary tract will show the abnormalities.

History

Patients usually relate a history of one or more of the following situations:

1. Trauma with urinary extravasation
2. Abnormalities of urine
   a. Pyuria
   b. Hematuria
   c. Chyluria
   d. Pneumaturia
3. Abnormality in voiding
   a. Incontinence
      (1) Urgency
      (2) Paradoxic
      (3) Dribbling between normal urination
      (4) Stress
   b. Frequency
   c. Dysuria
   d. Oliguria
   e. Polyuria
   f. Small stream
   g. Retention
   h. Dribbling. Is it incontinence or is it associated with apparently normal voiding? The latter is pathognomonic of an ectopic ureteral orifice.
4. Tumors or swellings in urogenital area
   a. Scrotum
      (1) Painful
      (2) Tender
      (3) Associated redness
   b. Abdominal masses
      (1) In the flank
      (2) Suprapubic
      (3) In the groin
5. Pain and tenderness in region of genitourinary tract
   a. Infection
   b. Stone
   c. Trauma
   d. Congenital or acquired obstruction
6. Uremia—a blanket term used to designate the syndrome that results from renal insufficiency of any type—may be characterized by nausea, vomiting, stupor, coma, azotemia, oliguria, etc. The signs and symptoms vary with the myriad of variations in pathophysiology associated with renal insufficiency.
7. Azotemia may be part of the picture of renal insufficiency (uremia) but may be present with no underlying renal disease (dehydration, severe gastrointestinal tract hemorrhage).
8. Chills or fever may mean infection of the urinary tract.
9. Loss of weight may indicate urogenital malignant neoplasm, uremia, or chronic infection.

10. Evidence of metastases
    a. Osteoblastic lesions usually are metastases from carcinoma of the prostate in the male.
    b. Hypernephroma frequently metastasizes to the lungs, as does tumor of the testis.
    c. Pulsating bone tumors, osteolytic in nature, usually are metastases from hypernephroma.
11. Poor growth in children may be an indication of renal insufficiency, related to congenital urinary tract obstruction.
12. Sexual dysfunction: Impotence, total or partial, is a common symptom and is based on organic problems in over half the cases. Premature ejaculation is unrelated to organic disease, whereas retrograde ejaculation usually results from anatomic disturbances of either the lumbar sympathetic ganglia or bladder neck (internal sphincter).

Physical Examination

General Appearance

The general appearance of the patient frequently suggests urinary tract disease. However, many serious diseases of the urinary tract produce no external changes, even in their late stages. In children abnormalities of growth, particularly dwarfism, suggest disease of the urinary tract with associated renal insufficiency. In all ages edema, sallow complexion, shortness of breath, and anemia or dehydration may herald serious genitourinary tract disease.

Findings

These findings often justify careful evaluation of the urinary tract:

Fever. Fever may be an indication of urinary tract infection; it is usually high, erratic, and frequently associated with chills.

Hypertension. Hypertension is frequently associated with glomerular disease of the kidneys, late stages of chronic pyelonephritis, polycystic disease of the kidney, decreased perfusion of one or both kidneys or even a segment of one kidney, and acute ureteral obstruction.

Edema. Edema associated with urinary tract disease is of two types. It may be peripheral to venous or lymphatic obstruction caused by urinary tract neoplasm, or it may be generalized and associated with renal insufficiency or hypoproteinemia.

Abnormalities of growth. Abnormalities of growth in children may be associated with changes in adrenal function or severe renal insufficiency.

Secondary anemia. Secondary anemia is frequently seen with renal insufficiency and urinary tract neoplasm from bleeding and bone marrow involvement.

Evidence of metastasis. Neoplasms of the prostate, kidney, and testis frequently metastasize to the lungs, the brain, and the bones of the torso.

Neurologic findings. Diseases of the spinal cord frequently produce abnormalities in function of the bladder and the upper urinary tract, especially infection, stone formation, and residual urine in the bladder and kidneys. Early urologic workup is particularly important, since damage to the urinary tract caused by spinal cord disease may be so insidious that an irreversible change may occur before symptoms arise.

Loss of weight, dehydration. Loss of weight and dehydration are hallmarks of renal insufficiency and chronic urinary tract diseases.

Abnormal breathing. Abnormal breathing may herald acidosis accompanying renal insufficiency.

Abdominal masses. Abdominal masses require complete urinary tract investigation, including x-ray examination. A suprapubic mass may simply be a full bladder caused by obstruction of the bladder neck. A pelvic or abdominal mass may be ectopic kidney that should not be removed.

Local Examination and Findings

Careful examination in the region of the kidneys and ureters should be a part of every physical examination. The skin should be inspected for enlarged, dilated veins that indicate collateral circulation. Palpation of the costovertebral angle, for muscle spasm and tenderness should be carefully carried out. Suprapubic dullness and masses should be noted. The inguinal canals should be palpated while the patient stands for an undescended testis or hernia.

The scrotum should be carefully palpated. The vas deferens, the epididymis, and the testis should be examined separately, and abnormalities should be noted in their size, consistency, and form. Any mass in the scrotum should be transilluminated. A varicocele on the left side is not of great significance, but a varicocele on the right side may signal a mass in the retroperitoneal area. The patient should be examined in the standing position to allow filling of a varicocele.

The perineum, urethra, and penis should be palpated carefully and inspected for swelling, tenderness, and urethral discharge.

The rectal examination includes the following:

1. Anal sphincter tone should be noted; if lax, it may indicate neurologic disease.

2. Hemorrhoids may be caused by urinary or genital tract neoplasm producing vascular obstruction.

3. The prostate should be palpated carefully. Normally it is triangular with its apex caudad, each side measuring 1 inch, and its consistency is firm and rubbery. Hard areas should be noted; they may be caused by chronic inflammation (such as tuberculosis) but are more likely composed of prostatic neoplasms or calculi. The seminal vesicles are not normally palpable; if they are palpable, this may be evidence of inflammation (tuberculosis) or neoplastic invasion.

4. Prostatic secretion should be examined microscopically; it is obtained by digitally milking the prostate after the patient has urinated, so that as the prostatic secretion is discharged through the urethra it will not be contaminated with urethral secretion. Normally five to ten pus cells or fewer are visible in each high-power field. Tumor cells or large numbers of pus cells indicate prostatic neoplasm or infection, respectively. If bacterial prostatitis is suspected, the secretions should be cultured.

Instrumental Examination of the Urethra

Besides examining the urethra by palpation, one may examine it by means of a catheter, a bougie, a urethroscope, or urethrography. Urethral obstruction will prevent passage of a catheter; its precise cause (stricture, foreign body, or tumor) requires further work-up with urethroscopy and cystourethrography. Spasm of the external urethral sphincter must be differentiated carefully from organic obstruction.

Residual urine in the bladder may be determined as follows: The patient is asked to void, and the character of the stream is observed. A good strong stream producing 100 to 300 ml of urine usually eliminates the possibility of residual urine in the bladder. The patient then lies on his back on the examining table. Suprapubic percussion and palpation are carried out. Any lower abdominal mass, even if it is not in the midline, should be suspected of being a full bladder or an undrained diverticulum of the bladder. Aseptic catheterization should then be performed; more than 30 to 75 ml of urine in the bladder indicates significant residual. The cause of this should be ascertained.

Catheterization in the male. The patient to be catheterized should lie on his back with the thighs separated slightly. The penis, scrotum, and pubic area are cleaned thoroughly with antiseptic. In the average adult a No. 14 French catheter is used. A sterile tube of lubricant jelly is removed from the antiseptic solution in which it is stored, and the first teaspoonful or so is discarded. Then the nozzle of the tube is inserted into the urethral meatus, and with steady pressure the entire urethra is filled with jelly. Lubrication of the catheter tip alone is inadequate.

The operator stands at the right side of the patient, grasps the shaft of the penis between the third and fourth fingers and the glans penis at each side of the meatus with the thumb and index finger of the left hand, so as to open the meatal lips widely enough to admit the tip of the catheter. The penis is drawn gently forward and upward from the body so as to stretch it slightly and thus straighten the anterior urethra. When using soft rubber catheters, the penis is kept in the midline and the catheter is advanced to the bladder; the penile shaft is lowered as the catheter tip passes the external sphincter and enters the bladder. If the catheter does not enter the bladder easily, the tip is probably caught in the urethral bulb or is held by the contracted external sphincter. In the former instance the catheter is withdrawn a little and advanced again drawing the penis over it with the left hand, much as a glove is drawn over a finger, at the same time depressing the penile shaft between the thighs. If the external sphincter is in spasm, the tip of the catheter is held against it with gentle but continuous pressure for several seconds. The contraction generally relaxes partially, and the catheter enters the bladder. Larger instruments overcome the spasm of the sphincter more easily than small ones. Irrigation is then carried out, since the lubricating jelly may have plugged the lumen of the catheter.

Catheterization in the female. The same general principles apply in the female as in the male. Since the urethra is short, once the meatus is located, the catheterization is easily carried out.

Cystourethroscopic examination. The modern cystoscope is used to visualize the urinary bladder and urethra for diagnostic purposes. It allows operative procedures to be carried out under vision, without an incision being made into the bladder or urethra.

Cystoscopy and urethroscopy may be carried out with ease in patients of all ages, including infants. Ordinarily in the adult female patient, no anesthesia is necessary. In children and adult males, and in patients with severe inflammatory lesions, it may be necessary to carry out the procedure under general or regional anesthesia. When operative procedures are to be performed, anesthesia is, practically speaking, always necessary.

Asepsis is observed and then the instrument is introduced in much the same manner as a stiff catheter is introduced. After careful observation of the bladder neck, trigone, ureteral orifices, fundus, anterior and lateral walls of the bladder, and the urethra, any indicated operative procedure is carried out.

LABORATORY EXAMINATION OF URINE

Urinalysis is an integral part of the examination of any patient. However, important urinary tract abnormalities may be associated with relatively normal urine.

Under normal conditions the urine is formed by a process of filtration of the blood through the glomeruli, followed by selective or active reabsorption of a large part of the filtrate by the renal tubules. What is left, plus a few substances that are excreted by the tubules, is the urine.

Abnormalities of the urine may be classified in three separate categories: physical, chemical, and microscopic changes.

Physical Changes
Volume

The amount of urine excreted is very important, particularly in relation to fluid intake. One of the most important single duties of the person in charge of a patient who has a urologic condition is accurately measuring the intake and output, especially the urinary output. Normally, the adult excretes anywhere between 1 and 2.5 L of urine in 24 hours, depending on intake. Children excrete about three times as much as adults per kilogram of body weight. About two thirds of the urine is excreted during the daytime.

Anuria. *Anuria* is failure to excrete urine. Anuria from renal failure must be differentiated from acute *retention* of urine in which the kidneys secrete a normal amount of urine that cannot be voided because of obstruction somewhere in the transport system. Bladder outlet obstruction is most common and may readily be determined by urethral catheterization. Occasionally, anuria is caused by bilateral obstruction of the ureters. This is *not* relieved by bladder catheterization and instead mandates supravesical diversion.

Oliguria. When the adult secretes less than 400 to 500 ml of urine in a 24-hour period, the condition is called *oliguria*. It is definitely pathologic; the physician must ascertain its cause. It is *rarely* caused by an obstructive lesion in the urinary passageway.

Polyuria. Polyuria is a condition in which an excess amount of urine is excreted. Diabetes mellitus and insipidus and simply a large intake of fluids are the most common causes. Frequency of urination may occur, which must be distinguished from the much more common frequency of urination secondary to bladder outlet obstruction with overflow. Accurate measurement of the total amount of urine excreted in 24 hours will distinguish these two causes of frequency of urination. True polyuria is characterized by urine with low specific gravity.

Turbidity

Normally the urine is clear. The clarity of the urine may be disturbed by phosphates, fat, chyle, and pus. Most urine becomes cloudy on standing because of the action of bacteria, and therefore turbidity must be studied on the fresh specimen. Phosphaturia will clear when the urine is acidified.

Color

Urine is normally light amber in color. Occasionally it changes because of the administration of drugs, such as methylene blue. With hematuria, it may be smoky, red, or brown, depending on the amount, duration, and age of the blood in the urine. When the urine is brown and turns black on standing after alkalinization, the color may be caused by alkaptonuria (homogentisic acid), or it may be caused by melanin.

Odor

Urine has a characteristic odor. Urea-splitting organisms in the urine give it a distinct ammoniac odor. These organisms produce severe urinary tract infections and predispose to struvite stones; therefore an ammoniac odor to the urine requires investigation of the urinary tract. Some commonly prescribed drugs such as ampicillin impart a characteristic odor to urine.

pH

Normally pH of urine ranges from 5.0 to 8.0. Renal tuberculosis produces acid urine, but most other types of urinary tract infections are associated with an alkaline urine. Urine pH is important in the work-up of patients with urolithiasis, since certain types of stones (e.g., cystine, uric acid) tend to occur when the urine is acid, and others (e.g., calcium phosphate, calcium ammonium magnesium phosphate) when the urine is alkaline. Testing a fresh specimen with Nitrazine paper is the most practical way to study the urine pH. Urine pH often reflects the acid-base balance status of the patient. Many of the newer paper-strip indicators (Combistix, Hema-Combistix, and Labstix) afford the patient and the physician an opportunity to detect rather accurately glycosuria, proteinuria, pH, and other urinary changes simultaneously. Similarly, frequent pH testing can monitor a patient's response to therapy for infection or urolithiasis.

Specific Gravity

The specific gravity of urine varies from 1.001 to 1.030, according to the quantity of solutes in the urine. It is usually reduced in chronic renal disease, with a tendency to fixation at 1.010. Inability to concentrate after dehydration is a valuable clinical test indicating poor renal function.

Chemical Changes

The following chemical changes in the urine are important: albuminuria, glycosuria, hematuria, and abnormalities in the excretion of chloride, phosphates, and calcium (Tables 37-1 and 37-2). Albuminuria may be orthostatic in type and transitory because of changes in position that interfere with the circulation through the kidney. It may be renal in origin because of chronic disease of the kidney, or even extrarenal.

Table 37-1. Diagnostic Measures in Hematuria

Test	What it Detects
General examination (including eye grounds, blood pressure, cuff test, studies of bleeding and clotting mechanisms, etc.)	Nephritis, hemorrhagic diathesis, anticoagulant therapy
Urinalysis*	Verifies presence of blood
Plain radiograph (KUB)	Stone, enlarged kidney
Excretory urogram	Tumor, tuberculosis, stone
Cystoscopy (preferably during bleeding)	Source of blood (vesical tumor, stone, renal origin)
Retrograde pyeloureterogram	On side of bleeding; on both sides if not localized to side
Abdominal aortogram and renal arteriogram	Renal neoplasm, vascular malformation
Renal biopsy (open, percutaneous)	Glomerular, interstitial disease
Repeated studies at intervals	To discover lesion at first undetected

*Red urine does not necessarily contain red blood cells; so this point must be settled by microscopic examination unless clots are present. Other causes of red urine include hemoglobin (March's and cold hemoglobinuria), porphyria, and ingestion of certain azo dyes or large quantities of beets. Malingerers may add blood to the urine; this practice may be difficult to prove if the patient is clever.

Table 37-2. Origin of Hematuria in 2400 Cases

Cause	
Neoplasm	800
Inflammation	500
Miscellaneous (systemic, indeterminate, etc.)	400
Stone	425
Tuberculosis	275
TOTAL	2400
Site	
Vesical	860
Renal	840
Prostatic	300
Ureteral	250
Urethral	60
Systemic	20
Unidentified	70
TOTAL	2400

Microscopic Changes
Examination

Careful microscopic examination of the urine for casts, red blood cells, leukocytes, epithelial cells, and other formed elements is of great value. Special stains allow study of urinary tract cytology; transitional cell tumors may be diagnosed by this means.

The microscopic examination should always include a thorough search for organisms. Grossly, this is possible in the freshly voided, unstained specimen, but if more information is desired, the sediment should be studied with Gram stain. *Staphylococcus, Streptococcus, Gonococcus,* or gram-negative bacilli may be distinguished in this manner. Cultures of the urine are confirmatory and inform the selection of the proper antibiotic. In cases of "sterile pyuria," particularly in an acid urine, cultures for tubercle bacilli should be done (Table 37-3).

ESTIMATION OF RENAL FUNCTION

Evaluation of renal function is an extremely important part of the examination of any patient but of particularly the patient with urologic disease. Moreover, the renal function is variable from one time to another, justifying serial evaluations in many patients.

The most common ways by which renal function is estimated are (1) history of loss of appetite or nausea and vomiting, (2) edema or severe dehydration—"uremic snow," (3) urinary output—quantity, specific gravity, (4) specific renal function tests—the most important of these are discussed below.

Mosenthal Specific Gravity Test

In progressive renal damage, one of the earliest changes in impairment of the concentrating power of the kidney. In the Mosenthal test fluids are omitted after 6 PM, and the first urinary specimen passed in the morning is tested for specific gravity. Normally the urine will be concentrated to 1.028. This test may be unreliable during diuresis.

Blood Urea Nitrogen and Creatinine

Normally, the blood urea nitrogen (BUN) is 10 to 20 mg/dl and the creatinine 0.6 to 1.5 mg/dl. Both values are elevated with intrinsic renal damage or obstructive disease causing impairment of function.

Urea Clearance Test

The term "clearance" is defined as the volume of blood in milliliters "cleared" by the kidneys in 1

minute. To carry out the test, one must collect the urine for a 2-hour period and obtain a blood urea determination at the end of the first hour.

Procedure. In the morning after breakfast the patient drinks at least 1 L of water to ensure maximum diuresis; the bladder is emptied and the specimen is discarded. The next 2-hour urine is the one that is studied. Normally about 75 ml of blood is cleared of urea per minute.

Excretory Urography

Excretory urography is the most *important single test of renal function* available today. It not only gives an estimation of total renal function, but it also differentiates each kidney and gives information about the urinary passageways. With renal impairment, the time of the appearance is delayed, excretion is prolonged, and there is less dense shadow cast on the radiograph. On the contrary, with incomplete obstruction, the shadow may be more dense than normal. Known sensitivity to iodinated contrast media is the main contraindication.

Differential Renal Function Tests During Cystoscopy

The urine emerging from the ureters at the time of cytoscopic examination may be observed after the intravenous injection of 5 ml of indigo carmine. Normally, the dye appears in 3 minutes and concentrates to a deep blue.

Endogenous Creatinine Clearance

The endogenous creatinine clearance test measures a patient's ability to clear the plasma of circulating creatinine. A 24-hour urine collection is made, and a serum creatinine concentration is drawn midway during the collection. The clearance is calculated using the formula $Cl_{cr} = \dfrac{U \times V}{P}$ where U represents the urine creatinine concentration, P the serum creatinine concentration, and V the 24-hour urine volume expressed in milliliters per 1440 minutes. Correction for body surface area variation should be made for children and large or small adults. The normal range of creatinine clearance is 70 to 130 ml/minute.

X-RAY EXAMINATION OF THE URINARY TRACT

X-ray examination of the urinary tract is just as important as a chest film in a general evaluation of a patient. No other single technique so clearly evaluates renal function or detects urinary tract disease. Early diagnosis is essential to avoid severe and irreparable damage to the urinary tract.

Examination of the urinary tract is carried out by a plain film, by cystograms, urethrograms, excretory urography, and retrograde pyelography. Retrograde pyelography is carried out after cystoscopic examination and the passage of ureteral catheters to the kidney pelves.

In interpreting the films, it is wise to establish a definite routine for each type of examination and to follow that pattern. This may seem tedious, but it produces the best results. The routine that I recommend is presented in the outline that follows:

Table 37-3. Diagnostic Measures for Pyuria

Test	What it Measures
Two-glass test	Exclusion of urethritis
Culture, Gram stain	Selection of antiseptic or antibiotic
Acid-fast culture	Tuberculosis (skin test, chest film)
Residual urine	Prostatism, neurogenic dysfunction, stricture of urethra
Plain radiography (KUB)	Stones, perinephric abscess
Excretory urography	Stasis, anomalies, tuberculosis, impaired function
Cystourethroscopy	Dilated prostatic ducts, diverticula, etc.
Ureteral catheterization	Source of pyuria, divided cultures
Retrograde pyelography	When excretory urogram fails or is not possible
Foci of infection	Prostate, cervix, Skene's glands

I. The plain, or scout, film (kidneys-ureter-bladder, or KUB)
  A. Procedure: The patient lies supine, and the film is taken to include the area from the lower ribs to the pubis.
  B. Bone survey
    1. Look for changes in the ribs, spine, sacrum, pelvis, and femurs (Fig. 37-1).
    2. Metastatic lesions of carcinoma are particularly important
      a. Osteoblastic bone lesions: carcinoma of the prostate
      b. Osteolytic bone lesions: carcinoma of the kidney, thyroid, lung, and urinary bladder
      c. Bone tumors such as multiple myeloma, sarcoma, etc.
    3. Other bone changes such as arthritis, Paget's disease, bone cysts, and fractures
  C. Soft tissue survey
    1. Kidney outline
      a. Size, shape, position
      b. Frequently not seen because of gas or poor detail
    2. Psoas shadow outline
      a. Are the outlines bilaterally the same?
      b. Notice whether the outline is sharp and distinct.
      c. Frequently is not seen because of gas or stool
    3. Other soft tissue shadows
      a. Liver, spleen, tumors

  D. Foreign bodies, stones
    1. Show up as opaque or radiodense shadows (Fig. 37-2)
    2. A phlebolith can be differentiated from a stone by its typical lucent center and location in the true pelvis
  E. Intestinal gas pattern
II. Excretory urography (intravenous pyelography; IVP)
  A. Procedure: Check for sensitivity to iodine. If possible, the patient is prepared previously by being dehydrated—no fluid or food for 12 to 18 hours before the films. (An important exception to the dehydration preparation is the patient with multiple myeloma. These patients should not be dehydrated lest they suffer renal failure.) First, a plain film (KUB) is taken. Then, 100 to 150 ml of radiopaque contrast material (Hypaque, Renografin, Renovist, Conray) is injected slowly intravenously. If injected too rapidly, it may cause flushing, abdominal distress, nausea, and vomiting. Exposures, covering the same area as the KUB are usually made at 5, 10, and 25 minutes. A fifth film, the excretory cystogram, is taken over the bladder region alone.

  Visualization of the urinary tract is improved by the technique of infusion urography. Here, the patient need not be dehydrated in advance. An infusion consisting of 1 ml of contrast per pound of body weight added to an equal volume of 5% dextrose in

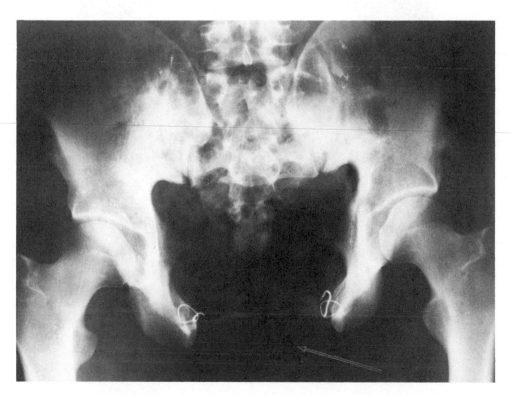

Fig. 37-1. Pelvic roentgenogram of young male with congenital bladder exstrophy and epispadias. *Arrow,* Typical associated defect in pubic symphysis. Metal sutures are seen in pubic arches.

water is administered intravenously over 15 or 20 minutes. Appropriate films are taken after the infusion is completed. This study is more expensive but results in improved filling of the collecting systems. Oblique and compression films are included.

B. Value of the excretory urogram
   1. It is useful when retrograde pyelograms would be difficult or dangerous to do, as with children, urethral or ureteral strictures, impassable stones, suspected rupture of the kidney, suspected anomalies, and poor-risk patients.
   2. It is a quick, simple, safe screening test to help rule out pathologic conditions of the urinary tract.
   3. It is a good indicator of kidney function. A normal kidney is visualized well; a nonfunctioning kidney will not be visualized.

C. The size, shape, and position of the drainage pathways of the tract are established (Fig. 37-3).

III. Cystography: The patient's bladder is entirely emptied by means of a urethral catheter. Any iodinated contrast medium can be used, depending on the effect desired, and there are times when air is used as the contrast medium. The cystogram may be taken in many different positions, depending on the nature of the lesion to be studied. One makes a voiding cystogram by having the patient void while the film is exposed.

IV. Opaque cystogram
   A. Procedure: The patient lies supine and an iodinated contrast solution is instilled into the bladder through a catheter until the patient complains of a feeling of fullness. This amount is usually less than 400 ml of solution. Anteroposterior and oblique exposures are taken.
   B. Size, shape, and location of the bladder
      1. The normal bladder configuration is a rounded shadow, centrally placed, about the size of a grapefruit.

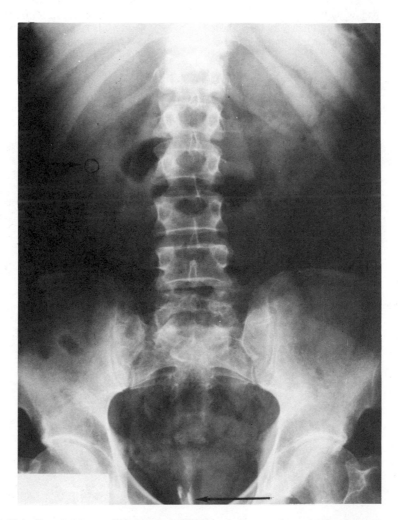

Fig. 37-2. Plain film of abdomen (kidneys-ureter-bladder) reveals extensive prostatic calcifications above pubic symphysis *(large arrow)* and small right renal calculus *(small arrow)*.

2. Chronic cystitis is characterized by an extremely small, spastic bladder; atony by an extremely large, flaccid bladder.
3. Pelvic tumors displace the bladder from the midline.

C. Character of the bladder wall
1. Normally it is smooth.
2. Long-standing obstruction causes a hypertrophied and greatly roughened bladder wall with many coarse trabeculations.

D. Diverticula
1. A diverticulum is a herniation of mucosa through the hypertrophied muscle fibers. This outpouching most commonly results from long-standing obstruction. The normal bladder has no diverticula.
2. Sometimes the diverticulum may be larger than the bladder itself, or there may be many diverticula, creating a problem of identifying the true bladder. Distinguishing features of the diverticulum are the following:

   a. It has smooth outline, whereas the obstructed bladder is slightly roughened.
   b. It is usually eccentrically located.
   c. The urethral catheter usually does not enter it.
3. Emptying: Does the diverticulum empty, or does urine stagnate? This may be distinguished by the position of the diverticulum or by a postevacuation film.

E. Vesicoureteral reflux
1. It is not normal to have the contrast solution pass up the ureters.
2. Ureteral reflux is attributable to incompetence of the ureterovesical junction, caused by infection, long-standing obstruction, congenital anomalies, surgery, or neurogenic disease.

F. Rupture of the bladder: The contrast medium extravasates from the bladder.

G. Bladder contents: The contrast cystogram may outline tumors or foreign bodies within the bladder, but this is better done with the air cystogram.

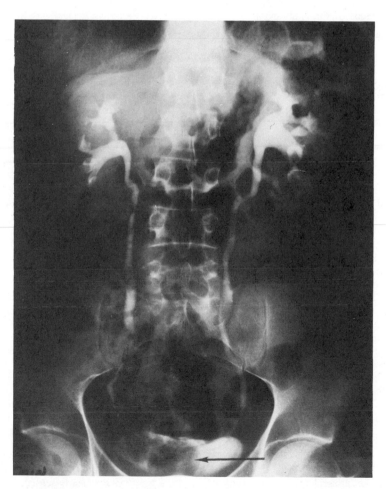

Fig. 37-3. Excretory urogram (intravenous pyelogram). Normal study; arrow indicates rectal gas superimposed on bladder.

V. Air cystogram
   A. Procedure: The bladder is emptied of the contrast medium and washed out. The patient is placed in the right oblique (semilateral) position. The bladder is filled with air, by catheter, until the patient complains of a feeling of fullness.
   B. The air acts as a lucent contrast medium and will help to visualize:
      1. Intravesical position of the prostate
      2. Bladder tumors
      3. Foreign bodies, especially radiolucent stones

VI. Retrograde urethrography
   A. Procedure: Urethrography is of great value in the study of trauma, strictures, contractures, congenital deformities at the bladder neck, and deformities of the prostatic urethra associated with prostatism. A urethrogram is made by emptying the bladder of fluid, filling it with air with the patient in the oblique position, and then filling the urethra with a mixture of iodinated contrast medium and sterile lubricating jelly. During the exposure of the film, 50 ml of this mixture is injected into the urethra. This gives a simultaneous air cystogram and opaque urethrogram and is particularly valuable for outlining the posterior urethra to evaluate the adequacy of prostatectomy. At times a voiding urethrogram is helpful. This is usually done by filling the bladder with contrast medium and exposing the film during micturition.
   B. The following landmarks should be observed
      1. The pendulous urethra
      2. The bulbous urethra—the usual seat of inflammatory strictures
      3. The external sphincter and the internal sphincter
      4. The prostatic urethra: elongation, widening, and anterior angulation are indicative of benign prostatic enlargement.
         a. Are there prostatic calculi?
         b. Are there periurethral abscesses?

VII. Retrograde pyelography
   A. Retrograde pyelography is a more exact method of visualizing the upper urinary tract. Its purpose is fourfold.
      1. Accurate visualization of the anatomic structure of the upper urinary tract
      2. Procurement of segregated specimens of urine from each kidney for culture, cytology, and microscopy
      3. When the ureteral catheters are in place, the differential function of each kidney is determined accurately by the intravenous injection of methylene blue or indigo carmine
      4. Relief of ureteral obstruction
   B. Procedure: A cystoscope is introduced into the bladder, and after cystoscopy has been completed, the ureteral orifices are entered with catheters that are advanced gently into each renal pelvis. Specimens of urine are

then obtained from each renal pelvis for the examinations mentioned previously.

After this, plain films are taken to mark the course of the ureters and to locate any radiopaque density, such as stones. Either air or an iodinated contrast is injected into the kidney pelvis, and radiographs are made to visualize the pelvis and calyces accurately. Alternatively the procedure may be performed with fluoroscopic guidance.

If visualization of the ureters is desirable, the catheters are withdrawn to the lower portion of the ureter and contrast is injected for a ureteropyelogram. Air is used instead of contrast to show nonopaque calculi or other relatively nondense filling defects of the ureter. Retrograde pyelography is not an innocuous procedure; reflex anurias and pyelonephritis are rare complications.

Most cystoscopies and retrograde pyelograms are done without any anesthesia whatsoever, and the patients experience no undue discomfort.

VIII. Special x-ray studies
   There are many special studies that have limited use:
   A. Perirenal air and gas injections are used to outline the kidneys and possible adrenal tumors. This is not an innocuous procedure but does, at times, give sufficient additional information to justify its risk. Ultrasound and computed tomography have eliminated the need for these studies.
   B. Gastric air injections: Air introduced into the stomach may aid in demonstrating a renal mass, especially in children.
   C. Nephrotomography: Very valuable, particularly to outline masses in the renal area; most uroradiologists now include nephrotomography routinely in excretory urography.
   D. Abdominal aortography: Contrast medium injected into the aorta outlines the renal arterial system. Uses:
      1. The main advantage of aortography is to differentiate malignant lesions of the kidney from benign cysts. Contrast medium fills the vascular spaces within a neoplasm but outlines only the periphery of a cyst.
      2. The nephrogram demonstrates certain parenchymal lesions before they are large enough to encroach on the calyces or pelvis or to produce detectable reduction of renal function. This is particularly true in early tuberculous and neoplastic renal lesions.
      3. Visualization of the renal artery may help diagnose renovascular hypertension (some obstructive mechanism of the arterial supply to the kidney). Massive renal infarct may also be detected by this procedure.
      4. The question of renal ptosis versus ectopia is clearly settled, but these usually can be distinguished by retrograde pyelograms.

5. Ectopic vessels that obstruct the ureteropelvic junction in congenital hydronephrosis may be documented by aortography. This may be demonstrated better if one does a retrograde pyelogram immediately preceding the arteriogram, superimposing one on the other.

6. Selection of renal donors.

E. Selective renal angiography: Very useful for visualizing renal artery lesions and renal tumors and has in many instances supplemented aortography. Angiographic infarction of renal tumors is now used instead of, or as a preoperative adjunct to, surgery.

OTHER SPECIAL DIAGNOSTIC STUDIES

Other special diagnostic studies include the following:

Radioactive renography
Renal scanning
Needle biopsy
Cinefluorography
Urodynamic studies: ureters, kidney pelvis, bladder, and urethra
Endocrine function studies
Chromatin test for somatic sex and chromosomal analysis (karyotype)
Bone scanning
Ultrasound
CT
Magnetic resonance imaging (MRI)

KIDNEY
Anomalies

The congenital anomalies of the renal parenchyma may be classified as abnormalities of number, position, form, structure, and vascularization.

Number

The most common anomaly, that of number, usually is asymptomatic. Obviously, if both kidneys are absent, life is impossible. Congenital *solitary kidney* does occur. This means that whenever nephrectomy is to be considered, the possibility that the other kidney may be absent or hypoplastic makes preoperative study mandatory. Occasionally a true *supernumerary kidney* may be present. The most common type of abnormality of number is *duplication* of the pelvis and ureter. Some are associated with ectopic ureteral openings, usually of the ureter draining the upper kidney pelvis, which is the source of the symptoms. (See discussion of congenital anomalies of the ureter, below.) Many are also associated with anomalies of vascularization that produce partial urinary obstruction.

Position

Anomaly of position occurs when the embryonic process of ascent and rotation of the kidney is interfered with at any point. Usually failure of rotation is associated with compression of the pelvis or ureter, or both, by renal vessels, producing obstruction. The *ectopic kidney* can easily be recognized by its short ureter and anterior position of its pelvis. Sometimes *crossed ectopia* with fusion occurs, resembling a large tumor

mass. This may actually be all the renal parenchyma the patient has, and removal of such a fused kidney would be lethal.

Form

Anomalies of form occur during embryonic ascent of the kidneys. Their lower poles may fuse to form a *horseshoe kidney*. After fusion one kidney may ascend and pull the other to the opposite side *(crossed ectopia with fusion)*. The anterior surface of one may be fused to the posterior surface of the other, and they remain in the pelvis (so-called disk kidney). These anomalies frequently are confused with other masses or are associated with obstruction to the outflow of urine from their pelves from ectopic renal arteries. Treatment is tailored to the exact difficulties each produces.

Structure

Anomalies of structure may be unilateral or bilateral and are characterized by *hypoplasia* or *cyst formation*. If hypoplasia is unilateral, no symptoms may occur. If hypoplasia is bilateral, renal insufficiency will result. Cyst formation may be asymptomatic, but massive replacement of remaining renal tissue will produce renal insufficiency (Fig. 37-4). Multicystic kidney is usually associated with an atretic ureter.

Congenital polycystic disease. Congenital polycystic disease is one of the important anomalies of the kidney. It is usually *bilateral* and *familial* and seems to be caused by a lack of fusion of most of the renal elements with the excretory elements of the tubules. This produces a large number of varying-sized cysts in each kidney that grow slowly, destroy renal substance, and

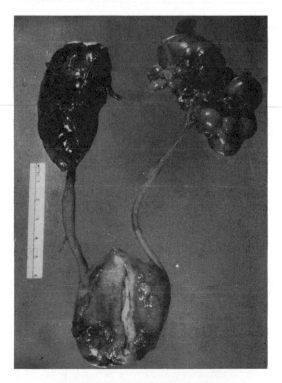

Fig. 37-4. Multicystic kidney, on left.

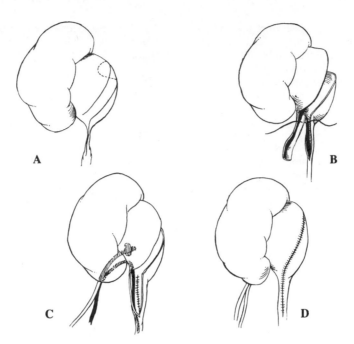

Fig. 37-5. Congenital stricture of ureteropelvic junction and its surgical correction. **A,** Outlined is incision that crosses stricture and raises flap from kidney pelvis. **B,** Flap swung down to widen strictured area. **C,** Nephrostomy tube and ureteral catheter splint inserted. **D,** Result.

produce gradual renal insufficiency. Bilateral palpable masses usually result. The cysts distort the kidney outlines and the kidney pelves to produce a characteristic radiographic appearance.

If polycystic disease is unilateral, it cannot be readily differentiated from hypernephroma.

When bilateral, the diagnosis is usually easily made. Hypertension with red and white cells and casts in the urine heralds the gradual onset of renal insufficiency. The treatment is symptomatic and operative. *Symptomatic treatment* consists essentially in avoiding trauma and infection to the kidneys, since massive hemorrhage may result. *Surgical treatment* consists in aspirating as many of the cysts as possible to reduce the pressure on the normal-functioning renal substance. This, of course, is purely palliative. The prognosis varies with the rapidity with which renal insufficiency and hypertension develop, which in turn probably depends on the extent of the renal involvement. Some patients live only a few years, most die in middle age, and a few live out their normal span. A small percentage of cases are associated with cystic disease of the liver and lungs and cerebral artery aneurysms. Hemodialysis and renal transplantation have been effective in the treatment of the chronic renal insufficiency related to polycystic kidney disease. Bilateral nephrectomy is indicated to make room for the renal graft or for relief of hypertension.

Vascularization

Anomalies of vascularization may occur in otherwise normal kidneys. They are hazards during operative procedures on the kidney, or they may produce ob-

struction at the ureteropelvic junction that requires correction.

Abdominal masses, renal insufficiency, abdominal pain, or urinary symptoms may indicate a congenital anomaly of the kidney. This is true no matter what the age of the patient.

Congenital anomalies of the renal pelvis are essentially *obstructive* from bands, high insertion of the ureter, or stricture at the ureteropelvic junction (Fig. 37-5). They may produce enormous hydronephrotic sacs with renal atrophy. They are bilateral in over 50% of the cases and should be differentiated from renal cysts, renal neoplasms, and obstructive uropathy originating lower in the urinary tract. They may be silent or produce an ache or pain in the side or evidence of severe infection. They may produce a large abdominal mass. The treatment is surgical—removal or repair—with the surgeon always keeping in mind that the condition is frequently bilateral. The pathognomonic findings are demonstrated readily with intravenous and retrograde pyelography.

Urolithiasis

Stones in the urinary tract are common disorders with distinct geographic variations in incidence (Fig. 37-6). So-called stone belts occur in various parts of the world, in which certain types of stone predominate (e.g., in the southern part of the United States, calcium oxalate stones are common). In the United States as a whole, about 75% to 80% are calcium oxalate, calcium phosphate, or magnesium ammonium phosphate stones. Of the remaining, four fifths are uric acid stones, and the others are cystine stones. Magnesium

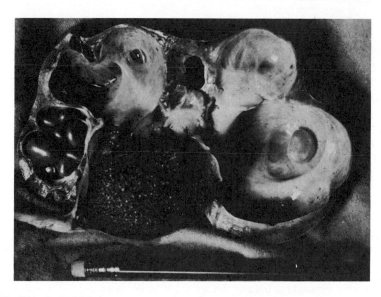

Fig. 37-6. Urolithiasis. Multiple large stones (cystine) have obstructed and totally destroyed kidney.

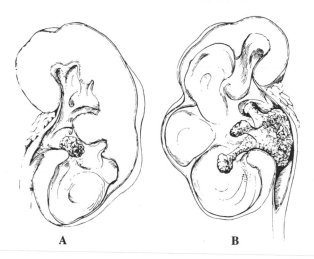

A   B

Fig. 37-7. A, Single calculus obstructing and dilating lower renal calyx. **B,** "Staghorn" calculus obstructing and dilating all renal calyces.

ammonium phosphate stones commonly occur after infection in the urinary tract with urea-splitting organisms (Fig. 37-7).

Stones in the urinary tract are the result of a series of predisposing factors. Elucidation of these factors is necessary for correct therapy. Renal calculi are a result of one or more of the following: a foreign body in the urinary tract, vitamin A deficiency, urinary tract infection (UTI), urinary tract stasis, metabolic disturbances causing increased crystalloid excretion (cystinuria, hyperparathyroidism, etc.), and changes in the urine that lessen the solubility of the crystalloids in the urine. In some instances a matrix, or nucleus, acts as a template for further precipitation of crystalloids. However, in certain types of recumbency calculi, such a matrix is obviously not necessary. Some factors are important in the formation of a nucleus, and others facilitate precipitation of the various stone-forming crystalloids. Some factors that are precursors of calculi should be emphasized.

Foreign Body

Any *foreign body* in the urinary tract favors the formation of calcium phosphate and ammonium magnesium phosphate stones. Nonabsorbable suture material used in operations on the bladder or renal pelvis will act as a nucleus around which precipitation of the supersaturated calcium salts occurs. Ulcerating lesions and papillary tumors in the urinary tract act similarly.

Vitamin A Deficiency

In man the relationship of *vitamin A deficiency* to urinary calculi is debatable, but in animals it may produce urinary stones in several ways: (1) by producing ulceration of the epithelium of the urinary tract, (2) by causing desquamation of the epithelium (the desquamated epithelium acts as a nucleus), and (3) by predisposing the urinary tract to infection that may change the precipitability of the stone-forming crystalloids.

Urinary Tract Infection

UTI is believed to be the most important single cause of urolithiasis. It may produce a stone by creating a nucleus in a manner similar to vitamin A deficiency, by changing the pH of the urine, or by altering the protective colloids of the urine.

Urinary Stasis

Urinary stasis from acquired or congenital obstruction of the urinary passageway is an important predisposing cause of urolithiasis. In a series of 60 patients with obstruction at the ureteropelvic junction without infection, the incidence of urolithiasis was 10 times higher than it was in a series of patients without such obstruction. If other causes for urolithiasis exist and a tiny stone forms, it may pass without becoming clinically manifest if obstruction is not present. If recurrent urolithiasis is to be prevented, urinary stasis must be corrected.

Metabolic Disturbances

Certain metabolic disturbances produce qualitative and quantitative changes in the urinary crystalloids that predispose to the formation of calculi, particularly if a nucleus has formed, if urinary stasis and infection occur, or if changes in the urine aid in the precipitation of such crystalloids. The most frequent of these metabolic changes are cystinuria and alterations of calcium and uric acid metabolism.

Cystinuria is a familial abnormality of renal tubular absorption of the amino acid cystine characterized by the excretion of a large amount of cystine in the urine. Normally, 10 to 100 mg of cystine excreted in the urine in 24 hours. With abnormal cystine reabsorption, 300 to 1500 mg may be excreted in 24 hours. At present, no method for altering this abnormality is known. The following measures are helpful: forced administration of fluids, correction and avoidance of all factors that lead to the formation of a nucleus, correction of urinary stasis if present, and alteration of the hydrogen ion concentration of the urine so that it will be continuously alkaline (cystine is insoluble in acid urine and highly soluble in alkaline urine). The urine usually is made alkaline by administration of sodium bicarbonate, or sodium citrate and potassium citrate. The chelating agent D-penicillamine (Cuprimine) is also indicated in cystinuria. The drug forms a complex with cystine that is more soluble than the cystine alone. Large cystine calculi have been dissolved by such therapy.

Metabolic conditions that predispose to an increased excretion of *calcium phosphate* are very common. The most important of these is recumbency. If other factors that predispose to the formation of urinary calculi can be avoided by a proper regimen, the precipitated calcium salts can be washed out readily before irreparable renal damage occurs. Tiny stones can be demonstrated

on x-ray studies of the kidneys even in the first few months of recumbency.

Hyperparathyroidism from adenoma or hyperplasia of the parathyroid glands may be the underlying cause of urolithiasis. Up to 50% of patients with hyperparathyroidism have renal stones. Hyperparathyroidism is characterized by localized or generalized osteoporosis, urinary calculi, and a high serum calcium and low serum phosphorus in the early stage of the disease before renal insufficiency develops. The serum alkaline phosphatase usually is increased. In most cases treatment of the hyperparathyroidism should precede treatment of the urinary calculi. Exceptions to this are cases in which acute urinary obstruction or infection is present.

Other metabolic diseases may be important in the formation of urinary calculi. *Uric acid stones* are seen with hypersecretion of uric acid associated with a disturbance of purine metabolism. The medical management and prevention of these calculi are very similar to those utilized in cases of cystinuria (i.e., an alkaline pH of the urine and a low-purine diet). The xanthine oxidase inhibitor allopurinol (Zyloprim) is useful in that it decreases both serum and urine uric acid concentrations. With improved chemotherapy for various malignancies, more cancer patients are at risk for the hyperuricemia and subsequent hyperuricosuria related to increased cell destruction and release of nucleic acids.

Changes in the Urine that Predispose to Crystalloid Precipitation

At the time a urinary stone is formed, the hydrogen ion concentration of the urine is the final factor that determines the chemical composition of the stone. Infection of the urinary tract plays an important role, since urea-splitting organisms alkalinize the urine to favor the precipitation of calcium phosphate. Treatment includes control of urinary infection and acidification of the urine by the administration of sodium acid phosphate. In addition, this drug decreases the urinary excretion of calcium by as much as 50%. Ascorbic acid (vitamin C) is also useful to acidify the urine.

Other Etiologic Factors

In some cases a primary renal defect may be associated with hyperexcretion of oxalates and calcium phosphate. In such cases diets relatively low in oxalates and phosphorus may be useful.

The prolonged administration of ACTH and corticosteroids produces osteoporosis and an accompanying hypercalciuria. Renal calculi should be considered in any case in which either of these drugs is administered for a long time.

Many patients, particularly young males with recurrent calcium oxalate calculi, have only hypercalciuria (daily excretion of more than 250 mg of calcium). Newer methods of testing have allowed the subdivision of this category into at least two types: hypercalciuria caused by (1) *gastrointestinal hyperabsorption* and (2) *renal tubular hyperexcretion*. The latter form is best treated by thiazide diuretics, which reduce renal tubular loss of calcium; patients with hyperabsorption should be treated with low-calcium diets and the newer calcium binders.

Ureteral Stones

Ureteral stones essentially are renal stones that have passed down into the ureter. They rarely arise in the ureter itself, except when a foreign body, such as a ureteral suture, acts as a nucleus for precipitation of calcium and magnesium ammonium phosphate salts (Fig. 37-8).

In general, stones under 5 to 6 mm pass spontaneously. Those over that diameter usually must be removed, whether they are causing symptoms or not. Uric acid calculi are nonopaque on radiography and show up as filling defects in the pyeloureterogram; they must be differentiated from blood clots and tumors of the ureter.

Bladder Stones

Bladder stones are becoming less common. They are associated with infection and obstruction at the bladder neck, neurogenic disease, or ulcerating lesions or foreign bodies in the bladder itself. Vesical calculi therefore are found in the bladder itself, though some of them are actually stones that have passed down from the kidney and have been retained in the bladder because of bladder neck obstruction. They may be removed suprapubically or transurethrally by cystolitholapaxy or cystolithotripsy, depending on their size, consistency, and the condition of the bladder itself. Calculi may form in bladder diverticula because of increased stasis. Here treatment must be directed against the underlying cause of the diverticulum and removal of the stone as well.

Nonopaque uric acid stones require differentiation from bladder tumors, large subcervical prostatic lobes, or blood clots. Opaque calculi are readily recognized on the radiograph. Since many of them are associated with ulcerative lesions of the bladder or bladder neck obstruction, these accessory or predisposing conditions must be treated simultaneously.

Surgical treatment of renal calculi is shown in Figs. 37-9 and 37-10. Two new methods for treatment of renal calculi short of major open surgery are worthy of mention: percutaneous ultrasonic lithotripsy and extracorporeal shock-wave (ESWL) lithotripsy. In the former method, after a percutaneous nephrostomy tract is obtained and dilated, renal calculi can be either directly removed or shattered by a special ultrasonic probe. In the latter method (ESWL) with the patient placed in a waterbath to allow passage of the energy

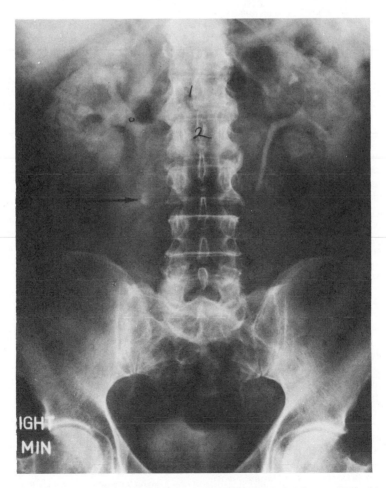

Fig. 37-8. Excretory urogram (I.V.P.) demonstrates right hydroureteronephrosis associated with two opaque calculi in proximal ureter (*arrow*); left upper urinary tract and bladder are normal.

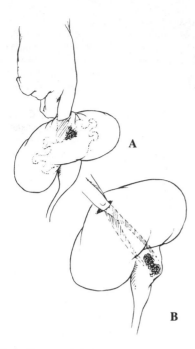

Fig. 37-9. A, Transrenal digital removal of stone from calyx. **B,** Transrenal removal of stone from kidney pelvis by instrument.

beam, finely focused shock waves are pulsed at the stones. The calculi are fragmented into many tiny particles, which are passed spontaneously down the ureter.

Renal Neoplasms

Neoplasms of the kidney are common and are generally malignant. The best clinical classification is related to age. Most tumors in children under 8 years of age are Wilms' tumors, or nephroblastomas. Generally, few malignant tumors occur between 8 years and about 25 or 30 years of age. About 95% of renal tumors in adults are malignant neoplasms of the renal parenchyma, the hypernephroma (renal cell carcinoma). The other 5% are tumors of the renal pelvis: transitional cell, squamous cell, or adenocarcinoma.

The general trend in the treatment of malignant renal neoplasms favors more radical surgery. Preoperative or postoperative x-ray therapy is not helpful for hypernephroma, though irradiation may be part of the therapy for Wilm's tumor.

Childhood Neoplasms

Renal neoplasms of childhood are mixed mesenchymal tumors (Wilms' tumors, or nephroblastoma). They appear very early in life and constitute one of the most frequent malignant tumors of childhood, rivaled in incidence by neuroblastoma, which frequently invades the kidney and resembles Wilms' tumor. Wilms' tumors grow rapidly and metastasize early through the bloodstream and lymphatics, with the lungs being frequently involved. Over 30% of patients have metastases when first seen: the most common sign is a large abdominal mass. The urine is often normal, and there are generally no urinary symptoms. Gastrointestinal disturbances

and pain are frequent because of the weight and bulk of the tumor. Metastatic lesions produce a variety of symptoms and signs. The diagnosis is usually readily made by means of urography; intravenous pyelograms show a mass deformity or no function from the involved kidney, and retrograde pyelograms show a distorted and deformed pelvis. Wilms' tumors must always be differentiated from congenital hydronephrosis and cystic disease of the kidney, which are frequently bilateral and in which removal of a kidney might be contraindicated. A differential diagnosis between neuroblastoma and Wilms' tumor should also be made, since therapy is different: a very fine stippled calcification is seen in the neuroblastoma, which involves the kidney only indirectly (by pushing it down and involving the cortex or a portion of the cortex so that the intravenous pyelogram shows good function in a portion of the kidney); (Fig. 37-11). On the other hand, Wilms' tumor usually involves the entire kidney and usually has no calcification.

In addition Wilms' tumor must be distinguished from a fetal hamartoma (mesoblastic nephroma), a benign developmental renal mass presenting in the first year of life and generally in the newborn period. Fetal hamartoma requires only simple nephrectomy as therapy.

Treatment. The treatment of Wilms' tumor consists of three modalities: surgical removal of the primary tumor, irradiation therapy, and chemotherapy. For Wilms' tumors, actinomycin D seems to be almost specific. Treatment must be carried out over a long period of time so that metastatic lesions are destroyed. Results have been steadily improving, so that in patients who do not have obvious metastases an 80% 5-year survival can be expected. Vincristine sulfate and doxorubicin (Adriamycin) are also useful in chemotherapy for Wilms' tumor.

Adult Neoplasms (Fig. 37-12)

A. General
 1. All neoplasms are malignant, with rare exceptions.
 2. There is no definite agreement on the pathologic classification of these tumors, but for practical purposes they are all hypernephromas (renal cell carcinoma, clear cell carcinoma, adenocarcinoma).
 3. Treatment is surgery
B. Metastases
 1. Most frequent to the lung; x-ray evidence is characteristic (snowball lesion)
 2. Almost as frequent to bone (osteolytic lesion)
 3. 30% have metastases when first seen
C. Cardinal signs and symptoms
 1. Pain
 2. Unilateral mass
 3. Hematuria
D. Diagnosis
 1. Suspicion is aroused by
    a. Any of the preceding cardinal signs or symptoms
    b. Unexplained fever
    c. Unexplained weight loss
    d. Unexplained anemia
 2. However, diagnosis at the stage when these signs and symptoms appear is usually too late for curative therapy.
 3. Cytologic studies of the urine show promise of aiding early diagnosis in tumors that develop close to the urothelium.

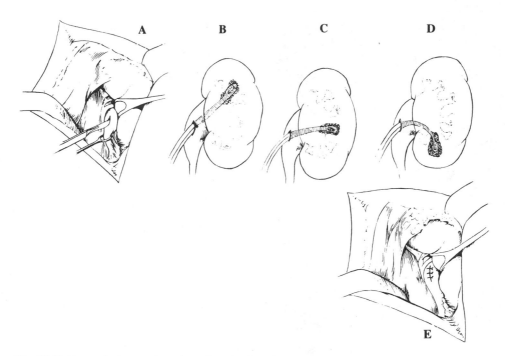

Fig. 37-10. Removal of stones through renal pelvis. **A,** Incision into renal pelvis. **B** to **D,** Extraction of stones from various locations in renal calyces by stone forceps. **E,** Closure of incision in renal pelvis.

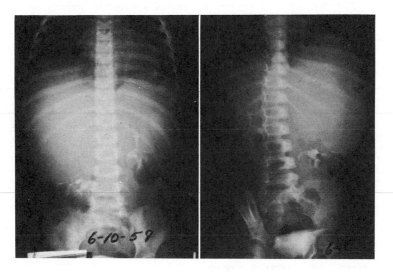

Fig. 37-11. Mass above right kidney in child, depressing and distorting kidney. Oblique view on right. Neuroblastoma.

4. Endocrinopathies (paraneoplastic syndromes): erythrocytosis, hypercalcemia, hyperreninemia
5. X-ray diagnosis
  a. Characteristic urogram (Fig. 37-13)
    (1) Splaying or spiderlike deformity of calyces
    (2) Asymmetric enlargement of kidney substance on film
    (3) Obscuring of the renal outline
    (4) Irregular calcifications
  b. Renal ultrasound
    (1) Echogenic mass lesion
    (2) Any mass that is not clearly echolucent (cystic)
  c. CT

    (1) Mass lesion more dense than normal renal parenchyma
    (2) Obliteration of perinephric space
    (3) Retroperitoneal lymphadenopathy
    (4) Renal vein or inferior vena cava involvement
    (5) Identification of hepatic masses as possible metastases
  d. Aortography (renal arteriography; see Fig. 37-13)
    (1) Hypervascular or neovascular pattern in mass
    (2) Parasitic (collateral) vessels
    (3) Arteriovenous fistula
    (4) Nodal or hepatic metastases may be visualized
  e. Chest film

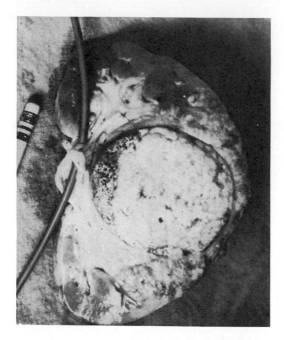

Fig. 37-12. Carcinoma of kidney parenchyma.

    (1) Pulmonary metastasis
    (2) Mediastinal lymphadenopathy
  f. Bone films
    (1) Osteolytic metastatic lesions
    (2) Pathologic fractures
E. Differential diagnosis
  1. Congenital lesions
    a. Cysts
      (1) Polycystic—usually bilateral
      (2) Solitary—cannot tell by radiographic examination, calcification less frequent, radiolucent center, smooth wall
      (3) Multiple solitary—same as for solitary
  2. Trauma: hematoma—history, blood clot is not smooth in outline, clot is generally mobile in the pelvis and will gradually disappear.
  3. Infection
    a. Renal carbuncle—tenderness, renal mass, chills and fever, white blood cell count elevated, history of diabetes mellitus
    b. Tuberculosis—history of pulmonary disease
    c. Parasites (e.g., hydatid disease)
  4. Stone—smooth, movable, does not disappear, x-ray evidence, blood chemistry studies

Treatment. Surgical removal (nephrectomy) is indicated; 40% to 70% 5-year survival is expected if there are no metastases when the diagnosis is made. Radical nephrectomy with regional lymphadenectomy is the procedure of choice.

Neoplasms of the Urothelium

Tumors arising from the urothelium are relatively uncommon but present a serious diagnostic problem (Fig. 37-14). The most common symptoms are gross hematuria and pain that simulates a renal calculus. Retrograde pyelography shows filling defects or distortions of the calyces that are quite characteristic but need to be distinguished from nonopaque stone and blood clot.

They frequently metastasize along the ureter or into the bladder. Sometimes this causes a problem in differential diagnosis in that the tumor blocks the ureter and presents itself in the bladder. Separate bladder tumors are seen in about half the patients with renal pelvic or ureteral tumors.

The treatment is surgical (nephroureterectomy). Cytology of the urine from the ureters is helpful in differential diagnosis.

Renal Injuries

Renal injuries may be divided into two types: *penetrating* and *blunt.* The former are caused by bullet or knife wounds and the latter by indirect injury. With regard to the latter type, a kidney that is already the seat of a pathologic lesion is more easily injured because inflamed or tumor tissue is more friable and the increased size of the diseased kidney makes it more accessible to the forces producing the injury. Renal injuries may also be classified according to the extent of the injury: (1) a slight tear or *contusion,* (2) a large tear of the renal substance, (3) a tear of the kidney substance involving the renal pelvis, (4) a hematoma about the kidney, and (5) injuries (including avulsion) to the vascular pedicle or ureter.

The ensuing symptoms, signs, and pathologic changes depend on the nature and extent of the lesion. Extravasation of urine into the kidney substance may occur, producing necrosis and subsequent infection. Massive hemorrhage or renal infarction may result. Serious late sequelae to kidney trauma can occur, including scarring and caliectasis with poor drainage from portions of the kidney, leading to hypertension, stone formation, and renal infection.

Symptoms and Diagnosis

After the history of injury, pain, hematuria, a mass on the injured side, strong muscle spasm, and tenderness with shock may appear. Physical, urine, blood, and radiographic examinations, including CT, should be done immediately. The findings are varying degrees of shock, hemorrhage, a mass with tenderness in the area of the renal injury, and abdominal distension. Hematuria is variable, depending on whether the blood has access to the ureter. Intravenous and retrograde pyelograms confirm the diagnosis, though intravenous pyelograms are useless if the patient is in shock. Abdominal aortography plus renal arteriography and even celiac axis injection are most helpful in the identification of the site and character of vascular injuries. Pyelography may be required in the operating room. Careful consideration of both kidneys and all the renal substance involved is necessary. The best surgical approach is transabdominal to allow evaluation of all other intraabdominal organs as well as both renal arteries and both kidneys. The surgical procedure is tailored to the precise injury, from simple suture to nephrectomy (Fig. 37-15).

Postinjury examinations should be done every 3 months for at least a year (with intravenous pyelography) to evaluate possible permanent damage to the kidney. Ultrasound and CT examinations are helpful in monitoring blood or urine accumulation resulting from trauma.

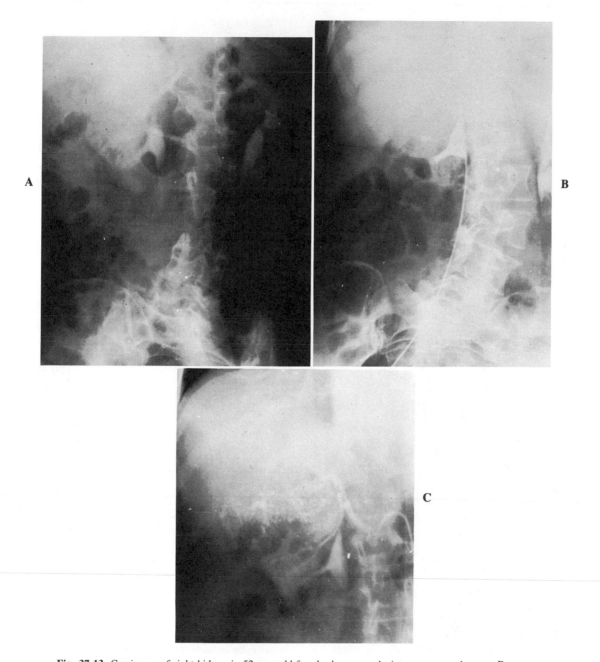

Fig. 37-13. Carcinoma of right kidney in 52-year-old female shown on, **A,** intravenous pyelogram, **B,** retrograde pyelogram, and, **C,** selective renal arteriogram. Notice metastasis to third lumbar vertebra.

One other complication associated with trauma, called *crush syndrome,* must be considered. Massive amounts of crushed tissue can cause severe oliguria and acute tubular necrosis. Fluids must be managed carefully (see Chap. 3). In severe cases peritoneal or hemodialysis may be required.

Renal Tuberculosis

Renal tuberculosis is decreasing in incidence with more effective general control of the disease by public health measures and antituberculosis drugs, since it is part and parcel of hematogenous dissemination from a primary focus in the lung or gastrointestinal tract. The primary focus produces a temporary bacteremia of tubercle bacilli, which are filtered out in the cortex of both kidneys and produce lesions that usually go on to repair themselves. Occasionally, however, they progress and involve the collecting system to produce an open renal tuberculosis. Before the advent of specific chemotherapy, this condition became bilateral in nearly 100% of the cases and required prolonged sanatorium care. With gross unilateral involvement, nephrectomy was the treatment of choice. At the present time, with the use of isoniazid (INH), ethambutol, and rifampin,

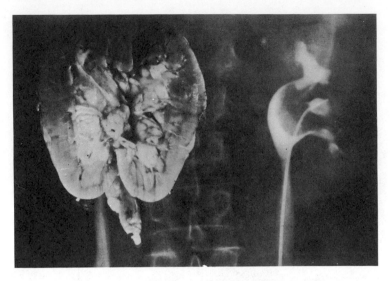

Fig. 37-14. Carcinoma of renal pelvis; pyelogram and specimen.

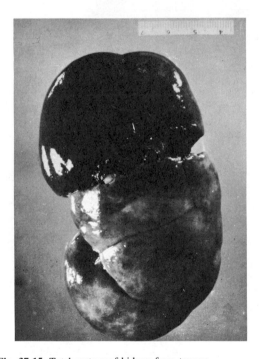

Fig. 37-15. Total rupture of kidney from trauma.

most of these cases can be controlled if massive lesions can be removed surgically.

Hematuria or pyuria is present with no evidence of pyogenic organisms, but with tubercle bacilli in the urine detected by acid-fast stains and cultures. Any patient with severe pyuria, with no obvious organisms on smear or ordinary culture, should be suspected of having renal tuberculosis. This is particularly true if there is a history of pulmonary tuberculosis, even though it is inactive and completely healed. Urography usually shows the typical lesion: scarring and obliteration of some of the infundibula of the calyces and distortion and irregularity of several of the calyces in a kidney (Fig. 37-16). Tuberculous lesions frequently calcify. In fact, renal tuberculosis can be first seen in so many different ways that it might be called "the great masquerader." If there is no substantial destruction of renal tissue or abscess formation, the treatment should be conservative and medical. If surgery is contemplated, chemotherapy before and after the surgical procedure for 6 months to 2 years is indicated.

Nontuberculous Infections of the Urinary Tract

Renal infections are common and may arise as primary lesions, with entrance of the organisms into the kidney from a *hematogenous* source, much as described in renal tuberculosis. On the other hand, they may be associated with *ascending infection,* starting with lesions primarily in the urethra and prostate in the male, the urethra in the female, and the bladder in both. They may also arise from *infections outside the urinary tract,* producing lesions that allow the entrance of organisms into the perirenal and periureteral lymphatics. If the ureterovesical junctions are incompetent because of bladder infection, congenital anomaly, or neurogenic involvement, renal infection is almost sure to ensue because of reflux of the infected urine into the renal pelvis.

Symptoms and Signs

UTI may manifest itself in many different ways. It may be discovered in an asymptomatic patient whose urinalysis shows bacteriuria or pyuria. It may produce disturbances of urination or pain over the region of the bladder or kidney. It may be associated with chills, fever, and leukocytosis, indicative of a general reaction. The history is important to rule out previous infections elsewhere in the body that might have acted as a primary source or some other pathologic lesion in the urinary transport system. Thus excretory urography, cystography (to evaluate ureteral reflux), careful examination and culture of the urine, and cystourethroscopy may all be necessary for complete evaluation.

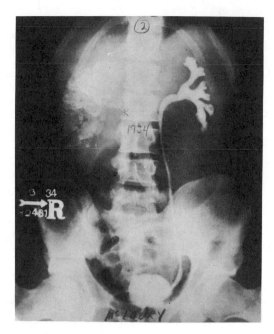

Fig. 37-16. Pyelogram showing tuberculosis of right kidney ("putty kidney").

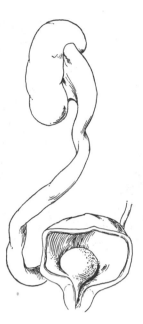

Fig. 37-17. Right ureterocele.

General supportive therapy, specific antibiotics for the organism that is cultured, and correction of urinary tract obstruction or other lesions that predispose to infection are keystones of treatment. An ulcerated bladder tumor, stones, bladder neck obstruction, benign prostatic hypertrophy in the adult male, and urethral stenosis in the elderly female produce obstruction that sustains the infection. These lesions *must* be corrected if the infection is to be eliminated. Pyuria or bacteriuria does not mean pyelonephritis. It means simply that an infection exists somewhere in the urinary passageway or the kidney. Newer methods detecting presence of antibody coating may better localize the source of UTIs. Intelligent management demands a thorough quest for contributory anatomic deformities. The eventual sequelae of uncontrolled UTI are loss of renal function (renal failure) and destruction of the urinary transport system.

URETER

Congenital Anomalies

Anomalies of the ureter are frequently associated with anomalies of the kidney, which have been discussed previously. They include duplications, fused ureters, and aberrant course.

Ureterocele

Ureterocele is a cystic dilation of the vesical end of the ureter caused by a congenital narrowing of the ureteral orifice (Fig. 37-17). It is asymptomatic until obstruction leads to hydronephrosis, stone formation, and infection. Diagnosis is made by cystoscopic examination and urography. Cystoscopy reveals a thin-walled cystic body that intermittently fills and balloons with urine and then collapses as the urine is discharged from the tiny orifice. Urograms may show the cystic radiolu-

cent mass in the bladder and the secondary damage to ureter and kidneys. Treatment consists of removal of the ureterocele with ureteral reimplantation.

Megaureter

Megaureter is a tremendously atonic and dilated ureter (Fig. 37-18). The cause is obscure, though a functional disturbance of the neuromuscular mechanism of the ureter is the most likely. The condition is asymptomatic until hydronephrosis, infection, and stone formation occur.

Diagnosis is made by cystoscopy and urography. On cystoscopy the ureteral orifice may be normal. Urograms reveal a dilated and tortuous ureter. The essence of treatment is to secure good drainage and relieve stasis, which may require ureterovesical reimplantation with ureteral reconstruction.

Ectopic Ureteral Orifices

Ectopic ureteral orifices are often associated with other congenital anomalies of the genitourinary passageways. In the female the aberrant opening of the ureteric orifice may be found in the vesical trigone, urethra, vagina, or even perineum. In the male the ectopic ureter opens proximal to the external sphincter. The symptoms affecting micturition vary greatly. In the female, sphincter control of the ectopic ureter is absent, and urinary incontinence is always present.

Diagnosis is made by history, urography, and cystoscopy. If the abnormality is discovered before renal damage is serious, the ureter may be implanted into the bladder, but if it is discovered after hydronephrotic atrophy and infection have occurred, nephrectomy is indicated if adequate renal function remains on the other side.

Other relatively rare congenital anomalies of the ureter include valves, diverticula, postcaval ureter, and stricture. Postcaval ureter is actually an anomaly of the

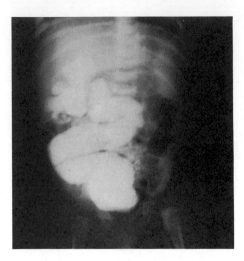

Fig. 37-18. Pyelogram showing right-sided megaloureter and hydronephrosis.

vascular system, for the vena cava forms in front of, instead of behind, the ureter. The ureter is compressed by this overlying vena cava, causing a hydronephrosis that may later become infected. True congenital strictures are rare; they result in hydroureter and hydronephrosis.

Injuries

Injuries from external violence are relatively infrequent because of musculoskeletal protection and relative mobility of the ureter. When injury does occur, it is accompanied by other injuries of great severity, such as shattered pelvis, and generally involves complete division of the lower ureter. In addition a fracture of one or more lumbar vertebral transverse processes must raise the possibility of trauma to the ureter.

Injuries from instrumentation are most frequently perforations made while attempting to extract a stone or to pass a catheter.

Injuries from surgery, particularly gynecologic pelvic surgery, are the most common cause of ureteral injury. Normally the uterine artery and ureter are only 2.5 cm apart, but neoplastic or inflammatory disease distorts this relationship and makes identification difficult. Injuries include incision, complete transection, occlusion, and necrosis from interference with blood supply.

Symptoms with unilateral injury include urinary fistula, progressive silent hydronephrosis, or pyonephrosis after infection. Symptoms with bilateral injury include anuria, uremia, and death.

Diagnosis

Indications of ureteral injury are the following:

1. Urinary fistula exists without bladder injury.

2. If methylene blue solution is introduced into the bladder and no dye appears through the fistula but dye does appear through the fistula when methylene blue is given intravenously, ureteral fistula must be suspected.

3. Further confirmation is obtained by cystoscopy and pyelographic studies.

Treatment

Treatment varies with the extent of injury to the ureter and the location of the lesion. Small incisions or minor damage to the ureteral wall may require to repair. Large incisions or transections should be repaired over a ureteral catheter, if possible, and the catheter left in place for 8 to 10 days. Other procedures include ureterovesical anastomosis, ureterointestinal anastomosis, cutaneous ureterostomy, transureteroureterostomy, autotransplantation, or even nephrectomy.

Calculus
Etiology

A ureteral calculus is usually a small stone that has passed down from the kidney pelvis. It rarely starts in the ureter, though an impacted fragment may grow larger there. The majority are composed of uric acid or calcium oxalate, since the phosphatic and cystine stones rapidly grow too large to pass down the ureter. The etiologic factors responsible for stones in the kidney pelvis are also responsible for ureteral stones, particularly those of stasis associated with strictures and congenital hydroureter.

Symptoms

The types of symptoms produced by ureteral calculi are the same as those produced by a stone in the kidney. However, pain, hematuria, evidences of obstruction, infection, and renal insufficiency are more common with ureteral stones than they are with renal stones. Rarely ureteral calculi may be present for long periods of time without producing symptoms. They may produce gradual destruction of the urinary tract above because of obstruction.

Diagnosis

History, particularly of the known predisposing factors, chemical examination of the blood and urine, and dramatic relief of pain when a ureteral catheter is passed beyond the obstruction are important in diagnosis. Radiographic examination is important, particularly oblique films that will show the relationship of the stone to the course of the ureter (Fig. 37-8).

Differential diagnosis. Calcified lymph nodes, phleboliths, pills, gas in the bowel, and skin moles must be distinguished radiographically from ureteral calculi. Of course, all other causes of acute abdominal disease must be ruled out.

Treatment

Generally all stones over 1 cm in diameter anywhere in the ureter, whether or not they are causing symptoms, should be treated.

Stones under 6 mm in diameter may pass spontaneously. Antispasmodics and narcotics are given as needed, and fluids are forced. If the stone does not pass, a ureteral catheter is inserted above the stone for 48 hours. The catheter is then removed for another trial at passing the stone. If the stone is already down in the lower one third of the ureter, an extractor is used to attempt to remove it under general or spinal anesthesia after dilating the ureter with an indwelling ureteral catheter for 2 to 3 days. Attempted basket extraction of calculi in the upper or middle third of the ureter is associated with a significantly increased complication rate. Ureterolithotomy and ESWL usually are safer procedures.

Carcinoma

Carcinoma of the ureter may be either primary, arising from the urothelium, or secondary, arising from such organs as the ovary or the gastrointestinal tract. The reported age incidence varies from 22 to 89 years. There seems to be no sex difference or preference for either side. The lower third of the ureter is the most common site of primary carcinoma.

Pathology

The most striking characteristic of ureteral tumors is their ability to seed elsewhere on the urothelium (Fig. 37-19). The primary growth may be in the renal pelvis, and the secondary "seedlings" may appear in the ureter, the bladder, or even the urethra. Some investigators believe that carcinogens are the cause of these new growths, or there may be a multifocal instability of the urothelium. Ureteral tumors characteristically are slow growing and confined to the urinary tract. Two general types of tumor are recognized: *papillary transitional cell carcinoma*, which may either be pedunculated or have a base as large as the tumor mass itself, and the *squamous cell* type, which is nonpapillary, more solid, less cellular, and tends to be invasive. Metastases occur in the areas drained by the lymphatics of the ureter.

Symptoms

Hematuria is the initial symptom in 70% of patients with ureteral neoplasms; renal colic or a mass in the flank area are less common heralding complaints. The hematuria is usually painless and may be accompanied by "fishworm" or "shoestring" clots. Pain may be colicky because of obstruction of the ureter but is more commonly dull and aching in character. The mass usually is a hydronephrotic kidney and not the tumor itself. Weight loss, easy fatigue, and a general rundown feeling are late symptoms of ureteral tumors.

Diagnosis

The urine consistently contains red blood cells, either grossly or microscopically. Cystoscopy is indicated to locate the source of the bleeding: bleeding from a ureteral tumor is usually continuous, not episodic, and the tumor may protrude from the meatus at each efflux of the urine. The drip from the ureteral catheter may be bloody initially and then suddenly clear as the catheter rises above the source of the bleeding. On the other hand, vigorous hemorrhage may be provoked by the passage of a ureteral catheter. All of these signs point toward a tumor of the ureter.

The intravenous urogram may show nonfunction or hydronephrosis on the involved side. The retrograde pyelogram may indicate hydronephrosis and hydroureter, but the most reliable sign of ureteral tumor is a constant filling defect in the ureter.

Nonopaque stones or a blood clot must be distinguished from ureteral tumors. The nonopaque stone is usually sharp in outline; its position may move from time to time as progressive x-ray studies are made. A

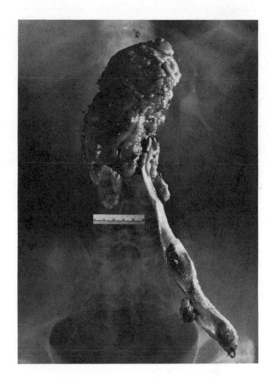

Fig. 37-19. Pyelogram and specimen of multiple tumors of ureter.

blood clot may also change position or disappear, indicating that the lesion is not constant.

One of the more recent and reliable methods of differentiating a ureteral tumor from a nonopaque stone or blood clot is cytologic examination of the urinary sediment for abnormal cells. Characteristically, the neoplastic cells have an increased nucleus-to-cystoplasm ratio, a thickened nuclear membrane, and prominent and bizarre nucleoles, and often the cells are tadpole-like, indicating their origin from transitional cell epithelium. Cytologic detection of abnormal cells in the urine is a useful adjunct but does not replace any of the standard diagnostic procedures.

Treatment

The classic treatment of ureteral neoplasia is early nephroureterectomy, with extirpation of the entire upper urinary tract, including a cuff of the bladder at the ureterovesical junction. (Remember that these tumors tend to seed themselves on the urothelium.) A single-stage procedure is usually employed.

An attractive alternative treatment is local resection of the neoplasm and adjacent ureter with end-to-end ureteroureterostomy. This therapy obviously conserves renal function in a disease that tends to be bilateral and recurrent. Follow-up includes interval urine cytology, excretory urography, and cystoscopy.

Prognosis

The prognosis of ureteral tumor is good in the papillary type, especially if the tumor is small, if the pathologic sections show noninvasive characteristics, and if the involved ureter is completely removed with the ac-

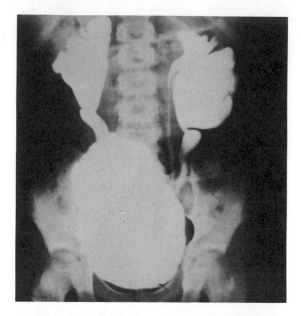

Fig. 37-20. Cystogram showing congenital bladder neck stricture with dilated bladder, bilateral ureteral reflux, and hydronephrosis.

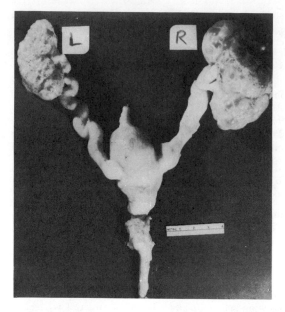

Fig. 37-21. Specimen of congenital bladder neck stricture.

companying kidney. The squamous cell type has a poor prognosis; invasion and metastases occur early.

Reflux

Ureteral reflux (Figs. 37-20 and 37-21) has captured the interest of urologists. Although the relationship of ureteral reflux to chronic bladder infection has been known for many years, the common occurrence of ureteral reflux in many other conditions was not generally recognized until recently. Ureteral reflux plays a major role in renal infection and gradual renal deterioration in patients with neurogenic bladder and in children with bladder infections from undetected causes. Renal failure may result from neglected bilateral reflux.

In some instances ureteral reflux is associated with a congenital patulous state of the ureteral orifice with failure of the ureterovesical valvelike mechanism to prevent ureteral reflux. Urinary tract obstruction or infection may well predispose to ureteral reflux. Many operative procedures have been devised for its correction, the most common being the submucosal "tunneling procedure." This is usually successful in patients who do not have greatly dilated ureters and in whom infection can be controlled satisfactorily. Ureteral reflux is usually readily demonstrated by cystography or by voiding cystourethrography.

URINARY BLADDER

The function of the bladder is twofold: to store urine and to remove it from the body. Any pathologic condition that changes these functions will usually be accompanied by frequent, difficult, and painful urination, nocturia, hematuria, and pyuria. These symptoms are discussed thoroughly under the primary pathologic conditions responsible for producing them.

A distended bladder is percussible or palpable on abdominal examination. A midline suprapubic mass should always suggest the possibility of a distended bladder, which may also be palpated rectally as fullness above the prostate. Evaluation of the size of the prostate by rectal examination is hindered by a distended bladder.

Bladder function may be accurately assessed by simple tests. Catheterization yields a great deal of information. *Residual urine,* the amount of urine remaining in the bladder after voiding, is diagnostically important. Residual urine in the bladder in any amount is significant of abnormal bladder function.

X-ray examination of the bladder may reveal valuable information. Stones and radiopaque foreign bodies will be seen on the plain film. The injection of radiopaque medium through a catheter into the bladder (cystography) outlines the size and shape of the bladder, trabeculation, diverticula, and ureteral reflux. Extravasation of radiopaque medium indicates bladder rupture. Micturition cystograms (radiographs of the bladder taken after the patient voids after instillation of radiopaque medium into the bladder) pinpoint the presence and location of residual urine (which may reside in a diverticulum). Air cystograms best demonstrate filling defects from tumors, nonradiopaque stones, and foreign bodies.

Examination of the interior of the bladder by cystoscopy allows precise evaluation of the mucosa for inflammation, trabeculation, stones, ulcers, tumors, scars, and fistulous tracts. Cystoscopy is also valuable in determining the source of hematuria (i.e., whether it is coming from the bladder or the right or left ureteral orifice).

Cystometry is useful in determining the neuromuscular function of the bladder.

Congenital Anomalies

Complete aplasia of the bladder is rare and is usually diagnosed at autopsy. *Double bladder* is also rare;

it may be complete or incomplete, transverse or sagittal. An hourglass bladder with a constricting fibrous band in the midportion has also been described. *Exstrophy of the bladder* occurs about once in every 50,000 births. Complete exstrophy of the bladder is characterized by a lack of the anterior bladder wall with a fasciomuscular defect in the anterior abdominal wall. The posterior wall of the bladder and the trigone occupy this defect. Exstrophy in the male is usually accompanied by complete epispadias, undescended testes, and a bifid scrotum. In the female the clitoris is bifid, the labia are separated, and the urethra is epispadic. In both sexes the symphysis is absent, with a wide separation of the pubic bones (Fig. 37-1). This creates the characteristic waddling gait of these children. Incomplete exstrophy of the bladder presents only a defect in the upper or lower portion of the anterior bladder wall. About 90% of exstrophies occur in males. The bladder wall is basically defective and often is associated with hydroureteronephrosis or even reflux.

Clinical Picture

The diagnosis of exstrophy of the bladder is easy. The exstrophied bladder is seen as a red outpouching of mucous membrane on the anterior abdominal wall in which the ureteral orifices and the interureteric ridge are clearly visible. The patient is constantly urine soaked and is physically and socially miserable.

The anomaly is not compatible with long life because upper urinary tract damage leads to renal failure. Another complication of exstrophy of the bladder is malignant change of the epithelium, which occurs in about 5% of the cases. An adenocarcinoma is the most common malignancy developing in an exstrophied bladder.

The management of bladder exstrophy consists of diversion of the urinary stream and resection of the exstrophied bladder. Attempts to close and reconstruct the bladder have been generally unsatisfactory. Diversion of the urinary stream is carried out either into the sigmoid colon (ureterosigmoidostomy), or into a rectal bladder from which feces have been diverted. This is a very successful operation if the anal sphincters are functioning. Otherwise an ileal conduit urinary diversion is indicated.

Results of treatment by this method are uniformly good and offer the patient comfort, social acceptability, and a good prognosis. At a later time the associated epispadias and undescended testes are surgically corrected. In all female patients and in some male patients, adequate sexual function and procreation can be achieved.

The *urachus* may give rise to anomalies that create definite clinical entities. Patent urachus is characterized by a fistula that drains urine at the umbilicus or in the midline between the symphysis and the umbilicus. The urachus may obliterate at the upper end only, forming a pouch off the bladder that may harbor stones and infection. Both ends of the urachus may obliterate, leaving a blind pouch in which calculi may also form. Adenocarcinoma and sarcoma in these urachal cysts also have been reported. Diagnosis of these lesions is confirmed by (1) cystography and (2) endoscopic examination of the lower urinary tract. The treatment consists of surgical removal.

Hernias of the bladder are uncommon. They are usually found in "sliding" direct inguinal hernias.

Injuries

Traumatic perforations of the urinary bladder result in two different pathologic entities: intraperitoneal or extraperitoneal urinary extravasation. Rupture of the bladder is caused by a variety of agents: instrumentation, penetrating wounds, and direct or indirect blows. The most common causes of ruptured bladder are comminuted fracture of the bony pelvis and operative damage incurred during transurethral manipulation or open pelvic operations. Penetrating wounds of the bladder are commonly associated with damage to other abdominal viscera. Sudden changes in directional force when the bladder is full may cause rupture of the urethra at the junction of the prostatic and membranous portion.

Diagnosis

The diagnosis of bladder or urethral rupture is not always simple. A history of trauma followed by hematuria and pain suprapubically with voiding abnormalities is suggestive of a ruptured bladder. Extraperitoneal extravasation of urine may produce only moderate tenderness and rigidity of the lower abdomen, though later a mass becomes apparent on the anterior abdominal wall that may extend upward to the umbilicus and laterally to the inguinal ligament, or may be felt as a mass above the prostate on rectal examination. By this time the patient is extremely ill with fever, chills, nausea, and vomiting. Urinalysis reveals gross or microscopic hematuria. Leukocytosis is also present.

If the rupture is intraperitoneal, the patient will have generalized abdominal tenderness and rigidity, paralytic ileus, shock, and the other well-known signs of generalized peritonitis.

Final diagnosis rests on visualization of the bladder extravasation by cystography with radiopaque media. Differentiation between rupture of the bladder and of the prostatic urethra is important; if a catheter passes easily into the bladder, it is presumptive evidence that the urethra is intact.

Treatment

The treatment of a ruptured bladder is prompt surgical closure of the rent with perivesical drainage. The bladder itself is drained with an indwelling urethral or suprapubic catheter. Supportive treatment and antibiotic therapy are vitally important. To temporize by catheter drainage alone in a suspected rupture of the bladder invites disaster.

Foreign Bodies

Foreign bodies arrive in the bladder in a number of different ways. They may come through the bladder wall, through the urethra, or through fistulous openings into the bladder from some other viscera. The variety and number of foreign bodies introduced into the bladder through the urethra by children and adults are amazing (e.g., paraffin, chewing gum, hairpins, matches, insects, worms, snakes, rubber tubing, and balloons).

The clinical features are those of pronounced bladder irritation; frequency, dysuria, tenesmus, hematuria, and pyuria are prominent. The diagnosis of foreign bodies rests on demonstration by radiographic and cystoscopic studies.

Treatment is removal either transurethrally or through a suprapubic cystotomy.

Inflammatory Disease

Inflammatory disease of the bladder is very common in women of all ages, but particularly in young girls and elderly women. It is associated with frequency, dysuria, aching in the suprapubic area, and bacteria and pus cells in the urine in abnormal quantities.

Extravesical sources for the infection must be ruled out, as must vesical tumor, vesical stones, and obstructions.

Ureteral reflux is evaluated by cystography. Cystoscopy will distinguish a vesical infection from some other underlying lesion such as a diverticulum, neurogenic bladder, stone or tumor, or bladder neck contracture. The urethra must be calibrated to rule out urethral stenosis. Careful study of the bladder neck is indicated to rule out congenital bladder neck contracture, valves at the bladder neck, or some other bladder neck obstruction. Prostatitis in the male is a common cause. When these conditions are eliminated, the diagnosis of primary bladder infection is made. The treatment is straightforward. Culture and sensitivity tests indicate the proper antibiotic to be used, generally one with a broad spectrum of effect because colon bacilli of various kinds are almost invariably responsible. Vaginal infections and cervical infections must be treated because the short female urethra allows reinfection from these adjacent areas.

Interstitial cystitis or *Hunner's ulcer* is a peculiar type of cystitis found much more frequently in women than in men. It is characterized by sterile, clear urine, without inflammatory cells but with painful and frequent urination. Cystoscopic examination reveals areas of hemorrhage and cracking of the vesical mucosa, usually in the fundus, when the bladder is distended. This lesion responds to increasing strength of silver nitrate solution instilled into the bladder, starting with 1 to 1,000 and going up to about 1 to 500. The cause of this lesion is unknown, though current research points to either a quantitative or qualitative difference in the normal protective layer of mucopolysaccharides (glycosaminoglycans) lining the urothelium.

Other treatments include anticholinergic drugs and hydraulic dilation performed under anesthesia. The antiinflammatory agent dimethylsulfoxide (DMSO), when instilled intravesically as a topical treatment, relieves symptoms of interstitial cystitis at least temporarily in about half the patients. An unfortunate sequela of inter-

Table 37-4. The Neurogenic Bladder

Type	Voluntary Control	Condition of Bladder; Muscle Tone	Bladder Capacity	Micturition
Sensory paralytic	Present early	Flaccid and distended; myogenic tone decreased	Considerably increased	Early stage—complete emptying Late stage—overflow incontinence; dribbling
Motor paralytic	Absent	Flaccid and distended; myogenic tone decreased	Considerably increased	Early stage—incomplete emptying; sense of distention Late stage—overflow incontinence; dribbling
Autonomous	Absent	Myogenic tone preserved	Variable—may be increased or somewhat reduced	Early stage—inability to void; distended bladder Late stage—dribbling and straining
Reflex (automatic)	Absent	Variable—may be below normal, normal, or above normal	Variable—may be reduced or increased	Early stage—inability to void Late stage—reflex and precipitous urination
Uninhibited	Maintained by external sphincter but often insufficient to preserve continence	Normal to increased	Decreased	Precipitous and frequent

stitial cystitis is the small-capacity, contracted, fibrotic bladder. Carcinoma in situ may masquerade as interstitial cystitis.

Enuresis

All patients 5 years of age or older with enuresis should be studied radiographically—and often endoscopically—to rule out an underlying lesion. Ectopic ureteral orifices, urethral diverticulum, foreign body in the bladder, congenital obstructions to the outflow of urine, and other bladder lesions are often the cause of enuresis. If a search for anatomic abnormality is unrewarding, therapy consists of anticholinergic agents and general psychological support for both child and parents. Many children with enuresis have delayed maturation of their central nervous systems, resulting in persistent infantile, small-capacity bladders.

Neurogenic Bladder

In the adult, function of the normal bladder is controlled by conditioned reflexes, the highest center of which is in the cortex; any break in the pathway or derangement affecting the cortical center produces some type of neurogenic vesical dysfunction.

In infancy the bladder is controlled by a simple reflex arc that synapses in the sacral cord (S2-S4). Sensory stimulation from distension of the bladder is carried to this sacral center, triggering motor impulses over the efferent limb that cause the detrusor muscle to undergo a series of contractions of increasing amplitude until a massive contraction occurs and the bladder evacuates its contents. This pattern is influenced by training and environment until, in a normal child, the bladder is completely controlled by the conditioned reflex mechanism arising in the cortex. The contractions occurring in an infant bladder may be termed uninhibited contractions and do not occur in the normal adult bladder.

The bladder may be evaluated neurologically much as any other portion of the nervous system, for perception of temperature, pain, touch, contraction, and filling. The motor function of the bladder is examined by cystometry (CMG). Table 37-4 lists the types of neurogenic bladders and summarizes the features.

Diverticulum

Diverticula and trabeculation of the bladder are produced by obstruction to the outflow of urine from the bladder itself. Urethral stricture, bladder neck contracture, benign prostatic hypertrophy, urethral stenosis, and congenital valves are the most common causes. Diverticula of the bladder may occur at any age, and the

Residual Urine	Infection	Etiology	Responsible Conditions	Comment
Large volume	Common	Loss of sensory supply of bladder, as in lesions of posterior roots and columns	Acute (shock) stage of spinal injury; tabes dorsalis; diabetic radiculitis; subacute combined sclerosis	With the subsidence of spinal shock this type will merge into the reflex bladder unless severe myogenic disturbance has occurred through overdistension
Large volume	Common	Loss of motor supply to bladder, as in lesions of anterior horns and roots of sacral segments 3 and 4	May be part of the picture of spinal shock or occur in acute poliomyelitis	This type of bladder is also susceptible to myogenic disturbance, as above, but usually not to such severe degree
Present, usually in small or moderate amounts	Generally present	Complete interruption of reflex arc when both the sensory and motor components are destroyed	Trauma of sacral cord or conus; spina bifida manifesta; trauma of nervi erigentes	Patient may be able to express some urine by straining or manual compression
Present in variable amounts, depending on muscle tone of bladder	Often present	Complete interruption of upper motor neuron control; spinal arc present	Trauma of spinal cord above sacral level (after period of shock); spinal cord tumor; multiple sclerosis	Patient may discover "trigger areas" for induction of micturition
None in absence of infravesical obstruction	Absent	Loss of cerebral inhibitory control	Cerebral arteriosclerosis; brain tumor; brain injury, incomplete lesions of spinal cord; delayed development of cerebral inhibitory mechanism	This type shows least variance from normal bladder activity

large ones should be removed surgically and their cause eliminated. They occur in at least 10% of the patients with benign prostatic hypertrophy.

Carcinoma

Carcinoma of the bladder is the second most common genitourinary neoplasm. The fact that most of these cancers occur near the trigone and ureteral orifices, is suggestive of the action of a carcinogenic agent in the urine acting on the bladder mucous membrane. No proof of this hypothesis exists, except in patients who are exposed to hydrocarbons, as in the chemical industry. One carcinogen is β-naphthylamine. Chronic irritation, vesical calculi, and chronic cystitis are not present in any sizable portion of the cases. Studies are being carried out to see whether tryptophan derivatives may be related to vesical cancer.

Fig. 37-22 shows the four classifications (degree of invasion) of bladder tumors. Cure and survival rates are related directly to the stage and grade of lesions.

Signs and Symptoms

Although gross total painless hematuria is the cardinal sign of carcinoma of the bladder, some patients do not manifest hematuria at all or only in the latter stages. Any disturbance of micturition or change in the urine may be a manifestation of carcinoma of the bladder. In many instances patients have been referred to the hospital with a mistaken diagnosis of chronic prostatitis or cystitis. Therefore any patient over 40 years of age who has any disturbance of micturition should have a cystoscopic examination to rule out carcinoma of the bladder. Early diagnosis makes a tremendous difference in the type of therapy recommended and the result of treatment. In one series of 540 patients the average time interval between the occurrence of the first symptom and the diagnosis was 1½ years.

Diagnosis

Absolute diagnosis is based on cystoscopic examination with biopsy of suspicious tissue. The lateral air cystogram and the intravenous pyelogram may visualize a bladder tumor, particularly if it is large and papillary or if it obstructs a ureter (Figs. 37-23 and 37-24).

Cytology studies of the bladder urine may reveal suspicious cells; bladder washings increase the yield of positive cytologic tests.

The differential diagnosis between transitional cell carcinoma of the bladder, urachal rest tumor, carcinoma of an adjacent organ invading the bladder (sigmoid colon, prostate, cervix, uterus), and intense chronic cystitis may be difficult even after microscopic study of sections of the tumor. All these lesions require thorough investigation.

Treatment

The treatment of carcinoma of the bladder is summarized as follows: *destruction* by means of electrocoagulation, either through the resectoscope transurethrally or through an open cystostomy; removal by *open surgical procedure* (partial cystectomy or total cystectomy with diversion of the urinary stream) to include the removal of the regional lymph nodes; *palliative treatment* (transurethral resection (TUR), high-energy radiotherapy, or diversion of the urinary stream).

TUR or fulguration is well-suited for low-grade, early-stage papillary tumors. Although 40% to 70% recur given enough time, the treatment can be repeated successfully because most of the new tumors continue to have a similar histologic appearance. On the other hand, the high-grade, late-stage (invasive, solid) tumors require aggressive treatment. Even so, only about 50% of patients with tumors invading the bladder muscle wall will live 5 years free of disease. Most treatment failures are attributable to previously undetectable distant metastases.

In recent years surgical treatment has been greatly aided by the ileal conduit (ureteroileal cutaneous anastomosis) and colon conduit for supravesical diversion. They have proved to be superior to ureterosigmoid anastomosis, particularly in patients treated with irradiation. External beam irradiation is a valuable therapeutic aid. Systemic chemotherapy (MVAC) continues to be studied. Local application of thiotepa and BCG for recurrent superficial tumors have proven value.

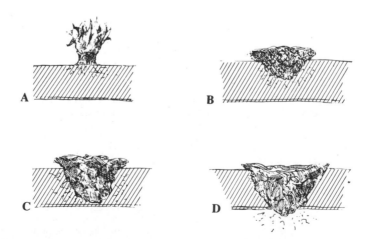

Fig. 37-22. Bladder tumors. **A,** Papillary, noninvasive. **B,** Partially invading bladder wall. **C,** Invading bladder wall completely. **D,** Invading perivesical tissue, generally with metastases.

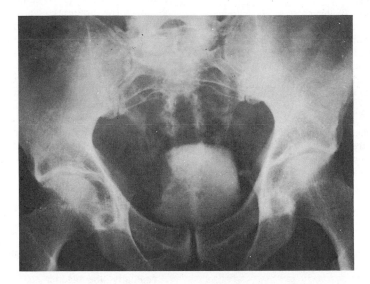

Fig. 37-23. Cystogram of tumor producing defect in right side of bladder.

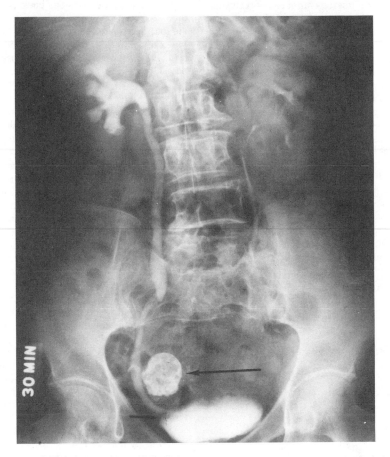

Fig. 37-24. Excretory urogram (I.V.P.) demonstrates right hydroureteronephrosis associated with infiltrating bladder tumor seen as filling defect *(small arrow)*. Calcified uterine fibroid is also present *(large arrow)*.

PROSTATE
Congenital Anomalies

Congenital anomalies of the prostate are extremely rare and are found only in association with other anomalies of the genitourinary tract, such as hypospadias. Congenital cysts of müllerian duct remnants arise between the lobes of a normal prostate. They may be felt on bimanual (rectal and abdominal) examination and are treated by complete excision.

Inflammatory Lesions

Inflammatory lesions of the prostate are quite common, particularly during middle life. They are caused by enteric bacteria, gonorrhea, or tuberculosis. They may be acute or chronic and can produce abscesses. The signs and symptoms vary, depending on the organism, the stage of the infection, and whether an abscess has formed. Acute prostatitis is characterized by dysuria (frequency, burning, pain) and retention of urine if a large abscess or an acutely swollen gland compresses the urethra. On the other hand, a dull, aching sensation in the perineum may be the only symptom of chronic prostatitis.

Treatment consists of general supportive care, prostatic massage, drainage (if an abscess is present), and appropriate antimicrobial therapy after the organisms have been cultured. Tuberculous prostatitis justifies a search for a primary tuberculous focus elsewhere in the body, and appropriate antituberculosis therapy.

Prostatic calculi may be an underlying cause for chronic prostatitis and may need to be removed transurethrally or by open prostatectomy.

Frequently prostatitis is associated with impotence and infertility. Both problems improve once the infection has been cleared.

Benign Prostatic Hypertrophy
Etiology

Benign prostatic hypertrophy is a common disease, probably the second most common disease of the aged male (Fig. 37-25); generalized arteriosclerosis is first. It is of tremendous importance in geriatric practice; 75% of all males over 60 years of age have benign prostatic hypertrophy, which causes complete bladder outlet obstruction in 50% of them (i.e., 38% of the total).

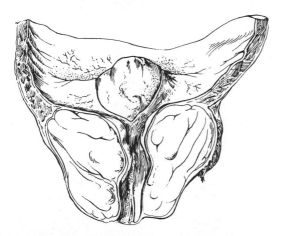

Fig. 37-25. Benign prostatic hypertrophy (trilobar).

The prostate is a compound structure composed of 100 or more outer (paraurethral) glands and 100 or more inner (periurethral) glands. A true capsule surrounds the entire gland. In benign prostatic hypertrophy the inner glands hypertrophy as nodules of fibroadenomatous tissue. These nodules push inward to distort the prostatic urethra and outward to compress the outer glands. Thus the outer (paraurethral) glands are not involved in benign prostatic hypertrophy. The hyperplasia so distorts the urethra as to cause a ball-valve effect leading to urinary retention. The disease first manifests itself as small spheroids of hypertrophy beneath the mucosa of the prostatic urethra that interfere with urination, not by constricting the urethra but by acting as a valve.

With long-standing obstruction in the prostatic urethra, the bladder muscle hypertrophies and the bladder wall becomes trabeculated. Later, small herniations of vesical mucosa are pushed outward between these hypertrophied muscle bundles, forming diverticula. Stagnation of urine, infection, and sometimes stone formation occur in these diverticula.

Eventually, the bladder can no longer compensate by hypertrophy, and the bladder wall becomes stretched and atonic. The ureterovesical junctions become impaired by constant back pressure; reflux, hydroureter, hydronephrosis, destruction of kidney tissue, uremia, and death result. *The most common cause of a lower abdominal mass in males over 50 years of age is a full bladder obstructed by benign prostatic hypertrophy.*

Symptoms and Signs

Urinary obstruction from prostatic hypertrophy has many clinical manifestations, including frequency, nocturia, hesitancy, urgency, inability to empty the bladder completely, episodes of complete retention, hematuria, pyuria, dysuria, episodes of chills and fever, back pain, renal colic, and a progressive history of slowing of the stream and diminution in its caliber. Oddly enough, hematuria is more common in benign prostatic hypertrophy than in carcinoma of the prostate: about 25% of patients complain of initial or terminal hematuria.

Long-standing bladder obstruction with renal damage also produces nonspecific complaints of poor appetite, anemia, general weakness, and at times excessive thirst and spells of disorientation.

The residual urine that remains after the patient attempts to empty his bladder is the most conspicuous sign of urinary obstruction. True, rectal examination can estimate the size of the prostate, but it cannot determine the degree of obstruction. Frequently, a huge gland will cause no obstruction, whereas a tiny, strategically located nodule, can cause complete retention.

Differential Diagnosis of Obstructive Uropathy of the Bladder

Many conditions, outlined as follows, produce obstruction to the outflow of urine from the bladder. In adult males benign hypertrophy of the prostate is the most common.

A. Conditions of the prostate that cause obstruction
   1. Acute prostatitis
   2. Prostatic abscess

3. Tuberculous prostatitis
4. Prostatic cyst
5. Prostatic calculi
6. Benign hypertrophy
7. Carcinoma of the prostate
8. Sarcoma of the prostate

B. Conditions about the prostatic urethra that cause obstruction
   1. Perirectal abscess
   2. Carcinoma or sarcoma adjacent to the urethra

C. Conditions of the prostatic urethra that cause obstruction
   1. Congenital conditions
      a. Urethral valve
      b. Congenital stricture
   2. Urethral stone
   3. Traumatic stricture of the prostatic urethra

D. Conditions in the bladder that cause obstruction
   1. Vesical stone
   2. Ureterocele
   3. Bladder neck contracture

E. Conditions of the bladder that cause obstruction
   1. Disturbances of position—prolapse
   2. Diverticulum
   3. Neurogenic
      a. Upper motor neuron
      b. Lower motor neuron
   4. Spasm of the sphincters
   5. Myogenic atony
   6. Carcinoma of the bladder

F. Conditions outside the bladder that cause obstruction
   1. Abscess in the pelvis
   2. Carcinoma of the cervix
   3. Diverticulitis of the sigmoid colon
   4. Carcinoma of the sigmoid colon

Disturbances of urination are the chief symptoms of diseases that involve any portion of the urinary tract and not just those originating in the bladder or prostate. Thus the characteristic symptoms of obstructive uropathy must be regarded merely as evidence of nonspecific urogenital disease, until definite abnormality of the bladder or prostate is proved. Only complete urologic investigation will differentiate among the many conditions that produce obstruction to the outflow of urine from those conditions that give symptoms of bladder dysfunction without obstruction.

Diagnosis

The following procedures are necessary for diagnosis.

Rectal examination. The prostate is smooth, usually symmetric, elastic, and mobile. On rectal examination it is usually graded from 0 to 4 +, 0 being a gland of small size and 4 + being one so large that the examining finger cannot go over it.

Residual urine. After voiding, the patient is catheterized and the amount of urine remaining in the bladder is measured. The normal bladder is able to empty itself to less than 1 ml of urine. But on practical clinical grounds residual urine volumes of less than 50 to 75 ml are not considered "significant" unless complications such as infection, calculi, or severe voiding difficulty supervene. The urine obtained in this manner should be examined for pH, specific gravity, blood, protein, sugar, and microscopic elements.

Cystourethrograms, cystoscopy, pyelography, renal function tests. Cystourethrograms, cystoscopy, pyelography, and renal function tests are used as follows (Fig. 37-26):

Urinary flow rate. A fairly recent yet simple test to study the balance between bladder detrusor activity and the resistance of the outflow tract (the bladder neck and all structures distal to it) is uroflowmetry (uroflow test, urinary flow rate measurements). The total urine volume voided and the time required for this voiding are measured by devices as simple as a stopwatch and calibrated beaker or by pressure transducer equipment. The minimal information gained is the average or mean urinary flow rate (milliliters per second); the pressure-transducer equipment also records on graph paper the peak or maximum urinary flow rate and the pattern of voiding. Abnormally low peak and average flow rates are compatible with both obstructive and neurogenic diseases and are helpful in monitoring response to any therapy utilized.

General physical examination, particularly cardiac status. The patient must be fully evaluated to determine whether he will benefit from surgical relief of his bladder neck obstruction.

Treatment

Treatment includes nonsurgical and surgical treatment of acute retention.

Nonsurgical. In mild cases with an acute episode of retention, conservative measures are often successful for a time. Prostatic massage, hot sitz baths, urinary antiseptics, antibiotics, bed rest, and catheter drainage may take the patient through an acute episode and avoid surgery. Hormonal agents to "shrink" the prostate are still being investigated.

Acute retention. The essence of treatment of acute retention is to drain the bladder slowly enough to prevent hemorrhage and bladder spasm but rapidly enough to draw off more urine than is being formed. Should the patient develop bladder spasms or hemorrhage, fluid is immediately replaced into the bladder and the patient is watched carefully. Once equilibrium has been achieved, surgical treatment is carried out.

Surgical. The four surgical approaches to the prostate for the treatment of benign prostatic hypertrophy are (1) *transurethral,* (2) *suprapubic,* (3) *perineal,* and (4) *retropubic* prostatectomy. Although called "prostatectomy," they are truly only adenectomy, or partial prostatectomy. The end result of each approach is identical—removal of the adenoma to the plane of cleavage at the surgical capsule, with the outer prostatic glands left undisturbed. In none of these methods is the entire prostate removed. The operation called the radical (total) prostatectomy is not performed for benign prostatic hypertrophy (see discussion of cancer, below).

TUR. In TUR the resectoscope is introduced into the urethra, and under direct vision the adenomatous tissue is cut away with a high-frequency current until the plane of the surgical capsule is reached (Fig. 37-27). *Advantages* are (1) low mortality and morbidity with (2) short and mild convalescence, average postoperative hospital stay is 3 to 5 days, (3) the disadvantages of open surgery are avoided, and (4) damage to the rectum is avoided. *Disadvantages* are that (1) the procedure is technically difficult to learn and to perform and (2) hemolytic reactions, urethral trauma, and stricture sometimes occur.

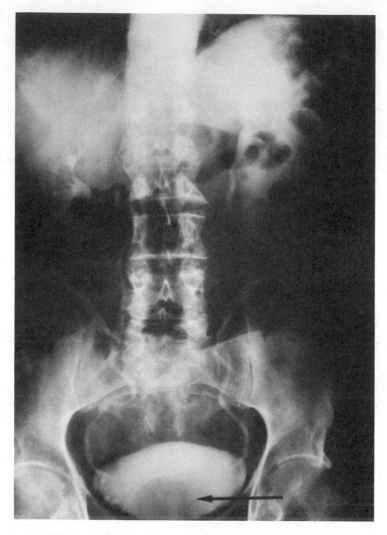

Fig. 37-26. Excretory urogram (I.V.P.) in older male with prostatism. Study is normal except for large filling defect in bladder base *(arrow)* consistent with intravesical prostatic enlargement.

Suprapubic (transvesical) prostatectomy. In suprapubic prostatectomy the bladder is opened extraperitoneally through an incision above the pubis, and the adenoma is enucleated with the finger. *Advantages* are that (1) this is an easy operative technique, best suited for the surgeon who does prostatic surgery infrequently and (2) it avoids the rectum and external sphincter. *Disadvantages* are (1) relatively high mortality and morbidity and (2) delayed healing with urinary fistula and long hospitalization (up to 2 weeks).

Perineal prostatectomy. The approach in perineal prostatectomy is through the perineum (Fig. 37-28). The prostate is detached from the rectum when the rectourethralis muscle is cut. The plane of cleavage is established, and the adenoma is enucleated. *Advantages* are (1) low mortality and morbidity and a mild convalescence second only to that following TUR and (2) dependent drainage. The *disadvantage* is that the operation is technically difficult and occasionally damages the rectum and external sphincter.

Retropubic prostatectomy. In retropubic prostatec-

tomy an incision is made just above the symphysis. The prostate is exposed in the prevesical space beneath the pubic arch. The plane of cleavage is established distal to the bladder neck, and the adenoma is enucleated through an incision in the anterior prostatic capsule. *Advantages* are (1) relatively low mortality and morbidity and a relatively short hospital stay and (2) a simple anatomic approach that avoids the rectum and external sphincter. *Disadvantages* are the hemorrhage from the prostatic venous plexus is not infrequent, and osteitis pubis may complicate the convalescence.

Vasectomy. Many clinics perform vasectomy before prostatectomy in hopes of preventing epididymitis. I have found approximately the same incidence of epididymitis with or without vasectomy. Probably bilateral vasectomy has its greatest place in preventing postprostatectomy epididymitis when it is performed *prior* to any urethral instrumentation. The scrotal route is most often employed, but an intrapelvic vasectomy can be achieved at the time of open prostatectomy.

Prognosis and results. The overall mortality in re-

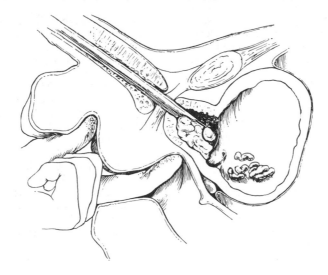

Fig. 37-27. Transurethral prostatic resection.

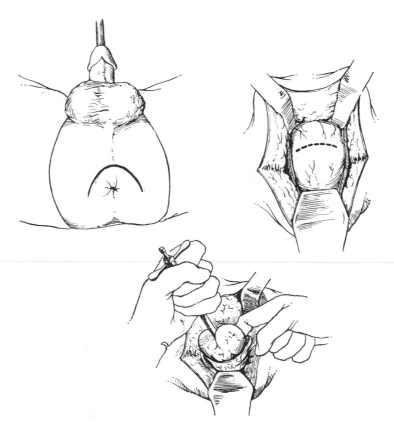

Fig. 37-28. Perineal prostatectomy.

cent years for all types of prostatic reaction in this country is less than 1%. Patients void well after resection, and only a small percentage suffer from incontinence or regrowth sufficient to cause prostatic obstruction to recur.

Cancer

Cancer of the prostate is the most common malignant growth in older males, and next to carcinoma of the lung it is the most frequent cause of death from cancer in males in the United States. It is relatively rare before 40 years of age but occurs in 20% of all white males over the age of 50. About 40% of all elderly males suffer from urinary obstruction, and one fifth of these cases are attributed to carcinoma of the prostate. There is no causal relationship between prostatic carcinoma and other lesions of the gland such as benign prostatic hypertrophy or chronic inflammatory disease. The cause is unknown.

Unlike benign prostatic hypertrophy, carcinoma arises in the periphery of the prostate (in the outer glands). Thus rectal examination may detect a carcinomatous nodule before it gives symptoms of obstruction and frequently before metastases have occurred, if rectal examination is carried out routinely. The neoplasm may remain limited to the gland itself for a relatively long period; then by direct invasion it involves the inner glands, the seminal vesical area, and the vas deferens. Later it breaks through the capsule to involve the urethra and bladder, rectum, periurethral tissues and the lymph nodes along the internal and external iliac vessels. Blood-borne metastases carry the malignancy to the bones, primarily the spine and pelvis, and to the lung.

Grossly, carcinoma of the prostate is a firm, white-yellow, irregular mass. Histologically, it is an adenocarcinoma, which characteristically produces an increase in the serum acid phosphatase when it has disseminated. Bony metastases are usually osteoblastic and associated with an elevation of the serum alkaline phosphatase as well.

Signs, Symptoms, and Diagnosis

Carcinoma of the prostate produces no symptoms until there is a spread to the urethra or until the bones are involved, causing pain. Urethral involvement produces dysuria, hematuria, and difficulty in urination. Detection of a hard prostatic nodule palpable on rectal examination requires confirmatory biopsy of the nodule. Chronic inflammatory disease of the prostate and prostatic calculi may mimic prostatic carcinoma. Once the biopsy findings confirm prostate cancer, the following studies are performed for staging: radionuclide bone scan, excretory urogram (IVP), serum acid and alkaline phosphatases, prostate-specific antigen, and in some patients CT of the abdomen and pelvis or pedal lymphangiogram.

Clinical staging is as follows: Stage A is defined as prostatic cancer discovered coincident to surgery performed for clinically benign disease; stage B, nodular areas confined to the substance of the prostate gland on rectal examination; stage C, evidence of periprostatic infiltration (rectum, seminal vesicles, bladder) on rectal examination; stage D, distant metastatic disease, most commonly skeletal.

Treatment

The treatment for prostate carcinoma depends on the stage. Stage A lesions, when low-grade and focal, need no further treatment, only observation. High-grade or diffuse stage A lesions, on the other hand, require aggressive treatment, either radical surgery or definitive radiotherapy. If the lesion is localized completely to the prostate area, a total (radical) prostatectomy can be car-

ried out with a high incidence of cure (80% to +90% 5-year survival free of disease). On the other hand, once the lesion has invaded the capsule, the base of the bladder, or the area around the seminal vesicles, there is a 50% chance that the regional lymph nodes are involved and a 10% to 15% chance of vascular metastases. External irradiation (linear accelerator) also is used as therapy for this type of patient. If dissemination has occurred, local therapy to relieve obstructive symptoms must be supplemented by systemic treatment. The local therapy usually is by transurethral prostatic resection.

Palliative systemic therapy of disseminated prostatic cancer consists essentially in altering the hormonal environment of the lesion by orchiectomy or the administration of estrogens or GNRH-agonists. Progesterone-like agents and alkylating agents have some effect on disseminated prostatic carcinoma. Controlled clinical trials to evaluate the efficacy of chemotherapeutic agents in this disease are now being conducted at several institutions. Recently open cryosurgical destruction of the malignant prostate has been utilized to destroy the large local lesion and alleviate pain from bone metastases. As yet there is no good objective evidence of regression of metastases or of an enhanced immunologic defense mechanism.

URETHRA
Congenital Anomalies
Male Urethra

Congenital valves of the posterior urethra may obstruct the passage of urine and, if not detected early, will produce strong back pressure with hydroureter, hydronephrosis, and, ultimately, renal insufficiency. Treatment consists of destruction of the valve leaflets by the resectoscope, to relieve the obstruction. Reconstructive procedures on the bladder, ureters, and kidney pelvis may be required to correct the effects of long-standing back pressure on the urinary transport system.

Hypospadias. The urethra opens on the ventral surface of the penis in hypospadias, the distal urethra having failed to form. In addition, there is pronounced ventral curvature, or *chordee,* of the penis. The corrective operations must first straighten the penis by removal of the fibrous band causing the chordee; then, a tube is fashioned of skin leading from the intact urethra to the glans penis. The untreated patient must urinate in the sitting position and is sterile, even if the chordee is mild enough to permit coitus, since ejaculation occurs outside the vagina.

Epispadias. In epispadias the urethra opens dorsally on the penis, appearing as a flat strip of mucous membrane on the upper surface of the penis between the separated corpora cavernosa. The severe forms involve the sphincters, causing incontinence of urine, and often are associated with exstrophy of the bladder. Treatment consists of closure of the urethral groove by urethroplasty.

Diverticulum of the urethra. Urethral diverticulum is rare; treatment is surgical excision.

Female Urethra

The female urethra is homologous with the posterior urethra in the male. Congenital anomalies are associated with defective development of the bladder, as in exstrophy and epispadias. In epispadias the urethra appears as a trough in the mons veneris.

Urethral stenosis. Congenital urethral stenosis is a possible cause of urinary obstruction in the female. The obstruction must be corrected, usually by dilation.

Infections

Infections of the urethra are common. They may produce prostatitis in the male and stricture formation in both the male and the female, with back-pressure effects on the urinary transport system. They are the result of various types of organisms (pyogenic, *Trichomonas vaginalis,* pleuropneumonia-like organisms) and tuberculosis.

Treatment centers around identification of the specific organism and administration of appropriate antibiotics. Obstruction to urine drainage must be relieved.

Gonococcal urethritis, caused by venereally transmitted *Neisseria gonorrhoeae,* continues to be the most common specific urethral infection. Symptoms in the male are an intense dysuria and a yellow-green purulent urethral discharge, whereas the female is usually asymptomatic. Diagnosis can be made in addition by identification of gram-negative intracellular diplococci on a Gram-stained urethral discharge or by new culture techniques. Treatment in nonallergic persons consists of high-dose parenteral penicillin G (4.8 to 9.6 million units) plus probenecid, given orally, to further increase tissue drug levels. A combination of oral ampicillin and probenecid is an alternative: Patients allergic to penicillin can be given either spectinomycin, administered intramuscularly, or tetracycline, administered orally. Treatment of sexual contacts as well will reduce the reinfection rate.

Stricture

Stricture of the urethra narrows the urethral channel and is generally caused by cicatrix from old inflammation. It is seen in both sexes but is more common in the male. It develops gradually, months or years after the initial episode of urethritis.

The urethral stricture is evaluated by radiographs or cystourethroscopy, with its length noted and the size of the lumen calibrated. Minor strictures may respond to dilations, but severe ones require surgical therapy to restore the natural size of the lumen. Unless this is done, there is gradual persistent damage to the proximal portion of the urinary transport system. Periurethral abscess, urinary fistulas, and infertility are other complications of urethral structure.

Urethral structures that are not easily managed by simple dilation and yet are symptomatic can now be treated by two new methods. The simpler of the two is *direct visual internal urethrotomy,* and endoscopic procedure that allows the operator to incise the stricture under visual control. Failures of this and other more conservative measures can be handled by *patch graft urethroplasty,* in which the stricture is incised through an open approach and a free graft or pedicle of preputial or penile skin is sutured into the resulting urethral defect.

Injuries

Simple contusion may be caused by forcible instrumentation, false passage, or acts of sexual violence. There is slight to moderate bleeding. Treatment generally is by splinting the area of injury with an indwelling catheter or suturing the area if accessible.

If *severe trauma* occurs, one must differentiate among ruptures of the anterior urethra, posterior urethra, and bladder.

Rupture of the anterior urethra is most frequently caused by forcible use of urethral instruments or lacerating wounds (Fig. 37-29). Injuries to the bulbous urethra are generally caused by straddle injuries or direct blows to the perineum. In both of these injuries there is a continuous drip of blood from the urethral meatus. A hematoma may form under Buck's fascia. The patient has no desire to urinate and later develops lower abdominal pain. He may have difficulty urinating, and urine may extravasate into the scrotum. Treatment is by antibiotic administration, immediate drainage of the area of extravasation, and splinting of the urethra with an indwelling catheter.

Rupture of the posterior prostatic urethra is usually associated with fractures of the pelvis, severe physical trauma, and occasionally instrument perforations during TUR. The patient becomes just as ill and "toxic" as in rupture of the anterior urethra, but there is no dripping of blood from the urethra, no hematoma under Buck's fascia, and no scrotal swelling; instead the urine extravasates posteriorly into the ischiorectal fossa or anteriorly into the suprapubic area. The urethral catheter passes easily but may go through the false passageway rather than into the bladder (Fig. 37-30). Injection of contrast medium determines whether the catheter is really in the bladder. The patient will not void spontaneously even though the bladder is distended with urine because of spasm. Many of these patients die of shock or sepsis if treatment is neglected.

Treatment of rupture of the posterior urethra is by a suprapubic cystostomy, with drainage of the prevesical

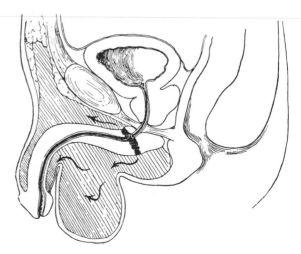

Fig. 37-29. Traumatic rupture of anterior urethra; *shaded areas,* routes of extravasation. Treatment consists in catheter splinting and drainage.

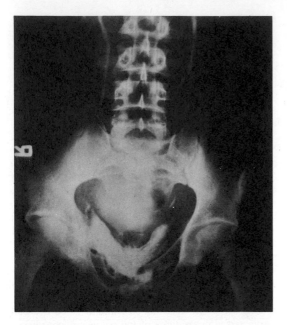

Fig. 37-30. Cystourethrogram with intravenous pyelogram showing rupture of posterior (prostatic) urethra with fractured pelvis. Notice extravasation of contrast medium about base of bladder, which has been displaced upward.

space. Later, plastic procedures may be necessary if fibrosis and scarring produce urethral stricture leading to chronic infection and calculi formation (Fig. 37-31). Long-term complications of posterior urethral injuries include impotence, urinary incontinence, and stricture.

Rupture of the bladder occurs from severe external trauma, usually with associated fracture of the pelvis, or from operative trauma. There is no immediate suprapubic extravasation or scrotal swelling, and frequently the patient is able to void. Diagnosis is suspected when saline solution injected into the bladder by catheter is not returned, and it is readily confirmed by cystography. Treatment is by immediate suprapubic drainage with surgical repair of the wound.

Neoplasms

Benign

Benign neoplasms of the urethra are rare in both sexes. They are usually papillomas or adenomatous polyps. Initial hematuria is the most frequent early complaint. Treatment is by electrocoagulation through the panendoscope or by direct excision.

Malignant

Etiology. Primary carcinoma of the urethra is a very rare disease that occurs in both circumcised and uncircumcised men. A history of chronic urethral stricture is common.

Pathology. This neoplasm is usually epidermoid carcinoma but may be adenocarcinoma; it is a relatively fast-growing neoplasm that arises with equal frequency in the anterior and posterior urethra. Urethral carcinoma spreads to the inguinal, external iliac, hypogastric, and common iliac nodes. Spread to the pelvic nodes should be suspected if there is pronounced local extension into the corpora or metastases to the inguinal nodes.

Symptoms. The symptoms result from progressive narrowing of the urethra and associated infection: diminution in size and caliber of the stream, dysuria, pyuria, and hematuria.

Diagnosis. Diagnosis is made by palpation of an indurated urethral mass and confirmed by panendoscopy.

Treatment. If there are no pelvic node metastases, I advocate wide surgical excision. Palliative treatment consists in providing a free passageway for urine and amputation of the penis for cosmetic purposes in neglected cases.

PENIS

Anomalies

The most common anomalies of the penis are associated with hypospadias and epispadias (see above). Anomalies of absence or multiplicity are extremely rare, as are micropenis and macropenis.

Phimosis may be either congenital or acquired and consists of a long, narrow prepuce with a minute orifice that limits the urinary flow and causes local irritation and inflammation. Treatment is by circumcision with or without a preliminary dorsal slit.

Paraphimosis results from the retraction of the prepuce behind the glans. The prepuce becomes so edematous that replacement becomes difficult, and local ulceration or gangrene may result. Again the treatment is by reduction and circumcision. A dorsal slit may be required if manual reduction is unsuccessful.

Inflammatory Lesions

Inflammatory lesions of the penis are relatively common. They consist essentially of balanitis, chancre, granuloma inguinale, chancroidal infection, and lymphogranuloma venereum. These are all venereal in nature and improved hygiene to accurate diagnosis, and proper antimicrobial therapy. Serologic testing may be necessary to rule out syphilis. Yeast or fungal infections may not respond completely to antiinfective agents until circumcision is performed. Condylomata acuminata can be eradicated by topical podophyllin or by excision. Herpes progenitalis, caused by the herpes simplex virus, is usually self-limited with proper hygiene and prevention of secondary bacterial infection. Recent clinical studies have demonstrated the efficacy of the antiviral agent acyclovir in initial cases of herpes progenitalis. The drug has proved useful for the vexing problem of recurrent herpetic infection.

Neoplasms

Neoplasms of the penis are not uncommon. Venereal warts are probably caused by a viral infection and are associated with poor hygiene and a redundant foreskin. They are readily treated by circumcision, coagulation of the papillomatous areas, or topical podophyllin. They may be precursors to carcinoma and should be cleared up at all costs.

Carcinoma of the penis is very rare in patients who have been circumcised in childhood or adolescence. Uncircumcised people who live in a hot, humid climate and have poor genital hygiene are predisposed to carcinoma of the penis. It is a slow-growing, painless, fun-

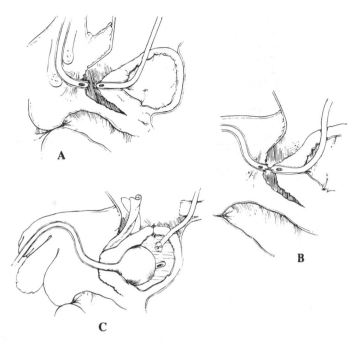

Fig. 37-31. Diagram showing traumatic rupture of posterior (prostatic) urethra and its repair. **A,** Catheter passed from urethra and bladder to meet at point of rupture. **B,** Catheter ends joined, and urethral catheter pulled on into bladder. **C,** Urethral catheter bag inflated and pulled down to splint urethra; perivesical space drained, suprapubic catheter placed.

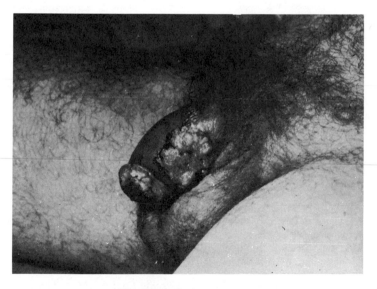

Fig. 37-32. Carcinoma of penis

gating epidermoid carcinoma that usually begins as a small pimple or wart on the glans, prepuce, or shaft of the penis (Fig. 37-32). Diagnosis is readily made by biopsy; certain types of chronic inflammatory lesions (chancre and chancroid) need to be differentiated. The treatment is by penectomy (partial or total), sometimes with inguinal lymphadenectomy. The prognosis is good if the regional lymph nodes are not involved.

Small premalignant and malignant lesions (e.g.,

erythroplasia of Queyrat, carcinoma in situ) can be successfully treated by wide local excision and circumcision. Alternative therapies include topical 5-fluorouracil and external beam irradiation using special penile molds.

Idiopathic Lesions

A fairly common lesion identifiable in middle-aged and older males is that of Peyronie's disease, or idiopathic penile fibrosis. Symptoms include penile curvature with erection (sometimes to the extent that vaginal penetration is impossible), localized pain, or the presence of subcutaneous penile nodules. Characteristically, variable areas of induration are palpable in the corpora cavernosa. Histologically, these penile plaques develop deep to the tunica albuginea covering each of the paired corpora but do not involve the corpus spongiosum or urethra. Treatment is exasperating; vitamin E is used for its antifibrotic activity in mild to moderate cases. Severely symptomatic men may require plaque incision or excision with the placement of a penile prosthesis, since impotence is a long-term result of the disease.

SCROTUM AND SCROTAL CONTENTS
Anomalies

Anomalies of the scrotum are rare and have little significance. A bifid scrotum usually is seen with congenital anomalies of the urethra such as epispadias, severe hypospadias, and intersex conditions. Congenital deformities of the scrotum are of importance only for cosmetic reasons.

Diseases

Carcinoma of the scrotum is seen occasionally as a soft, warty growth that soon becomes ulcerated. *Sebaceous cysts* of the scrotum are common; they are yellowish, rounded, firm and may grow to the size of a marble. The cysts are asymptomatic unless secondarily infected; then they should be treated by excision rather than by incision.

TESTIS
Anomalies

Anomalies of position of the testis are common, but anomalies of number are very rare. There are two types of anomalies of position: failure of descent (cryptorchidism) and abnormal location (ectopia).

Cryptorchidism is usually unilateral but may be bilateral; it occurs in approximately 1 out of every 25 boys and is commonly associated with an inguinal hernia. The cause of undescended testis is not completely understood, but it is probably related to maldevelopment of the structural route along which the testis must descend, to an abnormal testis, or to atrophy of the gubernaculum testis. Cryptorchidism is frequently associated with atrophy and alteration in the composition of the testis itself; degenerative changes of the seminiferous tubules are progressive with sterility resulting unless the testis is surgically brought into the scrotum (orchidopexy) early in childhood.

Failure of the testis to enter the scrotum is not abnormal until after the first year of life; after this, orchidopexy should be seriously considered and in all cases should be carried out before 5 years of age. The use of gonadotropic hormones from the anterior lobe of the pituitary gland has many advocates, particularly in bilateral cryptorchidism. However, I believe it is better to bring the testis down surgically than to depend on hormones.

Inflammation of the Testis and Epididymis
Orchitis

Orchitis may be acute or chronic. Chronic orchitis is usually associated with tuberculous epididymitis and is discussed later. Acute orchitis, too, may be associated with infection of the epididymis, vas deferens, and seminal vesicles, or it may be primary, in which case it does not involve the cord structures. Primary orchitis is seen most commonly in adults who develop mumps and other contagious diseases more characteristic of childhood. The diagnosis is made by palpation of an acutely tender, swollen testis, with or without involvement of the epididymis and vas deferens.

Mild cases of orchitis are treated conservatively and symptomatically with bed rest, analgesics, elevation of the scrotum, and application of heat. However, severe orchitis is treated surgically by incision and drainage of the tunica vaginalis and albuginea; this will prevent the severe testicular atrophy that otherwise might occur. Corticosteroid therapy is indicated in postpubertal mumps orchitis to prevent postinflammatory fibrosis and subsequent sterility.

Acute Epididymitis

Etiology. Acute epididymitis may be gonorrheal or nonspecific in origin. In either case the pathogenesis and treatment are generally the same. Usually epididymitis is associated with infection of the lower urinary tract from prostatitis, urethral manipulation, or too vigorous prostatic massage. The infection travels by a direct route from these structures up the seminal vesicles, through the vas deferens, and to the tail of the epididymis.

Diagnosis. The diagnosis is made by palpation of a greatly inflamed, hot, tender, and swollen epididymis, with or without involvement of the testis. Usually, the epididymis can be palpated separately from the testis. Accompanying these findings are systemic reactions with chills, fever, and leukocytosis.

Treatment. The treatment of acute epididymitis, be it gonorrheal or nonspecific, is medical. The use of large doses of antibiotics, elevation, bed rest, and local heat will usually arrest the process within a few days. However, it may be a matter of months before the swelling and induration subside completely. One should eradicate the focus of infection in the lower urinary tract to prevent the opposite epididymis from subsequently becoming involved.

Complications. The principal complication of acute epididymitis is sterility, caused by obliteration of the epididymal canals and lumen of the vas deferens. Complete aspermia is commonly found after bilateral epididymitis, even though testicular biopsy reveals entirely normal testicular tissue.

Chronic Epididymitis—Tuberculosis

Etiology. Chronic epididymitis is often tuberculous in origin and should be considered such until proved otherwise. Whether epididymal tuberculosis is primary or secondary is in dispute. Many believe that it arises from the prostate and seminal vesicles just as acute epididymitis does, traveling to the epididymis through the vas deferens. Others believe that it arrives in the epididymis by embolic metastases and spreads down along the genital tract into the testis.

Signs and symptoms. Tuberculous epididymitis begins in the globus minor as a painless mass and may reach an advanced stage before the patient is aware of its presence. Palpation reveals a hard, irregular, and commonly fixed mass involving a part or all of the epididymis; the vas deferens is often irregular and beaded, and there may be a secondary hydrocele. Chronic epididymitis may be bilateral and associated with one or many draining scrotal sinuses.

Diagnosis. The diagnosis is often difficult. A history of pulmonary tuberculosis (usually arrested) is helpful. Careful palpation of the vas deferens and rectal examination may disclose tuberculous involvement of other genital organs. One must rule out testicular tumor. A spermatocele will frequently cause confusion, but spermatoceles usually can be transilluminated. Tumors of the epididymis are rare.

Treatment. The treatment of tuberculous epididymis continues to be surgical. Prompt removal as soon as the diagnosis is made frequently prevents testicular involvement by direct extension. It may also prevent involvement of the other side. Simple epididymectomy usually suffices.

Chemotherapy has not yet proved itself capable of curing any but the superficial tuberculous lesions, but it is helpful as an adjunct in the treatment of genitourinary tuberculosis. Treatment for up to 2 years is indicated.

Torsion

Etiology

Torsion of the testis is caused by a sudden twisting of the spermatic cord that produces an acute partial or total obliteration of the vascular supply. Torsion may occur in a normal testis, but it is more frequently seen in the cryptorchid. It frequently follows minor trauma and may be confused with an acute epididymitis. The immediate and mechanical cause of the torsion is believed to be spastic contraction of the cremasteric muscle. The combination of an abnormal attachment of the testis, a deficiency in the gubernaculum, or an unusually large tunica vaginalis more frequently leads to a partial or complete rotation with subsequent vascular obstruction.

Diagnosis

Sudden pain usually occurs, followed by swelling, induration, and tenderness. It may be extremely difficult to differentiate from an acute epididymitis, but usually careful history will assist in clinching the diagnosis. Elevation of the testis relieves the pain of acute epididymitis but does not help in testicular torsion. The testis undergoing torsion may assume a more horizontal axis and superior position because of shortening of the spermatic cord. Newer diagnostic modalities used for identifying torsion include radionuclide testis scanning and evaluation of the vascular supply utilizing the Doppler principle.

Treatment

Torsion of the testis is a serious, distinct emergency, and, if relief is not prompt, infarction and subsequent atrophy will occur. The scrotum should be explored as soon as the diagnosis is even suspected. If, after straightening of the cord, the testis regains its normal color, it should be fixed securely in the scrotum. Unfortunately, by the time the diagnosis is made the testis is often infarcted, and the only recourse is surgical extirpation. In either event the contralateral scrotum should be explored and orchiopexy carried out, since the tendency to testicular torsion is often bilateral.

Neoplasm

Incidence

In general, most tumors of the testis are malignant and should be removed if the diagnosis is suspected. Tumors of the testis constitute about 1% of all malignant tumors in males. Although uncommon, the significance of these tumors lies in the age of the group affected, which is 20 to 40 years.

In descending order of frequency, malignant tumors of the testis are seminoma, embryonal carcinoma, teratocarcinoma, adult teratoma, and, the least common, chorioepithelioma, or choriocarcinoma.

Etiology

Although the cause of testicular tumors is unknown, the undescended testis is distinctly a predisposing factor. All cryptorchid testes should be either removed or brought down into the scrotum in early childhood as prophylaxis against development of testicular tumor.

Pathology

There is no unanimity in the pathologic classification of testicular tumors. From a practical viewpoint, they are probably best understood when they are classified according to cells. They may develop from any cell type found in the testicular tissue but usually are from the germ cells.

The *seminoma* closely resembles the cells of the seminiferous tubules. Seminomas are believed to be derived from the primordial sex cells. They usually are unicellular tumors and are the most common of the testicular tumors. They are definitely malignant. Their hormone production is usually nil.

The *embryonal carcinoma* is a more highly malignant tumor, which grows rapidly and metastasizes readily. Grossly they are soft, often necrotic-looking and hemorrhagic in the cut specimen. They may be unicellular, in which case they are difficult to differentiate from the seminomas. Usually they are multicellular and may appear either papillary or adenomatous. These tumors are therefore often described as either embryonal *adenocarcinoma* or embryonal *papillary adenocarcinoma*.

The *teratocarcinoma* is a mixture of fairly well-differentiated teratoid structures. This tumor is definitely malignant, unlike the adult teratoma. The teratoid structures are seen intermingling with masses of malignant cells recognized as embryonal carcinoma, seminoma, or chorioepithelioma. Grossly, they are solid and contain many cystic areas. The solid areas contain the malignant tissue.

The adult *teratomas* are believed to arise from isolated blastomeres. They are a mixed cell type, relatively benign, and uncommon. They cause no gonadotropic hormone to be excreted in the urine; grossly they may be solid or cystic. They are encapsulated. The cysts contain sebaceous and mucoid material. Microscopically they are characterized by a variety of well-differentiated structures.

The most malignant, and fortunately the rarest, of the testicular tumors is the *chorioepithelioma*. These tumors elaborate large quantities of gonadotropic hormone. Grossly, the primary lesion may be small and often hidden until postmortem examination, at which time there may be metastases throughout the body. The tumors are soft, extremely hemorrhagic, and necrotic, because of the tumor's propensity to outgrow its own blood supply. Microscopically it is distinguished by cytotrophoblasts and syncytiotrophoblast cells.

Metastases

The mode of metastases is primarily lymphatic, pressing up along the cord to the regional nodes: the paraaortic, mediastinal, and supraclavicular nodes. These tumors may, in addition, metastasize through the bloodstream; lung metastases have occasionally been excised with apparent cure and no systemic treatment.

Signs and Symptoms

Testicular tumors arise insidiously. The initial symptoms are usually a painless swelling of the testis and a sensation of increased weight. Because of the tumor's insidious onset, minor trauma to the area frequently directs attention to the mass. The mass enlarges slowly and continues to be painless. However, all too frequently the testicular mass goes unnoticed until widespread metastases have developed with weight loss, abdominal mass, abdominal or back pain, edema of the lower extremities, or pulmonary complaints. Lastly, gynecomastia is suggestive of chorioepithelioma.

Diagnosis

Testicular tumors must be differentiated from hydroceles. Differentiation is often very difficult since a hydrocele frequently accompanies the tumor. Usually the mass cannot be transilluminated, but if any doubt remains, the scrotum should be explored from an inguinal approach. Hematocele may be ruled out by palpation. Chronic or acute epididymitis is frequently confused with testicular tumors. Scrotal ultrasound exam may be helpful.

Biologic markers. It is now well established that many nonseminomatous testicular tumors secrete substances that can be fairly easily measured in serum. The two most helpful of these tumor markers are α-fetoprotein (AFP) and the beta subunit of human chorionic gonadotropin (β-hCG). The presence of either or both of these markers in abnormal concentrations, along with the presence of a scrotal mass, generally indicates an embryonal cell carcinoma, teratocarcinoma, choriocarcinoma, or some combination of these with or without seminoma. The return of these markers to normal levels after therapy (e.g., high inguinal orchiectomy and retroperitoneal lymphadenectomy) is helpful in assessment of the adequacy of treatment. Follow-up serum measurements of such markers are indicated to detect recurrences that otherwise would remain silent for many weeks to months.

Prognosis

The prognosis of testicular tumors depends largely on the type of tumor and the time that elapses between its onset and adequate treatment. The cure rate for early seminoma should approach 100%.

Treatment

The treatment of seminoma of the testis is high inguinal orchiectomy followed by irradiation therapy over the common routes of metastasis. In all other types of malignant testicular neoplasms, high inguinal orchiectomy plus complete node dissection of the iliac and paraaortic nodes up to the renal arteries is indicated. Irradiation therapy is not used for lesions other than seminoma. Chemotherapy is the treatment of choice in disseminated testicular tumors, and the effective agents are vinblastine sulfate, bleomycin, cisplatin (Einhorn regimen), and etoposide.

VARICOCELE

Etiology

Varicocele is the name given to varicosities of the pampiniform venous plexus. The veins become distended, elongated, and tortuous; 97% of varicoceles are found on the left side, and 5% are bilateral. Although the cause is unknown, the high incidence of left-sided varicoceles indicates that the 90-degree angle by which the left spermatic vein enters the renal vein may be, in some way, causative. On the right side the spermatic vein empties into the inferior vena cava at an oblique angle. Since obstruction of the inferior vena cava may produce a varicocele on the right side, all right-sided varicoceles must be thoroughly investigated to rule out this cause. Defective valves in the spermatic venous system may also cause varicocele.

Varicoceles are usually seen between 15 and 30 years of age. Frequently they are asymptomatic. Some patients complain of a dragging sensation or neuralgia of the testis. Each male evaluated for infertility needs to be examined for the presence of an asymptomatic varicocele, since this lesion is often implicated in the "stress-pattern" seminogram: poor motility, increased numbers of abnormal spermatozoa, and a sperm concentration that may be normal to decreased. The pathogenesis of this form of infertility is yet unknown; because of cross circulation of the scrotal contents, the unilateral varicocele results in bilateral spermatogenic changes.

Diagnosis

The diagnosis of a varicocele is simple. The involved testis hangs distinctly lower than its mate, and its cord has a "bag of worms" sensation to palpation. The distended veins empty when the patient is supine, and the "bag of worms" sensation disappears, only to return when the patient stands. If the varicocele does not disappear with scrotal elevation, an intraabdominal tumor or vena cava obstruction must be suspected. The Doppler stethoscope can detect varicoceles that are otherwise not obvious.

Treatment

The treatment of varicocele is controversial. In some instances varicoceles tend to disappear spontaneously with time. Furthermore, surgical ligation of the involved veins rarely relieves the neuralgia and may be followed by atrophy of the testis, hydrocele, hemorrhage, thrombosis, and epididymitis, leaving the patient worse off than before surgery. Therefore I recommend a scrotal support as the only treatment of simple varicocele. However, infertility associated with varicocele may respond to ligation of the spermatic veins. Improvement in sperm count, motility, and morphology with subsequent reproductive success has been reported in up to 50% of men so treated. Although this surgery can be performed at the scrotal or inguinal level, I prefer the retroperitoneal route to expose the internal spermatic veins superior to the internal inguinal ring.

SPERMATOCELE
Etiology

Spermatoceles are retention cysts of the vasa efferentia or epididymis, and they contain spermatozoa. Most spermatoceles are believed to arise from scarring and deformity of the epididymis because of inflammatory obliteration of the lumen of the vasa efferentia, though some are traumatic in origin.

Signs and Symptoms

Spermatoceles are manifest as slowly enlarging cystic masses of the scrotum in young and old men, and generally they produce only mild local discomfort.

Diagnosis

A spermatocele is palpable as a cystic mass separate and distinct from the testis, usually arising from the globus major. It can be transilluminated as well as a hydrocele, the fluid contents being gray-white and containing inactive spermatozoa.

Treatment

Spermatoceles usually require no treatment. When they become large, they may be excised.

HYDROCELE
Etiology

A hydrocele is an accumulation of fluid within the serous sac of the scrotum lying between the tunica vaginalis and the tunica albuginea. Hydroceles are classified as idiopathic or congenital , acute or chronic, and may involve the testis or the cord.

By far the most common hydrocele is the idiopathic variety, which may occur at any age. Congenital hydrocele occurs in the infant with an imperfect closure of the processus vaginalis; it may be associated with a congenital type of inguinal hernia, depending on the size of the opening into the peritoneal cavity.

Hydrocele of the cord may also be congenital. In this case there is obliteration of the funicular process proximally and distally, leaving an intervening lumen in which fluid accumulates. Hydrocele of the cord presents as a cystic mass along the cord, which transilluminates and is separate from both the testis and the epididymis.

Diagnosis

Diagnosis of hydrocele is established by palpation and transillumination, which will usually rule out hernia and hematocele. It must then be differentiated from spermatocele. In a hydrocele the testis is either not felt or is palpated within the hydrocele sac. The spermatocele is felt as a mass distinct from the testis.

Treatment

The treatment of hydrocele may be medical or surgical. The hydrocele may be aspirated from time to time; infection is the most likely complication of this conservative form of treatment. Surgical treatment is by excision of the redundant portion of the hydrocele sac or a plication procedure that enhances reabsorption of fluid produced by the tunica vaginalis testis.

DISEASES OF THE VAS DEFERENS

The vas deferens is afflicted by the same diseases as the epididymis. Vasitis may be of gonorrheal or nonspecific origin, as well as tuberculous. The acute pyogenic infections cause pain, swelling, and tenderness on deep palpation over the vas deferens and the lower quadrants of the abdomen. Systemic manifestations are nausea, vomiting, fever, and leukocytosis.

The treatment of vasitis is the same as for epididymitis: bed rest, heat applications, and antibiotics. The prognosis is usually good, with infection subsiding in approximately a week to 10 days. However, obliteration of the lumen is a distinct possibility, leading to sterility.

Chronic infection of the vas is usually tuberculous in origin and has been discussed in the section on tuberculous epididymitis.

DISEASES OF THE SEMINAL VESICLES

Seminal vesiculitis may be of gonorrheal, nonspecific, or tuberculous origin. Gonorrheal and nonspecific vesiculitis are often associated with prostatitis and epididymitis and are simply a part of a general infection of the genital tract. The posterior urethra is the most frequent source of infection, which involves the vesicles by direct extension.

The acute phase of seminal vesiculitis begins with pronounced engorgement of the vesicles, which may progress to suppuration and abscess formation if the process fails to resolve. Later, a chronic stage develops with thickening and induration of the vesicles. This accounts for the ease with which they are palpated on rectal examination in the chronic stage of seminal vesiculitis.

Acute seminal vesiculitis may begin with systemic manifestations of chills and fever, with or without urinary disturbances. Pain is variable; when present, it is referred to the suprapubic and inguinal regions but rarely as high as the kidney. In nongonorrheal seminal vesiculitis the onset is more insidious, with few systemic manifestations and little discomfort. Chronic vesiculitis is frequently asymptomatic except for pain in the perineum, hip, and low back area. Because it is frequently associated with prostatitis, there may be increased urinary frequency, dysuria, and the symptoms of prostatitis.

On examination one finds tenderness, induration, and thickening of the vesicles, in addition to epididymitis and vasitis. Seminal vesiculitis will frequently be followed by aspermia, oligospermia, or even a complete lack of ejaculate.

Treatment of acute seminal vesiculitis is by massive doses of antibiotics, bed rest, and sedation. Chronic vesiculitis is treated with antibiotics and massage or stripping of the vesicles. No treatment is needed if the patient is asymptomatic. Surgical excision is rarely needed.

STERILITY IN THE MALE
Etiology

Fertility in the male requires (1) normal, actively motile spermatozoa formed within the testis, (2) free transport of the spermatozoa through the epididymis, vas deferens, and ultimately out the urethra, and (3) deposition of the sperm into the vaginal fornix.

There is a multitude of causes for sterility. *Impotence* may produce a relative state of sterility because of the inability to deliver spermatozoa into the vaginal vault. Impotence may be either neurologic or psychogenic in origin. If the lesion is psychogenic, the prognosis is good with proper psychiatric care, but if it is neurologic, the prognosis is usually poor.

Hypospadias frequently results in sterility on the same basis as impotence, the chordee and foreshortened urethra precluding delivery of the ejaculated specimen into the vaginal vault.

Stricture of the urethra produces aspermia or oligospermia if the lumen is so narrow as to prohibit the extremely viscid semen from passing.

Prostatitis and *seminal vesiculitis* are believed by many to cause sterility by altering the pH of the prostatic secretions to decrease seriously the motility and longevity of otherwise healthy spermatozoa.

The most common cause of sterility in the male is bilateral *epididymitis*. It may be acute, gonorrheal, or nonspecific, perhaps resulting from a prostatitis. In any case, after the acute inflammatory reaction, scarring of the tubules results with either total or partial obliteration of their lumen.

Orchitis is another common cause of sterility. Mumps orchitis usually occurs during or after puberty and may result in extreme atrophy of the seminiferous tubules. Since the Leydig cells are much more resistant to injury, impotence usually does not occur.

Patients with cryptorchidism after the age of puberty are sterile on the involved side, and complete aspermia is the usual finding if the disease is bilateral. Secondary sex characteristics will develop normally, since the testicular atrophy does not involve the interstitial cells.

Diagnosis

The examination for sterility should include a careful history of past or present prostatitis, seminal vesiculitis, epididymitis, or orchitis.

The testes, epididymides, vasa deferentia, seminal vesicles, prostate, and urethra are examined carefully because a pathologic condition anywhere along the genital tract may eventuate in partial or complete sterility.

Examination of the Semen

After a complete history and physical examination, the semen is examined. It must be obtained after at least 3 days of sexual abstinence, so that the sperm count can return to its optimal level. Most clinics obtain the semen specimen by having the patient masturbate, and it is extremely rare that the patient complains of this method. There are other less satisfactory methods of obtaining semen specimens. Coitus interruptus may result in a partial loss of the fluid, making the

count unreliable. The semen may be obtained from the vaginal vault of the female partner, but this, too is an unsatisfactory method, since it is impossible to obtain the total volume of ejaculate. The use of a condom to collect the ejaculate is contraindicated since the latex rubber is impregnated with solutions designed to act as spermicides.

The semen is first checked grossly. Normal semen is milky in appearance, of a thick consistency, and has a high viscosity. The volume averages 3 to 4 ml; the pH varies from 7.7 to 8.5. Any appreciable alteration from these norms should be noted; a low pH will result in decreased motility and longevity of the spermatozoa. A positive fructose test indicates the presence of seminal vesicle fluid; this function is extremely sensitive to even low concentrations of plasma testosterone.

The specimen is studied best microscopically about 30 minutes after delivery. By this time it has lost its high viscosity and can be diluted easily for an accurate count; little change in the motility of the sperm occurs during this interval of time. Normally, 80% or more of the sperm are actively motile; any decrease of the motility percentage lowers fertility.

A cell count of the semen, which normally averages 40 to 150 million spermatozoa per mililiter, is next done.

Although great reliance is placed on the total sperm count, it has little practical significance inasmuch as only the actively motile spermatozoa can impregnant the ovum. Many clinics classify their degree of fertility on the actively motile count obtained by this formula: % motility × sperm count per mililiter × volume of specimen in milliliters. At least three seminograms are required for a baseline value in any patient.

Medical Treatment

Thyroid extract, vitamin E, steroids, and gonadotropins have been found on careful evaluation to produce no significant increase in sperm count. Parenteral testosterone therapy predictably results in a decreased sperm count. Some authors have described a subsequent "rebound" phenomenon to justify the treatment, but most studies do not bear this out. Furthermore, and more importantly, since the entire process of spermatogenesis requires 75 to 90 days, any attempt to assess the efficacy of a treatment modality on the seminogram should be postponed until about 3 months after the initiation of the therapy.

Men with infertility and oligospermia should have measurements made of their plasma levels of both luteinizing hormone (LH) and follicle-stimulating hormone (FSH). Men who demonstrate significant elevations of FSH and LH probably have primary testicular failure with expected increased pituitary hormone levels. On the other hand, men with normal LH and FSH levels may have hypothalamic or anterior pituitary dysfunction with secondary testicular impairment. This latter group of subfertile men may benefit from long-term cyclic administration of the drug clomiphene citrate, which in turn stimulates the hypothalamus-pituitary-testis axis.

Surgical Treatment

Surgical treatment of male sterility is disappointing. The surgery may be divided into prophylactic and therapeutic. Prophylactic surgery is of vital importance: undescended testes should be brought into the scrotum in early childhood, and patients with severe orchitis associated with mumps may be saved from sterility by prompt opening and draining of the tunica vaginalis and tunica albuginea or by corticosteroid therapy. Urethral strictures should be dilated, and hypospadias with chordee should be corrected by appropriate plastic surgery.

Surgery has little to offer aspermic patients. Epididymis-vas deferens anastomosis has been attempted in patients with sterility associated with old epididymitis with little success. Vasovasostomy is successful in 50% to 80% of patients previously rendered sterile by bilateral vasectomy.

Bilateral testicular biopsy is recommended for patients with aspermia. This procedure may be done under local anesthesia. The biopsy specimen is fixed in Bouin's solution, stained, and studied microscopically to determine the degree of spermatogenesis and to lend some insight into the cause of the sterility. Biopsy allows a more accurate prognosis of fertility.

Treatment of Low-Fertility Patients

Discouraging as the medical and surgical approaches to male sterility are, definite progress is being made in the management of low-fertility males. The date of ovulation must be determined accurately to allow the maximum number of spermatozoa to be ejaculated at the most opportune time. Spermatozoa are rarely viable fore more than 48 hours in the uterus. The date of ovulation may be estimated by a sharp drop in the daily basal temperatures, taken just after awakening. This method will usually localize the time of ovulation to within 48 hours. It has proved a definite boon to the subfertile males, even though its accuracy is limited. Recent tests may be accurate to within 6 to 12 hours of ovulation.

Instructions to the Low-Fertility Groups

After determining the exact time of ovulation, I am able to suggest the following course: sexual abstinence for a week before the date of ovulation; then coitus the day before, twice during the 8-hour period of ovulation, and daily for the next 3 days. By this method the husband will be able to concentrate the maximum number of spermatozoa at the most crucial period. Strict adherence to this routine has produced encouraging results in subfertile couples.

Men with documented high-volume ejaculates (6 to 10 ml) usually have their spermatozoa concentrated in the first portion of the ejaculate, whereas the overall sperm count may be normal or low. Instruction about the technique of coitus interruptus at the time of expected ovulation to deliver the undiluted active spermatozoa has resulted in pregnancies in this select group of subfertile couples.

Artificial Insemination

The initial successes with artificial insemination occurred at the University of Iowa. Two general types are now practiced: artificial insemination by husband (AIH) and artificial insemination by donor (AID). The former is indicated when physical abnormalities make normal sexual intercourse impossible or in the use of pooled or split ejaculates when coitus interruptus is unsuccessful. Unidentified donor insemination (AID) has many medicolegal ramifications, and the exact status of this technique may vary from state to state. Presumably its use would benefit those couples in which the husband is sterile, the wife is fertile, and adoption is considered less attractive.

The newer techniques of in vitro fertilization and embryo transfer are under the aegis of the obstetrician-gynecologist specializing in infertility. However, the close cooperation of a urologist in evaluating the potential father's fertility status must be emphasized.

IMPOTENCE
Definition

Impotence is best defined as any impairment of erectile function that prevents completion of sexual intercourse. Thus impotence includes diminished penile tumescence and rigidity and difficulty in maintaining an erection throughout sexual activity.

Etiology

Current research demonstrates that most instances of erectile impotence are primarily organic and the minority are due to functional causes. Common causes of impotence include arteriolosclerosis, diabetes mellitus, cigarette smoking, antihypertensives and other drugs, hypogonadism, radical pelvic surgery, Peyronie's disease, and aging. Vasculogenic disease may be reflected in diminished blood supply (arteriogenic) and/or enhanced venous leakage (venogenic). The lack of nocturnal erections along with normal libido and ejaculatory function suggests an organic etiology.

Evaluation

Physical examination may identify causative factors such as prostatitis or Peyronie's disease. Urinalysis and blood chemistry analysis may uncover diabetes mellitus or other chronic illness. Measurements of plasma testosterone, follicle-stimulating hormone, luteinizing hormone, and prolactin may point to an endocrine abnormality. Special testing may be required: nocturnal penile tumescence and rigidity monitoring, Doppler or ultrasonic measurements of penile blood flow, intensive neurologic examination, cavernosography, and pelvic arteriography and cavernosometry. A new clinical method employs a test dose of papaverine and phentolamine injected intracavernosally to produce an erection.

Treatment

Any underlying disease should be treated. Men with testicular failure and hypogonadism can be treated with parenteral testosterone replacement. Cessation of smoking is recommended. The drug yohimbine may be effective in mild cases of vasculogenic impotence by increasing relaxation of corporal vascular smooth muscle and thereby diminishing venous drainage. Men who respond to intracavernosal papaverine and phentolamine injections may wish to continue this method as treatment. Certain types of arteriogenic and venogenic impotence can be repaired surgically or transluminally. And finally, many men with impotence will best be rehabilitated with the implantation of a penile prosthesis, either of the semirigid or inflatable design.

38

Gynecologic Surgery

John T. Soper
Claude L. Hughes, Jr.
Daniel L. Clarke-Pearson

Gynecology is the medical and surgical specialty that is concerned with the study of the female genital tract. Although this specialty may appear to be restricted, the gynecologist participates in the evaluation and therapy of normal reproductive function and a variety of benign and malignant diseases of pelvic structure and function. Diseases of the pelvic organs may affect other organ systems. In addition, the gynecologist deals with gynecologic symptoms arising from localized or systemic diseases. The gynecologist must also screen women for nongynecologic diseases, since many women seek primary medical care from gynecologists. Finally, many gynecologic disorders may directly affect the patient's psychological self-image or, conversely, genital symptoms may reflect psychopathologic problems.

HISTORY

Similar to all medical histories, the gynecologic history is developed from the women's chief complaint to her total history, emphasizing menstrual, obstetric, and sexual function. Key gynecologic symptoms include abnormal vaginal bleeding or discharge, pelvic relaxation, coital dysfunction, abdominopelvic pain, and urinary and gastrointestinal tract symptoms. Previous pelvic examinations, genital cytology, obstetric and contraceptive histories, and abdominopelvic operations also provide important data for constructing a thorough gynecologic history.

EXAMINATION

The gynecologic examination is an integral part of the complete physical examination of a woman. Ultrasonic or computed tomography (CT) scans are poor substitutes for a physical examination of the pelvis. The gynecologic examination most conveniently follows the general examination after the patient has emptied her bladder and rectum. This allows optimal palpation of the pelvic organs and improves rapport with the patient.

Basic equipment consists of a table with foot stirrups, an adequate light source, a bivalve speculum, gloves, lubricating jelly, and equipment necessary for obtaining a Papanicolaou smear. Additional useful items include ring forceps with cotton balls, tenaculum, cervical and endometrial biopsy instruments, material for endometrial cytology, cotton swabs with normal saline for vaginal smears, Thayer-Martin culture plates, local anesthetics, instruments for vulvar biopsies, and silver nitrate sticks or Monsell's solution for hemostasis. Lugol's solution and acetic acid are useful for staining the cervix for directed biopsies. A colposcope is invaluable for directing the examination of patients with abnormal cytologic or gross pathologic disorders of the cervix, vagina, or vulva.

The external genitalia are examined and carefully palpated for abnormalities of the mons, labia, clitoris, perianal region, and Bartholin's and vestibular glands. The urethra, perineum, and hymenal ring are carefully palpated. A warm speculum is inserted into the introitus, and the entire vaginal canal and cervix are visualized (Fig. 38-1, *A*). Findings are recorded in relation to the patient's right and left or anterior and posterior. A convenient method of recording cervical lesions is in reference to the face of the clock (e.g., 12 o'clock corresponds to the anterior position and 6 o'clock to the posterior). Papanicolaou smears are obtained from the cervix; both direct smear from the cervical portio and endocervical swab or aspirate are utilized. Any abnormal discharge is sampled for microscopic evaluation. Grossly visible lesions of the vulva, vagina, or cervix are biopsied. The bimanual examination (Fig. 38-1, *B*) is utilized to assess the pelvic structures systematically.

Cervical consistency, mobility, and tenderness with motion are noted first. The uterine position, size, shape, and contour are determined. Each adnexal region is palpated to determine the size and shape of the ovaries and to search for tenderness, masses, or nodularity. Normal fallopian tubes are usually not palpable. Finally, a bidigital rectovaginal examination (Fig. 38-1, *C*) is performed to palpate the posterior aspect of the uterus, adnexal structures, cul-de-sac, and the cardinal and uterosacral ligaments. Stool is tested for occult blood.

Pelvic findings are described in terms of conventional units of measurement (centimeters). The shape, consistency, mobility, and tenderness of the structures are described. Uterine size is usually expressed in terms of gestational size (weeks). Experience in performing the pelvic examination increases the ability to appreciate subtle variations in normal pelvic anatomy and detect pathologic pelvic disorders.

DIAGNOSTIC TESTS AND PROCEDURES
Papanicolaou Test

The Papanicolaou (Pap) test utilizes smears of scrapings of exfoliated cells from the external cervical os and the cervical canal for cytologic evaluation (Fig. 38-2). Smears can also be obtained from the posterior vaginal fornix, directly from lesions of the vagina and vulva, or aspirates or brushings from the endometrial cavity. In general usage, Pap smear refers to endocervical and cervical samples. After microscopic examination, the smear is reported as negative, containing cells suggestive of inflammation, containing atypical cells suggestive of dysplasia, or containing cells consistent with carcinoma. We believe that sexually active women should have an annual pelvic examination including Pap smear, regardless of age. The optimal accuracy rate for detection of invasive cervical carcinoma probably exceeds 90%, but it is less efficient for the detection of endometrial or ovarian carcinoma or other endometrial lesions. A major purpose for obtaining the

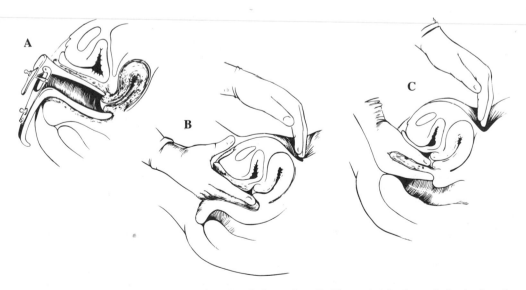

Fig. 38-1. Pelvic examination. **A,** Insertion of vaginal speculum. **B,** Bimanual abdominovaginal palpation of uterus and adnexa. **C,** Bidigital rectovaginal exam (forefinger in vagina and middle finger in rectum).

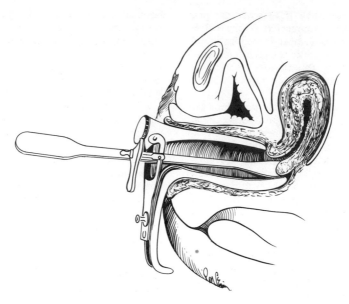

Fig. 38-2. Pap test—cervical scraping smear.

Pap smear is to screen for premalignant cervical lesions (dysplasia and carcinoma in situ), which can be treated conservatively. The management of the patient with an abnormal cervical Pap test is considered in detail later.

Wet Vaginal Smears

Direct microscopic evaluation of a wet-smear vaginal discharge (leukorrhea) often will be diagnostic in determining the cause of vaginitis, as in the following.

Trichomonas vaginitis. A mixture of vaginal discharge and normal saline solution examined immediately under the microscope may reveal motile, flagellated, pear-shaped parasites. The *Trichomonas* is intermediate in size between a white blood cell and an epithelial cell.

Candida vaginitis. One drop of 10% potassium hydroxide solution on the wet prep slide will dissolve squamous epithelium but not yeast forms. The identification of long thin septate hyphae and oval yeast buds is pathognomonic for *Candida*. The vaginal aspirate may be incubated on Nickerson's medium and produces dark brown colonies in a few days.

Bacterial vaginosis. Formerly known as nonspecific vaginitis, this mixed infection of *Gardnerella vaginalis* and anaerobes is diagnosed by identifying multiple white blood cells and bacteria with white blood cells containing intracellular bacteria (clue cells).

Atrophic vaginitis. Few quantified superficial cells and many basal epithelial cells are seen in the wet prep, a feature of estrogen deficiency. Superimposed vaginitis of a different cause may also produce many white blood cells, bacteria, trichomonads, or fungal forms.

Schiller's test. The normal squamous epithelium of the vagina and cervix contains a large amount of glycogen and stains a dark brown when exposed to concentrated iodine solution. Areas that do not stain are abnormal, and the test is considered positive. The Schiller-positive areas may be caused by epithelial ab-

normalities and should be biopsied for histologic analysis. Cervical biopsies usually require no anesthesia, and vaginal biopsies may be performed with a small amount of local anesthetic. In the past, this test was utilized to evaluate abnormal Pap smears but has been largely replaced by colposcopy.

Colposcopy

(See discussion of evaluation of abnormal Pap smear, page 514.)

Pregnancy Tests

Pregnancy tests are biologic, immunologic, and radioimmunologic assays that detect portions of human chorionic gonadotropin (hCG). Biologic assays have been replaced by immunologic and radioimmunologic assays. Radioimmunologic assays for hCG may become positive 6 or 7 days after ovulation at the time of implantation of the fertilized ovum. Less sensitive latex agglutination inhibition tests of urine are reliable approximately 2 weeks after the first missed menstrual period.

Dilation and Curettage (D&C) and Endometrial Biopsy

Cervical dilation with separate endocervical and endometrial curettage (fractional D&C) is both a diagnostic and therapeutic procedure. It is utilized in the evaluation of abnormal, most frequently postmenopausal or perimenopausal, vaginal bleeding. The D&C is most adequately performed under general anesthesia. After examination under anesthesia the endocervical canal is curetted, the uterine cavity is sounded, and the endocervical canal is dilated. The endometrial cavity is explored for polyps with forceps, and endometrial curettage is performed. Specimens are submitted separately for histologic evaluation.

Endometrial biopsy or aspirate is a simple outpatient

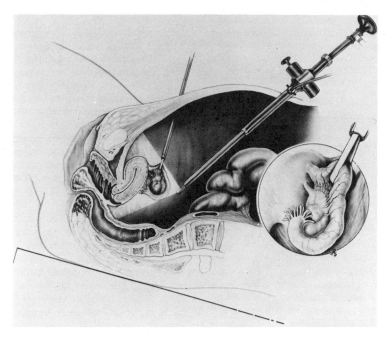

Fig. 38-3. Laparoscopy showing laparoscope and grasping forceps. Inset shows placement for tubal sterilization by coagulation.

procedure that can be utilized as the initial diagnostic test for evaluation of women with abnormal uterine bleeding. It is more than 90% accurate in the diagnosis of endometrial carcinoma when compared to D&C. However, negative endometrial biopsy results must be confirmed by D&C in women with perimenopausal or postmenopausal bleeding who have persistent symptoms.

Laparoscopy

The laparoscope is used to visualize pelvic organs and perform simple operative procedures. General anesthesia is usually required. The peritoneal cavity is insufflated with carbon dioxide through a verres needle, and the laparoscopic trochar is introduced through a small periumbilical incision. A fiberoptic light source is passed through the trochar sheath, and pelvic and abdominal contents are visualized (Fig. 38-3). Often a probe or instrument is introduced through a second suprapubic incision. Simple surgical procedures such as tubal sterilization may be performed through the laparoscope. The incidence of complications decreases with operator experience, but many severe complications from this seemingly minor surgical procedure have been reported. Some indications, operative procedures, complications, and contraindications of laparoscopy are listed below:

Indications
  Pelvic pain
  Infertility
  Suspected ectopic pregnancy or pelvic inflammatory disease
  Selected genital anomalies and amenorrhea
Operative procedures
  Tubal sterilization
  Lysis of adhesions
  Fulguration of endometriosis

Evaluation for residual carcinoma after primary therapy of ovarian carcinoma
Complications
  Hemorrhage, hematoma, large vessel injury
  Bowel perforation
  Electrical burns
  Gas embolism
  Cardiorespiratory problems
  Infection
  Anesthetic complications
Contraindications
  Peritonitis
  Ileus
  Abdominopelvic mass or ascites
  Aortic aneurysm
  Failed pneumoperitoneum
  Ventral hernia
  Previous abdominal surgery (relative)

INFECTIONS AND BENIGN DISORDERS OF THE LOWER GENITAL TRACT AND VULVA

Vulva

Vulvar Dystrophy

Vulvar lesions may be elevated or flat, white, hyperpigmented, or erythematous and are associated with changes caused by chronic irritation such as fissures, weeping, lichenification, ulceration, and excoriation. Pruritus and discomfort are the main symptoms. Since gross appearances are rarely diagnostic, biopsies should be made of all abnormalities with local anesthesia to exclude carcinoma in situ or invasive carcinoma. Colposcopic examination of the vulva or evaluation of the vulva with toluidine blue staining may help to direct biopsies.

Lesions of the vulva have been described by a variety of confusing terms in the past. Classification of these disorders has been simplified to take into account both atrophic and hypertrophic changes resulting from disordered epithelial growth:

1. Vulvar dystrophies
   a. Hyperplastic dystrophy
      (1) Without atypia
      (2) With atypia
   b. Atrophic dystrophy (lichen sclerosis)
   c. Mixed dystrophy
      (1) Without atypia
      (2) With atypia
2. Vulvar atypia (with or without dystrophy)
   a. Mild
   b. Moderate
   c. Severe

Benign vulvar dystrophy may be treated conservatively with improved local hygiene, treatment of coexistent vaginitis, and topical medications. Hyperplastic dystrophies are best treated with topical corticosteroids. Topical 2% testosterone proprionate in a petroleum base is effective treatment of lichen sclerosis. Mixed lesions may require both topical agents. Treatment with testosterone preparations may result in clitoral growth, hirsutism, and increased libido as a result of systemic absorption. Atypical and carcinomatous lesions require special therapy as discussed later.

Bartholin's Cyst

Bartholin's gland cysts result from inflammation and infection of the Bartholin's gland and occlusion of Bartholin's duct. When the cyst is infected, an extremely painful and tender Bartholin's abscess should be incised and drained. After treatment of acute inflammation, the cyst may be totally excised or marsupialized to form a new duct opening. Any Bartholin's cyst in a menopausal woman should be biopsied to exclude a rare adenocarcinoma arising in Bartholin's gland.

Vagina

Trichomonas Vaginitis

The trichomonad is a venereally transmitted parasite. The diagnosis of *Trichomonas* vaginitis is confirmed by visualization of the organism on wet smear. Patients complain of a thin, irritating, malodorous vaginal discharge. Metronidazole is the treatment of choice. Both the patient and sexual partner need simultaneous treatment, since the male is often an asymptomatic carrier. Metronidazole is contraindicated in pregnancy because of the risk of congenital malformation. Topical vaginal medications such as furazolidone or diiodohydroxyquin may be used during pregnancy.

Candidal Vaginitis

Candidal (formerly monilial) vaginitis is seen frequently in patients who are pregnant, diabetic, immunosuppressed, or taking oral contraceptives or broad-spectrum antibiotics. The vaginal discharge resembles cottage cheese and may cause a severe erythematous vulvovaginitis. Topical imodazole antifungal agents or nystatin are the treatment of choice. Occasionally, patients may require treatment with topical gentian violet painting of the entire vaginal wall.

Atrophic Vaginitis

Estrogen deficiency in postmenopausal or surgically castrate women results in thinning of the vaginal mucosa. This predisposes to infection, synechial formation, and symptoms of pruritus without significant discharge. The atrophic epithelium is susceptible to coital injury. Associated atrophy of the bladder epithelium may produce symptoms of cystitis. Systemic or local estrogen therapy is the treatment of choice and will alleviate systemic symptoms of estrogen deficiency simultaneously. Topical estrogen cream is absorbed systemically across the vaginal mucosa and should not be considered "topical" treatment only.

Bacterial Vaginosis

Formerly known as nonspecific vaginitis, bacterial vaginosis is a mixed infection caused by *Gardnerella vaginalis* and anaerobic bacteria. It is the most common vaginal infection. The symptoms are leukorrhea and vaginal odor. Topical therapy with sulfonamide-containing cream is ineffective. Metronidazole systemic therapy is the treatment of choice; however, bacterial vaginosis frequently recurs.

Vulvovaginitis in Children

A common cause of a purulent or bloody vaginal discharge in children is a vaginal foreign body. Often, a vaginal foreign object can be palpated on rectal examination or detected on plain film of the abdomen. Urethroscopic examination of the vagina is valuable and manual extraction of the foreign object can frequently be performed without anesthesia. Pinworm infestation may also cause vulvovaginal discharge and pruritus. Rarely, a gonococcal infection of the vagina can cause a purulent vaginal discharge. When a gonococcal infection is diagnosed, the child should be evaluated for sexual abuse. Another common cause of vaginal discharge is bacterial infection resulting from poor hygiene.

Gartner's Duct Cyst

Gartner's duct cysts arise in the lateral vaginal wall from wolffian duct remnants. These are frequently asymptomatic. Total excision for histologic assessment is recommended.

Vaginal Changes from Diethylstilbestrol

Several gross and microscopic changes of the upper vagina and cervix have been noticed in female offspring of mothers who received diethylstilbestrol (DES) or other estrogen during early pregnancy. These changes include vaginal adenosis, cervical erosion, and malformations of the vaginal fornices and cervical shape. These changes are not necessarily related to clear cell carcinoma of the vagina and cervix, which may also develop in children exposed in utero to DES. Initial evaluation of women with a history of exposure to DES should include complete physical evaluation with colposcopy and cytological smears from the cervix and upper vagina. The vaginal tube should be carefully palpated to detect any abnormal masses. Women exposed in utero to DES have an increased incidence of abnormalities of the uterine cavity, which may predispose to infertility or pregnancy loss.

Fistulas

Rectovaginal, vesicovaginal, and urethrovaginal fistulas may result from obstetric and surgical trauma, carcinoma, and pelvic radiation. Enterovaginal fistulas generally occur after radiation therapy. Traumatically induced fistulas are surgically repaired several months after fistula formation to allow resolution of inflammation. Total parenteral nutrition will maintain adequate nutrition while the small bowel is put to rest preoperatively. Occasionally an enterovaginal fistula will close during nutritional support therapy. A temporary colostomy may be required for colovaginal and rectovaginal fistulas. Fistulas resulting from radiation therapy often require repair with a vascularized pedicle transposed into the defect to allow healing. Larger postradiation fistulas or enterovaginal fistulas require diversion of the urinary or gastrointestinal tract.

Cervix

Cervicitis

The majority of sexually active women develop some degree of infection involving the columnar epithelium of the endocervical canal. This may become prominent if the squamocolumnar junction is located on the ectocervix with an eversion of the columnar epithelium. Most often, cervical eversions are asymptomatic but occasionally they produce a malodorous, mucopurulent discharge. Cytologic screening should be utilized. Sexually transmitted diseases such as gonorrhea and chlamydia are common causes of mucopurulent cervicitis. Screening tests are recommended for these diseases. Tetracycline is the best antibiotic therapy.

BENIGN DISEASES OF THE UTERUS
Leiomyomas (Fibroids)

Leiomyomas are benign tumors of smooth muscle origin arising from the myometrium. Leiomyomas are, to a certain extent, hormonally responsive. The highest incidence of leiomyomas is found in blacks and nulligravidas and during the later years of reproductive life. The majority of leiomyomas regress after menopause. Leiomyomas may remain confined to the uterine wall (intramural) or may bulge into the endometrial cavity (submucosal) or peritoneal cavity (subserosal). Subserosal fibroids may extend into the broad ligament (intraligamentous) or become pedunculated. Rarely, they may draw blood supply from adjacent tissues with regression of the uterine blood supply (parasitic). Less than 10% arise from the cervix. Benign degenerative changes of hemorrhage, calcification, or liquefaction are frequently seen. Leiomyosarcomas develop in less than 1% of uterine leiomyomas.

Clinical manifestations of leiomyomas include crampy menstrual pain, excessive menstrual or intermenstrual bleeding, and symptoms of pelvic pressure. Occasionally degenerative changes may cause enlargement or acute pelvic pain. Rarely, a fibroid may impede labor and delivery during pregnancy. Uterine leiomyomas are usually diagnosed by pelvic examination. A pedunculated subserosal fibroid may mimic an adnexal mass.

The majority of uterine fibroids are small and asymptomatic and require no therapy. Most gynecologists recommend that a fibroid uterus larger than a gesta-tional size of 12 weeks should be removed to exclude the possibility of uterine sarcoma or ovarian neoplasia. Total abdominal hysterectomy is indicated if the patient has significant symptoms of pelvic pain, develops significant anemia from menorrhagia, or has ureteral obstruction. Occasionally, leiomyomas can be "shelled out" (myomectomy) if they appear to cause infertility.

Adenomyosis

Adenomyosis is occasionally referred to as endometriosis interna. It is characterized by projections of endometrial tissue deep into the myometrium. Microscopically, this appears as diffuse or localized areas of endometrial glands and stroma interdigitated between normal myometrium. The symptoms and signs are menorrhagia, progressive dysmenorrhea, and an enlarged, softened uterus. Adenomyosis is most frequently seen in multiparous women during the fifth decade of life. The diagnosis is usually made after hysterectomy is performed to relieve symptoms.

Endometriosis

Endometriosis is characterized by hormonally responsive endometrial tissue implants in extrauterine sites. Most common sites for endometriosis are the ovaries, peritoneal surfaces of the pelvis including the uterosacral ligaments, cul-de-sac, and posterior part of the uterus, and occasionally the fallopian tubes (Fig. 38-4). Less common sites are the bowel, umbilicus, cervix, external genitalia, abdominal and episiotomy scars, and, rarely, distant sites such as the lungs. Probably the most common mechanism responsible for the development of endometriosis is retrograde menstruation through the fallopian tubes. More distant implants of endometriosis are presumably from lymphatic or hematogenous dissemination.

Endometriosis is usually not detected in teenage women. The disease may progress throughout reproductive years but usually disappears after menopause. While the classic symptom complex includes progressive dysmenorrhea, dyspareunia, or cyclic bowel and bladder pain, many patients who present with infertility but little or no pain in their late twenties or early thirties have endometriosis.

Physical examination may reveal tenderness and nodularity of the cul-de-sac and uterosacral ligaments, retroflexion and fixation of the uterus, ovarian enlargement, or nonspecific pelvic tenderness.

Although the diagnosis is suggested by history and physical examination, laparoscopy is generally required for a diagnosis. Typical endometriosis implants have a "powder-burn" appearance, although chocolate cysts can develop from larger deep-seated implants within the ovaries. Differential diagnosis includes pelvic inflammatory disease, uterine leiomyomas, and other causes of adnexal mass.

Regression of endometriosis often occurs during pregnancy. Hormonal manipulation such as combination oral contraceptives may be appropriate for mild endometriosis. For more severe cases, a pseudopregnancy regimen consisting of increasing doses of combination progestin-estrogen alone is used to cause amenorrhea for 6 to 9 months. Side effects may include weight gain, fluid retention, nausea, and breakthrough bleed-

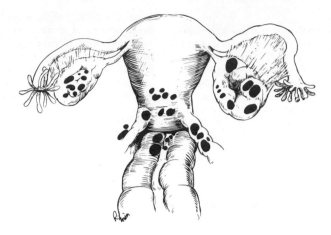

Fig. 38-4. Common sites of pelvic endometriosis.

ing. Hormonal manipulation is generally not curative but may result in sufficient atrophy of endometriosis to provide relief of symptoms. Danazol is an androgen with antigonadal activity that produces regression of endometrial tissue by suppressing gonadotropins and ovarian steroid output. Side effects are those of a weak androgen. While these medical regimens give good pain relief in a majority of patients, fertility rates following medical therapy of endometriosis are discouraging. The chance of conception per menstrual cycle is at most only slightly improved when medical therapy alone is compared to no therapy for endometriosis.

For more severe endometriosis, conservative surgical therapy does improve the per cycle rate of conception modestly. For these patients, preoperative treatment for 3 to 6 months with medical therapy for endometriosis does seem to make conservative resection operations technically easier. These conservative operations often include excision or fulguration of peritoneal implants, resection of ovarian endometriomas, lysis of adhesions, suspensions of the uterus and ovaries, and occasionally presacral neurectomy for relief of pain. When symptomatic endometriosis exists and fertility is no longer desirable, appropriate treatment is total abdominal hysterectomy with bilateral salpingo-oophorectomy. Retention of an ovary will result in a 25% to 30% recurrence of endometriosis, but residual endometriosis is rarely stimulated by exogenous hormone replacement.

PELVIC INFLAMMATORY DISEASE AND VENEREAL DISEASES
Gonorrhea

Gonorrhea is one of the most common communicable bacterial diseases, with an estimated 1 to 3 million cases per year. It is epidemic among men and women in the 16- to 24-year age group.

Although most males develop symptoms of urethritis, approximately 80% of women are clinically asymptomatic. Most of these asymptomatic carriers will have complaints of vaginal discharge or mild urethritis. The gonoccoccus invades columnar and transitional epithelium. The most common sites of infection in females are endocervical canal, urethra, Bartholin's and Skene's glands, and the rectum. Gonococcal pharyngitis is also a form of uncomplicated gonococcal infection. Approximately 15% to 25% of patients with untreated gonorrhea develop complications, including pelvic inflammatory disease (PID) and disseminated gonococcemia with septic arthritis and meningitis.

Culture of the endocervical canal is most effective for screening asymptomatic persons. Ideally, cultures should be obtained from the endocervix, urethra, oral pharynx, and rectum in symptomatic patients or patients with a history of exposure. The gonococcus is a fastidious organism requiring a high carbon dioxide content and special culture medium (Thayer-Martin medium). Despite the emergence of relative penicillin-resistant strains and penicillinase-producing strains of gonorrhea, aqueous procaine penicillin G remains the treatment of choice for uncomplicated gonorrhea. One half hour before treatment, 1 gram of probenecid is given orally to decrease renal excretion of penicillin. Aqueous procaine penicillin G, 4.8 million units, is then given intramuscularly (this will also treat incubating syphilis). Alternatively, a large dose of ampicillin or amoxicillin may be given as a one-time oral treatment. Tetracycline, spectinomycin, or erythromycin is used in patients who are allergic to penicillin. After treatment of uncomplicated gonorrhea, cultures are repeated. Antibiotic sensitivity testing is done to rule out penicillinase-producing gonorrhea or reinfection if cultures are positive. Resistant gonorrhea can be treated with spectinomycin, cefoxitin, or cefotaxime.

PID

PID is a spectrum of infections involving the uterus, tubes, and ovaries along with the pelvic peritoneum. In the United States, approximately 30% to 80% are associated with gonococcal infections. *Chlamydia trachomatis* may be isolated from 30% to 50% of salpingitis cases. The majority of cases of PID will have several pathogenic aerobic and anaerobic bacteria isolated from the fallopian tubes. Pelvic tuberculosis is rarely a cause of PID.

Frequently PID is caused by an ascending infection occurring at the time of menses when the cervical mucous barrier is breeched. Patients usually present with

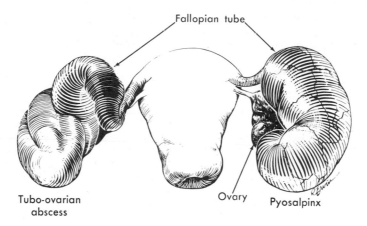

Fig. 38-5. Chronic pelvic inflammatory disease. On biological right, tubo-ovarian abscess. On biological left, pyosalpinx.

pelvic pain and fever. The clinical diagnosis of PID is made in a patient with symptoms, signs, and laboratory findings of acute pelvic peritonitis. The uterus and cervix are exquisitely tender to motion. Bilateral adnexal tenderness is present and tubal enlargement or bilateral adnexal masses may be palpated. Differential diagnosis includes other acute abdominal infections such as appendicitis, diverticulitis, pyelonephritis, and cystitis. Laparoscopy will aid in the early diagnosis of pelvic inflammatory disease.

Treatment is by broad-spectrum antibiotics. Patients should be treated with regimens that will be curative for gonococcus and also cover anaerobic bacteria. Clinical response usually occurs in 1 to 3 days, but antibiotics are continued for 7 to 10 days after the disappearance of fever. Frequent evaluation including pelvic examination during therapy is necessary to detect pelvic abscesses. Aggressive management of acute PID is mandatory to preserve tubal patency and fertility.

Before the advent of broad-spectrum antibiotics, pelvic abscesses were frequently drained vaginally through the posterior cul-de-sac. The development of a tuboovarian or cul-de-sac abscess refractory to antibiotic therapy will require surgical removal and drainage. Traditionally, this has entailed total abdominal hysterectomy with bilateral salpingo-oophorectomy. However, some patients may be selected for more conservative resection of unilateral abscesses in an attempt to preserve fertility.

Repeated episodes of acute PID lead to chronic PID (Fig. 38-5), characterized by tubal destruction and formation of hydrosalpinx or pyosalpinx, tubo-ovarian abscess, and chronic tubal adhesions. Patients with chronic PID may develop chronic pelvic pain, recurrent fever, and infertility. Although conservative tuboplasty may be employed to preserve fertility, the majority of patients with chronic PID and pelvic pain require total abdominal hysterectomy with bilateral salpingo-oophorectomy for definitive treatment.

Occasionally, patients with gonococcal or chlamydial PID develop an acute perihepatic peritoneal inflammation (Fitz-Hugh and Curtis syndrome). Rarely, this syndrome may be mistaken for acute cholecystitis. Occasionally, such patients require lysis of "violin-string" adhesions between the diaphragm and liver for treatment of chronic right upper quadrant pain.

Other Venereal Diseases

Other venereal diseases include syphilis, herpes progenitalis, chlamydial infections, condyloma accuminata, and the less common diseases of chancroid, lymphogranuloma venereum, and granuloma inguinale.

Syphilis is much less common than gonorrhea. The causative organism, *Treponema pallidum,* is a spirochete that can be demonstrated by dark-field microscopy of luetic lesions. The primary stage is characterized by an infectious hard chancre and secondary stage by generalized rash, systemic symptoms, and mucocutaneous patches. Tertiary lues may involve the central nervous system, cardiovascular system, and soft tissues. History, dark-field microscopy, serologic tests (RPR, VDRL), and clinical manifestations of tertiary lues establish the diagnosis. Penicillin remains the antibiotic of choice.

Herpes progenitalis is caused by the herpes simplex virus types I and II. Approximately 3 to 5 million new cases occur each year in the United States. Manifestations of primary herpes include painful vesicles on an erythematous base that involve the lower genital tract. Other symptoms include fever, inguinal lymphadenopathy, and urinary retention. Disseminated herpes virus infection or aseptic meningitis are rare manifestations. After a primary herpes infection, the virus enters into a latent phase of infection where viral particles can be demonstrated in the lumbosacral dorsal nerve root ganglia. Secondary recurrences are frequently observed, though the manifestations are generally not so severe as during the primary infection. Systemic acyclovir is effective in reducing the duration and severity of the symptoms of primary herpes. Oral acyclovir may reduce the frequency and severity of recurrent symptoms in patients who have frequent exacerbations. Otherwise, therapy is by use of analgesics, sitz baths, and other symptomatic measures.

The exact incidence of significant chlamydial infections of the genital tract is unknown because of insufficient culture techniques. *Chlamydia* species may cause symptomatic infections of the cervix, endometrium, fallopian tubes, urethra, and bladder. Previously, chlamydial urethritis was recognized as sterile nonspecific urethritis after successful eradication of gonorrhea. Treatment of choice is tetracycline.

Toxic shock syndrome (TSS). This syndrome is a spectrum of multisystem diseases mainly affecting menstruating women and is associated with vaginal infection with *Staphylococcus aureus.* The majority of affected women are tampon users. Clinical manifestations of TSS include fever, orthostatic hypotension, and rash in association with multisystem signs and symptoms. Patients may develop nausea and vomiting, diarrhea, myalgias, mucous membrane ulceration, renal or hepatic failure, thrombocytopenia, or neurologic symptoms. Treatment is by aggressive intravenous fluid hydration and β-lactamase-resistant antibiotics. Vasopressors, steroids, dialysis, and artificial ventilation may be required in selected patients. A range of mortality from 2% to 13% has been reported. Patients are at a 20% to 30% risk for a later recurrence. It is recommended that patients who develop TSS have follow-up cultures to ensure that vaginal colonization of *Staphylococcus* has been eradicated. They should discontinue use of tampons indefinitely.

DISORDERS OF PELVIC SUPPORT AND URINARY STRESS INCONTINENCE

Pelvic relaxation commonly results from obstetric trauma with resultant stretching and thinning of the pelvic supporting tissues. Postmenopausal atrophy of hormone-sensitive tissues caused by estrogen deficiency may accentuate pelvic relaxation. A cystocele or urethrocele is caused by weakening of the anterior vesicovaginal fascia so that the bladder and urethra bulge into the vagina. Relaxation of the posterior rectovaginal fascia results in a rectocele. A true hernia of the posterior cul-de-sac may occur through the apex of the vagina or along the rectovaginal septum. This peritoneum-lined sac generally contains loops of small intestine and is termed an enterocele. Relaxation of pelvic supporting tissues is often accompanied by uterine descensus. In its extreme form, the uterus may prolapse through the vaginal introitus. Abnormalities of pelvic support usually coexist.

The descent of the bladder neck and distortion of the normal posterior urethrovesical angle produced by cystocele and urethrocele causes urinary stress incontinence. This is involuntary loss of urine accompanying increased intraabdominal pressure from Valsalva maneuvers such as laughing, coughing, or straining. Stress incontinence must be differentiated from other types of incontinence that cannot be cured by surgical therapy including unstable bladder (detrusor dyssynergia), urgency incontinence produced by cystitis, overflow incontinence from neurogenic bladder, and continuous incontinence from a vesicovaginal fistula. A careful history and physical examination often allow the physician to distinguish these entities. Not infrequently, patients have a combination of anatomic urinary stress incontinence and detrusor dyssynergia. Cystometric and cystoscopic evaluation may help distinguish these entities. Before surgical correction of urinary stress incontinence, patients with mixed disorders should be treated with anticholinergic drugs to determine the true extent of stress incontinence.

Other components of pelvic relaxation may produce symptoms of pelvic pressure. Rectoceles are usually asymptomatic but may cause constipation. Incarcerated enteroceles may rarely produce bowel obstruction and infarction.

The key to surgical management of pelvic relaxation is to identify and correct all components of pelvic relaxation. Frequently, this is best accomplished by the vaginal route: vaginal hysterectomy, cul-de-sac plication, and posterior colporrhaphy correct uterine descensus, enterocele, and rectocele. Restoration of the normal posterior urethrovesical angle can be accomplished vaginally by Kelly plication of the urethrovesical angle and anterior colporrhaphy.

An alternative to the vaginal surgical correction of stress incontinence is retropubic urethropexy, which can be combined with abdominal hysterectomy and vaginal repair of a rectocele. Colpocleisis, obliteration of the vaginal canal, can be used in a small number of patients who are no longer sexually active and who are not candidates for a more definitive operative procedure because of medical complications.

Frequently, patients develop vaginal prolapse with or without associated cystocele or rectocele after a vaginal or abdominal hysterectomy. In the majority of these patients, a small enterocele was not corrected at the time of the primary procedure. Surgical repair includes obliteration of the enterocele and suspension to the sacrospinous ligament as a transvaginal procedure, or transabdominal suspension of the vaginal vault to the sacral periosteum using Marlex mesh.

Some patients will develop recurrent urinary stress incontinence after one or more surgical procedures. These patients may require a combined vaginal and abdominal approach to correct the incontinence. Often a sling of synthetic material or fascia is utilized to support the posterior vesicourethral angle.

ABORTION

Abortion is the spontaneous or induced termination of pregnancy during the first 24 weeks of gestation. Spontaneous abortion usually occurs in the first 12 to 14 weeks of gestation and is frequently caused by a blighted or chromosomally abnormal ovum. Spontaneous abortion is clinically recognized in approximately 15% of gestations, whereas the actual incidence is probably higher. *Threatened abortion* refers to spotting, cramping, or bleeding in early pregnancy without cervical dilation. This may progress to cervical dilation *(inevitable abortion)* or passage of products of conception *(incomplete abortion).* The dilated cervical os predisposes to uterine infection, and bleeding associated with abortion may be sufficient to cause hypovolemic shock. Treatment is by suction D&C to prevent further hemorrhage or infection. Only rarely is complete expulsion of the products of conception *(complete abortion)* observed.

Habitual abortion refers to three consecutive spontaneous abortions, usually occurring in the first trimester. Metabolic disorders such as diabetes and thyroid disease, chronic infection, uterine anomalies, and parental chromosomal anomalies should be excluded in the evaluation of habitual abortion. The majority of causes for habitual abortion are never determined, but a treatable disorder must be ruled out.

Second trimester abortions may result from uterine anatomic anomalies or incompetent cervix. The classical history for incompetent cervix is repetitive painless second-trimester cervical dilation and premature rupture of the amniotic sac or second trimester delivery of an immature fetus after a relatively short labor. Frequently, the pregnancy terminates at an earlier gestational age with each successive pregnancy. Placement of a nonabsorbable encircling suture at the level of the internal cervical os before significant cervical dilation corrects an incompetent cervix. The cerclage should not be placed after labor has begun or after significant cervical dilation or rupture of membranes has occurred, since under these circumstances the chance of success is low and the chance of inducing an infection of the intrauterine contents is high. After attainment of term gestation, the cerclage suture may be removed to allow vaginal delivery or may be left in place and delivery accomplished by cesarean section.

Elective abortion has become more common since liberalization of abortion laws in the early 1970s. Elective abortion is performed by suction D&C in the first trimester. Intraamniotic instillation of saline solution or prostaglandins are often used for second trimester abortions. Dilation and evacuation of the uterine contents (D&E) is also performed in some centers for the elective termination of second-trimester gestations. Although the risk of complications such as uterine perforation increases with gestational age, second trimester D&E is a safe procedure when employed by skilled practitioners.

The legalization of elective abortion has resulted in a lower incidence of septic abortion caused by unsterile termination of pregnancy either by self-manipulation or instrumentation by nonmedical personnel. Septic abortion is a fulminant mixed gram-negative and anaerobic infection of the products of conception, endometrium, and myometrium, a life-threatening emergency that requires aggressive management with broad-spectrum antibiotics, fluid resuscitation, and often vasoactive agents. Uterine evacuation by D&C is necessary after stabilization and initiation of antibiotics. Occasionally hysterectomy may be required to remove infected or necrotic tissues.

ECTOPIC PREGNANCY

Ectopic pregnancy results when a fertilized ovum fails to migrate and implant normally in the endometrial cavity. Most ectopic pregnancies involve the ampullary region of the fallopian tube (95%), but implantation may occur in the isthmic or cornual regions of the tube, on or in the ovary, in the abdominal cavity, or in the endocervical canal. Combined intrauterine and extrauterine pregnancies may rarely coexist. The most common predisposing factor for ectopic pregnancy is salpingitis with resultant tubal agglutination and adhesions. Other factors that mechanically interfere with normal tubal transport of fertilized ovum may cause ectopic implantation, such as endometriosis, adhesions from previous gynecologic or infertility surgery, or tubal ligation. The ectopic implantation site lacks the stroma necessary for normal placental development. Usually, the pregnancy undergoes abortion or the trophoblastic tissue invades into adjacent vessels resulting in hemorrhage. The incidence of ectopic pregnancy has

increased alarmingly in the last 10 years, paralleling an increase in the incidence of gonococcal and nongonococcal salpingitis.

Signs of hemorrhagic shock indicate tubal rupture. Aspiration of the cul-de-sac may yield nonclotting blood indicating intraperitoneal hemorrhage. After stabilization of the patient the ectopic pregnancy must be removed, most frequently by salpingectomy or linear salpingostomy. The ipsilateral ovary is not removed. Elective reconstructive surgery of the contralateral adnexal structures is deferred until hemorrhage and inflammation from the ectopic pregnancy have resolved.

With the employment of serum hCG testing and laparoscopy, unruptured tubal pregnancies are being diagnosed more frequently. Conservative surgical management of unruptured tubal pregnancies includes linear salpingostomy and segmental resection of the involved tube. These procedures may preserve the potential for normal pregnancies in patients with a damaged or absent contralateral tube and do not seem to increase the incidence of repeat ectopic pregnancies compared to salpingectomy. In any event, future prospects for normal pregnancy are limited. Approximately 15% of patients have a second ectopic pregnancy, and only one third have a subsequent normal viable intrauterine pregnancy.

Most often the classical historical and physical findings are absent. The patient may relate episodes of vaginal bleeding interpreted as normal menses and may not have distinct physical findings. Often, routine urinary pregnancy tests are negative because of low-level hCG secretion from the abnormally implanted placenta, but more sensitive serum β-hCG assays are usually positive. Other conditions that must be differentiated from ectopic pregnancy include early threatened abortion, bleeding or pain associated with a functional ovarian cyst, and pelvic inflammatory disease. The laparoscope may be useful in evaluating patients with atypical findings and, coupled with serum hCG assays, may detect unruptured ectopic pregnancies.

BENIGN OVARIAN TUMORS AND ADNEXAL MASSES

The ovary contains many components that can give rise to both benign and malignant neoplasms, functional cysts, and other lesions that simulate ovarian neoplasms (Table 38-1). Additionally, the adnexal regions may contain masses related to uterine, tubal, or bowel diseases. Therefore the management of an adnexal mass is aimed at exclusion of ovarian or tubal malignancy, prevention of acute complications of benign neoplasms (torsion or rupture), and avoidance of surgical intervention for benign functional events associated with the menstrual cycle. Functional cysts of the follicle or corpus luteum are frequently found in menstruating women. They rarely exceed 5 cm in diameter or persist for more than one menstrual cycle. Benign epithelial neoplasms occur during or after reproductive years. Cystic mature teratomas (dermoid cysts) are the most common ovarian germ cell tumor. They may contain tissue from all germinal cell layers: endoderm, mesoderm, and ectoderm. Teeth, hair, and a thick, greasy sebaceous material are frequently present in the cyst. Occasionally, calcifications resembling teeth may be detected on a plain film of the pelvis, which is a finding

Table 38-1. Histogenic Classification of Ovarian Tumors

Epithelial	Serous
	Mucinous
	Endometrioid
	Brenner
Germ cell	Dysgerminoma
	Teratoma
	Immature
	Mature
	Endodermal sinus
	Embryonal carcinoma
	Choriocarcinoma
	Gonadoblastoma
	Mixed forms
Sex cord-stromal	Granulosa
	Theca
	Sertoli-Leydig
Miscellaneous	Lymphoma
	Sarcoma
	Metastatic tumors

indicative of a benign dermoid cyst. Ovarian stromal neoplasms may produce either estrogen or androgen and systemic symptoms related to hormonal excess. Other conditions may produce an adnexal mass indistinguishable from an ovarian mass and include endometriosis, hydrosalpinx, pedunculated leiomyomas or paraovarian cysts. Nongynecologic conditions such as chronic appendicitis and diverticulitis may also give rise to adnexal masses.

Often benign causes of adnexal mass cannot be distinguished clinically from malignancy. The management of an adnexal mass depends on the patient's age and findings on pelvic examination. Asymptomatic, smooth, cystic adnexal masses less than 7 or 8 cm in a woman of reproductive age may safely be followed with serial pelvic examination for one or two menstrual cycles. Persistent masses, masses greater than 8 cm in diameter, or masses associated with ascites must be further evaluated and require surgical exploration with extirpation. Any ovarian enlargement in premenarcheal or postmenopausal women is abnormal and should prompt surgical intervention.

Preoperative evaluation includes routine laboratory blood studies, intravenous pyelography to evaluate the location of the ureters, and chest film. Data from barium enema and upper gastrointestinal series should be obtained if the patient has significant gastrointestinal symptoms. A pelvic ultrasound scan may be helpful if the patient is obese and examination unsatisfactory or if intrauterine pregnancy is suspected. In general, ultrasound is not more accurate than a careful pelvic examination in determining the size, location, or consistency of adnexal masses and does *not* yield a histologic diagnosis. A few patients may be evaluated with laparoscopy to determine whether surgical extirpation is required, but most patients should undergo exploratory laparotomy through a midline incision to allow surgical removal and staging of a possible ovarian malignancy.

CONGENITAL ANOMALIES
Vaginal Anomalies

An imperforate hymen or a transverse vaginal septum may result from failure of the urogenital sinus to fuse with the mullerian duct systems. These anomalies are usually detected after menarche when accumulation of menstrual flow collects above the obstruction causing pain and an abdominopelvic mass. Patients with these anomalies must be distinguished from those with other causes of primary amenorrhea because surgical removal of the septum is curative.

Congenital absence of the upper two thirds of the vagina often coexists with an absent or anomalous uterus and normal ovaries. Infrequently a normal uterus, cervix, and small segment of upper vagina are present. Since there is no prospect for normal fertility if the cervix is absent, the major therapeutic goal is creation of a functional vagina. At the time of sexual maturity, a space is created surgically between the bladder and rectum and lined with a split-thickness skin graft sutured around a vaginal mold. The vaginal mold is removed postoperatively, and the vaginal canal is kept patent through sexual activity and mechanical dilation. An alternative to surgical creation of a neovagina is the Frank method of progressive elongation of the rudimentary vaginal dimple using pressure with silicone rubber dilators. If a relatively normal cervix and uterus is lacking, the uterus and tubal structures should be removed to prevent reflux menstruation and development of endometriosis.

Total absence of the ovaries, tubes, uterus, and vagina is rare. Testicular feminization (androgen-insensitivity syndrome) should be suspected and gonads removed if the patient has a male (46, XY) karyotype.

Uterine Anomalies

The fallopian tubes, uterus, cervix, and upper vagina are created by fusion of the paired mullerian ducts. Failure of fusion can result in a wide spectrum of anomalies ranging from a uterus with a small intrauterine septum in the upper fundus to complete duplication with separate uterine horns, cervices, and vaginas. An isolated vaginal septum may exist. These anomalies may cause no problems or may result in repeated abortions, premature labor, or infertility. If a uterine septum is the cause of repeated pregnancy wastage or infertility, the uterus may be reunified surgically by excision of the septum. A vaginal septum should be removed to prevent difficulties with delivery. In all anomalies of the female reproductive tract except for an imperforate hymen, a preoperative intravenous pyelogram should be performed to rule out frequently associated urinary tract malformations.

PREMENSTRUAL SYNDROME

Although clinically recognized for many years, premenstrual syndrome (PMS) remains an inadequately defined and poorly understood spectrum of symptoms associated with the luteal phase of the menstrual cycle. A large segment of the female population is affected by this syndrome in one form or another. Clinical manifestations of premenstrual syndrome include cyclic headache, breast swelling and tenderness, abdominal bloating, fluid retention, mood alterations, skin eruptions, and gastrointestinal symptoms. Symptoms usually worsen during the second half of the menstrual cycle and abate after menstruation begins. Symptoms vary greatly in severity ranging from mild to incapacitating. Many causes have been proposed for premenstrual syndrome, including estrogen excess, progesterone deficiency, vitamin deficiency, and neuroendocrine abnormalities. Since the cause is poorly understood and the spectrum of illness encompasses many symptoms, it is understandable that a variety of different therapies are employed in the management of this syndrome. Oral contraceptives, vaginal progestin, diuretics, and analgesics may provide relief of some of the symptoms of premenstrual syndrome for selected women.

DYSMENORRHEA

Primary dysmenorrhea is defined as pain with menstruation in the absence of a definite cause (e.g., endometriosis). Symptoms are cramping pelvic pain beginning immediately before or at the onset of menses and gradually decreasing over several days after the onset of menstruation. Primary dysmenorrhea is most commonly observed in younger women and may improve after pregnancy or with the use of oral contraceptives. Since the syndrome is caused by production of local prostaglandins, prostaglandin synthetase inhibitors (e.g., indomethacin) have been successfully used in treating primary dysmenorrhea. Persistent dysmenorrhea despite an adequate trial of prostaglandin synthetase inhibitors or abnormalities detected on serial pelvic examinations warrant further investigation to rule out other causes of pelvic pain and dysmenorrhea.

PELVIC PAIN

The symptom of pelvic pain may result from many organic and functional causes. Initial evaluation of the patient with pelvic pain of short duration should be directed toward ruling out acute organic disease. Managing the patient with chronic pelvic pain requires patience and diligence to determine the cause. Frequently psychiatric counseling is helpful in determining psychological causes for pelvic pain. Often, laparoscopy is required to exclude organic pelvic disease and to reassure the patient who requires long-term psychiatric therapy. Without clear organic cause, surgical removal of the uterus and ovaries rarely resolves these chronic pelvic symptoms.

GYNECOLOGIC ONCOLOGY

Vulvar Intraepithelial Neoplasia

Vulvar dysplasia, carcinoma in situ, and Paget's disease of the vulva are intraepithelial proliferative vulvar diseases. Vulvar dysplasia and carcinoma in situ are squamous vulvar intraepithelial neoplasias (VIN) similar in histologic appearance to cervical and vaginal intraepithelial neoplasias. The lesions of VIN generally occur in younger women than frankly invasive vulvar carcinoma. Lower genital intraepithelial neoplasias coexist at multiple sites in approximately 25% of cases. Recent evidence indicates a strong association with infection by subtypes of the human papilloma virus subtypes, although these have not been proven as causative agents.

Carcinoma in situ and VIN may appear as raised, white or hyperpigmented lesions. They may be asymptomatic but often cause discomfort or pruritus. Lesions of VIN are often multifocal and often involve perianal skin. Paget's disease of the vulva has a similar gross appearance to Paget's disease of the breast, often presenting as an erythematous pruritic plaque. Histologi-

cally, Paget's disease is characterized by large polygonal clear cells infiltrating through the epidermis. Normal-looking skin is frequently involved beyond the visible margins of the lesion. Unlike Paget's disease of the breast, the vulvar lesion is infrequently associated with an underlying malignancy of the apocrine glands. Since many lesions of the vulva have similar gross appearances and carcinoma in situ is frequently associated with invasive carcinoma, biopsy should be used liberally to establish the diagnosis and exclude invasion. Toluidine blue staining or colposcopy may aid in directing biopsies. Wide local excision is the therapy of choice. In multifocal disease, a skinning vulvectomy with split-thickness skin grafting of the operative bed maintains normal vulvar appearance and clitoral function. Laser vaporization of VIN also has excellent cosmetic and functional results although no specimen is available for histologic study. Therefore liberal biopsy is indicated before performing laser vaporization to rule out invasion. Topical 5-fluorouracil cream is an alternate therapy that is usually poorly tolerated by patients owing to a high incidence of local irritation. Despite apparently adequate therapy, these lesions have a high recurrence rate and patients should be closely followed for life.

Invasive Vulvar Carcinoma

Invasive vulvar carcinomas account for 4% of all female genital malignancies. A rising incidence of vulvar carcinoma has been observed recently and parallels increased life expectancy. The average age of patients with invasive vulvar carcinoma is in the midsixties; the majority are over 60 years of age.

Although this disease occurs on the body surface and is amenable to early diagnosis, many patients delay seeking treatment because of false modesty or a reluctance to undergo pelvic examination. Physician delay caused by treatment of vulvar lesions without biopsy is unfortunately also common. Because of the advanced age of patients with vulvar cancer, many have associated medical diseases such as diabetes, hypertension, and cardiovascular disease. Approximately 25% of patients have second primaries, most frequently carcinoma of the cervix.

Symptoms and Diagnosis

The initial lesion is usually a small nodule that eventually enlarges and ulcerates. Occasionally the carcinoma may mimic a condyloma in appearance. Pruritus and discomfort are frequent symptoms. The majority of lesions arise on the labia majora (Fig. 38-6). The diagnosis is established by either incisional or excisional biopsy. Small lesions may be completely excised under local anesthesia for assessment of the depth of invasion. Biopsy should be obtained from the worst-appearing portion of any vulvar lesion.

Approximately 85% to 90% of vulvar malignancies are well-differentiated squamous cell carcinoma; melanoma, sarcoma, and adenocarcinoma are less common.

Pattern of Spread and Treatment

Vulvar carcinoma is usually indolent, locally invasive, and metastasizes primarily through the lymphatics. Lymphatic drainage begins with interconnecting subepithelial and subdermal plexuses that form larger

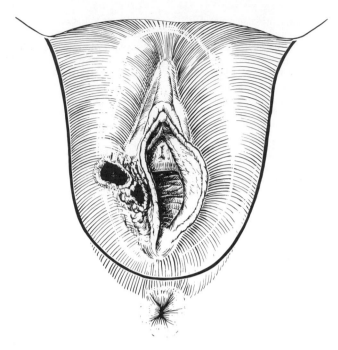

Fig. 38-6. Gross appearance of vulvar carcinoma. *Solid line,* Perineal resection margin of radical vulvectomy.

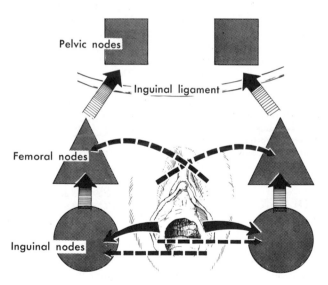

Fig. 38-7. Lymphatic dissemination of vulvar carcinoma. *Solid arrows,* Most common routes; *broken arrows,* less common routes.

subcutaneous channels that drain to the superficial inguinal and femoral lymph nodes. The channels run anterolaterally, medial to the labiocrural fold, and do not extend into the thigh. Lymph node involvement is usually orderly, with initial involvement of the superficial inguinal nodes located above the cribriform fascia before involvement of the femoral and finally external iliac nodes (Fig. 38-7). Cloquet's node is the last node of the deep femoral group: pelvic nodal involvement is rarely seen without involvement of Cloquet's node. Although lymphatics from the clitoris may drain directly

to the deep pelvic lymph nodes, the clinical significance of this route of drainage appears to be minimal.

Surgical management of invasive vulvar carcinoma is based on the lymphatic drainage of the vulva. Historically the treatment of choice has been dissection en block or radical vulvectomy with inguinal and femoral lymphadenectomies (Fig. 38-8). This removes the mons, clitoris, labia, and underlying tissues to the periosteum of the symphysis, the efferent lymphatics, and both primary and secondary lymph nodes. With this therapy, 5-year survival rate for early vulvar carcinoma

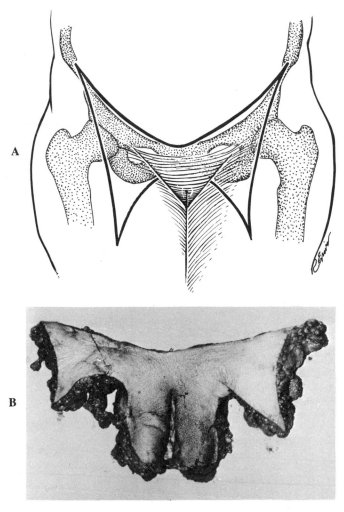

Fig. 38-8. A, Marshall incision for radical vulvectomy and bilateral groin dissection. **B,** Radical vulvectomy specimen with en bloc dissection of vulva, efferent lymphatics, and groin.

is approximately 90%. If femoral lymph nodes are involved, the operation can be extended to include a deep pelvic lymphadenectomy or the patient may be treated with whole pelvic radiation therapy. As expected, the morbidity from this procedure is significant: wound breakdowns are frequent and removal of the deep femoral lymph nodes often results in significant chronic lymphedema of the extremity.

An alternative approach to the surgical therapy of small(<2 cm) early invasive vulvar carcinoma is the combination of bilateral superficial inguinal lymphadenectomy with wide local excision of the vulvar lesion. The superficial inguinal nodes are submitted for immediate frozen-section analysis, and a radical vulvectomy with complete inguinal and femoral lymphadenectomies is performed if metastases are present. For properly selected patients, this procedure would appear to reduce the morbidity without significantly compromising survival. Occasionally, patients will have extensive disease involving the vagina or rectum, and exenterative surgery or radiation therapy may be required.

The survival of patients with vulvar carcinoma mirrors lymphatic involvement. Early vulvar carcinoma without regional metastases has a 5-year survival of approximately 90%, which is reduced to approximately 40% when regional lymph nodes are involved. Only 20% of paitents with positive pelvic nodes survive 5 years or more.

Evaluation of Abnormal Pap Smear

The cervix and lower genital tract of the female are uniquely accessible for direct observation and cytologic screening. Data from several studies indicate that premalignant lesions of the cervix (cervical intraepithelial neoplasia, CIN) are detected reliably by cytologic means. Although many patients with early CIN will have spontaneous regression of the abnormal cytologic condition to a normal pattern, a significant proportion develop invasive squamous cell carcinoma of the cervix if left untreated. Once CIN has been identified, progression can usually be prevented by simple outpatient therapy and continuing surveillance. "Cervical intraepithelial neoplasia (CIN)" has generally replaced the

Table 38-2. Classification of Cervical Intraepithelial Neoplasia

Type	Degree	Extent of Atypia
CIN I	Mild dysplasia	Basal third
CIN II	Moderate dysplasia	Lower two thirds
CIN III	Severe dysplasia Carcinoma in situ	Full epithelial thickness

terms "dysplasia" and "carcinoma in situ" as terms referring to the histologic characterization of premalignant cervical epithelial changes (Table 38-2). In lesions of CIN I and CIN II, the basal cell layer of the cervical squamous epithelium undergoes proliferation with nuclear atypia, changes in the nuclear-cytoplasmic ratio, and loss of polarity (Fig. 38-9). The upper layers of the epithelium undergo maturation, and often a few layers of stratified epithelium are present on the surface. When the architecture of the epithelium is completely disrupted and loss of polarity through all cell layers has occurred without invasion of underlying cervical stroma, the lesion is referred to as CIN III (Fig. 38-9). Exfoliated cells from the surface of the epithelium are detected cytologically and form the basis for the Papanicolaou smear.

Many epidemiologic studies have inferred associations of CIN and cancer of the cervix with multiple interdependent social factors. These disorders are more common in multiparous women with an early age of first coitus and multiple sexual partners. Cervical carcinoma is rare in celibate women. A male factor has been hypothesized. A viral cause has also been proposed, with both herpesvirus type II and human papilloma virus (HPV) having been associated with CIN and invasive carcinoma of the cervix. HPV DNA has been identified in most cases of CIN and cervical carcinoma, suggesting that HPV is a very important factor in the development of this disease.

Lesions of CIN are asymptomatic and not observed on routine examination. Thus, the Pap smear must be relied upon to detect these preinvasive changes. The natural history of early CIN is extremely variable. Frequently, lesions of CIN I or CIN II spontaneously revert to normal. Lesions of CIN III less frequently regress but frequently progress to invasive carcinoma over a variable length of time.

Screening for CIN and carcinoma of the cervix is by means of the cervical Pap smear. This test should be performed annually on all women who are sexually active. The Pap test is a screening mechanism only and is valid only in screening for cervical neoplasia. The cervix must be sampled at the squamocolumnar junction where most lesions originate. The Pap smear should evaluate both the endocervix and the ectocervix.

The interpretation of an abnormal Pap smear should take into account all possible explanations for the abnormal cytologic pattern. In the past, evaluation of a patient with an abnormal Pap smear included repeat cytology tests, random cervical biopsies, directed biopsies in areas that did not stain with Lugol's solution, and conization of the cervix (Fig. 38-10) to rule out invasive cancer. Recently colposcopy has led to a more conservative evaluation and therapy scheme for the pa-

tient with an abnormal Pap smear (Fig. 38-11). The colposcope is a binocular stereoscopic microscope with low magnification. The cervix is stained with 3% acetic acid, and the colposcope is utilized to visualize the entire portio of the cervix and the squamocolumnar junction. Acetic acid accentuates the difference between normal and abnormal colposcopic patterns. In most instances, the entire lesion can be visualized, and the most atypical area can be selected for biopsy. If the lesion extends into the endocervical canal or endocervical curettage reveals atypical cells, diagnostic conization will be necessary to define disease. The major advantage of colposcopy is that a skilled colposcopist can establish the definitive diagnosis by directed biopsy and avoid surgical conization. This is most important in the younger patient desirous of childbearing in whom cone biopsy may result in impaired fertility. Additionally, conization is a procedure that requires anesthesia and hospitalization. The majority of patients with CIN can thus receive appropriate outpatient treatment.

Patients selected for outpatient therapy are those in whom satisfactory colposcopy yields evaluation of the entire squamocolumnar junction, the entire lesion is visualized and biopsy is confirmatory of an abnormal cytologic pattern, and in whom the endocervical curettage is negative for dysplasia. Outpatient therapy for CIN includes cryotherapy and laser vaporization. All therapeutic modalities are successful in eradicating CIN in more than 90% of patients.

If colposcopy does not allow visualization of the entire lesion or the entire squamocolumnar junction, if the directive biopsy reveals questionable stromal invasion, or if the endocervical curettage is positive, cone biopsy is necessary for definitive diagnosis. The limits of the ectocervical incision can be delineated by use of the colposcope and the smallest possible cone obtained to excise all atypical epithelium. The depth of the incision as it tapers toward the endocervical canal is determined by the length of the cervical canal and suspected depth of involvement. Bleeding from the operative bed is controlled by hemostatic sutures. Cervical stenosis, cervical incompetence, infertility, and hemorrhage are possible but rare complications of cone biopsy. Cone biopsy may be therapeutic in patients whose lesion is contained in the cone biopsy specimen. Definitive therapy of CIN may also be attained with hysterectomy in patients who do not desire further childbearing.

Regardless of the therapeutic modality employed, patients with CIN are at a higher risk for recurrence of genital tract lesions and should be followed with genital cytology tests for the remainder of their lives.

Invasive Cervical Carcinoma

The incidence of invasive cervical carcinoma has decreased with the availability of routine cytologic screening in the United States. At the same time, the number of advanced cervical carcinomas has also decreased, along with the mortality from invasive cervical carcinoma. Approximately 16,000 new cases of cervical carcinoma occur annually in the United States, with approximately 7,000 deaths being attributable to cervical carcinoma. Squamous carcinomas account for 85% to 90% of invasive cervical cancers. Approximately 10% are adenocarcinomas with rare small cell carcino-

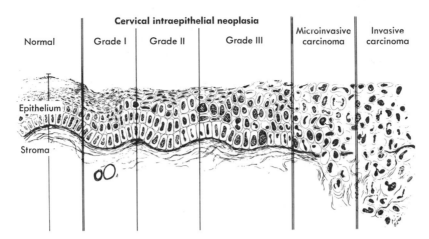

Fig. 38-9. Progression of histological changes from normal cervical epithelium through cervical intraepithelial neoplasia to invasive squamous cell carcinoma.

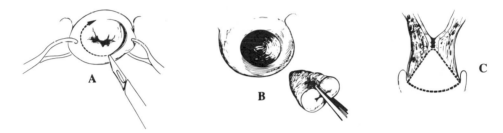

Fig. 38-10. Cone biopsy of cervix. **A,** Line of incision. **B,** Specimen removed. **C,** Frontal section of cervix and lower corpus demonstrating extent of conization.

mas, melanomas, and sarcomas comprising the remaining cases. The epidemiology of cervical squamous carcinoma is similar to the epidemiology of CIN in that squamous carcinoma is more frequently seen among patients with early onset of coital activity and numerous sexual partners.

The typical patient with invasive cervical carcinoma is between 45 and 55 years of age. The most common early symptom of cervical carcinoma, a thin bloody vaginal discharge, is frequently unrecognized. The classical symptom is abnormal intermenstrual bleeding, often occurring as postcoital spotting. Late symptoms of disease include flank or leg pain that is usually secondary to the involvement of ureters, pelvic wall, and sacral nerve roots. Some patients develop urinary and bowel symptoms because of local invasion. Distant metastases and persistent edema of the lower extremities are late manifestations of primary or recurrent disease. Occasionally patients present with profound genital hemorrhage or uremia from advanced pelvic disease.

Staging

Cervical carcinoma is clinically staged, preferably confirmed with examination under anesthesia. The international staging for cervical carcinoma allows limited diagnostic aids for determining the stage, including physical examination, routine chest radiographs, intravenous pyelogram, barium enema, colposcopy, cystos-

copy, and proctoscopy. Clinical staging allows a rough assessment of prognosis, and communication of treatment results between one institution and another. Staging does not limit the therapeutic plan, and therapy is tailored to the extent of disease in each patient. The clinical stages of cervical cancer are as follows:

Stage 0: Carcinoma in situ
Stage I: Carcinoma confined to the cervix
    Stage Ia: Focal stromal invasion
    Stage Ia$_2$: Stromal invasion <3 mm; with lesion >7 mm^2
    Stage Ib: All other cancers limited to cervix
Stage II: Involvement of upper vagina or infiltration of parametria, not involving pelvic sidewall
    Stage IIa: Upper two thirds of vagina but not parametria
    Stage IIb: Infiltration of parametria, not involving pelvic sidewall
Stage III: Involvement of lower vagina or parametria with extension to pelvic sidewall
    Stage IIIa: Lower third of vagina but not to pelvic sidewall if parametria are involved
    Stage IIIb: Infiltration of one or both parametria to the pelvic sidewall; obstruction of one or both ureters by intravenous pyelogram
Stage IV: Extension outside of reproductive tract
    Stage IVa: Involvement of bladder or rectal mucosa
    Stage IVb: Distant metastases

The major routes of spread for cervical carcinoma (Fig. 38-12) are: (1) into the vaginal mucosa, (2) into

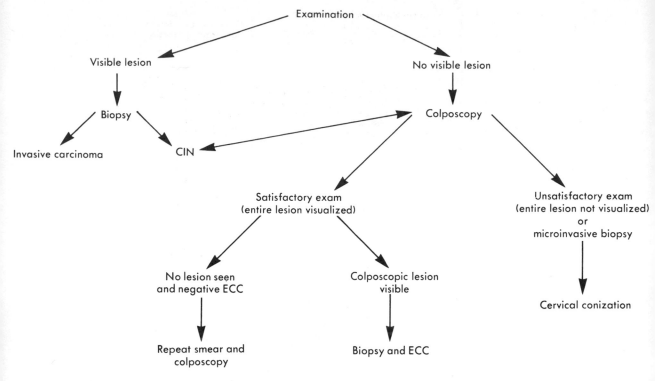

Fig. 38-11. Evaluation of abnormal cervical smear. *CIN,* cervical intraepithelial neoplasia; *ECC,* endocervical curettage.

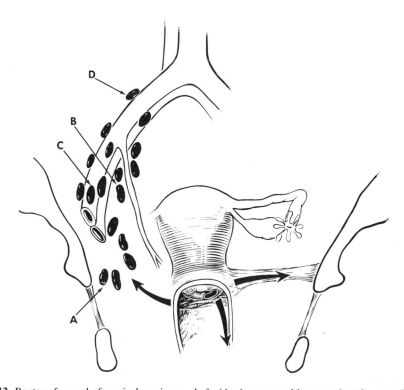

Fig. 38-12. Routes of spread of cervical carcinoma. Left side shows spread by extension along cardinal ligaments to lateral pelvic wall and into vagina. Right side demonstrates commonly involved pelvic lymph nodes. **A,** Obturator; **B,** hypogastric; **C,** external iliac; **D,** common iliac.

the lower uterine segment, (3) direct extension into the paracervical and parametrial tissues, (4) into the paracervical lymphatics and pelvic lymph nodes, and (5) directly into the bladder or rectum. Pelvic lymph node metastases are well correlated with the stage of disease. The incidence increases from 10% to 20% in stage I disease to greater than 50% in stage III disease. The primary lymphatic drainage of the cervix is along the cardinal and uterosacral ligaments to the pelvic lymph nodes with secondary involvement of the common iliac, paraaortic, and inguinal lymph nodes. Systemic dissemination is frequently present when the paraaortic nodes are involved.

Treatment

Therapy of cervical carcinoma is tailored to the extent of disease (Table 38-3). The primary modality of therapy is radiation; however surgery is appropriate for early lesions. Since the incidence of nodal metastases is extremely low in microinvasive lesions confined to a depth of 3 mm or less without lymphatic or vascular space involvement, patients with these lesions may be appropriately treated with simple vaginal or abdominal hysterectomy. Younger patients who are acceptable surgical risks may have radical surgical therapy of selected stage Ib and IIa cervical carcinomas. The radical hysterectomy involves removal en block of the uterus, lateral paracervical and uterosacral ligaments to the pelvic sidewalls, cervix, and a portion of the upper vagina. The ureters are preserved and must be carefully dissected from the cardinal ligaments. The pelvic lymph nodes are removed completely from the external iliac and obturator nodes. Presacral, common iliac, and para-aortic lymphadenectomies are also performed. The ovaries may be retained in younger patients to permit normal ovarian function until menopause. With modern surgical techniques the operative mortality and morbidity of radical surgery are extremely low; long-term survival for patients with stage Ib cervical carcinoma after radical hysterectomy is approximately 90%.

Otherwise, the therapy of cervical carcinoma at stages Ib through IVa is based on external radiation combined with intracavitary radium or cesium brachytherapy. The normal pelvic tissues are able to tolerate an extremely high dose of radiation therapy, particularly the cervix and upper vagina. Intracavitary brachytherapy is ideally suited to the treatment of cervical carcinoma because it is possible to place a radiation source in proximity to the lesion and thus deliver high central doses approaching 15,000 to 20,000 cGy (rad) to the surface of the cervix. This is combined with external radiation therapy to increase the dose to the pelvic sidewall for treatment of parametrial and retroperitoneal disease. The addition of radiation sensitizers such as hydroxyurea, 5-fluorouracil, or cisplatin increases the effects of radiation on malignant cells.

Acute treatment complications occurring during radiation therapy include irritation of the rectum, small bowel, bladder, skin, and mild bone marrow suppression. Radiation produces chronic obliterative endarteritis and fibrosis in normal tissues. Late radiation complications include fibrostenotic changes of the intestinal and bladder walls with atrophic gastrointestinal and genitourinary mucosa. Chronic complications can be progressive and manifest several months or years after completion of radiation therapy. Occasionally, such complications may require small bowel bypass, colostomy, or urinary diversion. In general, serious morbidity of pelvic radiation is low if external radiation is below 5000 cGy.

Approximately 35% of patients with invasive cervical carcinoma have recurrent or persistent disease after therapy. The triad of weight loss accompanied by leg edema and back or pelvic pain is ominous and indicative of pelvic sidewall recurrence. Vaginal bleeding or discharge is strongly suggestive of central recurrence. Patients with central recurrence after radiation therapy are occasionally candidates for ultraradical exenterative surgical therapy. Reirradiation for recurrent disease inside previously radiated fields is generally not possible because of the radiation tolerance of normal tissues. Cisplatin (*cis*-diaminodichloroplatinum) is the most active single agent in the chemotherapy of metastatic or recurrent cervical carcinoma.

Endometrial Carcinoma

Endometrial carcinoma is the most common malignancy of the female reproductive organs. Approxi-

Table 38-3. Therapy of Cervical Carcinoma

Stage	Whole Pelvis (cGy)	Brachytherapy Applications	Optional Surgery
Ia	—	—	Simple extrafascial hysterectomy
Ib	2000-4000	2	Radical hysterectomy with pelvic lymphadenectomy
IIa	4000	2	
IIb	4000-5000	2	
IIIa	5000-6000	1 or interstitial implant	
IVa	6000	2	
IVb	1000 pulse for central palliation		

Recurrent cervical carcinoma:
1. Central—consider pelvic exenteration
2. Distant metastases—chemotherapy

mately 37,000 new cases occur in the United States annually, while approximately 3500 patients die from endometrial carcinoma. The majority of patients are postmenopausal, and the average age at diagnosis is 60 years. Adenocarcinoma of the endometrium accounts for 95% of uterine corpus malignancies, the balance being sarcomas.

Unopposed endogenous or exogenous estrogen has been implicated as an etiologic factor in endometrial carcinoma. Endometrial carcinoma occurs more frequently in women with unopposed estrogen as in polycystic ovary disease, hormone-secreting ovarian tumors, and unopposed exogenous estrogen replacement therapy. In general, women who develop endometrial carcinoma have low parity, menstrual irregularity, and late menopause. Patients are frequently obese with associated hypertension and diabetes mellitus. Obese patients have a high rate of peripheral conversion of adrenal and ovarian androstenedione to estrone. This also results in unopposed endogenous estrogen exposure.

Diagnosis

Early symptoms of endometrial carcinoma include a thin, serosanguineous vaginal discharge, but postmenopausal or intermenstrual vaginal bleeding generally brings the patient to the physician's attention. Any episode of postmenopausal bleeding requires investigation with endometrial biopsy or D&C. The routine Pap smear is ineffective in detecting endometrial carcinoma. Although cytologic studies of the endometrial cavity may prove useful in some patients, a histologic technique such as endometrial biopsy or D&C is preferred for the diagnosis of endometrial carcinoma. Staging of endometrial carcinoma requires sounding of the uterus and endocervical curettage in addition to routine pelvic examination and histologic diagnosis of endometrial carcinoma.

Pathology

Adenocarcinomas of the endometrium may produce a varied pattern including adenocanthoma, adenosquamous, papillary, and clear cell patterns. A well-differentiated tumor retains glandular differentiation (grade 1). A moderately differentiated tumor has a mixture of solid and glandular areas (grade 2), and a poorly differentiated tumor (grade 3) loses glandular differentiation. Homologous sarcomas arise from tissues normally found in the uterus (e.g., leiomyosarcomas) while heterologous sarcomas are composed of elements not normally found in the uterus (e.g., rhabdomyosarcomas). In general, patients with uterine sarcomas have a worse prognosis than patients with uterine adenocarcinomas.

The premalignant precursors of endometrial carcinoma are less well characterized than those of cervical carcinoma. Adenomatous hyperplasia can progress under estrogen stimulation; approximately 20% develop into endometrial carcinoma if untreated. Adenomatous hyperplasia frequently responds to progestin therapy. Adenomatous hyperplasia with cellular atypia is less likely to respond to hormone therapy and requires hysterectomy both for treatment and to rule out a coexisting endometrial carcinoma. Cystic hyperplasia of the endometrium has an extremely low malignant potential.

Staging

Initially, endometrial carcinoma spreads along the surface of the uterine cavity and locally invades the myometrium. Deeply invasive and poorly differentiated lesions can metastasize through hematogenous or lymphatic routes to adnexal structures and the pelvic or paraaortic lymph nodes. Involvement of the endocervical canal results in more frequent extension into the lateral parametria and pelvic lymph node metastases. Intraperitoneal metastases may occur through seeding of peritoneal surfaces by free-floating malignant cells, which can be detected by peritoneal cytology tests. Hematogenous spread to lungs, liver, and brain are late manifestations. Survival is roughly correlated with clinical stage of endometrial carcinoma. The stages of endometrial carcinoma follow:

Stage I: Carcinoma confined to the corpus
   Stage Ia: Length of uterine cavity 8 cm or less
   Stage Ib: Length of uterine cavity more than 8 cm
Stage I carcinomas are subgrouped according to histologic grade:
   Grade 1: Highly differentiated adenocarcinoma
   Grade 2: Differentiated adenocarcinoma with partly solid areas
   Grade 3: Predominantly solid or undifferentiated carcinomas
Stage II: Carcinoma involving the corpus and cervix
Stage III: Carcinoma extending outside of the uterus but not outside the true pelvis
Stage IV: Carcinoma extending outside of the true pelvis or involving the bladder or rectal mucosa

The most significant prognostic factors in early endometrial carcinoma are histologic differentiation, depth of myometrial invasion, and the presence or absence of malignant cells in peritoneal washings. Pelvic and paraaortic lymph node metastases are associated with lack of histologic differentiation, deep myometrial invasion, and adnexal metastases.

Treatment

The majority of endometrial carcinomas are treated by total abdominal hysterectomy with bilateral salpingo-oophorectomy and examination of peritoneal cells. Sampling of pelvic and para-aortic lymph nodes are performed in cases with deeply invasive grade 1 lesions and all grade 2 or grade 3 lesions. The surgical findings dictate the necessity for adjuvant therapy. Intraperitoneal instillation of radioactive chromic ^{32}phosphate is effective therapy for patients with malignant peritoneal cells as the only poor prognostic factor. Adjuvant whole pelvic radiation therapy of 4500 to 5000 cGy is usually given to patients with deep myometrial invasion, cervical involvement, pelvic metastases, or pelvic lymph node metastases. Radiation fields may be extended to include involved paraortic lymph nodes.

Using individualized therapy selected on the basis of surgical staging, 5-year survival rates are approximately 90% to 95% for patients with disease limited to the uterine fundus. Stage II endometrial cancers have a much poorer prognosis if true invasion of cervical stroma is present, with a 50% to 60% survival. Survival for patients with stage III and stage IV cancers depends on the sites of metastatic involvement and response to progestin therapy. Cisplatin and doxorubicin (adriamycin) are active chemotherapeutic agents against endometrial carcinoma, but overall survival in advanced endometrial cancer is less than 10% to 15%.

Ovarian Carcinoma

Ovarian carcinoma is the second most common gynecologic malignancy with approximately 18,000 new cases annually, but it is the leading cause of death among gynecologic malignancies with approximately 12,000 deaths per year. The incidence of ovarian carcinoma is increasing in industrialized nations for unknown reasons. The risk of developing ovarian carcinoma approaches 1%, with the peak incidence in the fifth and sixth decades. From 85% to 90% of all ovarian carcinomas are derived from celomic epithelium. Germ cell tumors are the second most frequent type of ovarian malignancy and are more frequently found in patients under 25 years of age.

Unfortunately, the majority of ovarian carcinomas are detected at a late stage because of insidious, nonspecific symptoms of early ovarian carcinoma. No effective techniques are available to detect early stage ovarian carcinoma. Immunologic techniques aimed at detection of tumor-associated antigens are at present too nonspecific to serve in this capacity.

Diagnosis and Therapy

Most symptoms caused by ovarian carcinoma are related to intestinal involvement, ascites, or pleural effusion when the malignancy is far advanced. Therefore even asymptomatic adnexal masses must not be ignored. Frequently patients have nonspecific complaints of early satiety, bloating, or constipation. Increasing abdominal girth may be attributable to ascites. Abdominal pain and nausea or vomiting may reflect intestinal obstruction.

A woman with ascites in the 40- to 70-year age group, without other evidence of liver or cardiac disease, should be considered to have ovarian carcinoma until proved otherwise. Diagnostic paracentesis is not recommended, since a peritoneal cytologic examination may not establish the diagnosis and malignant cells may seed the needle tract. Occasionally, a large contained cyst mistaken for ascites ruptures during attempted paracentesis.

Preoperative evaluation of a patient suspected of having ovarian carcinoma should include a chest film to screen for pulmonary metastases or effusion and an intravenous pyelogram and small bowel series or barium enema if bowel involvement is suspected. Abdominal CT and ultrasound scan do not yield a histologic diagnosis and are rarely valuable in staging these patients.

Ovarian carcinoma is surgically staged as follows:

Stage I	Growth limited to the ovaries
Stage Ia	Growth limited to *one* ovary; no ascites
Stage Ib	Growth limited to *both* ovaries; no ascites
Stage Ic	Tumor either stage Ia or stage Ib, but with ascites* present or positive peritoneal washings, tumor on surface, or capsular rupture
Stage II	Growth involving one or both ovaries with pelvic extension
Stage IIa	Extension or metastases to the uterus or tubes
Stage IIb	Extension to other pelvic tissues
Stage IIc	Tumor either stage IIa or stage IIb, but with ascites* present or positive peritoneal washings, tumor on surface, or capsular rupture
Stage III	Growth involving one or both ovaries with intraperitoneal metastases outside the pelvis or positive retroperitoneal nodes
Stage IIIa	Tumor limited to the true pelvis with histologically proved malignant extension to small bowel or omentum
Stage IIIb	Upper abdominal implants less than 2 cm
Stage IIIc	Upper abdominal implants larger than 2 cm or lymph node involvement
Stage IV	Growth involving one or both ovaries with distant metastases
	If pleural effusion is present, there must be positive cytology tests to allot a case to stage IV
	Parenchymal liver metastases
Special category	Unexplored cases which are believed to be ovarian carcinoma

Therefore laparotomy establishes the diagnosis and determines the extent of disease. Two thirds of patients have stage III or stage IV disease at the time of diagnosis. Exploration for ovarian carcinoma includes sampling ascites or peritoneal washings for cytologic examination, examination and biopsy of the right hemidiaphragm, and visual or palpatory examination of all serosal and peritoneal surfaces with biopsies of suspicious areas. Even in the absence of gross involvement, partial omentectomy should be performed to detect occult metastases.

In early disease, total abdominal hysterectomy with bilateral salpingo-oophorectomy and omentectomy should be performed with sampling of pelvic and paraaortic lymph nodes. Young patients who desire to retain fertility may have more conservative extirpation of disease if the tumor is of borderline malignant potential or is well differentiated and there is no extraovarian spread. In the presence of more advanced disease, every attempt is made to reduce the tumor burden by surgical resection. "Debulking" appears to enhance a response to chemotherapy and survival.

Early-stage ovarian carcinoma is usually treated with adjuvant single-agent alkylating chemotherapy, since overall survival is approximately 60% in patients treated with surgery alone. Intraperitoneal radioactive isotopes (e.g., chromic ^{32}phosphate) may also be used. Results with these two modalities are equivalent. This has the advantage of requiring only a single application with fewer side effects than with chemotherapy.

Recently, advanced stage ovarian carcinoma has been treated with combination chemotherapy, usually based around cisplatin in combination with alkylating agents and doxorubicin. Multiple-agent chemotherapy improves the response when compared to single-agent alkylating therapy, and the duration of survival appears to be longer. Intraperitoneal chemotherapy with cisplatin has been introduced in an effort to increase the dose to peritoneal implants while limiting systemic toxicity. Often a "second look" laparotomy is performed to as-

---

*Ascites is peritoneal effusion that in the opinion of the surgeon is pathologic or clearly exceeds normal amounts.

sess the response to a planned course of chemotherapy. However, the ultimate cure rate for advanced-stage ovarian carcinoma is less than 15%.

External-beam radiation therapy to the whole abdomen is limited by the radiosensitivity of the liver, kidneys, and bowel. Ovarian carcinoma has a propensity to spread over all peritoneal surfaces; therefore radiation therapy directed at the pelvis alone is rarely successful.

Prognosis of ovarian epithelial carcinoma is most closely related to stage of disease. The histologic grade of the tumor affects the prognosis within each stage. The estimated 5-year survival rates range from 90% in stage Ia (i) borderline or well-differentiated lesions, to less than 15% for disease at stages III and IV.

Ovarian Germ Cell Malignancies

Ovarian germ cell carcinomas include both pure and mixed tumors of embryonal and extraembryonal origin. These malignancies occur most frequently in young adolescents and in women under 25 years of age. Before the development of effective chemotherapy, patients with ovarian endodermal sinus tumor, choriocarcinoma, immature teratoma, or mixed lesions had an extremely poor prognosis, even with Stage I disease. Although patients with ovarian dysgerminoma have a more favorable prognosis, the germ cell malignancies tended to be rapidly progressive, most patients dying less than 2 years following diagnosis after surgical resection. Fortunately, these ovarian malignancies are extremely sensitive to a variety of combination chemotherapy regimens. Currently the majority of patients with early stage and many patients with advanced stage germ cell malignancies of the ovary are cured of their disease with a combination of surgery and aggressive chemotherapy. Most patients with early germ cell malignancies can be treated adequately with unilateral salpingo-oophorectomy and adjuvant chemotherapy, thus retaining childbearing capacity.

Carcinoma Metastatic to Ovary

Endometrial adenocarcinoma frequently metastasizes to the ovary. The most common extragenital carcinomas that metastasize to the ovary are from gastrointestinal and breast primaries. Bilateral ovarian enlargement from metastatic mucinous carcinoma (generally of gastric origin) is frequently called "Krukenberg tumors," an imprecise term.

Gestational Trophoblastic Neoplasia

Gestational trophoblastic neoplasia (GTN) is a term applied to the rare placental neoplasms called hydatidiform mole, chorioadenoma destruens, and choriocarcinoma. In contrast to primary choriocarcinoma of the gonad, these neoplasms are essentially disorders of pregnancy and contain paternal genetic material. Normal trophoblast is locally invasive and also has the ability to metastasize. Normal villi are found in maternal lungs during many normal pregnancies, particularly in the third trimester of pregnancy. The viability of normal trophoblastic tissue is self-limited, probably under the influence of hormonal or immunologic controls.

Hydatidiform Mole

The incidence of hydatidiform mole in the United States is approximately 1 in 1500 to 2000 pregnancies. "Complete" moles are usually of karyotype 46,XX and contain paternal chromosomal material. "Partial" moles have a less frequent incidence of malignant sequelae and are generally triploid. Vaginal bleeding in the first half of pregnancy is the most frequent sign, with passage of molar tissue in the second trimester. Molar tissue is composed of multiple translucent vesicles ranging in size up to 1 cm. Approximately half the patients have a uterus that is large for gestational age, but one fourth will have a small-for-dates uterine size. Unilateral or bilateral theca lutein cysts (Fig. 38-13) are present in approximately 20% of cases, resulting from ovarian hyperstimulation by high levels of circulating

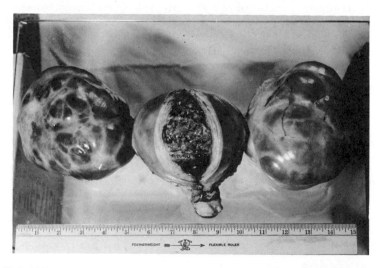

Fig. 38-13. Hydatidiform mole. Surgical specimen showing molar tissue in uterine cavity and bilateral theca-lutein cysts.

hCG. Fetal heart tones are absent. Approximately 20% to 25% of patients have hyperemesis. Toxemia of pregnancy before 24 weeks of gestation is highly suspicious for mole.

Slightly more than 50% of molar pregnancies are diagnosed before the expulsion of vesicles. The diagnostic method of choice is ultrasound (Fig. 38-14), which demonstrates a mixed echogenic diffuse pattern in the uterus without fetal parts. This is preferred to arteriography, amniography, or radiography, since ultrasound is noninvasive and poses no threat to mother or fetus. After the diagnosis of hydatidiform mole, the patient is screened for systemic metastases with a chest-film, and a baseline serum hCG level is obtained. The uterus is evacuated by suction curettage. If the patient desires sterilization, hysterectomy is performed. The lutein cysts require no therapy and regress spontaneously-when hCG stimulation is removed. Prophylactic chemotherapy is not recommended, since it does not elim-

inate the need for postmolar surveillance and may result in serious toxicity.

After evacuation, the patient is followed with serial hCG titers at 1- or 2-week intervals. Serum radioimmunoassays for β-hCG are preferred, since they do not cross react with serum luteinizing hormone and are sufficiently sensitive to detect small amounts of viable trophoblastic tissue. After remission, levels are followed for 12 months at 1- to 2-month intervals. During this time, contraception is employed. If the hCG titer rises or plateaus for more than three successive hCG levels, the patient is considered to have malignant gestational trophoblastic neoplasia and appropriate therapy is warranted. After remission of one year, the patient may become pregnant.

Malignant Gestational Trophoblastic Neoplasia

Malignant GTN was previously a devastating, rapidly progressive malignancy of young women with an

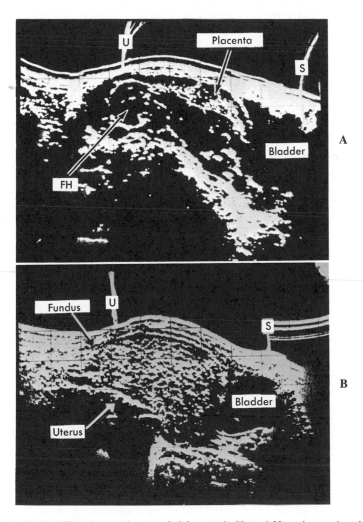

Fig. 38-14. Longitudinal midline ultrasound scans of abdomen. **A,** Normal 22-week gestation showing fetal head, *FH,* and placenta. *U,* Umbilicus; *S,* symphysis. **B,** Hydatidiform mole showing diffuse homogeneous echo pattern in uterus enlarged to 22-week size with absence of fetal parts.

almost uniformly fatal outcome when metastases were present. However, the advent of effective chemotherapy and hCG level surveillance have made malignant GTN one of the most curable of human malignancies.

Approximately 20% of molar pregnancies develop malignant sequelae. On the other hand, one third to one half of malignant GTN cases are preceded by nonmolar gestations. Histologically, malignant GTN can be divided into chorioadenoma destruens (invasive mole) and choriocarcinoma. Chorioadenoma destruens demonstrates maintenance of villous architecture with pronounced trophoblastic proliferation and direct invasion of the myometrium and may metastasize. Choriocarcinoma is histologically characterized by sheets of malignant trophoblastic cells without villous architecture. The prognosis and treatment of both entities are similar depending on the presence or absence of metastases and clinical features suggestive of poor response to single-agent chemotherapy. Before the advent of chemotherapy, the cure rate for nonmetastatic malignant GTN was less than 50% in patients treated by hysterectomy alone. Several chemotherapeutic regimens are effective for the treatment of malignant GTN, and therapy is monitored through the use of serum hCG levels as a tumor marker.

After the diagnosis of malignant GTN, the patient should be staged with a baseline (pretherapy) serum hCG level, chest film, brain scan or CT of the brain, and liver-spleen scan or liver CT to screen for high-risk metastases. The most common sites of metastases are lungs, vagina, brain, and liver. Brain and liver metastases have a poorer prognosis than metastases in other sites.

Nonmetastatic Gestational Trophoblastic Neoplasia

Patients with nonmetastatic GTN are managed with single-agent chemotherapy utilizing methotrexate or actinomycin D. Cycles of chemotherapy are repeated until hCG levels become negative. The reported cure rates for nonmetastatic GTN utilizing this approach are excellent; virtually all patients are cured. The majority of patients can be treated without hysterectomy, though hysterectomy may be combined with chemotherapy to shorten the duration of chemotherapy.

Metastatic Gestational Trophoblastic Neoplasia

Patients with metastatic GTN are divided into good-prognosis and poor-prognosis groups on the basis of whether one or more high-risk clinical features is present, which would predict failure of single-agent chemotherapy. If a patient has none of the following, she has good-prognosis metastatic GTN, if one or more, she has poor-prognosis metastatic GTN:

Pretherapy hCG level greater than 40,000 mIU/ml
Duration of disease greater than 4 months
Brain or liver metastases
Antecedent term pregnancy
Previous unsuccessful single-agent chemotherapy

Patients with good-prognosis metastatic GTN are treated with repetitive cycles of single-agent methotrexate or actinomycin D, and cure rates in excess of 90% have been reported (Fig. 38-15). Patients with poor-prognosis metastatic GTN should be treated initially with multiagent chemotherapy, since the expectations for cure with single-agent chemotherapy are low and the risk of severe toxicity when secondarily treated with combination chemotherapy is high. Surgical resection of isolated metastases or hysterectomy to remove intrauterine disease is useful in treating selected patients. Adjuvant radiation therapy to cerebral or hepatic metastases is given to control hemorrhage, since metastases are highly vascular.

Chemotherapy is individualized according to the hCG level response and is recycled on a frequent basis. Patients are monitored closely for toxicity including bone marrow depression, stomatitis, nausea and vomiting, and alopecia. When hCG level remission is achieved, patients are followed with frequent hCG levels for 1 year. If the patient remains in prolonged hCG remission, surveillance is performed at 6-month intervals indefinitely. Fertility is excellent after successful therapy of malignant GTN. There has been no increase in congenital anomalies among the offspring of women who have been successfully treated.

ENDOCRINOLOGY AND CONTRACEPTION
Conception and Sterilization

Currently the most effective method of contraception is the oral combination estrogen-progestin pill. The oral combination pill results in continuous therapeutic levels of estrogen and progestin, causing hypothalamic suppression of releasing factors with decreased gonadotropin secretion leading to inhibition of ovulation. Therapeutic levels of estrogen and progestin affect many physiologic and metabolic processes. Common side effects include nausea, spotting, minor psychological disturbances, and weight gain. More serious but rare side effects include thromboembolism, increased serum lipids, hypertension, and altered liver function. Rare liver neoplasms have been caused by oral contraceptives. Since the majority of these serious metabolic effects are associated with estrogen, it is recommended that pills containing less than 50 μg of estrogen be prescribed initially. Patients over the age of 35 years should employ some other form of contraception, since there is an increased incidence of coronary artery disease and cerebrovascular accidents associated with oral contraceptives. This risk is further increased among smokers. The theoretical effectiveness of combination oral contraception approaches 99%. The minipill consists of a low dose of progestin that is taken daily. A higher failure rate and frequent breakthrough bleeding are observed with its use.

Barrier methods of contraception include the diaphragm combined with spermicidal jelly, cervical cap, vaginal contraceptive foam, and condom. These are less effective contraceptive techniques than oral contraceptives but have no systemic side effects.

The intrauterine device (IUD) is an effective mode of contraception that is no longer readily available in the United States, although this method of contraception remains popular elsewhere. The only device presently available in the United States is impregnated with progesterone, and insertion of the device involves an extraordinary antecedent informed consent procedure.

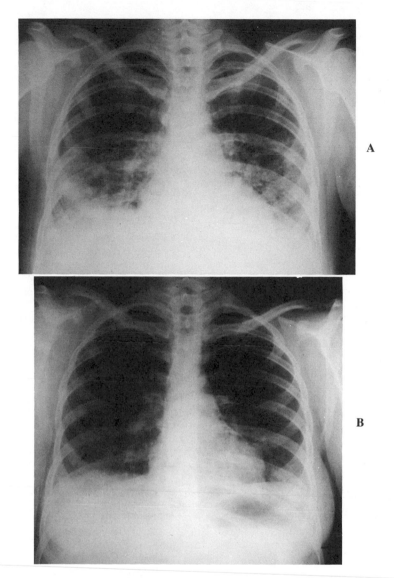

Fig. 38-15. Regression of pulmonary metastases of choriocarcinoma after treatment with methotrexate. **A,** Chest film before chemotherapy. **B,** Appearance after three courses of methotrexate.

Several inert plastic IUDs and plastic IUDs wrapped with copper wire, which have good safety records, were withdrawn from the U.S. market by manufacturers owing to the threat of costly litigation. These devices continue to be judged safe and effective contraceptives by physicians and patients in most of the world.

The contraceptive mechanism of the IUD appears to depend on induction of a low-grade chronic endometritis and possibly alteration of cervical mucus. The IUD does not usually prevent fertilization but prevents implantation of the fertilized ovum. Problems associated with the IUD include uterine perforation, dysmenorrhea, menorrhagia, uterine expulsion, and pelvic inflammatory disease. A string is usually attached to the end of the IUD which passes through the cervical canal and is visualized in the vagina. If the string of an IUD is not visualized, the patient should be evaluated with ultrasound or abdominal plain film to confirm intrauter-

ine placement of the IUD and exclude the possibility of late perforation or IUD expulsion. Since the IUD protects against intrauterine conception, there is a relatively higher incidence of ectopic pregnancy in women who become pregnant with an IUD in place.

Permanent contraception may be achieved by surgical sterilization. Although tubal ligation may be performed by either the abdominal or the vaginal route with low morbidity or mortality, vasectomy in the male is a less morbid procedure and should be seriously considered for a couple who desire permanent sterilization. Tubal sterilization by laparoscopy has become the most frequently performed sterilization procedure. It can often be performed on an outpatient basis but should be considered a major surgical procedure. Although tubal ligations are performed with the intent of permanence by both surgeon and patient, requests for reversal of sterilization do arise often after a change in life circumstances, such as remarriage. The reversibility of a "permanent" sterilization hinges on the extent of tubal injury incurred by the initial ligation procedure. Obviously, if the amount of initial tubal injury was minimal, then an attempt at subsequent microscopic reanastomosis is feasible. If only a small portion of the tubal isthmus was occluded or destroyed by application of a plastic clip, a small segmental resection, or limited cautery, then a majority of those patients can expect at least one patent tube from microscopic reanastomosis. The "reversals" have an excellent chance of conception. On the other extreme, aggressive tubal ligation procedures up to and including bilateral salpingectomy drastically reduce the chance of successful reanastomosis to nil and leave in vitro fertilization as the only option for fertility.

Endocrinology and Infertility

While there are many areas of overlap with endocrine disorders that are common to both men and women, gynecologic endocrinology generally focuses on the hormonal aspects of female reproduction and its disorders. As a result, gynecologic endocrinology and management of female infertility are intimately associated. Abnormal vaginal bleeding patterns are often the first sign of an endocrine problem. Before presuming that an abnormal bleeding pattern is due to hormonal factors, structural abnormalities must be excluded. Congenital absence of the vagina or other developmental abnormalities can explain the absence of vaginal bleeding (amenorrhea) in postpubertal women, whereas benign or malignant neoplasms can often cause excessively heavy or frequent vaginal bleeding (menorrhagia). Endocrine causes of abnormal uterine bleeding are most simply considered to result from failure to initiate normal ovulatory cycles at puberty or development of conditions that result in anovulation or more subtle perturbations of hormone levels associated with cyclic ovarian activity. Some of the terminology and diagnoses for these disturbances are described below.

Primary Amenorrhea

Primary amenorrhea is defined as the absence of menses by 14 years of age in the absence of secondary sexual development or absence of menstruation by 16 years of age. In general, true primary amenorrhea will be due to one of four causes.

Congenital Anomalies. Patients with congenital anomalies of the mullerian tract have normal secondary characteristics and normal karyotype. Pelvic examination should show the abnormality (i.e., transverse vaginal septum) that prevents normal menses, as discussed above.

Gonadal Dysgenesis. Patients with gonadal dysgenesis range from the classical Turner's syndrome karyotype (45,XO) with short stature and other somatic abnormalities to mosaic variants with normal physical appearance but with secondary amenorrhea and early ovarian failure. Women with elevated gonadotropins (follicle stimulating hormone [FSH] >40 mIU/ml) should have a chromosome karyotype study to identify XY mosaicism. Gonadectomy is indicated in patients with a Y chromosome to prevent potential neoplasm formation. These patients are infertile and require estrogen replacement.

Intersex. Intersex patients have divergence of karyotype and phenotype. Patients with testicular feminization have an XY karyotype but look like normal females lacking pubic and axillary hair. The gonads are testicles, but androgen-sensitive tissues in these patients lack intracellular androgen receptors or are unable to convert testosterone to dihydrotestosterone. These patients lack a uterus and upper vagina because they did respond to antimullerian hormone secreted by the testes in utero. The gonads are either intraabdominal or located in the inguinal canal. They should be removed because of neoplastic potential. Estrogen replacement and formation of a neovagina are indicated to fulfill the female sexual identity of these patients.

Overproduction of androgens from adrenal or ovarian sources can cause hirsutism, acne, deep voice, and clitoral hypertrophy along with primary amenorrhea. Polycystic ovarian syndrome can occasionally develop similar manifestations. Rarely, adrenogenital syndrome with clitoromegaly may not be diagnosed until adolescence or adulthood if the enzyme defect is incomplete.

Hypothalamic Amenorrhea. Patients with normal female karyotype, low gonadotropins, and hypoestrogenism usually have inadequate production of hypothalamic releasing factors. Psychogenic and physical stress and certain drugs can alter the synthesis and metabolism of monamine neurotransmitters and produce functional alterations of the hypothalamic gonadotropin regulating centers. Pituitary or peripituitary tumors are rare but can also cause hypogonadotropic amenorrhea. Constitutional delay of onset of menarche with delayed maturation of the hypothalamic regulatory centers is another cause. Bone growth should be assessed, and low doses of estrogen may be employed to facilitate development of secondary sex characteristics.

Secondary Amenorrhea

Secondary amenorrhea is defined as absence of menses for three menstrual cycles in a previously menstruating woman. There are several causes.

Pregnancy. Pregnancy should be considered and excluded by examination and hCG testing.

Hyperprolactinemia. Many women with secondary amenorrhea have elevated prolactin levels, and many of them have galactorrhea. Pituitary prolactinoma should be ruled out by CT or MRI of the pituitary in women who have significantly elevated prolactin levels (>50 ng/ml). Slight elevations of prolactin (20 to 50 ng/ml) may be caused by stress, psychotropic medications (e.g., narcotics, major and minor tranquilizers), and hypothyroidism with elevated TSH. If a prolactinoma is present, bromocriptine, a dopamine agonist, is utilized for conservative suppressive therapy. Occasionally, transsphenoidal microsurgery or radiotherapy is required for management.

Excess Androgen Syndrome. Polycystic ovarian disease with chronic anovulation and mild androgen excess is a common cause of anovulation. Signs of virilization such as clitoral hypertrophy, temporal balding, and deepening of the voice are indicative of an androgen-producing tumor and can be initially confirmed by elevated ovarian (testosterone) or adrenal (dehydroepiandrosterone sulfate) androgen levels. Laboratory findings of polycystic ovarian disease include withdrawal bleeding with progesterone administration, elevated serum LH, slightly elevated testosterone or dehydroepiandrosterone sulfate levels. As discussed in the section on polycystic ovarian disease, management depends upon the goal and includes ovulation induction, cycling with combination estrogen-progestin contraceptive pills, or monthly administration of progestin.

Hypothalamic Amenorrhea. Patients with disruption of normal hypothalamic-pituitary-ovarian function may secrete enough gonadotropin to stimulate the ovary, resulting in low levels of estrogen but without a midcycle estradiol peak and luteinizing hormone (LH) surge. Some patients have extremely low levels of FSH and LH, resulting in no follicular development and minimal estrogen output. These patients are hypoestrogenic and do not respond to a progesterone challenge test. Many causes for hypothalamic amenorrhea have been documented, including acute and chronic stress, weight loss, and psychogenic causes. Since nonfunctioning pituitary tumors can cause hypothalamic amenorrhea, these must be ruled out. Management depends on the cause and desires of the patient. Treatment may include estrogen supplementation, weight gain, removal of stress, and psychotherapy.

Ovarian Failure. Cessation of menses associated with an FSH level over 40 mIU/ml is diagnostic of ovarian failure. Causes include chromosomal mosaicism, autoimmune disorders, gonadotropin-resistant ovaries, and premature menopause. Patients with ovarian failure are sterile and require estrogen replacement. Chromosomal mosaicism should be excluded by karyotyping.

Estrogen Replacement Therapy. Perimenopausal and postmenopausal estrogen replacement relieves vasomotor symptoms (hot flashes), improves atrophic genital tissue, retards osteoporosis, and may have cardiovascular benefits. The most widely publicized risk of estrogen replacement therapy is increased risk for developing endometrial carcinoma in patients who have received exogenous estrogens. Estrogen replacement does not increase the risk of breast carcinoma but should not be used in a patient with a prior history of an estrogen-dependent tumor. Estrogen replacement should be administered at the lowest effective dose in a continuous manner, since that more closely mimics the secretory pattern of the premenopausal ovary. The addition of progestin for 10 to 14 days of each cycle in women who still have uterus in situ protects against endometrial hyperplasia and endometrial carcinoma. Endometrial biopsies should be employed liberally in these patients if they develop abnormal vaginal bleeding that does not conform to the expected withdrawal bleeding pattern.

Dysfunctional Uterine Bleeding. Abnormal bleeding associated with anovulatory or oligoovulatory states is termed dysfunctional uterine bleeding (DUB). Often episodes of DUB and long intervals of amenorrhea will occur in the same individual, demonstrating a common hormonal etiology for these different bleeding patterns.

Irregular and occasionally excessive anovulatory uterine bleeding is caused by uninterrupted estrogen effect. Prolonged exposure to estrogen may lead to endometrial hyperplasia. DUB is frequently seen at the extremes of reproductive life: in the adolescent before she develops consistent ovulation and in the perimenopausal woman as ovarian function declines. Excessive bleeding can be managed by cyclic estrogen-progestin hormone therapy, but older patients require endometrial sampling to rule out endometrial carcinoma.

Polycystic Ovarian Disease. Patients with polycystic ovarian disease (PCOD) may present with a wide range of symptoms suggestive of chronic anovulation and mild excess androgen. The classical Stein-Leventhal syndrome includes amenorrhea, hirsutism, and obesity, but these patients comprise only a relatively small number of patients with PCOD. Frequently, patients have an elevated LH and normal FSH. A small percentage have elevated prolactin. Continuous ovarian production of androstenedione with peripheral conversion to estrone may result in anovulatory bleeding or amenorrhea. Patients are infertile and do not demonstrate a normal basal body temperature rise indicative of ovulation if they are having regular menses. Ovarian production of testosterone and androstenedione may result in hyperandrogenism with hirsutism or acne. Patients with PCOD rarely have true virilism.

Management depends on the therapeutic goal. If fertility is desired, clomiphene citrate, an antiestrogen ovulation-induction agent, may be used. Some patients who fail to respond to clomiphene citrate ovulate in response to human menopausal gonadotropin therapy and other advanced ovulation-induction regimens. Ovarian wedge resections can be done in patients who are unresponsive to medical management, but this operation is only rarely indicated and may produce tubal or ovarian adhesions that compromise fertility.

Patients with PCOD who do not desire fertility should be cycled with either combination estrogen-progestin contraceptives or monthly progestin. This minimizes the long-term risk of endometrial hyperplasia and endometrial carcinoma caused by unopposed endogenous estrogenic stimulation of the endometrium. Cosmetic improvement of acne and hirsutism may be obtained with combination oral contraceptives that decrease the exposure of target tissues to free testosterone by increasing metabolic clearance of all steroids (including androgens) by inducing hepatic enzyme systems, increasing hepatic production of sex hormone-binding globulin, and decreasing ovarian production of testosterone through suppression of endogenous gonadotropin secretion from the pituitary. Spironolactone is also helpful in ameliorating hirsutism, acting on the cellular receptor as an antiandrogen. Successful medical management results in cessation of progression of hirsutism, however, a minority of patients note significant regression of excess terminal hair. Temporary hair removal by shaving or plucking is appropriate and does not increase regrowth. Electrolysis kills hair follicles and is a permanent treatment option for hirsutism.

INFERTILITY

Infertility is defined as 1 year of unprotected intercourse without pregnancy and affects approximately 15% of couples. In simple terms, conception requires sperm, eggs, and functional female upper genital tract anatomy. Disorders in one or more of these three general categories can cause infertility. While initial evaluation of infertility includes a complete medical and sexual history of the couple and physical examination (with pelvic examination) of the female partner, infertility diagnoses are almost always established by other tests. While most therapeutic options are diagnosis specific, some can be used appropriately for women with many causes of infertility and for multifactorial infertility. While many different tests and treatments have been tried in the management of infertility, Table 38-4 provides a contemporary summary of infertility tests and therapies.

The incidence for each diagnosis is very dependent on local or regional factors and patterns of referral for infertility care. The percentages shown in Table 38-4 seem to be reasonable general estimates based on the literature and experience. Perhaps owing to different impressions about the incidence of different infertility diagnoses, valid differences of opinion exist regarding priorities in testing and treatment of the infertile couple. There is certainly a consensus that testing should be systematic and complete enough to screen for major causes of infertility.

Therapy
Male

The infertile male should consult a urologist with expertise in male infertility. Artificial insemination may be required if semen analysis is unfavorable.

Cervical Factor

Thick, "hostile" cervical mucus at the time of ovulation may be improved with preovulatory estrogen. Many white blood cells in cervical mucus are suggestive of cervicitis and may be treated with antibiotics. The presence of antisperm antibodies in the cervical mucus is suggested when the sperm are nonmotile. There are many techniques for measuring antisperm antibodies, but unfortunately none has proven to be clinically reliable. Condoms can be utilized for 6 months in an attempt to reduce antisperm antibodies.

Tubal Factor

Tuboplasty is utilized in patients who have abnormalities of the tube identified on hysterosalpingography

Table 38-4. Infertility Diagnoses, Tests and Therapies

Diagnosis	Incidence* (%)	Common Tests	Diagnostic Results	Initial Therapy	Advanced Therapies
Multifactorial	40	Complete survey†	See individual tests	Treat one or more specific factors	IUI, GIFT IVF-ET‡
Endometriosis	17	Laparoscopy	Characteristic implants and adhesions	Prospective observation, suppression with medication, or conservative resection at laparotomy	IUI, GIFT, IVF-ET
Male factor	12	Semen analysis	<20 million normal motile sperm per ejaculation	Prospective observation or donor insemination	IUI, GIFT IVF-ET
Ovulatory dysfunction	11	Midluteal serum progesterone; late luteal endometrial biopsy	Progesterone <15 ng/ml is suspect; <10/ml is abnormal; biopsy lag ≥2	Directed therapies for endocrine diseases; otherwise clomiphene	Human menopausal gonadotropin or gonadotropic releasing hormone
Tubal factor/ pelvic adhesions	8	Laparoscopy with hydrotubation; hysterosalpingography	Tubal occlusion/ presence of adhesions at laparoscopy. Hysterosalpingography does not show adhesions	Laser laparoscopy or lysis of adhesions and tuboplasties at laparotomy	IVF-ET
Cervical factor	1	Postcoital test	<5 motile sperm/HPF in late follicular phase mucus	Prospective observation	IUI, GIFT IVF-ET
Uterine factor	1	Hysteroscopy; hysterosalpingography	Septum, polyp, fibroid seen; hysterosalpingography has a significant false-negative rate	Hysteroscopic resection	Metroplasty at laparotomy
Idiopathic	10	Complete survey	See individual tests	Prospective observation, empirical clomiphene or empirical antibiotics	IUI, GIFT IVF-ET

*Approximate
†Minimum of semen analysis, midluteal serum progesterone, and laparoscopy/hysteroscopy with hydrotubation
‡IUI, washed intrauterine insemination with husband's sperm, usually in superovulation cycles; GIFT, gamete intrafallopian transfer; IVF-ET in vitro fertilization with embryo transfer

or laparoscopy. If the woman does not have bilateral tubal occlusion, the couple should undergo a complete evaluation of other factors before employing surgery for lesser degrees of tubal injury. Tuboplasty procedures include salpingolysis, fimbrioplasty, salpingostomy, tubal anastomosis, and cornual implantation. Intraperitoneal high-molecular-weight dextran is employed to reduce postoperative adhesions. Microsurgical techniques with meticulous attention to hemostasis and minimizing tissue trauma improve pregnancy rates.

Ovulatory Factor

Clomiphene citrate is the most commonly used agent for inducing ovulation. Clomiphene has an antiestrogenic effect on the hypothalamus resulting in increased output of gonadotropin-releasing factors and, in turn, increased production of gonadotropins. An intact hypothalamic-pituitary-ovarian axis with endogenous estrogen production is necessary for ovulation induction with clomiphene. The dose of clomiphene is escalated during succeeding cycles until ovulation is achieved. Ovulation as evidenced by conception can be achieved in approximately 40% of anovulatory patients. The incidence of spontaneous abortion and twin gestation is increased. Ovarian hyperstimulation may result in ovarian cysts, which are treated conservatively.

Menopausal gonadotropins (Pergonal) and hCG (acting as a substitute for the endogenous LH surge) may be used in patients who are resistant to clomiphene or who lack an intact hypothalamic-pituitary-ovarian axis. Pergonal requires daily injections and frequent monitoring of the patient with ovarian ultrasound and estradiol levels to avoid hyperstimulation of the ovaries. Multiple pregnancies are often observed. Gonadotropin-releasing hormone analogs are not yet available for routine ovulation induction.

Modern Reproductive Technologies

Previously, options for infertile couples unable to achieve pregnancy by any of the aforementioned treatments were limited to adoption. Currently, the application of techniques utilized in animal husbandry for *in vitro* fertilization (IVF) and embryo transfer offer new options to these couples. IVF is achieved by producing ovarian hyperstimulation using menopausal gonadotropins. Ova are harvested by laparoscopy or by transvaginal ultrasonic aspiration and are fertilized with sperm. After appropriate maturation, the embryo is transferred into the endometrial cavity.

The gamete intrafallopian transfer (GIFT) procedure involves retrieval of oocytes, which are mixed with washed sperm and then transferred directly into the fallopian tube at laparoscopy. The use of the fallopian tube as the natural "incubator" for fertilization may yield a higher pregnancy rate in patients who have relatively healthy fallopian tubes.

Washed intrauterine insemination in superovulatory cycles appears to be appropriate therapy for patients otherwise being considered for the GIFT procedure, since the success rate is good and the regimen deletes the requirement for repetitive laparoscopies in treatment cycles.

Assessment of Infertility Therapy

Evidence of successful treatment of an infertile couple is, quite simply, a baby. All other parameters of response to treatment may be reassuring or encouraging, but these couples want a baby, not "a good cycle" or "a nice operation." Evaluation of treatment strategies for groups of patients with any particular diagnosis can be difficult, but some assessment of outcome can be made by estimation of fecundability.

Fecundability (or monthly fecundity) is the chance of conception in a single cycle of exposure, which for unscreened populations of humans is initially 15% to 20%. This fraction is not simply additive, so roughly 60% of couples conceive within 6 cycles and 85% of couples, within 12 cycles. Follow-up for 24 cycles or more yields only a few percent more conceptions. This basic pattern of human fertility is the "gold standard" by which to judge therapies. If normal fecundity is 15% per cycle, any treatment that increases fecundity *toward* that rate per cycle can be considered efficacious if the underlying fecundity in that diagnostic group is low. If the infertility factor, such as mild endometriosis, has a modest associated fecundity (perhaps 5% to 7% per cycle) then it may be extremely difficult to conclude that a therapy is effective if treated patients have a fecundity of 8% to 11%. On the other hand, if the diagnosis is bilateral tubal occlusion (<1% fecundity), an IVF cycle fecundity of 7% to 10% is clearly superior to no therapy but certainly not equal to normal fecundity.

39

Pediatric Surgery

Robert T. Soper
Ken Kimura

Fifty years ago, medical (infectious) disorders accounted for most hospitalizations and deaths of children. Today in industrialized countries more than half of hospitalized children have disease with surgical overtones and one fourth of all surgical patients are children. Since there are approximately 70 million people under 14 years of age in the United States, these figures have staggering logistic and professional implications. Surgical disease in children is becoming more important for two reasons: antibiotics, immunizations, and good medical care have dramatically decreased the infectious diseases that were responsible for most hospitalizations and deaths of children a half-century ago and new drugs, instruments, and better training now allow routine correction of abnormalities hitherto considered inoperable, transplant surgery being a prime example.

Ill infants and children cannot be treated as small adults. There are enough differences in the etiology, course, and pathophysiology of disease in the very young to adequately justify special consideration and training. The obvious problems imposed by the small size of the patient, the different maintenance requirements, inability to give a history, and the magnitude of certain corrective operations all add to the need for a chapter devoted to the very young surgical patient.

THE NEONATAL SURGICAL PATIENT

The newborn infant epitomizes the profound differences that exist between the adult and the pediatric surgical patient. These differences become less striking and important as the baby grows into childhood and adolescence. About 0.5% (1 out of 200) of live-born babies require emergency neonatal surgery, generally because of congenital anomalies obstructing flow through one of the vital body conduits (food through the gastrointestinal tract, cerebrospinal fluid through the central nervous system, blood through the heart or major vessels).

In certain ways newborns tolerate operations surprisingly well. The body systems that have developed correctly function remarkably well, despite measurable anatomic and physiologic evidence of immaturity. The cardiovascular system is perhaps the outstanding example: the heart muscle is hypertrophied at birth because during gestation it pumps 20% to 30% more blood (through the placental circuit) than the postnatal circulatory volume. The heart therefore possesses relatively more functional reserve at birth than it will have later.

The newborn infant enjoys a higher relative circulating blood volume than he will have subsequently because (a) of return of extra blood to the baby from the placenta at the time of delivery and (b) relative to weight, the newborn has 50% more extracellular fluid, part of which is blood, than the adult does.

The newborn's blood has a higher oxygen-carrying capacity than it will have later, with hemoglobin and hematocrit levels often 50% higher than those in adults. A relative hypoxemia in the fetus (from inefficient transport of oxygen across the placental barrier) stimulates fetal blood production. Increased tolerance to hypoxemia is carried over into the neonatal period.

A strong heart pump, hypervolemia, and the high oxygen-carrying capacity of the blood combine to make the newborn a relatively good operative risk.

Fluid Therapy

The newborn has 10% to 15% more total body water relative to weight than the older child or adult does. This excess fluid is soon lost as urine. It dictates the low maintenance fluid requirement of 50 ml/kg for the first day, which progressively rises to 100 ml/kg/day by the end of the first week of life. Thus the daily maintenance fluid of the week-old infant is three to four times that of the adult when calculated per unit of body weight. These requirements must be computed carefully on the basis of body weight, surface area, or calories expended.

One of the simpler methods for calculating daily maintenance fluid requirements for children is as follows: about 100 ml/day is needed for each of the first 10 kg of body weight, about 50 ml/day for each of the second 10 kg (from 10 to 20 kg of body weight), and about 20 ml/day for each kilogram above 20 kg of body weight. The average adult requires about 30 ml/kg/day.

Another method of calculating daily maintenance fluid is on the basis of body surface area. Surface area is expressed in square meters (m^2) and is calculated from a nomogram with the patient's body length (height) in centimeters and body weight in kilograms. Daily fluid for maintenance normally is 1500 ml/m^2 of body surface area, a figure that does not vary with age. Representative body surface areas for babies of given body weights are as follows:

Body weight (kg)	Body surface area (m^2)
1.8	0.15
2.7	0.2
4	0.25
5	0.29
8	0.4
10	0.5
20	0.8
30	1

When a patient cannot be nourished enterally, the intravenous fluid that we prefer for maintenance purposes is N/5 saline in 5% dextrose solution. This solution contains 30 mEq/L of NaCl. To this is added KCl, 20 mEq/L, after adequate urinary output is assured.

Parenteral (intravenous) fluids must be calculated precisely for volume and content and should be given at a rather steady rate over the entire 24-hour period. Unusual body fluid loss such as vomiting, diarrhea, nasogastric suction, and sequestered body fluids must be measured or estimated accurately and added to maintenance requirements. Hyperthermia or exposure to a dry environment increase fluid requirements. Oral feedings are self-regulated.

A newborn infant weighing 3 kg has a total circulating blood volume of roughly 250 ml. Blood loss in the relatively modest amount of 25 ml (less than 1 ounce) constitutes a significant hemorrhage that proportionately in the adult would approach 600 ml.

Environment

The newborn infant is much more sensitive to environmental temperature and humidity than the adult is because (1) he has almost three times the amount of skin exposed to the environment in relation to weight and (2) he has a meager insulating blanket of subcutaneous fat. The neonatal surgical patient must be nursed in an incubator. Advantages gained from the incubator include (1) humidification of the air to nearly 100% to reduce insensible fluid loss; (2) oxygenation of air breathed to 30% to 35% concentration to facilitate adequate oxygenation of tissue; and (3) control of air temperature at about 85° F (29.5° C) that allows easy maintenance of normal body temperature. Lower air temperature induces body heat loss and requires expenditure of energy to generate more body heat.

The lack of subcutaneous fat in the neonate (in contrast to the adult) is significant for one other reason: fat provides calories when oral caloric intake is insufficient. Thus correcting factors that preclude oral intake of food in the newborn is vital, since adequate calories cannot be supplied by conventional parenteral fluids.

Respiration

Four factors unique to the newborn influence respiration. Air exchange in the lungs and blood flow through the pulmonary circuit have just been initiated, and commonly a few days elapse before lung function becomes optimal. The right upper lung lobe is predisposed to atelectasis for anatomic reasons (a dependent position of its bronchus). The newborn depends entirely on diaphragmatic descent for lung expansion, because the ribs are horizontal and cannot "lift" on inspiration as in the adult. Anything impeding free motion of the diaphragm jeopardizes respiration: congenital diaphragmatic hernia, faulty innervation of the diaphragm muscles, and increase in intraabdominal pressure (intestinal obstruction). Finally the newborn breathes by preference through the nose rather than the mouth, and anything narrowing or occluding the nasal passages (choanal atresia, mucus plugs, nasogastric tubes) impairs respiratory exchange.

These factors of inefficient early lung function, atelectasis, inhibition of diaphragmatic motion, and obstruction of nasal passages must all be diagnosed and managed promptly to assure normal respiratory function.

Types of Operations (Newborn versus Adults)

Congenital anomalies are the most frequent indication for operations on the newborn, in distinction to infection, trauma, and degenerative and neoplastic diseases in the adult. Thus neonatal intestinal obstruction is generally caused by webs, bands, membranes, faulty innervation, or other abnormalities of development, whereas in the adult it is generally caused by hernias, postoperative adhesions, and neoplasms.

Surgical Disease—Rapid Progression

The speed at which surgical disease progresses is often dramatically accelerated in the newborn patient and may result in death in just a few hours. Small actual volume of body fluids, low energy and nutritional reserves, and poor defenses against infection contribute to this rapid progression. Furthermore, the newborn must communicate his illness by indirect and often subtle signs such as changes in color and rates of pulse and respiration, inability to feed, irritability, and lethargy. The good pediatric nurse or physician must be an astute observer, for the baby is a poor historian. Time is truly of the essence in the newborn surgical patient.

THE NEWBORN AND THE OPERATING ROOM

Temperature

Body temperature must be monitored continuously. Body heat of the infant is conserved when the operating room air is warmed, the time periods out of the incubator before and after operation are shortened, large volumes of rapidly evaporating fluids to prepare the skin are avoided, and a heat exchange blanket on top of the operating table mattress is used. Infrared lamps also may be used to deliver radiant heat to the baby during operation.

During operations, body heat is lost rapidly when major body cavities such as the thorax or abdomen are opened, and this loss must be countered by lavages of normal saline solution heated to just above body temperature. Clear plastic adhesive drapes reduce convection loss of heat, provide a sterile barrier impervious to water, allow better visualization of the entire patient by the operating room team, and are therefore highly recommended.

Technique

Placing a plastic catheter in a vein by "cutdown" or percutaneous insertion must precede all major operations performed on infants, as a dependable route for administration of fluids and blood. Good surgical principles are never more important that in the neonate: precision (magnification is sometimes helpful), gentleness, protection of exposed viscera, miniaturized instruments, and fine suture material are essential. Subcuticular closure of the skin incision will avoid the need for later suture removal, and clear plastic sprayed on the wound obviates the use of restricting conventional dressings that prevent observation and easy examination of the area. Above all, the *proper* operation must be performed *correctly*. The margin for error in neonatal surgery is narrow.

Postoperative Care

Postoperative convalescence of the newborn surgical patient is generally gratifyingly rapid. The infant should be checked frequently visually through the transparent incubator, but manipulations should be held to a minimum (e.g., at regular 2-hour intervals).

Postoperative complications in the newborn patient are mainly those of the operation itself plus infection and aspiration of vomitus. The postoperative complications common in the adult patient (paralytic ileus, pneumonia, urinary retention, deep vein thrombophlebitis) are almost unheard of in the newborn surgical patient. Aspiration of vomitus, anastomotic leaks, adhesive postoperative intestinal obstruction, and wound infections are poorly tolerated by the infant; they are best prevented or diagnosed and treated early.

The results of surgical treatment are very gratifying when the anomaly is completely corrected, no other anomalies are present, and no complications ensue. Multiple anomalies, incomplete surgical correction, prematurity, and postoperative complications are discouraging features that favor morbidity and mortality. There is no greater satisfaction to the surgeon or nurse than a newborn patient who has been given a normal life expectancy, surgically cured of an otherwise lethal anomaly.

CONGENITAL ANOMALIES

Congenital anomalies are simply abnormalities of development that are present at birth. Location, magnitude, and mode of origin differ. They constitute about 80% of surgical problems in the newborn.

Cause

Congenital anomalies are the result of three basic causes: (1) abnormal genes or chromosomes of the sperm or egg; (2) abnormalities that develop in previously normal genes or chromosomes (mutations) often because of noxious environmental influences; and (3) unfavorable environment that prevents normal development of the fetus without any detectable chromosome or gene alteration

Abnormal Genes or Chromosomes

Some congenital disorders are caused by gross chromosomal abnormalities that can now be verified microscopically (Down's syndrome, Turner's syndrome, and various trisomy and deletion syndromes). These are characterized by multiple, widespread, and often severe changes in the developing fetus.

Other congenital anomalies are believed to result from an abnormality of a single autosomal gene (con genital cataract, achondroplasia, and syndactylism). Some of them are *dominant* (polydactylism, familial polyposis coli) and are expressed in the patient regardless of the fact that the other gene for this trait is normal. If the gene abnormalities are *recessive,* both members of the genic pair must be abnormal (albinism, cystic fibrosis) before it is expressed in the offspring. Some of the genetically determined abnormalities are sex linked (such as hemophilia), are exhibited only in the male offspring, and are merely carried or transmitted without expression in the female.

Environment

Far more common than these are congenital abnormalities induced by exposure of the developing fetus to harmful stimuli, usually in early gestation. Vulnerability is directly proportional to the rapidity with which the body systems are developing; therefore the first trimester of pregnancy is the time when these harmful stimuli have their greatest effect. Some of the noxious environmental stimuli that have been identified are the following:

Chemical
  Alcohol, cyclophosphamide, diethylstilbestrol, phenytoin, tetracyclines, thalidomide, valproic acid
Maternal metabolic disturbances
  Diabetes, hyperthermia, phenylketonuria, virilizing tumors
Infection
  Viruses, rickettsia and bacteria; especially, cytomegalovirus, herpesvirus, rubella, toxoplasmosis, *Treponema pallidum*
Irradiation
  X-rays, atomic fallout, radium (alpha particles), radioactive iodine, natural background irradiation
Mechanical
  Malposition of the fetus (extended knees, ankylosis), mechanical pressure (atrophic single extremities), hydraulic pressure (all four extremities atrophic).
Defective fertilization and implantation
  Tubal pregnancy
Parental age
  Down's syndrome is more frequent when parents are older
Anoxia
  Possible ultimate pathway in many of the above conditions
Accidents of timing of embryonic events
  During the first 8 weeks of gestation, the embryo progresses from a single fertilized cell to a recognizable fetus in whom the foundations of all organ systems have been laid. This phenomenal growth demands dovetailing of an infinite number of events that must occur precisely on time in order to achieve normal development. Misadventures in timing of these events may cause some congenital anomalies. For example, congenital diaphragmatic hernia seems to occur either when closure of the pleuroperitoneal canals is delayed or when the midgut returns early to the abdomen from its extracoelomic umbilical hernia.

Incidence

Over 25% of stillborn babies have congenital anomalies that caused the stillbirth; 3% of live babies are found to have congenital anomalies on immediate careful examination, and an additional 4% harbor occult abnormalities. Fortunately, most of these are minor and do not significantly affect growth, development, or life expectancy; 75% are single, but 25% are multiple—thus when one congenital anomaly is discovered in a baby, others must be anticipated. Anomalies are about 15% higher in males than in females. The incidence is 2.5 times higher in multiple than in single births. When one anomalous child is born into a family, there is a 25 times greater chance that subsequent children will have anomalies than if previous siblings were normally developed. With two malformed siblings in a family, there is about a 50% chance that the anomalies will be similar in location and severity. The central nervous system, cardiovascular, skeletal, and intestinal systems appear to be most commonly involved in abnormal development.

History

The history is most important in diagnosing congenital anomalies, with the preceding causes being kept in mind. Questions should be directed to anomalies in previous generations and the maternal health and habits during the pregnancy.

Abnormalities of amniotic fluid volume (polyhydramnios is excessive volume; oligohydramnios is too little fluid) are frequently associated with fetal anomalies and should be investigated carefully by midtrimester prenatal amniocentesis and fetal ultrasound studies.

Normally the fetus continually swallows amniotic fluid from the fifth gestational month until delivery. This fluid is absorbed from the proximal small intestine to circulate as tissue fluid, plasma, and cerebrospinal fluid. It is then partially excreted through the placental circuit into the maternal circulation and partially excreted by the fetal kidneys back into the amniotic sac. Interruption of this cyclic flow at any point in the fetus (proximal small bowel: atresia; central nervous system: anencephaly, hydrocephaly, myelomeningocele; urinary tract: atresia, renal aplasia) may upset the delicate balance of amniotic fluid to produce oligohydramnios or polyhydramnios.

Physical Examination

Physical examination must be meticulous and detailed. It should include inspection of the freshly cut umbilical cord to see whether one of the umbilical arteries is missing; this often is a clue to the presence of a hidden anomaly in the body. Small catheters passed into both ends of the gastrointestinal tract can allow rapid diagnosis of obstruction. Special tests are listed under specific congenital anomalies.

Treatment

The treatment of congenital anomalies must be individualized. No treatment is possible if the anomaly is so serious as to be immediately lethal or incorrectable, and none is necessary if the anomaly is so minor as to produce no significant change in function. Important aspects of the more common congenital anomalies are summarized in Table 39-1.

TRAUMA

A person is probably subjected to more trauma during childhood than at any later period of life. Some is self-occasioned by poor judgment and imperfect muscle and nerve coordination during the toddler years, and some results from poor parental supervision. Thanks to the resiliency of young tissue, most trauma is well tolerated, and few of the scars are carried into adulthood.

Text continued on p. 535

Table 39-1. Important Aspects of the More Common Congenital Anomalies

Type	Anatomic Deformity	Clinical Characteristics	Treatment, Age	Prognosis
Central nervous system				
Myelomeningocele	Defect in bony and soft-tissue coverings of neural canal, generally lumbar level	Protrusion of cord coverings in back; paralysis and no sensation in lower extremities, anus, and bladder; about 75% later develop hydrocephalus; meningitis a constant threat	Cover exposed nerve elements with tissue and skin in infancy	No improvement in nerve function
Hydrocephalus	Obstruction to flow or absorption of cerebrospinal fluid with increasing pressure of fluid	Enlarging head, deterioration of cerebral function, tense fontanels	Shunt cerebrospinal fluid from brain to bloodstream or body cavity through plastic tubing and valve system; done in infancy	Malfunction of shunt may require revisions
Craniosynostosis	Premature closure of skull sutures (growth lines)	Small head, progressive cerebral deterioration	Osteotomy of suture lines to prevent closure; done in infancy	Good; repeat operations may be necessary
Cardiovascular system				
Interatrial septal defect	Hole in wall between left and right atrium	Systolic precordial murmur, some decrease in growth and exercise tolerance	Closure by suture or patch during heart-lung bypass; done in childhood; some close spontaneously	Excellent
Ventricular septal defect	Hole in wall between left and right ventricle	Systolic precordial murmur; if neglected, cyanosis and serious lung complications	Closure by suture or patch during heart-lung bypass; done in childhood; some close spontaneously	Excellent if repaired early
Tetralogy of Fallot	Interventricular septal defect, stenosis of pulmonary outflow tract, and takeoff of aorta from both ventricles	Cyanosis and breathlessness with exercise, stunted growth, systolic precordial murmur	Closure of septum to right of aorta, enlargement of pulmonary valve during heart-lung bypass; done in childhood	Higher risk operation, results good if complete correction can be achieved early
Malformation of heart valves	Stenosis or imperfect valves that allow regurgitation of blood	Systolic or diastolic murmur; dilation, hypertrophy, and failure of heart with edema and breathlessness	Enlargement of stenotic valve, suture correction or replacement of deformed valve during heart-lung bypass; done in childhood	Good if complete correction can be achieved, guarded if not
Coarctation of aorta	Narrowing of descending aorta	Headache, heart enlargement, hypertension in upper body, hypotension in lower body, absent femoral pulses	Excision under hypothermia or during heart-lung bypass; done in childhood	Excellent
Patent ductus arteriosus	Retention of fetal vessel joining pulmonary artery to aorta (to bypass lungs in utero)	"Machinery" type of continuous murmur heard in chest and back; bounding pulses, left atrial enlargement, congestive heart failure in premature infants	Suture closure or ligation; in infancy or childhood	Excellent
Otolaryngological system				
Cleft lip or palate, or both	Cleft, or opening, in lip or palate; often seen together	Obvious cosmetic defects, difficulty in feeding and speech; dental malformations	Plastic surgical closure of lip in infancy, palate in young childhood	Good; generally requires large team of surgeons, dentists, speech and hearing experts for complete rehabilitation

Table 39-1. Important Aspects of the More Common Congenital Anomalies—cont'd

Type	Anatomic Deformity	Clinical Characteristics	Treatment, Age	Prognosis
Otolaryngological system—cont'd				
Branchial cleft abnormalities	Retention of part, or all, of the embryonic branchial structures	Cyst, sinus, or fistula of lateral part of neck	Complete excision at time of election	Excellent
Thyroglossal abnormalities	Retention of embryonic thyroid tract from base of tongue to low anterior neck	Cyst or tract in anterior midline of neck	Complete excision at time of election	Excellent
Gastrointestinal system				
Atresia: complete closure of intestinal lumen; rare in stomach and colon	Esophagus: generally has blind proximal pouch, plus fistula connecting distal esophagus to distal trachea	Blind pouch: saliva and feedings vomited. Fistula: air distending bowel, stomach; HCl bathing lungs to cause pneumonia	Division and closure of fistula, anastomosis of ends of esophagus in neonatal period	Good; often correctable stricture of anastomosis; frequent gastroesophageal reflux
	Anorectal: no anal opening, closed rectum; 70% have narrow fistula connecting rectum to vagina and perineum in females, or to bladder, urethra, and perineum in males	Abdominal distension, bilious vomiting; either no meconium passed, or (females) meconium through vagina or on perineum or (males) meconium in urine or on perineum	Division and closure fistula, pullthrough of end of rectum to perineum through anal muscles; may need preliminary colostomy in neonatal period	Good early results; ultimate fecal control is variable
	Ileum, jejunum: complete closure of lumen by membrane or with loss of continuity of bowel	Abdominal distension, bilious vomiting, scanty meconium rectally	Excision and end-to-end anastomosis; in neonatal period	Excellent if enough bowel remains to support nutritional needs
	Duodenum: complete closure by membrane beyond ampulla of Vater (where bile and pancreatic juice enter); 30% have Down's syndrome	Scaphoid abdomen, copious bilious vomiting, scanty meconium rectally	Surgical bypass of membrane by side-to-side anastomosis of duodenum above the block to duodenum below the block; done in neonatal period	Excellent
Stenosis: narrowing of intestinal lumen; rare in esophagus, stomach, or colon	Duodenum: partial obstruction by membrane with a hole in it; 30% have Down's syndrome	No distension, bilious vomiting of feedings, some diminution in stools	Surgical bypass of membrane by side-to-side anastomosis when discovered	Excellent
	Jejunum, ileum: partial obstruction by membrane with a hole in it	Moderate abdominal distension, bilious vomiting of feedings, some diminution in stools	Excision and end-to-end anastomosis when discovered	Excellent
Malrotation of midgut	Abnormal embryonic rotation of gut with extrinsic band across duodenum, small bowel in right side of abdomen and colon in left; 50% have volvulus, or twisting, of gut around vessels	Bilious vomiting when duodenum obstructed by band; symptoms may be vague, intermittent, or absent; volvulus produces pain, strangulation, and shock	Lysis of extrinsic duodenal band; derotation of volvulus, resection if bowel dead; operate whenever discovered or symptomatic	Excellent if no volvulus; strangulating volvulus may require massive small bowel resection resulting in short gut syndrome

Continued.

Table 39-1. Important Aspects of the More Common Congenital Anomalies—cont'd

Type	Anatomic Deformity	Clinical Characteristics	Treatment, Age	Prognosis
Gastrointestinal system—cont'd				
Meckel's diverticulum	Outpocketing on the surface of distal ileum, vestige of embryonic tract, seen in 2% of people; 15% contain stomach mucosa, secrete HCl acid, and produce symptoms of ulceration, inflammation, or bleeding	Many are asymptomatic; intermittent abdominal pain, distension, vomiting, and melena are characteristic symptoms	Excision and closure when diagnosed or symptomatic	Excellent
Hirschsprung's disease (congenital megacolon, or aganglionosis)	Absent autonomic nerve cells in wall of distal part of colon cause obstruction at this point because peristaltic waves are not propagated	Abdominal distension, constipation from birth	Excision or bypass of involved colon; may require preliminary colostomy	Good
Meconium ileus	Seen in 8% of babies with mucoviscidosis (fibrocystic disease of pancreas); undigested meconium obstructing small bowel	Abdominal distension, bilious vomiting, scanty meconium passed	Irrigation or bypass of obstructing meconium block; administration of pancreatic digestive enzymes; done in neonatal period	Poor because of generalized mucoviscidosis and pneumonia
Genitourinary system				
Congenital obstruction	Ureteropelvic junction (at kidney outlet): caused by extrinsic band or vessel, or intrinsic narrowing; may be unilateral or bilateral; results in hydronephrosis and often infection	Flank pain or mass, fever, pus in urine, uremia if bilateral	Plastic revision to relieve obstruction if kidney good; done whenever diagnosed	Good
	Ureterocystic junction (where ureter joins bladder): intrinsic or extrinsic narrowing, poor peristalsis; unilateral or bilateral; produces hydroureter, hydronephrosis, and often infection	Flank pain or mass, fever, pus in urine; uremia if bilateral	Excision of obstructed area, reimplantation of ureter into bladder; done whenever diagnosed	Good
	Bladder neck (outlet): intrinsic valve or membrane; produces enlarged bladder and often bilateral reflux and infection to both kidneys	Lower abdominal mass, flank pain, fever, pus in urine, uremia if neglected	Resection of valve or membrane, plastic widening of stenosis	Good
Undescended testes	One or both testes in or above inguinal canal, often associated with hernia	Empty scrotal sac on one or both sides with groin swelling	Surgical placement in scrotum; in early childhood	Good; fertility likely to be impaired when bilateral
Lymphatic and vascular systems				
Cutaneous capillary hemangioma "strawberry"	Pink-red, slightly raised skin lesion	Cosmetic deformity mainly; occasionally ulcerates and bleeds	None; 95% thrombose and disappear in early childhood after infant growth spurt	Excellent

Table 39-1. Important Aspects of the More Common Congenital Anomalies—cont'd

Type	Anatomic Deformity	Clinical Characteristics	Treatment, Age	Prognosis
Lymphatic and vascular systems—cont'd				
Cavernous hemangioma	Large venous channels with abnormal lymphatic and arterial connections	Enlarged, bulky, blue-red lesions with discomfort or dysfunction if extremity involved; occasionally ulcerates, bleeds, or becomes infected; gigantism may occur	Injection of sclerosing agents, partial excision with skin grafts or, rarely, amputation as symptoms necessitate	Poor; recurrence and progression common
Cystic hygroma	Enlarged lymphatic spaces that cannot empty watery tissue fluid	Cystic, soft, indentable mass of neck or axilla that transilluminates; rarely produces tracheal deviation and airway obstruction	Conservative excision at age of election	Excellent
Skeletal system				
Congenital dislocation of hip	Dislocation of femoral head out of shallow hip joint	Asymmetry of fat folds of leg and buttock; palpable "click" on passive abduction and external rotation of hip	Reduction by manipulation, plaster cast in neonatal period	Excellent
Clubfoot (talipes equinovarus)	Foot points downward and is twisted inward	Inability to elevate foot	Manipulation and plaster casts in increasing degrees of dorsiflexion in neonatal period	Excellent if begun early
Abdominal wall				
Umbilical hernia	Enlarged umbilical fascial ring with protrusion of intestines into sac covered by skin	Umbilical swelling, larger with straining; asymptomatic	None; almost all spontaneously disappear by the age of 7 years	Excellent
Omphalocele	Enlarged umbilical fascial ring with protrusion of intestines into thin translucent amniotic sac not covered by skin	Grayish sac filled with viscera bulging around base of umbilical cord at birth	If small, immediate excision and repair of abdominal wall; if large, prosthetic "silo" to house viscera 7 to 10 days until abdominal wall can be closed	Good
Gastroschisis	Small aperture in abdominal wall to right of umbilicus through which protrudes midgut: thickened, covered with exudate, aperistaltic	Grossly altered intestine protruding from abdominal wall defect; no covering whatsoever	Immediate reduction and closure of abdominal wall, if feasible; if not, temporary prosthetic "silo"	Good

However, accidents are still the most common cause of death in the United States during the first half of life, and one child in every four will be injured seriously enough to require medical care. Each year in this country, 50,000 are permanently disabled and about 10,000 die from trauma. Motor vehicle accidents, drownings, and burns accounted for three fourths of these deaths. The general heading of accidents includes (roughly in decreasing frequency) lacerations; contusions and abrasions; fractures; ingestion of poisons, drugs, and foreign bodies; bites; sprains; head injuries; puncture wounds; eye trauma; and burns.

Approximately two thirds of accidents occur in or near the home and can be prevented by intelligent parental supervision and removal of the more common hazards. Safer playthings, supervised playgrounds, less accessible and tasty medications, and the manufacture of nonflammable clothing are public health measures that can diminish this toll. Automobile and bicycle accidents injure or kill thousands of children. Improved automobile safety engineering (seat belts, accident-proof door locks) and education of the adult driver and the child pedestrian or bicycle rider are worthwhile efforts to lower the number of children injured in this manner.

Surgical treatment of all the traumatic wounds mentioned varies according to the type and location of the trauma.

CHILD ABUSE

It has been estimated that approximatley 1% of children in the United States are deliberately physically abused each year. Nearly 80% of child abuse is seen in children under 3 years of age (too young to communicate the cause of injury) and fully 90% is inflicted by caretakers of the child (parents, stepparents, babysitters, etc.). Often the abuse occurs in a family that is deprived socially, economically, and emotionally. The history of injury as given by the abuser is often vague and discrepant with the multiplicity and seriousness of the observed injury. Multiplicity of injuries is the rule: there are many fractures in different phases of healing and many ecchymoses and hematomas in various stages of resolution. The eyes, genitalia, and back are common targets for this kind of deliberate abuse. Occasionally fatalities occur. Almost all states in this country have enacted legislation to remove the threat of litigation (for false accusation) to the attending physician who reports a suspected case of child abuse to the proper authorities. In many states the physician who fails to report a suspected case of child abuse may be prosecuted.

CANCER

During the past 25 years, cancer has risen from twelfth to second place among the causes of death in young children in the United States. There is little to indicate an actual increase in the frequency of childhood malignancies, but rather other causes of death have declined, as described in the introduction to this chapter.

Comparison of Adult and Childhood Cancer

Many basic differences distinguish adult from childhood cancer. Cancer in the adult generally arises from epithelial tissue lining glands, external surfaces, or hollow organs of the body. In contrast, childhood cancer emerges most often from mesenchymal tissue or cells of very primitive embryonic origin. The organ systems involved are different; the adult has a high incidence of cancer arising from skin, breast, lung, prostate, and intestinal epithelium. Cancer of these structures is almost unheard of in the child. About half the malignancies of children arise from lymphoid tissue in the form of leukemias and lymphomas. Another 15% to 20% are located in the central nervous system, and 10% arise from the adrenal glands and 10% from the kidneys.

Causes of Cancer

A few tumors of childhood seem to have hereditary implications, including retinoblastoma, familial polyposis, and Hodgkin's disease. The incidence of cancer in the first decade of life exceeds that of the second decade, indicating that some of the malignancies may be congenital. Leukemia in the mother has been transmitted across the placenta to her fetus; cancers of the adrenal glands and kidney occur in newborns. Irradiation delivered to children for other causes has been incriminated in later development of some cancers, particularly of the thyroid gland and lymphoma family.

Treatment of Cancer

Until the past two decades the results of treating childhood malignancies were discouraging, partly because of their rapid growth rate, early spread, and a delay in diagnosis occasioned by either absence of symptoms or the inability of the child to communicate such symptoms. However, there is no room for a "defeatist" attitude in the treatment of childhood malignancy. The resiliency of the young and the occasional striking response to therapy in the face of seemingly hopeless odds justify an aggressive, confident approach to treatment. Recent cooperative studies and new chemotherapy drugs have spectacularly improved the prognosis of certain childhood cancers.

All the treatment modalities employed in adult cancer are used in children; chemotherapy shows particular promise in this age group. Combinations of therapy are the rule rather than the exception. This improvement has been so dramatic in some tumors (i.e., Wilms' tumor) that now the thrust of treatment is to select those patients with a good prognosis and give them as little treatment as possible. The more aggressive treatment protocols are reserved for patients with a poor prognosis based on histologic appearance and extent of disease.

Specific Types of Childhood Cancer

Lymphoma-Leukemia Family

Leukemia is the single most common malignant neoplasm seen in children. About 90% are of the acute lymphogenous type, with the peak incidence at about 4 years of age. Prognosis is guarded, though new drug and treatment protocols have remarkably increased remissions and cures. Chemotherapy is the treatment of choice at present; the surgeon is restricted to an occasional diagnostic node or bone marrow biopsy. The surgeon's role is more prominent in lymphoma: confirming diagnosis by biopsy, accurately mapping the extent of involvement by "staging" operations that allow the radiotherapist to better tailor treatment, and occasionally "debulking" large non-Hodgkin's lymphomas.

Neuroblastoma

Neuroblastoma is a malignancy arising in primitive elements of the sympathetic nervous system. Two thirds originate in or near the adrenal gland, about 20% in the posterior mediastinum, and about 5% each from the neck and pelvic areas. The average age at diagnosis is 18 months, and the growth rate is typically rapid.

Symptoms of neuroblastoma are nonspecific; bone pain and fever frequently herald bone marrow metastases. Diarrhea, weight loss, anemia, and irritability are often seen. About 80% of patients have an abdominal mass that often extends across the midline, occasionally associated with metastases palpable within the liver. Diagnosis is confirmed by plain films showing the mass (which often contains calcium stippling) displacing hollow viscera, and intravenous pyelograms that show kidney displacement. Ultrasound and CT pinpoint location and extent of the primary tumor and of liver metastases. Metastases to bone occur in about 30% and to the lungs in 10%.

The surest diagnostic test of neuroblastoma is the presence of specific catecholamine hormones (vanillylmandelic acid and homovanillic acid) in the urine or blood, representing metabolic end products of tumor origin. Treatment consists of surgical removal of as much tumor as possible, generally followed by low-dose irradiation. Chemotherapy in the form of vincristine and cyclophosphamide combinations may palliate neuroblastoma.

Onset within the first year of life or tumors primary in the neck, pelvis, or mediastinum command a favorable prognosis. Curiuosly, about 5% of neuroblastomas spontaneously transform into benign ganglioneuromas. Tumor antibodies have been demonstrated in some cured patients. Unfortunately, more than half of patients with neuroblastoma die of their disease. Treatment has not significantly improved prognosis during the past decade.

Wilms' Tumor

Wilm's tumor, or nephroblastoma, is a cancer arising in embryonal kidney cells that grows rapidly to destroy the normal kidney tissuc. Again, the symptoms are nonspecific and include vague abdominal discomfort, fever, and occasionally hematuria. Early direct spread to perirenal tissues is the rule, with metastases to lung and liver in one third of the patients by the time a diagnosis is established; 90% of patients have a mass in the abdomen on physical examination, and intravenous pyelograms, ultrasound studies, and CT scans differentiate from neuroblastoma. Regrettably, about 5% of patients develop Wilm's tumors of both kidneys. Treatment is combined surgical removal, x-ray therapy, and chemotherapy with actinomycin D and vincristine. Recent reports indicate a long-term survival or "cure" of 85% of these patients.

Central Nervous System Tumors

Most central nervous system tumors arise below the membrane, or tentorium, that separates the cerebrum from the lower centers. Most of these cancers stem from supporting tissues within the brain and produce symptoms by disturbing balance and motor activity or by blocking the flow of cerebrospinal fluid to increase intracranial pressure. Surgical excision is the most effective treatment at this time. In keeping with central nervous system tumors of all ages, no distant metastases are seen.

Connective Tissue Tumors

Osteosarcomas have a peak incidence later in childhood, probably because of increasing bone growth rates at this time of life. Striated muscle cancers (rhabdomyosarcoma) in infancy are most commonly located in the bladder or genital tract; in older children they are chiefly seen in the head and neck, but they may occur in any striated muscle. Surgical excision, x-ray therapy, and a number of therapeutic drugs are used in combination for treatment of these less common childhood malignancies. Prognosis is guarded, with salvage of the patient in less than one half of all cases. A notable exception is Ewing's sarcoma of bone, for which conservative surgical resection, x-ray therapy, and new chemotherapeutic drugs have remarkably improved the prognosis.

NEONATAL GASTROINTESTINAL OBSTRUCTION

Obstruction of the gastrointestinal tract in the newborn is both unique and serious enough to justify spe-cial consideration. Obstruction may occur anywhere from esophagus to anus, having a curious numerical predilection for both ends of the tract. All neonatal gastrointestinal obstructions are secondary to congenital anomalies that, however, arise from a host of different influences. Together they constitute by far the most common surgical emergency of the neonatal period of life.

Neonatal gastrointestinal obstructions are no exception to the rule that anomalies are often multiple. Two causes for intestinal obstruction may coexist at different levels (as exemplified by the association of esophageal atresia with duodenal atresia or anorectal atresia), or the associated anomaly may involve a totally different system, such as the major congenital heart defects that accompany esophageal or anorectal atresia. The intestine may be obstructed simultaneously by two different mechanisms at the same level (extrinsic duodenal obstruction resulting from malrotation, and intrinsic obstruction from duodenal membrane) or at different levels by the same mechanism (about 15% of patients with intestinal atresia have additional atretic areas downstream from the most proximal one). About one fourth of babies with neonatal gastrointestinal obstruction have other anomalies, which must be diagnosed and managed along with the primary obstructing lesion.

Prematurity (birth weight below 2500 g) is associated in about one third of babies with congenital gastrointestinal obstruction. Both prematurity and serious associated congenital anomalies greatly worsen prognosis. The mortality for full-term newborns with obstruction who have no other major anomalies is about 10%, contrasting unfavorably with an 80% to 90% mortality expected in the obstructed premature baby with other major anomalies. If the obstruction is complicated by peritonitis, mortality is 50%. If the intestine must be opened to relieve the obstruction, mortality (40%) is much higher than it is when the obstruction is extrinsic (5%). Overall, the salvage rate for neonatal gastrointestinal obstruction is about 75%.

Family and Pregnancy History

Some causes for neonatal gastrointestinal obstruction are familial or inheritable, so a carefully taken history of the genealogy is helpful. Fibrocystic disease of the pancreas (with meconium ilcus), congenital aganglionosis of thc colon (Hirschsprung's disease), and hypertrophic pyloric stenosis are all examples of this tendency. Down's syndrome has a familial tendency and a predilection for duodenal atresia (about 7%).

The maternal pregnancy history is important in terms of illnesses, ingestion of drugs, and exposure to irradiation or other noxious environmental influences associated with congenital anomalies. Polyhydramnios has a high association with obstructions of the proximal gastrointestinal tract, as explained above.

Patient History

Bile vomiting, abdominal distension, and obstipation arc the three cardinal signs of obstruction of the gastrointestinal tract at any age; however, exceptions to this rule occur frequently enough in the obstructed newborn baby to justify special attention. Thus esophageal atresia with tracheoesophageal fistula produces regurgitation of feedings and saliva unstained with bile;

the abdominal distension is profound but is associated with free passage of meconium. The newborn with duodenal obstruction will indeed have copious bile vomiting but only mild epigastric distension and may pass one or two normal meconium stools. Paradoxically, the functional (nonmechanical) type of colonic obstruction produced by congenital aganglionosis (Hirschsprung's disease) is sometimes associated with diarrhea and only late and infrequent vomiting, although abdominal distension is conspicuous. Notwithstanding these exceptions, any newborn baby who (1) fails to pass meconium rectally within 24 hours after birth, (2) vomits bile, or (3) exhibits abdominal distension should have a plain film of the abdomen taken in the supine and erect (or decubitus) positions as a minimal initial step to investigate intestinal obstruction.

Relative Incidence

Atresias of the esophagus and anorectal area are numerically the most common causes for neonatal gastrointestinal tract obstruction, each constituting roughly 25% of cases. An additional 20% are caused by atresia and stenosis of the small intestine, and another 25% are about equally divided among midgut malrotation, meconium ileus, and congenital aganglionosis; 5% of cases comprise a miscellaneous group of very diverse causes.

Diagnosis

The diagnosis of gastrointestinal obstruction may often be made in the newborn baby before symptoms occur, by gentle passage of a small, soft, plastic catheter into both ends of the gastrointestinal tract. If the tube passes into the stomach, esophageal and choanal atresia can be ruled out; if 10 ml or less of clear fluid is aspirated from the stomach, congenital obstruction of the small bowel is extremely unlikely. However, if more than 20 ml of bile-stained material is present in the stomach, the diagnosis of obstruction should be entertained seriously, and an upright radiograph of the abdomen should be taken. Passage of the catheter through the anus and into the rectum rules out anorectal atresia.

Plain films of the abdomen and chest in the supine and upright (or cross-table lateral) positions are the first step in diagnosis. Abnormal distribution or amounts of intestinal gas often allow a specific enough diagnosis that no additional radiographic procedures are necessary. Occasionally contrast enema is indicated, especially for showing the size and position of the colon. Upper gastrointestinal contrast studies are rarely needed—they are sometimes dangerous from the standpoint of aspiration of the contrast material.

Differential Diagnosis

There are many nonsurgical conditions that can simulate intestinal obstruction in the newborn baby. Some are very serious diseases in their own right, and it is tragic to compound an already grave medical problem by laparotomy undertaken with a mistaken diagnosis of intestinal obstruction. Examples of these nonsurgical conditions follow:

Feeding problems. Underfeeding, overfeeding, or improperly administered feedings are probably the most common cause for neonatal vomiting. Generally the material vomited consists simply of the feeding material itself or non–bile-stained material. Observation of a feeding or a carefully taken history of the feeding program should allow a proper diagnosis to be made.

Infections. Septicemia in the newborn can produce vomiting and abdominal distension, whether the infection is primary within the gastrointestinal tract or elsewhere. Cultures of the blood, pharynx, cerebrospinal fluid, urine, and stool plus detection of a source for the infection establish the correct diagnosis.

Increased intracranial pressure. Cerebral edema, hemorrhage caused by birth trauma, or hydrocephalus often cause vomiting in the newborn. Evaluation of fontanel pressure and careful neurologic examination should rule out these causes for neonatal vomiting.

Obstructive uropathy. Congenital obstruction of the urinary tract producing azotemia is associated with vomiting and difficult feeding of the baby. Observation of the urinary output, blood urea nitrogen determinations, and ultrasound studies are helpful clues in diagnosis.

Endocrine and metabolic. Congenital adrenal hyperplasia (adrenogenital syndrome), abnormalities of glucose metabolism (hypoglycemia, galactosemia, glycogenosis), maternal opiate addiction, and tetany from hypocalcemia can be associated with vomiting or abdominal distension in the newborn. Appropriate maternal history or studies of the serum and urine electrolyte and glucose levels establish the appropriate diagnosis.

Chalasia. Chalasia, or congenital incompetency of the esophagogastric sphincter, allows easy regurgitation of gastric contents and feedings and is occasionally confused with obstructive causes for vomiting. The non–bile-stained character of the regurgitated material and its relationship to the supine position are clues to the diagnosis, which is confirmed by upper gastrointestinal tract barium studies. Competence of the sphincter develops within a few weeks to months, and interim treatment consists in positioning the baby either prone or in the upright position in an appropriately constructed seat and offering thick feedings.

Embryology of the Gastrointestinal Tract

Misadventures that occur to the fetus resulting in abnormal development of the gastrointestinal tract are the most frequent cause for neonatal obstruction. This section reviews briefly the major stages of gastrointestinal tract development and some of the more common anomalies that occur.

For convenience and better understanding of its embryonic development, the gastrointestinal tract is divided into three subdivisions: (1) the foregut, which embraces the esophagus, stomach, and proximal duodenum (including the bile ducts, liver, and pancreas), vascularized largely by the celiac axis, (2) the midgut, running from the ampulla of Vater in the second portion of the duodenum to the splenic flexure of the colon and supplied with blood by the superior mesenteric artery, and (3) the hindgut, extending from the splenic flexure of the colon to the rectum and having as its major blood vessel the inferior mesenteric artery. The venous return from all three embryonic gut subdivisions is largely through the portal system to the liver.

In the early embryo the gastrointestinal tract is a

straight tube running in the midline from the oral cavity to the anus, suspended by both a dorsal and a ventral mesentery. The ventral mesentery is lost early, but the dorsal mesentery is retained with the blood supply to the developing gastrointestinal tract. By the fourth gestational week the lung anlage separates from the proximal end of the foregut; incompleteness of this splitting mechanism results in the various forms of esophageal atresia and tracheoesophageal fistula.

Beginning at the fifth week of intrauterine life, the stomach sacculates and the midgut begins to proliferate, enlarge, and elongate in a very accelerated manner. Epithelial proliferation tends to narrow the intestinal lumen; in lower animals the proliferation continues until the lumen is obliterated to form the so-called *solid cord stage*. In the human embryo the solid cord stage develops rarely and only in the duodenum; vacuolization and coalescence of vacuoles rapidly reestablish the internal lumen of the tract.

Linear growth of the midgut rapidly outstrips the volume of the peritoneal cavity, resulting in elongation of the mesentery and herniation of the entire midgut into the base of the umbilical cord. The resulting *extra-coelomic phase* (Fig. 39-1) of midgut development occurs during the sixth to the tenth week of intrauterine life.

As one views the fetus from the front, the midgut rotates 270 degrees in a counterclockwise direction around its vascular axis (the superior mesenteric artery); (Fig. 39-1, *A* to *D*) during this extracoelomic phase of development, after which an orderly return of the midgut to the enlarged peritoneal cavity occurs during the tenth to twelfth weeks of intrauterine life. Return of the midgut occurs in an aboral manner, from proximal to distal, the duodenum returning to the right upper abdominal quadrant after the first 90 degrees of rotation (Fig. 39-1, *B*), where it is fixed retroperitoneally. This forces the stomach to rotate 90 degrees, so that its original left side is now anterior and its right side the definitive posterior wall. This is correlated with elongation of its dorsal mesenteric surface into what we refer to as the greater curvature of the stomach.

As the proximal jejunum returns, the 270-degree counterclockwise rotation is completed (Fig. 39-1, *C* and *D*) so as to carry the distal portion of the duode-

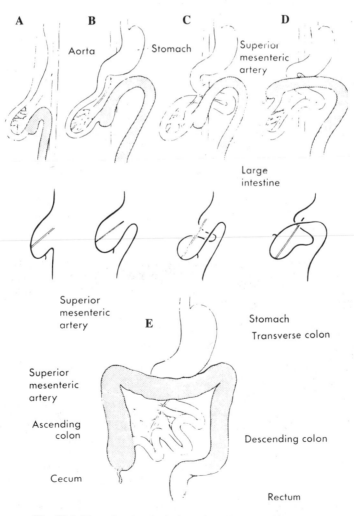

Fig. 39-1. Normal embryological rotation of midgut. (See text.)

num inferior (caudad) to the superior mesenteric artery and across the midline, where the duodenojejunal junction is fixed in a nearly retroperitoneal manner by the ligament of Treitz. The hindgut is pushed to the left by the returning small bowel (Fig. 39-1, *C*), and the cecum and the right colon are directed above (cephalad to) the superior mesenteric artery with the cecum ending in the right upper abdominal quadrant (Fig. 39-1, *D*). The embryonic changes in the midgut are completed leisurely during the succeding months of gestation and on into the first few weeks of postnatal life by the gradual descent of the cecum to the right lower abdominal quadrant (Fig. 39-1, *E*), where it becomes attached to the right posterior parietes in the normal adult position.

Two pathologic states involving the midgut are attributable to misadventures occurring during these critical fifth to twelfth weeks of gestational life. *Omphalocele* (exomphalos); Fig. 39-2 may be thought of as a retention of the extracoelomic phase of midgut development, with failure of both normal rotation and return of the midgut. It complicates about 1 in 10,000 live births. The midgut is contained extraperitoneally at the umbilicus in a sac composed of amniotic membranes devoid of skin. It is characterized by abnormalities of intestinal rotation and invariably is associated with a small peritoneal cavity, which has not been stimulated to enlarge by a normal return of the midgut viscera.

The omphalocele sac is friable and poorly vascularized; 10% rupture during intrauterine life or during or shortly after labor and delivery. In either event the exposed viscera must be covered immediately.

Treatment

Treatment of omphalocele is individualized.

Sac ruptured. Emergent surgical protection of exposed bowel is provided by either total repair of the abdominal wall defect (if the herniated viscera can be easily reduced back into the abdominal cavity) or coverage of viscera by a "silo" constructed of synthetic material (usually Dacron-reinforced Silastic) that is su-

tured to the edges of the defect and then over the exposed viscera. In 7 to 10 days the viscera can usually be easily reduced, so that removal of the prosthetic "silo" and suture closure of the abdominal wall can be carried out.

Sac intact. Nonsurgical treatment is generally restricted to poor-risk babies. The sac is painted with an astringent (0.5% merbromin [Mercurochrome]) to thicken and toughen it as the abdominal wall skin gradually overgrows and replaces the sac during the ensuing weeks. Surgical treatment when the sac is intact is to excise the sac and either close the abdominal wall in layers or cover exposed viscera with a prosthetic "silo."

A principle vital to the surgical treatment of all omphaloceles is to avoid excessively high intra-abdominal pressure when the bowel is being returned to the abnormally small peritoneal cavity. Elevated intraabdominal pressure is tolerated poorly by the newborn because of (1) reduced respiratory exchange from restricted motion of the diaphragm, and (2) impedance of venous return to the heart from the lower compartment by compression of the inferior vena cava. Effective decompression of the gastrointestinal tract and intraoperative manual stretching of the abdominal wall help avoid this disaster. When reduction of the viscera is impossible or dangerous, the aforementioned prosthetic "silos" are sutured to the edges of the abdominal wall defect to allow slow, progressive reduction of bowel back into the gradually enlarging abdominal cavity. Total parenteral feeding avoids early postoperative oral feedings, which are poorly tolerated in the crowded abdominal cavity.

Gastroschisis is an anomaly which complicates about one in 8,000 live births in which the midgut protrudes through a small paraumbilical aperture in the abdominal wall, generally on the right side, throughout gestation. The bowel suffers a chemical peritonitis which renders it foreshortened, matted, lusterless, and temporarily aperistaltic. Treatment principles are similar to those of omphalocele. The embryopathy that results in gastroschisis is not clear.

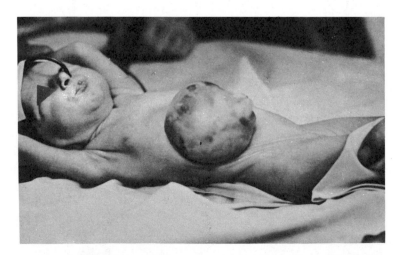

Fig. 39-2. Omphalocele—lusterless, semiopaque sac that contains herniated midgut.

Malrotation of the midgut is the second major problem resulting from faulty embryonic development of the midgut. It is characterized by various degrees of incompleteness of the rotation and fixation mechanism. Most commonly, rotation occurs only through the first 90-degree arc (Fig. 39-1, *B*) with a normal position of the stomach and the proximal duodenum. The duodenojejunum descends to the right of the superior mesenteric artery, and in general the entire small intestine lies in the right hemiabdomen, whereas the large bowel occupies the left hemiabdomen. The base or root of the midgut mesentery is invariably narrow.

With normal midgut rotation (Fig. 39-1, *E*), the base or root of the mesentery in the adult measures about 20 cm in length and extends from the ligament of Treitz (to the left of the second lumbar vertebra) obliquely downward to the ileocecal area in the right lower abdominal quadrant. With failure of normal midgut rotation, the mesenteric root or base is very narrow, measuring only the width of the superior mesenteric artery and vein (Fig. 39-1, *B*). The combination of a narrow mesenteric vascular axis and a very lengthy fan-shaped periphery (along which the midgut itself courses) provides the setting for the most significant and lethal complication of midgut malrotation, namely, twisting or *volvulus of the midgut*. Volvulus occurs in about 50% of patients with midgut malrotation. It involves a clockwise twist of the midgut around the very narrow vascular base, or axis, to produce varying degrees of occlusion of the lymphatic, venous, and arterial vessels of the mesentery. The volvulus always occurs in a clockwise direction for an unknown reason (perhaps because the liver developing in the right upper quadrant prevents an initial counterclockwise thrust)

and may involve twisting through several complete turns.

Two potentially lethal conditions occur, then, with volvulus of the midgut: the twist (1) closes off the midgut on both ends to produce *closed-loop intestinal obstruction* and (2) produces varying degrees of mesenteric vascular stagnation as venous outflow—and later arterial inflow—are occluded. These two features set the stage for midgut perforation and infarction, either of which can be fatal.

Midgut malrotation without volvulus is generally symptomatic because of some degree of duodenal obstruction. Extrinsic duodenal obstruction occurs from peritoneal bands *(Ladd's bands);* (Fig. 39-3) stretching from the right posterior parietes across the duodenum to the cecum and ascending colon in the left upper abdominal quadrant; they can be thought of as bands that would have fixed the cecum and ascending colon in the right gutter had normal rotation occurred. Approximately 15% of patients with extrinsic duodenal obstruction on this basis also have an intrinsic obstruction caused by a duodenal membrane. The duodenal obstruction is generally intermittent and partial, reflected by bouts of vomiting bile-stained material associated with epigastric distension. If volvulus ensues, the morbidity is sharply increased by trapping of fluid within the closed midgut loop, thereby producing more abdominal distension and obstipation, and perhaps less vomiting. Strangulation precipitates signs of peritoneal irritation progressing to shock and a critically ill patient within a matter of hours.

The diagnosis of midgut malrotation often must be made in the operating room, since it is difficult to distinguish duodenal obstruction occurring in young pa-

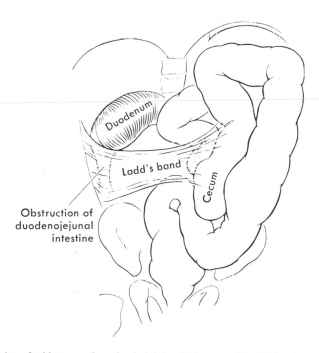

Fig. 39-3. Malrotation of midgut—entire colon in left hemiabdomen and Ladd's band running from cecum to right posterior parietes to cross and obstruct duodenojejunal intestine.

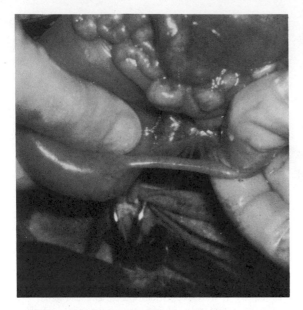

Fig. 39-4. Intestinal atresia with intrinsic membrane occluding lumen. Dilated and obstructed small intestine on left, and unused but patent "wormlike" bowel distal to membrane on right.

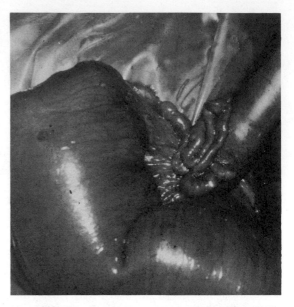

Fig. 39-5. Intestinal atresia with loss of intestinal continuity. Dilated and obstructed proximal bowel on left and below, and unused distal bowel on right.

tients on this basis from other causes, such as duodenal stenosis, atresia, and annular pancreas. Plain abdominal radiographs show a dilated stomach and duodenum without clear differentiation as to cause. Upper gastrointestinal contrast study performed with pressure on the stomach often forces barium past Ladd's bands and reveal the beaklike cutoff diagnostic of volvulus. When signs of intestinal strangulation are associated with duodenal obstruction in an infant or child, malrotation with midgut volvulus becomes the most likely cause and demands early laparotomy.

Surgical treatment of uncomplicated midgut malrotation involves (1) complete division of Ladd's bands, thereby allowing the cecum to lie freely within the left upper abdominal quadrant with the duodenum and jejunum proceeding down the right posterior parietes in an unobstructed manner, (2) prophylactic appendectomy so that left upper quadrant appendicitis will not later be a confusing clinical entity to diagnose, and (3) proof of intrinsic patency of the duodenum. If volvulus has occurred, the twist must be derotated completely in a counterclockwise direction, and necrotic bowel must be resected. Recurrent volvulus virtually never occurs, probably because of intestinal fixation from adhesions generated during the operation.

Origin of Intestinal Atresia and Stenosis

Gastrointestinal atresia implies total closure of the bowel lumen. It may be composed simply of a membrane or diaphragm stretched across the lumen (Fig. 39-4), or it may be extensive with total loss of continuity, and it may even be multiple (Fig. 39-5). Stenosis results in a narrowing of the lumen without complete obstruction, often represented by a diaphragm or membrane with a small aperture; it never involves loss of continuity of the intestine or complete obstruction.

Some dispute exists as to the embryogenesis of atresias and stenoses of the gastrointestinal tract. The traditional concept is that they represent a failure of canalization (vacuolization and coalescence of vacuoles) after the so-called solid core stage at about the fifth week of embryonic life, wherein the lumen of the developing intestine is occluded by hyperplasia of the mucosal epithelial cells. The basis for this solid core theory stems largely from embryologic studies done on lower animal forms. More sophisticated and recent studies of the human embryo demonstrate a somewhat abortive epithelial cell hyperplasia that produces total obliteration of the lumen (only rarely) in the duodenum. Therefore this mechanism is a logical explanation for congenital atresia and stenosis of the human duodenum only. The solid core theory does not explain many of the features of jejunal and ileal atresia: loss of bowel continuity, defects in the adjacent mesentery and visible remnants of volvulus, intussusception, and meconium peritonitis.

A more attractive explanation for congenital stenosis and atresia of the jejunum, ileum, and colon implicates occlusion of the mesenteric vessels sometime during gestation, which provokes a sterile infarction of that segment of developing intestine supplied by the vessels. Thrombosis of a small terminal artery (Fig. 39-6) would infarct only a short segment of gut, with the resulting granulation and scar tissue forming a membrane characteristic of stenosis or the minor forms of atresia. Occlusion of major vessels (Figs. 39-7 and 39-8) nourishing longer segments of developing intestine would better explain the more gross and extensive degrees of atresia. Spontaneous thrombosis or strangulating misadventures, such as intussusception or volvulus, might be the basic origin of the mesenteric vascular occlusion.

Deliberate experimental production of mesenteric

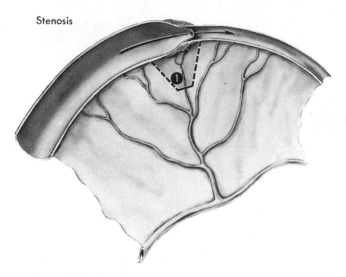

Fig. 39-6. Diagram of thrombosis of small mesenteric "end artery" of developing fetal intestine, producing sterile infarction of short segment of bowel nourished by this vessel. Resulting phagocytosis and repair reaction produce intrinsic diaphragm, which in diagram has small aperture through which some of intestinal content may pass.

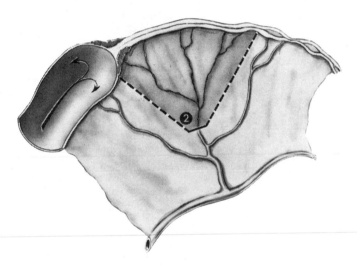

Fig. 39-7. Thrombosis of larger mesenteric artery of developing fetal intestine, producing sterile infarction of longer segment of bowel. External continuity of bowel is retained, but intrinsic membrane totally obstructs lumen. (See Fig. 39-4.)

vascular occlusion in unborn animal fetuses has successfully reproduced all degrees of stenosis and atresia of the intestine, lending experimental credence to this thesis of origin. Because of the short dorsal mesentery nourishing the esophagus and duodenum and the nonmesenteric collateral circulation to the developing rectum, this seems to be a less attractive and plausible explanation for the embryogenesis of atresia of the esophagus, duodenum, and rectum.

Esophageal Atresia with Tracheoesophageal Fistula

There are many anatomic variations of congenital esophageal stenosis and atresia, but approximately 80% have a blind proximal esophageal pouch extending to the upper thoracic level, with the distal esophagus connected to the tracheobronchial tree near the carina (Fig. 39-9). Because of its frequency, this is the only type that is discussed here.

A glance at Fig. 39-9 allows the student to predict the symptoms produced by this anatomic arrangement. Polyhydramnios is the earliest sign of esophageal atresia, which begins during the mid-trimester of gestation. Postnatally, the blind proximal esophagus fills with saliva, which is then regurgitated back into the mouth, producing a seemingly "mucusy" baby who seems to be salivating excessively. The first feeding provokes gagging and immediate regurgitation, with explosive coughing and cyanosis if any spills over into

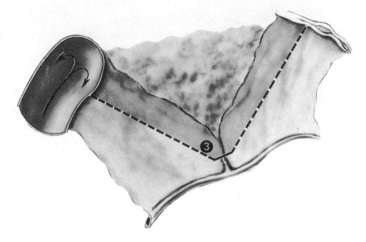

Fig. 39-8. Thrombosis of major mesenteric artery of fetal intestine, infarcting long segment of bowel and mesentery; sterile phagocytic reaction that this provokes causes loss of bowel and mesenteric continuity and total intestinal obstruction. (See Fig. 39-5.)

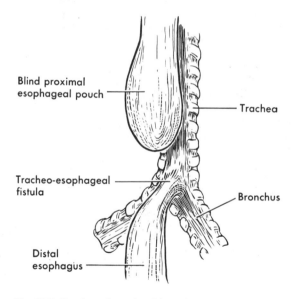

Blind proximal
esophageal pouch

Trachea

Tracheo-esophageal
fistula

Bronchus

Distal
esophagus

Fig. 39-9. Esophageal atresia with tracheoesophageal fistula.

the trachea. The fistula between the trachea and the stomach through the distal part of the esophagus is a two-way street. Some of the inspired air is diverted into the stomach and on downstream to produce unusual degrees of abdominal distension and tympany. When the infant is recumbent, hydrochloric acid from the stomach flows up into the lungs through the distal part of the esophagus to produce the most serious complication of this variety of esophageal atresia, namely, severe chemical pneumonitis.

Diagnosis is quickly made when one can pass a soft, small, plastic catheter through the nose and find that it meets an obstruction within 10 cm. A single upright radiograph outlines the blind proximal pouch and reveals pneumonitis and the unusually large accumula-

tion of intestinal gas characteristic of this disorder. Until further treatment can be carried out, the infant should be positioned upright, and continuous suction should be applied to the nasoesophageal tube to retrieve saliva.

Definitive treatment of esophageal atresia must be individualized according to the degree of pneumonitis, the weight of the baby, and the precise anatomic form of the anomaly. In good-risk babies, primary repair may be carried out either transpleurally or retropleurally, with ligation and division of the fistula and end-to-end anastomosis of the two esophageal ends. if the infant is premature and has other major anomalies or a severe pneumonitis, preliminary gastrostomy is carried out under local anesthesia to remove the threat of further chemical pneumonitis; the baby is then nourished parenterally until repair can be safely undertaken. If the proximal pouch is short, it may be elongated by daily dilations during this waiting period to facilitate primary anastomosis later.

Neonatal Duodenal Obstruction

Most neonatal obstructions of the duodenum occur distal to the ampulla of Vater, with bilious vomiting the outstanding clinical feature. If the obstruction is complete, plain films of the abdomen taken in the upright position show the classical "double-bubble" sign (Fig. 39-10), which results from air-fluid levels in the stomach and proximal part of the duodenum.

Duodenal atresia is the most common cause for complete duodenal obstruction; about one third of the babies also suffer from Down's syndrome. Malrotation of the midgut with or without volvulus can cause total neonatal duodenal obstruction but also is capable of producing intermittent obstruction at various times during infancy and early childhood. Duodenal stenosis is the most common cause for partial obstruction, and the most rare cause of all is annular pancreas. Diagnosis of partial or intermittent duodenal obstruction often requires an upper gastrointestinal tract barium series.

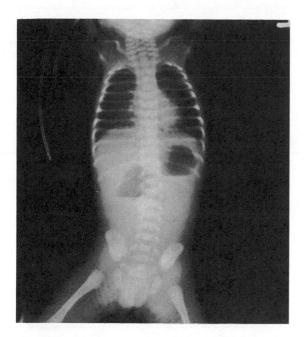

Fig. 39-10. "Double bubble" roentgenographic sign of complete duodenal obstruction in newborn. Air-fluid level in left upper quandrant is in dilated stomach; that to right of midline is in dilated and obstructed duodenum.

Duodenal atresia, stenosis, and annular pancreas are treated by surgical bypass; a side-to-side anastomosis is created between the duodenum proximal to the obstruction and the duodenum immediately beyond the obstruction. The treatment of malrotation with duodenal obstruction is discussed above in detail.

Jejunal and Ileal Obstruction

Neonatal obstruction of the jejunum and ileum is generally caused by congenital atresia or stenosis and less commonly by meconium ileus. Clinically the obstruction is manifested by bilious vomiting with abdominal distension proportionate to the level of the obstruction, its degree of completeness, and the time elapsed since delivery. Plain films of the abdomen taken in the upright position will diagnose the level and completeness of the obstruction but will not label the cause precisely. Resection and anastomosis is the preferred treatment of atresia and stenosis.

Meconium ileus complicates about 8% of children with generalized mucoviscidosis or fibrocystic disease of the pancreas. The obstruction is caused by extremely inspissated and tenacious meconium occluding the lumen because of insufficient digestive enzymes of pancreatic origin. A specific diagnosis may be indicated by a family history of cystic fibrosis of the pancreas and palpation of cordlike masses of meconium within the abdomen. Plain abdominal radiographs show variable-sized small bowel loops and a "soap-bubble" appearance of gas dispersed within tenacious meconium.

Because of the systemic (largely pulmonary) complications of cystic fibrosis, it is best to first try to relieve the obstruction of meconium ileus by nonsurgical means. This may be achieved by instillation of hypertonic, water-soluble contrast material (gastrografin) into the rectum and under direct vision (by cinefluoroscopy) controlling the progress of the contrast material retrogradely throughout the colon and on past the ileocecal valve into the obstructed terminal ileum. Fluids must be running intravenously while this is done because the hypertonic material draws fluids into the bowel to liquefy and break up the tenacious meconium enough to allow its expulsion rectally. Of course, this method of treatment can be undertaken only in uncomplicated cases (with no perforation), and reports indicate it is successful in only about two thirds of cases. If this method of therapy is unsuccessful, prompt surgical intervention must follow.

Surgical treatment consists in disimpacting the undigested meconium by irrigation with mucolytic agents, when possible. Alternate methods include temporary ileostomy through which proteolytic enzymes are instilled directly into the obstructed distal small bowel. The complicated forms of meconium ileus require appropriate resection and anastomosis or exteriorization of the perforated bowel. The prognosis is guarded from the standpoint of the intestinal obstruction itself, let alone problems with atelectasis and pneumonia to which the bronchial mucus predisposes the patient.

NEONATAL OBSTRUCTION OF THE COLON

Early in embryonic development, the hindgut and allantois are joined as the cloaca. Division into a urogenital sinus anteriorly and rectum posteriorly occurs during the sixth to eighth weeks of gestation by descent of the urorectal septum. Shortly thereafter, rupture of the cloacal membrane in the proctodeum produces separate genital and intestinal orifices. Defects in these mechanisms produce the many anatomic variations that characterize rectal atresia and imperforate anus.

The most common cause for congenital obstruction of the colon is the various forms of *anorectal atresia;* additional causes are the *meconium plug syndrome, congenital aganglionosis (Hirschsprung's disease),* and *congenital atresia* of the colon, in descending order of frequency.

There are many anatomic variations of *imperforate anus* and *rectal atresia,* but the common type consists of an absent anus with a dilated and obstructed rectum terminating somewhere in the pelvis. In *high rectal atresia* the rectum ends above the levator sling (the muscular plevic diaphragm through which the rectum normally courses and that contributes most to fecal control), and in *low rectal atresia* the rectum passes through the sling (anterior to the puborectalis muscle) before terminating. In 70% to 80% there will be a fistula that, in the male, connects the rectum to the bladder neck, urethra, or perineal skin. In the female the fistula opens into the vagina or perineum.

Obstipation with progressive abdominal distension and late bilious vomiting characterize the disorder clinically. Diagnosis can generally be made by inspection alone (Fig. 39-11). A plain film of the abdomen taken

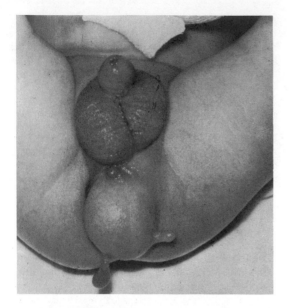

Fig. 39-11. Anorectal atresia, with abortive attempt at formation of perineal fistula marked by bluish, meconium-filled tract in scrotal raphe. Large lipoma occupies intergluteal cleft.

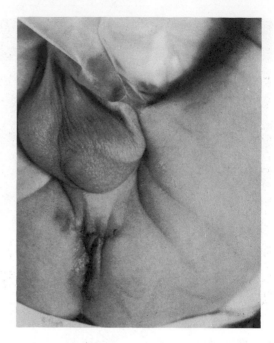

Fig. 39-13. Photograph taken 2 weeks after anoplasty repair of anorectal atresia in baby shown preoperatively in Fig. 39-11.

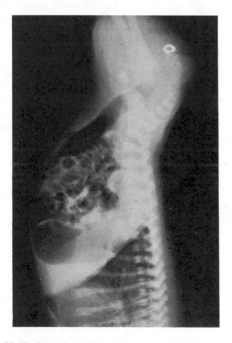

Fig. 39-12. Lateral roentgenogram taken after baby was inverted for several minutes, showing distance from perineum (radiopaque marker) to end of atretic, air-filled rectum.

after the infant has been inverted for several minutes (Fig. 39-12) gives a clue as to the distance between the end of the rectum and the perineum. Much more precise documentation of the abnormality is afforded when radiocontrast material can outline the atretic rectum after colostomy.

Probes are helpful in locating perineal and vaginal

fistulas, and meconium or air in urine is diagnostic of rectourethral or rectovesical fistula in male infants.

Relief of colonic obstruction is the first aim of treatment and can occasionally be satisfied by dilation of the larger perineal and vaginal fistulous tracts. Primary perineal anoplasty (Fig. 39-13) is carried out as definitive treatment of the low-lying rectal atresia. Colostomy is necessary with the higher rectal atresias or in poor-risk newborns to provide temporary relief of the obstruction. Later, the rectum is "pulled through" to the perineum by a posterior saggital approach. The most crucial aim of the operation is to draw the rectum in front of the puborectalis muscle and inside the external sphincter muscles to provide effective fecal continence.

Congenital aganglionosis of the colon (Hirschsprung's disease) may produce an acute obstruction in the neonatal period of life. It is characterized by abdominal distension with the passage of little or no meconium rectally and late bilious vomiting. Occasionally, paradoxical diarrhea may occur to confuse the diagnosis of obstruction. This diagnosis may be indicated by rectal digital examination that reveals a narrow rectal ampulla and often provokes explosive passage of gas and meconium when the finger is withdrawn. Barium enema reveals a narrow rectum that enlarges at some point proximally, with poor evacuation of barium. Anorectal manometry reveals that the internal anal sphincter does not relax when the rectum is distended. Absolute confirmation rests with biopsy demonstration of absent ganglia in the autonomic nerve plexuses in the submucosal and intermuscular planes on rectal wall biopsy.

Initial treatment consists in relieving the intestinal

obstruction. Usually colostomy (within ganglionated bowel) is necessary. Definitive corrective operation can occasionally be carried out primarily on a good-risk baby; it is best delayed in small or otherwise compromised babies until later in infancy.

The *meconium plug syndrome* consists of obstruction generally of the rectum or sigmoid colon by a long, pale, and stringy plug of inspissated meconium. Delayed passage of meconium rectally, gross and progressive abdominal distension, and late bilious vomiting are the clinical signs and symptoms. Plain radiographs show nonspecific dilation of multiple bowel loops with air and fluid.

Both diagnosis and treatment rest on barium enema examination, which reveals a long *filling defect* of the plug of meconium, proximal to which the colon is dilated and obstructed. Dissection of the barium around the plug commonly dislodges and allows passage of the obstructing bolus of meconium. Signs of obstruction are relieved promptly. A few of these babies later are found to have Hirschsprung's disease or cystic fibrosis. The cause of the inspissated meconium is unknown.

Besides the stomach, the colon is the least likely site for atresia or stenosis of the gastrointestinal tract to occur. It will produce complete (atresia) or partial (stenosis) obstruction at the site of the membrane, which must be distinguished from other causes of colonic obstruction by barium enema examination. Excision and anastomosis constitute proper surgical treatment.

NECK MASSES IN INFANTS AND CHILDREN

Cervical masses in infants and children are extremely common; a careful examiner is able to find neck nodules in virtually every youngster from 2 to 10 years of age. Fortunately, most of these are innocent lymph nodes that are simply residua of previous upper respiratory infections.

Lymph Nodes

Acute cervical lymphadenitis arises from a primary infection (usually in the pharynx) and in itself justifies no specific therapy other than that directed to the inciting primary inflammation. Less commonly, acute lymphadenitis becomes suppurative, manifested as a fluctuant, tender neck mass. Specific treatment in the form of warm soaks followed by surgical incision and drainage should be undertaken at this point, and cultures usually show *Staphylococcus* as the causative organism. The use of antibiotics depends on the organism, the status and site of the primary infection, and the general condition of the patient.

Chronic cervical lymphadenitis is less common than acute or subacute forms. In this country chronic cervical adenitis is rarely attributed to tuberculosis and is generally caused by atypical *Mycobacterium,* cat-scratch disease, or fungal infections.

Neoplasm

Cervical adenopathy in children can also herald a malignancy, generally primary and belonging to the lymphoma family, and less commonly cervical neuroblastoma or rhabdomyosarcoma. Metastatic carcinoma to cervical lymph nodes is much less common in the child than in the adult and is most likely to originate from a primary thyroid neoplasm.

The surgeon is frequently asked to perform a biopsy on a persistently enlarged cervical lymph node for histologic confirmation of diagnosis. Neck dissection for therapy of cervical malignancy is limited to localized cervical neuroblastoma or rhabdomyosarcoma and for the surgical treatment of thyroid carcinoma, commonly adjunctive to x-ray therapy and chemotherapy.

Branchial Remnants

Embryonic *remnants* of the *branchial arch system* produce *sinuses, cysts,* and *fistulas* that occur from the external pinna to the clavicular insertion of the sternocleidomastoid muscle in infants and children. Only the first two branchial arch systems are usually involved in these vestigial remnants.

The very common preauricular sinuses and skin tabs arise simply from misadventures occurring when the epithelial precursors of the external pinna merge together. They usually produce only cosmetic defects, but the sinuses can become infected. Either of these represents a valid indication for surgical excision.

First branchial remnants are only one tenth as common as second branchial remnants. They present as sinuses or fistulas, which commonly become infected, below or behind the ear or in the upper lateral part of the neck. Proper treatment requires complete excision, preferably performed when inflammation is quiescent and always in the operating room with proper anesthesia, light, and exposure, to avoid recurrences and injury to the facial nerve (cranial nerve VII).

Second branchial arch remnants present as cysts, sinuses, or fistulas in the anterior triangle of the neck. The cysts generally arise later in childhood as fluctuant swellings just anterior to the upper half of the sternocleidomastoid muscle. They represent approximately 10% of all branchial abnormalities. The cysts are prone to recurrent bouts of infection, thus justifying prophylactic complete excision.

Cervical fistulas and sinuses constitute the bulk of branchial remnants and in about 15% of patients are bilateral. The external ostia always open on the skin along the anterior border of the sternocleidomastoid muscle, usually in its lower one third (Fig. 39-14). The sinuses extend cephalad for varying distances to terminate blindly. The fistulas extend completely cephalad to empty into the pharynx at the tonsillar fossa; the tract invariably passes behind the posterior belly of the digastric muscle and between the branches of the carotid artery (in keeping with its second branchial arch derivation). Both cysts and fistulas are lined by epithelium and are prone to infection. Prophylactic total excision is the treatment of choice; long fistulas often require two parallel neck-crease incisions (stepladder incisions) to allow the exposure necessary for their safe and total removal. Recurrence is certain with incomplete excision.

Cystic Hygroma

Cystic hygroma (cavernous lymphangioma) is the classical developmental abnormality of the lymphatic system. It consists of multiloculated cysts filled with watery tissue fluid that may appear as relatively asymp-

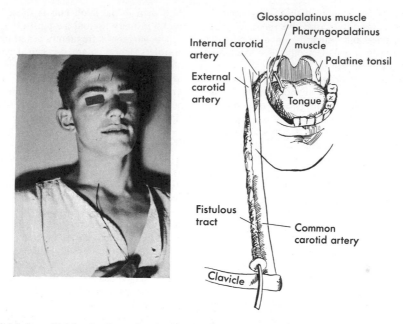

Fig. 39-14. Branchial fistula. Ureteral catheter passes from external ostium on up tract to tonsillar fossa.

tomatic masses anywhere on the body; however, 85% are confined to the lateral neck and face area (Fig. 39-15; the left side is slightly more common than the right side); 2% to 3% of the cervical cystic hygromas have extensions into the mediastinum. The axilla is the second most common location of cystic hygroma.

Cystic hygromas are generally present at birth and commonly enlarge rapidly during infancy. They tend to invade or displace surrounding structures, thereby producing their only serious symptoms: interference with deglutition and the airway. Pathologically, they are considered hamartomas rather than neoplasms. Cystic hygromas seem to represent lymphatic spaces that receive tissue fluid through afferent channels but do not establish the proper efferent connections to the venous system, resulting in accumulation of lymph. Correct diagnosis is made by palpation of a soft, cystic mass that does not change the color of the overlying skin, which is nontender and transilluminates brilliantly (Fig. 39-15).

Treatment by aspiration of cystic hygromas has been abandoned. The needle cannot penetrate into all the multiple cysts, and it carries the risk of introducing infection, which can be acute and fulminant. The most commonly accepted treatment of cystic hygroma is excision of as much of the lesion as possible without damaging vital neurovascular structures. Excision is carried out at an elective age, except in the rare instance when the airway is threatened by displacement or involvement.

Thyroglossal Duct Remnants

Thyroglossal duct remnants (Fig. 39-16) produce masses in the anterior midline of the neck, generally at about the level of the hyoid bone. They represent cystic dilation of remnants of the thyroglossal duct, the embryonic anlage of the thyroid gland that normally invo-

lutes and disappears. The thyroglossal tract arises as a midline diverticulum from the back of the tongue *(foramen cecum)* and moves caudad through the midportion of the hyoid bone before splitting into the two definitive lateral thyroid lobes in their normal position low in the anterior cervical area.

Thyroglossal cysts may appear anywhere along this tract but are most common in and around the hyoid bone. They must be differentiated from these other midline neck masses in children:

Submental lymph nodes are generally multiple, movable in a lateral plane, and not cystic in consistency.

Dermoid cysts are generally lower in the anterior midline of the neck than thyroglossal duct cysts, are more superficial, sometimes actually attaching to the skin, and are not elevated by protruding the tongue.

Ectopic thyroid tissue can arise anywhere along the thyroglossal tract, is solid rather than cystic, and concentrates iodine on diagnostic radioactive iodine uptake studies. Ectopic thyroid tissue should *not* be removed if it is the *only* thyroid tissue that the patient possesses.

Thyroglossal duct cysts are fairly deep seated, are cystic in consistency, are not tender unless secondarily infected, and move cephalad on protrusion of the tongue. Treatment is surgical excision of the cyst and the remnant of the thyroglossal tract that connects the cyst to the foramen cecum of the tongue; this obligates the removal of a 1-cm block of midline hyoid bone and the entire tract up to the base of the tongue.

VASCULAR ANOMALIES
Hemangiomas

The *capillary hemangioma (strawberry mark, raspberry mark)* is the most common peripheral vascular abnormality in infants and children. It is generally present at birth but can appear after a few weeks or

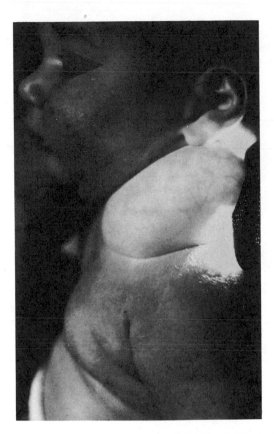

Fig. 39-15. Cystic hygroma of neck. Notice how brilliantly it transilluminates.

even months of life. Histologically it is composed of numerous tiny vascular channels. Grossly the capillary hemangioma is a bright red mass that may be small and flat or quite elevated and nodular but that retains the characteristics of blanching with compression, best observed when a glass slide is pressed firmly over the lesion. About 70% of the lesions are confined to the upper torso, head, and neck.

Although initially small, capillary hemangiomas almost uniformly display a growth spurt for the first 6 to 12 months of life, often at an alarming rate, with a slowing of growth during early childhood. Well over 90% begin to regress spontaneously during the middle childhood years, with progressive diminution in size by thrombosis of the vascular channels. The thrombosis typically begins centrally as whitish areas that appear within the pink-red lesion; these whitish areas then coalesce and spread peripherally to encompass the entire lesion.

Because of their tendency to regress spontaneously, active treatment of capillary hemangiomas is not recommended unless they compromise a vital function by virtue of their location or if their growth rate is continuous and entirely out of proportion to body growth rate. Surgical excision is often more disfiguring than the ultimate result of the untreated lesion. Systemic steroids sometimes control a lesion that is growing rapidly.

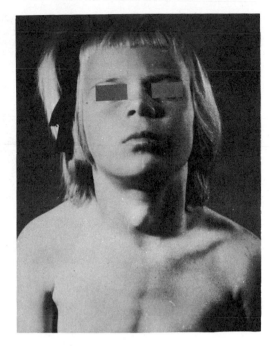

Fig. 39-16. Thyroglossal duct remnant.

Cavernous hemangioma (Fig. 39-17) is numerically only about one tenth as common as its capillary counterpart. It consists principally of larger-sized vascular channels that often contain some lymphatic elements and abnormal connections with the arterial vascular tree. Cavernous hemangiomas most commonly involve the dermis and subcutaneous tissues of the extremities to produce an irregular, soft mass that imparts a red to blue discoloration to the overlying skin. They may diminish in size on compression, reverting quickly to their former size on release of pressure and enlarging during periods of increased venous pressure (Valsalva effect, crying, straining).

Cavernous hemangiomas are much more serious than the capillary type because (1) they infrequently involute, (2) they are cosmetically more disfiguring, and (3) local gigantism results when the member is extensively involved, probably because of the increase in blood flow to the tissue. Treatment is generally unsatisfactory, whether by injection of sclerosing agents, excision and skin grafting, or irradiation. Complete surgical excision is performed safely only on small cavernous hemangiomas. Extensive lesions must be approached cautiously and conservatively, with therapy individually tailored to forestall or treat ulceration, infection, and hemorrhage and to ablate gigantism.

OTHER COMMON PEDIATRIC SURGICAL DISEASES
Tonsils and Adenoids

Tonsils and adenoids are part of the lymphatic system of the body. The tonsils are paired clumps of lymphoid tissue lying on each side of the pharynx at the base of the tongue, and the adenoid tissue is in the nasopharynx behind and above the uvula. As with lymphoid tissue elsewhere in the body, they enlarge with

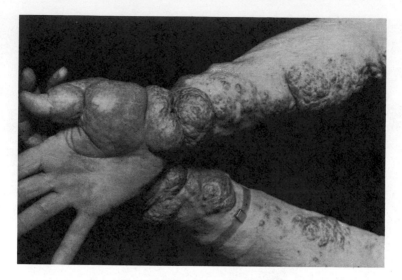

Fig. 39-17. Cavernous hemangiomas.

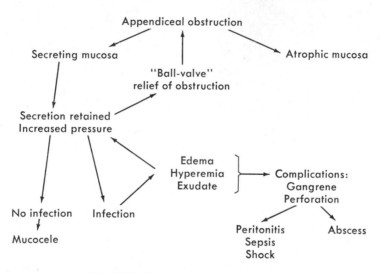

Fig. 39-18. Pathophysiology of appendicitis.

infections as mechanisms of defense. Because of the frequency of upper respiratory tract infections in children, they are commonly enlarged at this age.

Tonsils are not removed because of their size alone. Untreated tonsillitis can result in peritonsillar abscesses or bloodstream infections. Enlargement of the adenoids blocks nasal respiration and obstructs drainage of the eustachian tube connecting the middle ear with the pharynx to produce recurrent bouts of otitis media. Chronic adenoid enlargement encourages mouth-breathing, poor humidification of inspired air, and resultant episodes of bronchitis and cough.

Tonsillectomy and adenoidectomy are performed if tonsil and adenoid enlargement are associated with repeated middle ear infections, recurrent bouts of bronchitis or pneumonia, or a chronic habit of breathing through the mouth. Introduction of antibiotics has reduced the number of tonsillectomies and adenoidectomies performed in recent years.

Appendicitis

Appendicitis is the most common cause for emergency abdominal operation in children though its actual incidence appears to be declining. Extremely rare in the infant and unusual under the age of 5 years, its incidence increases rapidly thereafter with the peak incidence in the young teenager.

Obstruction of the lumen initiates appendicitis (Fig. 39-18). This occurs either from enlargement of the lymphoid tissue underneath the lining mucosa of the appendix (generally in the younger child) or by a concretion of feces and undigested vegetable matter called a fecalith (Fig. 39-19); (generally in the older child or adult). The obstruction traps the mucoid secretions of the appendiceal cells to progressively build up intraluminal pressure; intestinal organisms cause infection and abscess. Occasionally the obstruction relents and the attack of appendicitis is aborted; if it persists, the appendix becomes turgid, swollen, edematous, and inflamed,

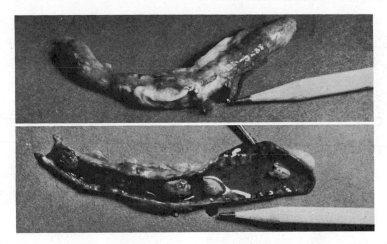

Fig. 39-19. Acute suppurative appendicitis. *Above,* Distended, injected, and edematous appendix. *Below,* Opened specimen shows obstructing fecalith to left and other fecaliths, pus, and debris filling lumen.

which then progresses by vascular thrombosis to gangrene and perforation. Perforation results in peritoneal contamination with rapid development of peritonitis with generalized abdominal pain, high fever, paralytic ileus, and abdominal rigidity (an acute surgical abdomen).

Very rare is the situation where there are no organisms resident in the appendix when its lumen becomes obstructed. The sterile mucoid secretions then gradually increase in volume to produce the so-called *mucocele of the appendix.* Vague right lower quadrant abdominal discomfort and a mass clinically herald the mucocele; its rupture is one of the causes of the condition known as *pseudomyxoma peritonei.*

The speed of progression from obstruction to perforation is rapid in the very young, since defense mechanisms are limited and the symptoms difficult to communicate. The complication rate of appendicitis in children under the age of 5 years is understandably high, approximately 80% by the time operation is undertaken. The older the child, the slower the progression, the more accurate the history, and the lower the complication rate.

Symptoms begin with epigastric pain that gradually migrates to the umbilical area and then localizes to the right lower abdominal quadrant as the parietal peritoneum in this area becomes involved in the inflammatory process. Anorexia, nausea and vomiting, low-grade fever, leukocytosis to a range of 9000 to 14,000 cells/mm^3, and malaise are common findings. Diagnosis can be difficult because of early nonspecificity of symptoms and findings. Localized tenderness in the right lower abdomen is the most accurate sign. Occasionally plain abdominal x-ray studies show an opacified obstructing fecalith.

Many nonsurgical illnesses mimic appendicitis; right lower lobe pneumonia, mesenteric lymphadenitis, and enterocolitis to mention only a few. A carefully performed barium enema examination carried out by a radiologist who is experienced with this technique may help in diagnosis: an appendix that does not fill completely, indentation of the cecum, displacement of ter-

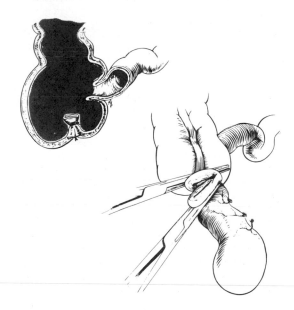

Fig. 39-20. Removal of inflamed appendix.

minal ileum, and mucosal inflammation of periappendiceal bowel are radiographic signs of acute appendicitis. Ultrasound may also be useful when it identifies a fluid-filled, thick-walled appendix. Because of its very serious potential complications, exploration is indicated whenever the possibility of appendicitis exists. The surgeon is wrong in about 15% of cases, but this is acceptable in order not to miss the difficult-to-diagnose case that, if untreated, would become complicated by perforation and peritonitis. Surgical treatment involves removal of the inflamed appendix, closure of the base of the appendix leading into the cecum, and drainage of localized pus (Fig. 39-20).

Intussusception

Intussusception is an invagination, or telescoping, of one segment of bowel into another (Fig. 39-21); its

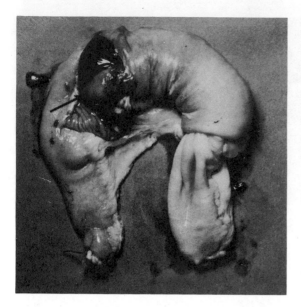

Fig. 39-21. Intussusception of small bowel. Notice telescoping of bowel toward left side of specimen, which has been opened in its midportion to disclose polyp *(arrow)* causing intussusception.

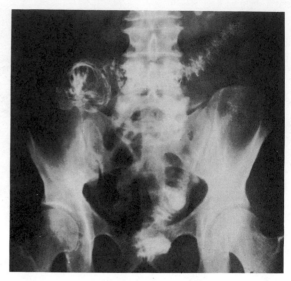

Fig. 39-22. Barium enema showing diagnostic "coil-spring" appearance of ileocolic intussusception at about hepatic flexure of colon in patient's right upper abdomen.

cause is often not known. Intussusception results in intestinal obstruction with the threat of strangulation of the involved bowel as its blood supply becomes compromised. The majority involve the distal ileum telescoping into the cecum with propagation around the colon to varying levels. Intussusception is characteristically seen in 3-month-old to 2-year-old well-nourished children. Abdominal pain occurs every 5 to 10 minutes (intestinal colic), during which the child cries and doubles up, followed by a period of disarming quiet. Vomiting of bile and the passage of bloody stools resembling currant jelly are classic features. The intussuscepted bowel can often be palpated as a tubular mass across the upper abdomen when the child relaxes between episodes of intestinal colic.

Barium enema (Fig. 39-22) confirms diagnosis and also can be used to reduce the intussusception safely (in about two thirds of the patients). This reduction is observed by fluoroscopy; the barium column is elevated no higher than 30 to 36 inches above the table to avoid perforation of the bowel or reduction of strangulated bowel. Signs of *intestinal obstruction* or *peritonitis* are related to bowel strangulation and mandate operative reduction. These signs contraindicate attempted barium enema reduction, since they are associated with an unacceptably high rate of perforation when hydrostatic reduction has been attempted. Surgical reduction (and sometimes bowel resection) is also required when barium reduction is ineffective.

Hypertrophic pyloric stenosis

Hypertrophic pyloric stenosis is the most common cause for intestinal obstruction in the baby 2 to 6 weeks of age (occurring once in 400 births). It occurs in males twice as often as in females. Forceful vomiting of gastric contents not discolored by bile is the outstanding

feature of the history. Prominent waves travel from left to right across the epigastrium; these represent forceful peristaltic contractions of the stomach attempting to squeeze gastric material through the narrowed pyloric channel. The pylorus, the muscle surrounding the outlet of the stomach, becomes thickened (Fig. 39-23, *A*). Its lumen (the pyloric channel) narrows, obstructing the outflow of material from the stomach. The basic cause for this hypertrophy is unknown.

The diagnosis is confirmed in about 80% of patients by palpation of the thickened muscle, the "olive" mass, in the right upper abdominal quadrant. If the age, history, or findings are atypical, an upper gastrointestinal series establishes the diagnosis by outlining the narrow pyloric channel. Ultrasound is also helpful in confirming diagnosis. Acute pyelonephritis, increased intracranial pressure, and the adrenogenital syndrome occasionally mimic the symptoms of pyloric stenosis.

Operative treatment is simple; the thickened pyloric muscle is incised and spread apart (Fig. 39-23, *B* and *C*) thereby enlarging the channel and relieving the obstruction. Pyloromyotomy (Ramstedt procedure) has perhaps the highest success rate and the lowest morbidity and mortality of any common operative procedure.

Inguinal Hernia, Hydrocele

Inguinal hernia in the male child results from retention of an embryonic outpocketing of peritoneum known as the *processus vaginalis,* which precedes testicular descent into the scrotum. The walls of this structure normally adhere to obliterate the sac (Fig. 39-24, *A*), but if obliteration fails, the sac will remain and allow bowel to enter as a hernia (Fig. 39-24, *B* and *C*).

Surgical correction is carried out when the diagnosis is made because of possible complications of incarceration of strangulation of the herniated bowel; this occurs in 5% to 15% of babies with a hernia. Hernia re-

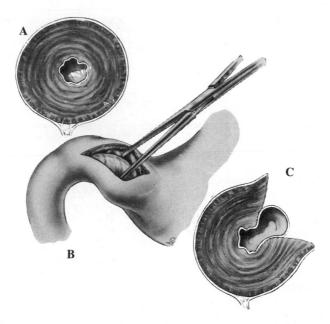

Fig. 39-23. Hypertrophic pyloric stenosis. **A,** Cross section of thickened pyloric muscle and narrow channel. **B,** Ramstedt pyloromyotomy showing instrument spreading muscle apart after it has been incised longitudinally, allowing intact mucosa to bulge outward as in **C** to greatly enlarge lumen of pyloric channel and relieve obstruction of stomach.

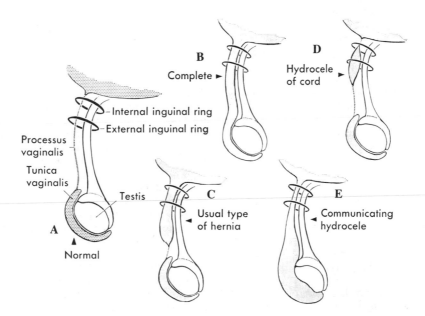

Fig. 39-24. A, Normally obliterated processus vaginalis. **B,** Complete failure of obliteration of processus vaginalis, with large opening into peritoneal cavity allowing bowel to enter as complete, or scrotal, hernia. **C,** Proximal part of processus vaginalis does not obliterate, allowing bowel to enter as usual type of indirect inguinal hernia. **D,** Hydrocele of cord. **E,** Communicating hydrocele; connection with peritoneal cavity is large enough to allow peritoneal fluid to enter sac, but not large enough for bowel to enter.

pair requires division and closure of the neck of the sac to remove the connection with the peritoneal cavity.

A hydrocele is embryonically related to the hernia (Fig. 39-24, *D* and *E*), the difference resting in the size of the connection of the patent *processus vaginalis* with the peritoneal cavity. In a hydrocele the connection is

large enough to allow fluid to gravitate into the unobliterated sac but not large enough to allow bowel to enter. The majority of hydroceles disappear spontaneously when the small peritoneal connection becomes obliterated, allowing no further peritoneal fluid to enter. Only rarely is surgical closure of this connection necessary.

About 15% of hernias are preceded by a hydrocele, the peritoneal connection having enlarged sufficiently to allow bowel to enter the sac.

Hirschsprung's Disease of the Older Child (Congenital Aganglionosis of the Colon, Congenital Megacolon)

Hirschsprung's disease is the most common functional congenital obstruction of the colon. The colonic obstruction is caused by absence of peristalsis within that segment of colon in which the autonomic ganglion cells (both intermuscular and submucosal) are congenitally absent. Proximal to the aganglionic segment, the colon dilates and hypertrophies to warrant the descriptive term "megacolon." The obstruction may be acute and relatively complete immediately after birth (discussed in the section of neonatal obstruction of the colon above.) Bouts of distension, vomiting, and paradoxical diarrhea interspersed with constipation characterize the disease during the first year of life. As the child grows older, chronic constipation emerges as the dominant complaint. Life-threatening complications of bowel perforation, enterocolitis, and sepsis accordingly bear an inverse relationship to age.

In about 80% of children aganglionosis is limited to the rectum and rectosigmoid but occasionally extends higher in the colon, and in nearly 5% of cases involves the entire colon. There are reported cases of aganglionosis of the entire gastrointestinal tract. Regardless of its proximal point of origin, the aganglionosis invariably extends from that point on down to include the internal anal sphincter, therefore allowing completely reliable diagnosis by the simple expedient of rectal wall biopsy carried out transanally. Abdominal distension and evidence of poor nutrition parallel the degree of obstruction. Children with Hirschsprung's disease are predisposed to acute necrotizing enterocolitis (Chap. 25), a complication that carries substantial mortality.

The history given by children with congenital aganglionosis may be extremely varied, though bowel dysfunction of some degree is present from birth. There often is a delay of 24 to 48 hours in the passage of meconium rectally after delivery, with varying degrees of constipation or explosive diarrhea thereafter. Abdominal distension, vomiting of feedings, and poor weight gain are common complaints. Invariably changes in formula and the use of laxatives, enemas, and suppositories have all been attempted for symptomatic control.

Physical examination reveals a somewhat pale and malnourished infant or child with soft abdominal distension. Loops of colon are often palpable, distended by gas and hard feces. Rectal digital examination reveals a small rectal ampulla. If the aganglionosis extends only to the rectosigmoid, the examining finger may reach the dilated and stool-filled sigmoid colon and provoke an explosive escape of liquid stool and gas on withdrawal of the finger.

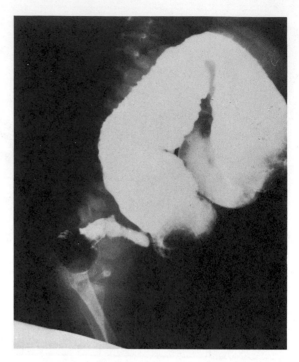

Fig. 39-25. Congenital aganglionosis (Hirschsprung's disease). Barium enema shows narrow, spastic rectum and rectosigmoid (aganglionic) flaring into megacolon (ganglionated bowel) at sigmoid colon.

Barium enema is helpful in diagnosis, characteristically showing a narrow or normal-sized rectum that flares into a megacolon above the point of obstruction (Fig. 39-25); only small amounts of barium should be used, and no effort should be made to fill the entire colon, since tardy expulsion of the barium is a second feature of the radiographic diagnosis. Confirmation of diagnosis rests on rectal wall biopsy, which can be achieved by a suction capsule without anesthesia; absent ganglion cells and an increase in acetyl cholinesterase staining are seen.

The treatment of Hirschsprung's disease is surgical, except in rare instances of a very short aganglionic segment that can be easily controlled by conservative methods (stool softeners and enemas). Initially efforts directed toward relief of the intestinal obstruction generally by performing a colostomy; the proximal extent of aganglionosis is determined histologically by seromuscular biopsy of the colon obtained at appropriate levels. The colostomy must be placed within an area of normal ganglion cells.

Definitive treatment consists of resection of the aganglionic colon to within 1 to 3 cm of the anus. Anastomosis of the ganglionated colon to the rectal pouch is achieved by one of a variety of abdominoperineal techniques. Prognosis is good.

40

Plastic and Reconstructive Surgery

David W. Furnas

Ivan M. Turpin

Free grafts
Pedicles
Z-plasty

The word "plastic" stems from the Greek word *plassein,* which means "to form." *Plastic operation* refers to a procedure that forms by means of *shifting* or *transplanting tissues.*

The branch of general surgery that is the specialty of *plastic surgery* deals particularly with the facial features (Fig. 40-1), the jaws and oral cavity, the hand, and the body surface in general, including the breasts and the external genitals. The plastic surgeon attempts to *restore a patient to his original state* after injuries, after removal of tumors, or after changes from aging; he attempts to *improve on the patient's original state* when there are congenital defects or body features that are believed to fall too short of ideal. The "four Cs" of plastic surgery are congenital deformities, calamities, cancer, and cosmesis. *Wound care, free grafts,* and *pedicles* are the foundation of the plastic surgeon's art and are fundamental to the craft of surgery in general. Craniofacial surgery and microvascular surgery are areas of recent rapid advances (Fig. 40-2).

FREE GRAFTS

A *free graft* is a piece of living tissue that is detached from one site and transplanted to another site where it survives as living tissue. Depending on the donor, it is termed *autograft* (self), *isograft* (identical twin), *allograft* (same species), or *heterograft* (different species).

Mechanisms of Graft Survival, or "Take"
Skin Graft

A skin graft appears white when first placed on a raw defect. It is nourished entirely by the host tissue

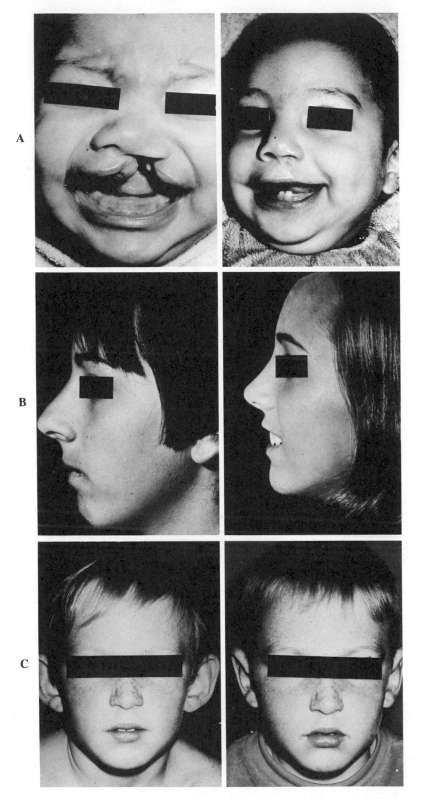

Fig. 40-1. A, Cleft lip. *Left,* Unilateral cleft lip in infant. *Right,* Lip closure several months postoperatively (scar minics left column of philtrum and will be scarcely noticeable in several years). **B,** Nasal hump and receding chin. *Left,* Preoperative. *Right,* Postoperative rhinoplasty and mentoplasty using cartilage and bone from nasal hump and septum. **C,** Prominent ears. *Left,* Preoperative. *Right,* Postoperative otoplasty.

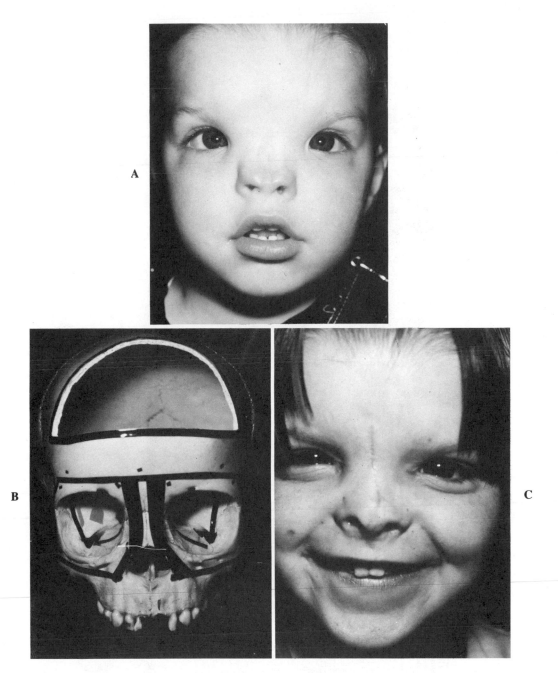

Fig. 40-2. A, Child with hypertelorism. **B,** Mock-up of bone cuts and bone removal for Tessier procedure. **C,** Postoperative status.

fluids that bathe its deep surface *(plasmatic circulation)*. After a few hours it becomes quite adherent, cemented in place by the formation of a fibrin coagulum. In less than a day the white graft becomes pink by *inosculation,* or linking up of the graft capillaries with host capillaries. After 1 or 2 days the graft is *penetrated* by new capillary buds that grow out from the host. As these develop, the graft's original vessels degenerate. The new vessels assume the entire circulatory load and the graft "takes" firmly. Final healing occurs by the same processes seen in other wounds.

Other Free Grafts

The "take" of grafts of other tissues (dermis, tendon, bone, fascia) is in some ways similar to that of skin; however, the process is much slower in bone, and fewer of the bone graft's cells remain alive; in cartilage a type of plasmatic circulation is the final form of nutrition.

Failure to "Take"

The three chief causes of failure of a skin graft to "take" are *bleeding* beneath the graft (Fig. 40-3), *infec-*

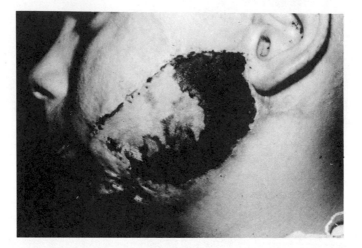

Fig. 40-3. Necrosis of skin graft from hematoma. Bleeding beneath this graft resulted after severe post-operative vomiting. Dark portion of graft is dead and must be replaced with another skin graft.

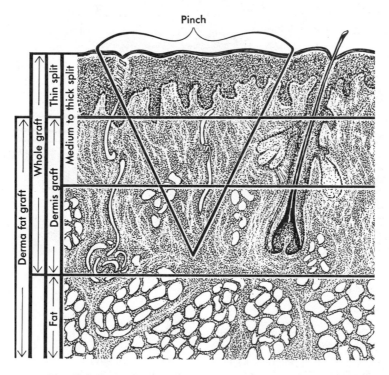

Fig. 40-4. Types of grafts taken from skin and subcutaneous tissue.

Table 40-1. Commonly Used Free Skin Grafts

Type	Common Donor Site	Uses	Comment
Split skin graft (thin, medium, or thick)	Thighs, abdomen, buttocks, back, and elsewhere	To close defects of integument almost anywhere on body	Donor sites epithelialize
Full-thickness skin graft (Wolfe or whole skin graft)	Retroauricular or preauricular area, supraclavicular area, groin	To close skin defects of limited size, particularly on face	Superior appearance and function; donor sites must be closed surgically
Dermis graft (whole graft with a thin graft removed from surface)	Abdomen or elsewhere	To fill our defects in contour or to bolster fascial defects	Buried beneath the skin surface
Dermafat graft (dermis graft with fat attached)	Abdomen, buttocks, on elsewhere	To fill out larger defects in contour	Loses ¼ to ½ of bulk after implantation
Hair follicle–bearing skin grafts	Scalp, eyebrow	To repair scalp, eyebrow, or lashes	Usually applied in small patches or strips
Composite skin grafts* (whole skin + cartilage; skin + fibrofat or bone)	Helix, anthelix, lobe of external ear	To repair defects of nose, ear, eyelid	Only small grafts survive Works best for children
	Fingertip (accident)	To replace finger part	

*Other composite grafts finding occasional use are nipple-areolar grafts and nailbed-nail grafts

Table 40-2. Commonly Used Autografts of Tissues Other Than Skin

Tissue	Common Donor Site	Uses	Comment
Fat + dermis	Buttock, abdomen	To fill out defects in contour	Easily reabsorbed; dermafat grafts are much better
Fascia	Fascia lata of thigh and elsewhere	To repair fascia, dura, or tendons; to lash or support other structures	May be used in sheets or strips
Tendon	Palmaris longus, plantaris, extensors of toes	To replace or elongate tendons; to bind other structures	Congenital absence of palmaris longus or plantaris is not infrequent
Bone	Ilium, ribs (especially in children), and sites on long bones	To replace missing bone and correct nonunion of fractures and skeletal contour defects	New ribs regenerate from donor defects in children if periosteum is left
Cartilage	Costal cartilage, nasal septum, conchal cartilage	To replace missing cartilage or bone; to correct contour defects	Tends to warp if not cut with a symmetrical section
Vessels	Veins in distal extremities; superficial temporal artery	To replace absent, thrombosed, or traumatized arteries; to patch arterial incisions	Valves must be placed in correct direction
Nerves	Sural, saphenous, greater auricular nerves	To replace absent or damaged nerve segments	The more peripheral the site of injury, the better the results

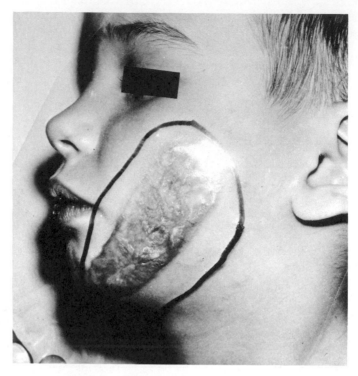

Fig. 40-5. Contraction of thin skin graft. Dark circle represents original granulating wound that resulted from full thickness burn. Very thin skin graft was the same size as this inked pattern, but over period of 3 months it has contracted to half the original size. Graft was later excised and replaced by advancement flap.

tion, and *movement* of the graft. If a hematoma forms, the graft is lifted from its bed and dies. *Hemolytic streptococci* form exotoxins that lyse the skin graft from its bed and destroy it. *Pseudomonas, Proteus,* and *Staphylococcus aureus* form pus that lifts the graft from the recipient bed. Excessive movement of graft shears the capillary connections between the graft and host, and the graft dies. Therefore meticulous hemostasis, aseptic technique, and adequate immobilization of the graft are important for success.

Clinical Use of Autologous Grafts

The factotum among skin grafts is the *split skin graft* (Tables 40-1 and 40-2 and Fig. 40-4). It can furnish viable cover for fresh wounds, granulating wounds, mucosal defects (mouth, vagina, nose), fascia, paratenon, periosteum, and even exposed lung, brain or pericardium. Split skin grafts do poorly if the vascularity of the recipient bed is poor, as in heavily scarred or irradiated wounds, or on bare bone, bare cartilage, or bare tendon. Large split skin grafts are cut with special knives, or *dermatomes,* small ones with ordinary scalpels. The donor sites heal by *epithelialization* in 1 to 4 weeks, depending on the thickness of the graft.

Thin split grafts are more likely to "take" in unfavorable circumstances, but they tend to contract and develop inferior appearance and durability (Fig. 40-5).

Thick split grafts are more likely to perish from excessive movement or from bacterial activity than are thinner grafts, but on surviving they furnish a more durable surface (Fig. 40-6).

Full-thickness grafts furnish a better quality coverage, but "take" is less reliable; the size of the graft is limited by the need to suture or graft (with split-thickness skin) the donor site (Fig. 40-7).

Split skin grafts may be cut in sheets, in strips, or in "postage stamps" (small squares). Sheet grafts furnish a superior surface; the smaller grafts are used to expand the area of coverage when donor sites are limited or to improve survival in the presence of infection, movement, or irregular contours.

Composite graft is skin plus other attached tissue. Only small blocks of composite tissue survive (Fig. 40-8).

Tissue expanders are inflatable silicone devices that stretch tissues. Research has shown that, in response to increasing pressure, epidermal cells multiply. Implanted under skin, muscle, or fascia, the silicone device is gradually inflated with sterile saline over several weeks, until the overlying tissue expands to the appropriate size. The excess, stretched tissue can then cover adjacent defects (scars, ulcers) or prostheses (breast implants). This technique is especially valuable because it mobilizes similar adjacent tissues, such as scalp, minimizing the cosmetic defect.

Replantation of a traumatically amputated part is the most complex clinical autograft in current surgical practice. These grafts, of course, depend for their survival on blood flow through major vascular anastomoses.

Recent advances have been made in allograft transplantation surgery using cyclosporine to prevent

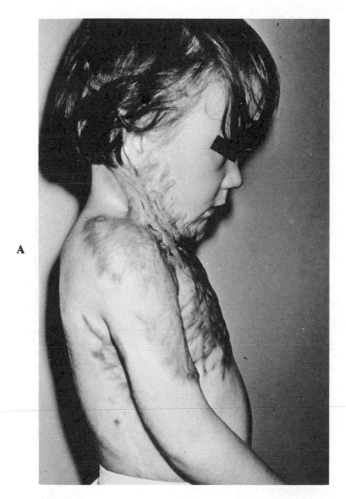

A

Fig. 40-6. Medium thickness split skin graft. **A,** Flaming nightgown caused burn scars that have contracted mandible tightly against sternum.   *Continued.*

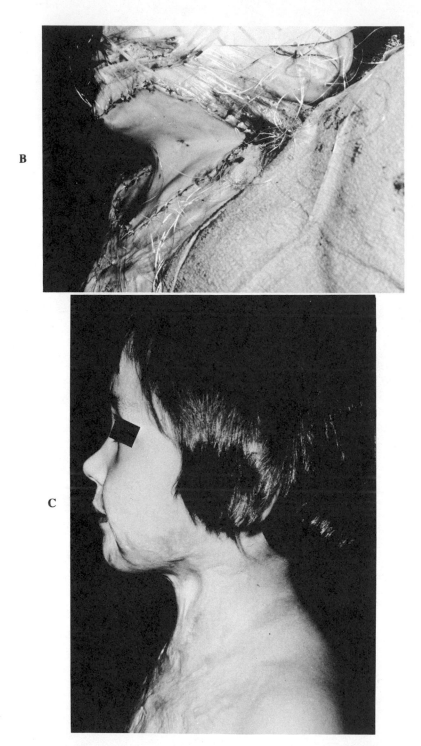

Fig. 40-6, cont'd. B, Raw surface is covered with single sheet of medium thickness split skin taken from abdomen, **C,** Graft has matured. Even though texture and color are not exact match, neck-chin angle has been restored and potential for deformity of skeletal growth has been greatly reduced.

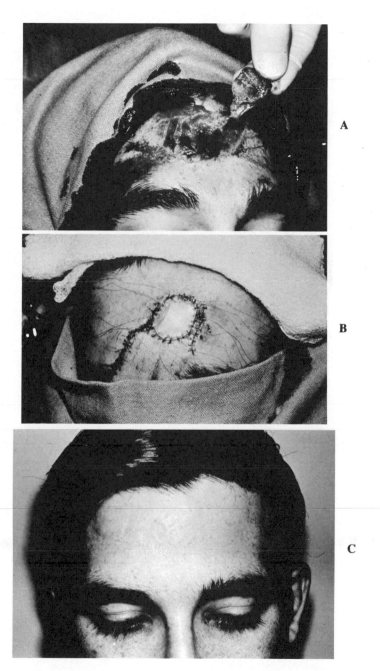

Fig. 40-7. Salvage of doomed flap by conversion into graft. **A,** Windshield injury to forehead has elevated a flap of skin. Pedicle attachment is too narrow for survival, and flap is rapidly becoming congested as blood flows in but fails to flow out. **B,** Flap is detached, trimmed, and replaced as full thickness skin graft. **C,** When mature, replaced graft is inconspicuous and gives perfect color match.

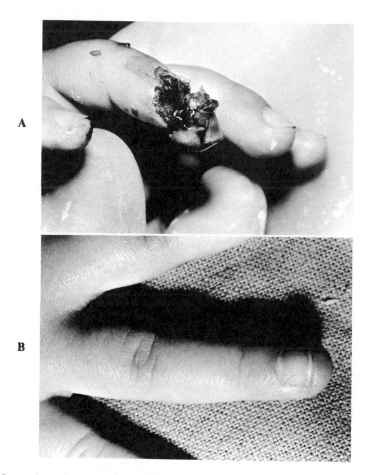

Fig. 40-8. Composite graft. **A,** Tip of ring finger of 3-year-old child was avulsed when caught in car door. It is held in place by tiny dermoepidermal remnant, but no active circulation is present and thus no congestion occurs. Fingertip was immediately sutured back into place with meticulous care. **B,** Survival of graft is complete. Results of this procedure are generally better in children that in adults.

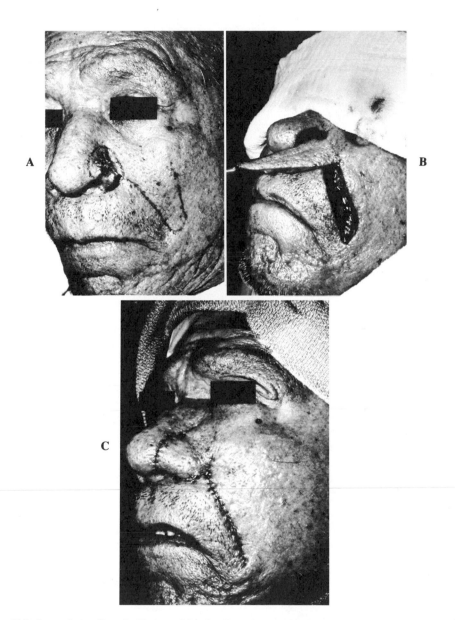

Fig. 40-9. Interpolation flap. **A,** Pigmented basal cell carcinoma of left nasal ala. Excision line and labial interpolation flap have been plotted with ink. **B,** Tumor has been excised. Frozen sections show that margins of specimen are free of tumor, and flap has been incised, undermined, and moved to nasal defect. **C,** Flap has been trimmed and doubled over to furnish interior lining for defect. Defect and donor site are closed.

LOCAL FLAPS

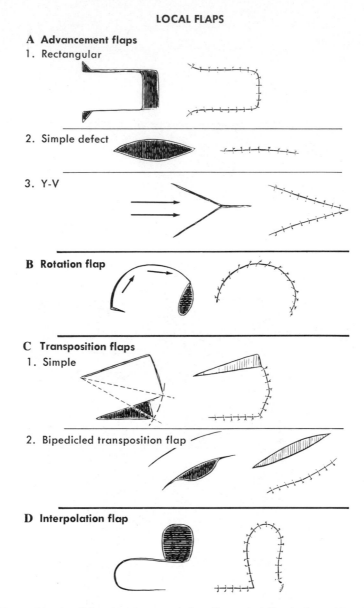

A Advancement flaps
1. Rectangular

2. Simple defect

3. Y-V

B Rotation flap

C Transposition flaps
1. Simple

2. Bipedicled transposition flap

D Interpolation flap

Fig. 40-10. Types of local pedicles. **A,** *Advancement flap:* (1) stretched directly forward into defect aided by excision of Burow's triangles; (2) advancement of edges of simple defect; (3) Y-V advancement flap. **B,** *Rotation flap:* stretched in arc toward defect; donor site closed without skin graft is four to five times bigger than defect; if ratio is smaller, split-skin graft may be required for defect. **C,** *Transposition flap:* (1) moved laterally into adjacent defect; split-skin graft may be required for donor site; (2) bipedicled transposition flap. **D,** *Interpolation flap:* moved over intervening tissue to reach defect, donor site closed with secondary flap or split-skin graft.

rejection of composite somatic tissues. Provocative results have been achieved with limb allograft transplantation in rats and primates and facial parts in rabbits and primates. Skin allografts in humans also show promise.

PEDICLES

Pedicle, flap, pedicled graft, and *pedicled flap* are synonyms for tissue (usually skin with attached subcutaneous tissue) that is transferred to a different site with

an intact blood supply. A pedicle is nourished by blood circulating through its own capillaries via a bridge of intact tissue, the base of the pedicle (Figs. 40-9 and 40-10), or circulation is reestablished by microvascular anastomoses (Fig. 40-11).

Use of Pedicles

Pedicles commonly surpass free grafts as the best procedure in the following instances: (1) where the defect to be treated is *poorly vascularized* (e.g., heavy

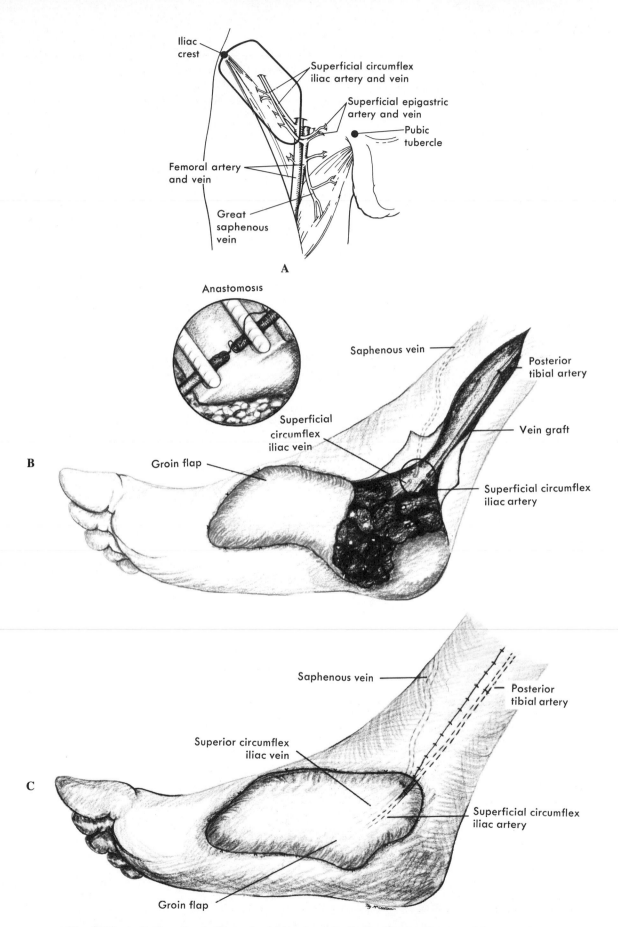

Fig. 40-11. A, Outline of groin flap and axial blood supply. **B,** Free flap transfers to recipient area: inset shows microvascular anastomosis of 1.5 mm. artery. **C,** Completed free flap transfer.

scar, radiation changes), (2) where *bare tendons, bare cartilage,* or *bare cortical bone* is exposed, (3) where *padding* is needed over the defect (e.g., pressure sores), (4) where *bulk* is required (e.g., replacement of a missing nose, filling out a sunken wound), (5) *where exact match of color, texture, and resilience* is desired (e.g., correction of a cheek defect with a pedicle from neighboring cheek and neck tissue), (6) where a *double facing* is required (e.g., replacement of full thickness defect of the cheek or mouth), (7) or where there is likelihood that the new surface will have to be temporarily elevated at a future time to permit further reconstructive surgery (e.g., in anticipation of secondary tendon grafts, tendon transfers, bone grafts, or nerve repairs).

Types of Flaps According to Blood Supply
Random Blood Supply

No named blood vessels are included in the flap. For hundred of years this has been the most common type of flap. Flaps can be created from tissue adjacent to the defect (local flaps). Terms such as rotation, advancement, transposition, or interpolation are added to describe the manner of movement (Fig. 40-9). Flaps may be brought from remote areas and applied directly to a defect (distant, *direct*) or *migrated* in stages.

Axial Blood Supply

A specific artery and vein are included in the flap and provide its circulation. Examples are the deltopectoral flap (internal mammary perforators) and the groin

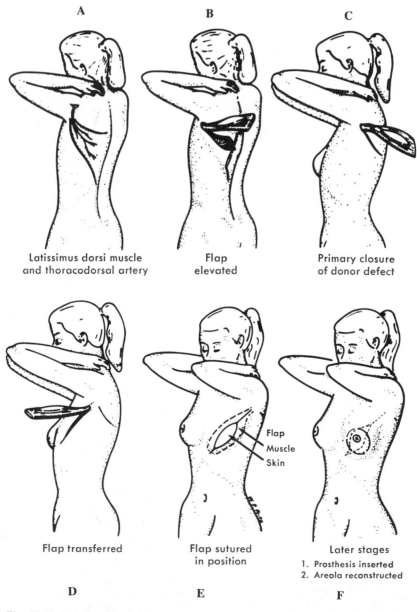

Fig. 40-12. Latissimus dorsi myocutaneous flap for breast reconstruction after mastectomy.

flap (superficial circumflex iliac vessels). Unfortunately, most vessels to the skin arise at right angles to vessels within the underlying muscles.

Myocutaneous Flap

A whole new family of axial flaps has now been described in which an entire muscle with its overlying skin is transferred (myocutaneous; Fig. 40-12). Examples include the pectoralis, gluteus, tensor fasciae latae, gracilis, and gastrocnemius muscles. Of course the muscle can be transferred without the skin and can then be skin grafted *(muscle flap)*.

Fasciocutaneous Flap

Described in 1981, this flap is based on a system of deep vessels which pass along the fibrous septa be-

tween the muscle bellies to form a superficial plexus of vessels at the level of the deep fascia. These vascular plexuses give off branches to the overlying skin. Advantages include easy elevation and less bulk and deformity. They are most useful in upper and lower extremity reconstruction; however, applications have been described for all regions of the body.

Island Flap

A complete island of skin is excised and elevated, but its subcutaneous connections with blood vessels are maintained. The artery is dissected free, and the island is burrowed subcutaneously to reach the recipient site with its arterial umbilicus trailing after. An eyebrow may be replaced with a temporal scalp island supported by the superficial temporal artery, or a thumb may be

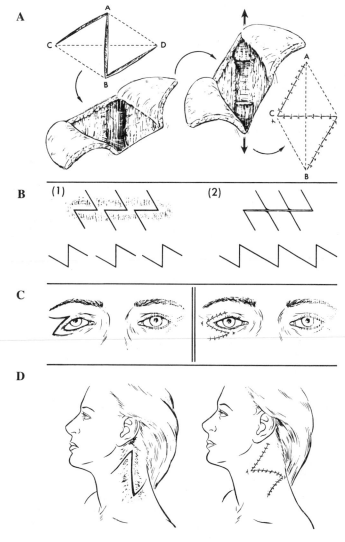

Fig. 40-13. Four functions of Z-plasties. **A,** Interpolation of two triangular flaps increases length along path *AB* at the expense of width along path *CD*. (In effect, dimensions are exchanged between *AB* and *CD*.) **B,** Interpolation of series of disconnected, *1*, or connected, *2*, series of Z's breaks up a straight line and also gives it increased length. **C,** Shift of topographic mark. Correction of contracted lateral canthus effected by Z-plasty; corner of mouth, eyebrow, or nasal ala may be similarly managed. **D,** Obliteration of secondary webbed scar contractures with a Z-plasty shifts the two planes of web so that they form planes of depression at base of neck.

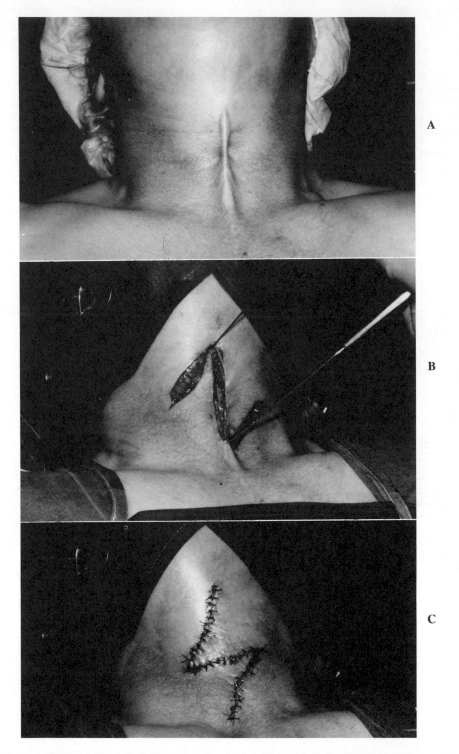

Fig. 40-14. A, Posttraumatic webbed-scar contracture of the anterior neck. **B,** Scar has been excised, and the flaps have been elevated. **C,** The flaps have been rotated into position and the vertical tension has been relieved.

given an area of normal sensation with an island of skin from the ring finger supported by a digital neurovascular bundle *(sensory island flap)*.

Free Flap

It is now possible to completely detach a flap, transfer it to its new location, and then, using microsurgery, anastomose the 1- to 2 mm vessels, reestablishing the circulation. Thus, what used to take many operations and several months can be accomplished in one day (Fig. 40-11).

Complications of Pedicle Surgery

Pedicle procedures are subject to the same problems as any other wound (e.g., hematoma, infection) plus special problems that can threaten the precarious circulation. If a pedicle is too narrow, if it is detached too early, if the blood flow is obstructed by external pressure (the patient's own weight, tight dressings, heavy bedding), or if it is kinked or twisted, the pedicle may die. If the newly incised free end of a pedicle is placed at a lower level than the base of the pedicle, the pedicle may become congested *(gravitational congestion)* and die from circulatory stasis.

Z-PLASTY

The Z-plasty is a useful surgical technique that may perform any of four basic functions: *increase length along a specific path* (Fig. 40-13 *A*), *break up and reorient a straight line scar* (Fig. 40-13, *B*), *shift topographic landmarks* (Fig. 40-13, *C*), and *deepen webs or obliterate clefts* (Fig. 40-13, *D*).

The Z-plasty is performed by elevating two triangular flaps in the form of a Z and *interpolating* them so that the final figure is a reversed Z. The incisions should be of approximately equal lengths. The angles may be unequal, but the most common form of a Z-plasty has two 60-degree angles. Z-plasties may be single or serial (Fig. 40-14).

41

Care of the Acutely Injured Patient

John F. Hansbrough
Ben Eiseman

The most important environmental health problem the United States faces is violent and accidental injuries. Deaths by trauma lead all causes of death in the first half of man's life span. In the United States trauma afflicts 50 million people each year, killing 165,000 and disabling at least 14 million others. The overall cost (including medical expenses, property loss, insurance claims, lost working hours, etc.) totals more than $97 billion yearly. Even though the general public tends to forget the enormity of this problem, the medical profession cannot, because accident victims occupy one of every eight beds in a typical general hospital.

This chapter introduces the student to the acutely injured patient and the early, life-saving procedures in the emergency room. Other chapters discuss the later, specialized care of these patients.

THE EMERGENCY ROOM

Every modern hospital provides emergency rooms equipped to receive and treat the injured. Readily accessible to ambulances and automobiles, some emergency services feature heliports as well. Probably more important, special centers train paramedics who travel to the accident site and begin immediate treatment. Programs in many areas have reaffirmed the worth of these ultramodern regional emergency centers that initiate treatment on the spot.

Emergency room physicians must become expert at triage—*sorting first things first*. They rapidly scan patients for life-threatening conditions: (1) airway and respiration, (2) heart and circulation, (3) active bleeding, (4) state of consciousness, and (5) obvious threatening injuries (i.e., sucking chest wound, flail chest, sharp bone fragments near major vessels). They know the conditions that threaten life, and they attack these problems rapidly and systematically, the most urgent ones first (see Fig. 41-1).

AIRWAY AND RESPIRATION

The airway is the first consideration in all emergency situations; the physician must determine immediately whether the patient is breathing adequately. Cyanosis with gasping chest movements and upper airway noise (stridor) indicates airway obstruction. The most common cause of obstruction in injured patients is posterior displacement of the tongue; the physician should force the mouth open and thrust the mandible forward. Any foreign matter should be removed with the finger or with suctioning. If there is any suspicion of a neck injury, the neck should not be extended but kept in a neutral position. An unstable cervical fracture must be assumed to exist until it is excluded by a cross-table lateral spine radiograph. An oral airway may be placed in the comatose patient but will not be tolerated if the patient is awake. If these procedures fail to relieve the obstructed breathing, tracheal intubation (orally, nasally, or through a tracheostomy) will bypass an obstructed larynx and assure an open upper airway.

Continuing cyanosis indicates lower respiratory problems; *pneumothorax,* usually resulting from fractured ribs, heads the list. Any fractured rib can puncture a lung, often without causing gross chest wall deformity. Characterized by a tympanitic hemothorax, absent breath sounds, tracheal displacement (to the opposite side), and subcutaneous emphysema, pneumothorax can become *tension pneumothorax* from a flutter-valve defect in the puncture site that forces air into the intrapleural space with each inspiration. As the air builds up, it compresses the opposite lung, sometimes fatally. Aspiration of the entrapped air by needle or thoracostomy tube reverses this process.

Crushing chest trauma that fractures several ribs at multiple sites results in *flail chest.* The shattered chest wall, lacking normal rigidity, moves paradoxically (in with inspiration and out with expiration). Although external bracing helps somewhat, intubation and mechanical ventilation continued until the chest wall solidifies (10 to 20 days) have proved most effective. Simple tamponade with an occlusive dressing temporarily repairs open "sucking" wounds of the chest wall while thoracostomy tubes drain out entrapped air.

Acute gastric dilation (from ileus and swallowed air) may impede diaphragmatic movement and thus hinder ventilation. Nasogastric suction provides instant relief and also helps prevent vomiting and aspiration pneumonitis. Removing gastric juice also decreases stress ulceration.

CIRCULATION

Once assured that the patient has an adequate airway, the physician checks circulation. Any serious bleeding sites should be tamponaded at once; a large intravenous catheter is inserted and crystalloid solutions are administered (after taking a blood sample for typing and matching).

Many patients in shock respond to this treatment alone, but if shock (cold clammy skin, weak rapid pulse) persists despite adequate fluid and blood replacement, one of the following causes is likely: cardiac tamponade, tension pneumothorax, internal bleeding (chest, abdomen, or fracture sites), bowel rupture, aortic tear, or, rarely, adrenal failure. At this point a central venous catheter immensely aids further evaluation.

Cardiac Tamponade

In patients with chest trauma, distant, muted heart sounds, low pulse pressure, and a high central venous pressure (CVP), and often a paradoxical pulse, indicate cardiac tamponade. Echocardiography, if available, can rapidly confirm these clinical signs. Needle aspiration of the pericardial blood, repeated if necessary, usually

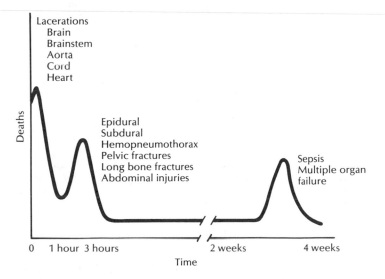

Fig. 41-1. Relationship of death to time after injury. Brain, heart, and aortic trauma cause most early deaths; sepsis and multiple organ failure most late deaths.

reestablishes normal heart action (see Chap. 30). Unresponsive cases may require thoracotomy and direct repair of any bleeding site.

Hemothorax

Because of two factors (collapsible lung tissue and low pulmonary blood pressure), bleeding from lung parenchyma rarely persists. Continued intrapleural bleeding usually comes from severed intercostal or internal mammary vessels. Needle aspiration or insertion of a thoracotomy tube (with suction) removes the blood and allows the lung to expand. Tube drainage provides a constant monitor to assess continued bleeding (see Chap. 29). Less than 10% of these patients require thoracotomy.

Hemoperitoneum

The neophyte physician can easily be misled by the relatively normal-appearing abdomen that contains 2000 ml of blood or more. Thus he should always suspect the abdomen as a likely source of continuing bleeding and persistent shock. Although four-quadrant, intraperitoneal aspiration with an 18-gauge needle serves as a rapid indicator of bleeding, a negative tap means nothing. With a sensitivity of about 98%, peritoneal lavage yields more reliable results. We instill 500 to 1000 ml of lactated Ringer's solution through a peritoneal dialysis catheter that enters the abdomen through a tiny skin incision in the lower midline. The bottle, placed on the floor, siphons the fluid from the abdomen. A pink tinge indicates bleeding. More than 100,000 RBCs/ml indicates significant bleeding. Bacteria, fecal material, or amylase indicates visceral perforation. Any one of these indicators signals the need for laparotomy. Abdominal computed tomography (CT), when readily available, will play a greater role in evaluating these patients (see Chap. 26).

Aortic Tears

Severe chest trauma may shear the aortic arch, causing dissection along the wall. A widening mediastinum on x-ray examination or absent or unequal peripheral pulses justifies emergency arteriography (see Chap. 29).

Adrenal Failure

Long-term steroid therapy suppresses normal adrenal response to stress. The physician should suspect adrenal failure in patients who give a history of steroid intake and in comatose patients with stigmata of arthritis, asthma, or chronic dermatoses.

COMA

Head trauma rarely causes shock. In fact, a person whose skull and brain sustain the shattering impact necessary to produce hemorrhagic shock seldom reaches the emergency room alive. But shock itself produces coma by depriving brain cells of oxygen. Thus initial efforts to restore airway and circulation aim most urgently at getting more oxygen to brain cells because cerebral cells, unlike other tissues, die within minutes from hypoxia. These efforts alone often restore consciousness as the brain receives its vital oxygen.

Brain cells suffer hypoxia from a second major cause after trauma—edema or hemorrhage within the skull depresses local cerebral circulation. Although slowing pulse and respiration, fever, and dilated pupils indicate increased intracranial pressure, the *level of consciousness* remains the most reliable sign. The physician must record early neurologic findings, especially noting state of consciousness, and immediately call for neurosurgical consultation (see Chap. 35). He should also note other possible causes of coma (alcohol, drugs, diabetes, epilepsy). The most important early treatment in minimizing brain edema is hyperventilation of the patient.

OTHER INJURIES

After the patient's cardiorespiratory function has been stabilized, the physician should systematically review other areas. He or she should question the patient or those who accompany the patient for pertinent information concerning the accident and the patient's health (diabetes, cardiac status, renal status etc.) while surveying the patient for pulses, bone abnormalities, hematuria (after catheterization), and other defects.

The same forces that cause head injuries also cause cervical spine injuries. All head injuries should direct attention to concurrent spine trauma. The conscious patient can move his digits and respond to pain stimuli from extremities, but the unconscious patient withdraws from these stimuli. These responses indicate an intact spinal cord. To lessen the chance of vertebral fractures or dislocations injuring the spinal cord, the patient must be moved cautiously and only when necessary.

TREATMENT PRIORITIES

One person, usually a general surgeon or traumatologist, must take charge, coordinate the consultants, and assign immediate priorities throughout this critical period. That person arranges priorities as follows: (1) restore cardiorespiratory function (stop bleeding, visible and hidden), (2) repair hollow viscera injuries (intestine, bladder), (3) repair vascular injuries, (4) treat head and spinal injuries, (5) repair open fractures, and (6) treat lacerations and closed fractures. When, for example, a patient sustains a skull fracture, femoral fracture, colon rupture, lacerations, and shock, the admitting surgeon treats the shock. stops external bleeding by pressure or ligation, and places a simple splint on the fractured femur. As soon as the patient's vital signs stabilize, the surgeon repairs the colonic tear in the operating room and thus interrupts lethal peritonitis at an early, curable stage. Other surgeons meanwhile clean and close the patient's lacerations. Skull and cervical spine films, taken en route to the operating room, show no displaced bone fragments, and echoencephalography reveals no midline shift; thus craniotomy can be deferred. Although the patient is unconscious before and during the operation, coma does not interdict the lifesaving laparotomy.

The team captain who must oversee the total care of acutely injured patients uses consultants for specialized problems and coordinates their diagnostic and treatment recommendations. Studies have proved that acutely injured patients treated in efficient emergency centers have the best chance of surviving.

SUMMARY

All emergency room personnel must keep clearly in mind the following steps for the care of acutely injured patients:

1. Assure airway and respiratory exchange.
2. Assure circulation.
   a. Stop bleeding.
   b. Treat shock.
   c. Prepare to treat cardiac arrest at any moment.
3. Determine need for operative control of internal bleeding or bowel rupture.
4. Determine need to restore peripheral circulation.
5. Determine need for operative decompression of spinal cord or brain.
6. Treat open fractures first, then repair lacerations, then treat closed fractures.

Because severe injury disrupts many vital functions, critically ill patients require a variety of conduits that connect them to outside supports. Life-sustaining substances flow in through some tubes; displaced bodily fluids (or gases) drain out through others. Some catheters serve mainly as monitors to help us alter, as necessary, this artificial flux. As a rapid reminder of these life-saving priorities, the student should picture a patient with five tubes in place, each serving a vital function.

Tube	Function
Oral airway or endotracheal tube	Assure adequate ventilation
Intravenous catheter	Restore fluids; treat shock
Central venous catheter	Monitor fluid load, hemopericardium, heart failure
Urinary catheter	Monitor renal perfusion; detect blood from urinary tract
Nasogastric tube	Prevent vomiting and aspiration pneumonia; prevent stress ulcers
Other tubes sometimes indicated	
Arterial catheter	Blood gas analyses
Thoractomy tube	Treat pneumothorax or hemothorax

42

Bites and Stings

Harold R. Mancusi-Ungaro, Jr.

Animal Bites
Snakebite
Stings

The surgeon's approach to an animal bite or sting is like that for any other soft tissue wound, with one exception: the surgeon must understand the animal and the mechanisms of injury, both physical and biological. Highlighting these mechanisms, this chapter focuses on the physiologic response to envenomation and treatment.

ANIMAL BITES

A bite is a wound inflicted by the mouth of an animal. Depending on the size of the animal and its teeth, the result is either a series of puncture wounds, perhaps compounded by a local crush injury, or a large open defect. In the case of a poisonous snake, fangs, not teeth, inflict the bite and introduce venom. Problems peculiar to animal bites determine the bacterial contamination. An inoculum of greater than 10^5 bacteria/g of tissue will predispose to infection, especially in wounds compromised by injured tissue, foreign bodies, or hematoma. Some of the organisms transmitted in animal bites are listed below:

Gram-positive organisms
    Streptococci
        β-Hemolytic
        S. viridans
        Others
    Staphylococcus
        S. aureus
        S. epidermidis
    Clostridium
        C. tetani
        C. perfringens
    Corynebacterium diphtheriae
Gram-negative organisms
    Pasteurella
        P. multocida
        P. tularensis
        P. pestis

Bacteroides
Fusobacter
Moraxella
Enterobacteriaceae
Pseudomonas
Vibrio
Fungi
  Candida
  Sporotrichosis
Spirochetes
  Leptospira

Initial wound care consists of careful examination in the emergency room or operating room. Obviously devitalized tissue requires débridement. The obvious bacterial contamination demands vigorous cleansing and irrigation of the wound by means of jet lavage (which can also kill the rabies virus). Prophylactic antibiotics are probably indicated for all animal bites, and *tetanus prophylaxis is always indicated* (see Chap. 6). The predominant flora for that animal, if known, dictates the choice of antibiotic. For example, dog bites feature *Pasteurella multocida,* certain marine organisms, and *Vibrio;* and human bites, both aerobic and anaerobic bacteria. Prophylaxis continues for about 5 days or until swelling subsides. Grossly contaminated and frankly contused wounds should be left open to drain.

Routine swab cultures of bite wounds are seldom helpful, but organisms seen on an initial Gram stain or wound biopsy should interdict wound closure. Initial antibiotic therapy can be guided by the predominant animal organisms and the victim's skin organisms,

staphylococci and streptococci. Closed wounds must be drained. Antibiotics should be adjusted according to culture and sensitivity reports. A topical antibacterial, such as bacitracin, polymixin, neomycin, or mafenide complements systemic therapy.

Rabies Prophylaxis

The clinical history helps determine whether to give prophylaxis against rabies. When symptoms develop, the disease is almost uniformly fatal. The vaccination process is time-consuming and uncomfortable. Local epidemiology can help in this decision: Has rabies been reported recently in the area or in the kind of animal that inflicted the bite? Wild animals, especially skunks, foxes, raccoons, and bats, are likely vectors; the vaccinated family dog is not. Rabies is transmitted through any open wound by contact with mucous membranes, saliva, or the tissues, of the infected animal. Not only bites, but scratches and abrasions can be a portal of entry. Table 42-1 outlines the current guidelines published by the Centers for Disease Control. Rabies immune globulin (RIG) or antirabies serum confers passive immunity.

Dog Bites

Dog bites are the most common of all animal bites, yet certain aspects of their treatment are debatable. They range from puncture wounds to wounds requiring major reconstruction. Unfortunately the height of a large dog often corresponds to the height of a child,

Table 42-1. Rabies Postexposure Prophylaxis Guide—July 1984

The following recommendations are only a guide. In applying them, take into account the animal species involved, the circumstances of the bite or other exposure, the vaccination status of the animal, and presence of rabies in the region. Local or state public health officials should be consulted if questions arise about the need for rabies prophylaxis.

Animal species	Condition of Animal at Time of Attack	Treatment of Exposed Person*
Dog and cat	Healthy and available for 10 days of observation	None, unless animal develops rabies†
	Rabid or suspected rabid	RIG§ and HDCV
	Unknown (escaped)	Consult public health officials. If treatment is indicated, give RIG§ and HDCV
Skunk, bat, fox, coyote raccoon, bobcat, and other carnivores	Regard as rabid unless proven negative by laboratory tests¶	RIG§ and HDCV
Livestock, rodents, and lagomorphs (rabbits and hares)	Consider individually. Local and state public health officials should be consulted on questions about the need for rabies prophylaxis. Bites of squirrels, hamsters, guinea pigs, gerbils, chipmunks, rats, mice, other rodents, rabbits, and horses almost never call for antirabies prophylaxis.	

All bites and wounds should immediately be thoroughly cleansed with soap and water. If antirabies treatment is indicated, both rabies immune globulin (RIG) and human diploid cell rabies vaccine (HDCV) should be given as soon as possible, *regardless* of the interval from exposure. Local reactions to vaccines are common and do not contraindicate continuing treatment. Discontinue vaccine if fluorescent-antibody tests of the animal are negative.

†During the usual holding period of 10 days, begin treatment with RIG and HDCV at first sign of rabies in a dog or cat that has bitten someone. The symptomatic animal should be killed immediately and tested.

§If RIG is not available, use antirabies serum, equine (ARS). Do not use more than the recommended dosage.

¶The animal should be killed and tested as soon as possible. Holding for observation is not recommended. (From: Morbidity and Mortality Weekly Report, July 20, 1984, Vol. 33, No. 28; "Rabies Prevention—United States, 1984.")

making bites about the delicate tissues of the face all too common in children.

Wound care includes débridement of crushed and devitalized tissues and lavage of open wounds. The controversy arises with regard to primary closure of the wound. The normal flora of the domestic dog's mouth consists of a relatively low concentration (10^4 organisms/g [or ml] saliva) of *Pasteurella multocida,* which is universally sensitive to penicillin. A fresh wound not compromised by crush or hematoma that is properly débrided, irrigated, and treated with penicillin should heal without infection. Generally, dog bites to the face should be débrided and closed primarily. Puncture wounds and wounds to the extremities more than 6 hours old should be left open. Topical antibacterial dressings may aid healing.

Cat Bites and Cat Scratches

Many of the considerations given to dog bites can be applied to cat bites and scratches. Cat bites are more likely to become infected, *Pasteurella multocida* being the predominant organism. Prophylaxis with penicillin is indicated, as is tetanus prophylaxis. Following adequate débridement and lavage, low-risk wounds are closed but wounds of more than 6 hours' duration are left open.

Cat-scratch fever is a systemic disease that probably originates from a pleomorphic gram-negative bacillus. Following an incubation period of about a week, malaise, fever, nausea, and vomiting usually accompany a regional lymphadenopathy proximal to the wound. The disease resolves spontaneously over several weeks. The organism has been seen in some lymph nodes, but no reliable diagnostic test exists.

Human Bites

The human mouth contains a plethora of organisms, both aerobic and anaerobic, in excess of 10^4 organisms/ml saliva. Human bites routinely produce infected wounds. Hands (especially knuckles) tend to be vulnerable during fist fights (Fig. 42-1). Human bites should seldom be closed. They should be debrided, lavaged,

and left open to heal by secondary intention, or, in critical areas, closed after several days' delay. Antibiotic therapy must be directed toward both anaerobic and aerobic coverage. Penicillin usually provides adequate coverage against one's own flora; however, the complex microbiology of alien organisms requires broader coverage. Such treatment should target the usual oral flora, staphylococci and gram-negative bacteria. Minimal initial therapy should consist of intravenous penicillin plus clindamycin (erythromycin or vancomycin in allergic persons). The addition of a broad-spectrum aminoglycoside completes therapy while awaiting sensitivity reports.

SNAKEBITE
Diagnosis

Diagnosis and treatment of snakebite requires identification of the snake and verification of the bite. In the United States, if a snake has a rattle, it is poisonous (Fig. 42-2). Other identifying physical attributes include the distinctive arrowhead-shaped or triangular head of the pit viper with its distinguishing pits, and the unique color sequence of the coral snake (Fig. 42-3). The poisonous snakes of the United States, distinguished by their markings, fall into two families, the *Crotalidae* and *Elapidae.*

The family of pit vipers, Crotalidae, which includes rattlesnakes and moccasins, is the most common. The genus *Crotalus* includes most of the species of rattlesnakes. The genus *Agkistrodon* includes the cottonmouth, or water moccasin, and the copperhead, or land moccasin.

The other family, Elapidae, is related to cobras. In the United States, it is represented by the Texas coral snake. The sequence of its colored bands distinguishes it from its nonpoisonous imitators. The coral snake has a yellow band on either side of its red band; the yellow band of the Mexican scarlet king snake (nonpoisonous) borders on black; thus: "Red on yellow, kill a fellow; red on black, venom lack" (Fig. 42-3). The snout of

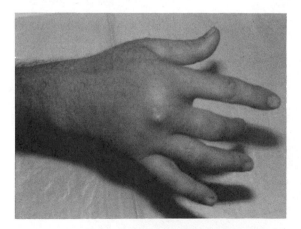

Fig. 42-1. Human bite to the knuckle of the middle finger sustained in a punch to the mouth required treatment of a resulting infection.

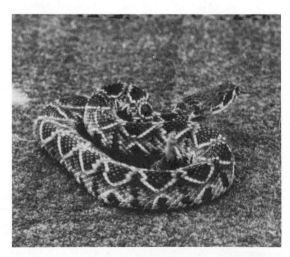

Fig. 42-2. Western diamondback rattlesnake coiled and ready to strike. Note the rattle and characteristic shape of the head. (Photograph courtesy Ted. T. Huang, M.D.)

the coral snake is also black. In Latin America, some species of coral snakes are all black.

There are some 7000 venomous snakebites a year, accounting for only 12 to 15 deaths annually. Texas, which leads all other states, records about 1500 snakebites each year. Rattlesnakes, copperheads, and cottonmouths account for 99% of all snakebites. Most happen between April and November, occur in the late afternoon, and usually afflict people under 20 years old, most often on the extremities.

To identify a venomous snakebite requires an appreciation of envenomation and the venom apparatus. The large rattlesnake strikes rapidly and forcibly with its jaws open, imposing contusion upon envenomation. Its large fangs penetrate and inject much like a hypodermic needle. While the snake has two rows of fangs, the fangs slough at variable intervals, so that the snake might have one mature fang with new fangs growing up from behind. Because of this moulting process, rattlesnake bites may vary from the classic paired fang marks. The encircling ecchymosis can result from crushing, envenomation, or both. While the snake may have up to 1 ml of venom, it usually injects only one tenth that amount. More important, as much as one third of the time, no envenomation occurs. Envenomation is even less common in certain exotic snakes, such as cobras.

Because of its small body and fangs, the coral snake lacks substantial impact. This snake must grasp the tissue to achieve envenomation. Assuming it can surround tissues to grasp, it leaves behind the imprint of its row of fangs. Not surprisingly, the coral snake's bite may not envenom.

Snake venom contains a mixture of enzymes that digest tissue, spread the venom, and disrupt coagulation and nerve tissues. The relative proportion of enzymes differs from species to species. The venoms of the rattlesnake and cottonmouth trigger tissue destruction and coagulopathy, while coral snake and cobra venom tend to be more neurotoxic. The first manifestations are local, severe pain. Despite the pain, the affected skin may be anesthetic, permitting excision without local anesthesia. Systemic manifestations follow, varying with the amount of venom. Diaphoresis, weakness, nausea, and vomiting are the chief symptoms, followed by dizziness and peripheral paresthesia. Emotional shock from the attack and consequent hyperventilation can mimic these symptoms.

Clinical evaluation of the patient begins with the basics: check the respiratory status, the systemic circulation and the circulation of the involved extremity; determine the extent of the systemic reaction and local ecchymosis and swelling. The local zoo can be most helpful in identifying the snake.

Laboratory studies help evaluate systemic toxicity. Prothrombin time and partial thromboplastin time assess clotting factors. Elevated serum fibrinogen and fibrin split products indicate the degree of hemolysis and fibrinolysis.

Envenomation can be estimated clinically. Minimal envenomation causes local pain and swelling, but no systemic symptoms. Moderate envenomation causes obvious local changes, usually ecchymosis, with mild systemic involvement and aberrations in clotting or a decreasing platelet count. Severe envenomation usually produces local necrosis, rapid swelling involving the entire extremity, advancing shock, and frank coagulopathy (Fig. 42-4).

First Aid and Initial Care

Despite some controversy, initial treatment should progress as follows: Expedite evacuation of the victim. Place the victim at rest, immobilize the bitten part level with the heart, and institute supportive measures. Perhaps most important is reassurance. Calm the patient and treat shock. Cold compresses over the bite reduce

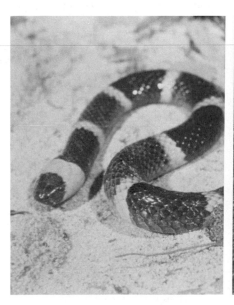
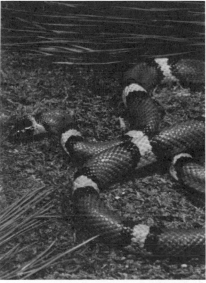

Fig. 42-3. *Left,* Poisonous Texas coral snake. *Right,* Nonpoisonous Mexican scarlet king snake. *Red on yellow, kill a fellow/Red on black, venom lack.*

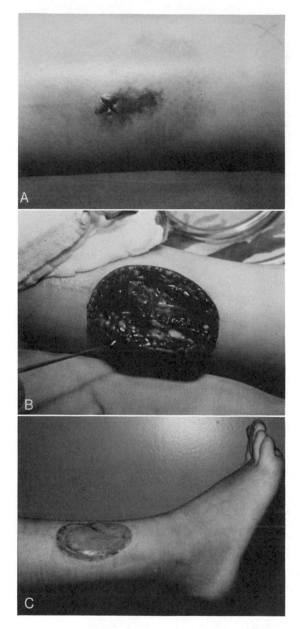

Fig. 42-4. Severe envenomation. **A,** The right leg was bitten by a rattlesnake. (An X incision was made at the scene to suck out the poison.) Note the central area of necrosis and surrounding ecchymosis and swelling, which was observed to be rapidly increasing. **B,** Exploration of the bite reveals deep subcutaneous hemorrhagic tissue but no penetration of the fascia and no muscle involvement. **C,** Healed wound following a delayed skin graft.

the blood flow, amount of reaction, and tissue destruction, but do not apply ice; do not exchange snakebite for frostbite. Do not apply a tourniquet. Venom is carried in the lymphatics, not the bloodstream. Any constricting band on the lymphatics will impede venous return as well, thus increasing swelling.

Initial hospital care consists of basic medical care. When there is any question of envenomation, establish intravenous access and restore third-space fluids. Administer oxygen. Keep the part level, and continue applying cold. As with any puncture wound or animal bite, update tetanus prophylaxis and administer prophylactic antibiotics. Oxygen with intubation and mechanical ventilation are given if needed. Medications for pain or sedation should be given intravenously in small titrated doses. *Steroids have no place in treatment.*

Antivenin

The routine use of antivenin remains highly controversial. Many never use it. Others prescribe massive doses. Antivenin should be withheld from anyone who does not display systemic signs or symptoms. No evidence exists that antivenin can reverse the local manifestations of snakebite. All antivenin is horse serum, and allergic reactions are common. Commercial antivenin is either polyvalent or species specific. Adrenalin must be readily available in case of anaphylaxis. A test dose should be given, preferably in the intensive care unit. The dose for minimum envenomation is 5 vials intravenously in solution over 1 hour; for moderate envenomation, 5 to 9 vials; and for severe envenomation, 10 to 15 vials or more, repeated until systemic symptoms subside. Remember that minimal envenomation has little systemic effect; lower doses may not justify the risk. Furthermore, the effectiveness of antivenin diminishes with delay; it provides minimal benefit after 24 hours. Some believe that coral snake antivenin has no benefit once systemic effects of the venom appear.

Surgical Therapy

Surgical excision of snakebite provides an alternate approach to the risk of antivenin. In the first 20 minutes, incising the bite aids diagnosis by revealing local hemorrhagic response within the tissues (Fig. 42-5); however, simple suction cannot remove a fluid that has been injected deeply into tissues. That injectate remains relatively well localized for up to 4 hours. Thus, using proper exposure and good surgical technique, it can be excised together with the tissues it has permeated. Muscle compartments may require exploration and fasciotomy. Excision of the venom-laden tissues limits local necrosis and systemic spread of the venom.

A fresh bite sometimes shows few signs of envenomation on the surface. Incision of the bite and identification of a local hemorrhagic response makes the diagnosis; excision effects the cure. A bite several hours old with minimal local response or none and no systemic or laboratory abnormalities is probably innocuous.

Nonpoisonous Snakes

The most important aspect of treating the bite of a nonpoisonous snake is to verify it as nonpoisonous. Local pain may be related to bruising. Some swelling may occur as an atopic or allergic reaction. Obviously, local signs do not progress, and no systemic symptoms occur.

STINGS

A sting is the wound resulting from venom-bearing animals such as insects and some marine life, excluding snakes. Basic care starts with wound care: cleans-

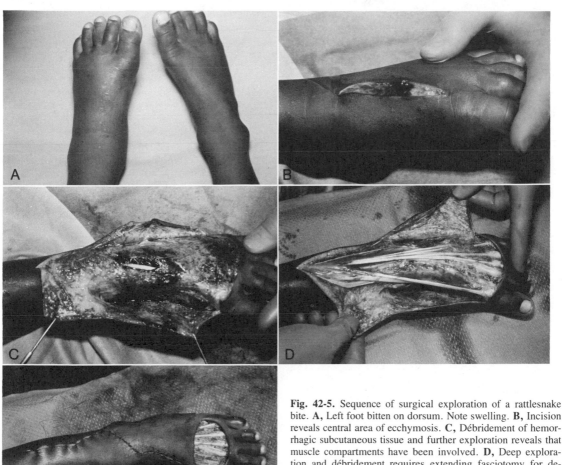

Fig. 42-5. Sequence of surgical exploration of a rattlesnake bite. **A,** Left foot bitten on dorsum. Note swelling. **B,** Incision reveals central area of ecchymosis. **C,** Débridement of hemorrhagic subcutaneous tissue and further exploration reveals that muscle compartments have been involved. **D,** Deep exploration and débridement requires extending fasciotomy for decompression of injured muscles of anterior compartment. **E,** Extent of final wounds following primary closure. A delayed skin graft was eventually required to close the defect.

ing and removal of the offending stinger or barb from the puncture site. The second step requires antidotes that neutralize the venom in the wound. As with bites, tetanus prophylaxis should be updated. Prophylactic antibiotics play a minor role; their usefulness depends on the size of the puncture wound and the origin of the sting. Allergic reactions frequently require antihistamines, less often anaphylactic treatment.

Spiders

Virtually all spiders are venomous, but only two require special medical attention in the United States: the black widow *(Latrodectus mactans)* and the brown recluse *(Loxosceles reclusa)*. The black widow's venom induces a systemic reaction; the brown recluse produces a problematic wound. Although the tarantulas *(Aphonopelma* and *Pamphobeteus)* have an infamous reputation, the enzyme content of their venom is less than the brown recluse's and has little cardiovascular effect.

Brown Recluse Spider

The brown recluse spider, or fiddle-back spider, native to the southern half of the United States, lives in woodpiles, timbers, basements, and storage areas. A dark brown spider, it measures about 2 to 3 cm, including its leg span; it is identified by a light brown violin outlined on its back (Fig. 42-6). Victims occasionally describe pain and itching at the time of envenomation, or, several hours later, they become aware of a small pustule or blister surrounded by a halo of erythema or rubor. By 24 hours, the central pustule becomes surrounded by an area of ecchymosis and an outer halo of rubor. If unattended, the sore progresses to chronic ulceration that does not heal or accept a skin graft (Fig. 42-7). Successful treatment depends on wide excision of the ulcer with primary closure or a skin graft. Some surgeons favor early excision, a treatment analogous to that for snakebite.

No brown recluse antivenin is commercially available. Dapsone, 50 mg b.i.d., appears to limit the local response and prevent ulceration. Patients must be monitored for dose-dependent blood dyscrasias. Dapsone loses some of its effect after 48 hours. Older bites should, therefore, be treated expectantly with prophylactic antibiotics against streptococci and staphylococci, tetanus prophylaxis, and surgical intervention as necessary.

Black Widow Spider

The black widow spider, indigenous to the southern United States, is found in its web under stones, woodpiles, in brush, and in sheds and other shelters. A dark black spider, it measures 2 to 3 cm, including its leg

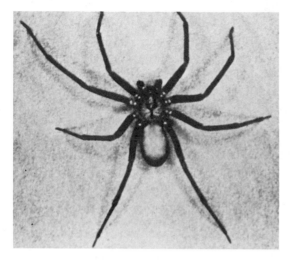

Fig. 42-6. Female brown recluse spider.
(Reprinted with permission from page 178, *Dangerous Plants, Snakes, Arthropods and Marine Life—Toxicity and Treatment,* edited by Michael D. Ellis. Published by Drug Intelligence Publications, Inc., 1241 Broadway, Hamilton, IL 62341.)

span; its trademark is a red-orange hourglass shape on its underbelly (Fig. 42-8).

Victims describe pain at the time of envenomation lasting for several hours, followed by local spasms or cramping that extends throughout the body. Blood pressure is usually elevated. Associated symptoms include headache, abdominal cramps, nausea, vomiting, diaphoresis, and weakness.

Muscle pain, cramps, and nausea can be controlled with the intravenous infusion of 10 ml of 10% of calcium gluconate, repeated once and then at hourly intervals, depending on the serum calcium. Symptoms usually decrease in 1 to 3 hours. Muscle relaxants and analgesics may also help. Black widow spider antivenin is given as follows for severe symptoms: after the test dose, one vial is administered with usual precautions. Children may require respiratory support. The wound is inconsequential; prophylactic antibiotics are not indicated.

Bees, Wasps, Hornets

Bee stings that induce anaphylaxis kill more people every year than snakebites. For the sensitized victim, major supportive measures include adrenaline, steroids, and at least *an initial dose of an antihistamine.* Some effects can be minimized by local care. The wound should be examined for the persistence of a stinger, and the stinger should be removed. While an ice cube or a topical steroid may ease the pain, the venom can be neutralized by sprinkling common *meat tenderizer* over the bite and massaging it into the area.

Ants

Ant bites induce allergic reactions similar to those of bee stings. Minimal treatment requires administering an antihistamine. One notorious offender is the fire ant *(Solenopsis).* When disturbed, a colony swarms upon the trespasser inflicting multiple stings, with intense burning pain (hence the name). The venom can be neu-

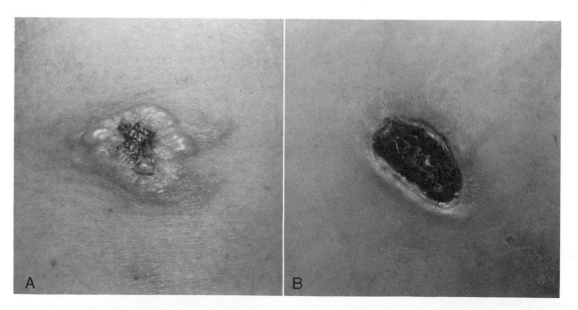

Fig. 42-7. Brown recluse spider bites in development. **A,** About 1 week old; **B,** chronic.

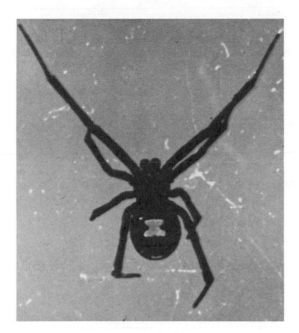

Fig. 42-8. Female black widow spider, ventral surface.
(Reprinted with permission from page 179, *Dangerous Plants, Snakes, Arthropods and Marine Life—Toxicity and Treatment,* edited by Michael D. Ellis. Published by Drug Intelligence Publications, Inc., 1241 Broadway, Hamilton, IL 62341.)

tralized with soaks of hypochlorite solution as a 1 to 10 dilution of household bleach until the pain subsides. Occasionally, resulting cellulitis requires topical antibacterials. Tetanus prophylaxis should be updated and the victim should be placed on antistreptococcal, antistaphylococcal antibiotics until the swelling subsides. Extremities should be elevated. Ancillary care includes antihistamines for persistent itching and analgesics.

Jellyfish and Man-o'-War Stings

The treatment of coelenterate stings parallels that of bee stings. Small papules appear where the tentacles inject their nematocysts. Topical application of *meat tenderizer,* massaged into the afflicted area, will resolve most symptoms. Antihistamines provide adjunctive care.

Sting Rays and Sea Skates

The sea skate favors the shallow waters of the Gulf of Mexico. When stepped on, the sea skate imbeds its spine in the sole of the foot. The protein in the spine induces severe pain, but its effect can be neutralized with heat. Initial care consists of placing the extremity under *hot running water* (104° to 111° F, 40° to 44° C) for up to 2 hours. Unfortunately, the spine usually breaks into several pieces making extraction difficult. Under local anesthesia, *without epinephrine,* the wound is explored. (Epinephrine compromises the wound's ability to resist infection and may cause ischemia.) Radiographs made with soft tissue technique may aid in localizing and extracting the spine. Tetanus prophylaxis and broad-spectrum antibiotic coverage are required, and the wounds should never be closed. Despite meticulous débridement, these wounds are invariably infected. Because of the preponderance of resistant strains of *Vibrio,* antibiotic treatment requires a 5- to 7-day course of an aminoglycoside. Hence, victims of these creatures generally require hospitalization for intravenous antibiotics, elevation of the extremity, and daily dressing changes that incorporate a topical antibiotic.

Lionfish

The spiny dorsal fin of the lionfish *(Scorpaenidae)* contains venom that produces a sting analogous to that of the sting ray or sea skate. By denaturing the protein, hot water eases the pain. Surgical exploration, tetanus prophylaxis, intravenous aminoglycosides, hospitalization, and elevation keynote the treatment. The major complication is infection, especially hand infections.

43

Thermal Injuries

Gerald P. Kealey
Albert E. Cram

Pathology
Pathophysiology
Types of Cutaneous Injury
Survival
Management
Cold Injury

Each year over 2 million Americans incur a burn injury that requires medical attention. While the great majority of them may be cared for as outpatients, approximatley 100,000 burn victims require hospitalization and over 6000 succumb to burn injuries yearly. Forty-one percent are under 19 years of age. Burn injuries are second to motor vehicle accidents as a cause of accidental death in the United States. Burn victims who survive their initial injury are faced with a painful rehabilitation and prolonged morbidity.

Two-thirds of all burns occur in the home environment, the rest in the workplace or a recreational setting. Flame burns account for 56% of all injuries, but scalding is most common in children under 3 years of age. The University of Iowa Burn Center treated 999 patients from 1976 to 1985. The average patient was a 26-year-old male with a 17% body surface area burn (BSAB). Mortality for this group of patients was 4.4%. A significant proportion of physicians are involved in family and emergency medicine, where they may come into contact with burn patients. Therefore, it is essential that the physician have a clear understanding of the initial assessment and treatment of such patients.

Appropriate care of a burn victim is based on an understanding of the tissue injury resulting from thermal trauma. Skin consists of two layers: *the epidermis,* a tough, dry, avascular outer layer that regenerates, and is relatively impervious to injury, and the *dermis,* a deeper layer, 0.5 to 3.0 mm thick, which does not regenerate and contains nerve endings, epidermal appendages, and blood vessels (Fig. 43-1). These two contiguous layers perform the following functions:

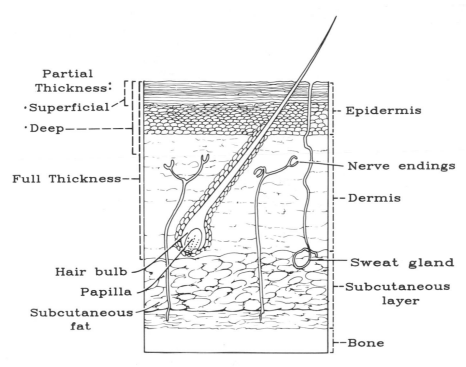

Fig. 43-1. Diagram of skin anatomy and classification of burn injury by depth.

Protect from injury and infection.
Regulate transcutaneous fluid loss.
Mediate sensation.
Regulate body temperature.

Burns that cause significant dysfunction of skin and other vital organs are major injuries.

PATHOLOGY

Thermal injury occurs when the ability of the physiologic system to dissipate heat is overwhelmed. Excessive thermal injury causes protein denaturation, coagulation, and cell death. This rarely occurs at temperatures under 44°C. Cell death rate doubles for each degree increment from 44° to 51°C. Short exposure times at extreme temperatures result in tissue destruction.

Cutaneous burn wounds are either partial-thickness or full-thickness injuries. Partial-thickness burns are injuries of varying depth in which epidermal and dermal elements remain viable. This allows spontaneous epithelialization from the depths of the wound. Full-thickness burns cause destruction of all epidermal and dermal elements.

Partial-thickness burns may be superficial or deep. Superficial partial-thickness burns involve epidermis and outer dermis, generally resulting in minimal physiologic and anatomic damage. Pain and erythema are major components of these injuries. Deep partial-thickness burn wounds involve injury to all surface epidermis and some portion of the deep dermis, leaving viable portions of epidermal skin appendages (hair follicles, sweat, and sebaceous glands). Viable epidermal remnants can reepithelialize the surface of the burn wound. Affected areas may be blistered and erythematous and blanch when touched. Injured areas are moist to the touch. These wounds are painful because dermal nerve endings are exposed. Full-thickness burn wounds involve complete destruction of both epidermis and dermis. The wound has a white or black appearance. It is dry and anesthetic to touch, and hair offers no resistance to removal. Full-thickness wounds cannot reepithelialize from epidermal remnants within the wound, and skin grafts may be required.

It is simple to distinguish between superficial partial-thickness and full-thickness burn wounds. Deep partial-thickness burn wounds represent a heterogeneous injury of irregular depth within a simple burn wound. It is not always possible to determine the exact depth of a given injury at initial examination. Observations over time are needed to determine the depth of a deep thermal injury.

PATHOPHYSIOLOGY

Thermal injuries cause increased capillary permeability within 15 minutes of injury. This results in translocation into the extravascular space of intravascular fluid, electrolytes, and proteins of molecular weight up to 150,000. This fluid shift is restricted to the burn wound in burns <30% BSAB. Translocation of fluid occurs in organs (skeletal muscle) not anatomically involved in the burn in larger burn injuries. Fluid shift is most rapid during the first 8 hours after injury and continues at a diminishing rate for 24 to 48 hours. Loss of intravascular volume results in hemoconcentration, hypovolemia, hypotension, decreased cardiac output, and reduced peripheral organ perfusion. Thrombosis of the burn wound microvasculature occurs resulting in cellular ischemia and death. This hypovolemia, if untreated, results in burn shock. Renal failure due to acute tubular necrosis may develop because of hypovolemia and inadequate cardiac output. The reduced cardiac output is due to hypovolemia and can be restored to normal by adequate fluid resuscitation.

Significant red blood cell hemolysis (up to 8%) may occur at the time of thermal injury. Burn injury–induced bone marrow depression results in decreased erythropoiesis, and circulating red blood cells have a reduced life span. The coagulation system characteristically displays a biphasic pattern of response to thermal injury. Initially, there is a depression in serum clotting factors and platelet levels with a concomitant rise in fibrinogen degradation products. This is followed by a postresuscitation rise to supranormal levels of coagulation components. Disseminated intravascular coagulopathy may occur if burn wound sepsis develops.

Abnormal ventilation patterns are common. Burn victims may exhibit an increased minute ventilation because of peripheral anoxia, hypovolemia, or increased pulmonary physiologic dead space. Inhalation of hot gases may result in edema and acute obstruction of the supraglottic airway. Carbon monoxide poisoning is a constant hazard. Chemical tracheobronchitis and pneumonia are the subacute sequelae of an inhalation injury.

The gastrointestinal tract responds to the burn injury in a classical manner. Mucosal hemorrhages due to decreased splanchnic blood flow may be seen in the stomach and duodenum within 3 hours of the acute burn injury. Paralytic ileus and acute gastric dilation occur frequently.

A catabolic endocrine response develops that is characterized by elevated levels of stress hormones (i.e., norepinephrine, epinephrine, growth hormone, cortisol, and glucagon). These abnormalities are amplified if sepsis or other complications of the burn injury develop. Circulating hormone levels return to normal after the burn wound is closed.

Burn wounds may have a profound effect on immune-system integrity and function, which appears to be related to burn size. Posttraumatic immunosuppression predisposes the host to overriding infectious complications associated with burn injury. Immunoglobulin and fibronectin levels are depressed immediately after the injury, returning to supranormal levels by the third week. Lymphocyte subpopulations change, resulting in relatively increased B cell and decreased T cell concentrations. Depression of leukocyte and lymphocyte function due to a circulating immunosuppressive factor has been described.

TYPES OF CUTANEOUS INJURY

Cutaneous injury occurs because of denaturation and coagulation of cellular proteins in the epidermis and dermis. A wide variety of noxious stimuli can initiate events leading to cell death. Excess ultraviolet energy, flame, scald, and heat contact cause cell damage and death by exposing cells to excessive heat energy. Extent and depth of injury are determined by duration and temperature of exposure.

Chemical agents also cause protein denaturation and coagulation. They may be classified as oxidative, reductive, corrosive, salt-forming, desiccant, or vesicant agents. Tissue injury is determined by (1) duration of exposure, (2) concentration and quantity of the chemical, and (3) mechanism of chemical action. Chemical agents continue to cause tissue destruction until removed by dilution or inactivated by tissue reaction. Acute care of chemical injuries must include immediate washing with copious volumes of water.

Electrical burns occur because heat is generated by the passage of electricity through resistance fields in the body. The amount of heat generated is a function of Joule's Law

$$Calories = 0.24 \times A^2 \times R$$
$$A = amperes$$

Classically, this entails an entrance wound (usually in an extremity or the skull) with extensive tissue necrosis of the involved extremity and an exit wound with tissue destruction around the site of exit. Larger conduits, like the torso, may show few changes after passage of high-voltage, high-amperage current. Transthoracic current may cause cardiac dysrhythmias and circulatory arrest. Electrical injuries to the skull may cause respiratory arrest, seizures, or loss of consciousness. Neurologic sequelae, such as peripheral neuropathy, progressive transverse myelitis, seizure disorder, or intellectual dysfunction, may develop up to 6 months after electrical injury. Ocular cataracts are a long-term complication of electrical injuries, occurring most frequently if the skull is directly involved. Electrical injuries can also cause release of the chromogen myoglobin from injured skeletal muscle or hemoglobin from lysis of red blood cells, resulting in acute tubular necrosis and renal failure. This is treated by vigorous fluid resuscitation and large-volume diuresis, allowing clearance of chromogens from the blood.

Deep muscle groups and, rarely, viscera may be devitalized as a result of heat generated by passage of electrical current. The viability of all injured tissues must be determined by direct inspection as soon as possible. All dead tissue must be removed. These débridements should be carried out when the patient is able to tolerate an operative procedure and before sepsis or metabolic derangements develop. Electrical injury may cause a compartment syndrome with resultant ischemic necrosis of compartment contents. These complications may be averted by early diagnosis and surgical release of the anatomic constriction.

SURVIVAL

Factors influencing survival of burned patients have been defined in general terms. Burn-related mortality is a function of the extent and depth of injury. This is best expressed as a percentage of total BSAB and the percentage of BSAB that is full-thickness injury. Fig. 43-2 shows the relationship between survival and total BSAB, and the lower curve shows the relationship between survival and full-thickness injury.

Age is a prime determinant of burn survival. Very young and elderly burn victims have a higher mortality than young adults with a similar injury. Females have a higher mortality than males with comparable burn injuries: this difference is statistically significant for all age groups, but the underlying cause is unknown.

Inhalation of hot, noxious fumes can result in acute upper airway obstruction, tracheobronchial mucosal injury, or chemical alveolitis. Addition of an inhalation injury to a thermal burn increases the predicted mortal-

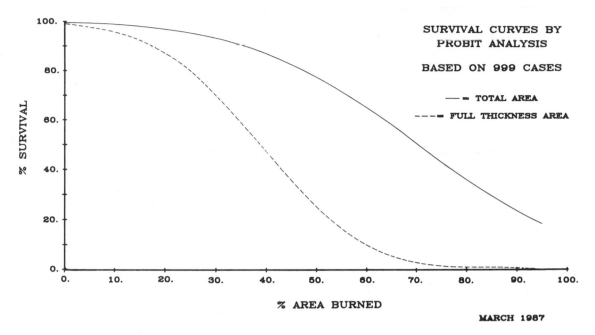

% SURVIVAL

% AREA BURNED

MARCH 1987

Fig. 43-2. Demonstration of the relationship between extent of burn injury and survival. Figures from study of burned patient survival at University of Iowa Hospitals, 1979 to 1986.

ity by 20%. Preexisting medical conditions (i.e., cardiopulmonary, renal, neurologic, or immunologic disease) imply a poor prognosis for the burn victim. All of these factors must be taken into account when a prognostic statement is made concerning the individual patient.

MANAGEMENT
Initial Assessment and Care

Major burn injuries rarely result in death in the first hour; however, other occult injuries may be missed owing to the distracting nature of the burn injury. Initial evaluation of the burn patient is identical to the assessment of any trauma patient. The primary survey must include assessment of airway, breathing, and circulation and cervical spine immobilization. Next, a secondary survey should be conducted—a head-to-toe examination to detect associated injuries. Every attempt must be made to obtain a pertinent history from the patient and accurate data about the accident. It is important to determine the cause of the injury, where it occurred, the presence of noxious chemicals, and any related trauma. The medical history should include identification of preexisting illness or disease; utilization of medications, drugs, or alcohol; allergies and drug sensitivities; and the patient's immunization status.

Supportive therapy is initiated while the assessment is being carried out. All burning clothing must be extinguished and removed. All jewelry is removed from extremities to prevent a tourniquet effect due to burn edema. The airway must be assessed, and, if necessary, the patient is intubated and ventilated. Oxygen should be administered to counteract the effects of hypoxia and possible carbon monoxide poisoning. Fluid shifts are greatest during the first 8 hours after injury and are related to the BSAB, the body mass, and the age of the patient. It is essential that the BSAB be carefully determined.

The Lund-Browder chart is used to determine BSAB. This nomogram relates body surface changes to age and is applicable to all patients (Fig. 43-3). The Rule of Nines is less accurate and should be used only for field assessment. The head and each upper extremity is 9%; the anterior and posterior torso are 18% each, and each lower extremity is 18% (Fig. 43-4). Small children have different body surface measurements, and Lund-Browder charts are more accurate in this group. Resuscitation fluid calculations are based on BSAB and body mass.

The Parkland Formula is used to calculate resuscitation fluid needs. The BSAB and body mass are entered into the equation. Total resuscitation fluid for the first 24-hour period after injury is then calculated. Half of this fluid is given in the first 8 hours after injury and the second half in the next 16 hours:

Fluid Resuscitation First 24 Hours after Injury

4 ml lactated Ringers/kg body mass/% BSAB
  (Parkland Formula)
Give half in first 8 hours
Give remaining half over next 16 hours*

It may be necessary to administer intravenous fluids at a higher hourly rate to compensate for time lost between injury and initiation of fluid therapy. Lactated Ringer's solution is a balanced, slightly hypotonic salt solution. It is the resuscitation fluid of choice for burn patients. Fluids containing dextrose should not be used in order to avoid hyperosmolality caused by rapid infusion of nonphysiologic quantities of dextrose. The objective of burn resuscitation is to maintain vital organ function and to avoid inadequate or excessive intrave-

---

*After Baxter CR: Crystalloid resuscitation of burn shock. In Polk HC Jr and Stone HH, eds: Contemporary burn management, Boston, 1971, Little, Brown & Co.

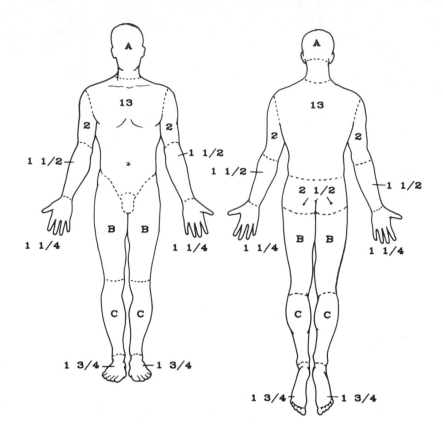

RELATIVE PERCENTAGES OF AREAS AFFECTED BY GROWTH

Area	0	1	5	10	15	Adult
A 1/2 of head	9 1/2	8 1/2	6 1/2	5 1/2	4 1/2	3 1/2
B 1/2 of one thigh	2 3/4	3 1/4	4	4 1/4	4 1/2	4 3/4
C 1/2 of one leg	2 1/2	2 1/2	2 3/4	3	3 1/4	3 1/2

Fig. 43-3. Modified Lund-Browder chart. This nomogram accounts for growth-related changes in body proportions.

nous fluid therapy. Fluids are administered using the Parkland Formula as a starting point for therapy. The patient's clinical and physiologic response to resuscitation is carefully monitored. Hourly urine output is a sensitive index of resuscitation. In the thermally injured adult, 30 to 50 ml urine/hour is evidence of adequate resuscitation. In children weighing up to 30 kgm, 1 ml/kg body mass/hour is an adequate urine flow. A Foley catheter must be inserted. A nasogastric tube is necessary to decompress the paralytic ileus and prevent gastric dilation, which are common in moderate and serious burn injuries. Adult and pediatric burn patients should have a clear sensorium during resuscitation. Tachycardia up to 100 beats/minute in adults and 120 beats/minute in children is to be expected. Blood pressure should be normal.

Burn pain is best treated with narcotics given intra-

venously in doses sufficient to control pain. The intravenous route is preferred for all medications (except tetanus toxoid) owing to erratic absorption of medication from subcutaneous tissue and muscle during fluid resuscitation.

A compartment syndrome may develop in circumferentially burned extremities. Edema developing under the inelastic burn eschar initially obstructs venous drainage from the extremity and finally impedes arterial inflow. This results in ischemia, necrosis, and tissue loss. Early signs include loss of pulses, pallor, paresthesia, pain on passive motion of the extremity, and delayed capillary refill. Circumferential burns of the chest and abdomen can cause restricted excursion of the abdomen and thorax leading to respiratory insufficiency. The patient's sensorium, respiratory rate, respiratory efforts, and arterial blood gases must be carefully mon-

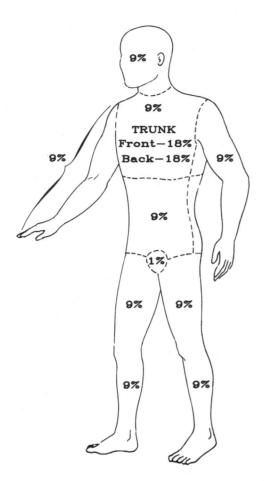

Fig. 43-4. Rule of Nines diagram for estimation of BSAB in adults.

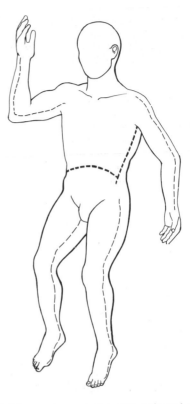

Fig. 43-5. Diagram demonstrating proper site and orientation of escharotomy incisions.
(redrawn from Sabiston, DC, Jr: Textbook of surgery, ed 13, Philadelphia, 1986, WB Saunders Co.)

itored. These complications must be diagnosed and treated before life or tissue is endangered. The burn wound is incised to release the constricting eschar and restore adequate ventilation or blood flow. Fig. 43-5 shows the proper anatomic sites for escharotomy incisions.

Wound Management

Initially, the burn wound can be covered with a clean, dry cloth. This minimizes contamination of the wound and helps to control pain by preventing casual contact. Cold substances should not be placed on large wounds, because of the risk of cold injury to underlying tissue and the metabolic stress of chilling.

Blisters may be débrided or left intact in small burns. They are a sterile and effective wound dressing. When these small blisters eventually rupture, residual dead skin must be débrided. Blisters and damaged loose skin are immediately débrided from all large burn wounds. A topical antimicrobial agent is applied only after the entire wound has been carefully débrided and cleansed using mild soap and warm water.

Topical agents are available that modify the type and concentration of microflora in the burn wound. Commonly used agents include 0.5% silver nitrate so-

lution, silver sulfadiazine cream, and Sulfamylon cream (mafenide). Each agent temporarily modifies wound microbial growth, but none can sterilize the burn wound indefinitely. Topical antimicrobials must not be seen as definitive burn wound management but as adjuvant therapy in wound care.

Silver sulfadiazine is a cream that is easily applied, has low incidences of allergic and toxic reactions, and exhibits a wide spectrum of antibacterial activity. It does not penetrate burn eschar and is not effective against penicillinase-producing *Staphylococcus aureus*.

Sulfamylon burn cream is bacteriostatic and freely soluble and rapidly diffuses, establishing effective concentrations in burn eschar. It has a broad spectrum of activity against gram-negative bacteria, in particular *Pseudomonas aeruginosa*. Sulfamylon's principal limitations are allergic reactions, pain upon application to partial-thickness burn wounds, and metabolic acidosis due to systemic inhibition of carbonic anhydrase enzymes.

One-half–percent silver nitrate solution has a broad spectrum of antimicrobial activity. It is applied as a soaked, bulk dressing, and thus minimizes wound pain, though large bulk dressings may impede patient mobility and complicate physical therapy. It does not penetrate burn eschar. It is a hypotonic solution and can cause significant losses of sodium, potassium, chloride, calcium, and magnesium across the burn wound. Transeschar movement of aqueous diluent into the burn patient also occurs. Careful management of fluid and electrolyte balance is essential when using this agent.

The burn wound is cleansed daily with soap and water, and topical antimicrobial is applied twice daily. Wounds are inspected daily for signs of invasive infection. Cultures of suspicious areas within the burn wound are obtained twice weekly. Penicillin is administered for 3 days from the time of admission to prevent invasion of the burn wound by Group A β-hemolytic streptococci. Systemic antimicrobials are then discontinued. If the diagnosis of burn wound sepsis is made on the basis of the appearance of the wound and the patient's symptoms, systemic antibiotics are instituted.

Clinical Manifestations of Septicemia

Core temperature greater than 39°C or hypothermia
Leukocyte count greater than 20,000 cells/mm³ or leukopenia
Thrombocytopenia
Gastrointestinal bleeding or paralytic ileus
Progressive renal failure
Deteriorating mental status
Increased body mass due to fluid retention
Unexplained reduction in PaO_2 or metabolic acidosis
(After Hartford)

Clinical Signs of Burn Wound Infection

Conversion of second-degree burn to full-thickness necrosis
Focal brown or black discoloration of wound
Unexpected rapid eschar separation
Hemorrhagic discoloration of subeschar fat
Erythematous or violaceous edematous wound margin
Metastatic infectious lesions in unburned tissue
(ecthyma gangrenosum characteristic of *Pseudomonas* burn wound sepsis) (After Pruitt)

Wound closure is the goal of burn care. Effective wound management will prevent invasive burn wound sepsis and allow spontaneous reepithelialization of superficial partial-thickness burns. Deep partial-thickness or full-thickness burn wounds of significant size require split-thickness skin grafts to expeditiously close the burn wound. Formal surgical débridement (tangential or fascial excision) is begun between the third and eighth day after the injury. Burn eschar is removed, and healthy subeschar tissue is exposed. Split-thickness autograft is harvested and applied to the débrided surface. Hands, feet, joint surfaces and cosmetically important areas are grafted initially in patients whose predicted mortality is less than 30%. Large, flat surfaces are initially excised and grafted in patients with higher predicted mortality. The size of the burn injury is reduced, and survival prospects are improved. A maximum of 20% of the body surface area is excised and grafted at one operation because of the large blood loss, anesthesia risk, and hypothermia associated with this aggressive surgical procedure. Sequential operations are necessary for patients with large body surface area burns. Donor sites can be reharvested when reepthelialization has occurred (approximatley every 2 weeks).

Biologic dressings are used to temporarily close large burn wounds when the patient has insufficient donor sites for autografting. Biologic dressings may be cadaver allograft, porcine xenograft, or synthetic skin substitutes. The advantages of these dressings are (1) reduction of pain and inhibition of bacterial growth, (2) reduction of fluid and protein loss from the burn wound, (3) wound adherence of a biologic dressing allows development of autograft recipient site, and (4) optimal autograft take.

Viable cadaver allograft vascularizes and is rejected in 1 to 3 weeks after transplantation. The burn wound is sterile, and sepsis is avoided during this period. Porcine xenograft must be changed every 4 days in order to prevent ingrowth of granulation tissue and incorporation of the xenograft.

Artificial skin and Biobrane are synthetic skin substitutes. They are bilaminar dressings consisting of a synthetic outer layer that is impervious to fluid and bacteria and a biodegradable inner layer. Débridement of necrotic, infected burn eschar is meticulously performed, and fluid collection beneath the biologic dressings is controlled prior to application. If these dressings become adherent, the wound is sterilized and a satisfactory granulation bed develops. The external plastic membrane is then removed, and split-thickness skin autograft is applied to the underlying granulation tissue. These synthetics have a long shelf life, are readily available, and do not transmit disease.

Surgical Management

Surgical procedures must be carefully planned and efficiently executed. The team members—burn surgeon, anesthesiologist, and operating room staff—must understand therapeutic goals and coordinate support efforts. Preoperative consultation and planning are essential.

Hypothermia is a constant threat because large body surface areas are exposed and intravenous fluids and cold transfusion products are rapidly infused. These fluids should be warmed, and uninvolved areas of the body should be covered with drapes to control radiant and evaporative heat loss. Operating room temperature is kept between 30° and 32° C.

Tangential excision of a burn wound results in blood loss of 100 to 150 ml. for every 1% of body surface area débrided. Donor site blood loss amounts to approximatley 25 ml per 1% of body surface area harvested. Operations should be planned so that transfusion requirements are less than one blood volume for the patient, avoiding clotting abnormalities due to dilutional thrombocytopenia or dilution of clotting factors. Adequate volumes of blood must be made available preoperatively, and the total area of the body tangentially excised at any one time should not exceed 20% of the body surface.

Split-thickness skin grafts are harvested from donor sites using a width- and depth-adjustable power dermatome. Grafts are made as thin as possible to minimize loss of donor site dermis. Grafts 12 to 14 one thousandths of an inch thick (0.012 to 0.014 inch) are easily handled without tearing. Donor sites are treated as a burn wound to prevent infection and loss of donor sites. Skin grafts may be expanded to cover a larger defect by the use of a mechanical device such as the Tanner-Vandeput mesher.

Initially skin grafts are held in place by fibrin clot. Graft viability depends on osmosis of nutrients from underlying recipient sites. Capillary ingrowth from recipient bed to skin graft occurs after 72 to 96 hours. The recipient site must be hemostatic and free of infected, necrotic tissue prior to application of the skin graft. Once applied, the skin graft must be stable in its position to maintain nutrient flow from recipient site to skin graft. If these criteria can be met (i.e., control of graft motion, absence of necrotic or infected tissue, and prevention of fluid and foreign material under the graft) the skin graft will vascularize, closing the burn wound.

Infection in Burn Patients

Infection remains the leading cause of death among burn patients. Cutaneous and enteric flora indigenous to patients are the initial sources of bacterial and fungal pathogens in critically ill patients. These bacteria and fungi normally coexist in a dynamic equilibrium with the host and with each other. When the host is seriously stressed, anatomic barriers are destroyed, or immunocompetence is attenuated, these fair-weather bacterial associates become pathogens that invade and destroy the host. Therapeutic manipulation of the host environment can result in selection and overgrowth of potential pathogens. These may be endogenous to the host or acquired from the hospital environment. Group A β-hemolytic streptococcus, a common skin inhabitant, induces fulminating cellulitis, lymphangitis, and death within a few days of injury as a result of overgrowth in the damaged tissues. It is effectively eliminated by penicillin; however, the patient's bacterial ecosystem changes upon exposure to penicillin, enabling penicillinase-resistant *S. aureus* to predominate. Every attempt must be made to prevent burn wound contamination and minimize antibiotic pressure on the host flora.

Surveillance cultures of the wound should be obtained on a systematic biweekly basis. Cultures of urine, sputum, and blood are performed as indicated by clinical findings. All foreign bodies (Foley catheters, endotracheal tubes and intravenous lines) are removed as soon as possible. Intravenous line insertion sites are changed every 48 hours to prevent development of septic thrombophlebitis.

Burn patients with signs and symptoms of septicemia are carefully examined, surveillance cultures are reviewed, and antibiotic therapy is begun. The burn wound must be inspected daily for signs of invasive sepsis. See page 590.

If the burn wound develops signs of invasive infection it is carefully débrided under general anesthesia and closed with a biologic dressing to prevent desiccation and destruction of exposed tissue. Systemic antibiotics are used for limited periods to control specific septic foci.

Nutritional Support

All burn patients exhibit a supranormal metabolic rate, which increases in a linear manner up to 40% to 50% BSAB and levels off thereafter. This suggests that the metabolic rate of patients with large burn wounds is near maximum. The hypermetabolism is due primarily to increased levels of catecholamine synthesis and utilization and secondarily to evaporative heat loss across burn wounds. Burn patients have abnormal protein losses across burn wounds. The magnitude of this loss is proportional to burn wound size. Additional protein losses are also due to increased gluconeogenesis and ureagenesis, reflecting the body's catabolism of protein in response to injury. Glucose kinetics are also altered to meet hypermetabolic demands imposed by burn injury.

Prevention of immunologic and structural consequences of protein and calorie malnutrition is an essential part of burn therapy. The Curreri Formula may be used to estimate calorie needs of adult burn victims:

$$\text{Caloric needs} = 25 \text{ Kcal} \times \text{lsg body mass} + 40 \text{ Kcal} \times \% \text{ BAAB}$$

This formula accounts for both basal and supranormal metabolic requirements imposed by a burn injury. Protein requirements are calculated as 2 g/kg body mass/day. The basal metabolic requirements of children and infants must be taken into account when using this formula for their specific needs. Nutritional support is begun as soon as possible after injury. Patients with significant burns exhibit anorexia after injury and do not eat enough food to fill their metabolic requirements. Hyperalimentation using the gastrointestinal tract or central venous nutrition is usually necessary. Dehydration and hyperosmolality must be prevented. Commercially prepared formulas are generally isosmolar and have low incidence of associated side effects such as diarrhea, hyperosmolality, and delayed gastric emptying. The patient's nutritional status must be reassessed frequently to assure that therapeutic goals are being achieved.

Physical Therapy

Burn wounds are metabolically and structurally dynamic for 2 years after wound closure. Burn scars go through phases of maturation. New wounds exhibit erythema (immaturity) due to increased density of capillaries and high-volume blood flow. Capillary density decreases and the color fades with time. Hypertrophic scars have a red, indurated surface. Hypertrophic scar development is related to the length of time the wound is open, the body area burned, and the patient's wound healing characteristics. Scar contracture occurs in all wound healing and may cause loss of body function.

Physical therapy is initiated within a few days to the burn injury and continued until wounds are mature and the scar contracture phase ends. Elastic pressure garments probably hasten maturation of burn scars. Aggressive splinting, range-of-motion, and strengthening exercises can optimize patient rehabilitation.

Partial-thickness or full-thickness burn wound injuries may exhibit alopecia, itching, dryness, abnormal sweating, decreased skin oils, abnormal sensitivity to ultraviolet light, or decreased sensory function. This is due to loss of epidermal appendages and dermal functions. These characteristics may not be completely amenable to therapy and can contribute to the victim's long-term disability. Burn patients should be instructed in protective therapy such as use of sunscreen, proper clothing, and skin lubrication. Casual trauma may result in significant cutaneous injury.

Psychosocial Aspects

Coping with burn injury is a multifaceted process. Patients must endure painful, physically demanding care routines, integrate the traumatic accidents into their lives, and contend with the psychological and emotional sequelae of disfigurement, loss, and disability. Burn patients frequently exhibit anger, depression, emotional lability, anxiety, phobia, and delirium.

Anxiety, insomnia, and pain are closely linked. Anxiety increases pain perception. Inadequate rest reduces pain tolerance and increases anxiety. This escalating cycle is best treated by an intelligent, flexible combination of pharmacologic and nonpharmacologic agents. Narcotics, nonnarcotic analgesics, and strategies such as distraction, relaxation, and guided imagery are useful combinations of pain management techniques. Anxiolytic and hypnotic agents should be utilized in appropriate doses.

Professional staff attuned to burn patients' problems are a key to providing pain control, anxiety control, and emotional support. Honest, compassionate communication between patient, staff, and family is essential. Families and friends must be made aware of the realities of the injury and be supportive. Family and social support is known to be a vital factor in burn recovery. Families must be extensively involved and educated in burn rehabilitation.

Psychological morbidity after hospital discharge appears to be determined by the preinjury emotional maturity of the burn victim; therefore, the prognosis for emotional recovery is based on the patient's previous life experiences. Children may sustain a signifi-cant long-term psychological disability owing to their immature physical and emotional development coupled with the attendant disfigurement of the burn. The posttraumatic stress disorder may occasionally occur in burn victims. Burn care after discharge should include careful assessment of physical and emotional status.

Pain control, emotional adaptation, and social reintegration are as important as fluid resuscitation, sepsis, and skin grafting. Careful consideration of these aspects of recovery is crucial to the comprehensive care of the burn patient.

COLD INJURY

Tissue injury from cold depends on the degree of cold, exposure time, and environmental conditions. Cold injury is divided into freezing (frostbite), nonfreezing (trench foot) injury, and systemic hypothermia. Intracellular ice crystal formation leads to cell injury after freezing. Nonfreezing cold causes endothelial damage resulting in microvascular thrombosis, capillary and venous obstruction, and tissue ischemia. Hypothermia results from excessive heat loss, lowering body core temperature below 34°C.

Cold injuries are treated by rapid rewarming of the affected tissue or individual. Immersion in 40°C water is most effective. Wounds are then carefully cleansed, and a topical antimicrobial is applied to suppress invasive infection.

44

Transplantation Surgery

Richard Weil III

Biology of Rejection
Patterns of Rejection
Diagnosis of Rejection
Prevention or Control of Rejection
Clinical Transplantation
Organ Preservation
Organ Donor Issues

The sixteenth-century Italian surgeon Tagliacozzi, often considered the father of plastic surgery, developed detailed techniques for rotating soft tissue pedicles for reconstruction of nasal mutilation caused by disease or trauma; however, free transfer of even skin was not considered feasible until the nineteenth century. The distinctions between autografts (grafts from one part of an individual to another part of the same individual), allografts or homografts (grafts from one individual to another of the same species), and heterografts or xenografts (cross-species grafts) were not clearly appreciated until well into the twentieth century. The technique for anastomosing small blood vessels with reliable patency was developed by Alexis Carrel in the first decade of this century and in part won him the 1912 Nobel Prize in physiology and medicine; this technique was a prerequisite for successful organ transplantation. The immunologic basis for graft rejection was established in the 1940s by Sir Peter Medawar, who also received the Nobel Prize in physiology and medicine, in 1960, for his contributions to transplantation immunology.

Although there were sporadic earlier efforts, the first systematic attempts at human organ transplantation were the kidney transplants carried out at the Peter Bent Brigham Hospital in Boston in the early 1950s. In 1954 a transplant between identical twins (isograft), in whom immunologic rejection of the transplanted organ was not at issue, was successful and lasting. In the late 1950s, in Boston and in Paris, total body irradiation of the recipient was used in an effort to prevent rejection of the transplant, but this form of immunosuppression was dangerous and was replaced in the early 1960s by pharmacologic immunosuppression, which has remained the principal immunosuppressive tool for preventing and treating rejection of all allografts. In 1963 the human liver was replaced by Dr. Thomas Starzl in Denver, Colorado. In 1966 pancreas transplantation was done by Drs. Kelly and Lillehei in Minneapolis, Minnesota. In 1967 the human heart was replaced by Dr. Christiaan Bernard in Capetown, South Africa. In 1981 heart-lung transplantation was carried out by Dr. Norman Shumway's team at Stanford University.

A considerable number of human tissue allotransplants are carried out: cornea transplants to restore vision, skin grafts to cover burn wounds, bone marrow infusions to restore hematopoietic function (in aplastic anemia or leukemia treated with massive doses of cytotoxic agents), bone chips for spine fusion, composite long bone-joint transplants to save limbs in patients with bone cancer, and others. Human hand transplants are currently under consideration. This chapter focuses mainly on transplantation of vascularized thoracic and abdominal organs.

BIOLOGY OF REJECTION

The immune system is a protection against foreign substances, or "nonself." The strength of the immune response to transplants increases with the genetic disparity between donor and recipient, but violent immune responses can occur even when donor and recipient are the same species, as in human cadaver kidney transplantation.

Graft rejection is initiated by foreign histocompatibility antigens on cell surfaces or free within the graft. Mismatched ABO blood group antigens can elicit strong graft rejections in recipients with natural isoantibodies. Vertebrate species have a major histocompatibility complex (MHC) that is primarily responsible for allograft rejection. The human MHC, located on chromosome 6, is the human leukocyte antigen (HLA) complex; it governs the production of cell surface antigens of major and minor strengths. The HLA complex, which has been divided into class I and class II, can be identified on cell surfaces by monospecific typing antisera (HLA typing). The class I antigens, such as HLA-A and HLA-B, were originally defined through the generation of cytotoxic allogeneic T lymphocytes. Usually these antigens are unable to initiate proliferation of allogeneic lymphocytes. The class II antigens, such as HLA-DR, can initiate allogeneic helper T lymphocyte proliferation.

When an allograft is revascularized in a patient, the donor histocompatibility antigens initiate an immune response in the recipient. Strong allograft-specific responses result from the direct presentation of donor antigens on the surfaces of "macrophage type" cells in the graft. Donor antigens also may be processed by recipient macrophages, monocytes, or dendritic cells, which activate helper T lymphocytes and B lymphocytes in the recipient's spleen and lymph nodes. The multiple steps in this activation process are incompletely understood, but the lymphokines interleukin-1 and interleukin-2 are almost certainly important intercellular activation messengers.

The T lymphocytes (thymus-dependent) primarily mediate cellular immune responses. T lymphocyte subclasses can be defined by antigenic markers (e.g., T_4 and T_8) that purport to identify functionally distinct subsets (T_4 helper and T_8 cytotoxic); however, such absolute functional distinctions are questionable. Currently T_4 is defined by its ability to recognize class II antigens, and T_8 is defined by its ability to recognize class I antigens.

The B lymphocytes are named after the avian *bursa of Fabricius,* the human functional analog of which is probably bone marrow and gut lymphoid tissue. B lymphocytes produce antibodies against donor antigens. These antibodies are not required for graft rejection, which can occur without antibody; however, alloantibodies against donor antigens participate in some forms of rejection.

PATTERNS OF REJECTION

The patterns of rejection vary among different tissues and solid organs. The clinical and corresponding histopathologic characteristics have been most fully described for kidney allografts. During the 1980s the histopathology of liver, heart, lung, and pancreas rejection have become better defined. The physiologic and microscopic characteristics of rejection are most clearly expressed in experimental animals that have received no immunosuppression; however, the clinician must work with immunosuppressed patients in whom the characteristics of rejection are less clear.

Hyperacute Rejection

When a kidney is transplanted into a patient who has circulating preformed cytotoxic antibodies against the histocompatibility antigens of the donor, there is a high probability of violent early rejection—within a few minutes to a few hours after revascularization of the kidney. The cause of these antibodies in the recipient may be prior pregnancies, transplants, or blood transfusions; but such antibodies also occur without evident previous exposure to foreign histocompatibility antigens.

In hyperacute rejection the reaction between preformed IgG antibody and the vascular endothelial antigens of the graft, in the presence of complement, results in irreversible activation of the clotting system and rapid thrombosis of the microcirculation of the graft, which infarcts. Hyperacute rejection has been observed many times in human kidney transplants. Human livers and hearts have been transplanted despite preformed recipient cytotoxic antibodies against the donor, and hyperacute rejection has rarely been documented in these transplants. The liver appears particularly resistant to hyperacute rejection

Acute Rejection

Many human transplants undergo at least one acute rejection episode after transplantation, mediated primarily by T lymphocytes that infiltrate the graft. Acute rejection usually is not detected until at least a few days after transplantation, but acute rejection episodes may occur months, or occasionally years, after transplantation. T lymphocytes are often visible by light microscopy in biopsied kidney allografts, but these round cell infiltrates do not always impair renal function. In some grafts, the infiltrating lymphocytes and other round cells, by direct cellular contact or by release of cytotoxic factors, physically damage the cells of the graft and thereby interfere with function. Acute rejections of liver and heart have histopathologic characteristics somewhat analogous to those of the kidney. The criteria for pancreas and lung rejection are still under development.

Chronic Rejection

Months or years after transplantation, some degree of slow rejection, mediated primarily, but not exclusively, by humoral antibody, usually leads to the destruction of graft function. The host immune system almost never fully accepts the graft, even though chronic low-dose immunosuppression is continued. It is unusual for cadaver kidney transplants to survive this process for more than 10 years; grafts seldom last a lifetime, even if initial function is excellent. In kidney transplants, chronic rejection is histologically manifested by thickening of glomerular basement membrane and damage to the intima of arterioles with resultant narrowing of the arteriolar lumen and, eventually, tissue ischemia. This process in almost all cases eventually causes cell damage and loss of graft function.

DIAGNOSIS OF REJECTION

Even after more than 30 years of study of graft rejection, the precise events of rejection are not clearly understood and methods for diagnosis are inexact. No single test can reliably establish a diagnosis of rejection of a kidney, liver, heart, lung, or pancreas. Biopsy information is often helpful but may be difficult to interpret. When a transplant does not function well, the physician initially attempts to rule out problems other than rejection, such as insufficient circulation to the graft or obstruction of excretory drainage (urine in kidney transplants, bile in liver transplants, exocrine fluid and enzymes in pancreas transplants) before making a working diagnosis of rejection. The clinical diagnosis of rejection remains to some extent a diagnosis of exclusion. Nuclear magnetic resonance spectroscopy, using phosphorus 31 or another isotope, noninvasively provides precise biochemical information that may in the future allow more definitive analysis of rejection and other reasons for graft dysfunction.

PREVENTION OR CONTROL OF REJECTION

Matching Recipient With Donor (Immunologic Testing)

ABO Blood Group

As with blood transfusions, a person with blood group O is a universal donor in organ transplantation and one with group AB is a universal recipient. Persons with blood group A (? group A2) or B should not donate kidneys to blood group O patients because of the high probability that recipient isoantibodies would result in violent early rejection of the transplant. Special immunologic preparation of the recipient (e.g., plasmapheresis, splenectomy) may sometimes allow ABO-incompatible kidney transplants to succeed. Breech of ABO blood group barriers is less dangerous in liver transplantation. The Rh system appears to be unimportant in organ transplantation.

Direct Cross-Match

The most predictive—and therefore most important—of the histocompatibility matching tests is the direct cytotoxic cross-match test for the presence of preformed cytotoxic antibodies in the recipient against cells of the potential donor. If the recipient has IgG antibodies that in the presence of complement are cytotoxic to the lymphocytes of the donor, hyperacute rejection is very likely to occur if a kidney is transplanted. Hyperacute liver rejection has only rarely been observed, even after transplantation in the presence of preformed cytotoxic antibodies. Dr. Paul Terasaki in Los Angeles, California, has recently developed a more sensitive direct cross-match test using flow cytometry, which may prevent some of the previously unappreciated early violent rejections that were labeled primary nonfunction of the transplant. In addition, a vascular endothelial cell cross-match may identify a small subset of presensitized patients who cannot be detected by more conventional tests.

HLA

Each person inherits from each parent one chromosome 6 and one haplotype of HLA. Siblings may therefore be perfectly matched or completely mismatched for HLA (Fig. 44-1). HLAs are present on all nucleated human cells. Clinical HLA testing is done by microcytotoxicity methods using monospecific typing sera, which then infer the antigen specificities of the person being tested. The force of the rejection response in kidney transplants from living relatives is to some extent governed by the degree of mismatch of donor and recipient HLA, but even nonidentical-twin kidney transplants or kidney transplants from siblings perfectly matched for HLA antigens can be violently rejected. Table 44-1 depicts a recipient and five potential donors, all with ABO blood group and direct cytotoxic cross-match compatible with the recipient, who have from none to four HLA-A and HLA-B matches.

For cadaver kidney transplantation, matching the HLA-A, HLA-B, and HLA-DR antigens has not had a powerful influence on graft success, especially in the United States, where the population is genetically heterogeneous. The HLA system has not been extensively evaluated in nonrenal solid organ transplantation but appears to exert only a minor influence on the outcome of these grafts.

Mixed Lymphocyte Culture (MLC)

For kidney transplantation (in contrast to bone marrow transplantation), the mixed lymphocyte culture usually tests the unidirectional reactivity of recipient lymphocytes against donor lymphocytes. This test correlates to some extent with HLA-DR matching. The MLC test generally requires 5 days of tissue culture for completion and can facilitate identification of the immunologically optimal living related donor among a group of relatives who are equally well-matched to the recipient at the HLA-A and HLA-B loci.

Immunologic Modification of Donor or Donor Organ

If it were possible to modify the donor organ before transplantation so that it did not elicit a strong immune response in the recipient, immunosuppression of the recipient could be reduced. Attempts at pretransplant treatment of the donor organ have been directed mainly

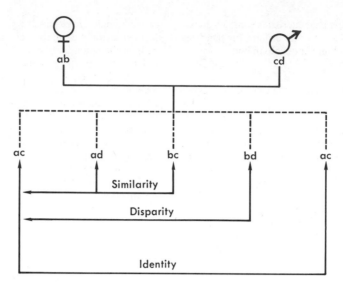

Fig. 44-1. Possible genetic relationships in a family. Since siblings inherit one haplotype from each parent, there is 1 in 4 chance of identity, 2 in 4 chances of similarity, and 1 in 4 chance of disparity.

Table 44-1. Simplified Scheme of HLA-A and HLA-B Typing Showing Some of the Antigens*

Donor or recipient	ABO	HLA A2	HLA A3	HLA A10	HLA A11	HLA A29	HLA AW33	HLA B8	HLA B13	HLA B16	HLA BW22	HLA BW35	HLA BW40	Cross-match
Recipient	A	+	+	–	–	–	–	+	–	+	–	–	–	
Donor 1	O	+	+	–	–	–	–	+	–	+	–	–	–	Neg.
Donor 2	A	+	–	–	–	+	–	+	–	+	–	–	–	Neg.
Donor 3	A	–	+	–	+	–	–	–	–	+	–	–	+	Neg.
Donor 4	O	–	–	–	+	+	–	–	+	+	–	–	–	Neg.
Donor 5	A	–	–	–	+	–	+	–	–	–	+	+	–	Neg

*Varying degrees of match and mismatch between recipient and donors 1 to 5 are present. Donor 1 is completely matched, whereas donor 5 is completely mismatched.

at decreasing antigen expression or outflow from the graft with pharmacologic agents such as cyclophosphamide or corticosteroids, by radiotherapy, and by long-term perfusion of the graft. These techniques have been intended partly to eliminate passenger leukocytes of donor origin that remain in any transplanted graft. Another means of removing these donor-origin passenger leukocytes from small grafts such as pancreatic islet fragments is temporary storage of the grafts in vitro in organ culture, particularly with a high ambient oxygen atmosphere. Such storage is more toxic to donor-origin passenger leukocytes than to donor endocrine tissue. Reduction of passenger leukocytes by any of these techniques reduces the immunogenicity of the transplant.

Recipient Immunosuppression

The goal of immunosuppression is to render the recipient specifically tolerant of the transplant without lowering defenses against infection or cancer and without any side effects. This goal has not yet been attained.

Immunologic Preparation of Recipient

Both splenectomy and total lymphoid irradiation decrease the amount of functioning central lymphoid tis-

sue. Neither splenectomy nor total lymphoid irradiation has been systematically evaluated in human nonrenal organ transplantation. Splenectomy may be carried out a few weeks before transplantation or concurrently; total lymphoid irradiation, originally developed for treatment of Hodgkin's disease, requires a few weeks for completion and is carried out before transplantation. Splenectomy, a major operation with perioperative risks, carries the late postoperative risk of overwhelming sepsis from encapsulated bacteria such as *Diplococcus pneumoniae* or *Haemophilus influenzae*. Total lymphoid irradiation has been associated with radiation sickness. In the 1980s, routine splenectomy has been abandoned in most transplant units; total lymphoid irradiation may be useful in immunologically difficult patients but is still under evaluation.

A third method of immunologic preparation, thoracic duct drainage, removes billions of lymphocytes from the circulation each day through a catheter inserted into the root of the left side of the neck, where the thoracic duct enters the confluence of internal jugular and subclavian veins. Thoracic duct drainage is most effective when done continuously for at least 4 weeks before transplantation, but this cumbersome and expensive form of therapy is rarely used.

A fourth, simpler but not entirely risk-free, method

of immunologic preparation is pretransplant blood transfusion. For many years blood transfusions were withheld from potential transplant patients on chronic dialysis, even very anemic patients, for fear of generating cytotoxic antibodies that would decrease the probability of finding a safe kidney donor. In the early 1970s, Dr. Paul Terasaki's UCLA kidney transplant registry showed that patients who had received at least a few blood transfusions in fact had less kidney transplant rejections than patients who had never received transfusions. Most patients waiting for cadaver kidney transplants in the late 1970s and early 1980s were immunologically prepared for transplantation by several transfusions from random donors, and many patients who received living relatives' kidney transplants were immunologically prepared by the administration of pretransplant donor-specific blood transfusions from the living relative who would subsequently provide the kidney transplant. The administration of immunologically nonspecific blood transfusions from blood banks carries a small risk of transmission of non-A, non-B hepatitis and smaller risk of transmission of acquired immunodeficiency syndrome (AIDS). A few patients who received transfusions (approximately 10% to 15%) became so highly sensitized by the transfusions that a safe donor could not easily be found. The introduction of more potent, pharmacologic immunosuppression, in the form of cyclosporine, in the middle 1980s, decreased the relative importance of pretransplant transfusions and the frequency of their use.

Pharmacologic Immunosuppression

Azathioprine (Imuran) and adrenal corticosteroids were the pharmacologic agents most commonly used for all organ transplants during the 1960s and 1970s. In the mid 1980s cyclosporine was released for general use by the U.S. Food and Drug Administration (FDA). Heterologous antilymphocyte serum or globulin, produced in animals, was widely used in the 1960s and 1970s as an adjunct to azathioprine and corticosteroids; in the 1980s monoclonal antilymphocyte antibodies made by cell hybridization techniques began to replace less precise antilymphocyte preparations. In many patients combinations of three to five pharmacologic agents are used concomitantly or sequentially in efforts to achieve optimal immunosuppression.

Azathioprine. The active portion of azathioprine is 6-mercaptopurine, which is liberated from the larger molecule by the liver. 6-Mercaptopurine is a purine-analog antimetabolite, which, in the form of 6-mercaptopurine ribonucleotide, interferes with intracellular purine metabolism in host cells that are actively dividing in response to donor antigen stimulation. Its main side effect is bone marrow toxicity.

Adrenal corticosteroids. The exact mechanism of corticosteroid immunosuppression is not known, but lymphocytolysis, particularly of T lymphocytes, is almost certainly one mechanism. Steroids have less effect on B lymphocyte function than on T lymphocyte function. Steroids also reduce the inflammatory activity of many cells, including macrophages and polymorphonuclear leukocytes, by stabilizing their lysosomal membranes. Adrenal corticosteroid toxicities are multiple and can be very debilitating: hypertension, moon facies, acne, peptic ulcer, pancreatitis, ocular cataract, aseptic necrosis of bone, diabetes mellitus, psychosis, and interference with growth in children.

Cyclosporine. This relatively new polypeptide extracted from fungus is a potent immunosuppressive agent that is not a bone-marrow depressant. It inhibits T lymphocytes from secreting interleukin-2, which is necessary for full activation of the T lymphocyte immune response. Cyclosporine inhibits the generation of cytotoxic T lymphocytes, but once cytotoxic T cells have been activated, cyclosporine will not inhibit expression of their cytotoxic activity. Its major side effect is nephrotoxicity; it has additional mild side effects of hirsutism, gastrointestinal disturbance, central nervous system toxicity, and hepatotoxicity. Cyclosporine is very hydrophobic and is administered orally in oil; intestinal absorption is often erratic.

Other. The Fujisawa Pharmaceutical Corporation in Japan has developed a compound (FK 506), extracted from *Streptomyces tsukubaensis,* that is a more potent immunosuppressant than even cyclosporine. This compound appears promising, although it has considerable gastrointestinal toxicity when administered to dogs.

Antilymphocyte preparations. Antilymphocyte (or antithymocyte) sera or globulins can be generated in animals against human T lymphocytes, B lymphocytes, lymphocyte subpopulations, cultured lymphoblasts, or thymocytes, by injecting these cells into the responding animal. If human lymphocytes are injected into a mouse, the sensitized mouse spleen cells can be fused with mouse myeloma cells to form hybridomas capable of producing a continuous supply of monoclonal mouse antihuman lymphocyte antibodies. OKT3 (Ortho Pharmaceuticals) is a monoclonal mouse–anti–human lymphocyte antibody that makes circulating blood lymphocytes essentially undetectable within a few minutes of intravenous administration; OKT3 has fewer side effects than its predecessor antilymphocyte-antithymocyte preparations and in the late 1980s has become the most frequently used antilymphocyte agent. Heterologous antilymphocyte preparations are often highly cytotoxic to circulating lymphocytes, but such lymphocytotoxicity is not necessarily associated with improved graft survival. Allergic reactions are not uncommon with these agents but rarely take the form of life-threatening anaphylaxis.

Disadvantages

The chief disadvantages of all the preceding methods of recipient immunosuppression are increased risks of infection and malignancy. The goal of immunosuppressive therapy is to provide just enough immunosuppression to permit graft acceptance without interfering with the patient's ability to resist infection or malignancy. Unfortunately this objective is not always attainable with current immunosuppressive tools. Immunologic monitoring techniques designed to guard against both underimmunosuppression and overimmunosuppression of the patient have generally been unreliable.

Infection is the main cause of death after transplantation; it reflects the imperfection of available immunosuppressive agents. The infections observed after transplantation are caused by bacteria, viruses, protozoa, and fungi, including saprophytes incapable of causing infection in nonimmunosuppressed hosts. Posttransplant infection can to some extent be reduced by elimination of all sites of infection before transplantation. One can partially reduce the consequences of infection by promptly decreasing or discontinuing immunosuppression in patients who develop signs of life-threatening infection, even though the graft may be rejected.

Malignancy occurs 60 to 100 times more frequently in transplant patients than in age-matched normal controls. In the 1960s and 1970s, squamous cell carcinoma of the skin was the commonest malignancy in kidney transplant patients and was usually curable. With the widespread use of cyclosporine in the 1980s, lymphoproliferative tumors, some of which are truly malignant, have become the most common tumor in transplant patients. Malignancy, like infection, probably reflects excessive immunosuppression. The precise mechanisms of tumor induction or facilitation in transplant patients are unclear, but depressed immune surveillance and increased propensity for virus-induced malignancy, particularly Epstein-Barr (EB) virus, are two possible pathways. Some lymphoproliferative tumors, particularly polyclonal ones, regress or disappear if immunosuppression is reduced.

CLINICAL TRANSPLANTATION

Tissue and organ autotransplants are common: skin, hair, teeth, digits, tendons, blood vessels, pericardium, nerves, bone, cartilage, parathyroid fragments, and intestinal segments are not infrequently transferred from one part of a patient's body to another part for reconstitution of appearance or function. Allotransplants of these structures have been attempted less frequently than autotransplants because of the probability of rejection in the absence of immunosuppression; however, allografts, and even xenografts, of skin serve as temporary coverage for large burn wounds, and allografts of blood (blood transfusions) are used extensively all over the world. Corneal allografts are not rejected unless the cornea, which normally is nourished by diffusion, develops an ingrowth of capillaries carrying host cells capable of rejecting the graft. Bone marrow allografts (infusions) are sometimes provided to patients with primary or secondary bone marrow failure; the bone marrow allografts are not only subject to rejection by the host but are also capable of attacking the host (graft-versus-host disease). Allograft or xenograft (porcine) heart valve replacements, in some ways superior to synthetic artificial heart valves, tend to deteriorate slowly, perhaps partly because of rejection.

Immunosuppression, invariably administered to recipients of bone marrow allografts, is occasionally appropriate for persons who have rejected multiple corneal grafts or for burn patients receiving skin grafts from living relatives; however, most tissue allografts or xenografts are not considered vulnerable enough to rejection to justify the risks of immunosuppression.

For patients who have vascularized organ allografts such as kidney, liver, pancreas, heart, heart-lung, or intestine, immunosuppression is initiated prophylactically at or before the time of transplantation to prevent rejection before it starts. For the recipient of a kidney transplant or partial pancreas transplant from an identi-

cal twin, immunosuppression for rejection is unnecessary because rejection does not occur between monozygotic twins, but immunosuppression in low doses is sometimes used to suppress recurrence of the original disease (glomerulonephritis or type I diabetes).

Kidney Transplantation

Patients with irreversible end-stage renal disease (ESRD) have two potential ways of replacing lost kidney function: chronic dialysis or kidney transplantation. A pretransplant period of peritoneal dialysis or hemodialysis is usually advisable to treat uremia and optimize the patient's general health before transplantation. Either a peritoneal dialysis catheter is inserted or an arteriovenous vascular access is established to carry out dialysis. Peritoneal dialysis, a slower exchange process than hemodialysis, can be carried out on a continuous ambulatory basis (CAPD) with three or four fluid exchanges per day or by a stationary mechanical pump for approximately 8 hours per night while the patient sleeps (IPD). The main difficulty with peritoneal dialysis is peritonitis; in addition, some patients' peritoneal cavities are so scarred from previous operations or previous intraperitoneal infections that peritoneal dialysis is impossible. Patients undergo hemodialysis for 4 to 5 hours three times per week, either in a dialysis facility or at home. The main difficulty with hemodialysis is thrombosis of vascular access, which occurs more often with synthetic arteriovenous vascular grafts than with autogenous arteriovenous fistulas.

In the early 1960s when kidney transplantation was just starting to be developed, there were very strict criteria for acceptance into transplant programs. In the 1980s kidney transplantations became a realistic option for most patients with irreversible end-stage renal disease; but patients over 60 years of age, who are sometimes debilitated and may be less able to tolerate immunosuppression, are transplanted less frequently than younger patients. A history of recent malignancy is a contraindication to transplantation because of the risk that immunosuppression will foster the growth and spread of any residual foci of cancer. In the United States in the middle 1980s, less than 10% of the chronic dialysis population (approximately 100,000) received kidney transplants each year; approximately one fourth of the kidneys were provided by living relatives and three fourths by cadaver donors.

The kidney transplant operation (Fig. 44-2) consists of performing three anastomoses: artery, vein, and ureter. Any of these anastomoses can become stenotic or occluded, but major technical anastomotic complications occur in less than 10% of kidney transplant patients.

In the 1980s, if donor and recipient were ABO compatible and if the recipient did not have preformed cytotoxic antibodies (IgG) against donor T lymphocytes (negative direct cross-match test), the 1-year cadaver graft survival rate in some transplant centers rose to a range of 80% to 85% and the 1-year patient survival rose to a range of 90% to 95%. The main cause of graft failure was still rejection, and the main cause of patient mortality was still infection. The long-term results with cadaver kidneys remained slightly inferior to the results with transplants from living relatives.

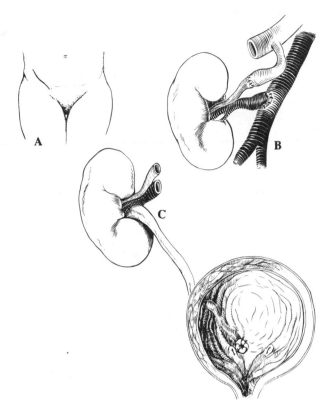

Fig. 44-2. Renal homotransplantation. **A,** Incision is made in recipient's groin. **B,** Renal artery is anastomosed end-to-end to hypogastric artery and renal vein end-to-side to external iliac vein. **C,** Donor ureter is implanted into recipient's bladder (ureteroneocystostomy). This anastomosis can be performed via intravesical or extravesical approach.

The majority of irreversible rejections of kidney transplants and the majority of patient deaths occur within the first 3 to 6 months after transplantation. A recipient's immune system almost never fully accepts a transplanted organ, and even a kidney transplant that is initially accepted may be rejected after a period of years. After the first year following transplantation, the rate of graft loss from rejection is approximately 5% per year. Infection continues to be a major cause of patient mortality, but atherosclerotic heart disease and other causes of death in the general population also take their toll.

Liver Transplantation

Liver transplantation is potentially life saving for patients with irreversible end-stage liver disease. The timing of liver transplantation is more critical than the timing of kidney transplantation because there is no mechanical support system for patients with liver failure comparable to dialysis for patients with kidney failure. A patient with fulminant irreversible liver failure rarely survives more than a few days. Liver transplantation, seldom recommended until a patient's predicted survival is less than a few months, should be carried out before the patient becomes moribund.

Congenital biliary atresia, cirrhosis caused by hepatitis, primary biliary cirrhosis, sclerosing cholangitis, and cirrhosis caused by inborn errors of metabolism are indications for liver transplantation. Alcoholic cirrhosis, a more common problem, is less amenable to treatment by liver transplantation because of the high probability of persistent alcoholism and its sequelae. Primary liver or bile duct cancer has been treated by liver replacement, but with the possible exception of fibrolamellar hepatoma, the cancer is likely to recur and metastasize under the influence of immunosuppression.

For nonmalignant liver disease, the heterotopic auxiliary liver transplant (Fig. 44-3) is an appealing concept because it spares the patient the risk of removal of the cirrhotic liver and provides the advantage of retaining potential functional hepatic reserve in the cirrhotic liver; however, the few human auxiliary liver transplants performed to date have been almost uniformly unsuccessful.

The majority of human liver transplants have been orthotopic liver replacements (Fig. 44-4). This operation is extremely difficult in patients with advanced cirrhosis because of the risk of massive intraoperative hemorrhage attributable to portal hypertension and impaired blood coagulation mechanisms. Autotransfusion by means of a venovenous shunt without heparin is used in most centers to reduce the risk of hemorrhage during the procedure. The liver replacement operation usually requires four vascular anastomoses: suprahepatic inferior vena cava, infrahepatic inferior vena cava, portal vein, and hepatic artery. The fifth anasto-

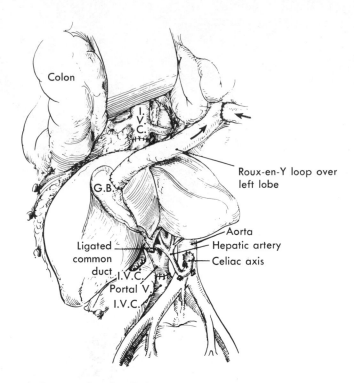

Fig. 44-3. Heterotopic liver transplantation. Patient's own liver is under retractor at top of illustration. Recipient's vena cava was transected below level of renal veins and donor liver was revascularized as follows: Donor portal vein was anastomosed to recipient's distal inferior vena cava; donor's suprahepatic vena cava was joined to recipient's proximal inferior vena cava; donor celiac axis was anastomosed to recipient's aorta. Donor subhepatic vena cava was closed with suture. Common bile duct was ligated below its junction with cystic duct, and biliary drainage was provided by anastomosis of gallbladder to Roux-en-Y loop of small bowel. Alternatively, recipient portal venous inflow may be provided to the graft portal vein, and choledochojejunostomy may be substituted for cholecystojejunostomy.

(From Starzl TE: Experience in Hepatic Transplantation, Philadelphia, 1969, W.B. Saunders Co.)

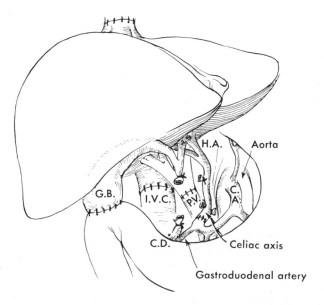

Fig. 44-4. Orthotopic liver transplantation. Host's diseased liver and related segment of inferior vena cava have been removed. Donor liver and related segment of inferior vena cava have been placed in position with anastomoses of vena cava above and below liver, portal veins, and hepatic arteries. Donor common bile duct was ligated and biliary drainage provided by anastomosis of gallbladder to duodenum. This older method of biliary drainage (cholecystoduodenostomy) has been replaced by choledochocholedochostomy over a T-tube stent or by choledochojejunostomy (Roux-en-Y) over a stent.

(From Starzl TE: Experience in Hepatic Transplantation, Philadelphia, 1969, W.B. Saunders Co.)

mosis, for bile drainage, has been the least reliable of the five anastomoses because of bile leakage and biliary obstruction. If the recipient's common bile duct is patent, choledochocholedochostomy over a T-tube stent is the preferred method of bile drainage. If the recipient's common bile duct is not usable, as in congenital biliary atresia, choledochojejunostomy and cholecystojejunostomy are alternatives.

At the University of Pittsburgh, with the world's most experienced surgical team using cyclosporine and prednisone immunosuppression, the 1-year survival after liver replacement in the 1980s rose to 74%, in contrast to 30% to 50% during the 1970s. Currently the patient who has survived longest is a 20-year-old woman who underwent liver transplantation more than 18 years ago.

Heart Transplantation

During the 1980s, in large part because of cyclosporine immunosuppression, heart transplantation became highly therapeutic. Three parts of the operative technique are illustrated in Fig. 44-5. The recipients have usually been relatively young adults with intractable heart failure from cardiomyopathy caused by viruses or unknown agents. An increasing number of older patients with secondary cardiomyopathy due to coronary artery disease are also receiving transplants. Severe irreversible pulmonary hypertension interdicts orthotopic cardiac replacement because of the inability of the donor right ventricle to pump effectively against high resistance, although pretransplant treatment can sometimes identify and treat reversible pulmonary hypertension in patients with severe congestive heart failure who might initially be considered untransplantable. A small number of critically ill cardiac patients have needed temporary artificial heart (Jarvik or Penn State) support until a human cadaver donor heart could be found. Percutaneous transjugular endomyocardial biopsy specimens of the right ventricle have been valuable guides to rejection. In the 1980s the 1-year patient survival after orthotopic heart transplantation (replacement) rose to approximately 85%, with a 5-year survival of approximately 70%. An increasing number of children with congenital heart defects are being transplanted, including a small number of newborns with hypoplastic left heart syndromes; however the number of brain-dead newborn infant heart donors is very small. Immunosuppression for most cardiac recipients is cyclosporine, azathioprine, and prednisone, plus antithymocyte globulin (ATG) or monoclonal antilymphocyte antibodies (OKT3) to treat severe rejection episodes. Recurrence of coronary artery disease may be delayed by dietary measures and antilipedemia medications, but it remains a serious problem in long-term transplant survivors. Most patients who survive heart transplantation, whose life expectancies were only a few months without transplantation, have been successfully rehabilitated.

Auxiliary (heterotopic) heart transplantation is an alternative to heart replacement in patients with protracted but reversible heart failure who cannot be maintained by intraaortic balloon assist pumps. Auxiliary heart transplantation may also apply to patients with end-stage heart disease whose pulmonary hypertension precludes heart replacement; however as with auxiliary liver transplantation, the therapeutic role of the auxiliary graft remains unclear.

Lung and Heart-Lung Transplantation

Between 1963 and 1980, approximately 25 patients had one lung replaced, and a few patients had transplantation of one pulmonary lobe. One patient in 1970 had transplantation of both lungs. The longest survival from this era, 10 months, was in a patient who had a single lung transplant in 1968 for silicosis. Most of the other patients died soon after transplantation.

In the 1980s, using cyclosporine plus other immunosuppressants, the Toronto lung transplant group resumed single lung, and occasionally double lung, transplantation in patients with end-stage primary lung disease, with promising results in more than 20 patients. The single lung transplant is used for end-stage pulmonary fibrosis, and the double lung transplant for nonfibrotic end-stage disease such as emphysema.

The three main problems for the early lung transplant patients were suboptimal quality of cadaver donor lung, disruption of bronchial anastomoses, and graft rejection. All brain-dead cadaver organ donors' lungs are ventilated mechanically and are often abnormal by the time of death. Bronchial anastomotic healing was often impaired by ischemia of the graft bronchus because of interruption of bronchial arteries. Lung allograft rejection was difficult to distinguish from pulmonary problems of nonimmunologic origin. The Toronto lung transplant group has made progress toward solving these problems, but pulmonary rejection and infection remain difficult to diagnose, even with transbronchial lung biopsy.

Combined heart-lung transplantation was undertaken initially at Stanford University in 1981 for patients with end-stage pulmonary hypertension of unknown cause (primary) or secondary to Eisenmenger's syndrome. These conditions remain the main indications for the procedure. The combined heart-lung transplant is much more complex and less successful than transplantation of the heart alone; nevertheless, it is more than 50% successful for at least 1 year as performed in experienced centers such as the University of Pittsburgh. Routine transbronchial lung biopsy has helped to identify pulmonary infection and rejection and has strengthened the concept that heart and lungs may be rejected independently.

Pancreas Transplantation

The pancreas is not essential to life. Transplantation of this organ is undertaken primarily to improve quality of life by alleviating the vascular complications of type I diabetes mellitus, which may cause blindness at an early age from retinopathy, loss of limb from peripheral arterial disease, or renal failure from glomerulopathy. The discovery of insulin in 1921 and its subsequent widespread use has usually prevented death from diabetic coma, but even constant infusion of insulin from portable pumps connected to subcutaneous delivery systems has not convincingly prevented the vascular complications of diabetes.

Although the precise cause of the vascular complications of diabetes is not known, experimental work in

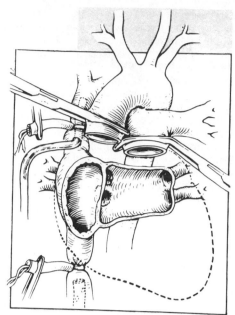

Fig. 44-5. Transplantation of heart. **A,** Using cardiopulmonary bypass recipient's heart has been excised with transected posterior portions of both atria, ascending aorta, and pulmonary artery being left behind. **B,** Entire donor heart has been removed. Superior vena cava has been ligated. Right atrium has been opened by incision from inferior vena cava opening extending toward atrial appendage, with care being taken to preserve sinus node and sinoauricular pathways. Left atrium has been opened by incision joining orifices of the four pulmonary veins. **C,** Donor heart is sewn into recipient. Left and then right atrial anastomoses are completed, followed by anastomosis of pulmonary artery and aorta.

(From Cooley DA: JAMA 205:479-486,1968.)

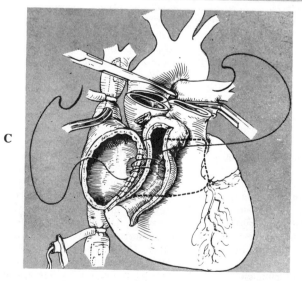

animals indicates that these complications can be prevented or arrested by transplantation of the endocrine part of the pancreas (the islets of Langerhans). It is mechanically difficult to separate adult human pancreatic islets from the surrounding exocrine pancreas tissue without damage to the islets, but islet transplantation is an attractive concept because of its simplicity: islets can be injected into a vein or implanted in tissue without a complex operation. Fetal human pancreas tissue is a potential but limited source of transplantable islet

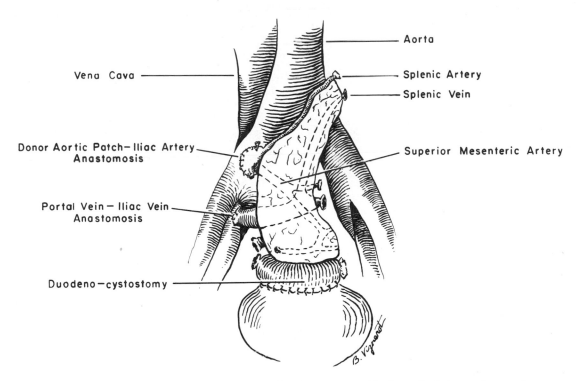

Vena Cava

Donor Aortic Patch—Iliac Artery Anastomosis

Portal Vein—Iliac Vein Anastomosis

Duodeno—cystostomy

Aorta

Splenic Artery

Splenic Vein

Superior Mesenteric Artery

Fig. 44-6. Transplantation of the whole pancreas with a short segment of duodenum for drainage of pancreatic exocrine secretions into the recipient's urinary bladder (duodeno-cystostomy).

tissue. Up to now no human islet transplant has completely eliminated the need for exogenous insulin.

A second more complex method of pancreas transplantation is revascularization of the whole pancreas (with or without duodenum) or the body-and-tail segment of the pancreas. More than 80% of these transplants have been done in association with kidney transplantation, but more than 150 pancreas transplants were performed in patients who had not yet developed severe renal failure. Such large grafts are rearterialized by donor celic axis and superior mesenteric artery in pancreaticoduodenal grafts, or by donor splenic artery in segmental body-and-tail grafts. Venous drainage is via the donor portal vein (Fig. 44-6). The proteolytic proenzymes in the exocrine pancreas can become activated by inflammation, causing serious intraabdominal complications. In order to avoid such complications, the pancreatic exocrine output has been blocked by injection of quick-setting polymers into the pancreatic duct system; alternatively the exocrine output has been drained into the free peritoneal cavity, stomach, Roux-en-Y jejunal limb, ureter, or bladder. None of these techniques has been an entirely safe or effective method for handling the exocrine secretions of large pancreas grafts.

Transplantation of whole cadaver pancreas and a short segment of duodenum, with duodenocystostomy for drainage of exocrine pancreatic secretions into the urinary bladder, currently appears to be the most successful technique for handling the exocrine pancreas. Experienced centers using this method achieve a 1-year pancreatic graft survival of approximatly 80%, and technical problems such as pancreatic leak of peripancreatic abscess have become uncommon. Nevertheless

the early diagnosis of rejection remains difficult, in spite of measurements of urinary amylase or urinary insulin or biopsy of the duodenum (via cystoscope) or even pancreatic biopsy.

Living donor segmental pancreas transplantation has been performed mainly at the University of Minnesota, usually using enteric, rather than bladder, drainage for the exocrine secretions. Some of these living donors have developed abnormal glucose tolerance tests after donation. Three segmental pancreas transplants from living donor identical twins performed without immunosuppression resulted in recurrent diabetes; a fourth identical twin transplant recipient treated with azathioprinc did not develop recurrent diabetes, supporting the concept that type I diabetes is an immunologically mediated disease. A controlled study from the University of Minnesota (1988) unfortunately showed that successful pancreas transplantation and subsequent normoglycemia neither reversed nor arrested diabetic retinopathy in 22 patients.

Intestinal Transplantation

There are a few children with intestinal atresia and a few adults with midgut infarction or extensive inflammatory bowel disease who could benefit from small-bowel transplantation if bowel rejection (with anastomotic disruption) and graft-versus-host disease from intestinal lymphoid tissue could be prevented. In the fall of 1987, at the University of Pittsburgh, a child with congenital intestinal atresia and severe liver damage from years of total parenteral nutrition, underwent transplantation en bloc of stomach, small bowel, colon, liver, and pancreas. Although current follow-up is only a few months, this imaginative operation may open the door to a new era of intestinal transplantation.

Multiple Organ Transplantation

In addition to the multiple pediatric organs described above, a small number of dual organ transplants for special indications also have been carried out, such as heart-liver transplantation for homozygous familial hypercholesterolemia and liver-kidney transplantation for end stage renal failure complicated by postnecrotic cirrhosis.

Retransplantation

When a transplant fails, retransplantation is a potential option. Patients with renal failure sometimes undergo multiple retransplantations if they prefer this form of therapy to chronic dialysis. Patients with end stage heart, lung, or liver failure whose transplants fail have no way of surviving other than retransplantation; however such patients are sometimes very ill, and retransplantation of these organs has been less successful than primary transplantation.

ORGAN PRESERVATION

Organ preservation, a vital component of transplantation technology, allows time for transport of the organ from donor to recipient. In kidney transplantation, the preservation also allows time for histocompatibility matching. The most important aspect of organ preservation is cooling, to retard metabolism and reduce oxygen demand. Prevention of cellular acidosis and prevention of cellular swelling are also very important. Balanced intracellular-type electrolyte solution containing potassium ion at approximately 115 mEq/L and sodium ion at 10 mEq/L is used to preserve most cadaver kidneys and livers. At 4° to 8° C, kidneys can be stored in this solution for 24 to 48 hours; longer storage periods are associated with greater than 50% initial nonfunction. Initial nonfunction, even for weeks, is acceptable in kidney transplantation because dialysis can support the patient until adequate function begins. In liver transplantation, where early function after transplantation is essential for survival, the safe cold storage time is currently 8 to 10 hours. In heart transplantation, where immediate function after transplantation is essential for survival, the safe cold storage time is currently less than 6 hours. When possible, heart-lung grafts are performed with donor and recipient in adjacent operating rooms to reduce transfer time to an absolute minimum; but 3 to 4 hour's cold storage of heart-lung blocks has also been successful, with or without mechanical lung inflation during storage. In 1987, Dr. F.O. Belzer introduced a new University of Wisconsin preservation solution for cold storage of extrarenal organs as well as kidneys. In this new solution, lactobionate replaces the lower-molecular-weight chloride ion and raffinose replaces the lower-molecular-weight glucose. Other additives are hydroxyethyl starch to increase oncotic pressure, allopurinol to reduce free oxygen radical formation, adenosine and phosphate to promote adenosine triphosphate formation, and glutathione as a reducing agent. Early trials suggest that this new solution can double the safe storage time for liver, and possibly other organs.

Organ preservation can also be accomplished by a pulsatile perfusion machine, which cools the organ to 4° to 8° C and at the same time pumps through it cryo-precipitated (to remove lipoproteins) plasma or a plasma substitute as well as oxygen. Pulsatile perfusion currently appears to have little advantage over simple cold storage for most clinical purposes.

Whichever of the two methods of organ preservation is used, the organ must be well perfused and well oxygenated in the brain-dead cadaver donor until the moment it is removed from the donor, so that irreversible warm ischemic damage is avoided.

ORGAN DONOR ISSUES

In the United States the concept of brain death is now well accepted, as reflected in brain death legislation or judicial precedent presently in force in most states. In the late 1980s, in response to the 1984 National Organ Transplant Act, federally controlled organ-sharing programs began to replace the less controlled but effective regional organ-sharing arrangements developed during the 1960s and 1970s. In the late 1980s in the USA, there were approximately 13,000 people waiting every day for cadaver kidneys. Some of these patients were so highly and broadly presensitized that a very small percentage of any donor pool—no matter how large—would be compatible; nevertheless the demand for cadaver kidneys and extrarenal organs has increased far beyond the available supply. Educational programs for the public and for health care providers, particularly in underdeveloped areas of the world, could increase the supply of transplantable cadaver organs; but the improving success rates in transplantation may sustain, or even increase, the disparity between cadaver organ supply and demand. Some otherwise suitable donors must be rejected because of risk of transmission of communicable disease such as hepatitis or AIDS. In the long run, cross-species grafts (xenografts) may become an acceptable alternative to human cadaver organs. In the meantime, Dr. Thomas Starzl of the University of Pittsburgh has proposed a national system for equitable allocation of kidneys and extrarenal organs based on regional primacy, physician responsibility, and patient free choice. The question of offering financial incentives to increase the number of cadaver donors continues to surface periodically, but most students of this complex field continue to favor a strictly charitable system. Many states are enacting legislation requiring the hospital to request tissue and organ donation from the decedent's next of kin whenever there is a death in hospital.

CONCLUSIONS

Approximately 10,000 organ transplants are done each year in the United States. This represents a very small percentage of the approximately 25,000,000 annual US operations. Nevertheless transplantation has emerged as one of the most highly visible and closely scrutinized undertakings in all of medicine. Ethical questions, such as whether anencephalic newborns will become cadaver donors, must be evaluated by carefully constituted panels representing the broad public interest. In the long run, the future of transplantation may depend less on biologic advances than on the willingness and ability of nations to pay for the application of these technologies.

Normal Laboratory Values

CHEMISTRY

Alanine aminotransferase (ALT)	Serum	7-30 units/L
Albumin	Serum	4.0-5.5 g/dl (40-55 g/L)
Alcohol (ethyl)	Blood	<0.1 g/L (2.2 mmol/L)
Aldolase	Serum	Male, 8.5-20 units/L, female, 7.0-14 units/L
Aldosterone	Urine	2-26 μg/24 hr. (6-72 nmol/24 h)
Amino acid nitrogen	Plasma	3.5-7.0 mg/dl (2.5-5.0 mmol/L)
	Urine	50-200 mg/24 hr. (3.6-7.2 mmol/24 h)
Ammonia	Blood	18-60 μg/dl (10-30 μmol/L)
Amniotic fluid		Net absorbance at 540 nm < 0.020, bilirubin, <0.25 mg/dl (4.3 μmol/L); L/S ratio > 2
Amylase	Serum	60-180 Somogyi units (110-330 U/L)
	Urine	35-260 units/hr; 80-5000 units/24 hr
Antistreptolysin titier	Serum	<200 Todd units; absence of rising titer
Ascorbic acid	Plasma	0.5-2.0 mg/dl (30-120 μmol/L)
Aspartate aminotransferase (AST)	Serum	12-30 units/L
Arsenic	Urine	<100 μg/L (1.3 μmol/L)
Barbiturates (therapeutic range)	Serum	
Short acting		0.05-0.15 mg/dl (0.5-1.5 mg/L)
Intermediate acting		0.1-0.5 mg/dl (1-5 mg/L)
Long acting		1.5-3.0 mg/dl (15-30 mg/L)
Bilirubin	Serum	Total, 0.2-1.3 mg/dl (3.4-22 μmol/L); direct, 0.1-0.4 mg/dl (1.7-7.0 μmol/L)
Blood urea nitrogen (BUN)	Serum	10-18 mg/dl (3.6-6.5 mmol/L as urea)
Bromide	Serum	<3 mg/dl (0.12 mmol/L)
Bromsulfphthalein (BSP)	Serum	<6% remaining after 45 min
Calcium	Serum	8.5-10.5 mg/dl (2.1-2.6 mmol/L)
	Urine	60-400 mg/24 hr (1.5-10 mmol/24 h)
Calcium, ionic	Serum	4.6-5.4 mg/dl (1.15-1.35 mmol/L)
Carbon dioxide (CO_2) content	Serum	24-32 mmol/L
	Venous blood	23-30 mmol/L
	Arterial blood	21-28 mmol/L
Carbon dioxide pressure (P_{CO_2})	Blood	38-49 mm Hg (torr) (5.1-6.5 kPa)
Carboxyhemoglobin	Blood	<5% of total hemoglobin
Cardio-Green (liver function)	Serum	<4% remaining after 20 min; disappearance rate of 18-26%/min
Carotene	Serum	50-250 μg/dl (0.93-4.7 μmol/L)
Catecholamines (total)	Urine	30-70 μg/24 hr (175-420 nmol/L as norepinephrine)

The values listed are those for adults (those differing for children are specifically mentioned). Caution should be used in interpreting these normal values in children (except where specifically noted) and in individuals over the age of 60. These differences in normal values are discussed in the interpretations given with the specific procedures. Therapeutic levels are given only for some of the most commonly used drugs.

*Competitive protein binding

†Radioimmunoassay

Ceruloplasmin (see Ferroxidase)		
Chloride	Serum	98-109 mEq/L (mmol/L)
	Spinal fluid	122-132 mEq/L (mmol/L)
	Sweat	10-35 mEq/L (mmol/L)
Cholesterol (total)	Serum	150-270 mg/dl (39-70 mmol/L)
Cholesterol esters	Serum	68-74% of total
Cholinesterase (pseudo)	Serum	9-12 units/L
Cold agglutinin	Serum	<1:32 dilution
Concentration test	Urine	Specific gravity of 1.025 or higher
Copper	Serum	75-155 μg/dl (12-25 μmol/L)
Coproporphyrin	Urine	20-100 μg/24 hr (30-150 nmol/24 h)
Corticosteroids, total (hydroxy-steroids as cortisol)	Urine	Male, 5-14 mg/24 hr (14-39 μmol/24 hr); female, 4-13 mg/24 hr (11-36 μmol/24 hr)
Cortisol	Plasma	8 AM, 10-25 μg/dl (300-700 nmol/L); 8 PM, 4-13 μg/dl (110-350 nmol/L)
	Urine	Male, 110-410 μg/24 hr (0.3-1.1 μmol/24 h); female, 80-360 μg/24 hr (0.22-0.90 μmol/24 h)
Creatine phosphokinase (CPK)	Serum	Male, 20-50 units/L; female, 10-40 units/L
Creatinine	Serum	0.6-1.2 mg/dl (53-106 μmol/L)
	Urine	Male, 1.0-1.4 g/24 hr (8.8-12.4 mmol/24 h); female, 0.8-1.2 g/24 hr (7.1-10.6 mmol/24 h)
Creatinine clearance		Males, 113-167 ml/min (1.88-2.78 ml/s); females, 92-132 ml/min (1.53-2.20 ml/s)
C'3 component	Serum	123-167 mg/dl (1.23-1.67 g/L)
Digoxin (therapeutic level)	Serum	1.0-2.25 ng/ml (1.3-2.9 nmol/L)
Diphenylhydantoin (phenytoin) (therapeutic level)	Serum	1-2 mg/dl (40-80 μmol/L)
Epinephrine	Urine	10-40% of the total catecholamines
Estrogens	Pregnancy urine	Gradually increasing from 3-7 mg/24 hrs (11-18 mmole/d) at 20 weeks to 15-45 mg/24 hrs (33-100 mmol/d) at term
Fat	Feces	<5 g/24 hr on normal diet
Fatty acids	Serum	
Esterified		7-14 mmol/L
Free		0.15-1.2 mmol/L
Fibrinogen	Plasma	0.2-0.4 g/dl (2-4 g/L)
Follicle-stimulating hormone	Urine	6-60 mU/24 hr
Gastric analysis		Free acidity 0-40 mmole/L, total acidity, 10-50 mmole/L, pH 1.5-4.0; volume, 30-100 ml
Globulins (see protein fractionation and Immunoglobulins)		
Glucose	Serum	85-110 mg/dl (4.4-6.0 mmol/L)
	Spinal fluid	40-80 mg/dl (2.2-4.4 mmol/L)
Glucose tolerance (oral)	Serum	Fasting, 80-110 mg/dl (4.4-6 mmol/L); 1 hr <180 mg/dl (8.3 mmol/L); 2 hr, <140 mg/dl (7.8 mmol/L)
Glucose-6-phosphate dehydroge-nase	Blood	5-10 U/g hemoglobin
Glutamic oxalacetic transaminase (see Alanine aminotransferase)		
Glutamic pyruvic transaminase (see Aspartate aminotransferase)		
Glutamyl transpeptidase	Serum	Males 10-50 units/L; females, about 20% lower
Haptoglobin	Serum	70-140 mg/dl (9.7-1.4 g/L)
Hydroxybutyric dehydrogenase	Serum	50-125 units/L
5-Hydroxyindoleacetic acid (5-HIAA)	Urine	2-14 mg/24 hr (11-75 μmol/d)
Hydroxysteroids (see corticoster-oids)		
Immunoglobulins	Serum	IgA, 100-400 mg/dl (1-4 g/L); IgG, 650-1600 mg/dl (6.5-16 g/L); IgM, 30-120 mg/dl (0.3-1.2 g/L)
Iron	Serum	Male, 80-160 mg/dl (14-28 μmol/L); female, 60-136 mg/dl (11-24 μmol/L)
Iron-binding capacity (total)	Serum	250-350 mg/dl (45-63 μmol/L)
Isocitric dehydrogenase (ICDH)	Serum	240-690 units/L
17-Ketosteroids (calculated as dehydroepiandrosterone)	Urine	Male, 10-18 mg/24 hr (35-63 μmol/24 h); female, 6-15 mg/24 hr (21-52 μmol/24 hr)
ACTH stimulation		Increase of 50% or more in ketosteroids; 100% increase in ketogenic steroids
Metyrapone test		Increase of 50% in ketosteroids; 100% increase in ketogenic steroids
Lactate	Blood	5-12 mg/dl (0.56-1.3 mmol/L)

Lactate dehydrogenase (LDH)	Serum	95-200 units/L
	Spinal fluid	10-30 units/L
	Urine	60-240 units/hr in overnight specimen
Lead	Blood	<40 μg/dl (1.9 μmol/L)
Leucine aminopeptidase (LAP)	Serum	11-30 units/L
	Urine	Male, 0.8-6.2 units in overnight specimen; female, 0.2-4.7 units/L in overnight specimen
Lipase	Serum	<1.0 units (<280 mU/L)
Lipids (total)	Serum	400-850 mg/dl (4.0-8.5 g/L)
Lithium (therapeutic range)	Serum	0.5-1.2 mEq/L (mmol/L)
Lysozyme (muramidase)	Serum	3-8 μg/ml (mg/L)
Magnesium	Serum	1.6-2.1 mEq/L (0.8-1.05 mmol/L)
Methemoglobin	Blood	<1.5% of total hemoglobin
3-Methoxy-4-hydroxymandelic acid (see VMA)		
Metyrapone test (see 17-Keto-steroids)		
Norepinephrine	Urine	60-90% of total catecholamines
Osmolality	Serum	275-295 mOsm/kg
	Urine	400-1000 mOsm/kg
Oxygen pressure (Po₂)	Arterial blood	60-80 mm Hg (torr) (8.0-10.7 kPa)
	Venous blood	30-50 mm Hg (torr) (4.0-6.3 kPa)
Oxygen saturation	Arterial blood	90-95% (0.90-0.95)
	Venous blood	60-85% (0.60-0.85)
pH	Arterial blood	7.32-7.42
	Venous blood	7.35-7.45
	Urine	4.8-7.6 (average 6.0)
Phenolsulfonphthalein (PSP)	Urine	25-50% excreted in first 15 min; 15-25% more in next 15 min; 10-15% in next 30 min; 60-85% total excreted in 1 hr
Phosphatase		
Acid	Serum	Male, 2.5-11 units/L; female; 0.3-9 units/L
Total		
Tartaric acid labile		Male, 0.2-3.5 units/L; female; 0.0-0.8 units/L
Alkaline	Serum	Adults, 20-90 units/L; children, 40-200 units/L
Heat labile, bone		>60% of total
Phospholipids	Serum	150-300 mg/dl (1.9-4.5 mmol/L)
Phosphorus (inorganic)	Serum	Adults, 2.5-4.8 mg/dl (0.8-1.55 mmol/L); children, 3.5-6.0 mg/dl (1.1-1.9 mmol/L)
Porphobilinogen synthase (aminolevulinate dehydratase)	Red cells	4-20 mmole/min/ml red cells
Porphyrins	Urine	Uroporphyrin <40 μg/24 hr (50 nmol); coproporphyrin < 200 μg/24 hr (250 nmol)
Potassium	Serum	3.5-5.6 mEq/L (mmol/L)
	Urine	25-100 mEq/L (mmol/L)
Protein (total)	Serum	6-8 g/dl (60-80 g/L)
	Spinal fluid	15-45 mg/dl (150-450 mg/L)
Protein fractionation		
Prealbumin	Serum	—
	Spinal fluid	2-7% of total
Albumin	Serum	52-68%
	Spinal fluid	52-72%
α₁-Globulin	Serum	2-6%
	Spinal fluid	1-7%
α₂-Globulin	Serum	5-11%
	Spinal fluid	3-12%
β-Globulin	Serum	8-16%
	Spinal fluid	7-23%
γ-Globulin	Serum	10-22%
	Spinal fluid	3-13%
Prothrombin time	Plasma	70-100% or 11-13 sec
Protoporphyrin	Red cells	15-100 μg/dl red cells (0.27-1.78 μmol/L)
Quinidine (therapeutic level)	Serum	0.2-0.5 mg/dl (6-15 μmol/L)
Renin level		
Normal diet	Plasma	Upright, 0.3-3.6 ng/ml; supine, 0.3-1.9 ng/ml
Low salt diet		Upright, 4.1-9.1 ng/ml; supine, 0.9-4.5 ng/ml
Salicylate (therapeutic level)	Serum	15-30 mg/dl (110-220 μmol/L)
Serotonin (see 5-Hydroxyindoleacetic acid)		
Sodium	Serum	125-145 mEq/L (mmol/L)
	Sweat	5-35 mEq/L
	Urine	130-260 mEq/24 hr

Sulfhemoglobin	Blood	<1% of total hemoglobin
T3, T4, TBI (see thyroid function tests)		
Testosterone	Serum	Male, 400-1000 µg/dl (14-35 µmol/L); female, 40-120 µg/dl (1.4-2.2 µmol/L)
Thyroid function tests	Serum	
Thyroxine (by column)		3.5-7.5 µg thyroxine iodine/dl = 5.5-11.6 µg thyroxine/dl (70-150 µmol/L)
Thyroxine (by CPB* or RIA†)		5.5-11.5 µg/dl (70-150 µmol/L)
T3 uptake		25-35%
TBI		1.10-0.90
Triglycerides	Serum	50-145 mg/dl (0.57-1.66 mmol/L)
Trypsin	Duodenal contents	150-600 µg/ml
Urea (see Blood urea nitrogen)		
Uric acid	Serum	Male, 3.5-8.0 mg/dl (210-475 µmol/L); female, 2.5-7.0 mg/dl (150-415 µmol/L)
Urobilinogen	Urine	0.4-1.0 mg/24 hr (0.7-1.7 µmol/24 h)
	Feces	40-280 mg/24 hr (68-475 µmol)
Vitamin A	Serum	25-75 µg/dl (0.85-2.65 µmol/L)
Vitamin C (see Ascorbic acid)		
VMA	Urine	2-14 mg/dl (10-70 µmol/L)
Xylose excretion	Urine	25 g dose, 16-36% excreted in 4 hr; 5 g dose, 20-45% excreted

HEMATOLOGY

Hemoglobin	Male, 14-18 g/dl (140-180 g/L); female, 12-16 g/dl (120-160 g/L)
Hematocrit	Male, 40-54% (0.40-0.54); female, 37-47% (0.37-0.47)
Red cell count	Male, 4.6-6.2 mil/mm^3 (4.6-6.2 × 10^{12}/L); female, 4.2-5.4 mil/mm^3 (4.2-5.4 × 10^{12}/L)
White cell count	5000-10,000/mm^3 (5-10 × 10^9/L)
Differential leukocyte count	
Neutrophils	60-70% (0.60-0.70)
Lymphocytes	20-30% (0.20-0.30)
Monocytes	2-6% (0.06-0.10)
Eosinophils	1-4% (0.01-0.04)
Basophils	0-0.5% (0.00-0.005)
Platelet count	150,000-350,000 (150-350 × 10^6/L)
Blood indices	
MCH	27-31 µµg (27-31 pg [picograms])
MCV	82-92 µm^3 (82-92 fl [femtoliters])
MCHC	32-36% (0.32-0.36 pg/fl)
Eosinophil count	100-300 mm^3 (100-300 × 10^6/L)

Suggested Readings

CHAPTER 1
Origin of Surgical Disease

Anson BJ and McVay CP: Surgical anatomy, Philadelphia, 1984, WB Saunders Co.

Davis JH: Clinical surgery, St. Louis, 1987, The CV Mosby Co.

Dunphy JE and Botsford TW: Physical examination of the surgical patient, Philadelphia, 1975, WB Saunders Co.

Greenfield L: Complications in surgery and trauma, Philadelphia, 1984, JB Lippincott.

Hardy JD: Textbook of surgery, ed 2, Philadelphia, 1988, JB Lippincott Co.

Maingot R: Abdominal operations, ed 7, New York, 1980, Appleton-Century-Crofts.

Nora PF: Operative surgery, ed 2, Philadelphia, 1980, Lea & Febiger.

Norton LW and Eiseman B: Surgical decision making, Philadelphia, 1986, WB Saunders Co.

Sabiston DC: Christopher's textbook of surgery, ed 13, Philadelphia, 1986, WB Saunders Co.

Schwartz SI et al, editors: Principles of surgery, ed 4, New York, 1984, McGraw-Hill Book Co.

Shackelford RT and Zuidema G: Surgery of the alimentary tract, ed 3, Philadelphia, 1982, WB Saunders Co.

Zollinger RM and Zollinger RM, Jr: Atlas of surgical operations, ed 6, New York, 1988, The Macmillan Co.

CHAPTER 2
Wounds and Wound Healing

Dineen P and Hildick Smith G: The surgical wound, Philadelphia, 1981, Lea & Febiger.

Falcone RE and Nappi JF: Chemotherapy and wound healing, Surg Clin North Am 64:779, 1984.

Hunt TK et al, editors: Soft and hard tissue repair: biologic and clinical aspects, ed 1, New York, 1984, Praeger Publishers.

McMurry JF: Wound healing with diabetus mellitus, Surg Clin North Am 64:769, 1984.

Nicoletis C, Bazin S, LeLous M: Clinical and biochemical features of normal, defective and pathologic scars, Clin Plastic Surg 4:347, 1977.

Peacock EE and Van Winkle W: Wound repair, ed 3, Philadelphia, 1984, WB Saunders Co.

Rudolph R: Contraction and the control of contraction, World J Surg 4:275, 1980.

CHAPTER 3
Fluids and Electrolytes

Cohen JJ and Jassier JP: Acid-base, Boston, 1982, Little, Brown & Co.

Davenport HW: The ABC of acid-base chemistry, ed 6, Chicago, 1974, The University of Chicago Press.

Kinney JM, Lister J, and Moore FD: Relationship of energy expenditure to total exchangeable potassium, Ann NY Acad Sci 110:711, 1963.

Kwun KB et al: Treatment of metabolic alkalosis with intravenous infusion of concentrated hydrochloric acid, Am J Surg 146:328, 1983.

Leaf A: The clinical and physiological significance of the serum sodium concentration, N Engl J Med 267:24, 1962.

Mason EE: Fluid, electrolyte and nutrient therapy in surgery, Philadelphia, 1974, Lea & Febiger.

Mundy GR and Martin TJ: The hypercalcemia of malignancy: Pathogenesis and management, Metabolism 31:1247, 1982.

Schrier RW, editor: Renal and electrolyte disorders, ed 3, Boston, 1986, Little, Brown.

Shapiro BA, Harrison RA, and Walton JR: Clinical application of blood gases, ed 2, Chicago, 1977, Year Book Medical Publishers, Inc.

CHAPTER 4
Disorders of Hemostasis: Diagnosis and Treatment

Coller BS: Von Willebrand disease. In Hemostasis and thrombosis—basic principles and clinical practice, ed 2, Philadelphia, 1987, JB Lippincott.

George JN, Nurden AT, and Phillips DR: Molecular defects in interaction of platelets with the vessel wall, N Engl J Med 311:1084, 1984.

Levine PH: Clinical manifestations and therapy of hemophilias A and B. In Hemostasis and thrombosis—basic principles and clinical practice, ed 2, Philadelphia, 1987, JB Lippincott.

White GC et al: Approach to the bleeding patient. In Hemostasis and thrombosis—basic principles and clinical practice, ed 2, Philadelphia, 1987, JB Lippincott.

Zimmerman TS and Plow EF: Disorders of blood coagulation. In Internal Medicine, Boston, 1983, Little, Brown.

CHAPTER 5
Shock

Bone RC et al: A controlled clinical trial of high-dose methylprednisolone in the treatment of severe sepsis and septic shock, N Engl J Med 317(11):653, 1987.

Brooks DK: Resuscitation: care of the critically ill, ed 2, Australia, 1986, Edward Arnold Ltd.

Chaudry IH, Clemens MG, and Baue AE: Alterations in cell function with ischemia and shock and their correction, Arch Surg 116:1309, 1981.

Chernow B and Roth BL: Pharmacologic manipulation of the peripheral vasculature in shock: clinical and experimental approaches, Circ Shock 18:141, 1986.

Folkow B and Neil E: Circulation, London, 1971, Oxford University Press.

Higgins TL and Chernow B: Pharmacotherapy of circulatory shock, Dis of the Mth June, 312, 1987.

Hinshaw L et al: Effect of high-dose glucocorticoid therapy on mortality in patients with clinical signs of systemic sepsis, N Engl J Med 317(11):659, 1987.

Holcroft JW and Blaisdell FW: Shock: causes and management of circulator collapse. In Sabiston DC, Jr: Textbook of surgery, ed 13, Philadelphia, 1986, WB Saunders Co.

Houston MC, Thompson WL, and Robertson D: Shock: diagnosis and management, Arch Intern Med 144:1433, 1984.

Luce JM: Pathogenesis and management of septic shock, Chest 91(6):883, 1987.

Mizock B: Septic shock: a metabolic perspective, Arch Intern Med 144:579, 1984.

Perkin RM and Levin DL: Shock in the pediatric patient, Part I, J Pediatr 101(2):163, 1982.

Perkin RM and Levin DL: Shock in the pediatric patient, Part II, J Pediatr 101(3):319, 1982.

Shoemaker WC: Circulatory mechanisms of shock and their mediators, Crit Care Med 15(8):787, 1987.

Shoemaker WC: Relation of oxygen transport patterns to the pathophysiology and therapy of shock states, Intensive Care Med 13:230, 1987.

Swan HJC et al: Catheterization of the heart in man with the use of a flow-directed balloon-tipped catheter. N Engl J Med 283:447, 1970.

CHAPTER 6
Surgical Infection

Alexander JW: Nosocomial infections, Curr Probl Surg 1973.

Ben-Shoshan M, Gius JA, and Smith IM: Exploratory laparotomy for fever of unknown origin, Surg Gynecol Obstet 132:994, 1971.

Coles B et al: Incidence of wound infection for common general surgical procedures, Surg Gynecol Obstet 154:557, 1982.

Cruse PJE and Foord R: The epidemiology of wound infection: a 10-year prospective study of 62,939 wounds, Surg Clin North Am 60:27, 1980.

FDA Drug Bulletin, vol 17, no 2, 1987.

Gozal D et al: Necrotizing fasciitis, Arch Surg 121:233, 1986.

Hart GB, Lamb RC, Strauss MD: Gas gangrene, J Trauma 23:991, 1983.

Hunt TK: Surgical wound infections: an overview, Am J Med 70:712, 1981.

Jacobson MA and Young LS: New developments in the treatment of gram-negative bacteremia, West J Med 144:85, 1986.

Laurence J: Tracking the transmission of HIV infection, Infect Surg 6:17, 1987.

McCabe WR et al: Pathophysiology of bacteremia, Ann J Med 75:7, 1983.

Oates, JA and Wood AJJ: Antimicrobial prophylaxis in surgery, N Engl J Med 315:1129, 1986.

Recommendations for prevention of HIV transmission in health-care settings, MMWR 36: 1987.

Robson MC, Krizek TJ, and Heggers JP: Biology of surgical infection, Curr Probl Surg 1973.

Simmons RL and Howard RJ, editors: Surgical infectious diseases, New York, 1980, Appleton-Century-Crofts.

Tetanus—United States, 1982-1984, JAMA 254:2873, 1985.

Wangensteen OH, Wangensteen SD, and Klinger CF: Surgical cleanliness, hospital solubrity, and surgical statistics historically considered, Surgery 71:477, 1972.

World Health Organization Committee and Rabies Fourth Report, Technical Series, No. 201, 1960.

CHAPTER 7
Surgical Nutrition

American College of Surgeons Committee on Pre- and Postoperative Care: Manual of preoperative and postoperative care, ed 3, Philadelphia, 1983, WB Saunders Co.

Baker JP et al: Nutritional assessment: a comparison of clinical judgement and objective measurements, N Engl J Med 306:960, 1982.

Cerra FB: Hypermetabolism, organ failure, and metabolic support, Surgery 101:1, 1987.

Delany HM et al: Postoperative nutritional support using needle catheter feeding jejunostomy, Ann Surg 186:165, 1977.

Fischer JE: Nutritional support in the seriously ill patient, Curr Probl Surg 17:1 (entire issue), 1980.

Freeman JB: Peripheral parenteral nutrition, Can J Surg 21:489, 1978.

Heymsfield SB et al: Enteral hyperalimentation: an alternative to central venous hyperalimentation, Ann Intern Med 90:63, 1979.

Johnson DG: Total intravenous nutrition in newborn surgical patients: a three-year perspective, J Pediatr Surg 5:601, 1970.

Mullen JL et al: Reduction of operative morbidity and mortality by combined preoperative and postoperative nutritional support, Ann Surg 192:604, 1980.

Mullen JL, editor: Surgical nutrition, Surg Clin North Am 61:427 (entire issue), 1981.

Müller JM et al: Indications and effects of preoperative parenteral nutrition, World J Surg 10:53, 1986.

Sheldon GF and Baker C: Complications of nutritional support, Crit Care Med 8:35, 1980.

CHAPTER 8
Preoperative Care

American College of Surgeons Committee on Pre- and Postop-

erative Care: Manual of preoperative and postoperative care, ed 3, Philadelphia, 1983, WB Saunders Co.

Brenowitz JB, Williams CD, and Edwards WS: Major surgery in patients with chronic renal failure, Am J Surg 134:765, 1977.

Bunker JP, and Wennberg JE: Operation rates, mortality statistics and the quality of life, N Engl J Med 289:1249, 1973.

Gaensler EA and Weisel RD: The risks in abdominal and thoracic surgery in COPD, Postgrad Med 54:183, 1973.

Goldman DR: Medical care of the surgical patient, Philadelphia, 1982, JB Lippincott Co.

Goldman L et al: Multifactorial index of cardiac risk in noncardiac surgical procedures, N Engl J Med 297:845, 1977.

Kyle J and Hardy JD: Scientific foundations of surgery, London, 1981, William Heinemann, Ltd.

Papper S: Manual of medical care of the surgical patient, ed 3, Boston, 1985, Little, Brown & Co.

Strunin L: Preoperative assessment of the patient with liver dysfunction, Br J Anaesth 50:25, 1978.

CHAPTER 9
Anesthesia

Kaplan JA: Cardiac anesthesia, vols 1 and 2, Orlando, 1987, Grune & Stratton.

Churchill-Davidson HC: A practice of anaesthesia, Philadelphia, 1984, WB Saunders Co.

Gray TC, Nunn JF, and Utting JE: General anaesthesia, Woburn, Mass, 1980, Butterworth Publishers.

Miller RD: Anesthesia, Edinburgh, 1986, Churchill Livingstone.

Tinker JH and Rapin M: Care of the critically ill patient, Berlin, 1983, Springer-Verlag.

CHAPTER 10
Postoperative Care

American College of Surgeons Committee on Pre- and Postoperative Care: Manual of preoperative and postoperative care, ed 3, Philadelphia, 1983, WB Saunders Co.

Fariello RG and Mutani R: Treatment of hiccup, Lancet 2:1201, 1974.

Freischlag J and Busuttil RW: The value of postoperative fever evaluation, Surgery 94:358, 1983.

Greenfield LJ: Complications in surgery and trauma, Philadelphia, 1984, JB Lippincott Co.

Papper S: Manual of medical care of the surgical patient, ed 3, Boston, 1985, Little, Brown & Co.

Shapiro BA, Harrison RA, and Trout CA: Clinical application of respiratory care, ed 2, Chicago, 1979, Year Book Medical Publishers.

CHAPTER 11
Intensive Care

Beal JM: Critical care for surgical patients, New York, 1982, Macmillan Publishing Co.

Berk JL and Sampliner JE: Handbook of critical care, Boston, 1982, Little, Brown & Co.

Condon RE, and Nyhus LM: Manual of surgical therapeutics, Boston, 1985, Little, Brown & Co.

Costrini NV and Thomson WM: Manual of medical therapeutics, Boston, 1977, Little, Brown & Co.

Czer LSC and Shoemaker WC: Optimal hematocrit in critically ill postoperative patients, Surg Gynecol Obstet 147:363, 1978.

Gilbert EM et al: The effect of fluid loading, blood transfusion and catecholamine infusion on oxygen delivery and consumption in sepsis, Am Rev Resp Dis 134:873, 1986.

Greenfield, L: Complications in surgery and trauma, Philadelphia, 1984, JB Lippincott Co.

Hill DW and Dolan AM: Intensive care instrumentation, New York, 1982, Grune & Stratton.

CHAPTER 12
Malignant Neoplasms

Bartlett GL: Milestones in tumor immunology, Semin Oncol 6:515, 1979.

Beahrs OH and Myers MH, editors: American Joint Committee on Cancer. Manual for Staging of Cancer, Philadelphia, 1983, JB Lippincott Co.

Bonadonna G et al: Are surgical adjuvant trials altering the course of breast cancer? Semin Oncol 5:450, 1978.

Carter RL: General pathology of the metastatic process. In Baldwin RW, editor: Secondary spread of cancer, New York, 1978, Academic Press Inc.

Fisher B and Gebhardt MC: The evolution of breast cancer surgery: past, present, and future, Semin Oncol 5:385, 1978.

Haagensen CD: An exhibit of important books, papers, and memorabilia illustrating the evolution of the knowledge of cancer, Am J Cancer 18:42, 1933.

Haskell CM: Drugs used in cancer chemotherapy. In Haskell CM, editor: Cancer treatment, ed 2, Philadelphia, 1985, WB Saunders Co.

Kaplan HS: Historic milestones in radiobiology and radiation therapy, Semin Oncol 6:479, 1979.

Morton DL and Giuliano AE: Cancer immunology and immunotherapy. In Haskell CM, editor: Cancer treatment, ed 2, Philadelphia, 1985, WB Saunders Co.

Pack GT and Ariel IM: The history of cancer therapy. In Cancer management, Philadelphia, 1968, JB Lippincott Co.

Salisbury AJ: The significance of the circulating cancer cell, Cancer Treat Rev 2:55, 1975.

Silverberg E and Lubera J: Cancer statistics, 1988, Ca 38:5, 1988.

Sim FH et al: A prospective randomized study of the efficacy of routine elective lymphadenectomy in management of malignant melanoma, Cancer 41:948, 1978.

Zubrod CG: Historic milestones in curative chemotherapy, Semin Oncol 6:490, 1979.

CHAPTER 13
Skin

Apfelberg DB, Maser MR, and Lash H: Argon laser treatment of cutaneous vascular abnormalities, Ann Plast Surg 1:14, 1978.

Breslow A: Thickness, cross-sectional areas and depth of invasion in the prognosis of cutaneous melanomas. Ann Surg 172:902, 1970.

Clark NH et al: The histogenesis and biologic behavior of primary human malignant melanomas of the skin. Cancer Res 29:705, 1969.

Cosman B: Experience in the argon laser therapy of port wine stains. Plast Reconstr Surg 65:119, 1980.

Edgerton MT: The treatment of hemangiomas with special reference to the role of steroid therapy. Ann Surg 183:517, 1976.

Fergin PE, Chu AC, and McDonald DM: Basal cell carcinomas complicating nevus sebaceus. Clin Exp Dermatol 6:111, 1981.

Friedman RJ, Rigel DS, and Kopf AW: Early detection of malignant melanoma: the role of physician examination and self-examination of the skin, Am Cancer Society, 1985.

Lever WF and Schaumberg-Lever G: Histopathology of the skin, ed 6, Philadelphia, 1983, JB Lippincott Co.

McGovern VJ et al: The classification of malignant melanoma and its histologic reporting, Cancer 32:1446, 1973.

Moschella SL and Hurley HJ: Dermatology, ed 2, Philadelphia, 1985, WB Saunders.

Pathak MA: Sunscreens: topical and systemic approaches for protection of human skin against harmful effects of solar radiation. J Am Acad Dermatol 7:285, 1982.

Williams HB: The use of dermabrasion in giant pigmented nevi. In Williams HB, editor: Symposium on vascular malformations in melanotic lesions, vol. 22, St. Louis, 1983, The CV Mosby Co.

Wisnicki JL: Hemangiomas and vascular malformations, Ann Plast Surg 12:41, 1984.

CHAPTER 14
Thyroid Gland

Block MA: Management of carcinoma of the thyroid, Ann Surg 185:133, 1977.

Bradley EL and Liechty RD: Modified subtotal thyroidectomy for Graves disease: a two institution study, Surgery 94:955, 1983.

Cady B: Surgery of thyroid cancer, World J Surg 5:3, 1981.

Clark OH: Endocrine surgery of the thyroid and parathyroid glands, St. Louis, 1985, The CV Mosby Co.

Degroot LJ and Larsen PR: Thyroid and its diseases, New York, 1984, John Wiley & Sons, Inc.

Hubert JP et al: Occult papillary carcinoma of the thyroid. Arch Surg 115:394, 1980.

Ingbar SH and Braverman LE: The thyroid, ed 4, Philadelphia, 1986, JB Lippincott Co.

Johnston IDA and Thompson NW: Endocrine surgery, London, 1983, Butterworth & Co.

Kaplan EL: Surgery of the thyroid and parathyroid glands, Edinburgh, 1983, Churchill Livingstone.

Liechty RD, and Zimmerman D: Solitary thyroid nodules, Arch Surg 112:59, 1977.

Lowhagen T, Willem JS, and Lundell G: Aspiration biopsy cytology in diagnosis of thyroid cancer, World J Surg 5:61, 1981.

CHAPTER 15
Parathyroid Glands

Clark OH: Endocrine surgery of the thyroid and parathyroid glands, St. Louis, 1985, The CV Mosby Co.

Haussler MR and McCain TA: Basic and clinical concepts related to vitamin D metabolism and action, N Engl J Med 297:974, 1041, 1977.

Johnston IDA and Thompson NW: Endocrine surgery, London, 1983, Butterworth & Co.

Kaplan EL: Surgery of the thyroid and parathyroid glands, Edinburgh, 1983, Churchill Livingstone.

Liechty RD and Weil R: The anatomy of parathyroid hyperplasia, Surgery 96:1099, 1984.

Purnell DC, Scholz DA, and Beahrs OH: Hyperparathyroidism due to single gland enlargement, Arch Surg 112:369, 1977.

Rothmund M and Wells SA: Parathyroid surgery, Basel, 1986, Karger.

Saxe AW and Brennan MF: Strategy and technique of reoperative parathyroid surgery, Surgery 89:417, 1981.

Wells SA et al: Transplantation of the parathyroid glands in man: clinical indications and results, Surgery 78:34, 1975.

CHAPTER 16
Adrenal Glands

Bigos ST et al: Cushing's disease: management by transsphenoidal microsurgery, J Clin Endocrinol Metabol 50:348, 1980.

Friesen SR: Surgical endocrinology: clinical syndromes, Philadelphia, 1978, JB Lippincott Co.

Grant CS et al: Primary aldosteronism, Arch Surg 119:585, 1984.

Johnston IDA and Thompson NW: Endocrine surgery, London, 1983, Butterworth & Co.

Prinz RA et al: Cushing's disease: the role of adrenalectomy and autotransplantation, Surg Clin North Am 59:159, 1979.

Sisson JC et al: Scintigraphic localization of pheochromocytoma, N Engl J Med 305:12, 1981.

Thompson NW and Vinik AI: Endocrine surgery update, New York, 1983, Grune & Stratton.

Welbourn RB: Some aspects of adrenal surgery, Br J Surg 67:723, 1980.

CHAPTER 17
Breast

Baum M: Nolvadex adjuvant trial organization: controlled trial of tamoxifen as single adjuvant agent in management of early breast cancer; analysis at 6 years, Lancet 1:836, 1985.

Bonadonna G et al: Ten-year experience with CMF-based adjuvant chemotherapy in resectable breast cancer, Breast Cancer Res Treat 5:95, 1985.

Fisher B et al: Five-year results of a randomized clinical trial comparing total mastectomy and segmental mastectomy with and without radiation in the treatment of breast cancer, N Engl J Med 312:665, 1985.

Harris J et al, editors: Breast diseases, Philadelphia, 1987, JB Lippincott Co.

Lippman M et al, editors: Diagnosis and management of breast cancer, Philadelphia, 1987, WB Saunders.

Veronese U et al: Results of guadrantectomy, axillary dissection, and radiotherapy (QUART) in TI NO patients. In Harris J, Hellman S, and Silen W, editors: Conservative Management of Breast Cancer, Philadelphia, 1983, JB Lippincott.

CHAPTER 18
Liver and Biliary Tract

Barone RM et al: Intra-arterial chemotherapy using an implantable infusion pump and liver irradiation for the treatment of hepatic metastases. Cancer 50:850, 1982.

Bennion LJ and Grundy SM: Risk factors for the development of cholelithiasis in man (2 parts), N Engl J Med 299:1161, 1221, 1978.

Bismuth H: Surgical anatomy and anatomical surgery of the liver, World J Surg 6:3, 1982.

Bodvall B: The postcholecystectomy syndromes, Clin Gastroenterol 2:103, 1973.

Burnstein MJ, Vassal KP, and Strasberg SM: Results of combined biliary drainage and cholecystokinin cholangiography in 81 patients with normal oral cholecystograms, Ann Surg 196:627, 1982.

Den Besten L and Berci G: The current status of biliary tract surgery: an international study of 1,072 consecutive patients, World J Surg 10:116, 1986.

Dietrick RB: Experience with liver abscess, Am J Surg 147:288, 1984.

Fischer JE: Amino acids in hepatic coma, Dig Dis Sci 27:97, 1982.

Gracie WA and Ransohoff DF: The natural history of silent gallstones: the innocent gallstone is not a myth, N Engl J Med 307:798, 1982 (also the delightful accompanying editorial).

Lees CD et al: Carcinoma of the bile ducts, Surg Gynecol Obstet 151:193, 1980.

LeVeen HH et al: Ascites: its correction by peritoneovenous shunting, Curr Probl Surg 16:1, 1979.

Lewis JW, Chung RS, and Allison JG: Injection sclerotherapy for control of acute variceal hemorrhage. Am J Surg 142:592, 1981.

Lindner HH and Green RB: Embryology and surgical anatomy of the extrahepatic biliary tract. Surg Clin North Am 44:1273, 1964.

McSherry CK and Glenn F: The incidence and causes of death following surgery for nonmalignant biliary tract disease, Ann Surg 191:271, 1980.

McSherry CK et al: The natural history of gallstone disease in symptomatic and asymtomatic patients, Ann Surg 202:59, 1985.

Pitt HA et al: Factors influencing outcome in patients with postoperative biliary strictures, Am J Surg 144:14, 1982.

Rattner DW and Warshaw AL: Impact of choledochoscopy on the management of choledocholithiasis experience with 499 common duct explorations at the Massachusetts General Hospital, Ann Surg 194:76, 1981.

Rikkers LF: Operations for management of esophageal variceal hemorrhage, West J Med 136:107, 1982.

Scharschmidt BF, Goldberg HI, and Schmid R: Current concepts in diagnosis: approach to the patient with cholestatic jaundice, N Engl J Med 308:1515, 1983.

Sherlock S: Diseases of the liver and biliary system, ed 6, Oxford, England, 1981, Basil Blackwell Publisher.

Sherlock S: Patterns of hepatocyte injury in man, Lancet 1:782, 1982.

Sugiura M and Futagawa S: Further evaluation of the Sugiura procedure in the treatment of esophages varices, Arch Surg 112:1317, 1977.

Thompson JE, Tompkins RK, and Longmire WP: Factors in management of acute cholangitis, Ann Surg 195:137, 1982.

Van der Linden W and Edlund G: Early versus delayed cholecystectomy: the effect of a change in management, Br J Surg 68:783, 1981.

Verlenden WL III and Frey CF: Management liver abscess, Am J Surg 140:53, 1980.

Walt AJ: The mythology of hepatic trauma or Babe revisited, Am J Surg 135:12, 1978.

CHAPTER 19
Pancreas

Bradley EL, Clements JL, and Gonzalez AC: The natural history of pancreatic pseudocysts: a unified concept of management, Am J Surg 137:135, 1979.

Deveney CW et al: Resection of gastrinomas, Ann Surg 198:546, 1983.

Ebid AM, Murray PD, and Fischer JE: Vasoactive intestinal peptide and the watery diarrhea syndrome, Ann Surg 187:411, 1978.

Frey CF, Child CG, and Fry W: Pancreatectomy for chronic pancreatitis, Ann Surg 184:403, 1976.

Friesen SR: Tumors of the endocrine pancreas, N Engl J Med 306:580, 1982.

Friesen SR: Treatment of the Zollinger-Ellison syndrome, Am J Surg 143:331, 1982.

Graham JM, Mattox KL, and Jordan GL: Traumatic injuries of the pancreas, Am J Surg 136:744, 1978.

Harrison TS et al: Current surgical management of functioning islet cell tumors of the pancreas, Ann Surg 178:485, 1973.

Jones RC: Management of pancreatic trauma, Ann Surg 187:555, 1978.

Kelly TR: Gallstone pancreatitis: pathophysiology, Surgery 80:488, 1976.

McCarthy DM: The place of surgery in the Zollinger-Ellison syndrome, N Engl J Med 302:1344, 1980.

Meinke WB et al: Gastric outlet obstruction after palliative surgery for cancer of head of pancreas, Arch Surg 118:550, 1983.

Miller TA et al: Pancreatic abscess, Arch Surg 108:545, 1974.

Prinz RA et al: Operative and chemotherapeutic management glucagon producing tumors, Surgery 90:713, 1981.

Prinz RA and Greenlee HB: Pancreatic duct drainage in 100 patients with chronic pancreatitis, Ann Surg 194:313, 1981.

Ranson JHC: Conservative surgical treatment of acute pancreatitis, World J Surg 5:351, 1981.

Ranson JHC and Spencer FC: The role of peritoneal lavage in severe acute pancreatitis, Ann Surg 187:565, 1978.

Ranson JHC et al: Prognostic signs and the role of operative management in acute pancreatitis, Surg Gynecol Obstet 139:69, 1974.

Ranson JHC and Spencer FC: Prevention, diagnosis, and treatment of pancreatic abscess, Surgery 82:99, 1977.

Ranson JHC: The timing of biliary surgery in acute pancreatitis, Ann Surg 189:654, 1979.

Safrany L and Cotton PB: A preliminary report: urgent duodenoscopic sphincterotomy for acute gallstone pancreatitis, Surgery 89:424, 1981.

Sankaran S and Walt AJ: The natural and unnatural history of pancreatic pseudocysts, Br J Surg 62:37, 1975.

Semel L, Schrieber D, and Fromm D: Gallstone pancreatitis, Arch Surg 118:901, 1983.

Thompson JC et al: The role of surgery in the Zollinger-Ellison syndrome, Ann Surg 197:594, 1983.

van Heerden JA, Edis AJ, and Service FJ: The surgical aspects of insulinomas, Ann Surg 189:677, 1979.

Warren KW et al: Current trends in the diagnosis and treatment of carcinoma of the pancreas, Am J Surg 145:813, 1983.

Weaver DW et al: A continuing appraisal of pancreatic ascites, Surg Gynecol Obstet 154:845, 1982.

CHAPTER 20

Spleen

Block GE and Exelby RP: In Nora PF, editor: Operative surgery, ed 2, Philadelphia, 1980, Lea & Febiger.

Burrington JD: Surgical repair of a ruptured spleen in children: report of eight cases, Arch Surg 112:471, 1977.

Claret I, Morales L, and Montaner A: Immunological studies in the post splenectomy syndrome, J Pediatr Surg 10:59, 1975.

Ein SH et al: Nonoperative management of traumatized spleen in children: how and why, J Pediatr Surg 13:117, 1978.

Erkalis AJ and Filler RM: Splenectomy in childhood: a review of 1413 cases, J Pediatr Surg 7:382, 1972.

Feliciano DV et al: A four-year experience with splenectomy versus splenorrhaphy, Ann Surg 201:568, 1985.

Green JB et al: Late septic complications in adults following splenectomy for trauma, J Trauma 26:999, 1986.

Hebeler RF et al: The management of splenic injury, J Trauma 22:492, 1982.

Kidd WT et al: The management of blunt splenic trauma, J Trauma 27:977, 1987.

Malangoni MA et al: Management of injury to the spleen in adults, Ann Surg 200:701, 1984.

Pearson HA: Splenectomy: its risks and its roles, Hosp Pract 8:85, 1980.

Pearson HA et al: The born-again spleen, N Engl J Med 298:1389, 1978.

Ratner MH et al: Surgical repair of the injured spleen, J Pediatr Surg 12:1019, 1977.

Scheele J, Gentsch HH, and Matteson E: Splenic repair by fibrin tissue adhesive and collagen fleece, Surgery 95:6, 1984.

Schwartz PE et al: Postsplenectomy sepsis and mortality in adults, JAMA 248:2279, 1982.

Sherman RT et al: Panel: splenic injuries, J Trauma 22:507, 1982.

Soper RT: Splenic salvage, Hosp Physician 19:73, 1983.

Traub AC and Perry JF: Splenic preservation following splenic trauma, J Trauma 22:496, 1982.

Velcek FT et al: Posttraumatic splenic replantation in children, J Pediatr Surg 17:879, 1982.

CHAPTER 21

Peritoneal and Acute Abdominal Conditions

Botsford TW and Wilson RE: The acute abdomen, ed 2, Philadelphia, 1977, WB Saunders Co.

Cope Z (revised by Silen W): The early diagnoses of the acute abdomen, ed 15, New York, 1987, Oxford University Press.

Deutsch A and Leopold G: Ultronsonic demonstration of the inflamed appendix: a case report, Radiology 140:163, 1981.

Jones PF and Dudley HA: Emergency abdominal surgery in infancy, childhood and adult life, Philadelphia, 1974, JB Lippincott Co.

Kirkpatrick J: The acute abdomen, diagnosis and management, Baltimore, 1984, Williams and Wilkins.

Requarth W: Indication for operation for abdominal trauma, Surgery 46:461, 1959.

Silen W: Cope's early diagnosis of the acute abdomen, ed 16, New York, 1983, Oxford University Press.

Simmons RL and Howard RJ: Surgical infectious diseases, ed 2, New York, 1987, Appleton-Century-Crofts.

Skucas J and Spataro R: Radiology of the acute abdomen, New York, 1986, Churchill Livingstone.

Warren KW: Acute surgical conditions of the abdomen in the aged and the poor risk patient, Surg Clin North Am 34:745, 1954.

CHAPTER 22

Abdominal Hernias

Anson BJ, Morgan EH, and McVay CB: Surgical anatomy of the inguinal region based upon a study of 500 body halves, Surg Gynecol Obstet 111:707, 1960.

Bartlett RH: Extracorporeal membrane oxygenation in newborn respiratory failure. In Ravitch M, editor: Pediatric surgery, ed 4, Chicago, 1986, Year Book Medical Publishers.

Bohn D et al: Ventilatory predictors of pulmonary hypoplasia in congenital diaphragmatic hernia, J Pediatr 111:423, 1987.

Bombeck GT and Nyhus LM: In Nora PF, editor: Operative surgery, ed 2, Philadelphia, 1980, Lea & Febiger.

Kaufman M, Weissberg D, and Bider D: Repair of recurrent inguinal hernia with Marlex mesh, Surg Gynecol Obstet 160:505, 1985.

Lictenstein IL: Herniorrhaphy: a personal experience with 6,321 cases, Am J Surg 153:553, 1987.

McGregor DB, Halverson K, and McVay CB: The unilateral pediatric inguinal hernia: should the contralateral side by explored? J Pediatr Surg 15:313, 1980.

Nyhus LM and Condon RE: Hernia, ed 2, Philadelphia, 1978, JB Lippincott Co.

Osebold WR and Soper RT: Congenital posterolateral diaphragmatic hernia post infancy, Am J Surg 131:748, 1976.

Ponka JL: Hernias of the abdominal wall, Philadelphia, 1980, WB Saunders Co.

Postlethwait RW: Recurrent inguinal hernia, Ann Surg 202:777, 1985.

Rignault DP: Properitoneal prosthetic inguinal hernioplasty through a Pfannenstiel approach, Surg Gynecol Obstet 163:465, 1986.

Ruff SJ et al: Pediatric diaphragmatic hernias, Am J Surg 139:641, 1980.

Safaie-Shirazi S et al: Proceedings: Nissen fundoplication without crural repair: a cure for reflux esophagitis, Arch Surg 108:424, 1974.

Shirazi SS: Hernias of the diaphragm and abdominal wall, Garden City, NY, 1981, Medical Examination Publishing Co.

Skinner D: Pathophysiology of gastroesophageal reflux, Ann Surg 202:546, 1985.

Smith LA et al: Treatment of defects of the anterior abdominal wall in newborns, Mayo Clinic Proc 58:797, 1983.

Soper RT: Hernia in infants and children, Postgrad Med 40:523, 1966.

Talbert JL: Surgical management of massive ventral hernias in children, J Pediatr Surg 12:63, 1977.

Young DV: Comparison of local, spinal, and general anesthesia for inguinal herniorrhaphy, Am J Surg 153:560, 1987.

Zimmerman LM and Anson BJ: The anatomy and surgery of hernia, ed 2, Baltimore, 1967, Williams & Wilkins.

CHAPTER 23
Stomach and Duodenum

Bushkin FL and Woodward ER: Postgastrectomy syndromes, Philadelphia, 1976, WB Saunders Co.

Busman DC, Brombacher PJ, and Munting JD: Highly selective vagotomy and serum gastrin levels, Surg Gynecol Obstet 165:397, 1987.

Diehl JT et al: Gastric carcinoma—a ten-year review, Ann Surg 198:9, 1983.

Donahue PE et al: Proximal gastric vagotomy: the first 25 years, Adv Surg 19:139, 1986.

Dragstedt LR: Gastric and peptic ulcer, Arch Surg 91:1005, 1965.

Driks MR et al: Nosocomial pneumonia in intubated patients given sucralfate as compared with antacids or histamine type 2 blockers, N Engl J Med 317:1376, 1987.

Feldman M: Peptic ulcer: complications. In Wyngaarden JB and Smith LH, Jr: Cecil textbook of medicine, ed 18, Philadelphia, 1988, WB Saunders Co.

Goligher JC: A technique for highly selective (parietal cell or proximal gastric) vagotomy for duodenal ulcer, Br J Surg 61:337, 1974.

Halverson JD: Gastric restriction procedures for morbid obesity, Surg Rounds 11:49, 1988.

Hoffmann J, Olesen A, and Jensen HE: Prospective 14- to 18-year follow-up study after parietal cell vagotomy, Br J Surg 74:1056, 1987.

MacLean LD, Rhode B, and Shizgal HM: Nutrition after vertical banded gastroplasty, Ann Surg 206:555, 1987.

Mason EE: Evolution of gastric reduction for obesity, Contemp Surg 20:1982.

Moody FG and McGreevy JM: Stomach. In Schwartz SI et al, editors: Principles of surgery, ed 4, New York, 1983, McGraw-Hill Book Co.

Moore FD: Surgery in search of a rationale: eighty years of ulcerogenic surgery, Am J Surg 105:304, 1963.

Mulholland MW and Debas HT: Chronic duodenal and gastric ulcer, Surg Clin North Am 67:489, 1987.

Nyhus LM et al: Complete vagotomy: the evolution of an effective technique, Arch Surg 115:264, 1980.

Penn I: Surgical and medical treatment of peptic ulcer disease, Contin Educa Fam Physician 11:39, 1979.

Peterson WL: Peptic ulcer: medical therapy. In Wyngaarden JB and Smith LH, Jr, editors: Cecil textbook of medicine, ed 18, Philadelphia, 1988, WB Saunders Co.

Roth SH and Bennett RE: Nonsteroidal anti-inflammatory drug gastropathy. Recognition and response, Arch Intern Med 147:2093, 1987.

Schein PS et al: Current management of advanced and locally unresectable gastric carcinoma, Cancer 50:2590, 1982.

Taylor TV: Parietal cell vagotomy: long-term follow-up studies, Br J Surg 74:971, 1987.

Thirlby RC: Peptic ulcer: surgical therapy. In Wyngaarden JB and Smith LH, Jr, editors: Cecil textbook of medicine, ed 18, Philadelphia, 1988, WB Saunders Co.

Traynor OJ et al: Diagnostic and prognostic problems in early gastric cancer, Am J Surg 154:516, 1987.

Wolfe MM and Jensen RT: Zollinger-Ellison syndrome. Current concepts in diagnosis and management, N Engl J Med 317:1200, 1987.

Zollinger RM and Ellison EH: Primary peptic ulcerations of the jejunum associated with islet cell tumors of the pancreas, Ann Surg 142:709, 1955.

CHAPTER 24
Gastrointestinal Hemorrhage

Boley SJ et al: The nature and etiology of vascular ectasias of the colon, Gastroenterology 72:650, 1977.

Brandt LJ and Boley SJ: The role of colonoscopy in the diagnosis and management of lower intestinal bleeding, Scand J Gastroenterol 19(Suppl 102):61, 1984.

Browder W, Cerise EJ, and Litwin MS: Impact of emergency angiography in massive lower gastrointestinal bleeding, Ann Surg 204:530, 1986.

Buchman TG and Bulkley GB: Current management of patients with lower gastrointestinal bleeding, Surg Clin North Am 67:651, 1987.

Clason AE, MacLeod DAD, and Elton RA: Clinical factors in the prediction of further hemorrhage or mortality in acute upper gastrointestinal haemorrhage, Br J Surg 73:985, 1986.

Collins R and Langman M: Treatment with histamine H_2 antagonists in acute upper gastrointestinal hemorrhage, N Engl J Med 313:660, 1985.

Fleischer D: Endoscopic therapy of upper gastrointestinal bleeding in humans, Gastroenterology 90:217, 1986.

Larson DE and Farnell MB: Upper gastrointestinal hemorrhage, Mayo Clin Proc 58:371, 1983.

Lau WY et al: Preoperative and intraoperative localization of gastrointestinal bleeding of obscure origin, Gut 28:869, 1987.

Lewis J, Chung RS, and Allison J: Sclerotherapy of esophageal varices, Arch Surg 115:476, 1980.

Lieberman DA et al: Arterial embolization for massive upper gastrointestinal tract bleeding in poor surgical candidates, Gastroenterology 86:876, 1984.

Murray WR: Surgical management of haemorrhage from peptic ulceration, Br J Surg 73:947, 1986.

Richter JM et al: Angiodysplasia: clinical presentation and colonoscopic diagnosis, Dig Dis Sci 29:481, 1984.

Rikkers LF: Operations for management of esophageal variceal hemorrhage, West J Med 136:107, 1982.

Rutgeerts P et al: Long-term results of treatment of vascular malformations of the gastrointestinal tract by neodynium:YAG laser photocoagulation, Gut 26:586, 1985.

Torres AJ et al: Somatostatin in the treatment of severe upper gastrointestinal bleeding: a multicentre controlled trial, Br J Surg 73:786, 1986.

Wara P: Endoscopic prediction of major rebleeding: a prospective study of stigmata of hemorrhage in bleeding ulcer, Gastroenterology 88:1209, 1985.

Zinner MJ et al: The prevention of upper gastrointestinal tract bleeding in patients in an intensive care unit, Surg Gynecol Obstet 153:214, 1981.

CHAPTER 25
Small Intestine

Colcock BP and Fortin C: Surgical treatment of regional enteritis: review of 85 cases, Ann Surg 161:812, 1965.

Colcock BP and Braasch JW: Surgery of the small intestine in the adult, Philadelphia, 1968, WB Saunders Co.

Kutscher AH et al: Peutz-Jeghers syndrome: follow-ups on patients reported on in the literature, Am J Med Sci 238:180, 1959.

McPeak CJ: Malignant tumors of the small intestine, Am J Surg 114:402, 1967.

Rankin GB and Turnbull RB, Jr: Transmural colitis: medical and surgical management, Hosp Practice 65, 1971.

Read JD: Intestinal carcinoma in the Peutz-Jeghers syndrome, JAMA 229:833, 1974.

Sherman NJ et al: Regional enteritis in childhood, J Pediatr Surg 7:585, 1972.

Skinner DB et al: Mesenteric vascular disease, Am J Surg 128:835, 1974.

CHAPTER 26

Large Intestine

Bacon IIE and Pezzutti JE: Granulomatous ileocolitis, JAMA 198:1330, 1966.

Beahrs OH: Colorectal tumors, Philadelphia, 1986, JB Lippincott.

Burkitt DP: Epidemiology of cancer of the colon and rectum, Cancer 28:3, 1971.

Coller FA, Ransom HK, and Regan WJ: Cancer of the colon and rectum, New York, 1956, American Cancer Society.

Crespi M et al: The role of proctosigmoidoscopy in screening for colorectal neoplasia, CA 34:158, 1984.

Goligher JC: Surgery of the anus, rectum, and colon, ed 5, New York, 1983, The Macmillan Co.

Goligher JD, De Dombal FT, and Watts FM: Ulcerative colitus, Baltimore, 1968, Williams & Wilkins.

Hawk WA, Turnbull RB, and Farmer RG: Regional enteritis of the colon, JAMA 201:738, 1967.

Miller FE and Liechty RD: Adenocarcinoma of the colon and rectum in persons under thirty years of age, Am J Surg 113:507, 1967.

Thomson JPS, Nicholls RJ, and Williams CB: Colorectal diseases, New York, 1981, Appleton-Century-Crofts.

Turnbull RB, Jr, et al: Cancer of the colon: the influence of the no-touch isolation technique on survival rates, Ann Surg 166:420, 1967.

Welch CE and Hedberg S: Polypoid lesions of the gastrointestinal tract, Philadelphia, 1975, WB Saunders Co.

Wilson SM and Beahrs OH: The curative treatment of colonic carcinoma of the sigmoid, rectosigmoid and rectum, Ann Surg 183:556, 1976.

Winawer SJ and Sherlock P: Surveillance for colorectal cancer in average-risk patients, familial high-risk groups, and patients with adenomas, Cancer 50:2609, 1982.

CHAPTER 27

Intestinal Obstruction

Davis S and Sperling L: Obstruction of the small intestine, Arch Surg 99:424, 1969.

Nelson RL and Nyhus LM: Surgery of the small intestine, Norwalk, Conn, Appleton & Lange, 1987.

Quan SHQ and Stearns MW, Jr: Early postoperative intestinal obstruction and postoperative intestinal ileus, Dis Colon Rectum 4:307, 1961.

Wangensteen OH: Intestinal obstruction, ed 3, Springfield, Ill, 1955, Charles C Thomas.

Wangensteen OH: Great ideas in surgery—understanding the bowel obstruction problem, Am J Surg 135:131, 1978.

Welch CE: Intestinal obstruction, Chicago, 1958, Year Book Medical Publishers, Inc.

CHAPTER 28

Anorectum

Beahrs OH: Complete rectal prolapse: an evaluation of surgical treatment, Ann Surg 161:221, 1965.

Buckwalter JA and Jurayj MD: Relationship of chronic rectal disease to carcinoma, Arch Surg 75:352, 1957.

Dunphy JE: Surgical anatomy of the anal canal, Arch Surg 57:791, 1948.

Dunphy JE and Pikula J: Fact and fancy about fistula-in-ano, Surg Clin North Am 35:1469, 1955.

Goligher JC: Surgery of the anus, rectum, and colon, ed 5, New York, 1983, The Macmillan Co.

Goligher JC, Leacock AG, and Brossy JJ: The surgical anatomy of the anal canal, Br J Surg 43:51, 1955.

Harkins HN: Correlation of the newer knowledge of surgical anatomy of the anorectum, Dis Colon Rectum 8:154, 1965.

Page BH: The entry of hair into a pilonidal sinus, Br J Surg 56:32, 1969.

Parks AG: Haemorrhoidectomy, Surg Clin North Am 45:1305, 1965.

Patey DH: A reappraisal of the acquired theory of sacrococcygeal pilonidal sinus, Br J Surg 56:462, 1969.

Thomson JPS, Nicholls RJ, and Williams CB: Colorectal disease, New York, 1981, Appleton-Century-Crofts.

CHAPTER 29

Thoracic and Pulmonary Surgery

Bates DV, Macklem PT, and Christie RV: Respiratory function in disease, ed 2, Philadelphia, 1971, WB Saunders Co.

Comroe JL, Jr et al: The lung, ed 3, Chicago, 1965, Year Book Medical Publishers.

Doty DB et al: Cardiac trauma: clinical and experimental correlations of myocardial contusion, Ann Surg 180:452, 1974.

Edwards FR: Foundations of thoracic surgery, Baltimore, 1966, Williams & Wilkins.

Effler DB, editor: Blades' surgical diseases of the chest, ed 4, St. Louis, 1978, The CV Mosby Co.

Flavell G: An introduction to chest surgery, New York, 1957, Oxford University Press.

Glenn W, editor: Thoracic and cardiovascular surgery, ed 4, East Norwalk, Conn, 1983, Appleton-Century-Crofts.

Johnson J and Kirby CK: Surgery of the chest, ed 4, Chicago, 1970, Year Book Medical Publishers.

Nelson AR: The surgical treatment of pulmonary coccidioidomycosis, Curr Probl Surg 1-48, 1974.

Robin ED: A clinical approach to the diagnostic management of pulmonary embolism. In Bang NU et al, editors: Thrombosis and atherosclerosis, Chicago, 1982, Year Book Medical Publishers.

Slonim NB and Hamilton LH: Respiratory physiology, ed 3, St. Louis, 1976, The CV Mosby Co.

West JB: Ventilation/blood flow and gas exchange, ed 2, Philadelphia, 1970, FA Davis Co.

Zavala DC and Rossi NP: Nonthoracotomy diagnostic techniques for pulmonary disease, Arch Surg 107:152, 1973.

CHAPTER 30

Cardiac Surgery

Congenital Heart Disease

Behrendt DM and Austen WG: Patients care in cardiac surgery, ed 4, Boston, 1985, Little, Brown, and Co.

Bender HW, Jr et al: Repair of atrioventricular canal malformation in the first year of life, J Thorac Cardiovasc Surg 84:515, 1982.

Coles JG et al: Surgical experience with the modified Fontan procedure, Circulation 76(Suppl III):III-61, 1987.

Coto EO et al: Modified Senning operation for treatment of transposition of the great arteries, J Thorac Cardiovasc Surg 78:721, 1979.

Doty DB and McGoon DC: Closure of perimembranous ventricular septal defect, J Thorac Cardiovasc Surg 85:781, 1983.

Hammon JW, Jr et al: Total anomalous pulmonary venous connection in infancy. Ten years' experience including studies of postoperative ventricular function, J Thorac Cardiovasc Surg 80:544, 1980.

Kirklin JW and Barratt-Boyes BG: Cardiac surgery, New York, 1986, John Wiley & Sons.

Kirklin JW et al: Surgical results and protocols in the spectrum of tetralogy of Fallot, Ann Surg 198:251, 1983.

Langman J: Medical embryology, ed 5, Baltimore, 1985, Williams & Wilkins.

Pigott JD et al: Palliative reconstructive surgery for hypoplastic left heart syndrome, Ann Thorac Surg 45:122, 1988.

Quaegebeur JM et al: The arterial switch operation. An eight-year experience, J Thorac Cardiovasc Surg 92:361, 1986.

Stark J and de Leval M: Surgery for congenital heart defects, London, 1983, Grune & Stratton.

Stewart S, Alexson C, and Manning J: Late results of the Mustard procedure in transposition of the great arteries, Ann Thorac Surg 42:419, 1986.

Trinquet F et al: Coarctation of the aorta in infants: Which operation? Ann Thorac Surg 45:186, 1988.

Tveter KJ et al: Long-term evaluation of aortic valvotomy for congenital aortic stenosis, Ann Surg 206:496, 1987.

Ullom RL et al: The Blalock-Taussig shunt in infants: standard versus modified, Ann Thorac Surg 44:539, 1987.

Acquired Heart Disease

Behrendt DM and Austen WG: Patient care in cardiac surgery, ed 4, Boston, 1985, Little, Brown, and Co.

Bonchek LI: Current status of mitral commissurotomy: indications, techniques, and results, Am J Cardiol 52:411, 1983.

Braunwald E: Heart disease, ed 2, Philadelphia, 1984, WB Saunders Co.

Cameron A, Kemp HG, Jr, and Green GE: Bypass surgery with the internal mammary artery graft: 15-year follow-up, Circulation 74(Suppl III):III-30, 1986.

Carpentier A: Cardiac valve surgery—the "French correction," J Thorac Cardiovasc Surg 86:323, 1983.

Cosgrove DM et al: Primary myocardial revascularization. Trends in surgical mortality, J Thorac Cardiovasc Surg 88:673, 1984.

Cox JL: The status of surgery for cardiac arrhythmias, Circulation 71:413, 1985.

Craver JM et al: What role should the intra-aortic balloon have in cardiac surgery? Ann Surg 189:769, 1979.

Gaudiani VA et al: Long-term survival and function after cardiac transplantation, Ann Surg 194:381, 1981.

Kirklin JW and Barratt-Boyes BG: Cardiac surgery, New York, 1986, John Wiley & Sons.

Ludmer PL and Goldschlager N: Cardiac pacing in the 1980s, N Engl J Med 311:1671, 1984.

O'Brien MF et al: A comparison of aortic valve replacement with viable cryopreserved and fresh allograft valves, with a note on chromosomal studies, J Thorac Cardiovasc Surg 94:812, 1987.

Pierce WS: Artificial heart and blood pumps in the treatment of profound heart failure, Circulation 68:883, 1983.

Roberts AJ: Myocardial protection in cardiac surgery, New York, 1987, Marcel Dekker.

Sabiston DC, Jr and Spencer FC: Gibbon's surgery of the chest, ed 4, Philadelphia, 1983, WB Saunders Co.

Teply JF et al: The ultimate prognosis after valve replacement: an assessment at twenty years, Ann Thorac Surg 32:111, 1981.

CHAPTER 31
Vascular Surgery: Peripheral Arteries

Anton GE et al: Surgical management of popliteal aneurysms: trends in presentation, treatment, and results from 1952 to 1984, J Vasc Surg 3:125, 1986.

Baker WH et al: Diagnosis of peripheral occlusive disease, Arch Surg 113(11):1308, 1978.

Barker WF: Peripheral arterial disease, ed 2, Philadelphia, 1975, WB Saunders Co.

Barnes RW: Hemodynamics for the vascular surgeon, Arch Surg 115:216, 1980.

Bergan JJ and Yao JST: Gangrene and severe ischemia of the lower extremities, New York, 1978, Grune & Stratton, Inc.

Blaisdell FW and Hall AD: Axillary-femoral artery bypass for lower extremity ischemia, Surgery 54:563, 1963.

Boley SJ et al: Initial results from an aggressive roentgenological and surgical approach to acute mesenteric ischemia, Surgery 82:848, 1977.

Brewster DC and Darling RC: Optimal methods of aortoiliac reconstruction, Surgery 84:739, 1978.

Burgess EM, Romano RL, and Zettl JH: The management of lower extremity amputations, TR 10-6, Washington, D.C., 1969, U.S Government Printing Office.

Council on Scientific Affairs (AMA): Percutaneous transluminal angioplasty, JAMA 251:764, 1984.

Dale WA and Lewis MR: Management of ischemia of the hand and fingers, Surgery 67:63, 1970.

Dean RH et al: Retrieval of renal function by revascularization: study of preoperative outcome predictors, Ann Surg 202:367, 1985.

Dent TL et al: Multiple arteriosclerotic arterial aneurysms, Arch Surg 105:338, 1972.

DePalma RG and Clowes AW: Interventions in atherosclerosis: a review for surgeons, Surgery 84:175, 1978.

Eastcott HHG: Arterial surgery, Philadelphia, 1969; JB Lippincott Co.

Eastcott HHG, Pickering GW, and Rob CG: Reconstruction of internal carotid artery in a patient with intermittent attacks of hemiplegia, Lancet 2:994, 1954.

Fairbairn JF et al, editors: Allen-Barker-Hines peripheral vascular disease, ed 4, Philadelphia, 1972, WB Saunders Co.

Fogarty TJ et al: A method for extraction of arterial emboli and thrombi, Surg Gynecol Obstet 116:241, 1963.

Leather RP, Powers SR, and Karmody AM: A reappraisal of the in situ saphenous vein arterial bypass, Surgery 86:453, 1979.

Linton RR: Atlas of vascular surgery, Philadelphia, 1973, WB Saunders Co.

Linton RR and Wilde WL: Modifications in the technique for femoral popliteal saphenous vein bypass autografts, Surgery 67:234, 1970.

Mannick JA: Femoro-popliteal and femoro-tibial reconstruction, Surg Clin North Am 59:581, 1979.

Nath RL et al: The multidisciplinary approach to vasculogenic impotence, Surgery 89:124, 1981.

Nitatori T et al: Whole body intravenous digital subtraction angiography, Radiology 156:829, 1985.

O'Donnell TF, Darling RC, and Linton RR: Is 80 years too old for aneurysmectomy? Arch Surg 111:1250, 1976.

Pilcher DB, Barker WF, and Cannon JA: An aortoiliac endarterectomy case series followed 10 years or more, Surgery 67:5, 1970.

Roederer GO et al: Natural history of carotid arterial disease in asymptomatic patients with cervical bruits, Stroke 15:605, 1984.

Russell JB et al: Digital subtraction angiography for evaluation of extracranial carotid occlusive disease: comparison with conventional arteriography, Surgery 94:604, 1983.

Stanley JC and Fry WJ: Surgical treatment of renovascular hypertension, Arch Surg 112:1291, 1977.

Stoney RJ and Wylie EJ: Surgical treatment of ruptured abdominal aneurysms, Calif Med 111:1, 1969.

Strandness DE: Peripheral arterial disease, London, 1969, J. & A. Churchill Ltd.

Szilagyi DE et al: Contribution of abdominal aortic aneurysmectomy to prolongation of life, Ann Surg 164:678, 1966.

Szilagyi DE et al: A thirty-year survey of the reconstructive surgical treatment of aortoiliac occlusive disease, J Vasc Surg 3:421, 1986.

Tawes RL, Jr et al: Arterial thromboembolism: a 20-year perspective, Arch Surg 120:595, 1985.

Taylor LM, Jr et al: Reversed vein bypass to infrapopliteal arteries: modern results are superior to or equivalent to in-situ bypass for patency and for vein utilization. Ann R Coll Surg Engl 68:134, 1986.

Veith FJ et al: Six-year prospective multicenter randomized comparison of autologous saphenous vein and expanded polytetrafluoroethylene grafts in infrainguinal arterial reconstructions, Surgery 98:799, 1985.

Weale FE: An introduction to surgical haemodynamics, Chicago, 1967, Year Book Medical Publishers, Inc.

Working Group on Renovascular Hypertension (National Heart, Lung, and Blood Institute, NIH, Bethesda): Detection, evaluation, and treatment of renovascular hypertension: final report, Ann Intern Med 147:820, 1987.

Wylie EJ and Ehrenfeld WK: Entracranial occlusive cerebrovascular disease: diagnosis and management, Philadelphia, 1970, WB Saunders Co.

CHAPTER 32
Vascular Surgery: Peripheral Veins

Bell WR and Meek AG: Guidelines for the use of thrombolytic agents, N Engl J Med 201(23):1266, 1979.

Bernstein EF, editor: Noninvasive diagnostic techniques in vascular disease, St. Louis, 1978, The CV Mosby Co.

Borrow M and Goldson H: Postoperative venous thrombosis: evaluation of five methods of treatment, Am J Surg 141:245, 1981.

Coon WW: Epidemiology of venous thromboembolism, Ann Surg 186(2):149, 1977.

Coon WW and Willis PW III: Recurrence of venous thromboembolism, Surgery 73:823, 1973.

Cranley JJ, Canos AJ, and Sull WJ: The diagnosis of deep vein thrombosis: fallibility of clinical symptoms and signs, Arch Surg 111:34, 1976.

Dale WA and Allen TR: Unusual problems of venous thrombosis, Surgery 78:707, 1975.

Dodd H and Cockett FB: Pathology and surgery of veins of the lower limb, ed 2, Baltimore, 1970, The Williams & Wilkins Co.

Donaldson GA, Linton RR, and Rodkey GV: A twenty-year survey of thromboembolism at the Massachusetts General Hospital, 1932-1959, N Engl J Med 265:208, 1961.

Donaldson MC, Wirthlin LS, and Donaldson GA: Thirty-year experience with surgical interruption of the inferior vena cava for prevention of pulmonary embolism, Ann Surg 191:363, 1980.

Fairbairn JF et al, editors: Allen-Barker-Hines peripheral vascular disease, ed 4, Philadelphia, 1972, WB Saunders Co.

Goldsmith HW, de los Santos R, and Beattie EJ, Jr: Relief of chronic lymphedema by omental transposition, Ann Surg 166:573, 1967.

Greenfield LJ et al: Greenfield vena cava filter experience: late results in 156 patients, Arch Surg 116:1451, 1981.

Gurewich V, Thomas DP, and Stuart RK: Some guidelines for heparin therapy of venous thromboembolic disease, JAMA 199:116, 1967.

Hobbs JJ, editor: The treatment of venous disorders, Philadelphia, 1977, JB Lippincott Co.

Kakkar VV, Corrigan TP, and Fossard PP: An international multicentre trial: prevention of fatal postoperative pulmonary embolism by low doses of heparin, Lancet 2:34, 1975.

Lansing AM and Davis WM: Five-year follow-up study of ileofemoral venous thrombectomy, Ann Surg 168:620, 1968.

Lofgren KA: Pitfalls in vein surgery, JAMA 188:17, 1964.

Madden JL and Hume M, editors: Venous thromboembolism, New York, 1976, Appleton-Century-Crofts.

Sabiston DC: Pathophysiology, diagnosis and management of pulmonary embolism, Am J Surg 128:384, 1979.

Salzman EW and Davies GC: Prophylaxis of venous thromboembolism: analysis of cost effectiveness, Ann Surg 191:207, 1980.

Salzman EW et al: Management of heparin therapy, N Engl J Med 292:1046, 1975.

Shepard JT and Vanhoutte PM: Role of the venous system in circulatory control, Mayo Clin Proc 53:246, 1978.

Stallworth JM et al: Phlegmasia cerulea dolens: a ten year review, Ann Surg 161:802, 1965.

CHAPTER 33
Orthopedic Surgery

American Orthopaedic Association: Manual of orthopaedic surgery, Chicago, 1966, the Association.

Blount WP: Fractures in children, Baltimore, 1955, The Williams & Wilkins Co.

Brashear HR and Raney RB: Shand's handbook of orthopaedic surgery, ed 9, St. Louis, 1978, The CV Mosby Co.

Cooper R: Fractures in children: fundamentals of management, J Iowa Med Soc 54:472, 1964.

Cooper R: Management of common forearm fractures in children, J Iowa Med Soc 54:689, 1964.

Edmondson AS and Crenshaw AH: Campbell's operative orthopaedics, ed 6, St. Louis, 1980, The CV Mosby Co.

Hart VL: Acute osteomyelitis in children, JAMA 108:524, 1937.

Jaffe HL: Metabolic, degenerative and inflammatory diseases of bones and joints, Philadelphia, 1972, Lea & Febiger.

Larson CB: Low back pain, Disease a Month, Chicago, 1957, Year Book Medical Publishers, Inc.

Lovell W and Winder R: Pediatric orthopaedics, Philadelphia, 1978, JB Lippincott Co.

Mercer W and Duthie RB: Orthopedic surgery, Baltimore, 1964, The Williams & Wilkins Co.

Ponseti IV: Congenital dislocation of the hip in the infant. In American Academy of Orthopaedic Surgeons: Instructional course lectures, vol 10, Ann Arbor, 1953, JW Edwards.

Ponseti IV: Legg-Perthes disease. Observations on the pathological changes in two cases, J Bone Joint Surg 38A:739, 1956.

Ponseti IV and Fricdman B: Prognosis in idiopathic scoliosis, J Bone Joint Surg 32A:381, 1950.

Ponseti IV and Smoley EN: Congenital club foot: the results of treatment, J Bone Joint Surg 45A:261, 1963.

Rockwood CA and Green DP: Fractures, ed 2, Philadelphia, 1983, JB Lippincott Co.

Stone DB and Bonfiglio M: Pyogenic vertebral osteomyelitis: a diagnostic pitfall for the internist, Arch Intern Med 112:491, 1963.

Turek SL: Orthopaedics: principles and their application, ed 2, Philadelphia, 1967, JB Lippincott Co.

CHAPTER 34
Hand Surgery

Beasley RW: Hand injuries, Philadelphia, 1981, WB Saunders Co.

Boswick JA, Jr, editor: Current concepts in hand surgery, Philadelphia, 1983, Lea & Febiger.

Carter PR: Common hand injuries and infections: a practical approach to early treatment, Philadelphia, 1983, WB Saunders.

Flatt AE: The care of minor hand injuries, ed 4, St. Louis, 1979, The CV Mosby Co.

Flynn JE, editor: Hand surgery, ed 3, Baltimore, 1982, The Williams & Wilkins Co.

Green DP, editor: Operative hand surgery, New York, 1982, Churchill Livingstone.

Tubiana R, editor: The hand, Philadelphia, 1985, WB Saunders.

CHAPTER 35
Neurologic Surgery

Friedman WA: Head injuries, Clin Symp 35:4, 1983.

Jennet B and Teasdale G: Management of head injuries, Philadelphia, 1981, FA Davis Co.

Koos WT et al: Color atlas of microneurosurgery, New York, 1985, Thieme-Stratton, Inc.

Milhorat TH: Pediatric neurosurgery, Philadelphia, 1978, FA Davis Co.

Omer GE and Spinner M: Management of peripheral nerve problems, Philadelphia, 1980, WB Saunders Co.

Schneider RC et al: Correlative neurosurgery, ed 3, Springfield, Ill., 1982, Charles C Thomas.

Shillito J and Matson DD: An atlas of pediatric neurosurgical operations, Philadelphia, 1982, WB Saunders Co.

Watkins RG and Collis JS, Jr: Lumbar discectomy and laminectomy, Rockville MD, 1987, Aspen Publishers.

Wirth FP and Ratcheson RA: Neurosurgical critical care, Baltimore, 1987, Williams & Wilkins.

Youmans JR: Neurological surgery, ed 2, Philadelphia, 1982, WB Saunders Co.

CHAPTER 36

Head and Neck Surgery

Anson BJ and Donaldson JA: Surgical anatomy of the temporal bone and ear, Philadelphia, 1973, WB Saunders Co.

DeWeese DD and Saunders WH: Textbook of otolaryngology, ed 5, St. Louis, 1977, The CV Mosby Co.

Jesse RH and Fletcher GH: Treatment of the neck in patients with squamous cell carcinoma of the head and neck, Cancer 39(2 suppl):868, 1977.

Jesse RH and Lindberg RD: The efficacy of combining radiotherapy with a surgical procedure in patients with cervical metastasis from squamous cancer of the oropharynx and hypopharynx. Cancer 35:1163, 1975.

Paparella MM and Shumrick DA, editors: Otolaryngology, Philadelphia, 1973, WB Saunders Co.

Schuller DE et al: Increased survival with surgery alone versus combined therapy, Laryngoscope 89(4):582, 1979.

Sessions DG: Surgical pathology of cancer of the larynx and hypopharynx, Laryngoscope 86(6)814, 1976.

Shambaugh GD, Jr and Glasscock ME III: Surgery of the ear, ed 3, Philadelphia, 1980, WB Saunders Co.

Suen JY and Myers EN, editors: Cancer of the head and neck, Edinburgh, 1981, Churchill Livingstone.

The Centennial Conference on Laryngeal Cancer, Toronto, Canada, May 24-31, 1974, papers presented, published in Laryngoscope, Feb.-Nov. 1975.

CHAPTER 37

Urologic Surgery

Banner MP and Pollack HM: Evaluation of renal function by excretory urography, J Urol 124:437, 1980.

Buchsbaum HJ and Schmidt JD: Gynecologic and obstetric urology, ed 2, Philadelphia, 1982, WB Saunders Co.

Cinman AC: Genitourinary tuberculosis, Urology 20:353, 1982.

Duckett JW: Hypospadias, Urol Clin North Am 8:371, 1981.

Flocks RH and Culp DA: Surgical urology, ed 4, Chicago, 1975, Year Book Medical Publishers, Inc.

Flocks RH and Kadesky MC: Malignant neoplasms of the kidney: an analysis of 353 patients followed five years or more, Trans Am Assoc Genitourin Surg 49:105, 1957.

Fonkalsrud EW and Mengel W: The undescended testis, Chicago, 1981, Year Book Medical Publishers, Inc.

Glenn JF: Urologic surgery, ed 3, Philadelphia, 1983, Harper & Row, Publishers, Inc.

Javadpour N: The role of biologic tumor markers in testicular cancer, Cancer 45:1775, 1980.

Johnson DE and Boileau MA: Genitourinary tumors: fundamental principles and surgical techniques, New York, 1982, Grune & Stratton.

Kaufman JJ: Current urologic therapy, ed 2, Philadelphia, 1986, WB Saunders Co.

Marshall VF: Symposium on bladder tumors, Cancer 9:543, 1956.

McDonald MW: Current therapy for renal cell carcinoma, J Urol 127:211, 1982.

Pak CYC: Medical management of nephrolithiasis, J Urol 128:1157, 1982.

Ransley PG: Vesicoureteric reflux: continuing surgical dilemma, Urology 12:246, 1978.

Ross LS: Diagnosis and treatment of infertile men: a clinical perspective, J Urol 130:847, 1983.

Scott WD, Menon M, and Walsh PC: Hormonal therapy of prostatic cancer, Cancer 45:1929, 1980.

Walsh PC et al: Campbell's urology, ed 5, Philadelphia, 1986, WB Saunders Co.

Walsh PC and Jewett HJ: Radical surgery for prostatic cancer, Cancer 45:1906, 1980.

Wein AJ: Classification of neurogenic voiding dysfunction, J Urol 125:605, 1981.

Williams DI and Johnston JH: Paediatric urology, ed 2, Sevenoaks, Kent, 1982, Butterworth & Co.

Witten DM, Myers GH, Jr, and Utz DC: Emmett's clinical urography, Philadelphia, 1977, WB Saunders Co.

CHAPTER 38

Gynecologic Surgery

Creasman WT et al: The abnormal Pap smear—what to do next? Cancer 48:515, 1981.

DiSaia PJ and Creasman WT: Clinical gynecologic oncology, ed 2, St. Louis, 1984, The CV Mosby Co.

DiSaia PJ, Creasman WT, Rich WM: An alternative approach to early cancer of the vulva. Am J Obstet Gynecol 133:825, 1979.

Dodson WC et al: Superovulation with intrauterine insemination in the treatment of infertility: a possible alternative to gamete intrafallopian transfer and in vitro fertilization. Fertil Steril 48:441, 1987.

Droegmueller W et al, editors: Comprehensive gynecology. St. Louis, 1987, The CV Mosby Co.

Hammond MG and Talbert IM: Infertility: a practical guide for the physician, ed 2, Oradell NJ, 1985, Medical Economics.

Judd HL et al: Estrogen replacement therapy, Obstet Gynecol 58:267, 1981.

Kolstad P and Stafl A: Atlas of colposcopy, Baltimore, 1977, University Park Press.

Olive DL and Haney AF: Endometriosis-associated infertility: a critical review of therapeutic approaches, Obstet Gynecol Surv 41:538, 1986.

Schwarz RH, editor: Sexually transmitted diseases, Clin Obstet Gynecol 26:109, 1983.

Sciarra JJ, editor: Gynecology and obstetrics, vol 5, Philadelphia, 1987, JB Lippincott.

Soper JT, Clarke-Pearson DL, Hammond CB: Metastatic gestational trophoblastic disease: prognostic factors in previously untreated patients. Obstet Gynecol 71:338, 1988.

Verkauf BS: The incidence and outcome of single-factor, multifactorial and unexplained infertility. Am J Obstet Gynecol 147:175, 1983.

Wager GP: Toxic shock syndrome: a review. Am J Obstet Gynecol 146:93, 1983.

CHAPTER 39

Pediatric Surgery

Avery GB: Neonatology, Philadelphia, 1987, JB Lippincott Co.

deVries PA and Shapiro SR: Complications of pediatric surgery, New York, 1982, John Wiley & Sons.

Ehrenpreis T: Hirschsprung's disease, Chicago, 1970, Year Book Medical Publishers.

Filston H: The surgical neonates; evaluation and care, ed 2, Norwalk, Conn, 1985, Appleton-Century-Crofts.

Gans SL: Surgical pediatrics, New York, 1973, Grune & Stratton.

Gray SW and Skandalakis JE: Embryology for surgeons, Philadelphia, 1972, WB Saunders Co.

Gross RE: The surgery of infancy and childhood, Philadelphia, 1953, WB Saunders Co.

Harrison M: Unborn patient: prenatal diagnosis and treatment, Orlando, Fl, 1983, Grune & Stratton.

Holder TM and Ashcraft KW: Pediatric surgery, Philadelphia, 1980, WB Saunders Co.

Mayer TA: Emergency management of pediatric trauma, Philadelphia, 1985, WB Saunders Co.

Raffensperger JG: Swenson's pediatric surgery, ed 4, New York, 1980, Appleton-Century-Crofts.

Rickman PP, Lister J, and Irving IM: Neonatal surgery, ed 2, Sevenoaks, Kent, 1978, Butterworth & Co.

Rickman PP, Soper RT, and Stauffer U: Synopsis of pediatric surgery, Stuttgart, 1975, George Thieme Verlag.

Spits L, Steiner GM, and Zachary RB: Color atlas of pediatric surgical diagnosis, Chicago, 1981, Year Book Medical Publishers.

Stephens FD and Smith ED: Ano-rectal malformations in children, Chicago, 1971, Year Book Medical Publishers.

Touloukian RJ: Pediatric trauma, New York, 1978, John Wiley & Sons.

CHAPTER 40

Plastic and Reconstructive Surgery

Achauer BM et al: Cyclosporine and the treatment of burns. Presented to American Burn Association annual meeting, San Francisco, 1984 (American Burn Association, Durham, N.C.).

Cormack GC and Lamberty BGH: The arterial anatomy of skin flaps, Edinburgh, 1986, Churchill Livingstone.

Daniel RR and Kerrigan CL: Skin flaps: an anatomical and hemodynamic approach, Clin Plast Surg 6:181, 1979.

Fudem GM et al: Growth of vascularized somatic tissue allografts in young rabbits given cyclosporine, Surg Forum 36:604, 1985.

Furnas DW et al: Cyclosporine and long-term survival of composite tissue allografts (limb transplants) in rats, Transplant Proc 15:3063, 1983.

Georgiade NG et al: Essentials of Plastic, Maxillofacial, and Reconstructive Surgery, Baltimore, 1987, Williams & Wilkins.

Grabb WC and Smith JW, editors: Plastic surgery, ed 3, Boston, 1979, Little, Brown & Co.

Harii K: Microvascular tissue transfer: fundamental techniques and clinical applications, Tokyo, 1983, Igaku Shoin.

Hoopes JE: Pedicle flaps: an overview. In Krizek TJ and Hoopes JE, editors: Symposium on basic science in plastic surgery, St. Louis, 1976, The CV Mosby Co.

McCraw JB and Vasconez LO: Musculocutaneous flaps: principles, Clin Plast Surg 7:9, 1980.

Serafin D and Georgiade NG: Pediatric plastic surgery, St. Louis, 1984, The CV Mosby Co.

Urbaniak JR, editor: Microsurgery for major limb reconstruction, St. Louis, 1987, The CV Mosby Co.

CHAPTER 41

Care of the Acutely Injured Patient

Ballinger WF, Zuidema GD, and Rutherford RB: The management of trauma, ed 4, Philadelphia, 1984, WB Saunders Co.

Shires GT: Care of the trauma patient, ed 3, New York, 1984, Blakiston Division, McGraw-Hill Book Co.

Walt AJ, editor: Early care of the injured patient, American College of Surgeons, Committee on Trauma, ed 3, Philadelphia, 1982, WB Saunders Co.

CHAPTER 42

Bites and Stings

Furste W: Tetanus prophylaxis in the United States. Bull Am Coll Surg 72:16, 1987.

The Committee on Trauma of the American College of Surgeons: A guide to prophylaxis against tetanus in wound management, Bull Am Coll Surg 69:22-24, 1984.

Ellis MD, editor: Dangerous plants, snakes, arthropods and marine life: toxicity and treatment, with special reference to the state of Texas, Hamilton, IL, 1978, Drug Intelligence Publications.

Huang TT et al: The use of excisional therapy in the management of snakebite, Ann Surg 179:598, 1974.

Immunization Practices Advisory Committee: Rabies prevention—United States, 1984. MMWR 33:395, 1984.

King LE and Rees RS: Dapsone treatment of a brown recluse bite, JAMA 250:648, 1983.

Kizer KW: Epidemiologic and clinical aspects of animal bite injuries, J.A.C.E.P. 8:134, 1979.

Rees R et al: The diagnosis and treatment of brown recluse spider bites, Ann Emerg Med 16:95, 1987.

Russell FE: Snake venom poisoning, Great Neck, NY, 1983, Scholium International.

CHAPTER 43

Thermal Injuries

Andreasen NJ and Norris AS: Long-term adjustment and adaptation mechanisms in severely burned adults, J Nervous Mental Dis 154:352, 1972.

Artz CP, Moncrief JA, and Pruitt BA: Burns, a team approach, Philadelphia, 1979, WB Saunders Co.

Asko-Seljavaara S: Granulocyte kinetics in burns, JBCR 8:492, 1987.

Baker CC et al: Interleukin-1 and T cell function following injury, JBCR 8:503, 1987.

Banes AJ et al: Biologic, biosynthetic, and synthetic dressings as temporary wound covers: a biochemical comparison, JBCR 7:98, 1986.

Baxter C: Pathophysiology and treatment of burns and cold injury. In Hardy JD, editor: Rhoads' textbook of surgery: principles and practice, Philadelphia, 1977, JB Lippincott Co.

Burns. In Cowley RA and Dunham CM, editors: Shock Trauma/Critical Care Manual Initial Assessment and Management, Baltimore, 1982, University Park Press.

Curreri PW et al: Dietary requirements of patients with major burns, J Am Dietetic Assoc 65:415, 1974.

Daniel RK et al: High-voltage electrical injury: acute pathophysiology, J Hand Surg 13A:44, 1987.

Demling RH: Burn injury, Acute Care 11:119, 1985.

Hansbrough JF et al: Immune response modulation after burn injury: T cells and antibodies, JBCR 8(6):509, 1987.

Hartford CE: Fluid resuscitation of the burned patient. In Mason EE, editor: Fluid, electrolyte and nutrient therapy in surgery, Philadelphia, 1974, Lea & Febiger.

Helzer JE, Robins LN, and McEvoy L: Post-traumatic stress disorder in the general population: findings of the epidemiologic catchment area survey, N Engl J Med 317:1630, 1987.

Herndon DN et al: Treatment of burns in children, Pediatr Clin North Am 32:1311, 1985.

Herndon DN et al: Treatment of burns, Curr Probl Surg 345, 1987.

Higgins TL and Chernow B: Pharmacotherapy of circulatory shock, Dis Month 312, 1987.

Konter-Thioulouse E et al: Circulating fibronectin depletion in burned patients: relationship to development of infection and prognostic value, J Burn Care 6:477, 1985.

Mosley S: Inhalation injury: a review of the literature, Heart Lung 17:3, 1988.

Ninnenann JL: Trauma, sepsis, and the immune response, JBCR 8:462, 1987.

Panke TW and McLeod CG: Pathology of thermal injury: a practical approach, Orlando, Fl, 1985, Grune & Stratton.

Pruitt BA and Goodwin CW: Burns: including cold, chemical, and electrical injuries. In Sabiston DC, editor: Textbook of surgery: the biological basis of modern surgical practice, Philadelphia, 1986, WB Saunders Co.

Zawacki BE, moderator: Round table discussion: temporary wound closure after burn excision, JBRC 7:138, 1986.

CHAPTER 44

Transplantation Surgery

Allen MA et al: Noninvasive assessment of donor and native heart function after heterotopic heart transplantation, J Thorac Cardiovasc Surg 95:75, 1988.

Calne R, editor: Liver transplantation, Orlando, Fl, 1987, Grune & Stratton.

Cerilli GJ, editor: Organ transplantation and replacement, Philadelphia, 1988, JB Lippincott Co.

Claman HN: The biology of the immune response, JAMA 258:2834, 1987.

Kaye MP: Registry: International Society for Heart Transplantation, Clin Transplant 1:177, 1987.

Kirkpatrick CH: Transplantation immunology, JAMA 258: 2993, 1987.

Land W and Landgraf R, editors: Clinical pancreas transplantation: the world experience, Transplant Proc 19:1, 1987.

Nossal GJV: Immunoregulation: the key to transplantation and autoimmunity, J Thorac Cardiovasc Surg 94:802, 1987.

Patterson GA et al: Experimental and clinical double lung transplantation, J Thorac Cardiovasc Surg 95:70, 1988.

Starzl, TE: International organ transplant forum, Transplant Proc 20:1, 1988.

Index